Pediatric Oncology

Series Editors

Gregory H. Reaman
Center for Drug Evaluation and Research
U.S. Food and Drug Administration
Silver Spring, MD, USA

Franklin O. Smith
Medpace
Cincinnati, OH, USA

This series provides up-to-date information on important topics in pediatric oncology, from the diagnosis and treatment of particular forms of disease through to, for example, radiation oncology, supportive care, and survivorship. The entire spectrum of clinical management is covered with the aim of equipping readers with the latest knowledge relevant to daily practice. In addition, clinical, methodological, and research issues are addressed. The series benefits from homogeneous design and consistently high quality of illustrations. The volume editors are internationally renowned authorities and contributing authors have been selected for their expertise in the subjects discussed. *Pediatric Oncology* will serve pediatric oncologists, fellows, and residents both as a comprehensive source of information and as a quick reference. The series will also be of interest to pediatricians and general practitioners.

More information about this series at https://link.springer.com/bookseries/5421

Dominik T. Schneider
Ines B. Brecht • Thomas A. Olson
Andrea Ferrari
Editors

Rare Tumors in Children and Adolescents

Second Edition

Springer

Editors
Dominik T. Schneider
Clinic of Pediatrics
Municipal Hospital Dortmund,
University Witten-Herdecke
Dortmund, Germany

Ines B. Brecht
Department of Hematology and Oncology
University Children's Hospital
Tübingen, Baden-Württemberg, Germany

Thomas A. Olson
Aflac Cancer and Blood Disorders Center
Children's Healthcare of Atlanta and Emory University
Atlanta, GA, USA

Andrea Ferrari
Pediatric Oncology Unit
Fondazione IRCCS Istituto Nazionale dei Tumori
Milano, MI, Italy

ISSN 1613-5318 ISSN 2191-0812 (electronic)
Pediatric Oncology
ISBN 978-3-030-92073-9 ISBN 978-3-030-92071-5 (eBook)
https://doi.org/10.1007/978-3-030-92071-5

This Springer imprint is published by the registered company Springer Nature Switzerland AG
The registered company address is: Gewerbestrasse 11, 6330 Cham, Switzerland

Preface

If you work on frequent cancer, do randomized trials.
If you work on rare cancers—FIND FRIENDS!

All pediatric cancers are rare events when viewed in the backdrop of all cancers. And within the scope of childhood cancers, there are several infrequent tumors that pediatric oncologists would classify as "rare pediatric tumors." Therefore, what is the point in working on a book that specifically focuses on cancers that are "almost never" diagnosed? The most important reasons may be the child who suffers from a specific tumor, the families of these children not knowing how to cope with these diagnoses, and the treating physicians who may be confronted with a tumor, for which no evidence-based recommendations are available. Thus, this book shall help to take a group of tumors into focus, which otherwise would remain orphan diseases.

In fact, rare cancers as a group are not as uncommon as their designation may suggest. They contribute to at least 5% of all childhood cancers. However, caring for children with such rare cancers requires a tremendous effort, primarily because sufficient information on diagnosis and therapy is missing. As a consequence, the effort for treating physicians is inadequately high. Advances in pediatric oncology have always been facilitated through sharing information and networking between experts. Networks first began among groups of institutions. Later, networks were developed on a national basis, fostered by national cooperative groups. Recently, more and more international pediatric collaborations have been established to advance prospective therapeutic trials for "more common pediatric cancers." However, since rare tumors present with extremely low incidence, international collaboration is even more essential for these patients. Otherwise, each patient with a rare tumor will remain a "first patient" that cannot benefit from experience gathered from other patients with the same diagnosis.

This book attempts to fill this information gap, by providing pediatricians, pediatric oncologists, radiotherapists, and pediatric surgeons all currently available information required for diagnostic assessment and therapy of such patients. The second edition includes detailed checklists for diagnostic procedures and updated information on multimodal therapy of rare cancers. Furthermore, it integrates up-to-date information that has emerged from recent molecular genetic studies. These have often contributed to more precise classification and better understanding of the tumor biology, and sometimes even offered new targeted therapeutic strategies.

For most chapters, authors from different national study groups have shared their knowledge and developed common recommendations. Thus, the book reflects the growing experience gained through international collaboration. As for some entities, consensus recommendations have recently been developed; these are also integrated into the updated chapters. For other entities, these chapters represent the first comprehensive review in this particular entity to date. Sometimes, this has been a slow and stepwise but finally successful process. The discussions have also provided a fruitful and fantastic learning experience. We hope this book may provide a framework for future evolution into internationally accepted guidelines. Finally, this book is also the result of better understanding, deeper collaboration, and growing friendship—because: it is networking, or not working.

Therefore, we would like to thank all authors for their tremendous effort in writing their chapters. We would also like to thank Springer for the opportunity to further develop this project. Last, we thank our families for their continuous and loving support and their patience.

Encouraged by the overwhelming feedback to the first edition of our book, we sincerely hope that this book will again find the interest of the international audience and will be taken to hand often, rather than rarely.

Dortmund, Germany — Dominik T. Schneider
Tübingen, Germany — Ines B. Brecht
Atlanta, GA, USA — Thomas A. Olson
Milano, Italy — Andrea Ferrari

Contents

Part I

Introduction

1 Rare Tumors: A Different Perspective on Oncology

Thomas A. Olson, Dominik T. Schneider, Ines B. Brecht, and Andrea Ferrari

1.1 What Defines a Rare Tumor?

Compared to cancer in adults, childhood cancer is rare, accounting for significantly less than 1% of all cancer diagnoses. A meaningful clinical definition of a rare childhood cancer has to be developed in the context of the development of childhood cancer therapy over time. The successful treatment of children has been a remarkable accomplishment of the last 50 years. Today, approximately 75% of children diagnosed in countries with highly developed healthcare systems can be expected to be "cured" (Smith et al. 2010). This has been accomplished through extensive scientific exploration and the development of collaborative national and international clinical trials. Evidence from these trials has been incorporated into treatment strategies, suitable and assessable for children in countries with limited economic resources.

While most early pediatric clinical trials were conducted as national studies, collaborations have evolved which have incorporated specific disease members of several national groups into consortia. These alliances were necessary to allow randomized trials that could be completed in a reasonable period of time. Examples include Ewing's sarcoma and osteosarcoma trials, as well as current germ cell tumor and hepatoblastoma trials.

However, there is a hierarchy in the studies of childhood cancers. Most pediatric clinical trials involve childhood cancers that are relatively more common than other childhood cancers. Hepatoblastoma and germ cell tumors are examples of rare tumors in which national studies have led to established international collaborative clinical trials (Mann et al. 2000; Ortega et al. 2000; Göbel et al. 2002; Cushing et al. 2004; Perilongo et al. 2004, 2009). Other infrequent childhood cancers were often not registered or reported. However, there have been significant recent advances in the study of these cancers with the emergence of collaborative groups. An excellent example is the European EXPeRT collaboration (Ferrari et al. 2019). After establishing a consensus for joint actions, the EXPeRT group have subsequently published collaborative articles on mesothelioma (Orbach et al. 2020), sex cord stromal tumors (Schneider et al. 2021), and pleuro-

T. A. Olson
Division Pediatric Hematology/Oncology, Children's Healthcare of Atlanta at Egleston, Atlanta, GA, USA

D. T. Schneider (✉)
Klinik für Kinder- und Jugendmedizin, Clinic of Pediatrics, Klinikum Dortmund, University Witten/Herdecke, Dortmund, Germany
e-mail: dominik.schneider@klinikumdo.de

I. B. Brecht
Pediatric Oncology and Hematology, University Children's Hospital Tuebingen, Tuebingen, Germany
e-mail: ines.brecht@med.uni-tuebingen.de

A. Ferrari
Pediatric Oncology Unit, Istituto Nazionale Tumori, Milan, Italy

D. T. Schneider et al. (eds.), *Rare Tumors in Children and Adolescents*, Pediatric Oncology,
https://doi.org/10.1007/978-3-030-92071-5_1

pulmonary blastoma (Bisogno et al. 2021). From a clinical and scientific perspective, these rare cancers might be classified as orphan diseases, indicating that no clinical structures have been developed to aid in diagnosis and treatment. There are also many cancers that are common in adults, yet infrequently seen in children. This phenomenon increases as children age through adolescence into young adulthood. For some of these cancers, no specific clinical studies have been designed, but patients have been treated according to the corresponding guidelines for adult patients. Figure 1.1 illustrates the different epidemiological patterns of rare childhood cancers. There are some tumor types (Fig. 1.1a) that are defined by their generally extremely low incidence; nevertheless, they constitute characteristic tumors of childhood that are not diagnosed in adult patients. Well-defined examples include pancreaticoblastoma (see Chaps. 28 and 35) or mesoblastic nephroma. In contrast, other types (Fig. 1.1b) may be diagnosed during both childhood and adolescents. Clinically and pathologically, they may be undistinguishable; however, molecular genetic studies may reveal biological differences, as it has been demonstrated, e.g., for germ cell tumors in children and adults (for details see Chaps. 31 and 39) (Schneider et al. 2004).

Adult cancers, such as colon cancer and malignant melanoma, may also be diagnosed during childhood and adolescence (Fig. 1.1c). In general, this epidemiological pattern is character-

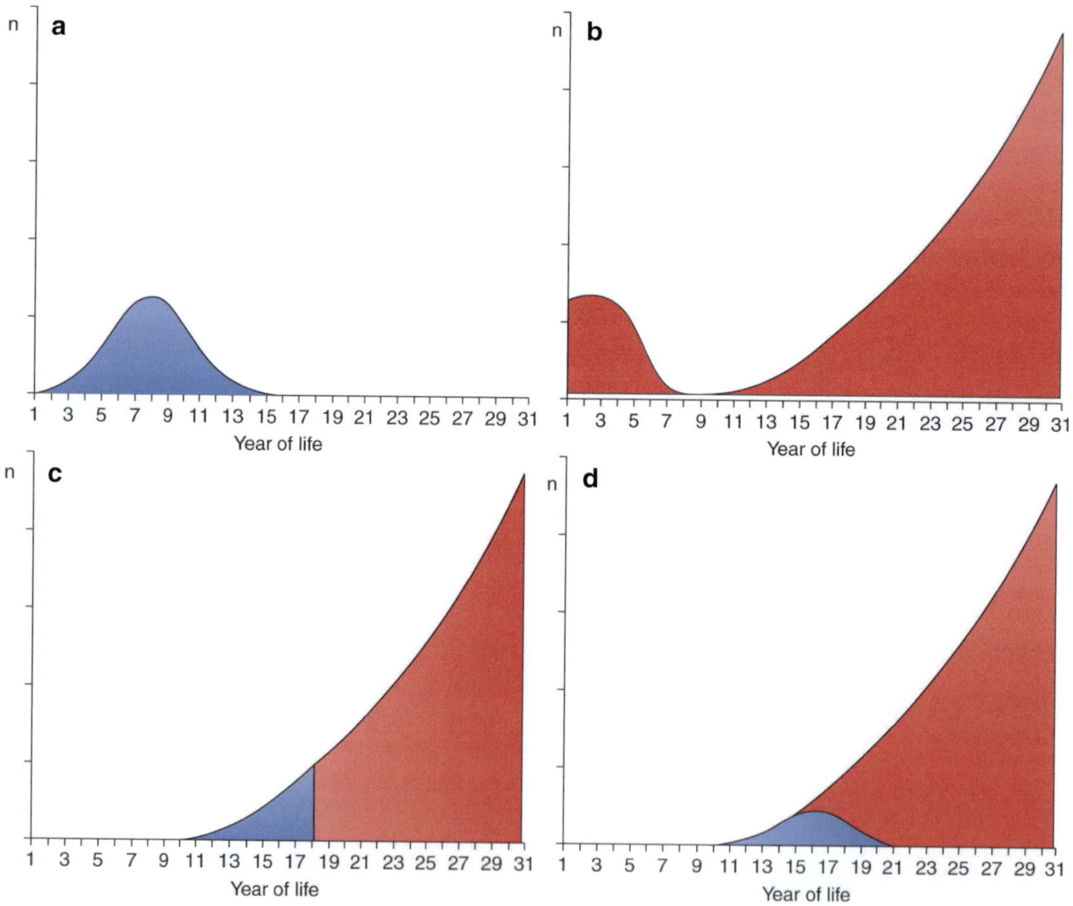

Fig. 1.1 Epidemiological patterns of rare childhood cancers: (**a**) low incidence tumor entity occurring exclusively in children. (**b**) A tumor entity with bimodal age distribution and age-dependent biology. (**c**) An adult-type tumor entity with rare occurrence during childhood and adolescence. (**d**) An adult-type tumor entity with rare occurrence during childhood and adolescence but with distinct biology

ized by a continuous increase of incidence over age. Thus, these rare childhood cancers constitute the left edge of the Gauss distribution curve of a frequent adult cancer. However, it should be noted that such cancers may also show biological and clinical characteristics that may distinguish such patients from others. Breast cancer and malignant melanomas are good examples. Both are frequent cancers in adults but infrequent in children and adolescents, and their presentation in young patients may be different from that in older patients (see Chaps. 33 and 40). Moreover, there are increased realization and identification of hereditary cancer and cancer predisposition syndromes in young patients (see Chap. 64).

Epidemiological investigations have formed the basis of our understanding of rare cancers. Most information on these "rare" tumors comes from national data sources such as Surveillance Epidemiology and End Results (SEER) database of the US National Cancer Institute (Ries et al. 1999), the German Childhood Cancer Registry, disease-specific registries (Schneider et al. 2004), or other national and international registries. The advancement of molecular profiling may enhance our understanding of these rare pediatric cancers. This book will focus on both rare pediatric cancers and cancers that commonly occur in adults, but only sporadically in children. Difficulties in diagnosis and treatment will be emphasized.

The first question to be addressed is what constitutes a "rare" disease? The National Institutes of Health in the USA defines a rare or orphan disease as one with a prevalence of fewer than 200,000 individuals in the USA (https://rarediseases.info.nih.gov). Subpopulations within a disease may also be considered "rare." In addition, the National Cancer Institute in the USA defines a "rare" cancer as one with an incidence less than 15/100,000 individuals. Of note, only 10,400 new cancer diagnoses are expected in 2010 among children up to 15 years of age in the USA (Table 1.1).

Though the incidence of childhood cancers is dwarfed by the numbers of most adult cancers, the individual impact on life expectancy is highest in children, in which a cancer diagnosis shortens life expectancy by approximately 70 years, compared to 9 years in prostate cancer. Thus, cancer remains the number one health-related cause of death in children beyond the neonatal period.

National pediatric groups have always understood that it was also their responsibility to care for children with "rare" tumors and to study the behavior of these childhood cancers. But the

Table 1.1 Incidence of selected cancer diagnoses in adult patients compared to age-related incidence rates of children and adolescents up to 19 years

Adult cancer		Childhood cancer	
Histology/site	Incidence (2003–2007)	Histology/site	Age-related incidence (2003–2007)
Resp. system/lungs	66.8	Leukemia	47.4
Digestive tract	87.0	Lymphoma	23.8
Breast (women)	152.9	Brain	41.4
Genital tract (women)	25.8	Neuroblastoma	10.2
Genital tract (men)	163.4	Gonadal tumors	11.6
Urinary system	36.0	Soft tissue	12.2
Skin	21.9	Bones	8.6
Endocrine system	10.9	Nephroblastoma	7.4
Oral cavity/pharynx	10.4	Thyroid	6.4
Soft tissues	3.2	Skin	5.8
Bones and joints	0.9	Others	5.1
Brain	6.5		
Lymphoma	22.4		
Leukemia	12.3		
Total	461.6	Total	183.2

Data from the US-SEER registry (http://seer.cancer.gov/csr/1975_2007/results_merged/sect_01_overview.pdf; http://seer.cancer.gov/csr/1975_2007/results_merged/sect_29_childhood_cancer_iccc.pdf)

development of clinical trials for infrequent childhood tumors has been limited. As a consequence, *the definition of a rare cancer in childhood does not simply reflect the low incidence but mainly refers to its status as an "orphan disease."* No standardized diagnostic and therapeutic guidelines are available to ensure that each patient is treated on an individual basis. For many of the more common childhood cancers, sophisticated risk stratification has led to further improvement of therapy. Many patients are treated on an individualized basis, determined by evidence-based risk assessment. But in rare pediatric cancers, limited risk assessment and treatment data are available. Therefore, networking, as demonstrated by the European EXPeRT Group, has as its goal the improved exchange of experience (and data) providing a method to increase understanding of these rare tumors. Finally, limited research opportunities exist for such rare cancers. This limits opportunities to collect further data that might speed up development of improved therapies. Current collection methods might not provide data on the true incidence of these tumors. Perhaps, the encouraging experience that has been gained with collaborative rare tumor groups might provide new perspectives for scientific evaluation and the development of guidelines based on better evidence.

1.2 The Issue of Adult Cancers in Children

Many adult cancers occur very infrequently in children. Gastrointestinal cancers, melanomas, lung cancer, breast cancers, and head and neck carcinomas cause millions of deaths each year. Yet, they are exceedingly rare in pediatric-aged patients. Nevertheless, parents and pediatric healthcare providers must be aware that these tumors can affect children because these children are rarely referred to a pediatric oncologist.

The question "Do adult-type cancers found in children have the same biological characteristics and behavior of the same cancer, isolated from an adult patient?" should be addressed (Ferrari et al. 2005). Are melanomas or epithelial cancers in children and adults the same disease? There are even more very important questions: "Why and how do pediatric patients develop adult tumors in a very short time period compared to protracted development in adults?" "Do they also develop through precancerous stages, as it has been extensively described, e.g., for intestinal polyps and colon carcinoma?" "How may these tumors arise in the obvious absence of environmental carcinogens such as ultraviolet light, tobacco smoke, asbestos, or others?"

One hypothesis is that pediatric tumors, which are classified as an adult-type tumor, such as adenocarcinoma of the colon, may not be biologically comparable to the histologically identical tumor in elderly patients. For some tumors, this hypothesis may be supported by different response rates to chemotherapy (e.g., gastrointestinal stromal tumors, GIST; see Chap. 27) (Demetri et al. 2006; Janeway et al. 2009). In this situation, pediatric patients would be expected to have decreased response rates when compared to adult patients. It is essential that if you administer treatments that have had success in adult patients, you collect data to support the hypothesis that this particular treatment will also save pediatric patients' lives.

In other entities, such as testicular and extragonadal germ cell tumors (GCT), different biological subgroups according to age have been clearly defined by genetic and molecular genetic analyses (see Chaps. 31 and 39). Even more importantly, there are well-defined biologic differences despite identical histology, e.g., yolk sac tumor. Of note, these biological differences may also translate into prognostic stratification, e.g., of mediastinal germ cell tumors according to age.

Comparable studies need to be performed for other adult cancers rarely occurring in children. However, such genetic studies have been hampered by the limited availability of appropriate tissue samples of these rare tumors. Therefore, central collection of tissue samples from rare tumors in central registries should strongly be advocated. This measure would provide researchers with the opportunity to advance the molecular understanding of rare cancer entities, with immediate impact on clinical diagnosis and follow-up (e.g., association of DICER1 mutations in pleuropulmonary blastoma and Sertoli-Leydig cell tumor (Hill et al. 2009)) and maybe even options for targeted treatment (C-KIT mutations in gastrointestinal stromal tumors (Demetri et al. 2006; Janeway et al. 2009)).

1.3 Clinical Issues in the Diagnosis and Treatment of Rare Pediatric Tumors

Rare pediatric tumors pose many challenges to pediatric oncologists. Some rare tumors, such as hepatoblastoma and GCT, are well known to pediatric oncologists. Pediatricians are also familiar with these tumors, even if they have never seen a patient with hepatoblastoma or GCT. However, the majority of tumors described in this book are tumors usually seen in adults. Diagnosis of these cancers in children can be difficult. Diagnostic approaches may not be familiar to pediatric oncologists. Once a diagnosis is established, treatments are often complex due to the lack of evidence to guide treatment in children. Moreover, some of the drugs or drug combinations applied in adult patients may not be familiar to pediatric oncologists, and toxicity in children has not yet been studied.

1.4 Delays in Diagnosis

Many pediatric providers may not be aware of the unusual presentations of rare tumors. An illustrative example is adenocarcinoma of the colon (see Chap. 32). Abdominal pain is a frequent complaint in children and adolescents. Most children with abdominal pain have gastrointestinal infections, and stool may often contain some blood. Another characteristic sign of adenocarcinoma of the right colon is iron deficiency. Iron deficiency constitutes another rather frequent diagnosis in children. In both situations diagnosis may be delayed. Several reports have suggested that colorectal carcinomas in children present with more extensive disease, more aggressive histiotypes, and poorer prognosis (Hill et al. 2007; Ferrari et al. 2008; Saab and Furman 2008; Sultan et al. 2010). These data may suggest that this disease may be biologically different in children (Durno et al. 2005). However, a delay in diagnosis may also contribute to the poorer prognosis. Education is important to identify patients at risk. We do have experience with screening as is well established in some childhood diseases, such as Beckwith-Wiedemann and familial polyposis (Half and Bresalier 2004; Erdman 2007). More must be done.

There are two decision points once a patient is referred for diagnosis. The appropriate laboratory and imaging studies must be completed. Diagnostic material must be acquired by appropriate surgery or biopsy. To ensure that adequate and complete material is collected for optimal diagnosis, both skilled (pediatric) surgeons and pathologists must collaborate. This expertise may be lacking at many institutions. This often results in further delays, and patients must be referred to other specialists. Patients often require subsequent surgery to collect more material.

Skilled pathologists are essential. One might require pathologists who specialize in both adult and pediatric tumors to be located in close proximity. Often, specimens must be sent to other pathologists for review, further delaying diagnosis.

Many pediatric tumors are treated on clinical trials. Central pathology review is mandated for some rare tumors such as hepatoblastoma and germ cell tumors. But for many rare pediatric cancers, central review does not exist; however it would urgently be required in order to avoid misdiagnoses.

1.5 The Challenge of Referral and Treatment

There is a great need for practical guidelines that can help physicians. Who to call, where to go, and what to do? There are few evidence-based studies because the numbers of patients are very small (Fig. 1.2). Pediatric oncologists will only

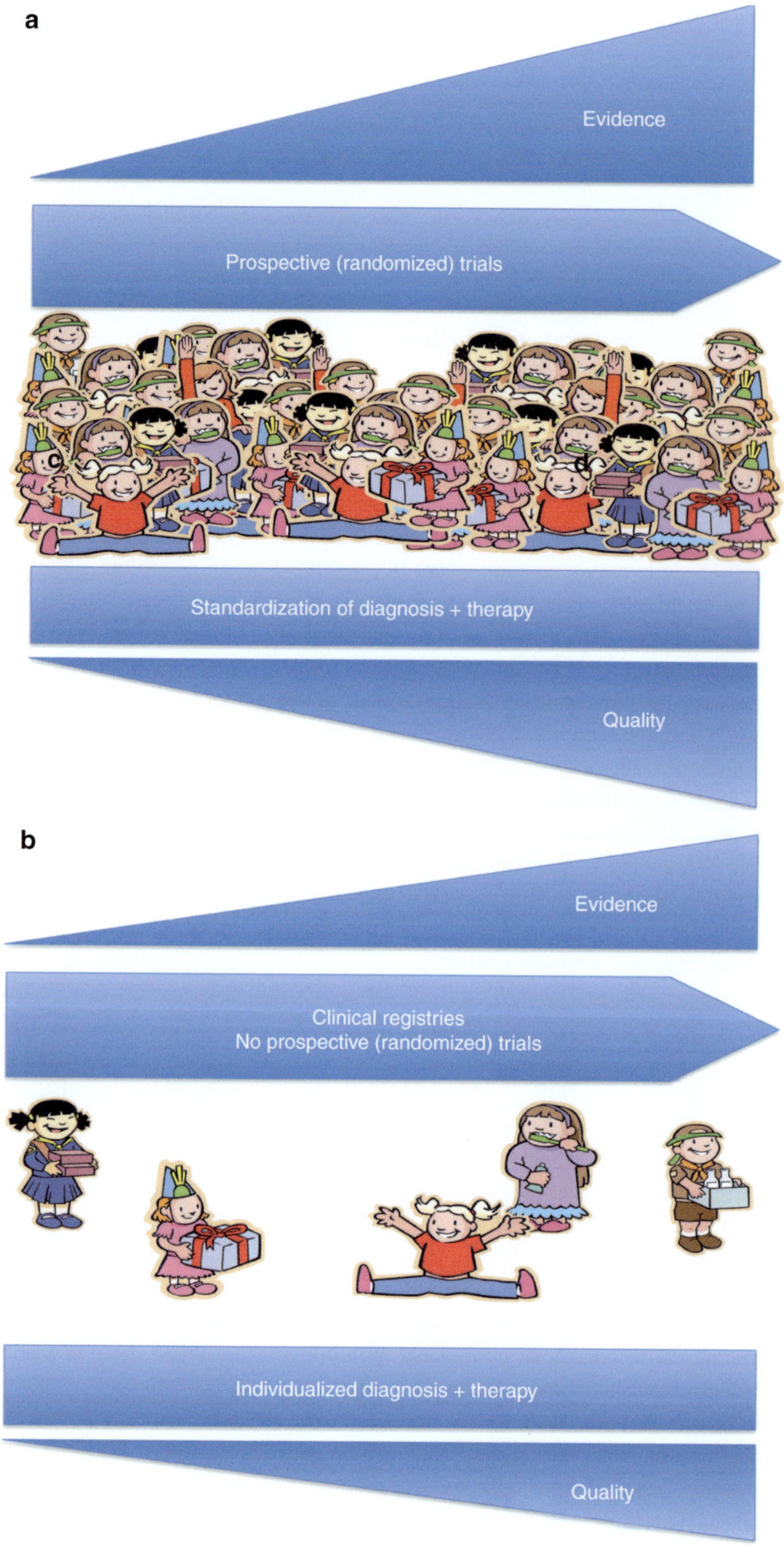

Fig. 1.2 Clinical standardization and development of increasing evidence in more frequent and rare childhood cancers. (**a**) The inclusion of large numbers of patients facilitates standardization of diagnosis and treatment. Clinical evidence is generated by the opportunity of "pattern recognition," thus identifying recurring clinical, pathological, and biological features that define prognostic and therapeutic groups. (**b**) In contrast, rare tumors are diagnosed and treated in a more individual approach. Therefore, and as a result of the low numbers, pattern recognition is impaired

manage a few patients with a specific diagnosis in their entire career.

It is crucial to develop a strategy for referral and treatment of children and adolescents with rare tumors. It is important that children and adolescents first have access to pediatric oncology treatment centers (Pastore et al. 2009). There are several considerations (Ferrari et al. 2010). There are comparison groups that, though not ideal, may be helpful. First, there are tumors that are very common in adults. Second, infrequent pediatric tumors that rarely occur in adults may also serve as a comparison group.

For children with adult-type tumors, one strategic option would be referral to an adult oncology facility. In the case of colorectal carcinoma, the presence of an experienced colorectal surgeon would seem beneficial. This might be appropriate in an older adolescent. Few pediatricians would be comfortable having a 10-year-old or even a 14-year-old treated in this manner. This may be "a good solution for the tumor, but not for the patient" (Ferrari and Sultan 2010). *Many children, both adolescents and young children, benefit from the family-focused care found in most pediatric oncology facilities*. The availability of psychologists, social workers, teachers, child life specialists, and volunteers contributes significantly to the well-being of the patients, parents, and other family members.

Another solution could be to treat these children in a pediatric setting with the contribution of experts who specialize in the treatment of adult tumors. This is often complicated by the physical separation of pediatric and adult treatment facilities. Though difficult, these obstacles have been overcome in many institutions, through collaboration at combined tumor boards, multidiscipline meetings, or clinics. Adolescent and young adult oncology centers have also been established. This collaborative strategy with medical oncologists may not always assure the best clinical management of children with adult cancers. Children are not small adults. They differ significantly from adults in physical, physiological, and cognitive functions. It is also important to emphasize that the description "child" is not uniform. Infants and old prepubertal children have immense differences in physiological, pharmacokinetic, and psychological characteristics. This knowledge and understanding of the developing child, however, is limited to the pediatrician and pediatric surgeon. One might argue that postpubertal adolescents and adults have similar physiological characteristics. However, no one would agree that their maturity and psychological states were similar. Gastrointestinal stroma tumor (GIST) in children may be one example of a complex integrated strategy. The National Cancer Institute in the USA has established a comprehensive pediatric GIST clinic that brings patients, clinicians, and scientists to the NCI clinical center for yearly study. The knowledge gained in this fashion has been very helpful in establishing that pediatric GIST differs from adult GIST. This effort benefits greatly from the strong commitment of patients, clinicians, and scientist as well as funding for NCI.

1.6 Biology

Pathological and biological studies are crucial to further success in the study of rare pediatric tumors. Clinicians and investigators must be prepared to apply new information to the study of rare pediatric tumors. This topic will be further developed in this book.

1.7 Possible Strategies in Pediatric Oncology Rare Tumors

1.7.1 Possible Solutions: "Collaboration, Find Friends!"

These tumors should no longer be viewed as "orphan" diseases, nor should they be the sole interest of small groups and experts. Rather, focused clinical/biologic studies should be promoted within the pediatric oncology community. Biology studies in pediatric rare tumors may also inform on biologic patterns in other pediatric tumors (Fig. 1.3).

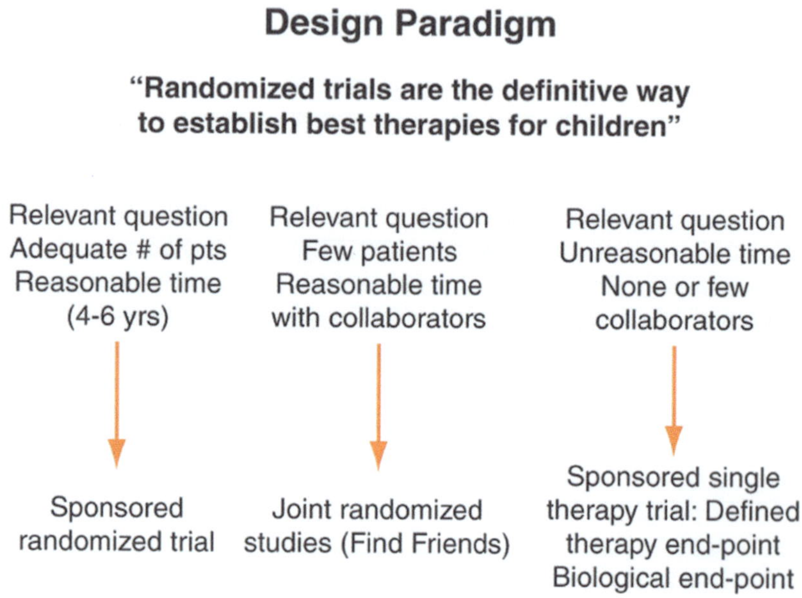

Fig. 1.3 Strategies for clinical trials in frequent and rare cancers

There have been recent movements to promote studies of patients with rare pediatric tumors. In Europe, several national groups established committees within their structures: the Italian Tumori Rari in Eta Pediatrica (TREP) (Ferrari et al. 2007) and Rare Tumor Group in the German Society of Pediatric Oncology and Hematology (GPOH) (Brecht et al. 2009). As detailed previously, the European Cooperative Study Group on Pediatric Rare Tumors (EXPeRT) has been very successful. In the USA, the Children's Oncology Group (COG) established the Rare Tumor Committee. Several collaborative groups for rare tumors, such as thyroid cancer, have also been established. Collaborations with national pediatric rare tumor groups could be established. One suggestion would be to develop specific guidelines for institutions that see only one to two new cases per year. The goal of such a study might be to collect biological specimens and minimal clinical data for correlation. These studies would require standard methodology to collect data.

It is essential that cooperative groups support efforts in advancing knowledge of rare pediatric tumors. However, these studies are hampered by lack of funding. In times of government cutbacks in research funding, priorities are established. Funding for infrequent childhood cancers may require innovative strategies.

There has been success recently in establishing clinical trials that accrue patients from childhood through adolescence, into young adulthood. Examples of these trials include leukemia, osteosarcoma, Ewing's sarcoma, and germ cell tumors. It is essential to determine a strategy for treating children and adolescents with adult-type cancers and referral institutions that have appropriate pediatric and internal medicine oncology collaboration. In addition, skilled oncology surgeons and pathologists are required.

1.8 Perspective

Despite the obstacles to the clinical management and research of rare cancers in childhood and adolescents, the field of rare cancers is one of the most fascinating aspects of pediatric oncology. Rare cancers may involve all different organ systems and many histological tumor types, including tumors of the spectrum of adult cancers. Thus, each patient broadens the perspective and deepens the knowledge of the responsible physician. In addition, the management of rare cancers poses specific challenges to the treating pediatric oncologist who must create a diagnostic and strategic concept for an individual patient rather than completing diagnostic algorithms proposed by a checklist within a study protocol. Lastly, in the perspective of no or only limited evidence, treatment decisions must be considered extremely carefully and in truthful and intensive discussions with the patient and his family. This is only possible in a trustful relation to the patient, which, on the other hand, makes the patient "special" not only in a medical and scientific but also in a very personal sense. Therefore, the "care for the rare" may constitute a very intensive and satisfying experience.

References

Bisogno G, Sarnacki S et al (2021) Pleuropulmonary blastoma in children and adolescents: the EXPeRT/PARTNER diagnostic and therapeutic recommendations. Pediatr Blood Cancer 68 Suppl 4:e29045. https://doi.org/10.1002/pbc29045

Brecht IB, Graf N et al (2009) Networking for children and adolescents with very rare tumors: foundation of the GPOH Pediatric Rare Tumor Group. Klin Pädiatr 221(3):181–185

Cushing B, Giller R et al (2004) Randomized comparison of combination chemotherapy with etoposide, bleomycin, and either high-dose or standard-dose cisplatin in children and adolescents with high-risk malignant germ cell tumors: a pediatric intergroup study—Pediatric Oncology Group 9049 and Children's Cancer Group 8882. J Clin Oncol 22(13):2691–2700

Demetri GD, van Oosterom AT et al (2006) Efficacy and safety of sunitinib in patients with advanced gastrointestinal stromal tumour after failure of imatinib: a randomised controlled trial. Lancet 368(9544):1329–1338

Durno C, Aronson M et al (2005) Family history and molecular features of children, adolescents, and young adults with colorectal carcinoma. Gut 54(8):1146–1150

Erdman SH (2007) Pediatric adenomatous polyposis syndromes: an update. Curr Gastroenterol Rep 9(3):237–244

Ferrari A, Brecht IB et al (2019) Defining and listing very rare cancers of paediatric age: consensus of the joint action on rare cancers in coordination with the European Cooperative Study Group for rare tumors. Eur J Cancer 110:120–126. https://doi.org/10.1016/j.ejca2018.12.031

Ferrari A, Sultan I (2010) When adult cancers occur in children. Expert Rev Anticancer Ther 10(11):1683–1685

Ferrari A, Bono A et al (2005) Does melanoma behave differently in younger children than in adults? A retrospective study of 33 cases of childhood melanoma from a single institution. Pediatrics 115(3):649–654

Ferrari A, Bisogno G et al (2007) The challenge of very rare tumours in childhood: the Italian TREP project. Eur J Cancer 43(4):654–659

Ferrari A, Rognone A et al (2008) Colorectal carcinoma in children and adolescents: the experience of the Istituto Nazionale Tumori of Milan, Italy. Pediatr Blood Cancer 50(3):588–593

Ferrari A, Casanova M et al (2010) Peculiar features and tailored management of adult cancers occurring in pediatric age. Expert Rev Anticancer Ther 10(11):1837–1851

Göbel U, Calaminus G et al (2002) Management of germ cell tumors in children: approaches to cure. Onkologie 25(1):14–22

Half EE, Bresalier RS (2004) Clinical management of hereditary colorectal cancer syndromes. Curr Opin Gastroenterol 20(1):32–42

Hill DA, Furman WL et al (2007) Colorectal carcinoma in childhood and adolescence: a clinicopathologic review. J Clin Oncol 25(36):5808–5814

Hill DA, Ivanovich J et al (2009) DICER1 mutations in familial pleuropulmonary blastoma. Science 325(5943):965

Janeway KA, Albritton KH et al (2009) Sunitinib treatment in pediatric patients with advanced GIST following failure of imatinib. Pediatr Blood Cancer 52(7):767–771

Mann JR, Raafat F et al (2000) The United Kingdom Children's Cancer Study Group's second germ cell tumor study: carboplatin, etoposide, and bleomycin are effective treatment for children with malignant extracranial germ cell tumors, with acceptable toxicity. J Clin Oncol 18(22):3809–3818

Orbach D, Andre N et al (2020) Mesothelioma in children and adolescents: the European cooperative study Group for Rare Tumors (EXPeRT) contribution. Eur J Cancer 140:63–70. https://doi.org/10.1016/j.ejca2020.09.011

Ortega JA, Douglass EC et al (2000) Randomized comparison of cisplatin/vincristine/fluorouracil and cisplatin/continuous infusion doxorubicin for treatment of pediatric hepatoblastoma: a report from the Children's Cancer Group and the Pediatric Oncology Group. J Clin Oncol 18(14):2665–2675

Pastore G, De Salvo GL et al (2009) Evaluating access to pediatric cancer care centers of children and adolescents with rare tumors in Italy: the TREP project. Pediatr Blood Cancer 53(2):152–155

Perilongo G, Shafford E et al (2004) Risk-adapted treatment for childhood hepatoblastoma. Final report of the second study of the International Society of Paediatric Oncology–SIOPEL 2. Eur J Cancer 40(3):411–421

Perilongo G, Maibach R et al (2009) Cisplatin versus cisplatin plus doxorubicin for standard-risk hepatoblastoma. N Engl J Med 361(17):1662–1670

Ries LA, Smith MAS, Gurney JG, Linet M, Tamra T, Young JL, Bunin GR (eds) (1999) Cancer incidence and survival among children and adolescents: United

States SEER Program 1975–1995, National Cancer Institute, SEER Program, NIH Publication No. 99–4649. Bethesda: National Cancer Institute

Saab R, Furman WL (2008) Epidemiology and management options for colorectal cancer in children. Paediatr Drugs 10(3):177–192

Schneider DT, Orbach D et al (2021) Consensus recommendations from the EXPeRT/PPARTNER groups for the diagnosis and therapy of sex cord stromal tumors in children and adolescents. Pediatr Blood Cancer 68 Suppl 4:e29017. https://doi.org/10.1002/pbc.29017

Schneider DT, Calaminus G et al (2004) Epidemiologic analysis of 1,442 children and adolescents registered in the German germ cell tumor protocols. Pediatr Blood Cancer 42(2):169–175

Smith MA, Seibel NL et al (2010) Outcomes for children and adolescents with cancer: challenges for the twenty-first century. J Clin Oncol 28(15):2625–2634

Sultan I, Rodriguez-Galindo C et al (2010) Distinct features of colorectal cancer in children and adolescents: a population-based study of 159 cases. Cancer 116(3):758–765

Part II

Epidemiology and Etiology of Rare Cancers

2 Epidemiology

Ines B. Brecht, Peter Kaatsch, and Annalisa Trama

2.1 Introduction

A rare disease affects a small percentage of the population. There had been several efforts to define rare diseases. Some characteristics of rare diseases have led to the expression "orphan disease" and influenced the definition of rare diseases: rare diseases often show a genetic origin, symptoms appear early in life, while the genetic predisposition lasts; rare diseases are often inadequately diagnosed and treated. The interest of the pharmaceutical industry to develop new drugs for rare diseases is generally low as the rarity of the disease leads to little financial incentive. Apart from this general consideration, a rare disease might be rare in a particular part of the world or in a specific group of people. The US Rare Disease Act of 2002 defines a rare disease as "any disease or condition that affects less than 200,000 persons in the United States," which is a prevalence of 1 in 1500 people or less (National Institutes of Health 2010).

However, this definition is based on prevalence and not incidence, as most rare diseases are chronic conditions. In contrast, cancer is a subacute disease; thus, its occurrence in a population should be measured by incidence. A consensus process within the European oncology community promoted by the RARECARE project defined rare cancers as those malignancies whose incidence is <6/100,000/year (Gatta et al. 2011). According to this definition, all childhood cancers are rare; however, there are some particularly rare pediatric cancers which have not benefited from advances made by the international pediatric oncology network. To establish a shared definition and produce a list of these entities, the European Union "Joint Action on Rare Cancers" (JARC) and the "European Cooperative Study Group for Pediatric Rare Tumors" (EXPERT) promoted a consensus effort. Rare pediatric tumors were listed and defined as those with an annual incidence of <2/1000,000 corresponding to 11% of all cancers in patients aged 0–14 years (Ferrari et al. 2019).

2.2 Classification

The specific spectrum of rare cancers in children is not well described through one of the existing classification systems. The International

I. B. Brecht (✉)
Department of Pediatric Hematology/Oncology, University Children's Hospital Tuebingen, Tuebingen, Germany
e-mail: ines.brecht@med.uni-tuebingen.de

P. Kaatsch
German Childhood Cancer Registry, Institute for Medical Biostatistics, Epidemiology and Informatics, Mainz, Germany

A. Trama
Evaluative Epidemiology Unit, Fondazione IRCCS Istituto Nazionale dei Tumori di Milano, Milan, Italy
e-mail: annalisa.trama@istitutotumori.mi.it

D. T. Schneider et al. (eds.), *Rare Tumors in Children and Adolescents*, Pediatric Oncology,
https://doi.org/10.1007/978-3-030-92071-5_2

Classification of Diseases for Oncology (ICD-O, third edition) is primarily developed for adult cancers and based on tumor site (Fritz et al. 2000). The International Classification of Childhood Cancer (ICCC, third edition) on the other hand is primarily based on morphology and histology (Steliarova-Foucher et al. 2005). A combination of both systems has to be used, the ICCC and ICD-O morphology and topography codes, in order to comprehensively describe rare tumors in children and adolescents. So far, no uniform classification system for rare pediatric tumor entities has been defined. Anyway, there have been efforts to develop a separate nosologic system for malignant entities occurring in adolescents and young adults (Birch et al. 2002). This system might be used as a basis for the development of a new classification for pediatric rare tumors, which mainly occur in adolescents and therefore show a similar spectrum.

2.3 How to Define Rare Tumors in Children and Adolescents?

Cancers rarely occur before the age of 14 years, and when they do, they raise a range of medical, psychological, ethical, and societal concerns. The age-standardized incidence rates of childhood cancer range from about 120 per million in southeast Asia to 150/160 per million in Europe and in the USA. However, the extent of the cancer burden in this young population is unknown in many low-income and middle-income countries (LMICs), where data on cancer incidence are not collected (Steliarova-Foucher et al. 2017). While according to the above definition of the RARECARE project all tumors are rare in childhood (incidence <6/100,000/year), pediatric oncologists realized that there are several cancers which they might only see once in their lifetime practice but present a major problem as no definite guidelines for diagnosis and treatment exist for pediatric age. Thus, realizing that we are actually dealing with not only very rare but also "orphan" entities, the Italian TREP project (Italian Study on Rare Tumors in Pediatric Age) pragmatically defined rare pediatric tumors as "any malignancies characterized by an annual incidence <2/million and not considered in other trials" (Ferrari et al. 2007). The German Rare Tumor group adopted this definition (Brecht et al. 2009).

However, due to the rarity of these tumors, problems arise in determining the exact incidence of rare pediatric tumors. Because of lacking experience with these tumor types, there might be diagnostic and coding inconsistencies and misclassification problems (Pastore et al. 2009). For example, the incidence of pleuropulmonary blastoma might be underestimated if they are registered as sarcomas. The risk of misclassification may inevitably be high in population-based cancer registries, because they are constructed on community-based pathological diagnoses and not exclusively on expert pathological diagnosis. Also, the classification of entities into benign, borderline, and malignant neoplasms might not be uniform (Stiller 2007). Some patients with rare tumors might not be reported to registries for reasons lying in the organizational structures of pediatric oncology within different countries. For example, an analysis from the population-based German Childhood Cancer Registry (GCCR) revealed 129 rare cases diagnosed between 1998 and 2007 and not being registered with one of the Society of Pediatric Oncology and Hematology (GPOH) studies (Brecht et al. 2010). This accounts for 1.2% of all malignancies or 3.8% of all malignant extracranial tumors registered within the GCCR. The authors concluded that rare pediatric cancers were underregistered due to different reasons lying in the status as an "orphan disease." In the UK, Brennan arbitrary defined rare pediatric tumors as those which have "an age-standardized annual incidence of less than 1 per million children in the U.K., excluding tumors of unspecified morphology" registering 766 patients under the age of 15 between 1991 and 2000 (Brennan and Stiller 2010). In the USA, the US Infrequent Tumor Initiative of the Children's Oncology Group basically deals with tumors "classified as other malignant epithelial neoplasms and melanomas in the International Classification of Childhood Cancer subgroup XI of the SEER database" being predominantly adult cancer occurring in pediatric age (Pappo et al. 2010). According to this definition, rare tumors compose approximately 15% of all cancers in the age group <15 years and 30% in <20 years (see chapter on national rare tumor groups).

Thus, traditionally, rare pediatric tumors are defined by incidence as well as their characteristics as an orphan disease:

Rare pediatric malignancies are characterized by an annual incidence <2/1,000,000 and/or are considered as "orphan" due to lack of pediatric trials and/or underestimation of incidence. Rare pediatric malignancies might be common in adult age or pediatric subpopulations like a specific age group, a country, or a gender, often an underlying genetic predisposition can be suspected, and they might be inadequately diagnosed and treated.

2.4 Incidence-Based Definition of Rare Tumors in Children and Adolescents

Recently, there have been efforts to define rare pediatric tumors according to incidence rates by using large databases. The Surveillance, Epidemiology, and End Results (SEER) database of the US National Cancer Institute registers patients with cancer of all age groups. Data is provided by 18 registries accounting for 10–14% of the US population during the study period from 1973 to 2004 (SEER 2007) and by 13 registries during the study period from 1992 to 2007 (SEER 2010). Data from the SEER database collected between 1992 and 2007 was used to get a more realistic overview of rare tumor entities in childhood and adolescence. According to the above-provided definition for rare pediatric tumors, all children and adolescents under the age of 20 years with an extracranial solid tumor and an incidence rate of <2/1,000,000 in the age group <15 years and/or <20 years were included in this analysis. Data was sorted by ICCC-3 and ICD-O3 (see Tables 2.1 and 2.2); 2887 patients with a rare solid extracranial tumor were identified within the age group 0–14 years and 6923 patients within the age group 0–19 years. The age-specific incidence rate of rare solid pediatric tumors in the USA was calculated to be 21.1/1,000,000 under the age of 15 and 37.6/1,000,000 under the age of 20. Table 2.1 shows age-specific incidence rates and percentages of rare pediatric tumors. In the age group 0–14 years, rare solid tumors account for 25% of all extracranial solid tumors and in the age group 0–19 years, 41%. Anyway, these numbers include germ cell tumors and rare soft tissue sarcomas, which are registered in pediatric clinical trials in most developed countries and therefore are not considered as rare pediatric tumors according to the above mentioned definition. If rare soft tissue sarcomas and germ cell tumors are excluded, the incidence rate of rare solid pediatric tumors usually not registered in clinical trials is 11.5/1,000,000 under the age of 15 and 21.3/1,000,000 under the age of 20. Consequently, surprisingly high numbers of children and adolescents with rare tumors can be identified through the SEER database.

In 2019, within the frame of a cooperative analysis of the European Union "Joint Action on Rare Cancers" (JARC) and the "European Cooperative Study Group for Pediatric Rare Tumors" (EXPeRT), a definition according to incidence rate could be found for very rare pediatric tumors by listing all pediatric cancers. Due to the strength of a profound epidemiological database, this consensus report succeeded to find a threshold below which a tumor entity is classified as rare – an annual incidence of 2/1,000,000. By doing this 11% of all cancers in patients aged 0–14 years were identified as rare (Ferrari et al. 2019). Within the population aged 0–19 years, three of these rare tumor types had an incidence rate which was >2/1,000,000 (i.e., thyroid and testicular cancers and skin melanoma); however, the consensus experts still considered them as "rare" according to their clinical needs (e.g., shortage of knowledge and clinical expertise as the other rare pediatric cancers) (Ferrari et al. 2019).

Table 2.1 Annual incidence of pediatric cancer and rare pediatric malignant tumors within different age groups (data from the US Surveillance, Epidemiology, and End Results database (1992–2007) (rare tumors defined as all extracranial solid tumors with an incidence rate of <2/1,000,000 in the age groups <15 years and/or <20 years)

	0–14 years		0–19 years		0–4 years		5–9 years		10–14 years		15–19 years	
US population	134,900,815		177,623,103		45,673,629		44,723,693		44,503,493		42,722,288	
	Rate	Count	Rate	Count	Rate	Count	Rate	Count	Rate	Count	Rate	Count
Incidence of all malignant cancer[a]	152.19	19,984	164.58	28,838	206.75	9445	110.57	4945	125.7	5594	207.25	8854
Incidence of all malignant solid tumors[b]	87.12	11,424	96.98	17,019	121.44	5552	58.49	2616	73.16	3256	130.96	5595
Incidence of rare malignant solid tumors[b]	21.06	2887	37.55	6923	20.94	958	11.46	516	31.7	1413	94.47	4036
Percentage of rare entities of all malignant solid tumors[b]	25		41		17		20		43		72	
Incidence of rare malignant solid tumors[b] excluding germ cell tumors and rare soft tissue sarcomas	11.53	1599	21.33	3952	10.04	459	6.77	305	18.72	835	55.08	2353
Percentage of rare entities[b] not registered in clinical studies of all malignant extracranial solid tumors	14		23		8		11		26		42	

[a] Including hematopoietic cancers and cranial tumors
[b] Excluding hematopoietic cancers and cranial tumors

Table 2.2 Rare tumors in children and adolescents: annual incidence rates and numbers of cases of all extracranial solid tumors (hematopoietic cancers excluded) with an incidence rate of <2/1,000,000 in the age group <15 years and/or <20 years sorted by ICCC (third edition) and registered within the US Surveillance, Epidemiology, and End Results database (1992–2007)

Age at diagnosis (years)	0–14 years		0–19 years		0–4 years		5–9 years		10–14 years		15–19 years	
International Classification of Childhood Cancer (third edition)	Rate	Count	Rate	Count	Rate	Count	Rate	Count	Rate	Count	Rate	Count
IV Rare tumors of the peripheral nervous cell												
IV (b) Other peripheral nervous cell tumors	0.19	26	0.26	47	0.15	7	0.18	8	0.25	11	0.49	21
VI Rare renal tumors												
VI (a.2) Rhabdoid renal tumor	0.20	24	0.16	24	0.50	23	0.02	1	0.00	0	0.00	0
VI (a.3) Kidney sarcomas	0.28	34	0.22	35	0.64	29	0.11	5	0.00	0	0.02	1
VI (b) Renal carcinomas	0.25	36	0.48	91	0.11	5	0.20	9	0.49	22	1.29	55
VII Hepatic tumors												
VII (a) Hepatoblastoma	**2.36**	282	1.83	282	**5.68**	260	0.40	18	0.09	4	0.00	0
VII (b) Hepatic carcinomas	0.36	52	0.59	110	0.18	8	0.27	12	0.72	32	1.36	58
VII (c) Unspecified malignant hepatic tumors	0.03	3	0.02	3	0.07	3	0.00	0	0.00	0	0.00	0
VIII Malignant bone tumors												
VIII (b) Chondrosarcomas	0.19	29	0.33	64	0.00	0	0.07	3	0.58	26	0.82	35
VIII (c.1) Ewing tumor and Askin tumor of bone	1.66	239	**2.27**	426	0.55	25	1.61	72	**3.19**	142	**4.38**	187
VIII (c.2) pPNET of bone	0.10	15	0.13	25	0.00	0	0.13	6	0.20	9	0.23	10
VIII (d.1) Malignant fibrous neoplasms of the bone	0.04	5	0.07	13	0.07	3	0.04	2	0.00	0	0.19	8
VIII (d.2) Malignant chordomas	0.15	21	0.23	43	0.11	5	0.20	9	0.16	7	0.51	22
VIII (d.3) Odontogenic malignant tumors	0.01	2	0.06	11	0.00	0	0.04	2	0.00	0	0.21	9
VIII (d.4) Miscellaneous malignant bone tumors	0.06	9	0.09	17	0.02	1	0.02	1	0.16	7	0.19	8
VIII (e) Unspecified malignant bone tumors	0.06	9	0.09	17	0.04	2	0.02	1	0.13	6	0.19	8
IX Rare soft tissue and other extraosseous sarcomas												
IX (b.1) Fibroblastic and myofibroblastic tumors	0.80	102	0.79	134	1.41	65	0.31	14	0.52	23	0.75	32
IX (b.2) Nerve sheath tumors	0.44	63	0.57	108	0.20	9	0.25	11	0.97	43	1.05	45
IX (b.3) Other fibromatous neoplasms	0.01	1	0.01	2	0.00	0	0.02	1	0.00	0	0.02	1
IX (c) Kaposi sarcoma	0.02	3	0.05	9	0.02	1	0.04	2	0.00	0	0.14	6
IX (d.1) Ewing tumor and Askin tumor of soft tissue	0.35	49	0.46	85	0.20	9	0.29	13	0.61	27	0.84	36
IX (d.2) pPNET of soft tissue	0.26	36	0.32	59	0.20	9	0.29	13	0.31	14	0.54	23
IX (d.3) Extrarenal rhabdoid tumor	0.22	27	0.17	28	0.44	20	0.04	2	0.11	5	0.02	1
IX (d.4) Liposarcomas	0.12	18	0.29	55	0.04	2	0.11	5	0.25	11	0.87	37
IX (d.5) Fibrohistiocytic tumors	0.94	133	1.33	247	0.59	27	0.65	29	1.73	77	**2.67**	114

(continued)

Table 2.2 (continued)

Age at diagnosis (years)	0–14 years		0–19 years		0–4 years		5–9 years		10–14 years		15–19 years	
International Classification of Childhood Cancer (third edition)	Rate	Count	Rate	Count	Rate	Count	Rate	Count	Rate	Count	Rate	Count
IX (d.6) Leiomyosarcomas	0.18	25	0.26	48	0.11	5	0.25	11	0.20	9	0.54	23
IX (d.7) Synovial sarcomas	0.59	88	0.96	184	0.11	5	0.29	13	1.57	70	**2.25**	96
IX (d.8) Blood vessel tumors	0.08	11	0.12	22	0.11	5	0.04	2	0.09	4	0.26	11
IX (d.9) Osseous and chondromatous neoplasms of soft tissue	0.08	11	0.11	21	0.02	1	0.07	3	0.16	7	0.23	10
IX (d.10) Alveolar soft parts sarcoma	0.08	12	0.12	23	0.04	2	0.04	2	0.18	8	0.26	11
IX (d.11) Miscellaneous soft tissue sarcomas	0.22	31	0.22	41	0.15	7	0.13	6	0.40	18	0.23	10
IX (e) Unspecified soft tissue sarcomas	0.77	108	1.03	190	0.55	25	0.49	22	1.37	61	1.92	82
X Germ cell tumors, trophoblastic tumors, and neoplasms of gonads												
X (b.1) Germinomas: extracranial/extragonadal	0.08	11	0.18	34	0.07	3	0.02	1	0.16	7	0.54	23
X (b.2) Malignant teratomas: extracranial/extragonadal	1.09	130	0.88	138	**2.70**	124	0.09	4	0.04	2	0.19	8
X (b.3) Embryonal carcinomas: extracranial/extragonadal	0.00	0	0.01	1	0.00	0	0.00	0	0.00	0	0.02	1
X (b.4) Yolk sac tumor: extracranial/extragonadal	0.54	65	0.45	70	1.31	60	0.04	2	0.07	3	0.12	5
X (b.5) Choriocarcinomas: extracranial/extragonadal	0.02	3	0.19	37	0.00	0	0.00	0	0.07	3	0.80	34
X (b.6) Other mixed germ cell: extracranial/extragonadal	0.09	11	0.14	25	0.20	9	0.00	0	0.04	2	0.33	14
X (c.1) Malignant gonadal germinomas	0.37	55	1.34	255	0.04	2	0.29	13	0.90	40	**4.68**	200
X (c.2) Malignant gonadal teratomas	0.85	121	1.86	348	0.52	24	0.60	27	1.57	70	**5.31**	227
X (c.3) Gonadal embryonal carcinomas	0.06	8	0.77	145	0.07	3	0.00	0	0.11	5	**3.21**	137
X (c.4) Gonadal yolk sac tumor	0.77	95	0.85	144	1.60	73	0.16	7	0.34	15	1.15	49
X (c.5) Gonadal choriocarcinoma	0.01	1	0.09	17	0.00	0	0.02	1	0.00	0	0.37	16
X (c.6) Malignant gonadal tumors of mixed forms	0.33	48	2.14	406	0.13	6	0.07	3	0.88	39	**8.38**	358
X (c.7) Malignant gonadal gonadoblastoma	0.00	0	0.01	1	0.00	0	0.00	0	0.00	0	0.02	1
X (d) Gonadal carcinomas	0.07	10	0.35	66	0.00	0	0.00	0	0.22	10	1.31	56
X (e) Other and unspecified malignant gonadal tumors	0.09	12	0.15	28	0.07	3	0.09	4	0.11	5	0.37	16
XI Other malignant epithelial neoplasms and malignant melanomas												
XI (a) Adrenocortical carcinomas	0.24	31	0.26	44	0.39	18	0.16	7	0.13	6	0.30	13
XI (b) Thyroid carcinomas	1.75	262	**5.18**	989	0.04	2	1.16	52	**4.67**	208	**17.02**	727
XI (c) Nasopharyngeal carcinomas	0.20	31	0.48	92	0.00	0	0.02	1	0.67	30	1.43	61
XI (d) Malignant melanomas	1.59	229	**4.63**	874	0.66	30	1.23	55	**3.24**	144	**15.10**	645
XI(e) Skin carcinomas	0.06	9	0.08	16	0.02	1	0.02	1	0.16	7	0.16	7
XI (f.1) Carcinomas of salivary glands	0.43	64	0.76	145	0.07	3	0.20	9	1.17	52	1.90	81

International Classification of Childhood Cancer (third edition)	Rate	Count	Rate	Count	Rate	Count	Rate	Count	Rate	Count	Rate	Count
XI (f.2) Carcinomas of colon and rectum	0.12	18	0.49	94	0.00	0	0.02	1	0.38	17	1.78	76
XI (f.3) Carcinomas of appendix	0.06	9	0.14	27	0.00	0	0.00	0	0.20	9	0.42	18
XI (f.4) Carcinomas of lung	0.11	16	0.25	47	0.02	1	0.04	2	0.29	13	0.73	31
XI (f.5) Carcinomas of thymus	0.04	6	0.06	11	0.00	0	0.04	2	0.09	4	0.12	5
XI (f.6) Carcinomas of breast	0.04	6	0.19	36	0.00	0	0.00	0	0.13	6	0.70	30
XI (f.7) Carcinomas of cervix uteri	0.02	3	0.23	43	0.00	0	0.04	2	0.02	1	0.94	40
XI (f.8) Carcinomas of bladder	0.02	3	0.08	15	0.02	1	0.00	0	0.04	2	0.28	12
XI (f.9) Carcinomas of eye	0.02	3	0.02	4	0.02	1	0.02	1	0.02	1	0.02	1
XI (f.10) Carcinomas of other specified sites	0.40	58	0.93	176	0.15	7	0.27	12	0.88	39	**2.76**	118
XI (f.11) Carcinomas of unspecified site	0.09	13	0.20	37	0.07	3	0.00	0	0.22	10	0.56	24
XII (a.1) Gastrointestinal stromal tumor	0.04	5	0.05	10	0.02	1	0.02	1	0.07	3	0.12	5
XII (a.2) Pancreatoblastoma	0.03	5	0.03	6	0.00	0	0.07	3	0.04	2	0.02	1
XII (a.3) Pulmonary blastoma and pleuropulmonary blastoma	0.10	12	0.08	13	0.22	10	0.00	0	0.04	2	0.02	1
XII (a.4) Other complex mixed and stromal neoplasms	0.03	4	0.05	9	0.00	0	0.02	1	0.07	3	0.12	5
XII (a.5) Mesothelioma	0.00	0	0.02	4	0.00	0	0.00	0	0.00	0	0.09	4
XII (a.6) Other specified malignant tumors	0.01	1	0.01	1	0.00	0	0.00	0	0.02	1	0.00	0
XII (b) Other unspecified malignant tumors	0.19	25	0.28	51	0.22	10	0.13	6	0.20	9	0.61	26
Sum	21.06	2887	37.55	6923	20.94	958	11.46	516	31.7	1413	94.47	4036

Incidence rates of >2/1,000,000 within specific age groups are marked in bold

2.5 Rare Pediatric Cancer Age-Specific Incidence

The overall incidence of rare pediatric tumors rises dramatically within adolescence (Table 2.1 and Fig. 2.1). As shown in Table 2.1, rare pediatric tumors account for 8% of all malignant solid extracranial tumors within the age group 0–4 years; within the age group of 15–19 years, this number rises up to 42%. Also, the European Automated Childhood Cancer Information System (ACCIS) reports an incidence of carcinomas of 3.4/100,000 in the age group 0–14 years, but 9.9/100,000 in children and adolescents up to 19 years (http://wwwdep.iarc.fr/accis.htm). While in younger age groups histotypes typically diagnosed in the pediatric age predominate (i.e., hepatoblastoma, pleuropulmonary blastoma, pancreatoblastoma), tumor types that frequently occur in adults, but rarely on children and adolescents (e.g., melanoma, carcinomas), prevail during adolescence.

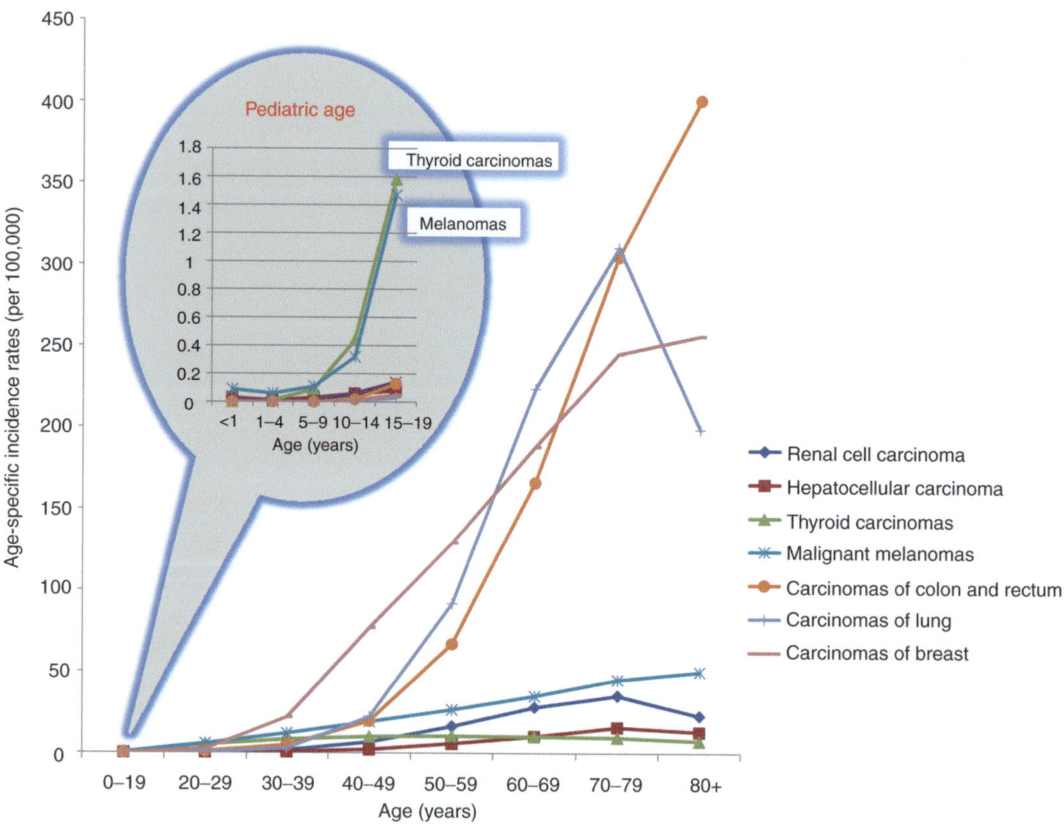

Fig. 2.1 Age-specific incidence rates (per 100,000 population) of selected adult cancers from the United States Surveillance, Epidemiology and End Results database (1973–2006). (Courtesy Dr. Sultan, Dr. Ferrari)

2.6 Conclusion

The JARC and EXPeRT consensus has provided a definition of very rare pediatric cancers based on incidence rates. However, this definition and the categorization and determination of incidence rates of rare tumors have to be considered "work in progress." For example, with the implementation of clinical and scientific structures for rare pediatric cancers, we see a rise in documented cases within registries. Moreover, new tumor entities are discovered by molecular characterization leading to a re-classification. Therefore, facilitated by sustainable clinical structures and scientific progress, the picture of rare pediatric tumors will develop continuously and hopefully become clearer over the next years.

References

Birch JM, Alston RD et al (2002) Classification and incidence of cancers in adolescents and young adults in England 1979–1997. Br J Cancer 87(11):1267–1274

Brecht IB, Graf N et al (2009) Networking for children and adolescents with very rare tumors: foundation of the GPOH pediatric rare tumor group. Klin Padiatr 221(3):181–185

Brecht I, Bremensdorfer C et al (2010) Incidence of rare malignant pediatric tumors in Germany 1998–2007: data from the German Childhood Cancer Registry. Pediatr Blood Cancer 55:909

Brennan B, Stiller C (2010) Rare tumors. In: Estlin EJ, Gilbertson RJ, Wynn RF (eds) Pediatric hematology and oncology. Blackwell Publishing Ltd, Hoboken

Ferrari A, Bisogno G et al (2007) The challenge of very rare tumours in childhood: the Italian TREP project. Eur J Cancer 43(4):654–659

Ferrari A, Brecht IB et al (2019) Defining and listing very rare cancers of paediatric age: consensus of the Joint Action on Rare Cancers in cooperation with the European Cooperative Study Group for Pediatric Rare Tumors. Eur J Cancer 110:120–126

Fritz AG, Percy C et al (2000) International classification of diseases for oncology (ICD-O), 3rd edn. World Health Organization, Geneva

Gatta G, van der Zwan JM, Casali PG et al (2011) Rare cancers are not so rare: the rare cancer burden in Europe. Eur J Cancer 47(17):2493–2511

National Institutes of Health (2010) National Institutes of Health. Office of rare disease research. Rare diseases and related terms. http://rarediseases.info.nih.gov/RareDiseaseList.aspx. Accessed 28 Feb 2011

Pappo AS, Krailo M et al (2010) Infrequent tumor initiative of the Children's Oncology Group: initial lessons learned and their impact on future plans. J Clin Oncol 28(33):5011–5016

Pastore G, De Salvo GL et al (2009) Evaluating access to pediatric cancer care centers of children and adolescents with rare tumors in Italy: the TREP project. Pediatr Blood Cancer 53(2):152–155

Surveillance, Epidemiology, and End Results (SEER) Program Populations (1973–2004) (2007) National Cancer Institute, DCCPS, Surveillance Research Program, Cancer Statistics Branch. www.seer.cancer.gov/popdata

Surveillance, Epidemiology, and End Results (SEER) Program Populations (1992–2007) (2010) National Cancer Institute, DCCPS, Surveillance Research Program, Cancer Statistics Branch. www.seer.cancer.gov/popdata

Steliarova-Foucher E, Stiller C et al (2005) International classification of childhood cancer, third edition. Cancer 103(7):1457–1467

Steliarova-Foucher E, Colombet M, Ries LAG et al (2017) International incidence of childhood cancer, 2001–10: a population-based registry study. Lancet Oncol 18(6):719–731

Stiller CA (2007) International patterns of cancer incidence in adolescents. Cancer Treat Rev 33(7):631–645

3 Biology and Etiology of Rare Pediatric Tumors

Ines B. Brecht and H. M. J. Merks

3.1 Introduction

Different malignant tumor types occur in children compared to adults. While in childhood we typically find leukemia, lymphoma, and various embryonal tumors, in adulthood, mainly gastrointestinal cancer, melanoma, malignancies of the head and neck, and lung and breast cancers occur. Not only tumor types and frequency differ, but also the pathogenetic origin and genetic factors in malignant childhood tumors are unlike those in adult cancer. Cancer biology changes over age as the inner and outer circumstances at the time of cancer initiating mutation vary according to state of development. Neoplasia in childhood and adolescence are mainly based on an intrinsic system error—mislead development within embryogenesis. These are often very simple but specific DNA, chromosome, or genomic rearrangements. Epithelial tumors and other adult-type tumors like secondary leukemia on the other hand show more complex genetic alterations. A long history of carcinogenic and mutagenic exposition and mislead differentiation, aging, and elimination processes are involved in carcinogenesis in adulthood. These differences might also explain why childhood cancer is more responsive to therapy than adult cancer (Haas 2004).

3.2 Rare Pediatric Tumors

Also in children, we rarely find malignancies of adult age (see Fig. 3.1). These are mainly carcinomas of the head and neck, malignancies of the gastrointestinal tract, and melanoma. Because of the rarity of these entities within childhood, most clinicians are unsure about the biological and clinical characteristics and thus management within young ages. We understand that we deal with four different groups of rare tumors in childhood (see Introduction and Fig. 3.1). These are:

(a) Characteristic malignant tumors of childhood with generally extremely low incidence, e.g., pancreaticoblastoma or mesoblastic nephroma
(b) Malignant tumors, which might be diagnosed both during childhood and adolescence, which might be clinically and pathologically undistinguishable but biologically different, e.g., germ cell tumors
(c) Characteristic adult cancers, which are rarely diagnosed during childhood or adolescence presenting as the left edge of the Gauss

I. B. Brecht (✉)
Pediatric Hematology and Oncology, University of Tuebingen, Tuebingen, Germany
e-mail: ines.brecht@med.uni-tuebingen.de

H. M. J. Merks
Emma Children's Hospital—Academic Medical Center, University of Amsterdam, Amsterdam, The Netherlands

D. T. Schneider et al. (eds.), *Rare Tumors in Children and Adolescents*, Pediatric Oncology,
https://doi.org/10.1007/978-3-030-92071-5_3

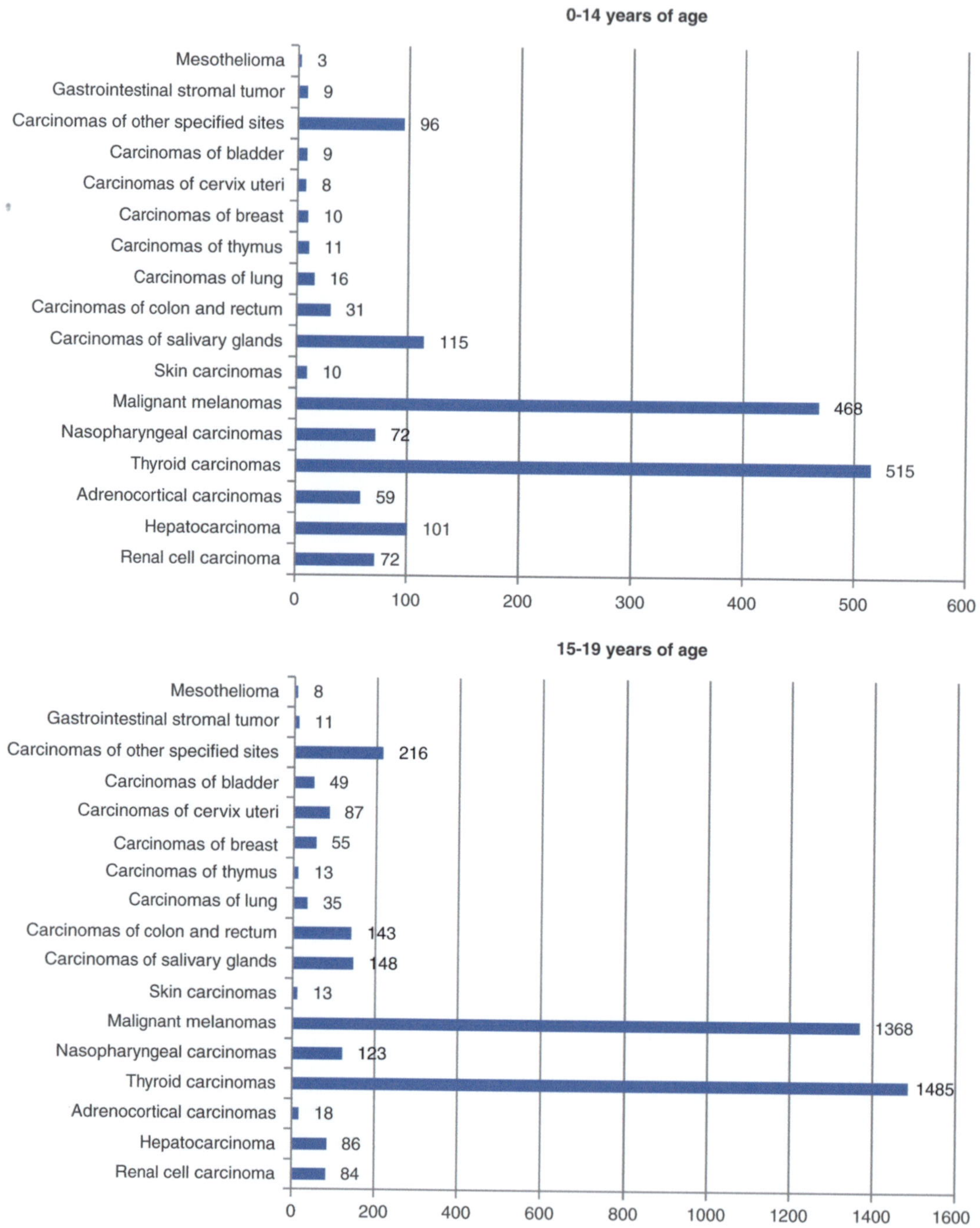

Fig. 3.1 Adult cancers occurring in childhood and adolescence: number of cases registered in the US Surveillance, Epidemiology and End Results (SEER) database (1973–2006)

distribution curve of a frequent adult cancer but still possibly showing biological and clinical characteristics different from adulthood, e.g., colon carcinoma and malignant melanoma

(d) Specific subentities of adult cancer types—hidden in the left edge of the Gauss distribution curve—with postulated distinct genetics and biology, e.g., underlying hereditary cancer syndromes

3.3 Etiological and Biological Characteristics of Rare Pediatric Tumors

Little is known about the etiopathogenesis of rare tumors as there are several barriers for biological studies resulting from the rarity. Anyway, for many reasons, it is likely that we deal with very different tumorigenic mechanisms in rare pediatric tumors compared to classical tumors of childhood or adulthood. While for most typical childhood cancers it seems that prognosis declines with age, as shown for acute lymphoblastic leukemia (ALL) and Ewing sarcoma (Rivera et al. 1993; Perentesis 1997; Cotterill et al. 2000), there is the impression that adult cancer shows a different behavior in childhood (Ferrari et al. 2010). For example, while survival and prognostic factors in pediatric malignant melanomas are generally comparable to adults (Brecht and Garbe 2015; Brecht et al. 2018; Offenmueller et al. 2017), pediatric spitzoid melanomas or so-called melanocytic tumors of uncertain malignant potential (MELTUMP) behave differently and diagnosis based on molecular analyses as well as clinical consultations is crucial to prevent overtreatment of children and adolescents.

In adulthood, these malignant tumors occur as a result of genetic changes following many years of exposure to carcinogens, but in young patients, cancer cannot be a result of long-term exposure. Typical childhood cancers are known to develop as a result of strong congenital and prenatal factors. In the same way the outer circumstances of cancer genesis change with age, we also see differences in the tissue environment over the phases in life. While in early life cell division and differentiation are dominant, in adulthood, we see a period of homeostasis and maintenance with cellular repair followed by a phase of degenerative changes with apoptosis and senescence at the end of life (Rubin et al. 2010). Tumorigenesis involves the escape from these mechanisms; and consequently, we see diverse types of cancer and different responses to therapy over the life span. Also, in the same way as a typical pediatric malignancy like acute lymphoblastic leukemia shows different genetic alterations according to pediatric age group (early age TEL-AML, later t(9;22)), it can be assumed that the genetic of adult-type cancer in children is unlike that seen in adults.

From these considerations results the interesting question, why we rarely observe adult-type tumors in childhood. Are they biologically the same tumors? Do they have the same characteristics? As cancer genesis is complex and multiple factors influence the process, the answer to these questions cannot be unilateral. We postulate that we find a combination of a genetic predisposition, immunological factors, and early exposure to environmental factors promoting cancer, which might be different from typical carcinogens of adulthood like asbestos and tobacco smoke. Anyway, there is increasing evidence that the biology and clinical characteristics of adult-type tumors in children are not the same as in adults. Several examples are given in individual disease-based chapters of this book. Here we want to give an overview of possible mechanisms.

3.3.1 Rare Typical Childhood Cancers

Rare typical childhood cancers are characteristic malignant pediatric tumors with generally extremely low incidence. In the phase of growth and development, mutations result in congenital defects or neoplasia. Hepatoblastoma is a typical malignant tumor of this category, arising usually in the first 2 years of life, with a mean age of onset of approximately 16–20 months (Darbari et al. 2003). The etiology is still matter of investigation; several studies suggest an interference with prenatal or postnatal exposure of the premature liver to different noxa like alcohol, oral contraceptive, and metals. Also, several genetic syndromes have been shown to be associated with hepatoblastoma: Beckwith–Wiedemann syndrome, familial adenomatous polyposis, Simpson–Golabi–Behmel syndrome, and trisomy of chromosome 8. Interestingly, even within childhood, different phases of rapid development of organs seem to coincide with variant malignancies of these organs (Rubin et al. 2010).

3.3.2 Rare Malignancies with Different Biology in Childhood and Adulthood

Malignant tumors, which might be diagnosed both during childhood and adolescence, might be clinically and pathologically undistinguishable but biologically different, e.g., germ cell tumors in children and adults (Schneider et al. 2004). Different biological subgroups were found and defined leading to a prognostic stratification according to age in the case of mediastinal germ cell tumors (Schneider et al. 2000). Jarzab proposes that thyroid cancer in children and adults constitutes a distinct disease. He describes a different histology (more papillary thyroid cancer), a higher prevalence of rEt/Ptc rearrangements, presentation at more advanced stages, a different pattern of tumor dissemination, and higher rates of recurrence in thyroid cancer of childhood compared to adult cases (Jarzab and Handkiewicz-Junak 2007).

3.3.3 Adult-Type Cancer in Children

In adulthood, mainly carcinomas occur, probably because of the epithelium being the most active tissue and therefore prone to malignant transformation by toxins, viruses, and radiation. Long-term exposure to toxins and failure in maintenance and repair lead to oncogenesis. This is rarely the case in childhood. Etiology is likely to be different as an exposure of carcinogens over decades was not possible before the occurrence in childhood. Anyway, if we postulate that a cumulative "dose" is necessary for the development of cancer, especially intense exposure could be the explanation for early occurrence. Examples are chemotherapy/radiation therapy in case of second malignancies or the Chernobyl accident in 1986 in case of thyroid cancer (Moysich et al. 2002). For unknown reasons, the thyroid gland is more susceptible to the carcinogenetic effect of ionization in children than in adults. A recent study revealed different molecular signatures in a rare subtype arising from congenital cutaneous nevi compared to the typical UV-related melanoma in elderly patients (Lu et al. 2015).

Oncogenic viruses lead to cancer in all age groups but show varying importance in different countries over the world. Carcinoma of the cervix and uterus, typical malignancies of older age, appear in young women in case of exposure to herpes simplex virus type 2 and human papilloma virus. Hepatitis B and C infections are the strongest risk factors for the development of hepatocellular carcinoma in children. Consequently, in endemic areas of Southeast Asia, where hepatitis B and C infection rates are high, a high rate of hepatocellular carcinoma is seen in children (Chang et al. 1997). The utilization of hepatitis B vaccine has significantly diminished the incidence of hepatocellular carcinoma. Chronic Epstein–Barr virus (EBV) infections play an important role in the malignant transformation of nasopharyngeal carcinoma cells (Raab-Traub 2002). While nasopharyngeal carcinoma is a rare malignancy in most parts of the world, it is one of the most common cancers in Southeast Asia due to specific environmental factors (certain herbs and salted fish), genetic factors, and early EBV infection (Ren et al. 2010).

For several rare tumors/adult-type tumors occurring in childhood, a genetic susceptibility or transcribed predisposition syndromes have been identified (see Chap. 4). In pediatric melanoma, etiology is not solely explained by UV exposure. Not only immunosuppression and radiotherapy have been described to play a role in carcinogenesis but also germline mutations in CDKN2A and CDK4 susceptibility genes as well as BRAF oncogene activation (Hayward 2003). Patients with Beckwith–Wiedemann syndrome, an overgrowth syndrome linked to chromosome 11p, are prone to rare (hepatoblastoma) and more frequent (Wilms' tumor and neuroblastoma) childhood tumors as well as adult-type tumors (adrenocortical carcinoma) (Clericuzio et al. 2003). Another study found alterations in the breast cancer susceptibility genes (including BRCA 1, BRCA 2, and TP53) in 20% of women diagnosed with carcinoma of the breast under the age of 30 (Lalloo et al. 2003). While heterozygous germline mutations in the human mismatch repair genes (MLH1, PMS2, MSH2, MSH6) predispose to the hereditary nonpolyposis colorectal cancer (HNPCC) syndrome, biallelic mutations in these genes have also been associated with occurrence of other gastrointestinal tumors in early childhood as well as childhood cancer (hematological malignancies and brain tumors) (Weber et al. 2016; Plaschke et al. 2006). So far, only few studies investigated the frequency of cancer susceptibility genes in early onset carcinoma.

Finally, there is evidence that translocation-triggered carcinomas are overrepresented among pediatric carcinomas as reflected by the predominance of MAML2-driven mucoepidermoid carcinomas as the most frequent salivary gland malignancy in children (Agaimy et al. 2021; Schwarz et al. 2011). Furthermore, recent evidence suggests that oncogenic gene fusions (some of them are novel therapeutic targets such as ALK, NTRK, and others) might be overrepresented in some pediatric epithelial malignancies and in mesotheliomas (Argani et al. 2021). In contrast to the primitive pediatric malignancies driven by simple genetic errors such as inactivating mutations of tumor suppressors (e.g., in AT/RT), the molecular background of epithelial malignancies is not understood yet.

3.3.4 Conclusion

Tumor biology and etiology change over the human life span. In consequence, clinical management cannot be transferred one-to-one from adult experience to pediatric oncology. It is crucial to learn more about the differences in biology of these tumors in order to guarantee the highest quality care for rare tumors in childhood and adolescence. Biological and epidemiological studies will have to be conducted in international cooperation in order to understand the processes underlying the differences of malignancies occurring according to age.

References

Agaimy A, Stoehr R et al (2021) YAP1-MAML2-rearranged poroid squamous cell carcinoma (squamoid porocarcinoma) presenting as a primary parotid gland tumor. Head Neck Pathol 15(1):361–367

Argani P, Lian DWQ et al (2021) Pediatric mesothelioma with ALK fusions: a molecular and pathologic study of 5 cases. Am J Surg Pathol 45(5):653–661

Brecht IB, Garbe C (2015) 443 paediatric cases of malignant melanoma registered with the German central malignant melanoma registry between 1983 and 2011. Eur J Cancer 51:861–868

Brecht IB, De Paoli A et al (2018) Pediatric patients with cutaneous melanoma: a European study. Pediatr Blood Cancer 65:e26974

Chang MH, Chen CJ et al (1997) Universal hepatitis B vaccination in Taiwan and the incidence of hepatocellular carcinoma in children. Taiwan Childhood Hepatoma Study Group. N Engl J Med 336(26):1855–1859

Clericuzio CL, Chen E et al (2003) Serum alpha-fetoprotein screening for hepatoblastoma in children with Beckwith-Wiedemann syndrome or isolated hemihyperplasia. J Pediatr 143(2):270–272

Cotterill SJ, Ahrens S et al (2000) Prognostic factors in Ewing's tumor of bone: analysis of 975 patients from the European Intergroup Cooperative Ewing's Sarcoma Study Group. J Clin Oncol 18(17):3108–3114

Darbari A, Sabin KM et al (2003) Epidemiology of primary hepatic malignancies in U.S. children. Hepatology 38(3):560–566

Ferrari A, Casanova M et al (2010) Peculiar features and tailored management of adult cancers occurring in pediatric age. Expert Rev Anticancer Ther 10(11):1837–1851

Haas OA (2004) Genetic diagnosis in pediatric oncology, de Gruyter

Hayward NK (2003) Genetics of melanoma predisposition. Oncogene 22(20):3053–3062

Jarzab B, Handkiewicz-Junak D (2007) Differentiated thyroid cancer in children and adults: same or distinct disease? Hormones (Athens) 6(3):200–209

Lalloo F, Varley J et al (2003) Prediction of pathogenic mutations in patients with early-onset breast cancer by family history. Lancet 361(9363):1101–1102

Lu C, Zhang J et al (2015) The genomic landscape of childhood and adolescent melanoma. J Invest Dermatol 135:816–823

Moysich KB, Menezes RJ et al (2002) Chernobyl-related ionising radiation exposure and cancer risk: an epidemiological review. Lancet Oncol 3(5):269–279

Offenmueller S, Leiter U et al (2017) Clinical characteristics and outcome of 60 pediatric patients with malignant melanoma registered with the German Pediatric Rare Tumor Registry (STEP). Klin Padiatr 229:322–328

Perentesis JP (1997) Why is age such an important independent prognostic factor in acute lymphoblastic leukemia? Leukemia 11(suppl 4):S4–S7

Plaschke J, Linnebacher M et al (2006) Compound heterozygosity for two MSH6 mutations in a patient with early onset of HNPCC-associated cancers, but without hematological malignancy and brain tumor. Eur J Hum Genet 14(5):561–566

Raab-Traub N (2002) Epstein-Barr virus in the pathogenesis of NPC. Semin Cancer Biol 12(6):431–441

Ren ZF, Liu WS et al (2010) Effect of family history of cancers and environmental factors on risk of nasopharyngeal carcinoma in Guangdong, China. Cancer Epidemiol 34(4):419–424

Rivera GK, Pui CH et al (1993) Progress in the treatment of adolescents with acute lymphoblastic leukemia. Cancer 71(10 suppl):3400–3405

Rubin P, Williams JP et al (2010) Cancer genesis across the age spectrum: associations with tissue development, maintenance, and senescence. Semin Radiat Oncol 20(1):3–11

Schneider DT, Calaminus G et al (2000) Primary mediastinal germ cell tumors in children and adolescents: results of the German cooperative protocols MAKEI 83/86, 89, and 96. J Clin Oncol 18(4):832–839

Schneider DT, Calaminus G et al (2004) Epidemiologic analysis of 1,442 children and adolescents registered in the German germ cell tumor protocols. Pediatr Blood Cancer 42(2):169–175

Schwarz S, Stiegler C et al (2011) Salivary gland mucoepidermoid carcinoma is a clinically, morphologically and genetically heterogeneous entity: a clinicopathological study of 40 cases with emphasis on grading, histological variants and presence of the t(11;19) translocation. Histopathology 58:557–570

Weber ML, Schneider DT et al (2016) Pediatric colorectal carcinoma is associated with excellent outcome in the case of cancer predisposition syndrome. Pediatr Blood Cancer 63(4):611–617

4 Childhood Cancer Predisposition

Johannes H. M. Merks, Illja Diets, Ines B. Brecht, and Marjolijn CJ Jongmans

4.1 Incidence

Each year, approximately 31,000 children (0–19 years) are diagnosed with cancer in Western Europe (Steliarova-Foucher et al. 2017). In most of these children, the cancer is sporadic, meaning that it is not caused by an inherited pathogenic variant in a cancer predisposition gene. However, in an estimated 10% of children with cancer, a cancer predisposition syndrome (CPS) is present. Children with such a syndrome have a germline pathogenic variant in a cancer predisposition gene, which leads to an increased risk of developing cancer.

J. H. M. Merks
Princess Máxima Center for Pediatric Oncology, Utrecht, The Netherlands
e-mail: j.h.m.merks@prinsesmaximacentrum.nl

I. Diets
Department of Human Genetics, Radboud University Medical Center, Nijmegen, the Netherlands
e-mail: Illja.Diets@radboudumc.nl

I. B. Brecht
Pediatric Oncology and Hematology, University Children's Hospital Tuebingen, Tuebingen, Germany
e-mail: ines.brecht@med.uni-tuebingen.de

M. CJ. Jongmans (✉)
Princess Maxima Center for Pediatric Oncology/Clinical Genetics, University Medical Center Utrecht, Utrecht, The Netherlands
e-mail: M.C.J.Jongmans-3@umcutrecht.nl

Until recently, it was unknown which proportion of childhood cancer results from a hereditary CPS. Multiple strategies have been used to estimate the hereditary fraction of childhood cancer. This was done for specific tumors but also for pediatric cancer in general. The tumor-specific hereditary fraction differs largely between tumors, with some being highly associated with genetic predisposition (e.g., germline *TP53* pathogenic variants in adrenocortical carcinoma) and others rarely being caused by CPSs. Recently, large studies investigating the hereditary fraction of two pediatric malignancies, Wilms' tumor and medulloblastoma, have been performed (Gadd et al. 2017; Waszak et al. 2018). For Wilms' tumor, 24 patients (20%) in the discovery set of 117 patients carried germline variants in the gene panel that was analyzed (Gadd et al. 2017). For medulloblastoma, 6% of patients carried a germline variant (Waszak et al. 2018).

The first research on the hereditary fraction of pediatric cancer in general dates back to 1991, when Narod et al. reviewed the clinical reports of 16,564 children with cancer for the presence of an underlying genetic disease (Narod et al. 1991). Merks et al. performed a clinical morphological examination on a series of 1073 children with cancer and diagnosed a syndrome in 42 patients (3.9%) (Merks et al. 2005). Knapke et al. reviewed clinical reports of 370 children with cancer (Knapke et al. 2012). Confirmed underly-

D. T. Schneider et al. (eds.), *Rare Tumors in Children and Adolescents*, Pediatric Oncology,
https://doi.org/10.1007/978-3-030-92071-5_4

ing CPSs were present in approximately 4% in all three studies. However, all studies state that these percentages are likely an underestimation of the true percentage, because of under-reporting. Knapke et al. considered 29% of their patients eligible for referral to a clinical geneticist (Knapke et al. 2012), and Merks et al. strongly suspected the presence of a syndrome in an additional 3.3% of patients (Merks et al. 2005). Furthermore, since the publication of these studies, multiple novel CPSs have been discovered, suggesting that the percentages identified are indeed higher.

The first prospective study to determine the hereditary fraction of childhood cancer was performed by Zhang et al. in 2015. They performed germline exome sequencing and whole genome sequencing (WGS) in 1120 children with cancer and found that 8.5% of these children harbored pathogenic or probably pathogenic variants in a pre-selected set of 60 genes known to be associated with autosomal-dominant cancer predisposition. The cohort was biased toward patients with tumors with poor prognosis (e.g., adrenocortical carcinoma and low-hypodiploid leukemia), and therefore this percentage is not a true representative for the general population of children with cancer. Two other large studies investigated the hereditary fraction in children with cancer. Mody et al. performed exome sequencing on tumor DNA and germline DNA of 102 children and young adults with relapsed, refractory, or rare cancer (Mody et al. 2015). They found that 10% of the children harbored germline variants causing the cancer. Finally, Parsons et al. performed tumor- and germline exome sequencing on 150 children with solid tumors and identified germline variants in 10% of the cases (Parsons et al. 2016).

4.2 Relevance

For multiple reasons, it is of utmost importance to recognize whether a child has a hereditary CPS.

First, the presence of a CPS might lead to changes in cancer treatment. Second, children with a CPS can be at risk of developing additional primary malignancies, requiring the need for instatement of specific surveillance protocols that may lead to early detection of subsequent malignancies and therefore reduction of morbidity and mortality.

Third, the CPS may also be present in family members of the child with cancer in some cases. Knowledge of a CPS in a family will enable genetic counseling and testing of family members and, if necessary, instatement of surveillance in family members as well.

Fourth, a CPS may include non-cancer-related problems like behavioral or immunologic disorders that may need specific attention and care.

Lastly, many parents of a child with cancer ask themselves the question: "why did our child develop cancer?" Identifying a genetic cause of cancer answers this important question.

To provide an overview of the consequences of diagnosing the most prevalent CPSs, Postema et al. performed a systematic review of the most commonly used clinical genetic databases, handbooks, and literature (Postema et al. 2018). In total, 33 syndromes were selected in which more than 100 individuals had been described and in which cancer occurred in 5% or more of affected individuals. Three additional syndromes were described in 50–100 individuals, with a cancer incidence of 10% or more. In 8 of the 36 syndromes, patients were known to be hypersensitive for ionizing radiation, where in 4 out of the 36 syndromes, caution was advised when administrating chemotherapy. Cancer surveillance was suggested in 21/36 syndromes, although opinions concerning the need, effectiveness, and potential unwanted side effects differ among countries. In almost half of the CPSs (15/36), developmental problems may arise, and in three CPSs, immunodeficiency was a frequent complicating problem. Knowledge of these consequences and their importance for optimal care underline the need for proper and timely recognition of CPS and referral to a clinical geneticist to ensure optimal care for each patient with childhood cancer.

4.3 Diagnostics of Childhood Cancer Predisposition

Although it is clear that recognizing a CPS in a child with cancer may have benefits for both the child and its family, the presence of a CPS is still often missed or goes unrecognized for years (Merks et al. 2005; Sherborne et al. 2017). In a study by Merks et al. on the incidence of malformation syndromes in children with cancer, the syndrome diagnoses were initially not recognized in 20 out of 42 patients (Merks et al. 2005). Additionally, in a cohort of childhood cancer survivors, it was shown that not all patients who met the clinical Chompret criteria for Li-Fraumeni syndrome were referred for testing of the *TP53* gene (Russo et al. 2017). Reasons for under-detection of CPSs are that many are very rare and that the phenotypes associated with the syndromes can be difficult to recognize. Furthermore, some genes are known to cause no other phenotypic features besides the tumor itself, such as Wilms' tumor predisposition gene *REST* (Mahamdallie et al. 2015), making the recognition of a CPS in these children especially challenging. This is further complicated by the fact that a family history of cancer is not always present, even though this is likely the most well-known indicator of genetic predisposition among pediatric oncologists. A study on childhood cancer predisposition showed that a family history of cancer is present in only 40% of the children diagnosed with a CPS (Zhang et al. 2015). Furthermore, in only half of the patients in whom a family history was present, the pattern of cancer in the family was compatible with the syndrome diagnosed (Zhang et al. 2015). Absence of a family history of cancer can be explained by incomplete penetrance, meaning that not every individual that carries the predisposing pathogenic variant will definitely develop cancer. An example is the *DICER1* tumor predisposition syndrome, for which incomplete penetrance has been reported in multiple studies (Doros et al. 1993; Hill et al. 2009; Rio Frio et al. 2011), and it is even suggested that approximately 95% of carriers of a pathogenic variant in *DICER1* will not have developed cancer by the age of 10 (Kim et al. 2017).

Another reason for the absence of a family history of cancer is the occurrence of de novo variants, meaning that the variant is not present in the parents but only in the child. For instance, in Li-Fraumeni syndrome the estimated percentage of de novo variants is between 7 and 20% (Gonzalez et al. 2009; Renaux-Petel et al. 2018). Furthermore, some CPSs inherit in an autosomal recessive way. In these families, the likelihood of a family history of cancer is lower, as carriers of a single pathogenic variant are generally not affected (e.g., the parents) and the chance that a sibling also carries two copies of the pathogenic variant is only 25%.

The identification of a CPS in a child with cancer relies heavily on the pediatric oncologists to recognize features suggestive of genetic predisposition and refer patients to a clinical geneticist. However, as stated above, the recognition can be difficult, and pediatric oncologists are not specifically trained for this. Therefore, efforts have been made to improve the recognition of childhood cancer predisposition by the development of referral criteria and screening instruments (Jongmans et al. 2016; Postema et al. 2017; Ripperger et al. 2017; Goudie et al. 2017). These referral tools select children with cancer in whom the suspicion of a CPS is particularly high, because of additional features pointing toward genetic predisposition, such as:

1. The presence of intellectual disability (ID) and/or additional features (e.g., congenital anomalies, growth disorders, dysmorphic features, excessive toxicity)
2. The presence of multiple primary malignancies
3. The presence of a family history of cancer
4. The presence of specific types of cancer or an adult type of cancer
5. Multiple of the above stated features

A clinical geneticist in general has three options when a child with cancer is referred for genetic testing: (1) refrain from genetic testing, either because the clinical suspicion of a CPS is low or because the patient refuses testing after adequate genetic counseling, (2) perform a targeted genetic test, or (3) perform exome- or genome-wide analysis like a SNP array analysis or whole exome sequencing (WES). In patients with a very clear clinical presentation of a specific CPS, a targeted genetic test is the most straightforward and cost-efficient approach to find the underlying genetic variant. However, when the differential diagnosis consists of multiple possible diagnoses, or when suspicion for a syndrome is high but the geneticist does not have a clue which specific syndrome could be involved, WES is an attractive option. Many centers are introducing whole exome or genome sequencing techniques in the diagnostic workup of pediatric cancers, meaning that tumor DNA is sequenced with germline DNA as a reference. The availability of germline WES or WGS data provides the opportunity to interrogate this data if molecular confirmation is sought for a clinical suspicion of a CPS. However, it also gives opportunities to perform germline genetic analysis in all patients, also in the ones without any features of genetic cancer predisposition. Several studies have shown that this approach results in identification of a germline pathogenic variant in approximately 10% of patients (Zhang et al. 2015; Mody et al. 2015; Parsons et al. 2016).

When the decision is made to perform WES, it is beneficial to add parental DNA or DNA of affected relatives to the analysis. Adding parental DNA enables the detection of de novo variants, and additionally the inheritance pattern of a certain variant can immediately be determined (Diets et al. 2018). A recently published paper highlights the benefits of trio-sequencing in children with cancer, versus sequencing of the affected child only (Kuhlen et al. 2019).

Analysis of WES data is usually performed in a two-step approach, the first being a cancer gene panel analysis. These cancer gene panels consist of genes that are already known to cause cancer. However, large differences exist in the composition of these gene panels. For example, the number of genes included in the panels is variable, ranging from 110 to 565 genes in published studies (Waszak et al. 2018; Zhang et al. 2015; Grobner et al. 2018). Furthermore, these gene panels are not designed specifically for pediatric cancer, so they also include genes that predispose primarily to adult cancer. This can be problematic, as the causality of a pathogenic variant in an adult cancer predisposition gene in children with cancer is unclear. To counter this problem, one could consider to develop a cancer gene panel specifically for childhood cancer. The main advantages of this approach are that it is easier to interpret the results from this childhood cancer gene panel and less incidental findings will be encountered. Nevertheless, several adult cancer predisposition genes still need to be included in this gene panel, as biallelic variants in these genes cause a recessive childhood CPS like Fanconi anemia.

An alternative approach that could be considered is the composition of tumor-specific gene panels. Again, the advantage of this approach is that the findings will be easier to interpret, and incidental findings will be less common. However, by performing a tumor-specific gene panel only, one could potentially miss causative variants, because the knowledge about associations between tumors and certain CPSs is still evolving. A proposition that covers all of this would be to start with a tumor-specific gene panel, followed by analysis of a complete childhood cancer gene panel if no causative variants are found. If this result then comes back negative as well, an exome-wide analysis could be performed. By using this step-wise approach, the risk of incidental findings is minimized.

4.4 Care for Children with Cancer Predisposition Syndromes

As said before, diagnosing a cancer predisposition syndrome in a child with cancer can have health benefits for the child and his or her relatives. This depends however on the availability of evidence-based guidelines to modify treatment protocols or to apply meaningful surveillance. A successful example is the advice to limit exposure to high doses of intravenous methotrexate and to apply intensified supportive care in children with Down syndrome, because of the well-recognized increased chemotherapy-associated toxicity in these children (Izraeli et al. 2014). Likewise, for some surveillance protocols prospective studies have shown benefits for the patients. A prospective analysis of patients with Li-Fraumeni syndrome, 59 of whom had surveillance according to the "Toronto protocol" and 30 who declined surveillance, found 5-year survival in those diagnosed with cancer through screening to be 88.8% compared with 59.6% in the patients diagnosed with cancer on the basis of clinical presentation (Villani et al. 2016). For many syndromes however, evidence in support of treatment modifications or cancer surveillance is lacking, and protocols are at best based on international expert opinions. Developing surveillance protocols is particularly challenging for syndromes known for low penetrance for a broad spectrum of malignancies, like the DICER1 syndrome (Doros et al. 1993; Hill et al. 2009; Rio Frio et al. 2011; Kim et al. 2017). To evaluate current surveillance and treatment protocols for children with CPSs and to develop novel protocols, international collaborations are crucial since overall these syndromes are extremely rare. A favorable development in this perspective is the recent institution of a SIOPE Host Genome Working Group of which the members will address these topics in the nearby future. At the level of a single pediatric cancer center, it is important to compile teams of pediatric oncologists, clinical geneticists, and radiologists who specialize in care for children with CPSs, since this will contribute to local expertise and high standards of care.

References

Diets IJ et al (2018) High yield of pathogenic germline mutations causative or likely causative of the cancer phenotype in selected children with cancer. Clin Cancer Res 24(7):1594–1603

Doros L et al (1993) DICER1-related disorders. In: Adam MP et al (eds) GeneReviews((R)). University of Washington, Seattle

Gadd S et al (2017) A Children's Oncology Group and TARGET initiative exploring the genetic landscape of Wilms tumor. Nat Genet 49(10):1487–1494

Gonzalez KD et al (2009) High frequency of de novo mutations in Li-Fraumeni syndrome. J Med Genet 46(10):689–693

Goudie C, et al 2017 The McGill interactive pediatric OncoGenetic guidelines: an approach to identifying pediatric oncology patients most likely to benefit from a genetic evaluation. Pediatr Blood Cancer 64(8)

Grobner SN et al (2018) The landscape of genomic alterations across childhood cancers. Nature 555(7696):321–327

Hill DA et al (2009) DICER1 mutations in familial pleuropulmonary blastoma. Science 325(5943):965

Izraeli S et al (2014) How I treat ALL in Down's syndrome: pathobiology and management. Blood 123(1):35–40

Jongmans MC et al (2016) Recognition of genetic predisposition in pediatric cancer patients: an easy-to-use selection tool. Eur J Med Genet 59(3):116–125

Kim J et al (2017) The prevalence of DICER1 pathogenic variation in population databases. Int J Cancer 141(10):2030–2036

Knapke S et al (2012) Hereditary cancer risk assessment in a pediatric oncology follow-up clinic. Pediatr Blood Cancer 58(1):85–89

Kuhlen M et al (2019) Family-based germline sequencing in children with cancer. Oncogene 38(9): 1367–1380

Mahamdallie SS et al (2015) Mutations in the transcriptional repressor REST predispose to Wilms tumor. Nat Genet 47(12):1471–1474

Merks JH, Caron HN, Hennekam RC (2005) High incidence of malformation syndromes in a series of 1,073 children with cancer. Am J Med Genet A 134A(2):132–143

Mody RJ et al (2015) Integrative clinical sequencing in the management of refractory or relapsed cancer in youth. JAMA 314(9):913–925

Narod SA, Stiller C, Lenoir GM (1991) An estimate of the heritable fraction of childhood cancer. Br J Cancer 63(6):993–999

Parsons DW et al (2016) Diagnostic yield of clinical tumor and germline whole-exome sequencing for children with solid tumors. JAMA Oncol 2(5):616–624

Postema FA et al (2017) Validation of a clinical screening instrument for tumour predisposition syndromes in patients with childhood cancer (TuPS): protocol for a prospective, observational, multicentre study. BMJ Open 7(1):e013237

Postema FAM et al (2018) Consequences of diagnosing a tumor predisposition syndrome in children with cancer: a literature review. Pediatr Blood Cancer 65(1)

Renaux-Petel M et al (2018) Contribution of de novo and mosaic TP53 mutations to Li-Fraumeni syndrome. J Med Genet 55(3):173–180

Rio Frio T et al (2011) DICER1 mutations in familial multinodular goiter with and without ovarian Sertoli-Leydig cell tumors. JAMA 305(1):68–77

Ripperger T et al (2017) Childhood cancer predisposition syndromes—a concise review and recommendations by the Cancer Predisposition Working Group of the Society for Pediatric Oncology and Hematology. Am J Med Genet A 173(4):1017–1037

Russo S et al (2017) Importance of updating family cancer history in childhood cancer survivors. Fam Cancer 16(4):605–610

Sherborne AL et al (2017) Somatic and germline TP53 alterations in second malignant neoplasms from pediatric cancer survivors. Clin Cancer Res 23(7):1852–1861

Steliarova-Foucher E et al (2017) International incidence of childhood cancer, 2001-10: a population-based registry study. Lancet Oncol 18(6):719–731

Villani A et al (2016) Biochemical and imaging surveillance in germline TP53 mutation carriers with Li-Fraumeni syndrome: 11 year follow-up of a prospective observational study. Lancet Oncol 17(9):1295–1305

Waszak SM et al (2018) Spectrum and prevalence of genetic predisposition in medulloblastoma: a retrospective genetic study and prospective validation in a clinical trial cohort. Lancet Oncol 19(6):785–798

Zhang J et al (2015) Germline mutations in predisposition genes in pediatric cancer. N Engl J Med 373(24):2336–2346

Part III

National and International Study Groups

5 National Initiatives in Europe

Andrea Ferrari, Daniel Orbach, Yves Reguerre, Ines B. Brecht, Dominik T. Schneider, Jan Godzinski, and Bernadette Brennan

For children affected by very uncommon malignancies, the very low incidence of their disease has often limited the interest in research capable of collecting significant clinical and biological data: as a consequence, it has always been difficult to produce evidence-based treatment guidelines, and physicians are forced to treat such patients only on an individual basis. Historically, the pediatric oncology community dedicated little resources to pediatric very rare tumors (VRTs), and research focused on them remained a challenge. In the first years of the new millennium, however, the situation changed; pediatric oncologists have increasingly recognized the necessity to develop specifically dedicated projects; and various national groups have launched national initiatives (in Italy first and then in Poland, Germany, and France).

5.1 The Italian TREP Project

The pioneering national-scale cooperative project on VRTs—the TREP project (Tumori Rari in Età Pediatrica [*Rare Tumors in Pediatric Age*])—was launched in Italy in 2000 under the auspices of the Associazione Italiana Ematologia Oncologia Pediatrica (AIEOP) and in cooperation with the Società Italiana Chirurgia Pediatrica (SICP) (Ferrari et al. 2007).

To clearly define its area of interest, the TREP group adopted a pragmatic definition of *rare pediatric tumors*, considering practical and clinical issues rather than epidemiological data and including "any solid malignancy characterized by an annual incidence <2 per million and not considered in other clinical trials." As a consequence of this definition, the TREP project did

A. Ferrari (✉)
Pediatric Oncology Unit, Fondazione IRCCS Istituto Nazionale Tumori, Milan, Italy
e-mail: andrea.ferrari@istitutotumori.mi.it

D. Orbach
SIREDO Oncology Center (Care, Innovation and Research for Children, Adolescents and Young Adults with Cancer), Institut Curie, PSL University, Paris, France
e-mail: daniel.orbach@curie.fr

Y. Reguerre
Pediatric Hematology and Oncology Unit, University Hospital, Saint Denis, Paris, France
e-mail: yves.reguerre@chu-reunion.fr

I. B. Brecht
Pediatric Hematology and Oncology, University of Tuebingen, Tuebingen, Germany
e-mail: Ines.Brecht@med.uni-tuebingen.de

D. T. Schneider
Klinik für Kinder- und Jugendmedizin, Clinic of Pediatrics, University Witten/Herdecke, Dortmund, Germany
e-mail: dominik.schneider@klinikumdo.de

J. Godzinski
Department of Pediatric Surgery, Marciniak Hospital, Wroclaw, Wroclaw, Poland

B. Brennan
Department of Pediatric Oncology, Royal Manchester Children's Hospital, Manchester, UK
e-mail: Bernadette.Brennan@mft.nhs.uk

D. T. Schneider et al. (eds.), *Rare Tumors in Children and Adolescents*, Pediatric Oncology,
https://doi.org/10.1007/978-3-030-92071-5_5

not include tumors with such a low incidence but already "covered" by other national studies, i.e., renal rhabdoid tumors were registered in the AIEOP Wilms Tumor Study, hepatoblastoma and malignant germ cell tumors had their own protocols, rare histotypes of soft part sarcomas (non-rhabdomyosarcoma soft tissue sarcomas) were covered by the cooperative study on soft tissue sarcomas, and so on. The definition adopted was considered suitable for classifying the "orphan" tumors in the Italian pediatric setting, i.e., in the sense that most pediatricians might encounter these tumors only once in their working lives, there were few or no published reports on clinical experiences, it was difficult to establish shared treatment guidelines (and there were no evidence-based therapeutic recommendations available), and few or no cooperative groups dedicated and structured projects or financial support for studies on these tumors.

An assortment of tumors was thus involved in the TREP project, including some neoplasms that are rare at any age, and also (and mainly) tumors that are rare in childhood and adolescence but more common in adulthood, e.g., nasopharyngeal carcinoma, adrenocortical tumors, pleuropulmonary blastoma (and other lung tumors), carcinoid tumors, cutaneous melanoma, renal cell carcinoma, pancreatoblastoma (and other pancreatic exocrine tumors), gonadal non-germ-cell tumors (ovary/testis), pheochromocytoma and paraganglioma, thyroid carcinoma, salivary gland tumors, breast carcinoma, carcinoma of the gastrointestinal tract, and carcinoma of the thymus.

The main aims of the TREP project were:

1. To develop diagnostic and therapeutic recommendations for each rare tumor
2. To collect and centralize clinical data by using specific printed forms for diagnostic workup, treatment, and follow-up
3. To identify one (or more) researcher(s) "dedicated" to each histotype who could act as an expert to consult
4. To create a network for cooperation with other specialists (adult oncologists and surgeons, endocrinologists, dermatologists, gastroenterologists, etc.) involved in managing these tumors
5. To organize pathological and biological studies

From September 2000 to September 2016, 964 patients <18 years of age were registered in the TREP database, which means a rate of more than 50 patients a year. Patients were registered by 39 different Italian centers, confirming the broad adhesion to the project. Patients range in age from 12 days to 18 years, with a median of 12 years (70% of cases were over 10 years old). Thyroid carcinoma proved the most common histotype (166 cases), followed by carcinoid/neuroendocrine tumors (154 cases), skin tumors including melanoma (123 cases), gonadal non-germ-cell tumors (109 cases), and nasopharyngeal carcinoma (63 cases).

Table 5.1 reports a list of the series published by the TREP group.

An analysis performed in cooperation with the AIEOP epidemiology group compared the number of cases actually registered (between 2000 and 2006) with the number of cases predicted in the light of incidence data in the Italian population-based cancer registries (AIRTum). The number of rare pediatric tumors predicted to occur in Italy between 2000 and 2006 was 305 among the 0 to 14-year-olds and 400 among the 15 to 17-year-olds (on average, 44 children and 57 adolescents are expected to develop a rare pediatric tumor each year), while the numbers of cases actually identified by the TREP were 261 and 75, respectively. For the 0 to 14-year-olds, the ratio of observed to expected cases was even 1:1 for several tumors (i.e., nasopharyngeal carcinoma, adrenocortical tumors, renal cell carcinoma, and gonadal non-germ-cell tumors), while for the adolescents, underreporting was statistically significant for all tumor types except nasopharyngeal carcinoma (Pastore et al. 2009). These findings were generally regarded as an indication of the TREP project's success (the vast majority of patients with rare pediatric tumors under 15 years of age were registered and treated according to TREP guidelines) and of the feasibility of cooperative protocols even for rare

Table 5.1 Various series published by the Italian TREP project

Series	Main results
Pleuropulmonary blastoma (Indolfi et al. 2007)	22 patients 5 cases on congenital lung cysts; 5-year EFS 44%, OS 49% Better prognosis with total resection, worse prognosis with extrapulmonary involvement
Pancreatic tumors (Dall'Igna et al. 2010)	21 patients 4 pancreatoblastomas, 2 pancreatic carcinomas, 3 neoplasms of the endocrine pancreas, 12 solid pseudopapillary tumors
Sex cord-stromal tumors of the testis (Cecchetto et al. 2010)	11 patients 4 Leydig cell tumors, 4 juvenile granulosa cell tumors, 1 Sertoli cell tumor, 1 incompletely differentiated tumor, 1 tumor with an intermediate pattern Sertoli cell tumor/mixed form All the patients are in first complete remission
Sex cord-stromal tumors of the ovary (Cecchetto et al. 2011)	23 cases, 9/23 cases with signs of hormonal secretion; 12 juvenile granulosa cell tumor, 6 Sertoli-Leydig cell tumor, 3 fibrothecoma, 2 sclerosing stromal tumor 22/23 alive; cisplatin-based chemotherapy seemed to be effective for locally advanced tumors
Epithelial thymic tumors (Carretto et al. 2011)	9 cases, 4 thymoma and 5 carcinoma; all patients with thymic carcinomas died of their disease despite of multidrug chemotherapy and radiotherapy
Nasopharyngeal carcinoma (Casanova et al. 2012)	46 patients (45 N1, 5 M1) 3 courses of cisplatin/5-fluorouracil induction chemotherapy followed by radiotherapy (doses up to 65 Gy) with concomitant cisplatin 90% response rate to primary chemotherapy 5-year PFS 79.3%, OS 80.9% 65% incidence of late sequelae The use of lower radiotherapy doses than those used in adults did not affect locoregional failure rates
Esthesioneuroblastoma (Bisogno et al. 2012a, b)	9 cases 3 Kadish stage B, 6 stage C; chemotherapy response in 5/7; 8/9 alive, 7 in first remission, 1 in second remission; treatment-related sequelae (endocrine dysfunctions, craniofacial growth impairments)
Adrenocortical tumors (Magro et al. 2012)	20 patients Wieneke scoring system: 7 tumors were classified as malignant, 12 tumors as benign, 1 tumor with "unpredictable behavior"; matrix metalloproteinase 2 was expressed in all malignant and in most benign tumors; HLA class II antigen immunoreactivity was absent in all benign tumors and restricted to rare isolated cells in most malignant tumors; unlike in adults, metalloproteinase 2 or loss of HLA class II antigens does not discriminate between benign and malignant tumors in children
Ovarian sex cord-stromal tumors (Virgone et al. 2012)	15 cases GATA-4 and FOG-2 expression: high expression of GATA-4 does not correlate with aggressive behavior as seen in adults
Salivary gland carcinomas (Chiaravalli et al. 2014)	17 patients (in 4/17 cases, it was a second tumor); 14 arising in the parotid gland; 14 low-grade tumors, often low-stage; all patients underwent surgical resection, with free margins in 9/17; adjuvant radiotherapy in 6 cases; 16/17 alive in first continuous remission
Myoepithelial carcinoma (Bisogno et al. 2014)	7 cases chemotherapy with ifosfamide, cisplatin and etoposide, radiotherapy; 6/7 alive in first remission (median follow-up, 2.5 years; range, 0.9–5)

(continued)

Table 5.1 (continued)

Series	Main results
Cutaneous melanoma (Ferrari et al. 2014)	54 patients 5-year EFS 75.2%, OS 84.6%; the variables influencing survival in children are the same as for adults
Adrenocortical tumors (Dall'Igna et al. 2014)	58 patients, stage II treated with mitotane, stage III–IV with mitotane + chemotherapy; 45 alive, 12 died of disease, 1 died because of cardiomyopathy; p53 mutation found in 7 cases
Appendiceal neuroendocrine tumors (carcinoid of the appendix) (Virgone et al. 2014)	113 patients 108/113 size <2 cm; 111/113 free excision margins; primary reexcision in 3 cases only; all 113 of 113 patients are alive in complete remission appendectomy alone should be considered curative for most patients, and a more aggressive surgical approach is warranted only in the cases with incompletely excised tumors
Epithelial tumors of the ovary (Virgone et al. 2015a, b)	16 patients 8 benign tumors (7 mucinous cystadenomas and 1 serous cystadenoma) and 8 borderline tumors (2 serous and 6 mucinous); 15/16 patients maintained the complete remission after surgical treatment alone; 1 died due to synchronous Wilms tumor (Proteus syndrome)
Atypical Spitz tumors (Massi et al. 2015)	50 cases Analysis of histological parameters associated with a diagnosis of atypical Spitz tumors over Spitz nevus; *minimal lethal potential; no data to support any clinical benefit for the sentinel lymph node biopsy procedure and completion lymphadenectomy*
Neuroendocrine tumors of the appendix (Virgone et al. 2015a, b)	5 cases with neuroendocrine tumor of the appendix associated with a parasitic bowel infection Possibility of inflammation-triggered carcinogenesis
Urothelial neoplasms of the bladder (Di Carlo et al. 2015)	12 patients Low-grade (11/12 G1), scarcely aggressive disease with an excellent prognosis; the role of intravesical chemotherapy is debatable
Papillary thyroid carcinoma (Spinelli et al. 2016)	250 patients 46% N1, 4% M1 90% total thyroidectomy, 10% lobectomy; 21% surgical complications (hypoparathyroidism, vocal fold palsy), all in case of total thyroidectomy group; 12% recurrent disease, 100% overall survival; pediatric patients are likely to benefit from a tailored surgical strategy; uniformly offering patients total thyroidectomy seems to be an overly radical approach
Gastrointestinal tract carcinoma (Indini et al. 2017)	15 cases, 12 colorectal carcinomas; all but one patient had advanced-stage disease and the majority had aggressive histological subtypes; 9 alive (but 3 with very few follow-up), 6 died due to disease
Solid pseudopapillary tumors (Crocoli et al. 2019)	43 patients One recurrence in a patient with intraoperative rupture; all alive

EFS event-free survival, *OS* overall survival, *PFS* progression-free survival, *N1* nodal metastases, *M1* distant metastases

diseases. The underreporting of adolescents was similar to what was seen also for the more common pediatric malignancies.

The key elements of the TREP project—and the lessons learned from it—were more than one. First is the dual need of the project, i.e., to prompt research and to provide all centers with practical patient management schemes. In Italy, there was a shortage of information on these rare pediatric tumors, and doctors were calling for treatment guidelines; the various experts involved in the project have been able to offer a real advisory service. Second—and consequently—is the importance of developing a network involving several centers and specialists from different branches of medicine and science. Third is the adoption of a common framework: the different working groups (one for each tumor type) developed their "protocols" in the context of the same structured manner, and this ensured homogeneous methods and guaranteed the discipline essential to the efficacy of cooperative clinical trials.

5.2 The Polish Paediatric Rare Tumours Study Group

The Polish Paediatric Solid Tumours Study Group (in Polish: Polska Pediatryczna Grupa Guzów Litych, PPGGL) was created in 1992 in Poznań. During the first 10 years of activity, the PPGGL developed, adapted, or joined international therapeutic programs for the majority of the common pediatric malignancies. In 2002, a specific initiative dedicated to pediatric VRTs was launched, named Polish Paediatric Rare Tumours Study Group. The interest of the group focused on those malignancies which had extremely low incidence and were not included in other already existing therapeutic protocols. Study started its activity with the call for retrospective data on VRTs from preceding decades in order to build a core database. This database served for a number of retrospective reviews on particular diseases presented and published widely (Bien et al. 2004; Bien et al. 2009a, b; Godzinski et al. 2004; Stachowicz-Stencel et al. 2010). Second objectives were the prospective registration of new cases and the building of an expert advice platform based on the experience gained thus far, on literature, and, to some extent, on the contacts with other experts identified for particular malignancies (e.g., International experts, experts in adult oncologists). The consultation platform and data bank organized by the Rare Tumours Study Committee served not only to the pediatric oncology centers cooperating within PPGGL but also to general pediatricians and other specialists, if requested.

5.3 The German STEP Project

In Germany, approximately 2200 children and adolescents are diagnosed with cancer each year (Kaatsch 2016). The 55 pediatric oncological centers cooperate within the clinical and scientific network of the German Society for Pediatric Oncology and Hematology (GPOH), which coordinates national and international clinical studies and registries. Compared to other countries, the infrastructure for pediatric rare tumors has a distinct history in Germany. Thus, some rare cancers have long been integrated into cooperative therapy optimization studies. Among others, these include endocrine cancers (e.g., thyroid cancers, adrenocortical carcinoma, carcinoids), nasopharyngeal carcinoma, and rare soft tissue sarcomas. With the advent of the EU regulation on clinical trials, these initiatives have developed into clinical registries that provide a therapeutic guidance based on consensus recommendations, central clinical data collection, and support of coordinated molecular genetic studies.

Apart from these, there remains a group of patients with VRTs that have not yet been cared for within the clinical network of GPOH until the foundation of the German Working Group in Pediatric Rare Tumors (Seltene Tumorerkrankungen in der Pädiatrie (STEP) in 2006 (Brecht et al. 2009). The work of this multidisciplinary working group focuses on all VRTs not registered to other studies or registries within the GPOH. Thus, some rare tumor entities such as rhabdoid tumors, nasopharyngeal carcinoma, endocrine cancers, or rare soft tissue sarcomas are explicitly excluded but reported to the respective diagnosis-specific registry. In 2012, the prospective registration of patients with VRTs into the STEP Registry started and will be continued in the STEP 2.0 registry in 2019 (www.seltene-tumoren.de). The annual accrual rate approaches 100 patients, i.e., 4% of all childhood cancer patients in Germany.

The patient registration is accompanied by a close consultation service for pediatric oncological centers (contact: step@klinikumdo.de). The working group also provides information on VRTs for physicians and affected families (www.

kinderkrebsinfo.de). In addition, the STEP working group studies potential associations of very rare cancers with hereditary cancer predisposition (Weber et al. 2016; Ripperger et al. 2017; Bauer et al. 2019). Lastly, the STEP registry provides access to tumor banking and molecular profiling platforms for the analysis of potential therapeutic targets in prognostically unfavorable situations (Ernestus et al. 2006; Worst et al. 2016).

By promoting these activities, STEP aims to providing children and adolescents with VRT access to optimal care within the clinical and scientific infrastructure of GPOH.

5.4 The French FRaCTurE

The French Group on Rare Tumors in Children (FRaCTurE; Groupe FRAnCais Des TUmeurs Rares de l'Enfant) was formally launched in 2007. It was developed in a context where the incidence of pediatric rare, malignant, or borderline tumors in France was difficult to evaluate, also due to the fact that only patients with severe, recurrent, or complicated forms were referred to oncology departments. In fact, also nowadays the incidence of a large number of rare diseases is severely underestimated, giving a false impression of the true incidence of the disease. The French Registry of Solid Tumours in Children—*Registre National des Tumeurs Solides de l'Enfant* (RNTSE)—provides epidemiological data on childhood cancers in France. However, certain rare tumors are not included in this registry, either because their malignant nature remains uncertain or because they are managed by adult oncology teams or pediatric specialities other than oncology, less accustomed to systematic patient registration. The RNTSE initially only recorded tumors occurring in children under the age of 15 years in metropolitan France and since 2011 extended to all patients less than 18 years old and living in overseas departments. Concomitant registration of borderline tumors is performed but is not comprehensive. The exceptional nature of these diseases and their heterogeneous management in terms of both the medical specialty involved (surgery, dermatology, ophthalmology, etc.) and the site of treatment (private clinic or public hospital, pediatric or adult medicine department) account for these difficulties (Réguerre et al. 2010).

The creation of a rare childhood tumor group by the *Société Française des Cancer de l'Enfant et de l'Adolescent* (SFCE) in November 2006 (and then launched few months later) was the first step designed to address these issues. This group, mainly composed of pediatricians, surgeons, radiotherapists, and pathologists, meets at least twice a year to discuss a specific theme, e.g., aggressive vascular tumors (Boccara et al. 2016), neuroendocrine tumors (de Lambert et al. 2015), mucoepidermoid carcinoma (Rebours et al. 2017), etc. Since the creation of the FRaCTurE group, diagnostic and treatment guidelines have been proposed for certain tumors such as adrenal cortical tumors (Picard et al. 2018, 2019), pleuropulmonary blastomas, pancreatic tumors (Irtan et al. 2016), melanomas (Reguerre et al. 2016), and nasopharyngeal carcinoma (Jouin et al. 2019), based on retrospective analyses of patients previously treated in France, data of the literature, and proposals from other European or international rare tumor groups. These clinical practice guidelines are then made available to clinicians via the SFCE website.

A local representative responsible for VRTs has been designated in each of the 30 SFCE centers throughout France to ensure diffusion of these guidelines. The presence of surgeons in the group also ensures close collaboration with the other members of the *Société Française de Chirurgie Pédiatrique* (SFCP). Another objective of this group is to improve the knowledge and treatment of pediatric VRTs by creating, in collaboration with the SFCE and the RNTSE, a national database for collection of medical information. Clinical, laboratory and radiological characteristics, the treatments administered, and outcome of the disease are recorded. Current treatment guidelines, initiated in the context of the FRaCTurE group, constitute the basis for setting up this database. This database therefore concerns diseases corresponding to various histologies, sharing in common their very low incidence (less than 2 cases per million children under the age of 18) and the absence of formal treatment guidelines. For practical purposes, tumors with an exceptionally low incidence, but for which treatment guidelines or data collection are already available in the context of the SFCE, will not be included in this group. It was also arbitrarily decided not to include in this rare childhood tumor group those rare hematological malignancies included in the "leukemia group." Consequently, the main diseases concerned by this group are undifferentiated nasopharyngeal carcinoma; pancreatoblastoma and Frantz's tumor (pseudopapillary tumor of the pancreas); pleuropulmonary blastoma; pseudo-inflammatory tumor; mesothelioma; thymoma (Rod et al. 2014); gastrointestinal stromal tumors; adrenal cortical tumor; malignant pheochromocytoma; carcinoid of the appendix; melanotic neuroectodermal tumor of infancy (Moreau et al. 2017); carcinoid of the small intestine; carcinoid tumor of the bronchus; midline carcinoma (Lemelle et al. 2017); aggressive giant-cell bone tumors; chondroblastoma; chondrosarcoma; malignant head and neck tumors, sialoblastoma, mucoepidermoid carcinoma, aggressive benign vascular tumor; lung carcinomas; urothelial carcinomas (Grapin-Dagorno et al. 2017); and chordomas.

From 2007 to 2018, overall 675 patients were registered from 34 centers and concerned 130 different histotypes. The most frequent tumors were neuroendocrine tumors of the appendix (55 cases, 8% of all), undifferentiated nasopharyngeal carcinoma (43 cases), pheochromocytoma/paraganglioma (34 cases), solid pseudo-papillary tumor of the pancreas (32 cases), salivary gland tumors (30 cases), pleuropulmonary blastoma (24 cases), and cutaneous melanoma (23 cases). National and international retrospective analyses on VRTs have been presented in 35 scientific congresses and published in 14 peer-reviewed journals.

5.5 The UK

In the UK, VRTs have been historically defined as those with an age-standardized annual incidence of less than 1 per million children, based on the categories of the International Classification of Childhood Cancer (Steliarova-Foucher et al. 2005) and the incidence rates from the UK National Registry of Childhood Tumours (NRCT). Overall, these tumors were considered to have an annual incidence rate of 6.8 per million, accounted for 16% of non-CNS malignant solid tumors, and accounted 5% of all childhood cancers. In both relative and absolute terms, they were most frequent in the age group 10–14 years, where their incidence was 12.4 per million and where they accounted for 35% of non-CNS solid tumors and 11% of all cancers. Carcinomas of all sites counted as rare tumors and collectively formed 50% of the total. Soft tissue sarcomas were the next most frequent histological group, representing 36% (Stiller 2007). It is important to note that the same diagnostic groups are not necessarily rare in all populations. Most strikingly, Kaposi sarcoma is one of the most frequent childhood cancers in parts of central and east Africa most severely affected by the AIDS epidemic, whereas malignant melanoma is rare throughout most of Africa and Asia.

The Rare Tumour Working Group of the Children's Cancer and Leukaemia Group (CCLG) initially focused on those pediatric VRTs that occurred only in childhood and had a poor prognosis. From about 1997, various members of the CCLG Rare Tumour Working Group took charge pulling together guidance for several rare tumors. The format consisted of the known data from the UK NRCT and an up to date review of the literature using this to conclude guidance around management, diagnosis, and treatment. Where possible, information regarding open International registries/protocols was also made available. The list of the Rare Tumour Guidelines was available to members on the CCLG website or incorporated into study protocols or published. In 2005, a multidisciplinary consensus statement of best practice for the management and treatment for pediatric endocrine tumors from a working group convened under the auspices of the BSPED (British Society of Paediatric Endocrinology and Diabetes) and CCLG was published as a booklet available to all members. The working group was multidisciplinary, consisting of pediatric endocrinologists, oncologists, and surgeons together with adult surgeons, oncologists, and clinical geneticists with pediatric expertise. The following endocrine tumors were covered in the booklet: craniopharyngioma, adrenocortical neoplasms, pheochromocytoma, thyroid carcinoma (differentiated), medullary thyroid carcinoma and multiple endocrine neoplasia type 2 (MEN 2) syndromes, parathyroid and pituitary tumors (including primary hyperparathyroidism), and multiple endocrine neoplasia type 1 (MEN1) syndromes.

Although the registration of these rare tumors continues in the UK in the NRCT for patients 15 years and under, it is less complete for older teenagers and contains limited details on treatment received and factors which may be important for prognosis such as tumor dimensions, sites of metastases, etc.

For over the last 5 years, the information on incidence, survival, prevalence, and mortality for cancer diagnosed among children under the age of 15 resident in England only has been published with data from the National Cancer Registration and Analysis Service (NCRAS) from the department of Public Health England, as advised by the Children, Teenagers and Young Adults Expert Advisory Group, NCRAS. This of course limits the completeness of the data by excluding the other countries in the UK. While the report has extensive details on the common cancers in childhood, the small numbers limit the analysis of the rare tumors, and hence they are grouped together. An example would be "other malignant epithelial neoplasms and malignant melanomas" from the ICCC-3 coding with a mean number in this category per year up to 2015 of 66 cases versus specific data for thyroid cancer of on average 12 cases per year. Malignant melanoma is also coded separately on average 10 cases per year. It is important to note that the cut-off is 15 years old. This of course limits the survival analysis, but we can say that 5-year survival from thyroid carcinoma was well over 90% throughout the study period 2001–2015. Survival from malignant melanoma was 78% for children diagnosed during 2001 to 2005 and around 90% for those diagnosed during 2006 to 2015. Whether the later improvement is due to better reporting or potentially over diagnosis of atypical spitzoid nevi, one cannot comment (Irvine and Stiller 2019).

5.6 From National Initiatives to a Comprehensive European Project

When dedicated schemes for pediatric VRTs began to appear on the scene, two different models emerged: the first focused on large cooperative projects that enrolled all rare tumors (or at least a lengthy list of them) within the same framework; the second (adopted for some tumor types in the USA) was based on the creation of ad hoc tumor registries for specific entities, like the International Pediatric Adrenocortical Tumor Registry (IPACTR) (Ribeiro et al. 2012) or the International Pleuropulmonary Blastoma Registry (IPPBR) (Messinger et al. 2015).

These pioneering European national projects were based on the first model. Though they had many similarities, each organization had its own characteristics, different registration/classification policies, different processes for central pathology review and data verification, and different forms of cooperation with other national disease-specific groups (Bisogno et al. 2012a, b). However, the rarity of the tumor entities always remained a key limitation, even on a national level: the small number of cases hinders the feasibility of randomized study that could test the treatment considered standard against an alternate arm of therapy. All the European groups dedicated to pediatric VRT, therefore, agreed that the low incidence, the heterogeneity, and the complexity of these tumors called for a broader, international cooperation. In 2008, the national VRT groups in Italy, France, the UK, Poland, and Germany thus joined forces to form the EXPeRT (European Cooperative Study Group for Pediatric Rare Tumors), the primary aim of which was to promote international clinical and biological research on these diseases (Bisogno et al. 2012a, b; Ferrari et al. 2013, 2021).

References

Bauer AJ, Stewart DR, Kamihara J et al (2019) DICER1 and associated conditions: identification of at-risk individuals and recommended surveillance strategies-response. Clin Cancer Res 25(5):1689–1690

Bien E, Stachowicz-Stencel T, Balcerska A et al (2004) Incidence, characteristics and outcome of the alimentary tract carcinomas (Atc) in children: report from the Polish Paediatric Rare Tumours Study. In: Chybicka A, Kazanowska B, Toporski J (eds) Advances in pediatric bone marrow transplantation and oncology. Medical University of Wrocław, Wrocław, pp 198–202

Bien E, Stachowicz-Stencel T, Balcerska A et al (2009a) Angiosarcoma in children—still uncontrollable oncological problem: the report of the polish paediatric rare tumours study. Eur J Cancer Care 18(4):411–420

Bien E, Stachowicz-Stencel T, Godzinski J et al (2009b) Retrospective multi-institutional study on hemangiopericytoma in polish children. Pediatr Int 51:19–24

Bisogno G, Ferrari A, Bien E et al (2012a) Rare cancers in children—the EXPeRT initiative: a report from the European Cooperative Study Group on pediatric rare tumors. Klin Padiatr 2012(224):416–420

Bisogno G, Soloni P, Conte M et al (2012b) Esthesioneuroblastoma in pediatric and adolescent age. A report from the TREP project in cooperation with the Italian Neuroblastoma and Soft Tissue Sarcoma Committees. BMC Cancer 5(12):117

Bisogno G, Tagarelli A, Schiavetti A et al (2014) Myoepithelial carcinoma treatment in children: a report from the TREP project. Pediatr Blood Cancer 61(4):643–646

Boccara O, Fraitag S, Lasne D et al (2016) Kaposiform Haemangioendothelioma-spectrum lesions with Kasabach-Merritt phenomenon: retrospective analysis and long-term outcome. Acta Derm Venereol 96:77–81

Brecht IB, Graf N, Schweinitz D et al (2009) Networking for children and adolescents with very rare tumors: foundation of the GPOH Pediatric Rare Tumor Group. Klin Padiatr 221(3):181–185

Carretto E, Inserra A, Ferrari A et al (2011) Epithelial thymic tumours in paediatric age: a report from the TREP project. Orphanet J Rare Dis 6:28

Casanova M, Bisogno G, Gandola L et al (2012) A prospective protocol for nasopharyngeal carcinoma in children and adolescents: the Italian Rare Tumors in Pediatric Age (TREP) project. Cancer 118(10):2718–2725

Cecchetto G, Alaggio R, Bisogno G et al (2010) Sex cord-stromal tumors of the testis in children. A clinicopathologic report from the Italian TREP project. J Pediatr Surg 45(9):1868–1873

Cecchetto G, Ferrari A, Bernini G et al (2011) Sex cord stromal tumors of the ovary in children. A clinicopathological report from the Italian TREP project. Pediatr Blood Cancer 56(7):1062–1067

Chiaravalli S, Guzzo M, Bisogno G et al (2014) Salivary gland carcinomas in children and adolescents: the Italian TREP project experience. Pediatr Blood Cancer 61(11):1961–1968

Crocoli A, Grimaldi C, Virgone C et al (2019) Outcome after surgery for solid pseudopapillary pancreatic tumors in children: report from the TREP project-Italian Rare Tumors Study Group. Pediatr Blood Cancer 66(3):e27519

Dall'Igna P, Cecchetto G, Bisogno G et al (2010) Pancreatic tumors in children and adolescents: the Italian TREP project experience. Pediatr Blood Cancer 54(5):675–680

Dall'Igna P, Virgone C, De Salvo GL et al (2014) Adrenocortical tumors in Italian children: analysis of clinical characteristics and P53 status. Data from the national registries. J Pediatr Surg 49(9):1367–1371

de Lambert G, Lardy H, Martelli H et al (2015) Surgical management of neuroendocrine tumors of the appendix in children and adolescents: a retrospective French multicenter study of 114 cases. Pediatr Blood Cancer 63:598–603

Di Carlo D, Ferrari A, Perruccio K et al (2015) Management and follow-up of urothelial neoplasms of the bladder in children: a report from the TREP project. Pediatr Blood Cancer 62(6):1000–1003

Ernestus K, Pietsch T, Gessler M et al (2006) Structure, use, and risks of biomaterial repositories of embryonal tumors. KlinPädiatr 218:132–138

Ferrari A, Bisogno G, De Salvo GL et al (2007) The challenge of very rare tumours in childhood: the Italian TREP project. Eur J Cancer 43:654–659

Ferrari A, Schneider DT, Bisogno G (2013) EXPeRT board. The founding of the European Cooperative Study Group on pediatric rare tumors—EXPeRT. Expert Rev Anticancer Ther 13(1):1–3

Ferrari A, Bisogno G, Cecchetto G et al (2014) Cutaneous melanoma in children and adolescents: the Italian Rare Tumors in Pediatric Age project experience. J Pediatr 164(2):376–382.e1–2

Ferrari A, Schneider DT, Bisogno G, et al (2021) Facing the challenges of very rare tumors of pediatric age: the European Cooperative Study Group for Pediatric Rare Tumors (EXPeRT) background, goals and achievements. Ped Blood Cancer 68(4):e28993

Godzinski J, Bien E, Pietras W et al (2004) Melanoma in children: same or different as in adults. In: Chybicka A, Kazanowska B, Toporski J (eds) Advances in pediatric bone marrow transplantation and oncology. Medical University of Wroclaw, Wroclaw, pp 223–225

Grapin-Dagorno C, Peycelon M, Philippe-Chomette P et al (2017) Urothelial tumors in children. Bull Cancer 104:195–201

Indini A, Bisogno G, Cecchetto G, et al (2017) Gastrointestinal tract carcinomas in pediatric and adolescent age: the Italian TREP project experience. Pediatr Blood Cancer 64(12)

Indolfi P, Bisogno G, Casale F et al (2007) Prognostic factors in pleuro-pulmonary blastoma. Pediatr Blood Cancer 8(3):318–323

Irtan S, Galmiche-Rolland L, Elie C et al (2016) Recurrence of solid Pseudopapillary neoplasms of the pancreas: results of a nationwide study of risk factors and treatment modalities. Pediatr Blood Cancer 63:1515–1521

Irvine L, Stiller C (2019) Childhood cancer statistics, England annual report 2018 report on behalf of the children, teenagers and young adults expert advisory group, National Cancer Registration and Analysis Service

Jouin A, Helfre S, Bolle S et al (2019) Adapted strategy to tumor response in childhood nasopharyngeal carcinoma: the French experience. Strahlenther Onkol 195(6):504–516

Kaatsch P (2016). Annual Report of the German Childhood Cancer Registry 2016

Lemelle L, Pierron G, Freneaux P, et al (2017) NUT carcinoma in children and adults: a multicenter retrospective study. Pediatr Blood Cancer 64

Magro G, Esposito G, Cecchetto G et al (2012) Pediatric adrenocortical tumors: morphological diagnostic criteria and immunohistochemical expression of matrix metalloproteinase type 2 and human leucocyte-associated antigen (HLA) class II antigens. Results from the Italian Pediatric Rare Tumor (TREP) Study project. Hum Pathol 43(1):31–39

Massi D, Tomasini C, Senetta R et al (2015) Atypical Spitz tumors in patients younger than 18 years. J Am Acad Dermatol 72(1):37–46

Messinger YH, Stewart DR, Priest JR et al (2015) Pleuropulmonary blastoma: a report on 350 central pathology-confirmed pleuropulmonary blastoma cases by the International Pleuropulmonary Blastoma Registry. Cancer 121(2):276–285

Moreau A, Galmiche L, Minard-Colin V et al (2017) Melanotic neuroectodermal tumor of infancy (MNTI) of the head and neck: a French multicenter study. J Craniomaxillofac Surg 46:201–206

Pastore G, de Salvo GL, Bisogno G et al (2009) Evaluating access to pediatric cancer care centers of children and adolescents with rare tumors in Italy: the TREP project. Pediatr Blood Cancer 53:152–155

Picard C, Orbach D, Carton M et al (2018) Revisiting the role of the pathological grading in pediatric adrenal cortical tumors: results from a national cohort study with pathological review. Mod Pathol 32:546–559

Picard C, Orbach D, Dijoud F (2019) Reply to “Pathological prognostication of pediatric adrenocortical tumors: is a gold standard emerging?”. Pediatr Blood Cancer 66:e27710

Rebours C, Couloigner V, Galmiche L et al (2017) Pediatric salivary gland carcinomas: diagnostic and therapeutic management. Laryngoscope 127:140–147

Réguerre Y, Lacour B, André N et al (2010) Epidemiology and management of rare paediatric tumours within the framework of the French society for children cancer. Bull Cancer 97(9):1041–1045

Réguerre Y, Vittaz M, Orbach D et al (2016) Cutaneous malignant melanoma in children and adolescents treated in pediatric oncology units. Pediatr Blood Cancer 63(11):1922–1927

Ribeiro RC, Pinto EM, Zambetti GP et al (2012) The international pediatric adrenocortical tumor registry initiative: contributions to clinical, biological, and treatment advances in pediatric adrenocortical tumors. Mol Cell Endocrinol 351(1):37–43

Ripperger T, Bielack SS, Borkhardt A et al (2017) Childhood cancer predisposition syndromes—a concise review and recommendations by the Cancer Predisposition Working Group of the Society for Pediatric Oncology and Hematology. Am J Med Genet A 173(4):1017–1037

Rod J, Orbach D, Verité C et al (2014) Surgical management of thymic epithelial tumors in children: lessons from the French society of pediatric oncology and review of the literature. Pediatr Blood Cancer 61(11):1910–1915

Spinelli C, Strambi S, Rossi L et al (2016) Surgical management of papillary thyroid carcinoma in childhood and adolescence: an Italian multicenter study on 250 patients. J Endocrinol Invest 39(9):1055–1059

Stachowicz-Stencel T, Bien E, Balcerska A et al (2010) Thymic carcinoma in children: a report from the Polish Pediatric Rare Tumors Study. Pediatr Blood Cancer 54(7):916–920

Steliarova-Foucher E et al (2005) International classification of childhood cancer, third edition (ICCC-3). Cancer 103(7):1457–1467

Stiller C (2007) Childhood cancer in Britain: incidence, survival, mortality. Oxford University Press, Oxford

Virgone C, Cecchetto G, Ferrari A et al (2012) GATA-4 and FOG-2 expression in pediatric ovarian sex cord-stromal tumors replicates embryonal gonadal phenotype: results from the TREP project. PLoS One 7(9):e45914

Virgone C, Cecchetto G, Alaggio R et al (2014) Appendiceal neuroendocrine tumors (carcinoid of the appendix) in childhood: a clinical report from the Italian TREP project. J Pediatr Gastroenterol Nutr 58(3):333–338

Virgone C, Alaggio R, Dall’Igna P et al (2015a) Epithelial tumors of the ovary in children and teenagers: a prospective study from the Italian TREP project. J Pediatr Adolesc Gynecol 28(6):441–446

Virgone C, Cecchetto G, Besutti V et al (2015b) Bowel parasitosis and neuroendocrine tumours of the appendix. A report from the Italian TREP project. Epidemiol Infect 143(7):1552–1555

Weber ML, Schneider DT, Offenmüller S et al (2016) Pediatric colorectal carcinoma is associated with excellent outcome in the context of cancer predisposition syndromes. Pediatr Blood Cancer 63(4):611–617

Worst BC, van Tilburg CM, Balasubramanian GP, al (2016). Next-generation personalised medicine for high-risk paediatric cancer patients—the INFORM pilot study. Eur J Cancer 65 91–101

6 EXPeRT: The European Cooperative Study Group for Pediatric Rare Tumors

Andrea Ferrari, Gianni Bisogno, and Dominik T. Schneider

During the first decade of the new millennium, the pediatric oncology community became increasingly aware that there was a neglected group of childhood cancers, the very rare tumors (VRTs). The improvements in knowledge and survival achieved over the years for many pediatric tumors (thanks to the propensity to develop national and international cooperative protocols) had not been historically seen for a number of very rare pediatric neoplasms, whose common denominator lies in the lack of interest and knowledge typical of orphan diseases. In fact, young patients with these rare malignancies paid the price for the rarity of their tumors and the shortage of dedicated studies or treatment guidelines (Ferrari et al. 2017).

With the increasing awareness, pediatric VRTs began to attract the attention of major pediatric cancer reference centers and cooperative groups of researchers. The first step forward saw the development of national cooperative programs, starting with the pioneering experience of the Italian TREP (*Tumori Rari in Età Pediatrica*, Rare Tumors in Pediatric Age) project (Ferrari et al. 2007) and culminating with the birth of the European VRT network called EXPeRT, i.e., the European Cooperative Study Group for Pediatric Rare Tumors (Ferrari et al. 2013; Bisogno et al. 2012).

The EXPeRT was established in 2008 by the national VRT working groups from Italy, France, Germany, Poland, and the United Kingdom, its stated aim being to improve the available treatments and promote research in the relatively uncharted territory of pediatric VRTs. The first goal of the group was to empower the research on pediatric VRTs by promoting collaboration between the founder national groups, to support the formation of similar groups in other countries and to foster international collaboration. Then, EXPeRT's founding members had a list of different specific objectives:

1. To pool national retrospective series of specific tumor types to obtain large series that enable the evaluation of risk stratified treatment strategies and to generate consensus therapeutic recommendations, using a shared research methodology and a common framework
2. To develop an organization with the double purpose of promoting research and serving as

A. Ferrari (✉)
Pediatric Oncology Unit, Fondazione IRCCS Istituto Nazionale Tumori, Milan, Italy
e-mail: andrea.ferrari@istitutotumori.mi.it

G. Bisogno
Hematology-Oncology Division, Department of Pediatrics, Padova University Hospital, Padova, Italy
e-mail: gianni.bisogno@unipd.it

D. T. Schneider
Klinik für Kinder- und Jugendmedizin, Klinikum Dortmund, University Witten/Herdecke, Dortmund, Germany
e-mail: Dominik.Schneider@klinikumdo.de

D. T. Schneider et al. (eds.), *Rare Tumors in Children and Adolescents*, Pediatric Oncology,
https://doi.org/10.1007/978-3-030-92071-5_6

an advisory network to help with difficult decisions regarding single clinical cases
3. To set up an international prospective case registry

The development of joint retrospective studies on specific VRTs was the first activity (also relatively easy to realize in the absence of financial support). For this purpose, harmonized core data sheet for uniform documentation of clinical data was developed. The group published joint series on pancreatoblastoma (Bien et al. 2011), Sertoli-Leydig tumors (Schneider et al. 2015), pleuropulmonary blastoma (Bisogno et al. 2014), thymic tumors (Stachowicz-Stencel et al. 2015), adrenocortical tumors (Cecchetto et al. 2017), and melanoma (Brecht et al. 2018) (Table 6.1). Overall, these publications firstly confirmed that cooperation on such topics on a European scale was not only feasible but also fruitful.

To achieve the further goals, however, the EXPeRT was able to activate different levels of cooperation, also thanks to the support from the European pediatric oncology community (i.e., the European Society for Pediatric Oncology, SIOPE). In fact, it soon became clear that it was crucially important to obtain dedicated funds and also to engage with figures outside the world of pediatric oncology: join forces, pool resources, boost collaborative efforts, involve everyone working on pediatric VRTs, be they international experts, specialists in various fields, care providers, families and patients, regulators, or providers of funding as well as work in synergy with the adult oncology community (Ferrari et al. 2019a, b).

The EXPeRT network was the prerequisite to obtain three consecutive important EU-funded collaborative efforts, i.e., the ExPO-r-Net, the JARC, and the PARTNER (Ferrari et al. 2021).

6.1 ExPO-r-Net

From 2014 to 2017, the EXPeRT was part of the 3-year ExPO-r-Net (European Expert Paediatric Oncology Reference Network for Diagnostics and Treatment) project. ExPO-r-Net was developed under an EU directive aiming to reduce inequalities across EU member states. This project focused on the need to improve access to highly specialized health care, particularly for patients with low-prevalence diseases who require special expertise. As part of the ExPO-r-Net project (and thanks to the financial support it provided), the EXPeRT had the chance to conduct its activities, strengthen cooperation with healthcare authorities, and adopt e-Health solutions to facilitate the exchange of information and knowledge rather than move patients, whenever possible.

In particular, three main activities were implemented. These included the development of consensus recommendations for some specific tumor types, the implementation of the website, and the virtual tumor board. A specific website was developed to inform families and the non-scientific community about rare pediatric malignancies (www.raretumors-children.eu). The website is currently under further development (in 2019) and will also include a section where professionals can find the harmonized recommendations/guidelines developed by the EXPeRT committee (e.g., on pleuropulmonary blastoma, pancreatoblastoma, thymic tumors, infantile fibrosarcoma).

The virtual tumor board and advisory desk was developed with the aim to offer a tool dedicated to professionals who need expert medical advice (https://vrt.cineca.it). This project was considered of major importance, because in the absence of clinical protocols or standardized therapeutic guidelines, clinical decisions for VRTs are often unprecedented for the physicians involved. Moreover, there is no or only limited validated experience to support such decisions, so that therapy must often be chosen based on an individual risk assessment. Since mid-2017, the virtual tumor board platform has been active, and professionals can ask advices by submitting anonymized documents, i.e., clinical data, reports, and images (including DICOM data). The EXPeRT has identified and established different virtual tumor panels (each focusing on specific tumor types) that embody the expertise available in various parts of Europe. The online discussion

Table 6.1 Published retrospective studies by EXPeRT (European Cooperative Study Group for Pediatric Rare Tumors)

Publication	Main results	Comments
Pancreatoblastoma (Bien et al. 2011)	20 patients (study period: 2000–2009) 5-year EFS, 58.8%; 5-year OS, 79.4% Rate of response to chemotherapy: 73% Outcome correlates with complete surgical excision	Development of a standardized approach to the diagnosis (staging system) and treatment (conservative surgery followed by cisplatin-doxorubicin chemotherapy, postponed aggressive surgery on primary tumor and metastases)
Sertoli-Leydig cell tumors (Schneider et al. 2015)	44 patients (study period: 1993–2008, depending on country) 5-year EFS, 70%; 5-year, OS 87% Stage, histopathological differentiation, and intra-/preoperative rupture or positive ascites determine prognosis Impact of chemotherapy in incompletely resected and advanced stages still to be assessed	Identification of possible prognostic factors, i.e., intraoperative tumor rupture and histological differentiation Development of diagnostic and treatment guidelines (including cisplatin-based regimen)
Pleuropulmonary blastoma (Bisogno et al. 2014)	65 patients (study period: 2000–2009) Type I: 5-year EFS, 83.3%; OS, 91.7% Type II/III: 5-year EFS, 42.9%; OS, 57.5% Favorable prognostic factors: complete tumor resection at diagnosis and absence of invasiveness Role of doxorubicin-based chemotherapy in type II/III (5-year EFS: 70% vs 31.3% in patients with or without doxorubicin-based regimens)	Identification of a common therapeutic approach Identification of prognostic factors
Thymoma and thymic carcinoma (Stachowicz-Stencel et al. 2015)	36 patients (study period: 2000–2012) 16 thymomas: 14 patients are alive with no evidence of disease 20 carcinomas: 5 patients alive; 5-year OS, 21% Surgical R0 resection: milestone of treatment	Common therapeutic guidelines in pediatric population have yet to be established. Surgical excision remains the milestone of treatment. The role of chemotherapy is unclear
Adrenocortical carcinomas (Cecchetto et al. 2017)	82 patients (study period: 2000–2013) 3-year EFS, 38.8%; OS, 54.7% Survival rates influenced by distant metastases, tumor volume, lymph node involvement, age, vascular involvement, and incomplete surgery For localized disease alone: EFS, 51.1%; OS, 73%	Identification of common treatment strategy (surgery alone if R0 achievable; if not, neoadjuvant chemotherapy) Issues: prognostic factors in adult population lack sensitivity and specificity Complete surgical resection is fundamental whenever possible. The impact of chemotherapy could not be ascertained

(continued)

Table 6.1 (continued)

Publication	Main results	Comments
Cutaneous melanoma (Brecht et al. 2018)	219 patients (study period: 2002–2012) 3-year EFS, 84%; OS, 91.4% Sentinel lymph node biopsy was performed in 112 patients and was positive in 37.5% Stage III cases: similar survival for patients who received (23 cases) or not (21 cases) adjuvant therapy Tumor site, tumor stage, and ulceration influenced survival rates	Patients treated by pediatric oncologists ($n = 140$) were more likely to have advanced disease than those treated by dermatologists ($n = 79$) The clinical history of melanoma in children and adolescents might resemble that of adult counterpart

EFS event-free survival, *OS* overall survival

of patients' data among the various panelists is moderated, and the conclusions and consensus recommendations are coordinated by each panel leader. Some aspects of this activity still need clarifications; among others, for example, the workload for the members of the various panels should be evaluated. The consulting work should be documented in terms of the amount of time these professionals spend on this activity. In principle, it should become possible or even necessary in the future, to consider some sort of compensation from public and private healthcare providers for the centers involved in this consulting process. In fact, the increasing visibility of EXPeRT and international initiatives such as EXPO-r-Net are expected to prompt an increasing demand for such consultations on pediatric VRTs (Ferrari et al. 2017).

Another initiative of EXPeRT within the EXPO-r-Net was to explore what action was taken on a national scale for children with VRTs in the various European countries. This was important for EXPeRT, because one of the goals of EXPeRT was to encourage other European countries to join the group. Accordingly, one of the EXPO-r-Net goals was to reduce inequalities in childhood cancer survival and healthcare capabilities in different EU member states. A survey (conducted by contacting the chairs of each European national pediatric oncology society/association) showed that a structured, national cooperative group focusing on VRTs existed, in 2014, in less than 30% of European countries (i.e., Italy, Germany, Austria, Poland, France, Spain, and the Netherlands). After the EXPO-r-Net project (and the invitation to cooperate), other VRT groups were set up (the first in Croatia and Israel).

As a major result of this project, EXPO-r-Net and EXPeRT's activities (the tumor board, for example, that opens the way to the development of other consultation desks involving other pediatric tumors) became a model for a subsequent, broader project to create the ERN PaedCan (European Reference Network for Paediatric Cancer) (http://paedcan.ern-net.eu/).

6.2 JARC

From 2016 to 2019, the EXPeRT was involved in the JARC (Joint Action on Rare Cancers) (http://www.jointactionrarecancers.eu/), promoted by the European Commission. JARC presented a natural framework for all stakeholders to work together, to prioritize rare cancer in the agenda of the EU and member states (with a view to national cancer plans), and to develop innovative and shared solutions. These goals should be implemented through the ERNs on rare cancers, in the areas of quality of care, research, education, and state of the art definition on prevention, diagnosis, and treatment of rare cancers. The JARC involved 12 different "families" of rare cancers (and so 12 different working groups), 11 on adult tumors (from head and neck cancers to sarcomas and neuroendocrine tumors) and 1 on pediatric cancers.

For the EXPeRT, working with the JARC provided two great opportunities. First, cooperation between pediatric oncologists and oncologists dealing with rare tumors in adults was put in place; second, links with researchers in cancer epidemiology were established that have proven essential to research on extremely rare tumors (e.g., RARECAREnet database, www.rarecarenet.eu).

In particular, in cooperation with the JARC, the EXPeRT promoted an effort to arrive at a consensus on the definition of pediatric VRTs, and therefore produced a list of these entities, that was not influenced by the different clinical practices or experience of different cooperative groups. According to the consensus, pediatric VRTs were identified as those with an annual incidence of <2/1000000 and corresponded to 11% of all cancers in patients aged 0–14 years. Using a lower threshold (<1 per million) excluded extragonadal germ cell tumors, cutaneous melanoma, hepatoblastoma, thyroid carcinoma, and non-epithelial tumors of the ovary from the very rare tumor list. Using higher cutoff led to the inclusion of classical pediatric tumors in the group of VRTs (e.g., rhabdomyosarcoma, bone sarcomas, medulloblastoma). The threshold of 2/million could also be adopted in populations aged 0–19 years: in this case, three tumor types had an incidence rate of >2/million (i.e., thyroid and testicular cancers and skin melanoma), but the consensus experts considered them as "very rare" according to their clinical needs (Ferrari et al. 2019a, b). The JARC consensus produced a definition and a list of pediatric VRTs which may represent a starting point for prioritizing research on these tumors, based on data and patients' clinical needs. In fact, if it is true that all childhood cancers are rare, it is important to differentiate very rare cancers, being true orphan diseases, from the other pediatric malignancies, in order to suggest dedicated methodological approaches for research. However, EXPeRT/JARC consensus authors highlighted how such a list should be used flexibly and considered as a "work in progress." New very rare entities, in fact, come to light every year, as researchers learn more about the molecular basis of many cancer types (e.g., NUT carcinoma or mammary analogue secretory carcinoma of the salivary glands). As examples, the authors explained that, while brain tumor groups would exceed the defined cutoff, newer and more refined classifications would reveal exceptionally rare entities such as the medulloblastoma SHH p53-mutated variant, with poor prognosis and no consensus on its standard treatment, or the ependymoma YAP1 variant, probably characterized by good prognosis (Ferrari et al. 2019a, b).

6.3 PARTNER

As part of the ERN PaedCan project, the EXPeRT is involved in the 2018–2021 PARTNER (Paediatric Rare Tumours Network-European Registry) project. Its main purpose is to set up a European registry of pediatric VRTs, thus establishing a common platform for registering cases (Orbach et al. 2021).

The value of this project is based on the capacity to set up a European registry able of gathering information on treatment of VRTs and provide this information to experts generating new guidance recommendations for daily practice. The platform that will be created using innovative IT tools to link the existing databases will enhance European collaboration and facilitate cross-border access to dedicated expertise.

One additional specific goal of PARTNER is to enlarge the network dedicated to VRTs involving the so-called European LHEAR (low health expenditure average rate) countries in the elaboration of treatment guidelines and the building of the registry. It is expected that the PARTNER project will strengthen the collaboration between countries involved and stimulate more European countries to join EXPeRT, with the aim of improving care for patients and reducing inequalities in cancer outcome across EU member states.

References

Bien E, Godzinski J, Dall'Igna P et al (2011) Pancreatoblastoma: a report from the European Cooperative Study Group for Paediatric Rare Tumours (EXPeRT). Eur J Cancer 47(15):2347–2352

Bisogno G, Ferrari A, Bien E et al (2012) Rare cancers in children—the EXPeRT initiative: a report from the

European Cooperative Study Group on Pediatric Rare Tumors. Klin Padiatr 224:416–420

Bisogno G, Brennan B, Orbach D et al (2014) Treatment and prognostic factors in pleuropulmonary blastoma: an EXPeRT report. Eur J Cancer 50(1):178–184

Brecht IB, De Paoli A, Bisogno G et al (2018) Pediatric patients with cutaneous melanoma: a European study. Pediatr Blood Cancer 65(6):e26974

Cecchetto G, Ganarin A, Bien E, et al (2017) Outcome and prognostic factors in high-risk childhood adrenocortical carcinomas: a report from the European Cooperative Study Group on Pediatric Rare Tumors (EXPeRT). Pediatr Blood Cancer 64(6)

Ferrari A, Bisogno G, De Salvo GL et al (2007) The challenge of very rare tumours in childhood: the Italian TREP project. Eur J Cancer 43:654–659

Ferrari A, Schneider DT, Bisogno G (2013) The founding of the European Cooperative Study Group on Pediatric Rare Tumors—EXPeRT. Expert Rev Anticancer Ther 13(1):1–3

Ferrari A, Schneider DT, Bisogno G et al (2017) The challenge of very rare childhood cancer in developed and developing countries. Expert Opin Orphan Drugs 5:331–341. https://doi.org/10.1080/21678707.2017.1298440

Ferrari A, Brecht IB, Gatta G et al (2019a) Defining and listing very rare cancers of pediatric age: consensus of the Joint Action on Rare Cancers (JARC) in cooperation with the European Cooperative Study Group for Pediatric Rare Tumors (EXPeRT). Eur J Cancer 110:120–126

Ferrari A, Schneider D, Bisogno G et al (2019b) Joining forces for pediatric very rare tumors. Oncotarget 10(33):3084–3085

Ferrari A, Schneider DT, Bisogno G, et al (2021). Facing the challenges of very rare tumors of pediatric age: the European Cooperative Study Group for Pediatric Rare Tumors (EXPeRT) background, goals and achievements. Pediatr Blood Cancer 68(l4):e28993

Orbach D, Ferrari A, Schneider DT, et al (2021). The European Padiatric Rare Tumours Network - European Registry (PARTNER) project for very rare tumors in children. Pediatr Blood Cancer 68(l4):e29072

Schneider DT, Orbach D, Cecchetto G et al (2015) Ovarian Sertoli Leydig cell tumours in children and adolescents: an analysis of the European Cooperative Study Group on Pediatric Rare Tumors (EXPeRT). Eur J Cancer 51(4):543–550

Stachowicz-Stencel T, Orbach D, Brecht I et al (2015) Thymoma and thymic carcinoma in children and adolescents: a report from the European Cooperative Study Group for Pediatric Rare Tumors (EXPeRT). Eur J Cancer 51(16):2444–2452

7 The United States

Farzana Pashankar and Carlos Rodriguez-Galindo

7.1 Introduction

In the United States, every year 12,000 children and adolescents less than 20 years old are diagnosed with cancer. The COG Rare Tumor Committee chose to define infrequent tumors within the context of a pediatric population as those neoplasms, which are generally classified as other malignant epithelial neoplasms and melanomas in the International Classification of Childhood Cancer subgroup XI of the SEER database.(Pappo et al. 2010) Thus included in the rare tumor group were a large number of tumors with a varied biology and clinical presentation as outlined in Table 7.1. Other tumors that are rare but were not included as they have their own clinical trials are malignant germ cell tumors, hepatoblastoma, renal rhabdoid tumors, and rare histiotypes of soft tissue sarcomas.

Although termed "rare tumors," these tumors are not so rare. Of all pediatric malignancies, the cumulative frequency of these tumors is around 4% in children younger than 14 years and 19.6% in adolescents between 15 and 19 years.(Ries et al. 1999)

F. Pashankar (✉)
Department of Pediatrics, Yale University School of Medicine, New Haven, CT, USA
e-mail: Farzana.pashankar@yale.edu

C. Rodriguez-Galindo
Department of Global Pediatric Medicine, St Jude Children's Research Hospital, Memphis, TN, USA

7.2 Children's Oncology Group (COG) Rare Tumor Group

There are considerable challenges associated with studying rare tumors (see Chap. 1).

In order to overcome some of these difficulties, the COG Rare Tumor Initiative was developed in 2002. Three subcommittees were established—germ cell, liver, and infrequent tumors. In 2008, the Retinoblastoma and Rare Tumors committees merged. In 2019, Germ Cell and Liver subcommittees were established as independent committees, and the current Rare Tumor Committee includes the Retinoblastoma and the Infrequent Tumor subcommittees.

Recognizing that small sample sizes and a broad array of diagnoses are a major limitation for the development of clinical trials, the focus of the infrequent tumor committee has been on international collaboration and development of feasible and novel multidisciplinary single-arm protocols that could maximize the likelihood of success. The other focus of the committee has been on developing therapeutic guidelines and a registry and rare tumor tissue bank. Apart from efforts within COG, several individual rare tumor registries have been developed in the United States that have significantly improved our understanding of some of these rare tumors.

D. T. Schneider et al. (eds.), *Rare Tumors in Children and Adolescents*, Pediatric Oncology,
https://doi.org/10.1007/978-3-030-92071-5_7

Table 7.1 Tumors included in the Rare Tumor Group

Infrequent tumors monitored by the COG Rare Tumor Committee
• Thyroid carcinomas
• Colorectal carcinomas
• Nasopharyngeal carcinomas
• Adrenocortical carcinomas
• Desmoplastic small round cell tumor
• Melanoma
• Pancreatoblastoma
• Gastrointestinal stromal tumors
• Gonadal stromal tumors
• Neuroendocrine tumors
• Other carcinomas
Rare tumors with clinical trials
• Malignant germ cell tumors
• Hepatoblastomas
• Renal rhabdoid tumors
• Rare histiotypes of soft tissue sarcomas

7.2.1 Infrequent Tumor Subcommittee Projects

7.2.1.1 Clinical Trials

The committee conducted two single-arm clinical trials with international collaboration. The ARAR0331 study was conducted in patients with nasopharyngeal carcinoma and sought to evaluate the impact of induction chemotherapy and concomitant chemoradiation. The study was conducted from 2006 to 2013 and enrolled 111 patients.

The ARAR0332 study was conducted in patients with adrenocortical carcinoma and sought to determine if extended surgery with retroperitoneal lymph node dissection can improve outcome for patients with stage II tumors and if intensive chemotherapy (mitotane and cisplatin-based) can improve outcome for patients with advanced (stages III and IV) disease. This study was conducted from 2006 to 2013 and enrolled 78 patients, 30 from Brazil. With the closure of these two clinical trials, new trials are in development.

7.2.1.2 Children's Oncology Group Registry and Rare Tumor Banking Protocol

Data from COG registry was analyzed from 2002 to 2007, for four infrequent tumors, melanoma, thyroid carcinoma, nasopharyngeal carcinoma, and adrenocortical carcinoma and compared to SEER registry. It showed significant underreporting, and only 7% of the expected numbers of rare cancers were registered.(Pappo et al. 2010) In 2007, a more robust registry called the Children's Cancer Research Network (CCRN) was developed to register all patients with childhood cancer under age 20 treated at COG institutions in the United States or Canada. Between 2008 and 2013, 1862 patients with rare cancers were registered, still with significant underreporting compared to SEER registry.(Pappo et al. 2015)

A tumor banking protocol (ABTR01B1) was also developed as part of the rare tumor initiatives in 2003. Rare tumors are banked on this protocol and are available to future investigators for study. The limitations of CCRN and ABTR01B1 were that there was no linking of phenotypic data to biospecimens.

In 2015, COG developed a registry called Project:EveryChild Protocol (APEC14B1). The goal of this registry is to prospectively collect biospecimens and key phenotypic data for all children diagnosed with cancer through a single study. This ability to link biological data to informative clinical data will allow for future research. For rare tumors, this registry will provide us a valuable resource to understand underlying biology, molecular targets, or prognostic factors. From November 2015 to January 2019, 285 patients with rare tumors have been enrolled (Fig. 7.1).

7.2.1.3 Diagnostic and Therapeutic Recommendations

The third major goal of the committee was to develop diagnostic and therapeutic recommendations for select rare tumors, by summarizing current literature reviews. A total of eight rare tumors were identified for the development of guidelines. These included thyroid carcinomas, colorectal carcinoma, melanoma, gastrointestinal stromal tumor, pancreatoblastoma, desmoplastic small round cell tumor, gonadal stromal tumors, and carcinoid tumors. In order to develop the guidelines, a working group was established, which consisted of pediatric oncologists, surgeons and pathologists, and radiation oncolo-

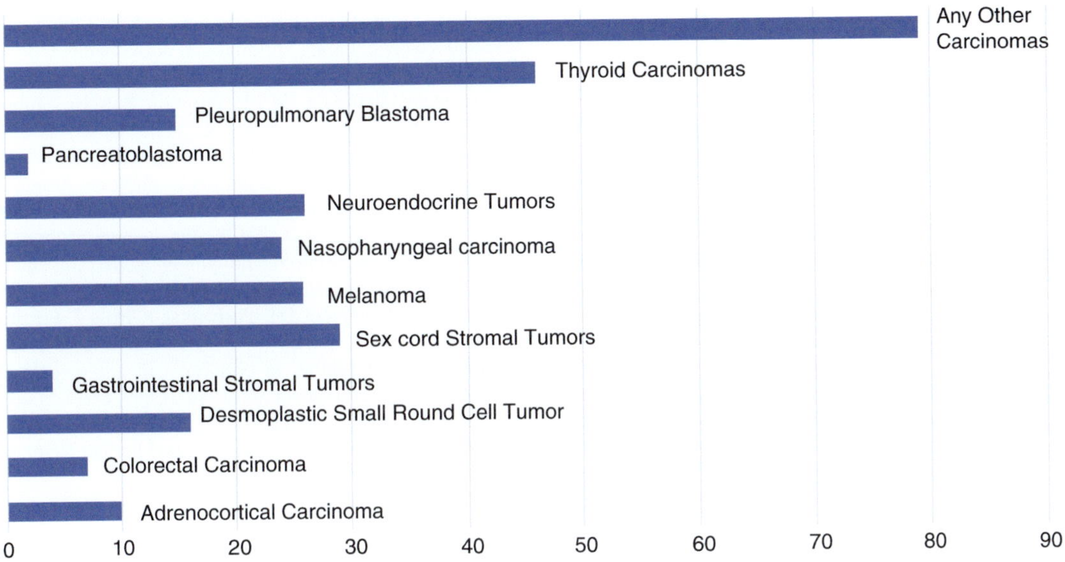

Fig. 7.1 Rare tumors registered in Project:EveryChild from November 2015 to January 2019

gists. For each tumor guideline, one or two investigators were identified with expertise in that tumor type. The guidelines were published as a special supplement in the *Journal of Pediatric Hematology and Oncology*, for wide dissemination to pediatric oncologists.(Rapkin and Pashankar 2012; Glick et al. 2012; Schultz et al. 2012; Neier et al. 2012; Howell and O'Dorisio 2012; Janeway and Pappo 2012; Jordan and Pappo 2012; Goldberg and Furman 2012) The authors of each rare tumor guideline also form a network of experts available to treating clinicians to help with the management of these rare tumors.

7.3 Rare Tumor Registries Outside of Children's Oncology Group

Apart from the rare tumor efforts through the Children's Oncology Group, several other efforts are ongoing in the United States for rare tumors. These include development of individual rare tumor registries and establishment of a Rare Tumors Tumor Board.

7.3.1 Individual Rare Tumor Registries

These registries have focused on one tumor type and have provided detailed invaluable information, on their clinical presentation, treatment, and outcome. More importantly, the individual tumor registries and tumor banks have made monumental discoveries and increased our understanding of the molecular pathogenesis of these tumors and serve as a model to understanding carcinogenesis. The individual rare tumor registries and contact information are outlined in Table 7.2.

Table 7.2 Rare tumor registries in the United States

Cooperative group rare tumor registries
• Project:EveryChild Protocol (APEC14B1) (www.childrensoncologygroup.org)
Individual rare tumor registries
• International Pediatric Adrenocortical Tumor Registry (IPACTR) (www.stjude.org/ipactr)
• Pleuropulmonary Blastoma Registry (PPB) (www.ppbregistry.org)
• International Ovarian and Testicular Stromal Tumor Registry (OTST) (www.otstregistry.org)
• NUT Midline Carcinoma Registry (www.nmcregistry.org)

7.3.2 Rare Tumors Tumor Board

The Rare Tumors Tumor Board is a teleconference tumor board that was established in 2018 by Baylor College of Medicine. It is held once a month. Rare tumors are presented by treating clinicians from across the United States. The members of the COG Rare Tumor Committee and other disease-specific experts are available to review the cases and provide treatment recommendations. This has been a very successful venture and has provided treating clinicians with a valuable resource and input from experts in rare tumors.

References

Glick RD, Pashankar FD, Pappo A, Laquaglia MP (2012) Management of pancreatoblastoma in children and young adults. J Pediatr Hematol Oncol 34(Suppl 2):S47–S50

Pappo AS, Krailo M, Chen Z, Rodriguez-Galindo C, Reaman G (2010) Infrequent tumor initiative of the Children's Oncology Group: initial lessons learned and their impact on future plans. J Clin Oncol 28(33):5011–5016

Ries LA, Smith MA, Gurney JG, et al Cancer incidence and survival among children and adolescents: United States SEER program 1975–1995. National Cancer Institute, Bethesda. SEER Program Pub No. 1999, 99–4649

Pappo AS, Furman WL, Schultz KA, Ferrari A, Helman L, Krailo MD (2015) Rare tumors in children: progress through collaboration. J Clin Oncol 33(27):3047–3054

Rapkin L, Pashankar FD (2012) Management of thyroid carcinoma in children and young adults. J Pediatr Hematol Oncol 34(Suppl 2):S39–S46

Schultz KA, Schneider DT, Pashankar F, Ross J, Frazier L (2012) Management of ovarian and testicular sex cord-stromal tumors in children and adolescents. J Pediatr Hematol Oncol 34(Suppl 2):S55–S63

Neier M, Pappo A, Navid F (2012) Management of melanomas in children and young adults. J Pediatr Hematol Oncol 34(Suppl 2):S51–S54

Howell DL, O'Dorisio MS (2012) Management of neuroendocrine tumors in children, adolescents, and young adults. J Pediatr Hematol Oncol 34(Suppl 2):S64–S68

Janeway KA, Pappo A (2012) Treatment guidelines for gastrointestinal stromal tumors in children and young adults. J Pediatr Hematol Oncol 34(Suppl 2):S69–S72

Jordan AH, Pappo A (2012) Management of desmoplastic small round-cell tumors in children and young adults. J Pediatr Hematol Oncol 34(Suppl 2):S73–S75

Goldberg J, Furman WL (2012) Management of colorectal carcinoma in children and young adults. J Pediatr Hematol Oncol 34(Suppl 2):S76–S79

Part IV

Rare Tumors of the Head and Neck

8 Epidemiology of Head and Neck Tumors

Jan Godzinski and Ines B. Brecht

Head and neck pathologies are frequent in childhood but rarely have malignant origin. Traumatic lesions, inflammatory enlargement of the lymph nodes, congenital malformations, cysts, hemangioma, lymphangioma, vascular malformations, and even infectious diseases may mimic malignant conditions. Though the incidence of head and neck cancer in pediatric patients is relatively low, recently, an increase in incidence of malignant head and neck cancer in pediatric patients was reported (Albright et al. 2002; Schwartz et al. 2015). The incidence rose from 1.1 per 100,000 in 1973–1975 to 1.6 in 2007–2009 (Schwartz et al. 2015). Twelve percent of all pediatric malignancies are located in the head and neck region (Albright et al. 2002). Lymphomas, rhabdomyosarcomas, and thyroid carcinomas are most often seen, followed by carcinomas of the salivary gland and nasopharyngeal carcinomas. However, the geographical region has an impact on the distribution of entities. For example, Burkitt lymphoma and nasopharyngeal carcinoma, which are associated with Epstein-Barr virus, are more often seen in Africa; on the other hand, Europe shows a predominance of lymphomas and sarcomas (Arboleda et al. 2020). In the subsequent chapters, the following unusual pediatric head and neck cancers are discussed: nasopharyngeal carcinoma, esthesioneuroblastoma, thyroid tumors, oral cancer, salivary gland cancer, and laryngeal carcinoma. Figure 8.1 shows the distribution of these rare head and neck tumors in children and adolescents.

J. Godzinski (✉)
Department of Pediatric Surgery, Marciniak Hospital, and Department of Paediatric Traumatology and Emergency Medicine, Medical University Wroclaw, Wroclaw, Poland

I. B. Brecht
Department of Pediatric Hematology/Oncology, University Children's Hospital Tuebingen, Tuebingen, Germany
e-mail: ines.brecht@med.uni-tuebingen.de

D. T. Schneider et al. (eds.), *Rare Tumors in Children and Adolescents*, Pediatric Oncology,
https://doi.org/10.1007/978-3-030-92071-5_8

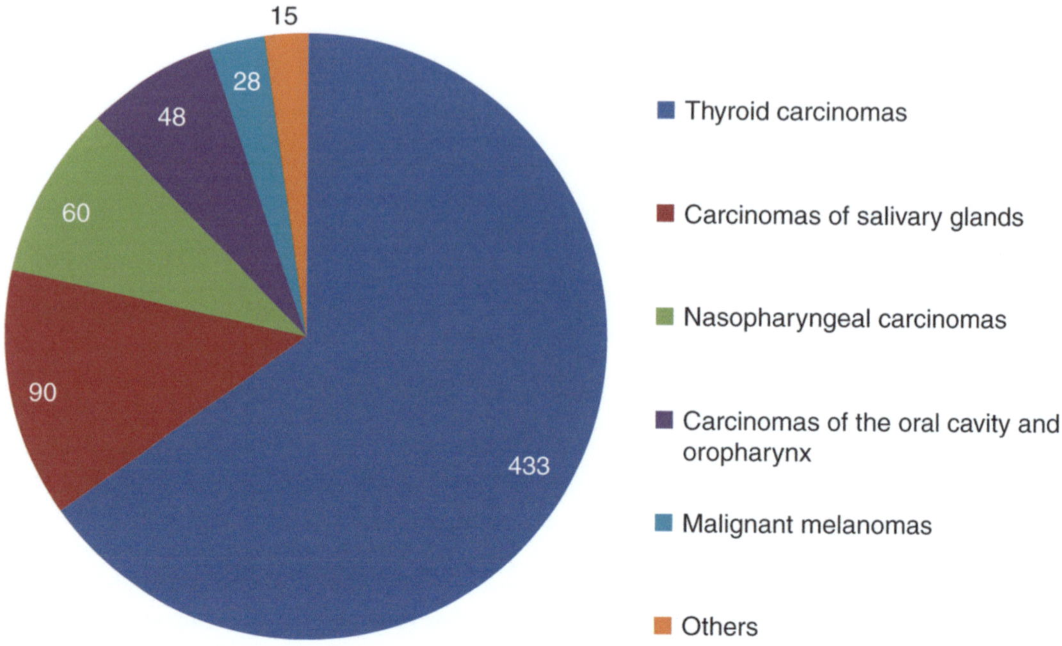

Fig. 8.1 Distribution of "other malignant epithelial neoplasms" of head and neck by ICD-3 code in children under the age of 15. Data from the US Surveillance and End Results Registry (SEER), 1973–2004

References

Albright JT, Topham AK, Reilly JS (2002) Pediatric head and neck malignancies: US incidence and trends over 2 decades. Arch Otolaryngol Head Neck Surg 128(6):655–659

Arboleda LPA, de Mendonça RMH, Lopez EEM, Araújo ALD, Palmier NR, de Pauli PM, Fonseca JM, Hoffmann IL, Cardinalli IA, Chaves ALF, Aranda S, Brandão TB, Lopes MA, Ribeiro ACP, Troconis CCM, Santos-Silva AR (2020) Global frequency and distribution of head and neck cancer in pediatrics, a systematic review. Crit Rev Oncol Hematol 148:102892

Schwartz I, Hughes C, Brigger MT (2015) Pediatric head and neck malignancies: incidence and trends, 1973-2010. Otolaryngol Head Neck Surg 152(6):1127–1132

Thyroid Carcinomas

9

Maura Massimino, Antje Redlich, Paola Collini, and Peter Vorwerk

9.1 Introduction

Thyroid cancers account for the most frequent tumors of endocrine glands in childhood and adolescence; however, these solid tumors are rare in this population. Currently, about 10% of all thyroid cancers occur in patients under 21 years of age (Buckwalter et al. 1981). The annual incidence as derived from the Surveillance, Epidemiology, and End Results (SEER) registry is 0.54 cases per 100,000 persons (Hogan et al. 2009).

Thyroid carcinoma represents approximately 7.5% of all invasive cancer in the 15- to 19-year-old age group and 10.6% of all invasive cancers in persons 20–24 years of age (Barr et al. 2016; Wu et al. 2003). In children younger than 15 years of age, it is a much rarer malignancy, and it has been reported that sporadic papillary thyroid carcinoma constitutes only 0.57% of all malignancies in children under 15 years old in Europe (Gatta et al. 2005). Fortunately, in young patients diagnosed with thyroid carcinoma, the overall 5-year survival rate is 98–100% (Gatta et al. 2005), assuring an excellent long-term prognosis in most cases. The classification of thyroid carcinomas follows the World Health Organization (WHO) Classification of Tumours of Endocrine Organs edited in 2017 (Lloyd et al. 2017), which considers both pathology and genetics together with clinical behavior in defining histotypes (Table 9.1). Due to their extremely low malignant potential if criteria are strictly applied, a part of tumors formerly put in the category of "carcinoma" are now classified as "tumors" or "neoplasms" with uncertain malignant potential. In childhood, the vast majority of follicular cell-derived thyroid cancers are differentiated thyroid carcinomas, i.e., papillary and follicular carcinomas. Both poorly differentiated and undifferentiated (anaplastic) carcinomas are practically absent in this age and are not discussed in this chapter.

Medullary thyroid carcinoma (MTC) arising from the parafollicular C cells and associated with inherited tumor syndromes will be also described.

M. Massimino (✉)
Pediatric Unit, Fondazione IRCCS Istituto Nazionale Tumori, Milan, Italy
e-mail: maura.massimino@istitutotumori.mi.it

A. Redlich · P. Vorwerk
Department of Pediatric Oncology, Otto-von-Guericke University Magdeburg, Magdeburg, Germany

P. Collini
Pathology Department, Fondazione IRCCS Istituto Nazionale Tumori, Milan, Italy

D. T. Schneider et al. (eds.), *Rare Tumors in Children and Adolescents*, Pediatric Oncology,
https://doi.org/10.1007/978-3-030-92071-5_9

Table 9.1 2017 WHO Classification of thyroid carcinomas

1. Papillary thyroid carcinoma (PTC)
1.1. Papillary carcinoma, not otherwise specified (NOS)
1.2. Follicular variant of PTC
1.3. Encapsulated variant of PTC
1.4. Papillary microcarcinoma
1.5. Columnar cell variant of PTC
1.6. Oncocytic variant of PTC
1.7. Diffuse sclerosing variant of PTC
1.8. Tall cell variant of PTC
1.9. Cribriform-morular variant of PTC
1.10. Hobnail variant of PTC
1.11. Papillary thyroid carcinoma with fibromatosis/fasciitis-like stroma
1.12. Solid/trabecular variant of PTC
1.13. Spindle cell variant
1.14. Clear cell variant of PTC
1.15. Warthin-like variant pf PTC
2. Follicular thyroid carcinoma (FTC), NOS
2.1. FTC, minimally invasive
2.2. FTC, encapsulated angioinvasive
2.3. FTC, widely invasive
3. Hurtle (oncocytic) cell carcinoma
4. Poorly differentiated thyroid carcinoma
5. Anaplastic thyroid carcinoma
6. Squamous cell carcinoma
7. Medullary thyroid carcinoma
8. Mixed medullary and follicular thyroid carcinoma
9. Mucoepidermoid carcinoma
10. Sclerosing mucoepidermoid carcinoma with eosinophilia
11. Mucinous carcinoma
12. Intrathyroid thymic carcinoma

9.2 Differentiated Thyroid Carcinoma

9.2.1 Epidemiology and Etiology

Differentiated thyroid cancer (DTC), which derives from follicular epithelial cells, includes papillary and follicular carcinomas and accounts for more than 90% of thyroid cancer in childhood (Danese et al. 1997). Among DTC, papillary thyroid carcinoma (PTC) is the most common type, with ionizing radiations appearing to be an important causal factor (Ron et al. 1989). Accordingly, a steep rise in the incidence of PTC was observed in the young population following the 1986 Chernobyl nuclear accident (Kazakov et al. 1992; Mettler Jr et al. 1992). Also, children treated with radiation therapy on the neck for malignant diseases, such as Hodgkin lymphoma or medulloblastoma, or in the past for benign pathologies such as thymic hyperplasia, are at risk for subsequent PTC (Bhatia et al. 2003). Other risk factors are Hashimoto thyroiditis or genetic syndromes, such as Gardner's syndrome (Bell and Mazzaferri 1993; Okayasu et al. 1995; Ott et al. 1985). The striking increase in new cases of "thyroid cancer" since 1990 has not affected the mortality rate of thyroid cancer, over all ages. Of the three major explanations, (1) the expected increase in the death rate has not yet occurred and will do so in the future, (2) current therapy is completely curative, and (3) the excess cases are overdiagnosed (nonlife threatening, not "cancer") and therapy is not necessary, the latter is most likely (Ahn and Welch 2015; Jegerlehner et al. 2017; Mathonnet et al. 2017; Sanabria et al. 2018). Again, the striking increase in new cases of "thyroid cancer" since 1990 did not affect the incidence of metastatic disease at diagnosis, which is most likely due to overdiagnosis. This "epidemic" has not included regional disease which indicates that more therapy, either more surgery, node dissections, and/or radiotherapy, was administered unnecessarily to those men and women who were overdiagnosed. Some authors also debate the differences in lifestyle as a cause of more thyroid tumors in this age group (Vergamini et al. 2014; Bernier et al. 2019). The preponderance of affected females throughout the literature is likely to be related to estrogen sensitivity of the thyroid gland (Hogan et al. 2009; Farahati et al. 1998; dos Santos and Swerdlow 1993). In fact, in prepubertal children, the gender influence is not that clearly detectable (Jarzab et al. 2005). Follicular thyroid carcinoma (FTC) are of the minimally invasive type, being the widely invasive type exceptional (Figs. 9.1, 9.2, and 9.3).

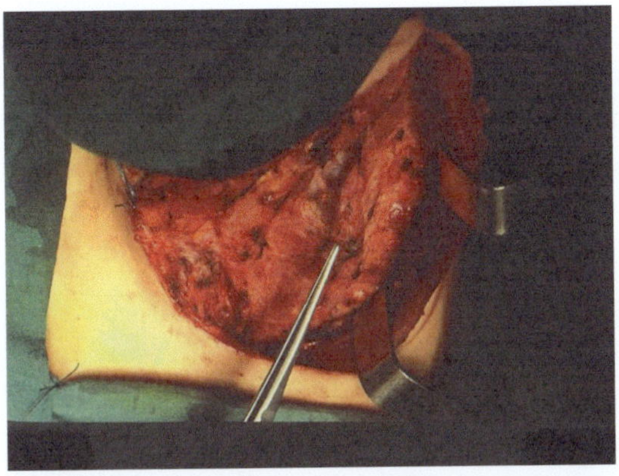

Fig. 9.1 Early operatory field showing secondary adenopathies

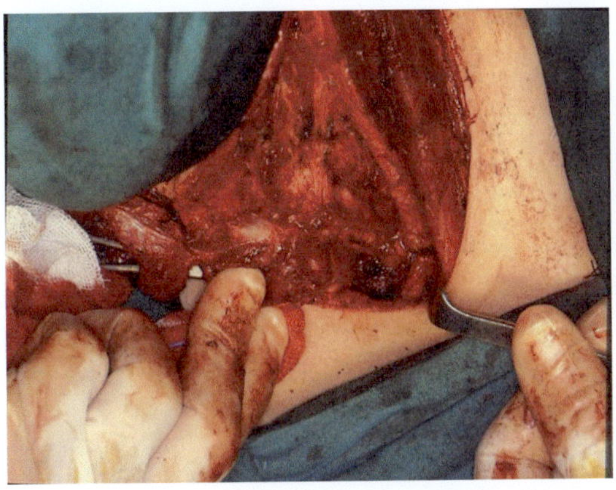

Fig. 9.2 During recurrent node resections

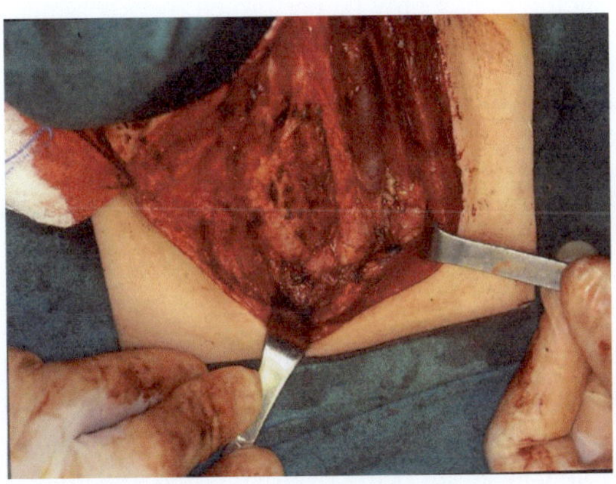

Fig. 9.3 Final result

9.2.2 Clinical Presentation and Diagnosis

Among DTC, PTC and FTC show a different presentation and biologic behavior. Both of them can present with a thyroid mass, and lung and bone metastases are possible. Nodal metastases are very frequent in PTC but practically absent in FTC.

Along these lines, children with DTC most commonly present with asymptomatic thyroid mass or palpable cervical lymphadenopathy (Danese et al. 1997; Chen et al. 1994; Chaukar et al. 2005). Hoarseness, dysphagia, and bronchial obstruction are not frequently found as initial symptoms.

Differentiating DTC from benign thyroid nodules challenges pediatricians, pediatric endocrinologists, and pediatric oncologists. Thyroid nodules are uncommon in childhood, affecting 0.5–0.7% of children and adolescents (Aghini-Lombardi et al. 1999; Liesenkotter et al. 1997). Since the frequency of malignancy in pediatric thyroid nodules is not quite clear, a carcinoma has to be ruled out as reliable in any case (Yip et al. 1994). In a meta-analysis, the mean incidence of DTC in pediatric thyroid nodules which were operated on was 26.4% (Niedziela 2006). Any nodule discovered in this age group should therefore be viewed with suspicion, and the diagnostic approach should be more extensive than in adults.

In the presence of a cervical mass, clinical assessment of the site of the nodule (thyroid vs node vs other), its characteristics (size, consistency, and mobility), and laryngeal or esophageal involvement (dysphonia and dysphagia) should be checked performed. Fixation of the mass to adjacent structures and lymphadenopathy are suspicious of malignancy (Lugo-Vicente and Ortiz 1998; Lassaletta et al. 1997).

In laboratory examinations, no preoperative marker is able to distinguish DTC from benign nodules. Nevertheless, laboratory evaluation of thyroid function and serum thyroglobulin is use-

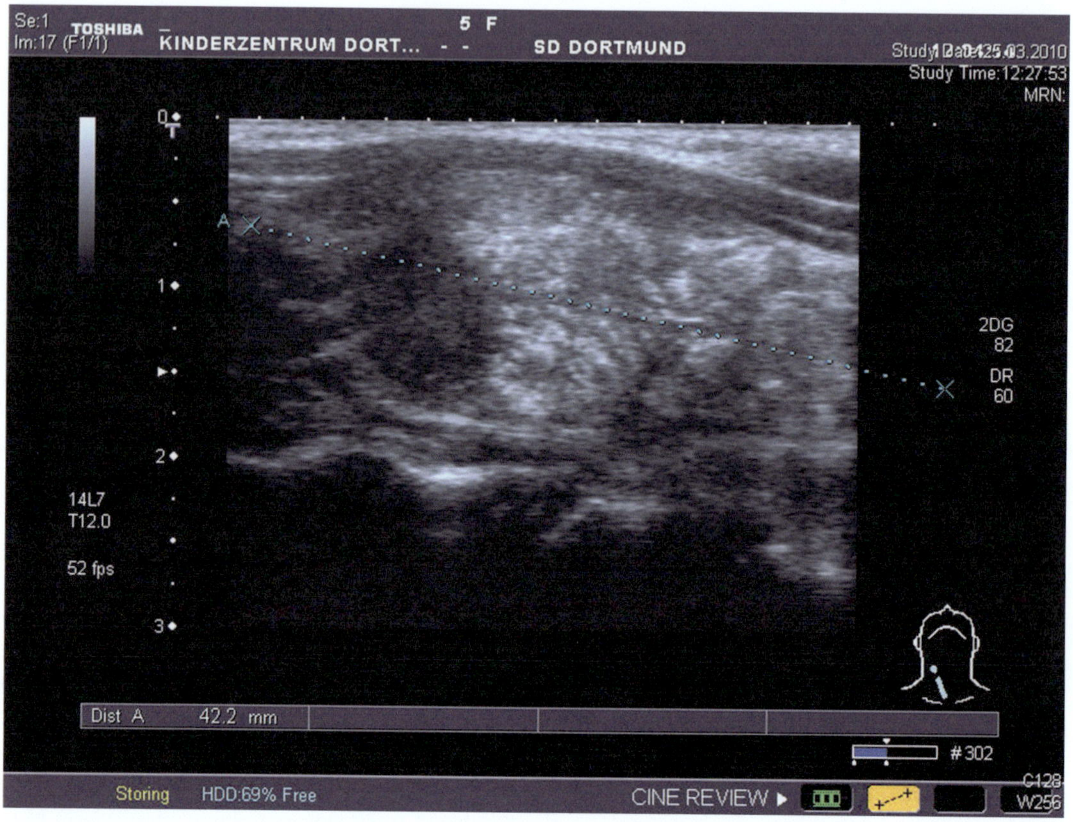

Fig. 9.4 Ultrasound of a thyroid carcinoma in the right lobe of the thyroid

ful. Thyroglobulin is used to detect recurrence of DTC after total thyroidectomy and ablative radioiodine therapy (Herle and Uller 1975; Ng Tang Fui et al. 1979).

Ultrasonography characterizes size and appearance of the gland and the nodules (see Figs. 9.4 and 9.5). The only reliable indicators for malignancy are invasive growth into surrounding tissue and metastases to cervical lymph nodes (Hegedus and Karstrup 1998). Other sonographic findings such as hypoechogenicity, solid composition, irregular margins, or microcalcifications are associated with an increased risk of malignancy but usually cannot distinguish benign from malignant nodules accurately.

In adults, numerous reports confirm that the introduction of fine needle aspiration biopsy (FNAB) reduced thyroid surgery (Gharib and Goellner 1993). In young patients FNAB is a sensitive diagnostic test and a useful tool in diagnosing malignancy in pediatric thyroid nodules (Stevens et al. 2009). In the analysis of the study GPOH-MET as a national registry, the sensitivity was 69.0% only—a central review was recommended (Redlich et al. 2012). The procedure should in fact only be performed by experienced physicians and cytologists.

9.2.2.1 Overdiagnosis/Disease Increase

The problem of overdiagnosis for thyroid cancer has been observed in the USA, Canada, Australia, and South Korea (Davies and Randolph 2014; Hall et al. 2014; Pandeya et al. 2016). The increase in incidence of thyroid cancer and lack of change in thyroid cancer mortality suggest that, especially in adolescent and young adult population, two of every three patients with thyroid cancer are being overdiagnosed, the highest rate of overdiagnosis of any cancer. The cause has been attributed to the increased availability and use of more sensitive imaging techniques such as ultrasound, CT scanning, and MRI

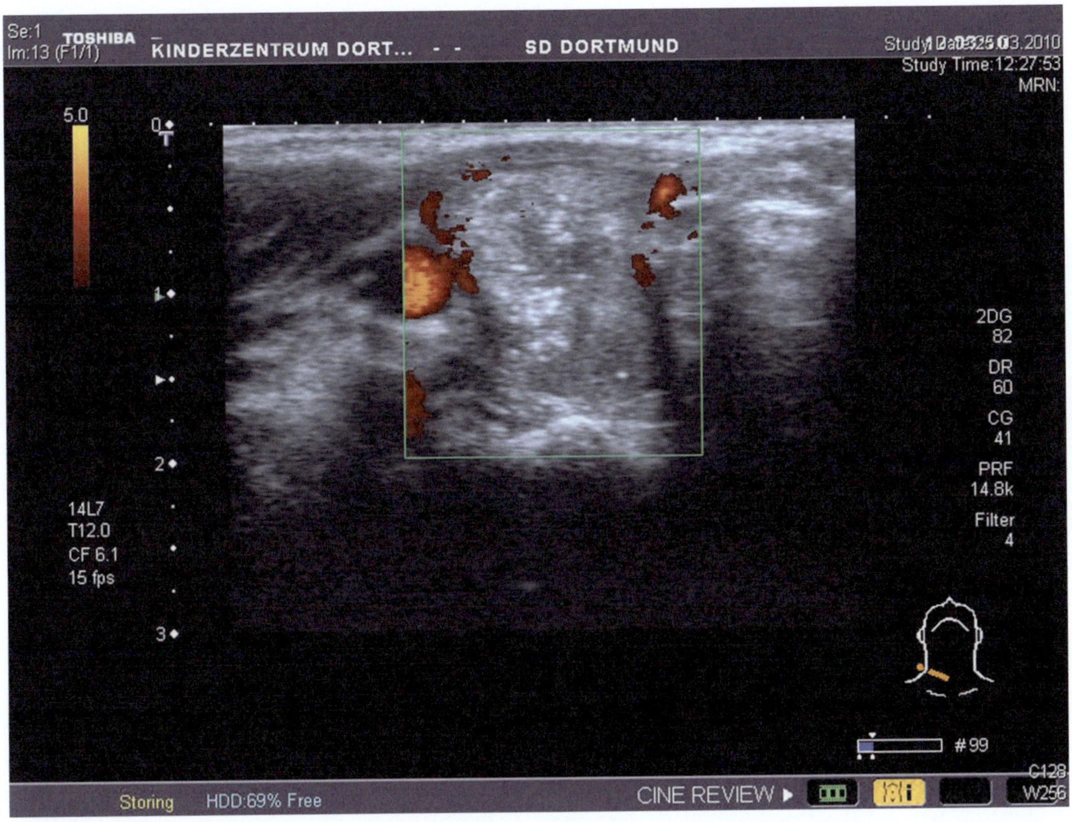

Fig. 9.5 Ultrasound of lymph node involvement of patient with thyroid carcinoma

scanning that detect subclinical nodules and that appear to pathologists as cancer but that do not affect the patient in her or his lifetime. Virtually all persons diagnosed with thyroid cancer are treated: roughly two thirds undergo radical thyroidectomy, and one third undergo subtotal thyroidectomy. The tumors being excised are getting smaller—at one center, the proportion of patients undergoing surgery for a tumor measuring less than 1 cm in diameter increased from 14% in 1995 to 56% 10 years later (Ahn and Kim 2014*).

9.2.3 Special Considerations

Several studies have shown that DTC in pediatric patients differs from that in adults with respect to its presentation and outcome (Table 9.2).

The malignant disease in childhood is associated with more locally aggressive behavior and more frequent distant metastases than its adult counterpart (Zimmerman et al. 1988; Jarzab and Handkiewicz-Junak 2007; Schlumberger et al. 1987). As the thyroid gland is smaller in children than in adults, earlier involvement of the thyroid capsule and the surrounding tissue of the neck is possible (Farahati et al. 1999). Recurrence rates tend to be higher in the pediatric population, but nevertheless, cause-specific mortality remains low.

9.2.4 Pathology

Nonmedullary, follicular-derived thyroid carcinomas, encompassing papillary thyroid carcinomas (PTC), follicular thyroid carcinomas (FTC), poorly differentiated carcinomas (PDC), and anaplastic carcinomas, represent biologically and genetically different and distinct entities (Lloyd et al. 2017).

While PTC is characterized by a prevalent lymphatic spread, FTC follows a vascular way of

Table 9.2 Differentiated thyroid cancer: differences in children and adults

	Children	Adults
Annual incidence (Hogan et al. 2009; Wiersinga 2001)	0.2–2:1,000,000	50–100:1,000,000
Staging at presentation		
Extrathyroidal tumor spread into the soft tissue of the neck (pT4)	52%	15% (low-risk variants) 45% (high-risk variants)
Lymph node metastases (Zimmerman et al. 1988; Farahati et al. 1997)	40–70% (–90%)	30–73%
Distant metastases at onset (Schlumberger et al. 1987; Ruegemer et al. 1988)	12–20% (lung, miliary; bone)	2–10% (lung; rarely bone)
Histology		
Histological subtype (Newman et al. 1998; Welch Dinauer et al. 1998)	PTC 80–90% (low-risk variants)	PTC 80% (also high-risk variants)
Multifocality (Spinelli et al. 2004)	50–80%	30–60%
Size (Wiersinga 2001; Chow et al. 2004; Miccoli et al. 2008)	Larger	Smaller
Outcome		
Event-free survival (5 years) (Jarzab and Handkiewicz-Junak 2007)	60%	80%
Overall survival (Jarzab and Handkiewicz-Junak 2007; Showalter et al. 2008; Parisi and Mankoff 2007)	95–100%	90%

diffusion. PTC shows a high tendency to intrathyroidal microscopic pluricentricity, intrathyroidal and nodal microscopic lymphatic diffusion, infiltration beyond the thyroid capsule into the soft tissue of the neck, and presence of nodal and distant metastases mainly in the lungs. FTC is characterized by vascular invasion, distant metastases in the bone and lungs, and absence of tendency to invade soft tissue of the neck or nodal metastases (Lloyd et al. 2017). Genetically, in PTC the most relevant genetic alterations are generally mutually exclusive and mainly cause activation of the MAPK pathway, being represented by point mutations in 75% of cases, gene fusions in 15% of cases, and copy number variations in 7% of cases. They mainly involve BRAF, RET, RAS, TERT promoter, NTRK1, NTRK3, and ALK. FTC shows a significantly higher rate of numerical abnormalities of chromosomes and loses and gains of specific chromosomal regions with respect to PTC. Somatic RAS point mutations and PPARG gene fusions are common. Mutations of the PI3K/PTEN/AKT pathway genes and TSHR and TERT promoter mutations also occur (Lloyd et al. 2017). Follicular-derived thyroid carcinomas can be divided into low- and high-risk histotypes and variants on the basis of overall survival (OS). In the low-risk group, the vast majority of PTC and the FTC with only capsular invasion show a very good outcome. In the high-risk group, the high-risk variants of PTC, the MIFC with extensive vascular invasion, the widely invasive FTC, PDC, and anaplastic carcinomas are included (Lloyd et al. 2017; Collini et al. 2004; Collini et al. 2006a, b). The vast majority of pediatric thyroid carcinomas are PTC. In these ages, FTC is exceptional and occurs as low-risk MIFC only. PDC is exceptional. Many thyroid carcinomas which have been diagnosed as FTC or PDC (i.e., insular carcinomas, solid/trabecular FTC, and moderately differentiated FTC) in the past are indeed low-risk PTC mainly of the solid/trabecular variants (Collini et al. 2006b; Lloyd et al. 2017; Volante et al. 2007). In childhood, high-risk histotypes of thyroid carcinomas such as widely invasive FTC and anaplastic carcinomas are practically absent.

9.2.5 Therapy

The management strategies for differentiated thyroid carcinoma in children remain to be debated. In general, the radical approach utilizing radical surgery (thyroidectomy plus lymph node dissection) followed by radioiodine therapy and TSH suppression aims for control of both macro- and microscopic diseases. This strategy has been adopted from corresponding trials in adult patients. However, considering potential long-term sequelae of this treatment, a more conservative approach might also be considered for selected patients. This strategy aims for control of only macroscopic disease with limited surgery (hemithyroidectomy plus limited neck dissection) without radioiodine therapy but always followed by TSH suppression. In the perspective of the excellent (almost 100%) overall survival with both approaches, these two options have to be carefully weighed in each patient, since no prospective studies are currently available that would provide definite evidence in favor of one or the other strategy. Both strategies are discussed in detail and summarized in Table 9.3.

9.2.5.1 Surgery

The development of a standard treatment strategy for the treatment of childhood thyroid cancer suffers from the same affliction that affects other rare pediatric tumors: the reliance on retrospective studies and the absence of prospective clinical trials (Spinelli et al. 2004; Dinauer et al. 2008; Collini et al. 2007; Massimino et al. 2018). Though the optimal primary surgical intervention is still unclear, future prospective trials comparing various procedures should be the goal. One very important factor for successful treatment of childhood thyroid cancer is the availability to receive treatment at a facility with the appropriate specialists with a large experience in the treatment of thyroid cancer. A multidisciplinary effort that may include surgeons, pediatric oncologists, medical oncologists, and nuclear medicine physicians would be ideal.

Table 9.3 Comparison between the radical and conservative approach in thyroid carcinoma of children and adolescents

Radical (same as for adults)	Therapeutic approach	Conservative [tailored for selected pediatric patients (tumors limited to one lobe, ± clinical evidence of monolateral N)]
Initial eradication of all clinical and subclinical neoplastic foci (at T, N, and M)	Strategy	Removal only of grossly detectable disease, without searching for microscopic disease after surgery
Improve progression-free survival by detecting and treating all tumor cells and preventing any dedifferentiation of occult neoplastic micro-foci	Aims	Contain treatment morbidity, without jeopardizing the zero mortality rate (the risk of tumor dedifferentiation from microscopic disease seems to be merely theoretical in children)
Total thyroidectomy (regardless of the tumor extent)	Thyroid resection	Removal of the thyroid lobe affected by clinically detectable disease and the isthmus (hemithyroidectomy)
Prophylactic lymphadenectomy	Lymphadenectomy	Selective neck dissection of only the clinically involved node levels
RAI scintigraphic scan to seek any subclinical metastases	Staging	No RAI scintigraphic scan (macrostaging instead of microstaging)
Treatment with 131I ablation, where necessary	Postoperative treatment	Lifelong TSH suppression therapy to control subclinical disease
Serum thyroglobulin level is a very sensitive marker of posttreatment relapse	Follow-up	Presence of thyroid tissue could prevent the effective use of thyroglobulin assay as a marker of tumor relapse, even if a higher cutoff than 0 could be used
Hypoparathyroidism (36%)	Risk of permanent morbidity	Very low, if ever
Recurrent laryngeal nerve paralysis and spinal accessory nerve paralysis (28%)		
Risk of iatrogenic effects of metabolic radiotherapy		

The vast majority of patients undergo total thyroidectomy with or without lymph node dissection. Advantages of this radical approach are:

- Upgrading progression-free survival (PFS).
- Ablative radioiodine therapy can be performed.
- Metastases can be sensitively detected by whole-body scintigraphy.
- Use of thyroglobulin as sensitive marker of posttreatment relapse.
- Numerous children with PTC have multifocal disease, so all thyroid tissue potentially at risk of containing multiple neoplastic foci is removed (Welch Dinauer et al. 1998; Miccoli et al. 1998; De Jong et al. 1992).

Some authors recommend total thyroidectomy even in microcarcinoma (Ogilvie et al. 2010). For selected cases, a more conservative approach is discussed (Massimino et al. 2006). A more conservative treatment approach has not been universally applied. This approach has been developed at several institutions and should be done as part of an organized clinical trial. Only selected patients with tumor limited to one lobe with or without clinical evidence of monolateral nodal metastases are eligible. The main argument for the conservative approach is the excellent prognosis of DTC in children and adolescents despite a more advanced stage at presentation and a more aggressive clinical course (Danese et al. 1997; Chow et al. 2004). The presence of lymph node or distant metastases does not influence mortality in children. The chance of dedifferentiation of microscopic disease over the years is only theoretical. More aggressive procedures, especially if applied in children under 16 years of age, are closely related to a morbidity increase (permanent hypoparathyroidism and recurrent nerve palsy) (La Quaglia et al. 1988; van Santen et al. 2004). Minimal approach is hemithyroidectomy consisting of lobectomy plus isthmectomy. If further surgery is required, no resection in an already operated bed associated with higher complications must be performed (Shaha 2008; Levin et al. 1992).

So as long as there are no prospective trials investigating different therapeutic regimes, the debate will continue. If a conservative approach is to be followed, the role of a pathologist, experienced in thyroid pathology and in particular in the diagnosis of pediatric thyroid carcinomas, becomes critical in the application of the conservative approach.

9.2.5.2 Radioiodine Therapy and Hormonal Manipulation

The radioactive isotope 131I can be administered for selective irradiation of remnant thyroid tissue, microscopic foci of carcinoma, and distant metastases if a radical surgical approach has been used. Radioiodine uptake in carcinoma cells depends on the expression of the sodium-iodide symporter (NIS). In pediatric DTC, the NIS is expressed stronger when compared with adult tumors (Jarzab et al. 2005). That may be one of the reasons why DTC in children is more sensitive to hormonal manipulation and has a better prognosis despite more advanced disease at diagnosis.

The first ablative radioiodine therapy (RIT) after total thyroidectomy is an adjuvant modality to eliminate regularly remaining thyroid tissue and increase sensitivity of thyroglobulin assay and whole-body scintigraphy in follow-up. RIT requires adequate TSH stimulation. It can be achieved endogenously via l-thyroxin withdrawal within 14 days in children (Kuijt and Huang 2005). The use of recombinant thyrotropin (rhTSH) in children is safe; well-tolerated and adequate TSH levels can be achieved (Luster et al. 2009; Ralli et al. 2005).

Functioning of the thyroid is dependent on TSH, whose synthesis and release depend on thyroid-releasing hormone (TRH), produced in the hypothalamus and secreted into the pituitary (Crile Jr 1966; Gharib et al. 1987). Suppression of TSH secretion (TSH < 0.1 mU/L) has the aim to prevent growth of hidden micro-foci, residual tumor, or metastases, respectively.

Used activities vary from 50 MBq/kg for ablation to 100 (−150) MBq/kg for metastatic disease (Franzius et al. 2007). Monitoring of the pulmonary function is recommended to detect radiation-induced pulmonary fibrosis, which is a rare sequela of RIT.

9.2.6 Follow-Up

Whole-body scintigraphy is repeated after 6–12 months from the metabolic treatment, and the RIT can be repeated in case of persistent disease. The goal of this strategy is to obtain a negative scan and a thyroglobulin with an undeterminable value. Thyroglobulin concentration after ablative RIT is a strong predictor of disease recurrence (Pelttari et al. 2010). Low-risk patients with undetectable basal thyroglobulin should receive at least one rhTSH-stimulated thyroglobulin because of the low predictive value for recurrence of basal thyroglobulin (Díaz-Soto et al. 2011).

9.2.7 Postoperative Complications and Their Treatment

Subsequently to radical surgery, high percentages of permanent postoperative complications are documented. After total thyroidectomy, permanent hypoparathyroidism and recurrent laryngeal nerve paralysis often occur, while after neck dissection, spinal accessory nerve paralysis is the major complication. In addition, iatrogenic effects of RAI therapy are reported. A recent report (Molenaar et al. 2018) has compared, in a cohort of 148.215 patients, the risk of developing second hematologic malignancies after thyroidectomy alone or thyroidectomy followed by RAI for well-differentiated thyroid cancer. The conclusion was a statistically increased risk of developing acute and chronic myeloid leukemia after RAI. Postoperative complications are high in almost all pediatric series, especially after total thyroidectomy, also if performed by pediatric surgeons or by neck surgeons devoted to thyroid surgery. Hypoparathyroidism accounts for 0–36% (Bargren et al. 2009; Machens and Dralle 2009; Massimino et al. 2006; Reeve and Thompson 2000) and recurrent nerve palsy from 0 to 28% (Crile Jr 1966; Verburg et al. 2009). Spinal accessory nerve paralysis may also complicate neck dissection. Age below 16 years is at risk of being accompanied by major complications. In children, recurrent nerves are at major risk of being injured, and parathyroid glands are very small, often hidden into the thyroid parenchyma, and difficult to recognize and with a light vascularization. These complications can be very severe in developing age. To make a pragmatic example, also, their support can be difficult and expensive. An adolescent girl around the age of menarche, when deprived of parathyroid normal function, needs frequent electrolyte assays, more than biweekly, to have a valid calcium, vitamin D, and/or parathormone support. Any calcium/phosphorus balance alteration can reflect in alteration of the body mass and in possible later consequences on the harmonic body growth. All these issues suggest that the management of children with thyroid carcinoma should be performed in selected centers.

9.2.7.1 Treatment at Relapse

The options, here again, are radical or conservative. The approach to local or nodal relapse or metastases after radical primary treatment remains the same as at diagnosis. For local or nodal relapses in conservatively treated patients, re-operation remains the standard of care. Even if there is no neoplastic lesion in the thyroid, completion thyroidectomy becomes necessary (instead of only resecting local relapses in the thyroid bed) in cases of contralateral relapse, with further node dissection in cases of radiologically evident metastases to enable RAI therapy. L-thyroxine should be continued at suppressive dosage (Francis et al. 2015).

9.2.8 Prognosis

Children and adolescents with DTC have an excellent prognosis despite the more aggressive behavior when compared with adults (Jarzab and Handkiewicz-Junak 2007). It is a well-known phenomenon that the outcome of pediatric PTC is independent of strong prognostic factors of

Table 9.4 Manifestations in MEN 2 syndrome and their frequencies

	MEN 2A (%)	MEN 2B (%)
MTC (Brandi et al. 2001; Iihara et al. 1997)	90–100	100
Pheochromocytoma (Brandi et al. 2001; Modigliani et al. 1998)	50	50
Hyperparathyroidism (Brandi et al. 2001; Modigliani et al. 1998)	20–30	–
Intestinal ganglioneuromatosis	–	40–100
Marfanoid habitus	–	>95
Stigmata	–	>95

Table 9.5 Timing of prophylactic thyroidectomy in MEN 2 (Machens and Dralle 2007; Brandi et al. 2001; Frank-Raue et al. 2006)

RET mutation	Time of surgery	Operation
Least high-risk level (609, 768, 790, 791, 804, 891)	<5–10 years or pPT	Total thyroidectomy
High-risk level (611, 618, 620, 630, **634**)	<5 years	Total thyroidectomy
Highest-risk level (883, **918**)	<1/2–1 years	Total thyroidectomy with central lymph node dissection

adults, such as low- versus high-risk histological subtype, extrathyroid local invasion into soft tissue of the neck, presence of distant metastases, site of distant metastatic spread, occurrence of relapse, and type of surgery (Verburg et al. 2009; Collini et al. 2006b).

9.3 Medullary Thyroid Carcinoma

Medullary thyroid carcinoma (MTC) arising from the parafollicular C cells is associated with inherited tumor syndromes. MTC derives from progenitor cells migrated from the neural crest during embryogenesis to the thyroid and is actually more a neoplasm of neural crest than of thyroid origin. The multiple endocrine neoplasia (MEN) types 2A and 2B and also familial medullary thyroid carcinoma (FMTC) are characterized by bilateral multifocal MTC invariably in a background of C-cell hyperplasia, the inherited predisposing abnormality. In MEN 2A, besides the calcitonin-producing thyroid tumor, pheochromocytoma and parathyroid adenoma/hyperplasia causing hyperparathyroidism are found. MTC, pheochromocytoma, and typical stigmata characterize patients suffering from MEN 2B (Table 9.4). The FMTC is diagnosed if at least four cases occur in a family in the absence of other MEN 2 manifestations.

MTC usually is the first tumor to develop in patients with MEN 2 and is the most common cause of death among these patients (Szinnai et al. 2007). The malignancy is particularly aggressive in patients with MEN 2B and may occur even in infancy (Yin et al. 2006). Different germline point mutations of the rearranged during transfection (RET) proto-oncogene are involved in the pathogenesis of MTC and MEN 2, respectively, with consequences on management of affected children (Raue and Frank-Raue 2009; Machens and Dralle 2007). Screening for MEN 2 of affected kindreds reveals children with MEN 2, who should undergo prophylactic thyroidectomy before developing MTC (Table 9.5). A strong genotype-phenotype correlation is known, leading to the discrimination in highest-, high-, and least high-risk mutations, respectively (Table 9.5). MEN 2A is frequently caused by mutation in codon 634 and MEN 2B by mutation in codon 918.

More than 90% of patients with MEN 2B harbor de novo mutations in the RET proto-oncogene. These index cases without any family history are at high risk for developing advanced MTC with high mortality. The distinct physical appearance of children with MEN 2B, e.g., mucosal neuromas of the tongue, lips, inner eyelids, marfanoid body habitus, is not appreciated before the occurrence of the thyroid tumor. Premonitory symptoms preceding metastatic MTC are constipation since infancy and inability to cry tears (Brauckhoff et al. 2004). Children with sporadic MTC commonly present with palpable thyroid nodule.

In MEN 2A, no accompanying visible signs are found. An association with Hirschsprung disease or cutaneous lichen amyloidosis is described (Cohen et al. 2002; Verga et al. 2003).

Calcitonin levels represent an accurate and sensitive marker for both preoperative diagnosis and follow-up of MTC (Cohen et al. 2000; Melvin et al. 1971). Pentagastrin testing may be helpful in differentiating C-cell hyperplasia from MTC in cases of moderately elevated basal calcitonin (Milone et al. 2010).

The most important therapeutic option is the radical approach, with the surgical resection of all tumor localizations, since no curative medical therapy is available (Kloos et al. 2009). In recent years, targeted therapy with small molecules such as tyrosine kinase inhibitors and RET kinase inhibitors has been studied in clinical trials with partial responses in up to 30% (Lanzi et al. 2009; Puxeddu et al. 2011; Sherman 2010). The most important prognostic factor is clinical stage at diagnosis. Patients with lymph node or distant metastases are at risk of relapse or fatal outcome (Bergholm et al. 1997).

Targeted receptor tyrosine kinase inhibitors (TKIs), including vandetanib, a RET, vascular endothelial growth factor receptor (VEGFR), and epidermal growth factor receptor inhibitor, have had some antitumor activity in TC patients. Some benefit has also been reported for other TKIs targeting RET and various VEGFR subtypes (sorafenib, sunitinib, pazopanib, and motesanib) (Wells Jr et al. 2012; Fox et al. 2013; Prazeres et al. 2011).

9.3.1 Pediatric Thyroid Cancer: A Model for Collaboration

The treatment of pediatric thyroid cancer is complex and should be managed by a medical team with appropriate experience and skills. The treatment of thyroid cancer in adult patients has been informed by several studies, and general guidelines exist. Pediatric oncologists have tried to extrapolate from these guidelines, but sufficient data do not exist. One aspect of the treatment debate is the fear of exposing children to potential late toxicity. It is known that pediatric thyroid cancer may be more aggressive than thyroid cancer in adults. However, pediatric patients respond well to hormonal manipulation with TSH suppression, and the mortality from pediatric thyroid cancer is very low. It is important to emphasize the need of developing guidelines for very rare cancers and that, as one develops guidelines, one must try to validate them with careful attention to outcomes. For this reason, the Italian approach to a more conservative approach serves as an excellent example (Table 9.3). Guidelines were established, and data are being collected that might inform future international collaborative trials.

References

Aghini-Lombardi F, Antonangeli L, Martino E et al (1999) The spectrum of thyroid disorders in an iodine-deficient community: the Pescopagano survey. J Clin Endocrinol Metab 84(2):561–566

Ahn HS, Welch HG (2015) South Korea's thyroid-cancer "epidemic"—turning the tide. N Engl J Med 373(24):2389–2390

Bargren AE, Meyer-Rochow GY, Delbridge LW, Sidhu SB, Chen H (2009) Outcomes of surgically managed pediatric thyroid cancer. J Surg Res 156(1):70–73

Barr RD, Ries LA, Lewis DR et al; US National Cancer Institute Science of Adolescent and Young Adult Oncology Epidemiology Working Group (2016) Incidence and incidence trends of the most frequent cancers in adolescent and young adult Americans, including "nonmalignant/noninvasive" tumors. Cancer 122(7):1000–8

Bell B, Mazzaferri EL (1993) Familial adenomatous polyposis (Gardner's syndrome) and thyroid carcinoma. A case report and review of the literature. Dig Dis Sci 38(1):185–190

Bergholm U, Bergstrom R, Ekbom A (1997) Long-term follow-up of patients with medullary carcinoma of the thyroid. Cancer 79(1):132–138

Bernier MO, Withrow DR, de Gonzalez AB et al (2019) Trends in pediatric thyroid cancer incidence in the United States, 1998–2013. Cancer 125(14):2497–2505. https://doi.org/10.1002/cncr.32125

Bhatia S, Yasui Y, Robison LL et al (2003) High risk of subsequent neoplasms continues with extended follow-up of childhood Hodgkin's disease: report from the Late Effects Study Group. J Clin Oncol 21(23):4386–4394

Brandi ML, Gagel RF, Angeli A et al (2001) Guidelines for diagnosis and therapy of MEN type 1 and type 2. J Clin Endocrinol Metab 86(12):5658–5671

Brauckhoff M, Gimm O, Weiss CL et al (2004) Multiple endocrine neoplasia 2B syndrome due to codon 918 mutation: clinical manifestation and course in early and late onset disease. World J Surg 28(12):1305–1311

Buckwalter JA, Gurll NJ, Thomas CG Jr (1981) Cancer of the thyroid in youth. World J Surg 5(1):15–25

Chaukar DA, Rangarajan V, Nair N et al (2005) Pediatric thyroid cancer. J Surg Oncol 92(2):130–133

Chen WK, Lee CH, Wang HC, Lui WY, Wei CF (1994) Thyroid cancer in children and adolescents. Zhonghua Yi Xue Za Zhi (Taipei) 54(6):400–406

Chow SM, Law SC, Mendenhall WM et al (2004) Differentiated thyroid carcinoma in childhood and adolescence-clinical course and role of radioiodine. Pediatr Blood Cancer 42(2):176–183

Cohen R, Campos JM, Salaun C et al (2000) Preoperative calcitonin levels are predictive of tumor size and postoperative calcitonin normalization in medullary thyroid carcinoma. Groupe d'Etudes des Tumeurs a Calcitonine (GETC). J Clin Endocrinol Metab 85(2):919–922

Cohen MS, Phay JE, Albinson C et al (2002) Gastrointestinal manifestations of multiple endocrine neoplasia type 2. Ann Surg 235(5):648–654

Collini P, Sampietro G, Pilotti S (2004) Extensive vascular invasion is a marker of risk of relapse in encapsulated non-Hurthle cell follicular carcinoma of the thyroid gland: a clinicopathological study of 18 consecutive cases from a single institution with a 11-year median follow-up. Histopathology 44(1):35–39

Collini P, Massimino M, Leite SF et al (2006a) Papillary thyroid carcinoma of childhood and adolescence: a 30-year experience at the Istituto Nazionale Tumori in Milan. Pediatr Blood Cancer 46(3):300–306

Collini P, Mattavelli F, Pellegrinelli A, Barisella M, Ferrari A, Massimino M (2006b) Papillary carcinoma of the thyroid gland of childhood and adolescence: morphologic subtypes, biologic behavior and prognosis: a clinicopathologic study of 42 sporadic cases treated at a single institution during a 30-year period. Am J Surg Pathol 30(11):1420–1426

Collini P, Mattavelli F, Spinelli C, Massimino M (2007) Treatment of sporadic nonmedullary thyroid carcinomas in pediatric age. Expert Rev Anticancer Ther 7(1):23–30

Crile G Jr (1966) Endocrine dependency of papillary carcinoma of the thyroid. JAMA 195(9):721–724

Danese D, Gardini A, Farsetti A, Sciacchitano S, Andreoli M, Pontecorvi A (1997) Thyroid carcinoma in children and adolescents. Eur J Pediatr 156(3):190–194

Davies L, Randolph G (2014) Evidence-based evaluation of the thyroid nodule. Otolaryngol Clin North Am. 47(4):461–474

De Jong SA, Demeter JG, Lawrence AM, Paloyan E (1992) Necessity and safety of completion thyroidectomy for differentiated thyroid carcinoma. Surgery 112(4):734–737

Díaz-Soto G, Puig-Domingo M, Martínez-Pino I, de Osaba MJM, Mora M, Rivera-Fillat F, Halperin I (2011) Do thyroid cancer patients with basal undetectable Tg measured by current immunoassays require rhTSH testing? Exp Clin Endocrinol Diabetes 119:348–352

Dinauer CA, Breuer C, Rivkees SA (2008) Differentiated thyroid cancer in children: diagnosis and management. Curr Opin Oncol 20(1):59–65

dos Santos SI, Swerdlow AJ (1993) Sex differences in the risks of hormone-dependent cancers. Am J Epidemiol 138(1):10–28

Farahati J, Bucsky P, Parlowsky T, Mader U, Reiners C (1997) Characteristics of differentiated thyroid carcinoma in children and adolescents with respect to age, gender, and histology. Cancer 80(11):2156–2162

Farahati J, Parlowsky T, Mader U, Reiners C, Bucsky P (1998) Differentiated thyroid cancer in children and adolescents. Langenbecks Arch Surg 383(3–4):235–239

Farahati J, Reiners C, Demidchik EP (1999) Is the UICC/AJCC classification of primary tumor in childhood thyroid carcinoma valid? J Nucl Med 40(12):2125

Fox E, Widemann BC, Chuk MK et al (2013) Vandetanib in children and adolescents with multiple endocrine neoplasia type 2B associated medullary thyroid carcinoma. Clin Cancer Res 19(15):4239–4248

Francis GL, Waguespack SG, Bauer AJ, Angelos P, Benvenga S, Cerutti JM, Dinauer CA, Hamilton J, Hay ID, Luster M, Parisi MT, Rachmiel M, Thompson GB, Yamashita S, American Thyroid Association Guidelines Task Force (2015) Management guidelines for children with thyroid nodules and differentiated thyroid cancer. Thyroid 25(7):716–759

Frank-Raue K, Buhr H, Dralle H et al (2006) Long-term outcome in 46 gene carriers of hereditary medullary thyroid carcinoma after prophylactic thyroidectomy: impact of individual RET genotype. Eur J Endocrinol 155(2):229–236

Franzius C, Dietlein M, Biermann M et al (2007) Procedure guideline for radioiodine therapy and 131iodine whole-body scintigraphy in paediatric patients with differentiated thyroid cancer. Nuklearmedizin 46(5): 224–231

Gatta G, Capocaccia R, Stiller C, Kaatsch P, Berrino F, Terenziani M, EUROCARE Working Group (2005) Childhood cancer survival trends in Europe: a EUROCARE Working Group study. J Clin Oncol 23(16):3742–3745

Gharib H, Goellner JR (1993) Fine-needle aspiration biopsy of the thyroid: an appraisal. Ann Intern Med 118(4):282–289

Gharib H, James EM, Charboneau JW, Naessens JM, Offord KP, Gorman CA (1987) Suppressive therapy with levothyroxine for solitary thyroid nodules. A double-blind controlled clinical study. N Engl J Med 317(2):70–75

Hall SF, Irish JC, Groome PA, Urbach DR (2014) Practice patterns in the management of patients with differentiated thyroid cancer in Ontario Canada 2000-2008. J Otolaryngol Head Neck Surg 43:29

Hegedus L, Karstrup S (1998) Ultrasonography in the evaluation of cold thyroid nodules. Eur J Endocrinol 138(1):30–31

Herle AJ, Uller RP (1975) Elevated serum thyroglobulin. A marker of metastases in differentiated thyroid carcinomas. J Clin Invest 56(2):272–277

Hogan AR, Zhuge Y, Perez EA, Koniaris LG, Lew JI, Sola JE (2009) Pediatric thyroid carcinoma: incidence and outcomes in 1753 patients. J Surg Res 156(1):167–172

Iihara M, Yamashita T, Okamoto T et al (1997) A nationwide clinical survey of patients with multiple endocrine neoplasia type 2 and familial medullary thyroid carcinoma in Japan. Jpn J Clin Oncol 27(3):128–134

Jarzab B, Handkiewicz-Junak D (2007) Differentiated thyroid cancer in children and adults: same or distinct disease? Hormones (Athens) 6(3):200–209

Jarzab B, Handkiewicz-Junak D, Wloch J (2005) Juvenile differentiated thyroid carcinoma and the role of radioiodine in its treatment: a qualitative review. Endocr Relat Cancer 12(4):773–803

Jegerlehner S, Bulliard JL, Aujesky D et al; NICER Working Group (2017). Overdiagnosis and overtreatment of thyroid cancer: a population-based temporal trend study. PLoS One 12(6):e0179387

Kazakov VS, Demidchik EP, Astakhova LN (1992) Thyroid cancer after Chernobyl. Nature 359(6390):21

Kloos RT, Eng C, Evans DB et al (2009) Medullary thyroid cancer: management guidelines of the American Thyroid Association. Thyroid 19(6):565–612

Kuijt WJ, Huang SA (2005) Children with differentiated thyroid cancer achieve adequate hyperthyrotropinemia within 14 days of levothyroxine withdrawal. J Clin Endocrinol Metab 90(11):6123–6125

La Quaglia MP, Corbally MT, Heller G, Exelby PR, Brennan MF (1988) Recurrence and morbidity in differentiated thyroid carcinoma in children. Surgery 104(6):1149–1156

Lanzi C, Cassinelli G, Nicolini V, Zunino F (2009) Targeting RET for thyroid cancer therapy. Biochem Pharmacol 77(3):297–309

Lassaletta AL, Melchor Diaz MA, Gavilanes PJ, Martin HG, de Vergas GJ (1997) Thyroid nodules: factors suggestive of malignancy. Acta Otorrinolaringol Esp 48(3):220–224

Levin KE, Clark AH, Duh QY, Demeure M, Siperstein AE, Clark OH (1992) Reoperative thyroid surgery. Surgery 111(6):604–609

Liesenkotter KP, Kiebler A, Stach B, Willgerodt H, Gruters A (1997) Small thyroid volumes and normal iodine excretion in Berlin schoolchildren indicate full normalization of iodine supply. Exp Clin Endocrinol Diabetes 105(Suppl 4):46–50

Lloyd RV, Osamura RY, Kloppel G, Rosai J (2017) WHO classification of tumours of endocrine organs. IARC, Lyon

Lugo-Vicente H, Ortiz VN (1998) Pediatric thyroid nodules: insights in management. Bol Asoc Med P R 90(4–6):74–78

Luster M, Handkiewicz-Junak D, Grossi A et al (2009) Recombinant thyrotropin use in children and adolescents with differentiated thyroid cancer: a multicenter retrospective study. J Clin Endocrinol Metab 94(10):3948–3953

Machens A, Dralle H (2007) Genotype-phenotype based surgical concept of hereditary medullary thyroid carcinoma. World J Surg 31(5):957–968

Machens A, Dralle H (2009) Age disparities in referrals to specialist surgical care for papillary thyroid cancer. Eur J Surg Oncol 35(12):1312–1317

Massimino M, Collini P, Leite SF et al (2006) Conservative surgical approach for thyroid and lymph-node involvement in papillary thyroid carcinoma of childhood and adolescence. Pediatr Blood Cancer 46(3):307–313

Massimino M, Evans DB, Podda M et al (2018) Thyroid cancer in adolescents and young adults. Pediatr Blood Cancer 65(8):e27025. https://doi.org/10.1002/pbc.27025. Epub 2018 Mar 12. Review

Mathonnet M, Cuerq A, Tresallet C et al (2017) What is the care pathway of patients who undergo thyroid surgery in France and its potential pitfalls? A national cohort. BMJ Open 7(4):e013589

Melvin KE, Miller HH, Tashjian AH Jr (1971) Early diagnosis of medullary carcinoma of the thyroid gland by means of calcitonin assay. N Engl J Med 285(20):1115–1120

Mettler FA Jr, Williamson MR, Royal HD et al (1992) Thyroid nodules in the population living around Chernobyl. JAMA 268(5):616–619

Miccoli P, Antonelli A, Spinelli C, Ferdeghini M, Fallahi P, Baschieri L (1998) Completion total thyroidectomy in children with thyroid cancer secondary to the Chernobyl accident. Arch Surg 133(1):89–93

Miccoli P, Minuto MN, Ugolini C et al (2008) Papillary thyroid cancer: pathological parameters as prognostic factors in different classes of age. Otolaryngol Head Neck Surg 138(2):200–203

Milone F, Ramundo V, Chiofalo MG et al (2010) Predictive value of pentagastrin test for preoperative differential diagnosis between C-cell hyperplasia and medullary thyroid carcinoma in patients with moderately elevated basal calcitonin levels. Clin Endocrinol 73(1):85–88

Modigliani E, Cohen R, Campos JM et al (1998) Prognostic factors for survival and for biochemical cure in medullary thyroid carcinoma: results in 899 patients. The GETC Study Group. Groupe d'etude des tumeurs a calcitonine. Clin Endocrinol 48(3):265–273

Molenaar RJ, Sidana S, Radivoyevitch T et al (2018) Risk of hematologic malignancies after radioiodine treatment of well-differentiated thyroid cancer. J Clin Oncol 36(18):1831–1839

Newman KD, Black T, Heller G et al (1998) Differentiated thyroid cancer: determinants of disease progression in patients <21 years of age at diagnosis: a report from the Surgical Discipline Committee of the Children's Cancer Group. Ann Surg 227(4):533–541

Ng Tang Fui SC, Hoffenberg R, Maisey MN, Black EG (1979) Serum thyroglobulin concentrations and whole-body radioiodine scan in follow-up of differentiated thyroid cancer after thyroid ablation. Br Med J 2(6185):298–300

Niedziela M (2006) Pathogenesis, diagnosis and management of thyroid nodules in children. Endocr Relat Cancer 13(2):427–453

Ogilvie JB, Patel KN, Heller KS (2010) Impact of the 2009 American Thyroid Association guidelines on the choice of operation for well-differentiated thyroid microcarcinomas. Surgery 148(6):1222–1226

Okayasu I, Fujiwara M, Hara Y, Tanaka Y, Rose NR (1995) Association of chronic lymphocytic thyroiditis and thyroid papillary carcinoma. A study of surgical cases among Japanese, and white and African Americans. Cancer 76(11):2312–2318

Ott RA, Calandra DB, McCall A, Shah KH, Lawrence AM, Paloyan E (1985) The incidence of thyroid carcinoma in patients with Hashimoto's thyroiditis and solitary cold nodules. Surgery 98(6):1202–1206

Pandeya N, McLeod DS, Balasubramaniam K et al (2016) Increasing thyroid cancer incidence in Queensland, Australia 1982-2008—true increase or overdiagnosis? Clin Endocrinol 84(2):257–264

Parisi MT, Mankoff D (2007) Differentiated pediatric thyroid cancer: correlates with adult disease, controversies in treatment. Semin Nucl Med 37(5):340–356

Pelttari H, Valimaki MJ, Loyttyniemi E, Schalin-Jantti C (2010) Post-ablative serum thyroglobulin is an independent predictor of recurrence in low-risk differentiated thyroid carcinoma: a 16-year follow-up study. Eur J Endocrinol 163(5):757–763

Prazeres H, Torres J, Rodrigues F et al (2011) How to treat a signal? Current basis for RET-genotype-oriented choice of kinase inhibitors for the treatment of medullary thyroid cancer. J Thyroid Res 2011:678357

Puxeddu E, Romagnoli S, Dottorini ME (2011) Targeted therapies for advanced thyroid cancer. Curr Opin Oncol 23:13–21

Ralli M, Cohan P, Lee K (2005) Successful use of recombinant human thyrotropin in the therapy of pediatric well-differentiated thyroid cancer. J Endocrinol Invest 28(3):270–273

Raue F, Frank-Raue K (2009) Genotype-phenotype relationship in multiple endocrine neoplasia type 2. Implications for clinical management. Hormones (Athens) 8(1):23–28

Redlich A, Boxberger N, Schmid KW et al (2012) Sensitivity of fine-needle biopsy in detecting pediatric differentiated thyroid carcinoma. Pediatr Blood Cancer 59:233–237

Reeve T, Thompson NW (2000) Complications of thyroid surgery: how to avoid them, how to manage them, and observations on their possible effect on the whole patient. World J Surg 24(8):971–975

Ron E, Modan B, Preston D, Alfandary E, Stovall M, Boice JD Jr (1989) Thyroid neoplasia following low-dose radiation in childhood. Radiat Res 120(3):516–531

Ruegemer JJ, Hay ID, Bergstralh EJ, Ryan JJ, Offord KP, Gorman CA (1988) Distant metastases in differentiated thyroid carcinoma: a multivariate analysis of prognostic variables. J Clin Endocrinol Metab 67(3):501–508

Sanabria A, Kowalski LP, Shah JP et al (2018) Growing incidence of thyroid carcinoma in recent years: factors underlying overdiagnosis. Head Neck 40(4):855–866

Schlumberger M, de Vathaire F, Travagli JP et al (1987) Differentiated thyroid carcinoma in childhood: long term follow-up of 72 patients. J Clin Endocrinol Metab 65(6):1088–1094

Shaha AR (2008) Revision thyroid surgery—technical considerations. Otolaryngol Clin North Am 41(6):1169–1183, x

Sherman SI (2010) Targeted therapy of thyroid cancer. Biochem Pharmacol 80(5):592–601

Showalter TN, Siegel BA, Moley JF, Baranski TJ, Grigsby PW (2008) Prognostic factors in patients with well-differentiated thyroid cancer presenting with pulmonary metastasis. Cancer Biother Radiopharm 23(5):655–659

Spinelli C, Bertocchini A, Antonelli A, Miccoli P (2004) Surgical therapy of the thyroid papillary carcinoma in children: experience with 56 patients<or =16 years old. J Pediatr Surg 39(10):1500–1505

Stevens C, Lee JK, Sadatsafavi M, Blair GK (2009) Pediatric thyroid fine-needle aspiration cytology: a meta-analysis. J Pediatr Surg 44(11):2184–2191

Szinnai G, Sarnacki S, Polak M (2007) Hereditary medullary thyroid carcinoma: how molecular genetics made multiple endocrine neoplasia type 2 a paediatric disease. Endocr Dev 10:173–187

van Santen HM, Aronson DC, Vulsma T et al (2004) Frequent adverse events after treatment for childhood-onset differentiated thyroid carcinoma: a single institute experience. Eur J Cancer 40(11):1743–1751

Verburg FA, Mäder U, Luster M, Reiners C (2009) Histology does not influence prognosis in differentiated thyroid carcinoma when accounting for age, tumour diameter, invasive growth and metastases. Eur J Endocrinol 160:619–624

Verga U, Fugazzola L, Cambiaghi S et al (2003) Frequent association between MEN 2A and cutaneous lichen amyloidosis. Clin Endocrinol 59(2):156–161

Vergamini LB, Frazier AL, Abrantes FL, Ribeiro KB, Rodriguez-Galindo C (2014) Increase in the incidence of differentiated thyroid carcinoma in children, adolescents, and young adults: a population-based study. J Pediatr 164(6):1481–1485

Volante M, Collini P, Nikiforov YE et al (2007) Poorly differentiated thyroid carcinoma: the Turin proposal for the use of uniform diagnostic criteria and an algorithmic diagnostic approach. Am J Surg Pathol 31:1256–1264

Welch Dinauer CA, Tuttle RM, Robie DK et al (1998) Clinical features associated with metastasis and recurrence of differentiated thyroid cancer in children, adolescents and young adults. Clin Endocrinol 49(5):619–628

Wells SA Jr, Robinson BG, Gagel RF et al (2012) Vandetanib in patients with locally advanced or metastatic medullary thyroid cancer: a randomized, double-blind phase III trial. J Clin Oncol 30(2):134–141

Wiersinga WM (2001) Thyroid cancer in children and adolescents–consequences in later life. J Pediatr Endocrinol Metab 14(Suppl 5):1289–1296

Wu XC, Chen VW, Steele B, Roffers S, Klotz JB, Correa CN, Carozza SE (2003) Cancer incidence in adolescents and young adults in the United States, 1992-1997. J Adolesc Health 32(6):405–415

Yin M, King SK, Hutson JM, Chow CW (2006) Multiple endocrine neoplasia type 2B diagnosed on suction rectal biopsy in infancy: a report of 2 cases. Pediatr Dev Pathol 9(1):56–60

Yip FW, Reeve TS, Poole AG, Delbridge L (1994) Thyroid nodules in childhood and adolescence. Aust N Z J Surg 64(10):676–678

Zimmerman D, Hay ID, Gough IR et al (1988) Papillary thyroid carcinoma in children and adults: long-term follow-up of 1039 patients conservatively treated at one institution during three decades. Surgery 104(6):1157–1166

10 Nasopharyngeal Carcinoma

Udo Kontny, Carlos Rodriguez-Galindo, Daniel Orbach, and Michela Casanova

10.1 Introduction

Nasopharyngeal carcinoma (NPC) is a rare malignant tumor in childhood not only in Europe but also in Asia, where the highest incidence of NPC in adult patients is seen. NPC represents one of the most frequent epithelial tumors of the child in intermediate-risk regions. However, distinguishing malignant tumors from the more common and numerous benign causes of neck masses in childhood is crucial, as many malignant conditions have an excellent prognosis with appropriate oncological management. The worldwide incidence of NPC in children and adolescents between 0 and 14 years is 0.1 per 100,000 and follows a bimodal age distribution with a first peak between 10 and 20 years and a second peak between the fourth and sixth decades (Bray et al. 2008; Wei and St Sham 2005). Males are more frequently affected than females, with a male to female ratio of 2:1. In the United States, the incidence is higher in African-American children than in children of other races, but this racial predilection is lost in older ages. While 10–15% of cases occur in patients younger than 30 years of age, it makes up only 1% of childhood malignancies. In pediatric series, median age is around 15 years (Dourthe et al. 2018). NPC has a distinct epidemiology, etiology, and clinical course compared with other head and neck squamous cell carcinomas, and its pathogenesis is multifactorial. Genetic predisposition and epigenetic alterations particularly related to Epstein-Barr virus (EBV) infection play a major role in the initiation and progression of NPC (Dittmer et al. 2008; Sultan et al. 2010; Cheuk et al. 2011; Huang et al. 2018).

10.2 Symptoms

Young patients with nasopharyngeal carcinoma frequently present with symptoms resulting from a mass effect from the primary tumor as well as frequent cervical lymph node metastasis (Fig. 10.1). Nasal symptoms, such as epistaxis and nasal obstruction, are almost always present and are secondary to the presence of the tumor in

U. Kontny (✉)
Division of Pediatric Hematology, Oncology and Stem Cell Transplantation, Department of Pediatrics, RWTH Medical Faculty, Aachen, Germany
e-mail: ukontny@ukaachen.de

C. Rodriguez-Galindo
Departments of Global Pediatric Medicine and Oncology, St. Jude Children's Research Hospital, Memphis, TN, USA

D. Orbach
SIREDO Oncology Center (Care, Innovation and Research for Children, Adolescents and Young Adults with Cancer), Institut Curie, PSL University, Paris, France

M. Casanova
Pediatric Oncology Unit, Fondazione IRCCS Istituto Nazionale Tumori, Milan, Italy

D. T. Schneider et al. (eds.), *Rare Tumors in Children and Adolescents*, Pediatric Oncology,
https://doi.org/10.1007/978-3-030-92071-5_10

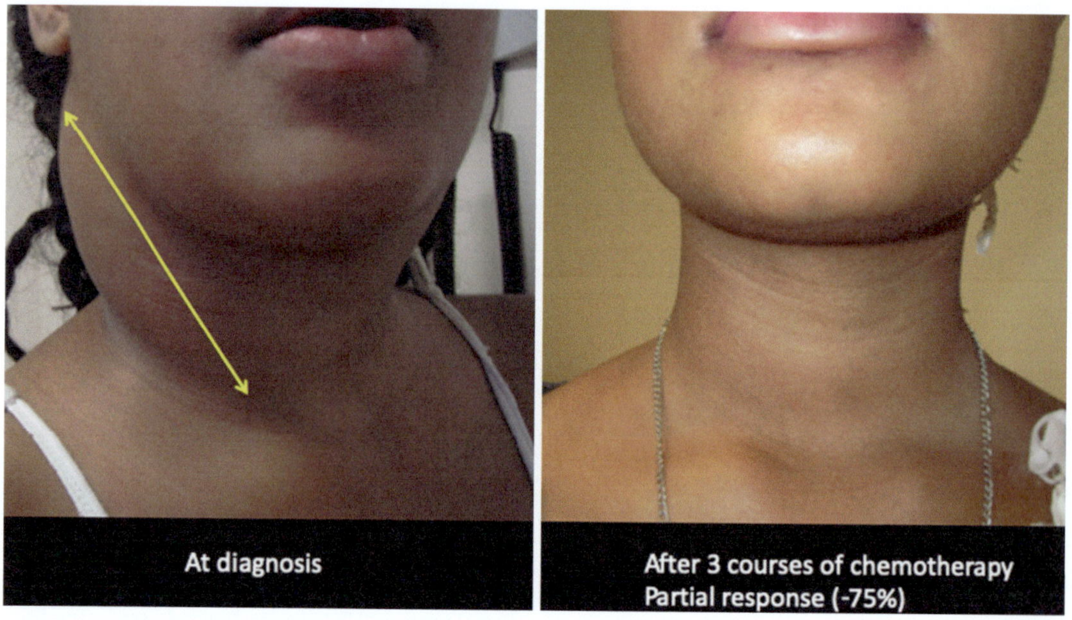

Fig. 10.1 Cervical lymphadenopathy in a 13-year-old girl with stage IV nasopharyngeal carcinoma

the nasopharynx. The second most common symptoms are otologic symptoms, such as hearing loss and tinnitus, which are related to the dysfunction of the Eustachian tube caused by the lateroposterior extension of the tumor into the paranasopharyngeal space. The third most common symptoms are cranial nerve palsies, mostly of the fifth and sixth cranial nerves, resulting from cranial extension of the tumor and skull base erosion; in addition, patients may experience headache, diplopia, facial pain, and numbness. A retrospective analysis of 4768 patients identified the following symptoms at presentation: neck mass (75.8%), nasal symptoms (73.4%), aural symptoms (62.4%), headache (34.8%), diplopia (10.7%), facial numbness (7.6%), weight loss (6.9%), and trismus (3.0%). The physical signs present at diagnosis were enlarged neck node (74.5%) and cranial nerve palsy (20.0%) (Lee et al. 1997). Since the nasal and auditory symptoms are nonspecific and a thorough examination of the nasopharynx is not easy, the majority of NPC patients are only diagnosed when the tumor has reached an advanced stage. Indeed, up to 90% of NPC patients present with lymph node metastases. Distant metastases are rare and can be detected in 5–10% of patients at diagnosis and most commonly involve bones (67%), liver (30%), bone marrow (23%), lungs (20%), and mediastinum (Altun et al. 1995; Ayan et al. 2003).

10.3 Pathogenesis

NPC presents as a complex disease caused by an interaction of the oncogenic gammaherpesvirus EBV chronic infection, environmental, and genetic factors, in a multistep carcinogenic process.

A monoclonal EBV infection is found in more than 98% of preinvasive lesions. The EBV-infected epithelial cells express the EBV antigens EBNA1, LMP1, and LMP2 as well as the EBERs. In vitro and in vivo models have shown that LMP1 and, in particular, LMP2 as well as viral miRNAs, especially BART miRNA, play a major role in the malignant transformation of the NPC cells (Lo et al. 2012).

While nasopharyngeal carcinoma is a rare malignancy in most parts of the world, it is one of the most common cancers in Southeast Asia. Epidemiologic studies conducted in that region have provided an invaluable insight into our current understanding of NPC pathogenesis. The pathogenesis of NPC is influenced by three major factors: environmental factors, such as certain herbs and salted fish consumed in regions with an elevated incidence of NPC; genetic factors, as documented by familial cases that suggest a genetically determined susceptibility; and infectious factors, as documented by the evidence of early EBV infection (Ren et al. 2010).

10.3.1 Environmental Factors

A large number of case control studies conducted in diverse populations in Southeast Asia, Alaska, the Mediterranean basin, and North America have shown that consumption of salted fish and other preserved foods containing large amounts of nitrosodimethylamine may predispose to the development of NPC (Chang and Adami 2006).

10.3.2 Genetic Factors

Three independent genome-wide association studies have consistently identified single nucleotide polymorphisms in the MHC region to be strongly associated with an increased risk for NPC (Su et al. 2013). A consistent association between NPC and the prevalent Chinese HLA-A2 subtype (HLA-A*0207) but not the prevalent Caucasian subtype (HLA-A*0201) has been detected (Hildesheim et al. 2002). The HLA types AW19, BW46, and B17 have also been reported to be associated with an increased risk, whereas HLA-A11 is associated with a decreased risk (Liebowitz 1994).

10.3.3 Epstein–Barr Virus

Epstein–Barr virus (EBV) or human herpes virus 4 (HHV4) is an oncogenic c-herpes virus. Under normal circumstances, EBV infection is restricted to humans, although some types of monkeys can be infected experimentally (Bornkamm 1984). EBV is consistently detected in NPC patients from regions of high and low incidence. Its ability to establish latent infection of host cells and to induce proliferation of the latently infected cells is directly involved in NPC pathogenesis (Niedobitek and Young 1994).

EBV-encoded RNA signal has been shown to be present in nearly all tumor cells, whereas EBV RNA is absent from the adjacent normal tissue, except perhaps for a few scattered lymphoid cells. Premalignant lesions of the nasopharyngeal epithelium have also been shown to harbor EBV RNA, which suggests that the infection occurs in the early phases of carcinogenesis. Detection of a single form of viral DNA suggests that the tumors are clonal proliferations of a single cell that was initially infected with EBV (Lo et al. 2000).

The EBV protein, latent membrane protein 2A (LMP2A), is expressed in NPC and can modulate epithelial proliferation, transformation, and differentiation and as such may promote malignancy (Huang et al. 2018). A key regulator of epithelial cell differentiation is the transcription factor p63, a member of the p53 family. The corresponding latent viral proteins (latent membrane proteins 1 and 2) have substantial effects on cellular gene expression and cellular growth, resulting in the highly invasive, malignant growth of the carcinoma (Fotheringham et al. 2010).

10.4 Pathology

In the past, NPC was called lymphoepithelioma, as the malignant epithelial cells of the nasopharynx frequently intermingled with lymphoid cells in the nasopharynx (Godtfredsen 1944). The histological classification of nasopharyngeal carcinoma proposed by the World Health Organization (WHO) in 1978 categorized tumors into three types. Type I are the typical keratinizing squamous cell carcinomas similar to those found in the rest of the upper aerodigestive tract. Type II includes nonkeratinizing squamous carcinomas and type III carcinomas are the undifferentiated carcinomas (Micheau et al. 1978; Shanmugaratnam 1980; Marks et al. 1998). In children and adolescents, the majority of NPC is WHO type III, whereas type I is not encountered (Ozyar et al. 2006; Jouin et al. 2019).

Table 10.1 WHO classification modified by Krüger and Wustrow

Squamous cell carcinoma (keratinizing)	Type I
Squamous cell carcinoma (nonkeratinizing)	
– Without lymphoid infiltration	Type IIa
– With lymphoid infiltration	Type IIb
Undifferentiated (anaplastic carcinoma)	
– Without lymphoid infiltration	Type IIIa
– With lymphoid infiltration	Type IIIb

Table 10.1 shows the WHO classification modified by Krüger and Wustrow indicating the varying degrees of lymphoid infiltration, whereby the undifferentiated NPC with lymphoid infiltration corresponds to the entities described in 1921 as lymphoepithelioma by Schmincke and nonkeratinizing epithelium carcinoma by Regaud. These histological variants are strictly associated with increased titers against EBV antigen (Krueger and Wustrow 1981).

10.5 Staging System

For staging, the classification of the American Joint Committee on Cancer Staging (eighth edition of the *AJCC stage groupings and TNM definitions*) is internationally accepted (Amin et al. 2017).

10.5.1 Primary Tumor (T)

T0	No tumor identified, but EBV-positive cervical node(s) involvement
T1	Tumor confined to nasopharynx, or extension to oropharynx and/or nasal cavity without parapharyngeal involvement
T2	Tumor with extension to parapharyngeal space and/or adjacent soft tissue involvement (medial pterygoid, lateral pterygoid, prevertebral muscles)
T3	Tumor with infiltration of bony structures at skull base, cervical vertebra, pterygoid structures, and/or paranasal sinuses
T4	Tumor with intracranial extension, involvement of cranial nerves, hypopharynx, orbit, parotid gland, and/or extensive soft tissue infiltration beyond the lateral surface of the lateral pterygoid muscle

10.5.2 Regional Lymph Nodes (N)

N0	No regional lymph node metastasis
N1	Unilateral metastasis in cervical lymph node(s) and/or unilateral or bilateral metastasis in retropharyngeal lymph node(s), 6 cm or smaller in greatest dimension, above the caudal border of cricoid cartilage
N2	Bilateral metastasis in cervical lymph node(s), 6 cm or smaller in greatest dimension, above the caudal border of cricoid cartilage
N3	Unilateral or bilateral metastasis in cervical lymph node(s), larger than 6 cm in greatest dimension, and/or extension below the caudal border of cricoid cartilage

10.5.3 Distant Metastasis (M)

M0	No distant metastasis
M1	Presence of distant metastasis

10.5.4 Definition of Risk Groups

Risk groups are defined by the AJCC (eighth edition). Staging directly correlates with outcome, and in general, two large groups of patients are identified based on rates of local control and risk of metastatic disease. Patients with stages I–II have an excellent outcome, with survival rates in excess of 80–90%, whereas patients with stages III–IV have lower survival (Lee et al. 2005a, b; Wee et al. 2005; Chen et al. 2011) (Table 10.2) (Figs. 10.2 and 10.3).

10.6 Diagnosis

Clinical examination, including endoscopic examination of the nasopharynx, can provide very valuable information on mucosal involvement and local tumor extension and allows nasopharyngeal tumor biopsy. A definitive histological diagnosis should require a positive biopsy taken from the tumor in the nasopharynx, although a cervical nodal biopsy in the appropriate context may also be diagnostic. Major differential diagnoses of malignant tumors in the nasopharyngeal region in children are rhabdomyosarcoma and lymphoma.

Table 10.2 Andrews staging system for juvenile nasopharyngeal angiofibroma (1989)

Stage	
I	Tumor limited to the nasal cavity and nasopharynx
II	Tumor invading the pterygopalatine fossa or maxillary, ethmoidal, and sphenoid sinuses; with bone destruction
III	Tumor invading the infratemporal fossa or orbital region:
	(a) Without intracranial involvement
	(b) With extradural intracranial involvement
IV	Tumor with intradural intracranial involvement:
	(a) Without or (b) with infiltration of cavernous sinus, pituitary fossa, or optic chiasma

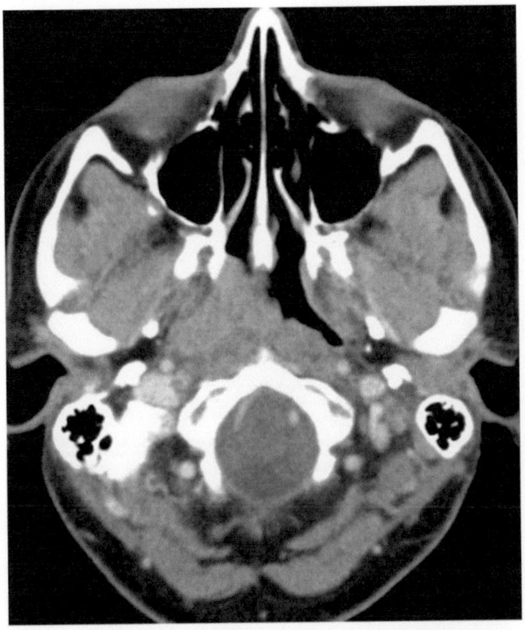

Fig. 10.2 Axial MRI shows the typical primary tumor of NPC (T3) extending into the right infratemporal fossa

Clinical examination cannot, however, determine a deep extension of the tumor, such as skull base erosion and intracranial spread (Colevas et al. 2018). Cross-sectional imaging has revolutionized the management of NPC. In terms of contribution to staging, MRI can identify the paranasopharyngeal extension as one of the most common modes of extension of NPC and perineural spread through the foramen ovale as an important route of intracranial extension (Sham et al. 1991). Perineural spread through the foramen ovale also accounts for the CT evidence of cavernous sinus involvement without skull base erosion (Chong et al. 1996). In addition, head and neck MRI helps to detect frequent cervical regional nodal involvement. Positron emission tomography (PET) may provide an additional tool for the initial diagnosis and staging and help in the evaluation of disease response after therapy (King et al. 2008; Buehrlen et al. 2012).

10.6.1 EBV DNA

Circulating free EBV DNA can be detected by polymerase chain reaction (PCR) in patients (Mutirangura et al. 1998). A significant EBV DNaemia in plasma but not in cellular compartments of the peripheral blood is observed, and it is assumed that the EBV DNA is directly released from the tumor tissue. Ninety-five percent of patients are positive for EBV DNA in plasma at diagnosis (Leung et al. 2006). Various clinical studies have demonstrated that circulating EBV DNA concentrations correlate positively with disease stage as well as exhibit prognostic importance in NPC (Leung et al. 2003; Chan et al. 2003; Lin et al. 2004; Wagner et al. 2009). A meta-analysis comprising 14 prospective and retrospective studies with a total of 7836 NPC patients found that high pre-DNA, detectable mid-DNA, detectable post-DNA, and slow EBV DNA clearance rates were all significantly associated with poorer OS, with hazard radios (HRs) equal to 2.81, 3.29, 4.26, and 3.58, respectively. Pre-DNA, mid-DNA, and post-DNA had the same effects on PFS, distant metastasis-free survival (DMFS), and local relapse-free survival (LRFS) (Zhang et al. 2015). Usually, patients achieving a complete remission become negative for EBV DNA in plasma, whereas patients with persistent or progressive disease remain positive or even show increasing EBV DNA plasma concentrations.

10.6.2 EBV Serology

Patients with EBV show an aberrant antibody response against EBV proteins. IgA antibodies against the EBV viral capsid antigen (VCA) and early antigen (EA) have been demonstrated to

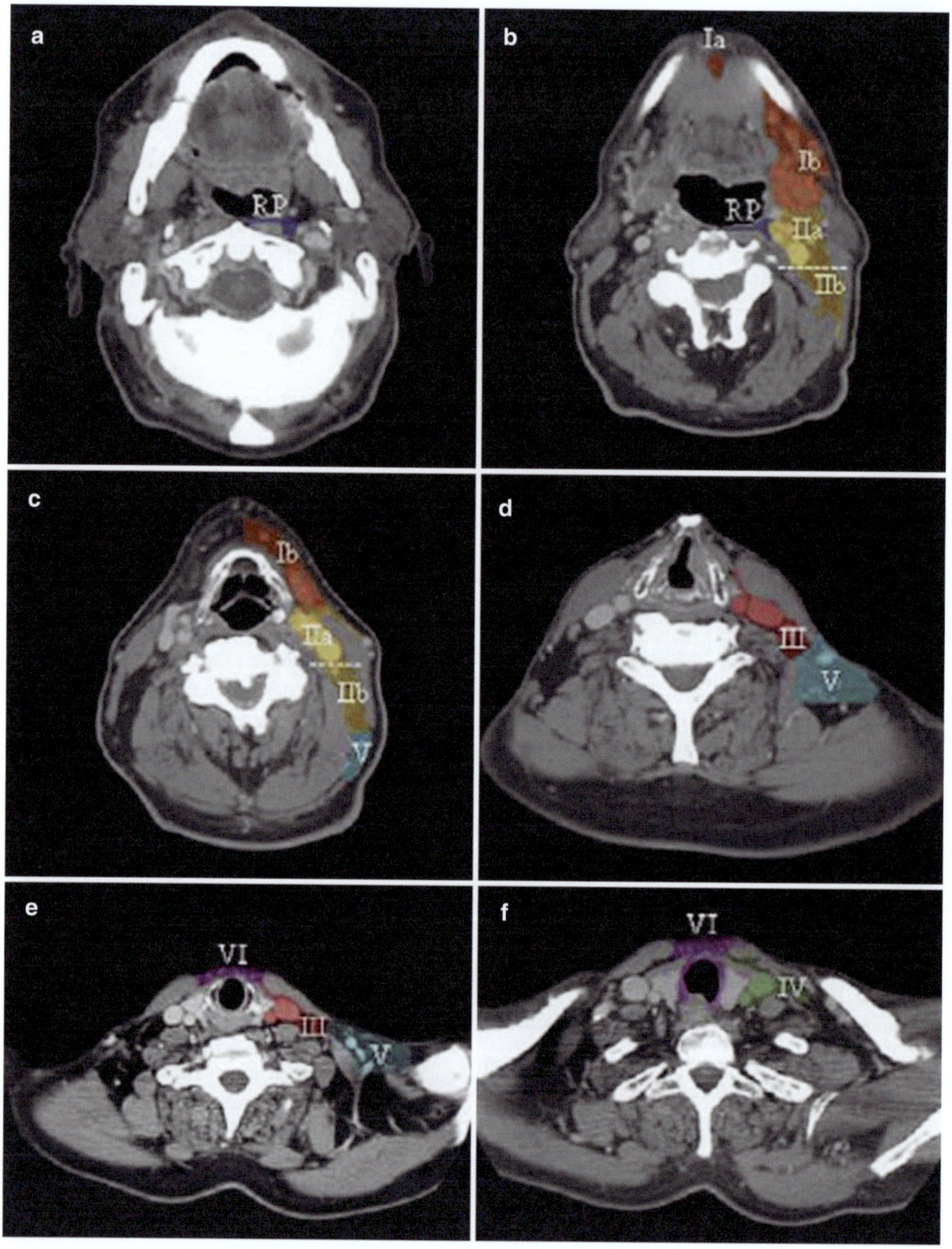

Fig. 10.3 (**a**) Parapharyngeal. (**b**) Level IIa + IIb: jugular LN. (**c** and **d**) Level III, IV: jugular LN. (**e**–**f**) Level V, supraclavicular LN; level VI, LN around the thyroid gland

precede the development of NPC. In a large prospective study in Taiwan, men from the general population who tested positive for IgA antibodies against the VCA protein had an increased risk of developing NPC compared to VCA IgA-negative men, an association that persisted even ≥5 years after antibody measurement (HR = 13.9; 95% CI 3.1–61.7) (Chien et al. 2001). Therefore, both antibodies have been used to screen for NPC in endemic regions. EBV-VCA IgA and EA IgA titers also correlate with tumor burden (Cai et al. 2010; Yao et al. 2017). Rising titers of EBV-EA IgA antibody have also been shown to predict relapse (de Vathaire et al. 1988).

10.6.3 Magnetic Resonance Imaging

The superior soft tissue resolution of MRI makes it an excellent modality in imaging of head and neck masses. It is particularly useful in delineating intracranial extension of disease and prepares further radiotherapy delineation. The examination is performed with the child supine in quiet respiration. Standard examination should include a T2-weighted fast spin echo (FSE) sequence in axial and coronal planes, a T2-weighted fat suppression or inversion recovery sequence, and a plain T1-weighted FSE or spin echo (SE) sequence (Lloyd and McHugh 2010). In evaluating mass lesions, a further fat-saturated T1-weighted SE sequence following gadolinium administration will often improve characterization of the mass. As MRI of the head and neck is nowadays the principal modality for delineation of the primary tumor and cervical lymph nodes, CT of the skull is only indicated if there is suspicion of bone invasion at the skull base (Colevas et al. 2018). Chest CT should be used for evaluation of pulmonary metastases either by itself or as part of FDG-PET/CT imaging.

10.6.4 Positron Emission Tomography

Various studies have investigated the use of [^{18}F]FDG PET/CT as imaging modality in patients with NPC. In the GPOH-NPC-2003 study, all tumors were PET positive at initial diagnosis or at time of relapse (Buehrlen et al. 2012). A comparison of PET/CT with MRI and CT for staging in children with NPC concluded that PET/CT may underestimate tumor extent and regional lymphadenopathy compared with MRI at the time of diagnosis, but it helps to detect metastases and clarify ambiguous findings (Cheuk et al. 2012). [^{18}F]FDG PET has been shown to be more sensitive than skeletal scintigraphy for detecting bone metastasis in endemic NPC at initial staging (Liu et al. 2008). A recent meta-analysis of 15 studies comprising 1938 patients with NPC confirms that high values of SUVmax, metabolic tumor volume (MTV), and total lesion glycolysis (TLG) predicted a higher risk of adverse events or death in patients with nasopharyngeal carcinoma, despite clinically heterogeneous nasopharyngeal carcinoma patients and the various methods adopted between these studies (Lin et al. 2017). In addition, the decrease in the standardized uptake value (SUV) during therapy has been shown to be of prognostic value in NPC (Xie et al. 2010) and may help to better delineate tumor after chemotherapy to prepare radiotherapy plans. Therefore, [^{18}F]FDG PET/CT is considered a valuable imaging modality for the evaluation and monitoring of NPC in pediatric patients.

10.7 Therapy

10.7.1 Chemotherapy

In children and adolescents with NPC, sensitivity to chemotherapy has been demonstrated as early as in the mid-70s (Ghim et al. 1998). Outcome has been analyzed in several retrospective studies, most of them with less than 50 patients, mostly heterogenous for the type of chemotherapy used and the dosage of radiotherapy applied; the reported 5-year overall and disease-free survival range between 41–94% and 47–85%, respectively, with more recent studies showing a better outcome than older ones (Zubarreta et al. 2000; Ozyar et al. 2006; Orbach et al. 2008;

Afquir et al. 2009; Tao et al. 2013; Yan et al. 2013; Jouin et al. 2019). NPC in children and adolescents has so far been prospectively studied only in eight clinical trials (Ghim et al. 1998; Mertens et al. 2005; Rodriguez-Galindo et al. 2005; Buehrlen et al. 2012; Casanova et al. 2012; Casanova et al. 2016; Rodriguez-Galindo et al. 2016; Zaghloul et al. 2016). Due to the low incidence of the disease in children and adolescents, only one of these studies included a randomized question to be answered.

The first prospective study was a single institutional study conducted at Emory University Medical Center in Atlanta, USA, treating 12 patients aged 6–20 years during years 1976–1995 (Ghim et al. 1998). Eleven patients had locally advanced tumors; one had systemic metastases at diagnosis. Chemotherapy contained doxorubicin, cyclophosphamide, and 5-fluorouracil (5-FU) and was given before radiotherapy in four patients and with or after radiation in eight patients in 3-week cycles for up to 2 years. Radiation dosages to the primary tumor site were between 59 Gy and 68 Gy and to the neck between 59 Gy and 66 Gy. Nine patients remained in complete remission with a median follow-up of 9 years, one patient developed a secondary osteosarcoma of the mandible, one patient died of tuberculosis, and one patient was lost to follow-up in remission. In the Pediatric Oncology Group Study 9486, 17 patients below 22 years with nasopharyngeal cancer were evaluable for analysis (Rodriguez-Galindo et al. 2005). One patient with stage II disease was only irradiated, 16 patients with stage III/IV NPC received four cycles of neoadjuvant chemotherapy with methotrexate, cisplatin, and 5-FU. Irradiation was given after the end of chemotherapy with a dose of 61.2 Gy to the primary tumor and positive lymph nodes, whereas 50.4 Gy were applied to non-involved lymph nodes of the upper neck and 45 Gy to non-involved ones of the lower neck. The 4-year EFS and OS rates were 77% and 75%, respectively. The NPC study of the Italian rare tumors in pediatric age project (TREP) treated 46 patients aged 9–17 during the years 2000–2009 (Casanova et al. 2012). Of these all but one patient had lymph node involvement and five had distant metastases. Patients received three cycles of neoadjuvant chemotherapy with cisplatin and 5-FU followed by radiotherapy. Radiation dosages were 65 Gy for the primary tumor and involved lymph nodes and 45 Gy for non-involved ones. The 4-year PFS and OS rates were 79.3 and 80.9%, respectively, including metastatic patients.

The NPC-91-GPOH study was the first multicenter study for the treatment of nasopharyngeal carcinoma in children, adolescents, and young adults (Mertens et al. 2005). Sixty-eight patients were registered, among them five patients with metastatic disease. Of the 59 protocol patients (58 "high-risk" patients and 1 "low-risk "patient, median age of 13, range: 8–25), high-risk patients were treated with induction chemotherapy consisting of three cycles of methotrexate, cisplatin and 5-FU, radiotherapy with a dosage of 59 Gy to the primary tumor and 45 Gy to locoregional lymph nodes, and maintenance therapy with interferon-β for 6 months. The estimated overall survival for the protocol patients after 9 years was 95% and the disease-free survival 91%. Therapy was complicated by severe mucositis requiring total parenteral nutrition in 46% of patients and dose reductions in subsequent cycles of chemotherapy in 30% of patients. In the NPC-2003 study, methotrexate was omitted because of increased toxicity in the NPC-91 study (Buehrlen et al. 2012). In addition, due to results on the benefit of concomitant radiochemotherapy in adults, cisplatin was given for 2 weeks during radiotherapy. A third change to the NPC-91 study was the reduction of the radiation dose of the primary tumor to 54 Gy in patients with complete tumor remission after induction chemotherapy. The study resulted in an overall survival of 97% after a median follow-up of 30 months and an event-free survival of 92% for non-metastatic patients. Follow-up after 52 months showed an overall survival of 93% and an event-free survival of 92% (unpublished).

The only randomized comparative prospective study in children and adolescent was an international study which involved 75 patients and was conducted in 13 countries from 2007 to 2008. The randomized question to be answered was whether the addition of docetaxel to the combination of cisplatin and 5-FU would increase the number of complete responses to induction chemotherapy. There was no significant difference in the overall response rates between the standard arm (ORR 80%) and the experimental arm (ORR 78%). Also, no significant difference in the 3-year overall survival was noted (Casanova et al. 2016).

In the COG study ARAR0331, 111 patients with NPC, aged 11 to 18, were treated between 2006 and 2013 with 3 cycles of 5-FU and cisplatin containing chemotherapy. This was followed by radiochemotherapy with a dose to the primary tumor of 61.2 Gy in patients with complete or partial tumor remission after induction chemotherapy and 70 Gy in patients whose tumor did not respond to induction chemotherapy. Cisplatin was given as a radiosensitizer during radiotherapy initially at a dose of 300 mg/m^2; however, it was subsequently reduced to 200 mg/m^2 because of toxicity. Five-year overall survival and event-free survival rates were 88.2% and 85.5%, respectively (Rodriguez-Galindo et al. 2016). A recent update of the study shows 5-year EFS and OS estimates of 84.3% and 89.2%, respectively. The 5-year EFS for stages IIb, III, and IV were 100%, 82.8%, and 82.7%, respectively. The 5-year cumulative incidence estimates of local, distant, and combined relapse were 3.7%, 8.7%, and 1.8%, respectively. Patients treated with 300 mg/m^2 of cisplatin during radiation therapy had improved 5-year post-induction EFS compared to those who received 200 mg/m^2 (90.7% vs. 81.2%, respectively, $p = 0.14$) (Carlos Rodriguez-Galindo, personal communication).

In adults, the standard of therapy for locally advanced NPC has been for many years concomitant radiochemotherapy (Colevas et al. 2018). However, in the last years several large randomized studies have shown a benefit for induction chemotherapy (IC) followed by concomitant radiochemotherapy (CCRT) versus radiochemotherapy alone. Recently, pooled analysis of 4 randomized studies comprising 1193 patients with locoregionally advanced NPC from endemic regions also demonstrated the superiority of additional IC over CCRT alone, with the survival benefit mainly associated with improved distant control.

10.7.2 Radiotherapy

Radiotherapy is the main treatment modality of NPC. The aims are to irradiate the primary nasopharyngeal tumor together with the initially involved lymph nodes as well as to prophylactically irradiate the remaining cervical lymph node regions. The major limitations of conventional 2D radiotherapy for NPC can now be overcome with three-dimensional (3D) conformal radiotherapy and intensity-modulated radiotherapy (IMRT). IMRT is an advanced form of 3D conformal radiotherapy, conforming high dose to tumor while conforming low dose to normal tissues (Wu et al. 2004; Wolden et al. 2006).

IMRT planning and dose optimization is fully computerized, a process known as inverse planning; thus, it is much preferred over the more expertise-dependent forward planning in 3D conformal radiotherapy (Hsiung et al. 2002; Jouin et al. 2019).

The use of IMRT in the treatment of NPC has multiple advantages. IMRT can be used for organ preservation, e.g., sparing the parotids of high-dose radiation will preserve salivary function after radiotherapy. IMRT can achieve good dose differential between the tumor and the dose-limiting organs and thus can achieve a high dose in the tumor without overdosing the normal organs. As the fractional dose will affect the biological effectiveness of radiation, there is a component of biological modulation of radiation besides just modulating the physical radiation dose in IMRT (Withers and Thames 1988).

Simultaneous modulated accelerated radiotherapy (SMART) employs this principle for accelerated radiotherapy with IMRT. IMRT resolves the problem of dose uncertainty at the junction between the primary tumor and neck lymphatic target volumes in conventional radiotherapy (Butler et al. 1999; Cheng et al. 2001).

Different series reported excellent local control of more than 90% in NPC achieved with IMRT, even among patients with advanced T3–4 diseases (Pow et al. 2006). Reports also showed preservation of salivary function and improved quality of life of survivors after IMRT (Wu et al. 2004). The superiority of IMRT versus conventional 2D radiotherapy was demonstrated in three prospective studies comparing the two treatment modalities in adult patients with NPC. Patients who underwent IMRT had significantly less late toxicities, especially hearing loss and xerostomia than patients who received conventional radiotherapy (Pow et al. 2006; Kam et al. 2007; Peng et al. 2012).

Considering the high incidence of severe late radiotherapy effects after NPC treatment even after IMRT, protons could be of interest in NPC, especially in children, adolescents, and young adults. The biological effect of protons is similar to photons, but the benefit expected is based on sharp dose fall-off, leading to a high therapeutic RT dose to the tumor with minimal exit dose, allowing for improved sparing of normal tissues (Taheri-Kadkhoda et al. 2008). The use of proton therapy, considered as the best technique for sparing critical organs, may induce less xerostomia and as a consequence less dental caries, as well as a potential reduction of ear and endocrine toxicities (Widesott et al. 2008). The place of this technique is still under investigation in pediatric NPC.

As cutting down late complications of treatment is one of the main objectives of pediatric clinical trials, another approach is adapting the dose of radiotherapy depending on the tumor response to induction chemotherapy. Such an approach has been taken by some national groups (French Group Fracture, German GPHO, or North American COG). Here, reduction of the dosage of radiation has been shown feasible in patients with a favorable response to induction chemotherapy, and it is assumed that this will lead to a decrease in long-term effects (Buehrlen et al. 2012; Rodriguez-Galindo et al. 2016; Jouin et al. 2019).

Radiotherapy in pediatric and adult NPC patients is nowadays combined with chemotherapy, usually cisplatin. This is based on several trials in adults which have confirmed the superiority of radiochemotherapy versus radiotherapy alone in advanced locoregional nasopharyngeal carcinoma. A meta-analysis comprising data on 1834 patients included in 7 adult trials showed that overall as well as progression-free survival was significantly improved in patients with radiochemotherapy versus radiotherapy alone (Blanchard et al. 2015). However, concomitant radiochemotherapy is associated with significant morbidity like severe mucositis requiring nutritional support, leading to lower dosages of cisplatin in most pediatric protocols compared to adult ones (Casanova et al. 2012; Buehrlen et al. 2012; Rodriguez-Galindo et al. 2016). As the benefit of concomitant radiochemotherapy has been established in adults who have not received previous induction chemotherapy, its role in pediatric NPC patients whose treatment concept includes induction chemotherapy for most patients is less clear.

10.7.3 Interferon Therapy

Interferon-β was introduced as a maintenance therapy into the GPOH studies after a boy with a second systemic NPC relapse went into a long-lasting complete remission with interferon-β alone, and response rates of around 25% were achieved in NPC patients with refractory disease treated with interferon-β (Treuner et al. 1980; Mertens et al. 1993). In the GPOH-NPC-91 and NPC-2003-GPOH studies, event-free survival rates were >90%, although radiation dosages were lower compared to other pediatric NPC protocols (Kontny et al. 2016). As NPC relapses are predominantly systemic, it is assumed that interferon-β improves systemic disease control. Recent preclinical data show that interferon-β induces the expression of tumor necrosis factor-related apoptosis inducing ligand (TRAIL) in NPC cells which subsequently elicits apoptosis via an intact TRAIL signaling pathway in an autocrine and paracrine manner (Makowska et al. 2018). Interferon-ß also activates natural killer cells and increases their killing of NPC cells in vitro (Makowska et al. 2019a). In NPC patients, interferon-ß increases the killing activity of NK cells against NPC cells and also increases levels of circulating soluble TRAIL which could contribute to the elimination of residual micrometastic disease (Makowska et al. 2019b).

In the German studies NPC-91-GPOH and NPC-2003-GPOH, all patients underwent 6 months of treatment with recombinant interferon-β or native interferon-β after completion of radiation therapy, receiving a dose of 10^5 U per kg body weight (max. dose: 6×10^6 U) intravenously (native interferon-β) or subcutaneously (recombinant interferon-β) three times a week. The favorable results of this strategy plead in favor of the use of this drug, but one should take into consideration that no comparative studies have proved the precise value of the maintenance therapy in this disease in young patients yet.

10.8 Metastatic Disease

Distant metastases are present in about 10% of patients with NPC at diagnosis. Although tumors and metastases usually respond to induction chemotherapy, most patients relapse and eventually die of their disease (Leong et al. 2008). However, patients with solitary or few osseous metastases or isolated lung metastasis have been shown to achieve long-term remissions, if they were treated with chemotherapy and radiotherapy to the primary tumor and the metastatic lesions (Fandi et al. 2000). Recently, a large, randomized study in adults with metastatic or relapsed NPC demonstrated that the combination of gemcitabine and cisplatin as induction chemotherapy was superior to the cisplatin/5-FU regimen as it significantly prolonged median progression-free survival (7.0 months versus 5.6 months) (Zhang et al. 2016).

10.9 New Treatment Strategies

10.9.1 T Cell Therapy

EBV-specific cytotoxic T cell (CTL) lines can readily be generated from individuals with NPC, notwithstanding patients' prior exposure to chemotherapy/radiation. In a pilot study, patients diagnosed with advanced NPC were treated with autologous CTLs. All patients tolerated the CTLs, although one developed increased swelling at the site of preexisting disease. The administration of EBV-specific CTLs to patients with advanced NPC was feasible, appears to be safe, and could be associated with significant antitumor activity (Comoli et al. 2005).

The EBV-specific CTLs used in this study were reactivated using LCLs that express all EBV latent antigens. LCLs are excellent antigen-presenting cells that are readily available for all patients, as only a limited amount of blood are required to establish an LCL line. As expected using this method, only a minority of the infused lines contained cytotoxic T cells specific for LMP2 (an EBV antigen usually expressed by NPC tumor cell mononuclear cells). Although there was no persistent rise in the frequency of circulating T cells specific for LMP2 after infusion, the CTLs appeared to show significant antitumor activity.

The EBV-specific CTLs were biologically active in vivo, reducing levels of EBV DNA in peripheral blood (Louis et al. 2010; Comoli et al. 2005).

10.9.2 Checkpoint Inhibition

As tumors of NPC patients from endemic regions and tumors from children show marked infiltration by lymphomononuclear cells, one could assume that measures to increase an immune response against NPC could lead to control of the disease. Inhibition of host tumor immune responses by negative checkpoints, such as the PD-1/PD-L1 checkpoint, has been demonstrated in various tumors, and blockade of immune checkpoints has led to impressive results in the treatment of various diseases such as melanoma and Hodgkin's lymphoma. NPC tumor cells express the immune effector cell inhibiting ligand PD-L1 in about 95% of tumors; therefore, blocking of the PD-L1/PD-1 interaction was also hypothesized to increase antitumor immunity in NPC. In two phase II trials in which patients with therapy-refractory nasopharyngeal carcinoma were treated with the anti-PD1 antibodies pembrolizumab or nivolumab, an overall response rate of 26% and stable disease rate of 42%, and 20% and 34.1%, respectively, were observed (Hsu et al. 2017; Ma et al. 2018). Currently, the addition of PD-1 checkpoint inhibition to standard treatment for NPC is evaluated in several randomized trials in adults with newly diagnosed NPC.

10.9.3 Targeted Therapy

Like other squamous head and neck carcinomas, NPC tumors mostly express epidermal growth factor receptor (EGFR) (Fujii et al. 2002). However, neither the EGFR-blocking antibody cetuximab nor the tyrosine kinase inhibitors (TKIs) gefitinib and erlotinib which inhibit the tyrosine kinase domain of the EGFR proved to have a significant effect on tumor growth in patients with recurrent or metastatic NPC in phase II trials (Perri et al. 2019). Vascular endothelial growth factor expression (VEGF-R) has been found in 60–70% of NPC tumors. Several VEGF-R-blocking TKIs have been investigated in phase II clinical trials in patients with recurrent or metastatic NPC with modest efficacy but significant toxicity (Elser et al. 2007; Hui et al. 2011; Lim et al. 2011).

10.10 Long-Term Sequelae

Survivors of NPC following radiotherapy or chemoradiation have impaired health-related quality of life. Patients may suffer from a variety of late complications, many of which result from the effects of radiation on dose-limiting organs situated adjacent to the nasopharynx and cervical lymph node (Huang et al. 1994). NPC survivors almost uniformly develop hypothyroidism secondary to neck irradiation and also are at risk for panhypopituitarism resulting from pituitary damage (Cheuk et al. 2011). A close endocrine follow-up is thus required for early diagnosis and intervention (Fang et al. 2002). Ototoxicity is also very common, and its incidence is particularly higher in patients receiving chemotherapy in addition to radiation, which often involved the auditory apparatus. A small proportion of the long-term sequelae represent the effects of unhealed residual damage by the tumor, such as residual cranial nerve palsies and serous otitis media resulting from persistent disturbance of the Eustachian tube function (McMillan et al. 2004).

In up to 8.5% of the NPC patients, subsequent malignancies developed 8.6–27 years after NPC diagnosis (Cheuk et al.2011). The 15-year cumulative incidence of any morbidity, sensorineural hearing loss, primary hypothyroidism, and growth hormone deficiency related to the stage were 84%, 53%, 43%, and 14%, respectively. There are dose-response relationships between radiotherapy dose and primary hypothyroidism and growth hormone deficiency (Ulger et al. 2007). In addition, three prospective studies comparing IMRT and conventional radiotherapy in patients with NPC all demonstrated that patients treated with IMRT had significantly less late toxicities than patients who underwent conventional radiotherapy (Pow et al. 2006; Kam et al. 2007; Peng et al. 2012). These frequent long-term toxicities associated with an overall nowadays good prognosis helped to propose adapted dose radiotherapy to induction chemotherapy in order to try to reduce sequelae in patients with favorable response.

10.11 Juvenile Nasopharyngeal Angiofibroma

10.11.1 Introduction

Juvenile nasopharyngeal angiofibroma (JNA) is a rare tumor with prominent vascularity and *benign histological* features. It originates from the superior margin of the sphenopalatine foramen, which is also a route for the sphenopalatine artery branching from the internal maxillary artery (Schuon et al. 2007; Tosun et al. 2006).

The reported incidence of JNA is between 1 in 6000 and 1 in 60,000 otolaryngology patients. It accounts for 0.5% of all head and neck neoplasms, and it is considered to be the most common benign neoplasm of the nasopharynx (Mann et al. 2004; Glad et al. 2007). JNA predominately affects male children and adolescents between the ages of 9 and 19 (Gullane et al. 1992). Although histologically benign in appearance, JNAs are locally aggressive and destructive, spreading from the nasal cavity to the nasopharynx, paranasal sinuses, and orbit skull base with intracranial extension in 10–20%.

10.11.2 Symptoms

The most common presenting symptom is persistent nasal obstruction with repetitive epistaxis.

Further classical clinical presentation is unilateral nasal block and/or rhinorrhea and occasionally pain. Because of its invasive nature, the tumor may cause facial deformity and proptosis, changes in visual acuity, and cranial nerve palsy if it reaches the orbit and intracranial region (Weprin and Siemers 1991; Tyagi et al. 2007). Differential diagnoses include parameningeal rhabdomyosarcoma, NPC, or diffuse lymphoma.

10.11.3 Pathogenesis

The gender selectivity of JNA, *with a high male-to-female ratio*, and the relatively young age at diagnosis suggest hormone-dependent development. Hormonal disorders have been reported in patients with JNA, and androgen and estrogen receptors have been identified in tumor tissue; however, a hormonal influence on JNA is controversial. Recent studies have attempted to further delineate the pathogenesis of JNA through analysis of genetic and molecular changes. While JNA is known to be sensitive to androgens, there are likely intermediary cytokines and/or growth factors that mediate aggressive stoma cell proliferation and angiogenesis. Transforming growth factor beta1 (TGF-beta1) is a polypeptide that is secreted in an inactive form, cleaved to produce an active form, and then deactivated in the tissues. The location of activated TGF-beta1 to the fibroblasts and endothelial cells within JNA tumors suggests that TGF-beta1 may play a role in the stromal cell proliferation and angiogenesis associated with JNA (Lee et al. 1980; Liang et al. 2000; Saylam et al. 2006; Ngan et al. 2008; Zhang et al. 2003).

10.11.4 Diagnosis

The diagnosis of JNA is based on a precise clinical history and examination of the patient and imaging (head and neck MRI or CT). Tissue biopsies should be avoided due to the highly vascular nature of the tumor. Angiography is used to define the feeding arteries of the tumor and to provide information for embolization (Nicolai et al. 2003; Jacobsson et al. 1989).

Various staging systems have been proposed. In the Andrews staging system (Table 10.3), JNA is classified as Type I when the tumor is restricted to the nasal cavity and the nasopharynx without bone destruction; Type II when the tumor invades the pterygomaxillary fossa and maxillary, sphenoidal, and ethmoid sinuses with bone destruction; Type III when the tumor invades the intratemporal fossa, the orbit, and the parasellar region but remaining lateral to the cavernous sinus; and Type IV when the tumor invades the cavernous sinus, the optic chiasma, and the pituitary fossa (Howard et al. 2001).

Table 10.3 Stage-related definition of risk groups (AJCC, eighth edition)

Stage grouping	
Stage I	T1 N0 M0
Stage II	T0-1 N1 M0, T2 N0-1 M0
Stage III	T0-1 N3 M0
	T3 N0-2 M0
Stage IVA	T4 N0-2 M0
Stage IVB	Any T N3 M0
Stage IVC	Any T Any N M1

10.11.5 Therapy

The management of JNA has changed during the last decades. It is generally agreed that surgery is the treatment of choice for all uncomplicated primary and recurrent JNA (López et al. 2017). Preoperative selective arterial embolization is almost always indicated as it helps to decrease the risk of intraoperative hemorrhage and facilitates the resection of large tumors. The management of JNA should be planned by an experienced head and neck surgeon, as part of a multidisciplinary team, preferably in a tertiary referral setting. Surgery aims for a complete and safe resection of tumor, with minimal morbidity and loss of blood. A transpalatal or transmaxillar (lateral rhinotomy or midfacial) approach is usually performed (Belmont 1988; Dubey and Molumi 2007).

For stages I and II, a transpalatal approach results in good outcome when the lesion is limited to the nasal cavity, nasopharynx, and paranasal sinuses. For patients with intracranial extension, the LeFort I surgical technique should be used. Involvement of the orbit, middle cranial fossa, and base of the pterygoid by the primary JNA results in a higher incidence of recurrent tumor (Borghei et al. 2006; Yiotakis et al. 2008).

Recurrence rates as high as 50% (ranging from 6 to 50%) have been reported (Reddy et al. 2001). Radiotherapy may be considered for advanced, incompletely resectable cases and cases with a high morbidity of resection (López et al. 2017). Chemotherapy has been suggested for recurrences and selected cases with aggressive growth (Goepfert et al. 1985). In postpubertal patients, hormonal therapy with flutamide, an androgen receptor antagonist, has been used preoperatively to achieve tumor regression and facilitate surgical resection; this approach was successful in some but not all patients treated (Labra et al. 2004; Thakar et al. 2011). Since strong vascularity is a common feature of JNAs, it has been suggested that antiangiogenic therapies ought to be considered in the management of selected cases; however, clinical data have been lacking so far (Hashizume et al. 2010; López et al. 2017).

References

Afquir S, Alaoui K, Ismaili N et al (2009) Nasopharyngeal carcinoma in adolescents: a retrospective review of 42 patients. Eur Arch Otorhinolaryngol 266:1767–1773

Altun M, Fandi A, Dupuis O, Cvitkovic E, Krajina Z, Eschwege F (1995) Undifferentiated nasopharyngeal cancer (UCNT): current diagnostic and therapeutic aspects. Int J Radiat Oncol Biol Phys 32(3):859–877

Amin MB, Edge SB, Greene FL et al (eds) (2017) AJCC cancer staging manual, 8th edn. Springer, New York, pp 103–111

Ayan I, Kaytan E, Ayan N (2003) Childhood nasopharyngeal carcinoma: from biology to treatment. Lancet Oncol 4:13–21

Belmont JR (1988) The Le Fort I osteotomy approach for nasopharyngeal and nasal fossa tumors. Arch Otolaryngol Head Neck Surg 114:751–754

Blanchard P, Lee A, Marguet S, Leclercq J, Ng WT, Ma J, Chan AT, Huang PY, Benhamou E, Zhu G, Chua DT, Chen Y, Mai HQ, Kwong DL, Cheah SL, Moon J, Tung Y, Chi KH, Fountzilas G, Zhang L, Hui EP, Lu TX, Bourhis J, Pignon JP, MAC-NPC Collaborative Group (2015) Chemotherapy and radiotherapy in nasopharyngeal carcinoma: an update of the MAC-NPC meta-analysis. Lancet Oncol 16(6):645–655

Borghei P, Baradaranfar MH, Borghei SH, Sokhandon F (2006) Transnasal endoscopic resection of juvenile nasopharyngeal angiofibroma without preoperative embolization. Ear Nose Throat J 85:740–743, 746

Bornkamm GW (1984) Virologisch-serologische Diagnostik des Nasopharynxkarzinoms. In: Nasopharynx-Tumoren. Urban & Schwarzenberg, München-Wien-Baltimore, pp 15–21

Bray F, Haugen M et al (2008) Age-incidence curves of nasopharyngeal carcinoma worldwide: bimodality in low-risk populations and aetiologic implications. Cancer Epidemiol Biomark Prev 17(9):2356–2365

Buehrlen M, Zwaan C, Granzen B et al (2012) Multimodal treatment, including interferon beta, of nasopharyngeal carcinoma in children and young adults. Cancer 118:4892–4900

Butler EB, Teh BS, Grant WH 3rd, Uhl BM, Kuppersmith RB, Chiu JK et al (1999) Smart (simultaneous modulated accelerated radiation therapy) boost: a new accelerated fractionation schedule for the treatment of head and neck cancer with intensity modulated radiotherapy. Int J Radiat Oncol Biol Phys 45(1):21–32

Cai YL, Zheng YM, Cheng JR, Wang W, Zhang YN, Wang WH, Wu YS, Zhong WM, Li J, Mo YK (2010) Relationship between clinical stages of nasopharyngeal carcinoma and Epstein-Barr virus antibodies Rta/IgG, EBNA1/IgA, VCA/IgA and EA/IgA. Nan Fang Yi Ke Da Xue Xue Bao 30(3):509–511

Casanova M, Bisogno G, Gandola L, Cechetto G, Di Cataldo A, Basso E, Indolfi P, D'Angelo P, Favini F, Collini P, Potepan P, Ferrari A (2012) A prospective protocol for nasopharyngeal carcinoma in children and adolescents. Cancer 118:2718–2725

Casanova M, Özyar E, Patte C, Orbach D, Ferrari A, Veyrat-Follet C, Errihani H, Pan J, Zhang L, Shen L, Grzegorzewski KJ, Varan A (2016) International randomized phase 2 study on the addition of docetaxel to the combination of cisplatin and 5-fluorouracil in the induction treatment for nasopharyngeal carcinoma in children and adolescents. Cancer Chemother Pharmacol 77:289–298

Chan KH, Gu YL, Ng F, Ng PS, Seto WH, Sham JS, Chua D, Wei W, Chen YL, Luk W, Zong YS, Ng MH (2003) EBV specific antibody-based and DNA-based assays in serologic diagnosis of nasopharyngeal carcinoma. Int J Cancer 105(5):706–709

Chang ET, Adami HO (2006) The enigmatic epidemiology of nasopharyngeal carcinoma. Cancer Epidemiol Biomark Prev 15(10):1765–1777

Chen QY, Wen YF, Guo L, Liu H, Huang PY, Mo HY, Li NW, Xiang YQ, Luo DH, Qiu F, Sun R, Deng MQ, Chen MY, Hua YJ, Guo X, Cao KJ, Hong MH, Qian CN, Mai HQ (2011) Concurrent chemoradiotherapy vs radiotherapy alone in stage II nasopharyngeal carcinoma: phase III randomized trial. J Natl Cancer Inst 103(23):1761–1770

Cheng JC, Chao KS, Low D (2001) Comparison of intensity modulated radiation therapy (IMRT) treatment techniques for nasopharyngeal carcinoma. Int J Cancer 96(2):126–131

Cheuk DK, Billups CA, Martin MG, Roland CR, Ribeiro RC, Krasin MJ, Rodriguez-Galindo C (2011) Prognostic factors and long-term outcomes of childhood nasopharyngeal carcinoma. Cancer 117(1):197–206

Cheuk DK, Sabin ND, Hossain M, Wozniak A, Najk M (2012) PET/CT for staging and follow-up of pediatric nasopharyngeal carcinoma. Eur J Nucl Med Mol Imaging 39:1097–1106

Chien YC, Chen JY, Liu MY, Yang HI, Hsu MM, Chen CJ, Yang CS (2001) Serologic markers of Epstein-Barr virus infection and nasopharyngeal carcinoma in Taiwanese men. N Engl J Med 345(26):1877–1882

Chong VF, Fan YF, Khoo JB (1996) Nasopharyngeal carcinoma with intracranial spread: CT and MR characteristics. J Comput Assist Tomogr 20(4):563–569

Colevas AD, Yom SS, Pfister DG, Spencer S, Adelstein D, Adkins D, Brizel DM, Burtness B, Busse PM, Caudell JJ, Cmelak AJ, Eisele DW, Fenton M, Foote RL, Gilbert J, Gillison ML, Haddad RI, Hicks WL, Hitchcock YJ, Jimeno A, Leizman D, Maghami E, Mell LK, Mittal BB, Pinto HA, Ridge JA, Rocco J, Rodriguez CP, Shah JP, Weber RS, Witek M, Worden F, Zhen W, Burns JL, Darlow SD (2018) NCCN guidelines insights: head and neck cancers, version 1.2018. J Natl Compr Cancer Netw 16(5):479–490

Comoli P, Pedrazzoli P, Maccario R et al (2005) Cell therapy of stage IV nasopharyngeal carcinoma with autologous Epstein-Barr virus-targeted cytotoxic T lymphocytes. J Clin Oncol 23:8942–8949

de Vathaire F, Sancho-Garnier H, de Thé H, Pieddeloup C, Schwaab G, Ho JH, Ellouz R, Micheau C, Cammoun M, Cachin Y et al (1988) Prognostic value of EBV markers in the clinical management of nasopharyngeal carcinoma (NPC): a multicenter follow-up study. Int J Cancer 42(2):176–181

Dittmer DP, Hilscher CJ, Gulley ML, Yang EV, Chen M, Glaser R (2008) Multiple pathways for Epstein-Barr virus episome loss from nasopharyngeal carcinoma. Int J Cancer 123(9):2105–2112

Dourthe ME, Bolle S, Temam S, Jouin A, Claude L, Reguerre Y, Defachelles AS, Orbach D, Fresneau B (2018) Childhood nasopharyngeal carcinoma: state-of-the-art, and questions for the future. J Pediatr Hematol Oncol 40(2):85–92. https://doi.org/10.1097/MPH.0000000000001054. PMID: 29300240

Dubey SP, Molumi CP (2007) Critical look at the surgical approaches of nasopharyngeal angiofibroma excision and "total maxillary swing" as a possible alternative. Ann Otol Rhinol Laryngol 116:723–730

Elser C, Siu LL, Winquist E, Agulnik M, Pond GR, Chin SF, Francis P, Cheiken R, Elting J, McNabola A, Wilkie D, Petrenciuc O, Chen EX (2007) Phase II trial of sorafenib in patients with recurrent or metastatic squamous cell carcinoma of the head and neck or nasopharyngeal carcinoma. J Clin Oncol 25(24): 3766–3773

Fandi A, Bachouchi M, Azli N, Taamma A, Boussen H, Wibault P, Eschwege F, Armand JP, Simon J, Cvitkovic E (2000) Long-term disease-free survivors in metastatic undifferentiated carcinoma of nasopharyngeal type. J Clin Oncol 18(6):1324–1330

Fang FM, Chiu HC, Kuo WR, Wang CJ, Leung SW, Chen HC et al (2002) Health-related quality of life for nasopharyngeal carcinoma patients with cancer-free survival after treatment. Int J Radiat Oncol Biol Phys 53(4):959–968

Fotheringham JA, Mazzucca S, Raab-Traub N (2010) Epstein-Barr virus latent membrane protein-2A-induced DeltaNp63 alpha expression is associated with impaired epithelial-cell differentiation. Oncogene 29(30):4287–4296

Fujii M, Yamashita T, Ishiguro R, Tashiro M, Kameyama K (2002) Significance of epidermal growth factor receptor and tumor associated tissue eosinophilia in the prognosis of patients with nasopharyngeal carcinoma. Auris Nasus Larynx 29(2):175–181

Ghim TT, Briones M, Mason P et al (1998) Effective adjuvant chemotherapy for advanced nasopharyngeal carcinoma in children: a final update of a long-term prospective study in a single institution. J Pediatr Hematol Oncol 20:131–135

Glad H, Vainer B, Buchwald C, Petersen BL, Theilgaard SA, Bonvin P, Lajer C, Jakobsen J (2007) Juvenile nasopharyngeal angiofibromas in Denmark 1981–2003: diagnosis, incidence, and treatment. Acta Otolaryngol 127:292–299

Godtfredsen E (1944) Chapter III: on the histopathology of malignant nasopharyngeal tumours. Acta Pathol Microbiol Scand 32(Suppl 59):38–56

Goepfert H, Cangir A, Lee YY (1985) Chemotherapy for aggressive juvenile nasopharyngeal angiofibroma. Arch Otolaryngol 111(5):285–289

Gullane PJ, Davidson J, O'Dwyer T, Forte V (1992) Juvenile angiofibroma: a review of the literature and a case series report. Laryngoscope 102(8):928–933

Hashizume H, Falcon BL, Kuroda T, Baluk P, Coxon A, Yu D, Bready JV, Oliner JD, McDonald DM (2010) Complementary actions of inhibitors of angiopoietin-2 and VEGF on tumor angiogenesis and growth. Cancer Res 70:2213–2223

Hildesheim A, Apple RJ, Chen CJ, Wang SS, Cheng YJ, Klitz W, Mack SJ, Chen IH, Hsu MM, Yang CS, Brinton LA, Levine PH, Erlich HA (2002) Association of HLA class I and II alleles and extended haplotypes with nasopharyngeal carcinoma in Taiwan. J Natl Cancer Inst 94(23):1780–1789

Howard DJ, Lloyd G, Lund V (2001) Recurrence and its avoidance in juvenile angiofibroma. Laryngoscope 111:1509–1511

Hsiung CY, Yorke ED, Chui CS, Hunt MA, Ling CC, Huang EY et al (2002) Intensity-modulated radiotherapy versus conventional three-dimensional conformal radiotherapy for boost or salvage treatment of nasopharyngeal carcinoma. Int J Radiat Oncol Biol Phys 53(3):638–647

Hsu C, Lee SH, Ejadi S, Even C, Cohen RB, Le Tourneau C, Mehnert JM, Algazi A, van Brummelen EMJ, Saraf S, Thanigaimani P, Cheng JD, Hansen AR (2017) Safety and antitumor activity of Pembrolizumab in patients with programmed death-ligand 1-positive nasopharyngeal carcinoma: results of the KEYNOTE-028 study. J Clin Oncol 35(36):4050–4056

Huang TS, Huang SC, Hsu MM (1994) A prospective study of hypothalamus pituitary function after cranial irradiation with or without radiosensitizing chemotherapy. J Endocrinol Invest 17(8):615–623

Huang SCM, Tsao SW, Tsang CM (2018) Interplay of viral infection, host cell factors and tumor microenvironment in the pathogenesis of nasopharyngeal carcinoma. Cancers (Basel) 10(4):106

Hui EP, Ma BB, King AD, Mo F, Chan SL, Kam MK, Loong HH, Ahuja AT, Zee BC, Chan AT (2011) Hemorrhagic complications in a phase II study of sunitinib in patients of nasopharyngeal carcinoma who has previously received high-dose radiation. Ann Oncol 22(6):1280–1287

Jacobsson M, Petruson B, Ruth M, Svendsen P (1989) Involution of juvenile nasopharyngeal angiofibroma with intracranial extension. A case report with computed tomographic assessment. Arch Otolaryngol Head Neck Surg 115:238–239

Jouin A, Helfre S, Bolle S, Claude L, Laprie A, Bogart E, Vigneron C, Potet H, Ducassou A, Claren A, Riet FG, Castex MP, Faure-Conter C, Fresneau B, Defachelles AS, Orbach D (2019) Adapted strategy to tumor response in childhood nasopharyngeal carcinoma: the French experience. Strahlenther Onkol 195(6): 504–516

Kam MK, Leung SF, Zee B, Chau RM, Suen JJ, Mo F et al (2007) Prospective randomized study of intensity-modulated radiotherapy on salivary gland function in early-stage nasopharyngeal carcinoma patients. J Clin Oncol 25(31):4873–4879

King AD, Ma BB, Yau YY, Zee B, Leung SF, Wong JK, Kam MK, Ahuja AT, Chan AT (2008) The impact of 18F-FDG PET/CT on assessment of nasopharyngeal carcinoma at diagnosis. Br J Radiol 81(964):291–298

Kontny U, Franzen S, Behrends U, Bührlen M, Christiansen H, Delecluse H, Eble M, Feuchtinger T, Gademann G, Granzen B, Kratz CP, Lassay L, Leuschner I, Mottaghy FM, Schmitt C, Staatz G, Timmermann B, Vorwerk P, Wilop S, Wolff HA, Mertens R (2016) Diagnosis and treatment of nasopharyngeal carcinoma in children and adolescents—recommendations of the GPOH-NPC Study Group. Klin Padiatr 228:105–112

Krueger GRF, Wustrow J (1981) Current classification of nasopharyngeal carcinoma at Cologne University. In: Grundmann E, Krueger GRF, Ablashi DV (eds) Nasopharyngeal carcinoma, vol 5. Gustav Fischer Verlag, Stuttgart, pp 11–15

Labra A, Chavolla-Magaña R, Lopez-Ugalde A, Alanis-Calderon J, Huerta-Delgado A (2004) Flutamide as a preoperative treatment in juvenile angiofibroma (JA) with intracranial invasion: report of 7 cases. Otolaryngol Head Neck Surg 130(4):466–699

Lee DA, Rao BR, Meyer JS, Prioleau PG, Bauer WC (1980) Hormonal receptor determination in juvenile nasopharyngeal angiofibromas. Cancer 46:547–551

Lee AW, Foo W, Law SC, Poon YF, Sze WM, O S K, Tung SY, Lau WH (1997) Nasopharyngeal carcinoma: presenting symptoms and duration before diagnosis. Hong Kong Med J 3(4):355–361

Lee AW, Lau WH, Tung SY, Chua DT, Chappell R, Xu L et al (2005a) Preliminary results of a randomized study on therapeutic gain by concurrent chemotherapy for regionally-advanced nasopharyngeal carcinoma: NPC-9901 trial by the Hong Kong Nasopharyngeal Cancer Study Group. J Clin Oncol 23(28):6966–6975

Lee AW, Sze WM, Au JS, Leung SF, Leung TW, Chua DT, Zee BC, Law SC, Teo PM, Tung SY, Kwong DL, Lau WH (2005b) Treatment results for nasopharyngeal carcinoma in the modern era: the Hong Kong experience. Int J Radiat Oncol Biol Phys 61(4):1107–1116

Leong SS, Wee J, Rajan S, Toh CK, Lim WT, Hee SW, Tay MH, Poon D, Tan EH (2008) Triplet combination of gemcitabine, paclitaxel, and carboplatin followed by maintenance 5-fluorouracil and folinic acid in patients with metastatic nasopharyngeal carcinoma. Cancer 113(6):1332–1337

Leung SF, Chan AT, Zee B, Ma B, Chan LY, Johnson PJ et al (2003) Pretherapy quantitative measurement of circulating Epstein-Barr virus DNA is predictive of posttherapy distant failure in patients with early-stage nasopharyngeal carcinoma of undifferentiated type. Cancer 98(2):288–291

Leung SF, Zee B, Ma BB, Hui EP, Mo F, Lai M, Chan KC, Chan LY, Kwan WH, Lo YM, Chan AT (2006) Plasma Epstein-Barr viral deoxyribonucleic acid quantitation complements tumor-node-metastasis staging prognostication in nasopharyngeal carcinoma. J Clin Oncol 24(34):5414–5418

Liang J, Yi Z, Lianq P (2000) The nature of juvenile nasopharyngeal angiofibroma. Otolaryngol Head Neck Surg 123:475–481

Liebowitz D (1994) Nasopharyngeal carcinoma: the Epstein-Barr virus association. Semin Oncol 21(3):376–381

Lim WT, Ng QS, Ivy P, Leong SS, Singh O, Chowbay B, Gao F, Thng CH, Goh BC, Tan DS, Koh TS, Toh CK, Tan EH (2011) A phase II study of pazopanib in Asian patients with recurrent/metastatic nasopharyngeal carcinoma. Clin Cancer Res 17(16):5481–5489

Lin JC, Wang WY, Chen KY, Wei YH, Liang WM, Jan JS et al (2004) Quantification of plasma Epstein-Barr virus DNA in patients with advanced nasopharyngeal carcinoma. N Engl J Med 350(24):2461–2470

Lin J, Xie G, Liao G, Wang B, Yan M, Li H, Yuan Y (2017) Prognostic value of 18F-FDG-PET/CT in patients with nasopharyngeal carcinoma: a systemic review and metaanalysis. Oncotarget 8:33884–33896

Liu FY, Chang JT, Wang HM, Liao CT, Kang CJ, Ng SK, Chan SC, Yen TC (2008) (18F) Fluorodeoxyglucose positron emission tomography is more sensitive than skeletal scintigraphy for detecting bone metastasis in endemic nasopharyngeal carcinoma at initial staging. J Clin Oncol 24:599–604

Lloyd C, McHugh K (2010) The role of radiology in head and neck tumours in children. Cancer Imaging 10:49–61

Lo YM, Leung SF, Chan LY, Chan AT, Lo KW, Johnson PJ et al (2000) Kinetics of plasma Epstein-Barr virus DNA during radiation therapy for nasopharyngeal carcinoma. Cancer Res 60(9):2351–2355

Lo AK, Dawson CW, Jin DY, Lo KW (2012) The pathological roles of BART miRNAs in nasopharyngeal carcinoma. J Pathol 227(4):392–403

López F, Triantafyllou A, Snyderman CH, Hunt JL, Suárez C, Lund VJ, Strojan P, Saba NF, Nixon IJ, Devaney KO, Alobid I, Bernal-Sprekelsen M, Hanna EY, Rinaldo A, Ferlito A (2017) Nasal juvenile angiofibroma: current perspectives with emphasis on management. Head Neck 39(5):1033–1045

Louis CU, Straathof K, Bollard CM et al (2010) Adoptive transfer of EBV-specific T cells results in sustained clinical responses in patients with locoregional nasopharyngeal carcinoma. J Immunother 33:983–990

Ma BBY, Lim WT, Goh BC, Hui EP, Lo KW, Pettinger A, Foster NR, Riess JW, Agulnik M, Chang AYC, Chopra A, Kish JA, Chung CH, Adkins DR, Cullen KJ, Gitlitz BJ, Lim DW, To KF, Chan KCA, Lo YMD, King AD, Erlichman C, Yin J, Costello BA, Chan ATC (2018) Antitumor activity of Nivolumab in recurrent and metastatic nasopharyngeal carcinoma: an international, multicenter study of the Mayo Clinic phase 2 consortium (NCI-9742). J Clin Oncol 36(14):1412–1418

Makowska A, Wahab L, Braunschweig T, Kapetanakis N, Vokuhl C, Denecke B, Shen L, Busson P, Kontny U (2018) Interferon beta induces apoptosis in nasopharyngeal carcinoma cells via the TRAIL-signaling pathway. Oncotarget 9:14228–14250

Makowska A, Braunschweig T, Denecke B, Shen L, Baloche V, Busson P, Kontny U (2019a) Interferon beta and anti-PD-1/PD-L1 checkpoint blockade cooperate in NK cell-mediated killing of nasopharyngeal carcinoma cells. Transl Oncol 12(9):1237–1256

Makowska A, Franzen S, Braunschweig T, Denecke B, Shen L, Baloche V, Busson P, Kontny U (2019b) Interferon-beta increases NK cell cytotoxicity against tumor cells in patients with nasopharyngeal carcinoma via tumor necrosis factor apoptosis-inducing ligand. Cancer Immunol Immunother 68(8):1317–1329

Mann WJ, Jecker P, Amedee RG (2004) Juvenile angiofibromas: changing surgical concept over the last 20 years. Laryngoscope 114:291–293

Marks JE, Phillips JL, Menck HR (1998) The National Cancer Data Base report on the relationship of race and national origin to the histology of nasopharyngeal carcinoma. Cancer 83(3):582–588

McMillan AS, Pow EH, Leung WK, Wong MC, Kwong DL (2004) Oral health-related quality of life in southern Chinese following radiotherapy for nasopharyngeal carcinoma. J Oral Rehabil 31(6):600–608

Mertens R, Lassay L, Heimann G (1993) Combined treatment of nasopharyngeal cancer in children and adolescents—concept of a study. Klin Padiatr 205:241–248

Mertens R, Granzen B, Lassay L, Bucsky P, Hundgen M, Stetter G, Heimann G, Weiss C, Hess CF, Gademann G (2005) Treatment of nasopharyngeal carcinoma in children and adolescents: definitive results of a multicenter study (NPC-91-GPOH). Cancer 104(5):1083–1089

Micheau C, Rilke F, Pilotti S (1978) Proposal for a new histopathological classification of the carcinomas of the nasopharynx. Tumori 64(5):513–518

Mutirangura A, Pornthanakasem W, Theamboonlers A, Sriuranpong V, Lertsanguansinchi P, Yenrudi S, Voravud N, Supiyaphun P, Poovorawan Y (1998) Epstein-Barr viral DNA in serum of patients with nasopharyngeal carcinoma. Clin Cancer Res 4(3):665–669

Ngan BY, Forte V, Campisi P (2008) Molecular angiogenic signaling in angiofibromas after embolization: implications for therapy. Arch Otolaryngol Head Neck Surg 134:1170–1176

Nicolai P, Berlucchi M, Tomenzoli D, Cappiello J, Trimarchi M, Maroldi R, Battaglia G, Antonelli AR (2003) Endoscopic surgery for juvenile angiofibroma: when and how. Laryngoscope 113:775–782

Niedobitek G, Young LS (1994) Epstein-Barr virus persistence and virus-associated tumors. Lancet 343:333–335

Orbach D, Brisse H, Helfre S et al (2008) Radiation and chemotherapy combination for nasopharyngeal carcinoma in children: radiotherapy dose adaptation after chemotherapy response to minimize late effects. Pediatr Blood Cancer 50:849–853

Ozyar E, Selek U, Laskar S et al (2006) Treatment results of 165 pediatric patients with non-metastatic nasopharyngeal carcinoma: a Rare Cancer Network study. Radiother Oncol 81:39–46

Peng G, Wang T, Yang KY, Zhang S, Zhang T, Li Q, Han J, Wu G (2012) A prospective, randomized study comparing outcomes and toxicities of intensity-modulated radiotherapy vs. conventional two-dimensional radiotherapy for the treatment of nasopharyngeal carcinoma. Radiother Oncol 104(3):286–293

Perri F, Della Vittoria Scarpati G, Caponigro F, Ionna F, Longo F, Buonopane S, Muto P, Di Marzo M, Pisconti S, Solla R (2019) Management of recurrent nasopharyngeal carcinoma: current perspectives. Onco Targets Ther 12:1583–1591

Pow EH, Kwong DL, McMillan AS, Wong MC, Sham JS, Leung LH et al (2006) Xerostomia and quality of life after intensity-modulated radiotherapy vs. conventional radiotherapy for early-stage nasopharyngeal carcinoma: initial report on a randomized controlled clinical trial. Int J Radiat Oncol Biol Phys 66(4):981–991

Reddy KA, Mendenhall WM, Amdur RJ, Stringer SP, Cassisi NJ (2001) Long-term results of radiation therapy for juvenile nasopharyngeal angiofibroma. Am J Otolaryngol 22:172–175

Ren ZF, Liu WS, Qin HD, Xu YF, Yu DD, Feng QS, Chen LZ, Shu XO, Zeng YX, Jia W (2010) Effect of family history of cancers and environmental factors on risk of nasopharyngeal carcinoma in Guangdong, China. Cancer Epidemiol 34(4):419–424

Rodriguez-Galindo C, Wofford M, Castleberry RP, Swanson GP, London WB, Fontanesi J, Pappo AS, Douglass EC (2005) Preradiation chemotherapy with methotrexate, cisplatin, 5-fluorouracil, and leucovorin for pediatric nasopharyngeal carcinoma. Cancer 103(4):850–857

Rodriguez-Galindo C, Krailo MD, Krasin MJ, McCarville MB, Hicks J, Pashankar F, Pappo AS (2016) Treatment of childhood nasopharyngeal carcinoma (cNPC) with neoadjuvant chemotherapy (NAC) and concomitant chemoradiotherapy (CCRT): results of the Children's Oncology Group ARAR0331 study. J Clin Oncol 34 (suppl; abstr 10513)

Saylam G, Yucel OT, Sungur A, Onerci M (2006) Proliferation, angiogenesis and hormonal markers in juvenile nasopharyngeal angiofibroma. Int J Pediatr Otorhinolaryngol 70:227–234

Schuon R, Brieger J, Heinrich UR, Roth Y, Szyfter W, Mann WJ (2007) Immunohistochemical analysis of growth mechanisms in juvenile nasopharyngeal angiofibroma. Eur Arch Otorhinolaryngol 264:389–394

Sham JS, Cheung YK, Choy D, Chan FL, Leong L (1991) Nasopharyngeal carcinoma: CT evaluation of patterns of tumor spread. AJNR Am J Neuroradiol 12(2):265–270

Shanmugaratnam K (1980) Nasopharyngeal carcinoma: epidemiology, histopathology and aetiology. Ann Acad Med Singap 9(3):289–295

Su WH, Hildesheim A, Chang YS (2013) Human leukocyte antigens and Epstein-Barr virus-associated nasopharyngeal carcinoma: old associations offer new clues into the role of immunity in infection-associated cancers. Front Oncol 3:299

Sultan I, Casanova M et al (2010) Differential features of nasopharyngeal carcinoma in children and adults: a SEER study. Pediatr Blood Cancer 55(2):279–284

Taheri-Kadkhoda Z, Björk-Eriksson T, Nill S, Wilkens JJ, Oelfke U, Johansson K-A et al (2008) Intensity-modulated radiotherapy of nasopharyngeal carcinoma: a comparative treatment planning study of photons and protons. Radiat Oncol 3(1):4

Tao CJ, Liu X, Tang LL et al (2013) Long-term outcome and late toxicities of simultaneous integrated boost-intensity modulated radiotherapy in pediatric and adolescent nasopharyngeal carcinoma. Chin J Cancer 32:525–532

Thakar A, Gupta G, Bhalla AS, Jain V, Sharma SC, Sharma R, Bahadur S, Deka RC (2011) Adjuvant therapy with flutamide for presurgical volume reduction in juvenile nasopharyngeal angiofibroma. Head Neck 33(12):1747–1753

Tosun S, Ozer C, Gerek M, Yetiser S (2006) Surgical approaches for nasopharyngeal angiofibroma: comparative analysis and current trends. J Craniofac Surg 17:15–20

Treuner J, Niethammer D, Dannecker G, Hagmann R, Neef V, Hofschneider PH (1980) Successful treatment of nasopharyngeal carcinoma with interferon. Lancet 12:817–818

Tyagi I, Syal R, Goyal A (2007) Recurrent and residual juvenile angiofibromas. J Laryngol Otol 121: 460–467

Ulger S, Ulger Z, Yildiz F, Ozyar E (2007) Incidence of hypothyroidism after radiotherapy for nasopharyngeal carcinoma. Med Oncol 24(1):91–94

Wagner HJ, Mertens R, Reiter A, Gauch C (2009) Molecular and serological monitoring of pediatric patients with nasopharyngeal carcinoma treated by the protocol NPC-2003-GPOH of the German Society for Pediatric Oncology. Pediatr Blood Cancer 53:751

Wee J, Tan EH, Tai BC, Wong HB, Leong SS, Tan T et al (2005) Randomized trial of radiotherapy versus concurrent chemoradiotherapy followed by adjuvant chemotherapy in patients with American Joint Committee on Cancer/International Union against cancer stage III and IV nasopharyngeal cancer of the endemic variety. J Clin Oncol 23(27):6730–6738

Wei W, St Sham J (2005) Nasopharyngeal carcinoma. Lancet 365:2041–2054

Weprin LS, Siemers PT (1991) Spontaneous regression of juvenile nasopharyngeal angiofibroma. Arch Otolaryngol Head Neck Surg 117:796–799

Widesott L, Pierelli A, Fiorino C, Dell'oca I, Broggi S, Cattaneo GM, Di Muzio N, Fazio F, Calandrino R, Schwarz M et al (2008) Intensity-modulated proton therapy versus helical tomotherapy in nasopharynx cancer: planning comparison and NTCP evaluation. Int J Radiat Oncol Biol Phys 72(2):589–596

Withers HR, Thames HD (1988) Dose fractionation and volume effects in normal tissues and tumors. Am J Clin Oncol 11(3):313–329

Wolden SL, Chen WC, Pfister DG, Kraus DH, Berry SL, Zelefsky MJ (2006) Intensity-modulated radiation therapy (IMRT) for nasopharynx cancer: update of the Memorial Sloan-Kettering experience. Int J Radiat Oncol Biol Phys 64(1):57–62

Wu VW, Kwong DL, Sham JS (2004) Target dose conformity in 3-dimensional conformal radiotherapy and intensity modulated radiotherapy. Radiother Oncol 71(2):201–206

Xie P, Yue JB, Fu Z, Feng R, Yu JM (2010) Prognostic value of 18F-FDG PET/CT before and after radiotherapy for locally advanced nasopharyngeal carcinoma. Ann Oncol 21:1078–1082

Yan Z, Xia L, Huang Y et al (2013) Nasopharyngeal carcinoma in children and adolescents in an endemic area: a report of 185 cases. Int J Pediatr Otorhinolaryngol 77:1454–1460

Yao JJ, Lin L, Jin YN, Wang SY, Zhang WJ, Zhang F, Zhou GQ, Cheng ZB, Qi ZY, Sun Y (2017) Prognostic value of serum Epstein-Barr virus antibodies in patients with nasopharyngeal carcinoma and undetectable pretreatment Epstein-Barr virus DNA. Cancer Sci 108(8):1640–1647

Yiotakis I, Eleftheriadou A, Davilis D, Giotakis E, Ferekidou E, Korres S, Kandiloros D (2008) Juvenile nasopharyngeal angiofibroma stages I and II: a comparative study of surgical approaches. Int J Pediatr Otorhinolaryngol 72:793–800

Zaghloul MS, Eldebawy E, Ahmed S, Ammar H, Khalil E, Abdelrahman H, Zekri W, Elzomor H, Taha H, Elnashar A (2016) Does primary tumor volume predict the outcome of pediatric nasopharyngeal carcinoma ? A prospective single-arm study using neoadjuvant chemotherapy and concomitant chemotherapy with intensity modulated radiotherapy. Asia Pac J Clin Oncol 12:143–150

Zhang PJ, Weber R, Liang HH, Pasha TL, LiVolsi VA (2003) Growth factors and receptors in juvenile nasopharyngeal angiofibroma and nasal polyps: an immunohistochemical study. Arch Pathol Lab Med 127:1480–1484

Zhang W, Chen Y, Chen L, Guo R, Zhou G, Tang L, Mao Y, Li W, Liu X, Du X, Sun Y, Ma J (2015) The clinical utility of plasma Epstein-Barr virus DNA assays in nasopharyngeal carcinoma: the dawn of a new era ? A systematic review and meta-analysis of 7836 cases. Medicine (Baltimore) 94(20):e845

Zhang L, Huang Y, Hong S, Yang Y, Yu G, Jia J, Peng P, Wu X, Lin Q, Xi X, Peng J, Xu M, Chen D, Lu X, Wang R, Cao X, Chen X, Lin Z, Xiong J, Lin Q, Xie C, Li Z, Pan J, Li J, Wu S, Lian Y, Yang Q, Zhao C (2016) Gemcitabine plus cisplatin versus fluorouracil plus cisplatin in recurrent or metastatic nasopharyngeal carcinoma: a multicentre, randomised, open-label, phase 3 trial. Lancet 388(10054):1883–1892

Zubarreta P, D'Antonio G, Gallo G et al (2000) Nasopharyngeal carcinoma in childhood and adolescence: a single-institution experience with combined therapy. Cancer 89:690–695

11 Esthesioneuroblastoma

Barbara Hero, Gianni Bisogno, and Dominik T. Schneider

Esthesioneuroblastoma (ENB), also often called olfactory neuroblastoma, is a rare tumor thought to arise from the olfactory neuroepithelium. It may occur at any age and accounts for 1–5% of intranasal tumors with an estimated incidence of 0.4 per million population (Broich et al. 1997; Ferlito et al. 2003; Thompson 2009). No strong sex predisposition has been reported. Recent reports favor a unimodal age distribution with the majority of patients diagnosed in the fifth to sixth decades of life and less than 10% of cases occurring in patients younger than 20 years old (Yin et al. 2018).

In children, ENB is rare with an estimated incidence of 0.1 per 100,000 children up to 15 years old, but it is the most frequent cancer of the nasal cavity in this age group. In a series of 47 patients with nasal cavity tumors in the SEER database from 1973 to 2002, ENB accounted for 28% of cases among patients younger than 19 years old (Benoit et al. 2008). Less than 100 cases have been reported during childhood with the youngest reported case being as young as 2 years old (Woerner et al. 1986; Dumont et al. 2020b).

11.1 Pathology

The diagnosis of ENB is difficult. In a substantial proportion of patients, the histological diagnosis has to be revised, when histology is reassessed according to current immunohistochemical criteria (Cohen et al. 2002). ENB is a tumor with small, round, blue tumor cells arranged in a lobular architecture in neurofibrillary stroma. Rosettes and pseudorosettes as well as calcifications may be found (Fig. 11.1). The Hyams histologic grading system is based on cytoarchitecture (lobular present or absent), mitotic rate (0, low, moderate, high), nuclear pleomorphism (absent, slight, moderate, marked), rosette (present or absent), and presence of necrosis (absent, mild, extensive) (Hyams 1988). It has been reported to have a significant impact on prognosis in adults (Bell et al. 2015; Van Gompel et al. 2012). In children, ENB tend to be classified as high-grade tumors more frequently than in adults, and this may explain its more aggressive biological behavior during childhood (Dumont et al. 2020b).

Immunohistochemically, ENB may stain positive for synaptophysin, chromogranin, CD56, LEU-7, neuron-specific enolase, neurofilament protein NFP, and S-100 protein but negative for

B. Hero
Children's University Hospital Cologne, Cologne, Germany

G. Bisogno (✉)
Haematology Oncology Division, Department of Women's and Children's Health, University of Padova, Padova, Italy
e-mail: gianni.bisogno@unipd.it

D. T. Schneider
Klinik für Kinder- und Jugendmedizin, Klinikum Dortmund, University Witten/Herdecke, Dortmund, Germany

D. T. Schneider et al. (eds.), *Rare Tumors in Children and Adolescents*, Pediatric Oncology,
https://doi.org/10.1007/978-3-030-92071-5_11

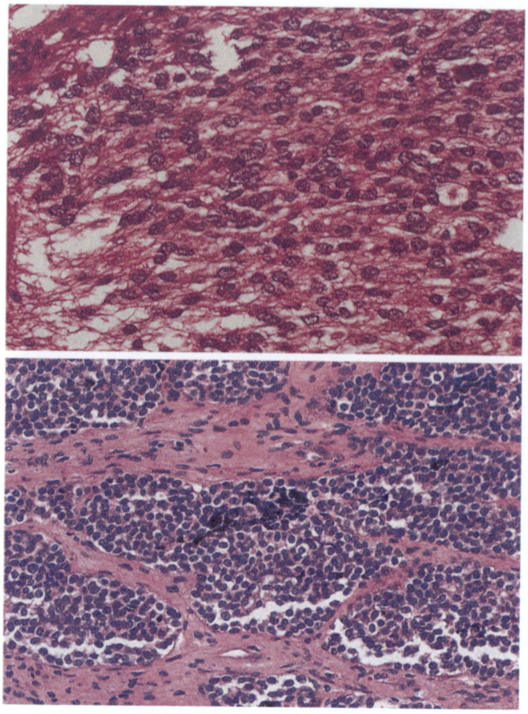

Fig. 11.1 Esthesioneuroblastoma, histology

desmin, myogenin, leukocyte common antigen, and CD99. S-100 protein can stain positive, mainly due to the presence of Schwann cells in the periphery of tumor lobules (Faragalla and Weinreb 2009; Thompson 2009). Immunohistochemical staining for calretinin has been reported to be helpful to differentiate from other small round blue cell tumors (Wooff et al. 2011).

Due to the rarity of the disease, histological evaluation by a second experienced pathologist should be obtained. Other small round cell tumors such as rhabdomyosarcoma, tumors of the Ewing tumor family, neuroblastoma, lymphoma, and, less common in childhood, neuroendocrine carcinoma, squamous cell carcinoma, and sinonasal undifferentiated carcinoma have to be ruled out. Although this has previously been discussed controversially, ENB does not belong to the Ewing tumor family, as CD99/MIC staining and the typical translocations are lacking (Nelson et al. 1995; Argani et al. 1998; Mezzelani et al. 1999). From the histopathological point of view, metastatic neuroblastoma would present with indistinguishable morphology as ENB. However, of note, amplification of the MYCN oncogene has not yet been reported in ENB.

Different genetic anomalies have been reported in ENB and some of them such as deletion of chromosome 11 or gain of 1p may correlate with impaired prognosis (Fiani et al. 2019). p-Akt, p- Erk, and p-Stat3 have been proposed as potential biomarkers for diagnosis of ENB (Peng et al. 2018). The recent finding that ENB frequently express the somatostatin receptor 2a suggests the possibility to investigate treatment with somatostatin analogues (Czapiewski et al. 2018).

11.2 Clinical Manifestations and Staging

The origin of ENB is confined to the olfactory mucosa involving the superior turbinate, cribriform plate, and the superior one-third of the nasal cavity. It may spread into the paranasal sinuses, into the orbits, and—through the lamina cribriformis—into the cranial cavity. Although dystopic sites of origin in the nasopharynx, in the maxillary sinuses, and intracranially have been reported (Holmes et al. 2016), a diagnosis of ENB outside the nasal cavity should only be made with great cautiousness (Mills 2002).

Symptoms are related to the site of origin and the local invasion (and therefore, patients may often first be seen by ENT specialists). Often symptoms may persist for several months prior to definite diagnosis. Sinusitis like symptoms, unilateral nasal obstruction, recurrent epistaxis, and—less common—a visible intranasal mass are observed, and patients may report anosmia (often only on testing). During inspection, the tumor presents as brownish, polypoid mass in the upper nasal cavity. Ophthalmic manifestations like periorbital pain, excessive tearing, visual disturbance, or ptosis have been reported to occur more commonly in children than in adults, because in this age group the tumor tends to arise more posterolaterally in the anterior cranial fossa and may invade ocular structures than in adults (Benoit et al. 2008).

Table 11.1 Esthesioneuroblastoma: (modified) Kadish staging system and prognosis

Stage		Stage distribution	Disease-specific survival rates (at 10 years)	Stage distribution	Proposed therapy in children
		As reported by Jethanamest et al. (2007) based on registry data, $n = 261$, all ages		As reported by Broich et al. (1997) based on systematic literature review, $n = 553$, all ages	
A	Tumor confined to the nasal cavity	17.2%	90%	18.3%	Resection
B	Tumors involving the nasal cavity and extending into the paranasal sinuses	49.8%	68.3%	32.3%	Resection + radiotherapy
C	Tumor extending beyond the nasal cavity and paranasal sinuses (includes involvement of orbit, base of skull, intracranial cavity)	3.8%	66.7%	49.4%	Resection + radiotherapy ± (neoadjuvant) chemotherapy
D	Any tumor with distant sites to cervical lymph nodes or distant sites	29.1%	35.6%		

Occasionally headache, nerve palsies due to involvement of cranial nerves, or hormone excess syndromes such as Cushing syndrome or inappropriate antidiuretic hormone secretion have been reported (Fiani et al. 2019).

In 1976, Kadish et al. proposed a staging system based on the pattern of spread (Table 11.1). Kadish A tumors are confined to the nasal cavity, while Kadish B tumors infiltrate the paranasal cavities. Kadish C tumors extend beyond the nasal and paranasal cavities (Kadish et al. 1976; Bell et al. 2015). Later, the system has been modified by adding the category Kadish D for tumors with metastases. The Kadish system correlates with prognosis and is still in use, although other systems based on the TMN classification have been proposed (Biller et al. 1990; Dulguerov and Calcaterra 1992; Dulguerov et al. 2001). Larger cohorts report that about one-third of the patients present with Kadish stage C (Fig. 11.2).

In pediatric patients with ENB, distant metastases are rare and may occur in less than 10% of patients. Metastases to the lungs, CNS, bone, liver, and bone marrow have been reported (Bradley et al. 2003; Eich et al. 2003; Bachar et al. 2008; Dumont et al. 2020a, b).

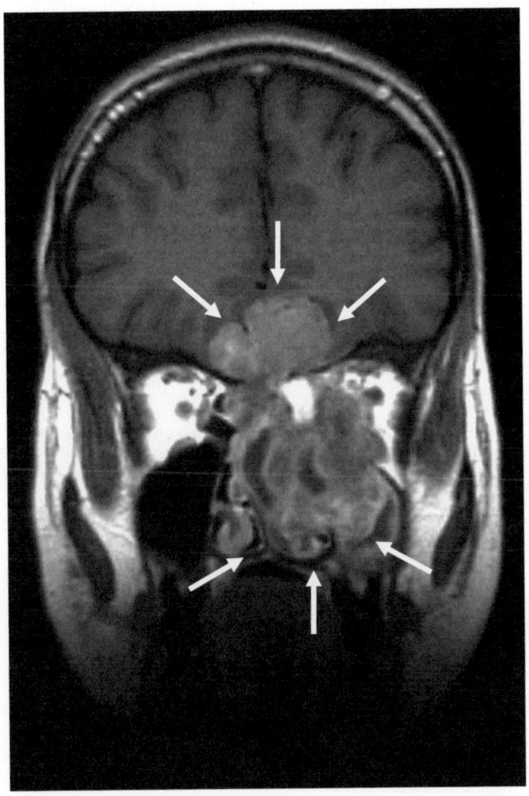

Fig. 11.2 Esthesioneuroblastoma, Kadish stage C, infiltrating the orbital, the nasal, and paranasal cavities and, through the lamina cribriformis, the brain (MRI)

Locoregional spread to cervical lymph nodes may occur in approximately 5–10% of adult patients but may be more frequent in children. In some pediatric series, up to 25% of patients had nodal involvement (Venkatramani et al. 2016; Lucas et al. 2015; Bisogno et al. 2012).

Investigations at initial workup include CT scan, which usually shows a homogenously enhancing lesion that extends across the cribriform plate to the anterior cranial fossa superiorly and to the nasal cavity inferiorly. Bone erosion may be seen, as well as invasion of the adjacent structures. Tumors may often present with calcifications. MRI images help to delineate the extent of the disease. Tumors appear isointense or hypointense to the brain on T1-weighted images and hyperintense on T2-weighted images and may show pronounced enhancement after gadolinium. MRI diffusion-weighted imaging (DWI) may be useful to differentiate ENB from other sinonasal masses presenting apparent diffusion coefficient (ADC) values significantly higher than other neoplasms and lower than benign lesions (Thompson 2009; Miracle et al. 2019).

Besides the imaging of the primary tumor site and the neck, the initial workup should include the search for distant metastases in the CNS, lung, liver, bone, and bone marrow. In bone marrow, multiple sites should be assessed as the diagnosis of neuroblastoma or rhabdomyosarcoma should be considered. Somatostatin receptor imaging has been reported to give positive results in patients with ENB and might be helpful in assessing the extent of the disease at diagnosis and during treatment (Ramsay et al. 1996; Freeman et al. 2005). Studies in adult suggested that PET can give additional information especially in detecting nodal involvement and metastatic disease and therefore upstaging the disease but with limitation in demonstrating intracranial metastasis (Nguyen et al. 2006; Broski et al. 2012).

Only a single patient with ENB has been reported to show positive mIBG uptake (Kairemo et al. 1998), but mIBG scintigraphy might be helpful in those cases where a metastatic lesion of a neuroblastoma is discussed as differential diagnosis. However, these imaging techniques have not been systematically addressed in larger cohorts of patients with ENB so far.

11.3 Prognosis and Therapy

Due to the rarity of the disease, the literature does not provide strong evidence on the prognosis of ENB, based on large, homogenously treated cohorts. Nevertheless, it seems quite clear that grading, staging, the presence of metastases, and the treatment received may have an impact on prognosis. Kadish et al. reported patients with advanced stage (Kadish stage C) to be younger at diagnosis (median age: 30.4 years) (Kadish et al. 1976). Vice versa older age at diagnosis correlated with better outcome in one series (<61 vs. >61 years) (Ozsahin et al. 2010). However, this observation was not confirmed by others (<20 vs. >20 years): (Eich et al. 2003, 2005; Dulguerov and Calcaterra 1992)).

In childhood, a high proportion of patients present with advanced stage (Lochrin 1989; Kumar et al. 2002, 2008). Therefore, it has been discussed whether ENB in childhood may show a more aggressive biology and clinical behavior compared to their adult counterparts. However, this has never been proven in larger comparative studies.

The amount of therapy needed is discussed controversially in the literature. Table 11.1 sets our proposal for the treatment in children in relation to the survival estimates as reported from a large cohort of 261 patients with ENB (Jethanamest et al. 2007).

Complete resection of the primary correlates with prognosis and is considered the backbone of all treatment strategies (Goldsweig and Sundaresan 1990; Devaiah and Andreoli 2009). Planning of the surgery may involve different subdisciplines (head and neck surgeons, neurosurgeons, ophthalmologists). Although most often open surgeries, preferably with a craniofacial approach, have been performed, endoscopic resections seem not to be inferior, as long as oncologic principles with clearance of margins are maintained. In some patients, endoscopic transnasal approach may be combined with a neurosurgical approach for intracranial components of the tumor (Lund and Wei 2015; Folbe et al. 2009; Snyderman et al. 2008). In locally advanced tumors, preoperative chemotherapy or radiotherapy has proven efficient to facilitate complete resection (Foote et al. 1993; Eich et al. 2003, 2005; El Kababri et al. 2014).

Kadish stage A tumors, especially when presenting with low-grade histology (Hyams grades I–II), seem to be sufficiently treated by resection only (with or without radiotherapy). However, these tumors account only for a small proportion of patients and have to be selected carefully. In higher stages, the addition of radiotherapy with doses ranging from 55 to 65 Gy is recommended (Foote et al. 1993; Chao et al. 2001; Dulguerov et al. 2001; Eich et al. 2001).

The planning of the radiotherapy should consider adjacent endangered structures as eye and CNS and requires, especially in children, modern radiation techniques such as intensity-modulated radiotherapy, proton irradiation, or stereotactic radiosurgery (Bhattacharyya et al. 1997; Walch et al. 2000; Zabel et al. 2002; Tselis et al. 2008; Sterzing et al. 2009).

Although some authors dispute the therapeutic effect of chemotherapy, most support the need for a multimodal treatment strategy including surgery, radiotherapy, and chemotherapy in tumors Kadish stage C (with or without metastases). Nevertheless, there is no evidence-based common consensus regarding the optimal regimen and cumulative dose of chemotherapy needed (Goldsweig and Sundaresan 1990; McElroy et al. 1998; Buckner et al. 1999; Oskouian et al. 2002; Eich et al. 2003, 2005; Loy et al. 2006; McLean et al. 2007; Kiyota et al. 2008; Dumont et al. 2020b; Venkatramani et al. 2016).

In children, chemotherapy regimen as used in soft tissue sarcoma or neuroblastoma protocols have been used most frequently. In adults, platinum- and etoposide-based regimens have been applied more often. In a report from the French working group, one cycle of preoperative chemotherapy was administered, followed by resection and postoperative irradiation, with long-term remission in 10 of 11 patients (El Kababri et al. 2014). Accordingly, a recent review reported an 84% response rate to preoperative chemotherapy in children with ENB (Venkatramani et al. 2016).

If cervical lymph nodes are involved, neck dissection and postoperative radiation therapy are discussed (Zanation et al. 2010). In contrast, cervical treatment is not considered necessary in N0 patients. However, to discover late evolving lymph nodes, adequate imaging of the neck should always be included in the follow-up of the patients (Gore and Zanation 2009).

Relapses and metastases usually develop within the first 2–3 years after diagnosis. However, late relapses even later than 5 years after therapy have been reported (Morita et al. 1993; Eden et al. 1994; Loy et al. 2006). This observation indicates the need for a long follow-up, which, in a childhood population, should always include the care for therapy-related sequelae. It should be considered that the need for local control including extensive surgical procedures and high-dose radiotherapy may pose specific problems in the pediatric age, when bone growth is not yet finalized. Thus, long-term sequelae in children may include impaired craniofacial growth and permanent dentition, endocrine dysfunctions of the thyroid and hypophyseal glands, and loss of sense of smell.

References

Argani P, Perez-Ordoñez B, Xiao H, Caruana SM, Huvos AG, Ladanyi M (1998) Olfactory neuroblastoma is not related to the Ewing family of tumors: absence of EWS/FLI1 gene fusion and MIC2 expression. Am J Surg Pathol 22:391–398

Bachar G, Goldstein DP, Shah M, Tandon A, Ringash J, Pond G, Gullane PJ, Perez-Ordonez B, Gilbert RW, Brown DH, Gentili F, O'Sullivan B, Irish JC

(2008) Esthesioneuroblastoma: the Princess Margaret Hospital experience. Head Neck 30:1607–1614

Bell D, Saade R, Roberts D, Ow TJ, Kupferman M, DeMonte F, Hanna EY (2015) Prognostic utility of Hyams histological grading and Kadish-Morita staging systems for esthesioneuroblastoma outcomes. Head Neck Pathol 9:51–59

Benoit MM, Bhattacharyya N, Faquin W, Cunningham M (2008) Cancer of the nasal cavity in the pediatric population. Pediatrics 121:e141–e145

Bhattacharyya N, Thornton AF, Joseph MP, Goodman ML, Amrein PC (1997) Successful treatment of esthesioneuroblastoma and neuroendocrine carcinoma with combined chemotherapy and proton radiation. Results in 9 cases. Arch Otolaryngol Head Neck Surg 123:34–40

Biller HF, Lawson W, Sachdev VP, Som P (1990) Esthesioneuroblastoma: surgical treatment without radiation. Laryngoscope 100:1199–1201

Bisogno G, Soloni P, Conte M, Podda M, Ferrari A, Garaventa A, Luksch R, Cecchetto G (2012) Esthesioneuroblastoma in pediatric and adolescent age. A report from the TREP project in cooperation with the Italian Neuroblastoma and Soft Tissue Sarcoma Committees. BMC Cancer 12:117

Bradley PJ, Jones NS, Robertson I (2003) Diagnosis and management of esthesioneuroblastoma. Curr Opin Otolaryngol Head Neck Surg 11:112–118

Broich G, Pagliari A, Ottaviani F (1997) Esthesioneuroblastoma: a general review of the cases published since the discovery of the tumour in 1924. Anticancer Res 17:2683–2706

Broski SM, Hunt CH, Johnson GB, Subramaniam RM, Peller PJ (2012) The added value of 18F-FDG PET/CT for evaluation of patients with esthesioneuroblastoma. J Nucl Med 53:1200–1206

Buckner JC, Peethambaram PP, Smithson WA, Groover RV, Schomberg PJ, Kimmel DW, Raffel C, O'Fallon JR, Neglia J, Shaw EG (1999) Phase II trial of primary chemotherapy followed by reduced-dose radiation for CNS germ cell tumors. J Clin Oncol 17:933–940

Chao KS, Kaplan C, Simpson JR, Haughey B, Spector GJ, Sessions DG, Arquette M (2001) Esthesioneuroblastoma: the impact of treatment modality. Head Neck 23:749–757

Cohen ZR, Marmor E, Fuller GN, DeMonte F (2002) Misdiagnosis of olfactory neuroblastoma. Neurosurg Focus 12:e3

Czapiewski P, Kunc M, Gorczyński A, Haybaeck J, Okoń K, Reszec J, Lewczuk A, Dzierzanowski J, Karczewska J, Biernat W, Turri-Zanoni M, Castelnuovo P, Taverna C, Franchi A, La Rosa S, Sessa F, Klöppel G (2018) Frequent expression of somatostatin receptor 2a in olfactory neuroblastomas: a new and distinctive feature. Hum Pathol 79:144–150

Devaiah AK, Andreoli MT (2009) Treatment of esthesioneuroblastoma: a 16-year meta-analysis of 361 patients. Laryngoscope 119:1412–1416

Dulguerov P, Calcaterra T (1992) Esthesioneuroblastoma: the UCLA experience 1970-1990. Laryngoscope 102:843–849

Dulguerov P, Allal AS, Calcaterra TC (2001) Esthesioneuroblastoma: a meta-analysis and review. Lancet Oncol 2:683–690

Dumont B, Fresneau B, Claude L, Defachelles AS, Couloigner V, Puget S, Brisse HJ, Fréneaux P, Lacour B, Orbach D (2020a) Pattern of loco-regional relapses and treatment in pediatric esthesioneuroblastoma: the French very rare tumors group (fracture) contribution. Pediatr Blood Cancer 67:e28154

Dumont B, Lemelle L, Cordero C, Couloigner V, Bernard S, Cardoen L, Brisse HJ, Jehanno N, Fréneaux P, Helfre S, Rouffiange L, Réguerre Y, Orbach D (2020b) Esthesioneuroblastoma in children, adolescents and young adults. Bull Cancer 107:934–945

Eden BV, Debo RF, Larner JM, Kelly MD, Levine PA, Stewart FM, Cantrell RW, Constable WC (1994) Esthesioneuroblastoma. Long-term outcome and patterns of failure—the University of Virginia experience. Cancer 73:2556–2562

Eich HT, Staar S, Micke O, Eich PD, Stützer H, Müller R (2001) Radiotherapy of esthesioneuroblastoma. Int J Radiat Oncol Biol Phys 49:155–160

Eich HT, Hero B, Staar S, Micke O, Seegenschmiedt H, Mattke A, Berthold F, Müller RP (2003) Multimodality therapy including radiotherapy and chemotherapy improves event-free survival in stage C esthesioneuroblastoma. Strahlenther Onkol 179:233–240

Eich HT, Müller RP, Micke O, Kocher M, Berthold F, Hero B (2005) Esthesioneuroblastoma in childhood and adolescence. Better prognosis with multimodal treatment. Strahlenther Onkol 181:378–384

El Kababri M, Habrand JL, Valteau-Couanet D, Gaspar N, Dufour C, Oberlin O (2014) Esthesioneuroblastoma in children and adolescent: experience on 11 cases with literature review. J Pediatr Hematol Oncol 36:91–95

Faragalla H, Weinreb I (2009) Olfactory neuroblastoma: a review and update. Adv Anat Pathol 16:322–331

Ferlito A, Rinaldo A, Rhys-Evans PH (2003) Contemporary clinical commentary: esthesioneuroblastoma: an update on management of the neck. Laryngoscope 113:1935–1938

Fiani B, Quadri SA, Cathel A, Farooqui M, Ramachandran A, Siddiqi I, Ghanchi H, Zafar A, Berman BW, Siddiqi J (2019) Esthesioneuroblastoma: a comprehensive review of diagnosis, management, and current treatment options. World Neurosurg 126:194–211

Folbe A, Herzallah I, Duvvuri U, Bublik M, Sargi Z, Snyderman CH, Carrau R, Casiano R, Kassam AB, Morcos JJ (2009) Endoscopic endonasal resection of esthesioneuroblastoma: a multicenter study. Am J Rhinol Allergy 23:91–94

Foote RL, Morita A, Ebersold MJ, Olsen KD, Lewis JE, Quast LM, Ferguson JA, O'Fallon WM (1993) Esthesioneuroblastoma: the role of adjuvant radiation therapy. Int J Radiat Oncol Biol Phys 27:835–842

Freeman SR, Mitra S, Malik TH, Flanagan P, Selby P (2005) Expression of somatostatin receptors in arginine vasopressin hormone-secreting olfactory neuroblastoma—report of two cases. Rhinology 43:61–65

Goldsweig HG, Sundaresan N (1990) Chemotherapy of recurrent esthesioneuroblastoma. Case report and review of the literature. Am J Clin Oncol 13:139–143

Gore MR, Zanation AM (2009) Salvage treatment of late neck metastasis in esthesioneuroblastoma: a meta-analysis. Arch Otolaryngol Head Neck Surg 135:1030–1034

Holmes M, Su SY, Bell D (2016) Ectopic primary olfactory neuroblastoma of the maxillary sinus. Ann Diagn Pathol 22:45–48

Hyams, VJ, Batsakis JG, Michaels L (1988) Olfactory neuroblastoma. In: Tumors of the upper respiratory tract and ear, Fascicle 25, Second Series. Armed Forces Institute of Pathology, Washington, DC, p 240–248.

Jethanamest D, Morris LG, Sikora AG, Kutler DI (2007) Esthesioneuroblastoma: a population-based analysis of survival and prognostic factors. Arch Otolaryngol Head Neck Surg 133:276–280

Kadish S, Goodman M, Wang CC (1976) Olfactory neuroblastoma. A clinical analysis of 17 cases. Cancer 37:1571–1576

Kairemo KJ, Jekunen AP, Kestilä MS, Ramsay HA (1998) Imaging of olfactory neuroblastoma—an analysis of 17 cases. Auris Nasus Larynx 25:173–179

Kiyota N, Tahara M, Fujii S, Kawashima M, Ogino T, Minami H, Hayashi R, Ohtsu A (2008) Nonplatinum-based chemotherapy with irinotecan plus docetaxel for advanced or metastatic olfactory neuroblastoma: a retrospective analysis of 12 cases. Cancer 112:885–891

Kumar M, Fallon RJ, Hill JS, Davis MM (2002) Esthesioneuroblastoma in children. J Pediatr Hematol Oncol 24:482–487

Kumar S, Shah JP, Bryant CS, Imudia AN, Cote ML, Ali-Fehmi R, Malone JM, Morris RT (2008) The prevalence and prognostic impact of lymph node metastasis in malignant germ cell tumors of the ovary. Gynecol Oncol 110:125–132

Lochrin C (1989) Esthesioneuroblastoma. Med Pediatr Oncol 17:433–438

Loy AH, Reibel JF, Read PW, Thomas CY, Newman SA, Jane JA, Levine PA (2006) Esthesioneuroblastoma: continued follow-up of a single institution's experience. Arch Otolaryngol Head Neck Surg 132:134–138

Lucas JT, Ladra MM, MacDonald SM, Busse PM, Friedmann AM, Ebb DH, Marcus KJ, Tarbell NJ, Yock TI (2015) Proton therapy for pediatric and adolescent esthesioneuroblastoma. Pediatr Blood Cancer 62:1523–1528

Lund VJ, Wei WI (2015) Endoscopic surgery for malignant sinonasal tumours: an eighteen year experience. Rhinology 53:204–211

McElroy EA, Buckner JC, Lewis JE (1998) Chemotherapy for advanced esthesioneuroblastoma: the Mayo Clinic experience. Neurosurgery 42:1023–1027; discussion 1027

McLean JN, Nunley SR, Klass C, Moore C, Müller S, Johnstone PA (2007) Combined modality therapy of esthesioneuroblastoma. Otolaryngol Head Neck Surg 136:998–1002

Mezzelani A, Tornielli S, Minoletti F, Pierotti MA, Sozzi G, Pilotti S (1999) Esthesioneuroblastoma is not a member of the primitive peripheral neuroectodermal tumour-Ewing's group. Br J Cancer 81:586–591

Mills SE (2002) Neuroectodermal neoplasms of the head and neck with emphasis on neuroendocrine carcinomas. Mod Pathol 15:264–278

Miracle AC, El-Sayed IH, Glastonbury CM (2019) Diffusion weighted imaging of esthesioneuroblastoma: differentiation from other sinonasal masses. Head Neck 41:1161–1164

Morita A, Ebersold MJ, Olsen KD, Foote RL, Lewis JE, Quast LM (1993) Esthesioneuroblastoma: prognosis and management. Neurosurgery 32:706–714; discussion 714

Nelson RS, Perlman EJ, Askin FB (1995) Is esthesioneuroblastoma a peripheral neuroectodermal tumor. Hum Pathol 26:639–641

Nguyen BD, Roarke MC, Nelson KD, Chong BW (2006) F-18 FDG PET/CT staging and posttherapeutic assessment of esthesioneuroblastoma. Clin Nucl Med 31:172–174

Oskouian RJ, Jane JA, Dumont AS, Sheehan JM, Laurent JJ, Levine PA (2002) Esthesioneuroblastoma: clinical presentation, radiological, and pathological features, treatment, review of the literature, and the University of Virginia experience. Neurosurg Focus 12:e4

Ozsahin M, Gruber G, Olszyk O, Karakoyun-Celik O, Pehlivan B, Azria D, Roelandts M, Kaanders JH, Cengiz M, Krengli M, Matzinger O, Zouhair A (2010) Outcome and prognostic factors in olfactory neuroblastoma: a rare cancer network study. Int J Radiat Oncol Biol Phys 78:992–997

Peng X, Liu Y, Peng X, Wang Z, Zhang Z, Qiu Y, Jin M, Wang R, Kong D (2018) Clinical features and the molecular biomarkers of olfactory neuroblastoma. Pathol Res Pract 214:1123–1129

Ramsay HA, Kairemo KJ, Jekunen AP (1996) Somatostatin receptor imaging of olfactory neuroblastoma. J Laryngol Otol 110:1161–1163

Snyderman CH, Carrau RL, Kassam AB, Zanation A, Prevedello D, Gardner P, Mintz A (2008) Endoscopic skull base surgery: principles of endonasal oncological surgery. J Surg Oncol 97:658–664

Sterzing F, Stoiber EM, Nill S, Bauer H, Huber P, Debus J, Münter MW (2009) Intensity modulated radiotherapy (IMRT) in the treatment of children and adolescents—a single institution's experience and a review of the literature. Radiat Oncol 4:37

Thompson LD (2009) Olfactory neuroblastoma. Head Neck Pathol 3:252–259

Tselis N, Heyd R, Baghi M, Zamboglou N (2008) Interstitial high-dose-rate-brachytherapy in advanced esthesioneuroblastoma. Laryngoscope 118:2006–2010

Van Gompel JJ, Giannini C, Olsen KD, Moore E, Piccirilli M, Foote RL, Buckner JC, Link MJ (2012) Long-term outcome of esthesioneuroblastoma: hyams grade predicts patient survival. J Neurol Surg B Skull Base 73:331–336

Venkatramani R, Pan H, Furman WL, Marron JM, Haduong J, Friedrich-Medina P, Mahajan A, Bavle A, Wu H, Chintagumpala M (2016) Multimodality treatment of pediatric esthesioneuroblastoma. Pediatr Blood Cancer 63:465–470

Walch C, Stammberger H, Anderhuber W, Unger F, Köle W, Feichtinger K (2000) The minimally invasive approach to olfactory neuroblastoma: combined endoscopic and stereotactic treatment. Laryngoscope 110:635–640

Woerner SJ, Lazerson J, Munn RJ, Turner EA (1986) Olfactory neuroblastoma (esthesioneuroblastoma) in a 2-year-old boy. Pediatr Hematol Oncol 3:167–174

Wooff JC, Weinreb I, Perez-Ordonez B, Magee JF, Bullock MJ (2011) Calretinin staining facilitates differentiation of olfactory neuroblastoma from other small round blue cell tumors in the sinonasal tract. Am J Surg Pathol 35:1786–1793

Yin Z, Wang Y, Wu Y, Zhang X, Wang F, Wang P, Tao Z, Yuan Z (2018) Age distribution and age-related outcomes of olfactory neuroblastoma: a population-based analysis. Cancer Manag Res 10:1359–1364

Zabel A, Thilmann C, Zuna I, Schlegel W, Wannenmacher M, Debus J (2002) Comparison of forward planned conformal radiation therapy and inverse planned intensity modulated radiation therapy for esthesioneuroblastoma. Br J Radiol 75:356–361

Zanation AM, Ferlito A, Rinaldo A, Gore MR, Lund VJ, McKinney KA, Suárez C, Takes RP, Devaiah AK (2010) When, how and why to treat the neck in patients with esthesioneuroblastoma: a review. Eur Arch Otorhinolaryngol 267:1667–1671

Germ Cell Tumors of the Head and Neck

12

Dominik T. Schneider and Thomas A. Olson

12.1 Introduction

The general aspects of germ cell tumors, common to all tumors, occurring at different sites, are discussed in the introduction chapter of germ cell tumors and genitourinary cancers (Chap. 39). Germ cell tumors of the head and neck region constitute rare but characteristic extragonadal germ cell tumors of childhood (Jordan and Gauderer 1988). They most commonly present in the neonatal period or during infancy (Bernbeck et al. 2009; Alexander et al. 2015; Brodsky et al. 2017). In this age group, virtually all tumors are mature or immature teratomas. A significant proportion of tumors are already diagnosed during prenatal ultrasound (Berge et al. 2004; Dunn et al. 1992).

In the perspective of the overall favorable prognosis, the diagnosis of a large, mostly cystic cervical tumor must not evoke therapeutic nihilism and lead to the recommendation of termination of pregnancy but should rather lead to a close follow-up during pregnancy and optimal planning of the perinatal management (Langer et al. 1992; De Backer et al. 2004; Bernbeck et al. 2009; Kerner et al. 1998).

Some tumors may include malignant yolk sac tumor components, sometimes only as microscopic foci. The risk of clinically relevant malignant yolk sac tumor components that are also associated with significant AFP secretion rises with age. Thus, among the rare head and neck germ cell tumors diagnosed beyond the first year of life, the majority show malignant yolk sac tumor as leading histology (Bernbeck et al. 2009). Other histologic subtypes of germ cell tumors only rarely develop at this site, and to the authors' knowledge, still no seminoma has yet been reported in the head and neck region. No genetic survey of these tumors has been reported so far. Rare single reports indicate for genetic aberrations characteristic of germ cell tumors of infancy and childhood. Moreover, these tumors have occasionally been reported in the context of a genetic syndrome such as CHARGE or Aicardi syndrome. In Aicardi syndrome, which is defined by several a pattern of malformations affecting the brain, the eyes, and the trunk skeleton, the association with head and neck germ cell tumors has already been reported in four patients, suggesting a biological link (Epperson et al. 2020).

D. T. Schneider (✉)
Klinik für Kinder- und Jugendmedizin, Clinic of Pediatrics, Klinikum Dortmund, University Witten/Herdecke, Dortmund, Germany
e-mail: dominik.schneider@klinikumdo.de

T. A. Olson
Division Pediatric Hematology/Oncology, Children's Healthcare of Atlanta at Egleston, Atlanta, GA, USA
e-mail: thomas.olson@choa.org

D. T. Schneider et al. (eds.), *Rare Tumors in Children and Adolescents*, Pediatric Oncology,
https://doi.org/10.1007/978-3-030-92071-5_12

12.2 Clinical Diagnosis

Most tumors are diagnosed during the perinatal period. In countries which promote prenatal ultrasound assessment of the fetus, the majority of tumors are diagnosed with fetal ultrasound (Alexander et al. 2015; Brodsky et al. 2017; Dunn et al. 1992). Tumors, in particular teratomas, present as partially solid and cystic lesions in the head and neck region, often in close association with the pharynx (Fig. 12.1). Vascular malformations and tumors such as lymphangioma constitute the most problematic differential diagnosis. Fetal MRI may assist in assessing the nature of the tumor and in evaluating the organ of origin of the tumor. Some tumors may develop within or in close anatomical proximity to the thyroid gland. If a head and neck tumor is diagnosed prenatally, a close follow-up schedule is mandatory in order to compare the growth kinetics of the tumor and the fetus, respectively. In addition, significant hemodynamic distress

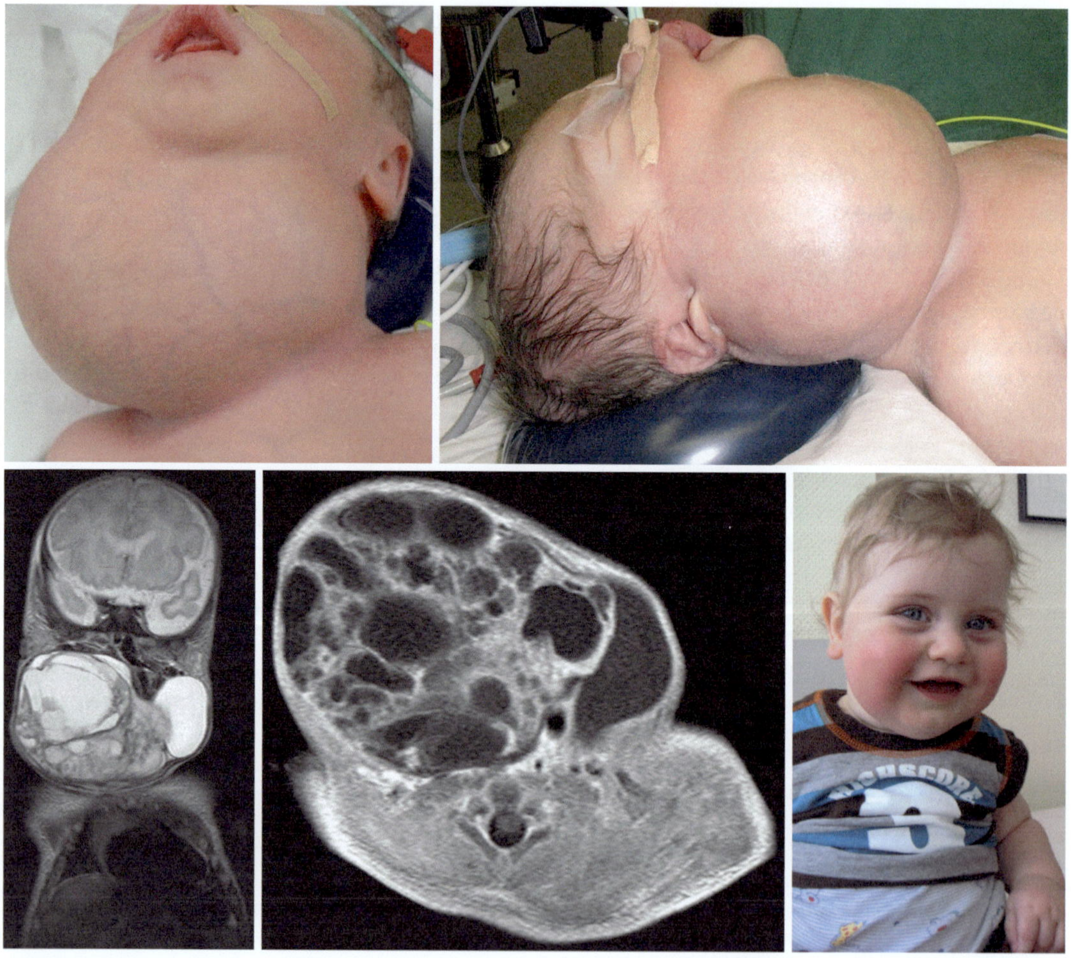

Fig. 12.1 Clinical images and magnetic resonance imaging of a neonate with a huge mature cervical teratoma involving the thyroids. The tumor was diagnosed with prenatal ultrasound. The patient was delivered with cesarean section and immediately intubated and ventilated after birth. At the second day of life, the tumor was completely resected including the thyroid gland which presented as the presumed site of tumor origin. After surgery, the patient showed intercurrent palsy of the vocal cords and hypocalcemia. Both resolved within weeks. The patient is on support of thyroid hormones. The boy is nicely developing without signs of neurocognitive deficits, apart from unilateral paresis of the hypoglossal nerve (the pictures are kindly provided by Dr. M. Albrecht and Dr. Schmitz-Stolbrink, Westfalian Children's Centre, Dortmund)

caused by increased blood flow through the tumor should be excluded. These parameters may assist in planning of the time of delivery.

At birth, head and neck teratomas commonly present as large tumors, covered by skin. Due to airway compression, neonates may have asphyxia, and severe respiratory distress may occur. In these patients, primary tracheal intubation and ventilatory support are mandatory ("EXIT (ex utero intrapartum treatment) strategy") (De Backer et al. 2004, #63299; Brodsky et al. 2017, #84990; Hullett et al. 2006, #95512).

During infancy and childhood, head and neck germ cell tumors present as circumscribed tumors, mostly arising in the pharyngeal region or the nasal sinuses. The majority of tumors are malignant yolk sac tumors. Nevertheless, metastases rarely occur and mostly involve the cervical lymph nodes or the lungs (Bernbeck et al. 2009).

In order to exclude malignant yolk sac tumor or choriocarcinoma, the measurement of AFP and β-HCG is recommended (Table 12.1). AFP levels must be compared to the age-related reference values (Blohm et al. 1998). In addition, the general considerations with regard to the diagnostic impact of tumor markers in germ cell tumors also apply to the head and neck germ cell tumors (see Chap. 39).

Prior to surgery, clinical assessment should include an endocrinologic workup, specifically focusing on the thyroid and parathyroid function.

Table 12.1 Specific diagnostic strategy in head and neck tumors, suspicious of germ cell tumors

Procedure	Specific questions
Clinical assessment	
Physical examination	Signs of upper airway obstruction
Laboratory assessment	
AFP (β-HCG)	Malignant germ cell tumor with yolk sac tumor—consider age-related reference range (or choriocarcinoma)
Catecholamines	Exclusion of neuroblastoma
Thyroid hormones	Hypothyroidism—pre- and postsurgery
Calcium, phosphate	Hypoparathyroidism—pre- and postsurgery
Radiographic assessment	
Prenatal ultrasound, fetal MRI	Site, organ of origin, cystic structures or calcification, observation of growth kinetics, timing of delivery
Head and neck MRI (+ angiography)	Site, size, organ of origin, cystic structures, calcification, involvement of larynx, pharynx, thyroid gland, proximity to large vessels and airways
Abdominal ultrasound	Liver metastases (if elevated AFP/YST)
Lung X-ray	Lung metastases (if elevated AFP/YST)
Histologic assessment	
H&E	Classification according to WHO
AFP	Yolk sac tumor (microfoci in teratoma)
(β-HCG)	Exclusion of choriocarcinoma
(CD-30)	Exclusion of embryonal carcinoma
(OCT3/4)	Exclusion of seminoma (embryonal carcinoma)

12.3 Therapy

In contrast to other teratomas and malignant germ cell tumors, the prognosis of head and neck germ cell tumors is primarily determined by the optimal management of local complications, which are primarily related to airway obstruction. Therefore, despite their benign histology, teratomas of the head and neck region constitute a life-threatening and potentially fatal disease. In a situation of suboptimal perinatal care, asphyxia may result in life-long neurological impairment. Therefore, careful planning of the perinatal management is absolutely mandatory, and treatment should be reserved to experienced neonatologic and pediatric surgical teams.

In the most comprehensive reviews by Jordan and Gauderer in 1988 and by Kerner et al. in 1998, a decrease in mortality from 37 to 25% has been described (Kerner et al. 1998; Jordan and Gauderer 1988). In most instances, patients died during the neonatal period as a result of respiratory failure caused by external airway obstruction. Different measures have been supposed to reduce perinatal risk, including intrapartum airway management (EXIT maneuver) or access to the airway in utero prior to delivery (Liechty et al. 1997; Hullett et al. 2006; De Backer et al. 2004; Dharmarajan et al. 2018). However, the combined data of more recent publications still report a high mortality in 5 of 16 cases (Martino et al. 2006) (Table 12.1). Two recent monoinstitutional series from large tertiary care centers confirm the low recurrence rate, even in patients with microscopically incomplete resection, and the overall excellent prognosis (Alexander et al. 2015; Brodsky et al. 2017) .

In a large series reported from the German MAKEI study group, none of the patients received an ante- or intrapartum airway management. Nevertheless, no newborn died perinatally, and significant asphyxia could also be avoided (Bernbeck et al. 2009). In 12 patients, repeated ultrasounds in short intervals demonstrated a marked enlargement of the tumor within a few days leading to preterm delivery during the 32nd to 37th week of pregnancy. Of note, the growth velocity after delivery was unpredictable. Six tumors showed dramatic tumor growth immediately after birth, while in others the growth velocity declined. As a consequence, three neonates were operated on soon after birth in an emergency situation. In tumors showing rapid growth, no beneficial short-time effects of chemotherapy have been reported, substantiating the central importance of timely planning and performance of tumor resection.

Notably, the tumor site has a significant impact on the therapeutic approach. Teratomas of the neck are usually better assessable to complete resection than pharyngeal tumors, in which microscopically complete tumor resection is often impossible (Bernbeck et al. 2009). In the latter patients, it might be helpful to postpone surgery until the infant's weight has significantly increased in order to facilitate complete resection. However this is only possible if tumor size and growth velocity do not argue against a further delay. Moreover, a delayed tumor resection may bear the potential risk of malignant overgrowth. In this context, it should be noted that tumors of newborns may already include some small foci of yolk sac tumor. It should be considered that in teratomas of different sites in particular at the sacrococcygeal region, YST may be the leading histology at relapse. Therefore, preoperative chemotherapy aiming for the elimination of potential YST microfoci may be considered in selected and very rare patients with unresectable tumors in whom delayed tumor resection is reasonable. Nevertheless, these patients presumably constitute absolutely rare exceptions from the general rule that surgery is the mainstay of treatment.

During infancy, the risk of malignant germ cell tumors increases with age but may vary according to tumor site (Schneider et al. 2004). In a large series of teratomas registered to the German MAKEI studies, all children older than 1 year suffered from malignant germ cell tumors with yolk sac tumor as the leading histology (Göbel et al. 1998). This observation supports the meta-analysis of Kerner et al. that included children with malignant cervical germ cell tumors (Kerner et al. 1998). However, the biological switch from histologically benign teratomas to mixed malignant germ cell tumors with yolk sac tumor elements remains to be elucidated for this specific tumor site. In sacrococcygeal germ cell tumors, which contribute about 40% of all germ cell tumors in pediatric registries, the risk for malignant overgrowth rises after the second month of life. Prior to the age of 2 months, the incidence of malignant germ cell tumors was 10% in males and 7% in females, whereas at 6 months two thirds of the boys and about half of the girls had malignant tumors. In contrast, all germ cell tumors of the vagina registered in the MAKEI registry occurred in early childhood (<2 years), and the exclusive histology was yolk sac tumor (Mauz-Körholz et al. 2000). Again, these site-specific patterns illustrate the varying malignant potential of germ cell tumors depending on age, sex, and primary site.

In conclusion, optimal pre- and perinatal management is essential for successful management of head and neck germ cell tumors. The recommended clinical approach to prenatally detected teratomas includes repeated ultrasound and fetal MRI (of available), allowing for an optimized timing of delivery. Rapid tumor growth in utero may then necessitate a premature elective cesarean section. It is apparent that children with suspected large head and neck germ cell tumors should be referred to tertiary care centers that may provide optimal interdisciplinary management, including experienced neonatologists, pediatric anesthesiologists, pediatric oncologists, and pediatric ear and nose surgeons. Infants should be delivered through cesarean section, and in case of respiratory distress, immediate laryngotracheal intubation is required. To our knowledge cricotomy is required infrequently.

12.4 Prognosis

With a multidisciplinary approach, patients with germ cell tumors of the head and neck region have a favorable chance of survival and cure from their tumors. The optimal perinatal and neonatal management, in particular postnatal life support in case of airway obstruction, strongly determines long-term outcome and presumably also neurological outcome if neonatal hypoxia can be avoided.

The oncologic prognosis is then determined by surgical experience and the ability to completely remove the tumor. Nevertheless, even with optimal management, patients may still suffer from late sequelae. These are predominantly related to local complications caused by the tumor or surgical therapy. Therefore, one important future issue will be to evaluate in how far early maybe even prenatal interventions or a centralization of the treatment to both neonatologic and pediatric oncologic centers will help to reduce or even avoid some of these handicaps.

References

Alexander VR, Manjaly JG, Pepper CM, Ifeacho SN, Hewitt RJ, Hartley BE (2015) Head and neck teratomas in children—A series of 23 cases at Great Ormond Street Hospital. Int J Pediatr Otorhinolaryngol 79:2008–2014

Berge SJ, von Lindern JJ, Appel T, Braumann B, Niederhagen B (2004) Diagnosis and management of cervical teratomas. Br J Oral Maxillofac Surg 42:41–45

Bernbeck B, Schneider DT, Bernbeck B, Koch S, Teske C, Lentrodt J, Harms D, Göbel U, Calaminus G (2009) Germ cell tumors of the head and neck: report from the MAKEI Study Group. Pediatr Blood Cancer 52:223–226

Blohm ME, Vesterling-Hörner D, Calaminus G, Göbel U (1998) Alpha 1-fetoprotein (AFP) reference values in infants up to 2 years of age. Pediatr Hematol Oncol 15:135–142

Brodsky JR, Irace AL, Didas A et al (2017) Teratoma of the neonatal head and neck: a 41-year experience. Int J Pediatr Otorhinolaryngol 97:66–71

De Backer A, Madern GC, van de Ven CP, Tibboel D, Hazebroek FW (2004) Strategy for management of newborns with cervical teratoma. J Perinat Med 32:500–508

Dharmarajan H, Rouillard-Bazinet N, Chandy BM (2018) Mature and immature pediatric head and neck teratomas: a 15-year review at a large tertiary center. Int J Pediatr Otorhinolaryngol 105:43–47

Dunn CJ, Nguyen DL, Leonard JC (1992) Ultrasound diagnosis of immature cervical teratoma: a case report. Am J Perinatol 9:445–447

Epperson MV, Born HL, Wang D, Myer CM (2020) Yolk sac tumors of the head and neck in Aicardi syndrome. Ann Otol Rhinol Laryngol 129:301–305

Göbel U, Calaminus G, Engert J, Kaatsch P, Gadner H, Bökkerink JP, Hass RJ, Waag K, Blohm ME, Dippert S, Teske C, Harms D (1998) Teratomas in infancy and childhood. Med Pediatr Oncol 31:8–15

Hullett BJ, Shine NP, Chambers NA (2006) Airway management of three cases of congenital cervical teratoma. Paediatr Anaesth 16:794–798

Jordan RB, Gauderer MW (1988) Cervical teratomas: an analysis. Literature review and proposed classification. J Pediatr Surg 23:583–591

Kerner B, Flaum E, Mathews H, Carlson DE, Pepkowitz SH, Hixon H, Graham JM Jr (1998) Cervical teratoma: prenatal diagnosis and long-term follow-up. Prenat Diagn 18:51–59

Langer JC, Tabb T, Thompson P, Paes BA, Caco CC (1992) Management of prenatally diagnosed tracheal obstruction: access to the airway in utero prior to delivery. Fetal Diagn Ther 7:12–16

Liechty KW, Crombleholme TM, Flake AW, Morgan MA, Kurth CD, Hubbard AM, Adzick NS (1997) Intrapartum airway management for giant fetal neck masses: the EXIT (ex utero intrapartum treatment) procedure. Am J Obstet Gynecol 177:870–874

Martino F, Avila LF, Encinas JL, Luis AL, Olivares P, Lassaletta L, Nistal M, Tovar JA (2006) Teratomas of the neck and mediastinum in children. Pediatr Surg Int 22:627–634

Mauz-Körholz C, Harms D, Calaminus G, Göbel U (2000) Primary chemotherapy and conservative surgery for vaginal yolk-sac tumour. Maligne Keimzelltumoren Study Group. Lancet 355:625

Schneider DT, Calaminus G, Koch S, Teske C, Schmidt P, Haas RJ, Harms D, Göbel U (2004) Epidemiologic analysis of 1,442 children and adolescents registered in the German germ cell tumor protocols. Pediatr Blood Cancer 42:169–175

13 Odontogenic Tumors

Jan Godzinski, Roberto Bianchi, and Marco Guzzo

Odontogenic tumors (OT) derive from epithelial, ectomesenchymal, and/or mesenchymal elements that still are or have been part of the tooth-forming apparatus. Therefore, they are found exclusively within the maxillofacial skeleton or in the soft tissue overlying tooth-bearing areas. These tumors are classified according to the fourth WHO histological classification published in 2017. In comparison with the previous edition, a number of significant change and simplifications have been introduced. Three new entities have been identified including the rare primordial odontogenic tumor that has been mainly reported in children (El Naggar et al. 2017) and the exceeding rare odontogenic carcinosarcoma reported by Chikosi (Schuch et al. 2018) in a 9-year-old child. It is also worth considering that the new classification reintroduced the terms odontogenic keratocyst (OKT) and calcifying odontogenic cyst (COC) since these lesions may be encountered in children. These entities behave clinically as non-neoplastic lesions and should be treated accordingly. There are few reports on OT in children (Adebayo et al. 2002; Asamoa et al. 1990; Guerrisi et al. 2007; Ulmansky et al. 1999). The literature shows these neoplasms accounted for between 1.0 and 28.8% of the oral lesion (Ulmansky et al. 1999; Soluk Tekkesin et al. 2016; Ataide et al. 2016).

Comparative studies of OT in children are difficult because various authors use differing classifications; age groups and patients are of different racial origins. Basically, all the defined histotypes can occur in children although most of them and particularly the malignant counterpart are rare in such patients.

The most common OT in children are reported in Tables 13.1 and 13.2. There appears to be a racial predilection for OT types.

13.1 Ameloblastoma

Ameloblastoma, or adamantinoma as this tumor was named before 1930, is a rare benign tumor originating from odontogenic epithelium with mature, fibrous stroma without odontogenic ectomesenchyme. It is one of the most frequent OT in all age group, but the peak incidence is in the third to fourth decades. About 10–15% of them occurred in children. The new edition (2017) of the WHO classification has simplified the terminology around ameloblastoma. The previous subclassification in four types (solid/multicystic, extraosseous/peripheral, desmoplastic, and

J. Godzinski (✉)
Department of Pediatric Surgery, Marciniak Hospital and Department of Paediatric Traumatology and Emergency Medicine, Medical University, Wroclaw, Poland
e-mail: jgodzin@wp.pl

R. Bianchi · M. Guzzo
Otolaryngology Unit, Istituto Nazionale Tumori, Milan, Italy
e-mail: roberto.bianchi@istitutotumori.mi.it; marco.guzzo@istitutotumori.mi.it

D. T. Schneider et al. (eds.), *Rare Tumors in Children and Adolescents*, Pediatric Oncology,
https://doi.org/10.1007/978-3-030-92071-5_13

Table 13.1 Odontogenic tumors in children and adolescent. Review of the literature

Authors	No. of cases	Geographic area	Histotype	%
Soluk Tekkesin et al. (2016)	149	Turkey	Odontoma	40
			Ameloblastoma	20
			Myxoma	16
			Ameloblastic fibroma	4.6
			Others	
Ataide et al. (2016)	137	Brazil	Odontoma	58
			Ameloblastoma	12
			Adenomatoid odontogenic tumor	7.2
			Odontogenic fibroma	6.5
			Others	
Adebayo et al. (2002)	78	Nigeria	Ameloblastoma	54
			Myxoma	19
			Adenomatoid odontogenic tumor	9
			Ameloblastic fibroma	8
			Odontoma	9
			Others	
Guerrisi et al. (2007)	153	Argentina	Odontoma	50
			Ameloblastoma	18.3
			Myxoma	8.5
			Adenomatoid odontogenic tumor	5.2
			Others	
Jones and Franklin (2006)	243	United Kingdom	Odontoma	79.4
			Adenomatoid odontogenic tumor	4
			Ameloblastoma	3.7
			Ameloblastic fibroma	3.3
			Others	
Ulmansky et al. (1999)	18	Israel	Myxoma	38.8
			Ameloblastic fibroma	22.2
			Ameloblastic fibro-odontoma	22.2
			Ameloblastoma	11
			Others	
Sato et al. (1997)	79	Japan	Odontoma	59.5
			Ameloblastoma	34
			Others	

unicystic) has been considered lacking in behavioral or biological significance. Ameloblastomas are now subdivided in three types: "conventional" ameloblastoma type which includes other variants such as desmoplastic, follicular, plexiform, and acanthomatous; extraosseous/peripheral; and unicystic ameloblastoma. Many studies reported that the unicystic type is the most common type in children (Ord et al. 2002; Bansal et al. 2015). Others show that the rate of solid type is higher than unicystic type (Zhang et al. 2010; Ord et al. 2002). Unicystic ameloblastoma is described as having three histological variants, two of these (luminal type and intraluminal type) are deemed to have better prognosis and rarely recur after enucleation. Conventional and unicystic types locate usually in the mandible (more than 90% of the cases). The mandible-to-maxilla ratio is 1:1 and 2.4:1 for desmoplastic and extraosseous type, respectively. In the mandible, the tumor has a marked predilection for the posterior region except in African Blacks in whom the tumor occurs in the symphysis (Chidzonga 1996). Localizations in other bones are described but very rarely (Kessler and Dominiquez 1986). Ameloblastomas in general grow slowly but may

Table 13.2 Diagnostic workflow of odontogenic tumors

Physical examination	In most benign tumors, signs and symptoms are scarce. Sometimes slow swelling of jaw and/or movement of teeth can be noted. Less frequently they can occur as painless exophytic-like lesion of the alveolar mucosa. In contrast, pain is the most frequent symptoms followed by rapid swelling of the bone in malignant odontogenic tumors
Laboratory assessment	None
Radiological assessment	
– First assessment	More often discovered incidentally during the course of routine intraoral dental (plain) radiographs or panoramic radiography
– Preoperative assessment	Panoramic radiography, CT
– FU	Panoramic radiography
Pathological assessment	Most odontogenic tumors are benign, and the diagnosis can be only achieved by clinical and radiological evaluations. Histological confirmation is often necessary and should be always obtained before planning a nonconservative surgery
Staging system (odontogenic carcinomas)	Usually, it is not applied
Grading system (odontogenic carcinomas)	Malignant odontogenic tumors are exceedingly rare in children and are usually highly aggressive. Grading is still defined by histotype
General treatment guidelines	Need for multidisciplinary approach
	Need for referral to center with expert physicians professionally dedicated to the management of this neoplasms in adults (or strict collaboration with them)
– Surgery	Keystone of treatment. Complete segmental bone resection, enucleation, or curettage according to histotypes. Immediate bone graft is recommended in order to prevent facial deformity
– Radiotherapy	High-grade tumors are very rare
– Chemotherapy	Palliative intent

markedly deform involved portions of the bone. Diagnosis based on clinical appearance may reveal swelling of the corresponding area of face and mandible or maxillary intraosseous mass. Pain or paresthesia is rare. Solid/multicystic types may be diagnosed as unilocular or multilocular (soap bubble-like) radiolucencies at panograph X-ray or CT scan. An unerupted tooth may be associated. The roots of the involved tooth may be eroded. Despite characteristic imaging, microscopic confirmation of diagnosis is recommended. Unicystic type radiographically presents as a unilocular, often pericoronal radiolucency that may also be associated with an unerupted tooth. Desmoplastic ameloblastoma shows a pronounced stromal component compressing the odontogenic epithelial component. Consequently, about 50% of them are radiographically present as a mottled, mixed radiolucency/radiopacity with ill-defined borders. Extraosseous ameloblastoma usually is located to the alveolar mucosa in edentulous area. This tumor grows as an exophytic-like lesion determining a superficial erosion of the bone crest due to pressure resorption (Stevenson and Austin 1990) (Figs. 13.1, 13.2, 13.3, 13.4, 13.5, 13.6, and 13.7).

Once the diagnosis is established, the treatment may be planned. Surgery is the treatment of choice. In children, the decision for treatment strategy should be made according to the patient's age, tumor size, location, and whether it is a primary or a recurring tumor. Resection usually creates fewer difficulties than reconstruction of the mandible. Although ameloblastoma is not a malignant disease, surgeons must keep in mind that complete excision of this locally aggressive tumor is the mainstay of treatment. Enucleation or curettage leads to risk of recurrence as high as 25–40%. The block resection of the tumor with subsequent reconstruction with bone graft is routinely recommended. In more advanced cases,

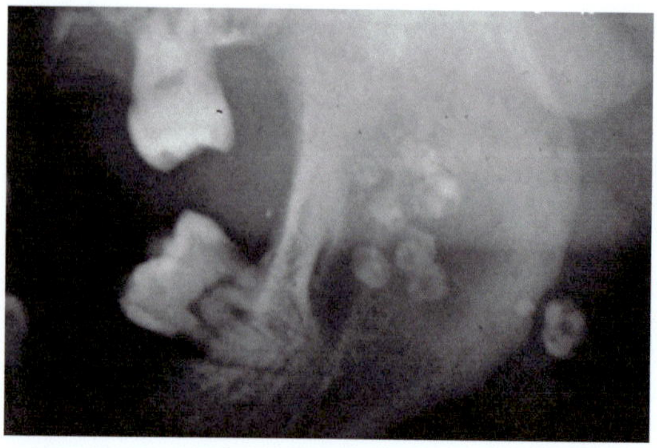

Fig. 13.1 Odontoma compound type in an 18-year-old girl

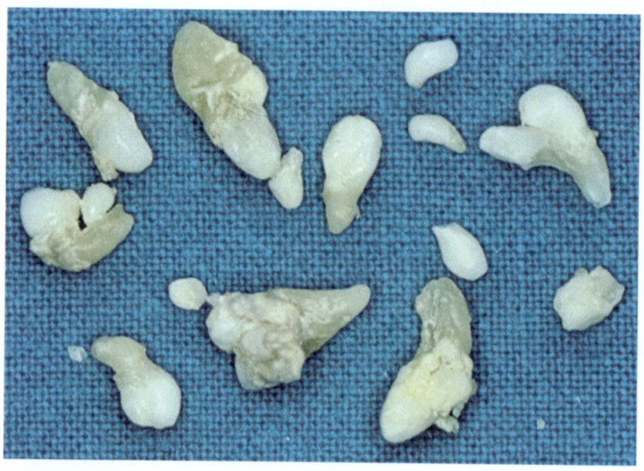

Fig. 13.2 Macroscopic specimen of odontoma compound type in an 18-year-old girl

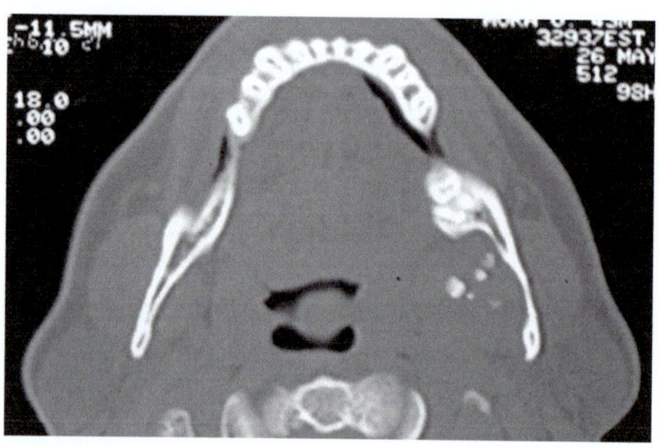

Fig. 13.3 Computed tomography of odontoma compound type in an 18-year-old girl

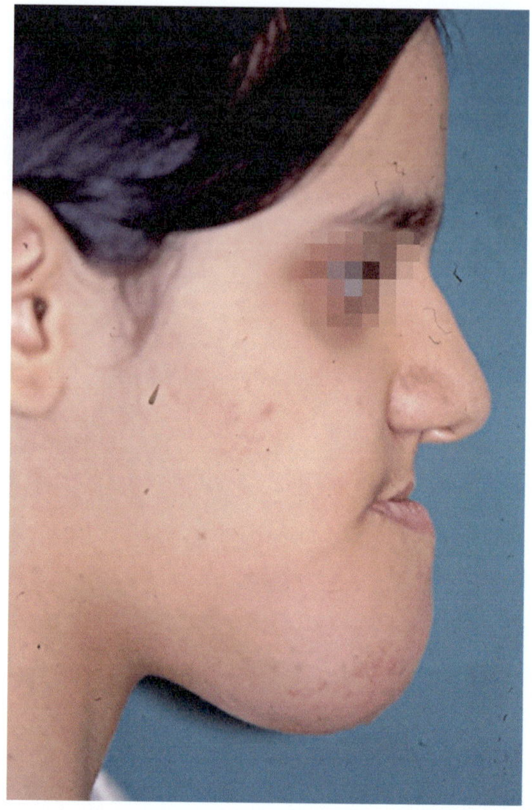

Fig. 13.4 Cementoblastoma in a 17-year-old girl

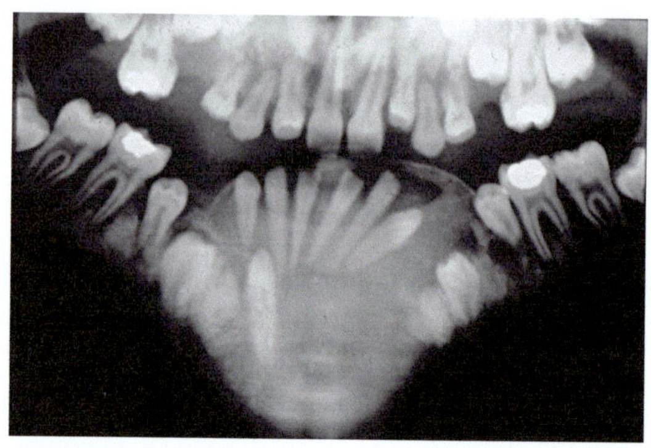

Fig. 13.5 Ortho-panoramic X-ray of cementoblastoma in a 17-year-old girl

the segmental resection of mandible followed by complete reconstruction may be necessary. Biopsy for histological confirmation is often necessary and should be always obtained before planning a nonconservative surgery (Zhang et al. 2010). Two variants of unicystic ameloblastoma are thought to recur less frequently than other subtypes; thus some authors advocate also less aggressive treatment in this form of tumor and reserve more aggressive surgery for any recurrence (Speight and Takata 2018).

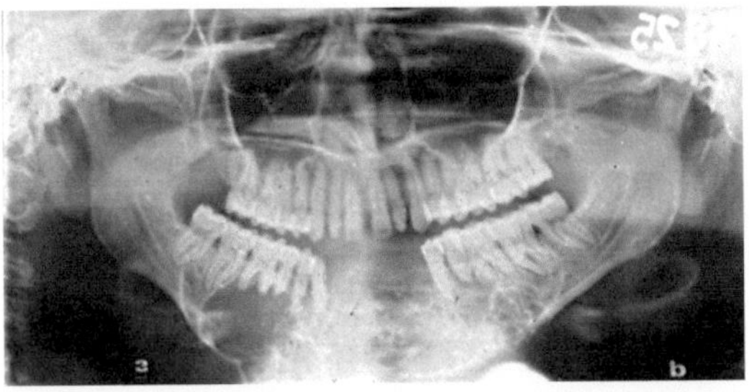

Fig. 13.6 Ortho-panoramic X-ray of ameloblastoma of the mandible extending from 4.7 to 3.7

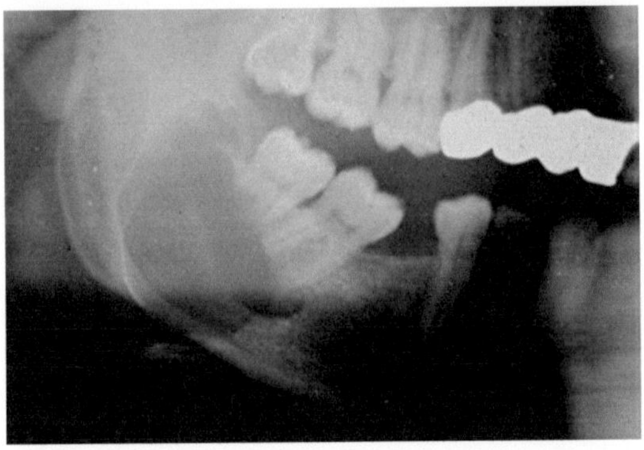

Fig. 13.7 Ortho-panoramic X-ray of ameloblastoma of the right mandible. Unilocular radiolucency resembling cysts with scalloped borders

The tumor usually recurs in between 1 and 15 years of follow-up with a peak within 5 years from surgery (Ord et al. 2002). Consequently, a long-term postoperative follow-up seems reasonable.

The complementary treatments, as chemotherapy or radiotherapy, are of limited value. In spite of a benign histologic aspect, some ameloblastoma may spread distant metastases, mainly to the lungs (metastasizing ameloblastoma). Moreover, an ameloblastic carcinoma may arise from a benign ameloblastoma either intraosseous or peripheral.

References

Adebayo ET, Ajike SO, Adekeye EO (2002) Odontogenic tumours in children and adolescents: a study of 78 Nigerian cases. J Craniomaxillofac Surg 30(5):267–272

Asamoa EA, Ayanlere AO, Olaitan AA, Adekeye EO (1990) Paediatric tumours of the jaws in northern Nigeria. Clinical presentation and treatment. J Craniomaxillofac Surg 18(3):130–135

Ataide AP, Fonseca FP, Santos Silva AR, Jorge Junior J, Lopes MA, Vargas PA (2016) Distribution of oral and maxillofacial lesions in pediatric patients from a Brazilian southeastern population. Int J Pediatr Otorhinolaryngol 90:241–244

Bansal S, Desai RS, Shirsat P, Prasad P, Karjodkar F, Andrade N (2015) The occurrence and pattern of ameloblastoma in children and adolescents: an Indian Institutional Study of 41 years and review of the literature. Int J Oral Maxillofac Surg 44:725–731

Chidzonga MM (1996) Ameloblastoma in children. The Zimbabwean experience. Oral Surg Oral Med Oral Pathol Oral Radiol Endod 81(2):168–170

El Naggar A, Chan J, Grandis J, Takata T, Slootweg P (2017) In: International Agency for Research on Cancer (IARC) (ed.) Classification of head and neck tumors, 4th edn. WHO OMS, Lyon

Guerrisi M, Piloni MJ, Keszler A (2007) Odontogenic tumors in children and adolescents. A 15-year retrospective study in Argentina. Med Oral Patol Oral Cir Bucal 12(3):E180–E185

Jones AV, Franklin CD (2006) An analysis of oral and maxillofacial pathology found in children over a 30-year period. Int J Paediatr Dent 16(1):19–30

Kessler A, Dominiquez FZ (1986) Ameloblastoma in childhood. J Oral Maxillofac Surg 44:609–611, ref type: generic

Ord RA, Blanchaert RH Jr, Nikitakis NG, Sauk JJ (2002) Ameloblastoma in children. J Oral Maxillofac Surg 60(7):762–770

Sato M, Tanaka N, Sato T, Amagasa T (1997) Oral and maxillofacial tumours in children: a review. Br J Oral Maxillofac Surg 35(2):92–95

Schuch LF, de Arruda JAA, Silva LVO, Abreu LG, Silva TA, Mesquita RA (2018) Odontogenic carcinosarcoma: a systematic review. Oral Oncol 85:52–59

Soluk Tekkesin M, Tuna EB, Olgac V, Aksakalli N, Alatli C (2016) Odontogenic lesions in a pediatric population: review of the literature and presentation of 745 cases. Int J Pediatr Otorhinolaryngol 86:196–199

Speight PM, Takata T (2018) New tumour entities in the 4th edition of the world health organization classification of head and neck tumours: odontogenic and maxillofacial bone tumours. Virchows Arch 472:331–339

Stevenson AR, Austin BW (1990) A case of ameloblastoma presenting as an exophytic gingival lesion. J Periodontol 61(6):378–381

Ulmansky M, Lustmann J, Balkin N (1999) Tumors and tumor-like lesions of the oral cavity and related structures in Israeli children. Int J Oral Maxillofac Surg 28(4):291–294

Zhang J, Gu Z, Jiang L, Zhao J, Tian M, Zhou J et al (2010) Ameloblastoma in children and adolescents. Br J Oral Maxillofac Surg 48(7):549–554

14 Salivary Gland Tumors

Marco Guzzo and Jan Godzinski

14.1 Introduction

Inflammatory tumors and benign cysts represent the major cause of salivary gland enlargements in children. In case of a tumor, hemangioma is the most common histotype within the salivary glands in these patients (Baker and Malone 1985; Lack and Upton 1988). The high percentage of vascular tumors reported by many authors exceeds the number of cases registered with the Armed Force Institute of Pathology (AFIP). In fact, the large experience of the AFIP reports benign mesenchymal tumors occurring in only 12.3% (8.1% hemangiomas) of all cases of salivary gland tumors under the age of 17 years, while 42.5% of these cases are benign and 42.9% are malignant epithelial tumors (Ellis et al. 1991).

14.2 Differential Diagnosis and Management of Rare Head and Neck Tumors

14.2.1 Hemangioma

Hemangiomas occur almost exclusively in the parotid gland with a female to male ratio of 2:1. This tumor usually evolves in three clinical phases: they may rapidly enlarge to reach their largest size over a period of 6–8 months. Then, after a second period of 22–24 months, they begin a last period of regression.

The adequate diagnosis is usually possible on the basis of clinical appearance and noninvasive diagnostic techniques. Open biopsy can be often avoided since ultrasound, computed tomography (CT) scan, and magnetic resonance imaging (MRI) are reported to give an accurate picture of the disease.

Management of hemangioma varies from surgical excision and/or systemic treatment with propranolol to wait-and-see policy expecting spontaneous regressions. Many authors recommend avoiding futile surgical removal of hemangioma from infant patient until after the patient has reached school age. In fact, it has been estimated that up to 80% of hemangioma in infants involute by the age of 7. Thus, no more than 20% of them need surgical treatment. Surgery should be only considered if medical therapy will be ineffective and for aesthetical purpose after medical treatment.

Up today a number of guidelines and consensus paper have been published ((Drolet et al. 2013; Ho et al. 2019) since propranolol was introduced to the treatment of hemangioma in 2008 (Leute-Labreze et al. 2008). Propranolol has been reported as the most promising drug for the treatment of hemangioma in infancy. The treatment is generally well tolerated; however,

M. Guzzo (✉)
Fondazione IRCCS Istituto Tumori, Milan, Italy
e-mail: marco.guzzo@istitutotumori.mi.it

J. Godzinski
Department of Pediatric Surgery, Medical University of Wroclaw, Wroclaw, Poland

D. T. Schneider et al. (eds.), *Rare Tumors in Children and Adolescents*, Pediatric Oncology,
https://doi.org/10.1007/978-3-030-92071-5_14

the side effect profile can include hypersomnolence, reflux, bronchospasm, hypotension hypoglycemia, and, rarely, failure to thrive. Although no relevant cardiac and hemodynamic changes were noted during β-blocker treatment, a safety protocol before starting the therapy, including cardiac ultrasonography and cardiac examination, is mandatory (Buckmiller 2009; Leboulanger et al. 2010; Schiestl et al. 2010). Steroids, interferon, and, to some extent, laser therapy have limited applications.

14.2.2 Epithelial Salivary Gland Neoplasms

Epithelial salivary gland neoplasms are infrequent both in adults and children, accounting for <3% of all head and neck tumors. About 5% of them occur in patients <18 years of age with mean and median age of 14.2 years old (Fig. 14.1). Compared to adults, a slight female preponderance (female to male ratio of 1:4) and a higher occurrence in black children/adolescents were observed. Childhood survivor of cancer treated with radio and chemotherapy had increased risk of developing secondary salivary gland cancer. Moreover, Thariat reported that 6% of secondary cancer in children are salivary gland mucoepidermoid carcinoma (Thariat et al. 2013). Over 30 histologic subtypes of salivary gland neoplasm have been described in adults; however a smaller number of these have been reported in the pediatric population (El Naggar et al. 2017; Zamani et al. 2019) Among benign tumors, pleomorphic adenomas account for more than 70% of pediatric cases, and mucoepidermoid carcinomas represent about 50% of malignant cases, followed by acinic cell carcinomas (34.6%) and adenoid cystic carcinomas (5.3%) (Sultan et al. 2011). Data collected from the literature (Tables 14.1 and 14.2) showed that in children, malignant tumors accounted for about 37% of cases and similar figure is also reported by the adult literature. Different in children is the distribution of benign and malignant histotypes among the sali-

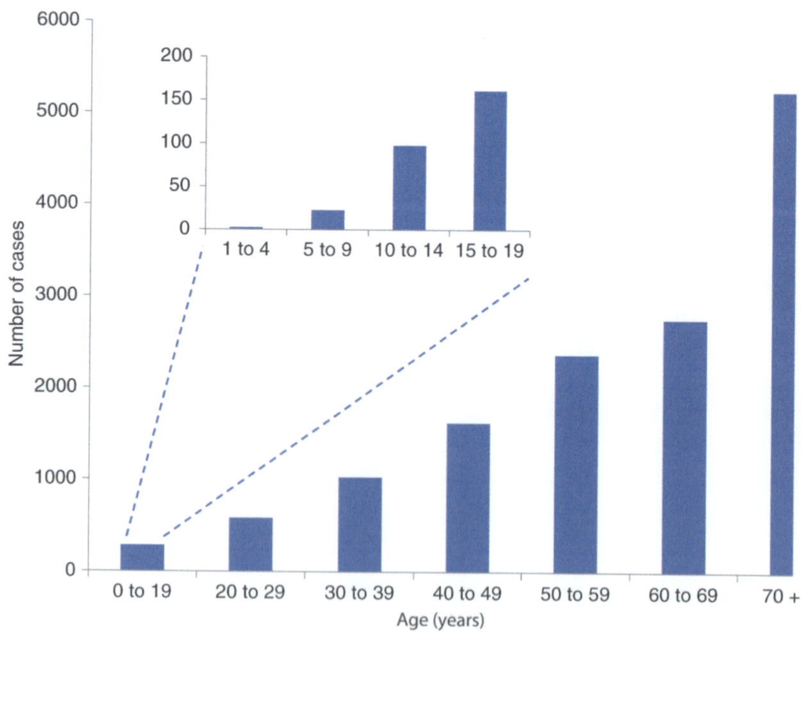

Fig. 14.1 Age distribution of patients with salivary gland tumors in the SEER 17 database (1973–2007). The window shows the age distribution of children/adolescents. (Courtesy of Dr. Iyad Sultan, King Hussein Cancer Center, Amman, Jordan)

Table 14.1 Epithelial salivary gland tumors in children. Review of series reported in the English literature. Distribution by site and histology

	No. of cases	Parotid		Submandibular gland		Others	
Authors		Benign tumors	Malignant tumors	Benign tumors	Malignant tumors	Benign tumors	Malignant tumors
Lack and Upton (1988)	25	5	13	4	–	1	2
Callender et al. (1992)	29	6	18	1	3	1	
De Cassia Braga Ribeiro et al. (2002)	38	4	20	5	2	2	5
Shikhani and Johns (1988)	21	14	2	4	1		
Baker and Malone (1985)	13	–	12	–	1		
Fonseca et al. (1991)	24	12	6	3		2	1
Rogers et al. (1994)	8	–	7	–	1		
Orvidas et al. (2000)	43	27	16	ND	ND	ND	ND
Ethunandan et al. (2003)	12	9	3	ND	ND	ND	ND
Kessler and Handler (1994)	15	6	6	1	2		
Guzzo et al. (2006)	52	32	9	4	1	1	5
Laikui et al. (2008)	79	25	9	13	3	22	7
Deng et al. (2013)	119	39	14	26	4	22	14
Fang et al. (2013)	122	73	15	21	0	11	2
Xu et al. (2017)	57	15	21	3	4	1	13
Total	657	267	171	85	22	63	49
Parotid	438 (67%)	61%	39%				
Submandibular gland	107 (16%)			79%	21%		
Others	112 (17%)						

ND no data, parotid tumors only

vary gland. Malignant tumors affected the parotid gland in about 40% of published pediatric series, while in the submandibular gland, benign neoplasms were four times as frequent as malignant tumors. In adults, malignant tumors comprised 25–32% of tumors of the parotid gland and 40–50% of submandibular gland neoplasms. In a large meta-analysis of 364 patients with cancer, 72% of the children had tumors in the parotid gland and 21% and 8% in the minor salivary gland and submandibular gland, respectively (Zamani et al. 2019) (Fig. 14.2).

It is of interest that in young patients, malignant tumors have been diagnosed as low to intermediate grade in about 87% of the cases (<50% in adults).

The leading symptom of epithelial salivary gland neoplasms is usually painless swelling within the parotid or—less frequently—the submandibular gland. Imaging includes ultrasound and MRI (CT) to define local-regional extension of the disease. Core biopsy seems better than fine-needle aspiration (Ramirez-Perez et al. 2017; Song et al. 2015) biopsy, and it may be helpful in pretreatment confirmation of the nature of the disease but is strongly suggested in the case of submandibular swelling since tumors are very rare in that region.

Surgery is the mainstay of treatment for both benign and malignant tumors. Parotidectomy (superficial or total) seems to be the best approach for achieving surgical resection of the neoplasms

Table 14.2 Salivary gland malignant tumor grading system

• Tumors in which grading is still defined by histotype:
– Low-grade carcinoma
Acinic cell carcinoma (frequent P)
Basal cell carcinoma (very rare SM)
Intraductal carcinoma (rare P)
Secretory carcinoma (very rare P)
Sialoblastoma (very rare P)
– High-grade carcinoma
Salivary duct carcinoma (very rare P)
Squamous cell carcinoma (very rare P)
• Tumors in which specific grading system is applied:
– Adenocarcinoma, NOS (not common SM MSG)
Grading according to the cytologic variability
– Adenoid cystic carcinoma (common P; SM)
Intermediate vs. high grade, depending on histologic patterns
– Mucoepidermoid carcinoma (very frequent P, SM; MSG)
Low vs. intermediate vs. high grade, depending on five histopathologic features
– Carcinoma ex pleomorphic adenoma (rare SM)
Grading correlated with histologic subtype of the carcinoma component

P parotid, *SM* submandibular gland, *MSG* minor salivary gland

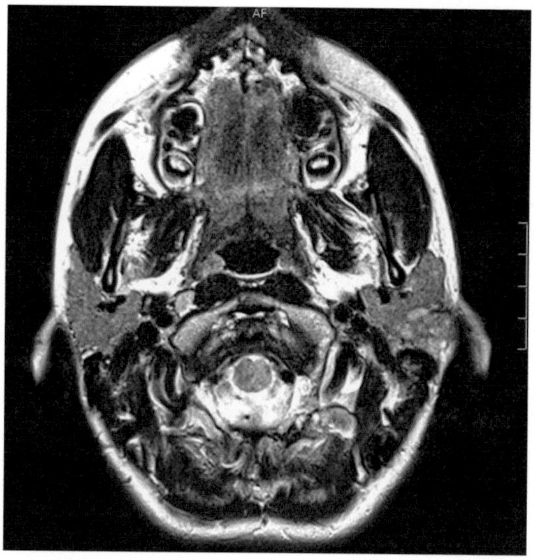

Fig. 14.2 Mucoepidermoid carcinoma of the left parotid gland in a 15-year-old girl

with clear margins. Since the tumors usually arise in the superficial glandular lobe, the formal identification and dissection of the facial nerve followed by the resection of the suprafacial portion of the gland (superficial parotidectomy) represent the safest approach both for nerve preservation and oncological purpose. In young patients, postoperative facial nerve injury is a critical risk in parotid surgery compared with adults. Tumor resection or limited excision of the parotid and submandibular gland is discouraged because of high risk of incomplete tumor removal. Moreover, high risk of nerve damage should be expected when the operation is performed without the formal identification of the facial nerve. The use of intraoperative facial nerve monitoring is a matter of debate all around the word. However, this procedure is increasing in Europe and in the United States. It seems to decrease the risk of immediate postoperative nerve weakness and to reduce the duration of surgery (Liu et al. 2015; Sood et al. 2015).

For benign tumors, local relapses after limited resection and superficial parotidectomy are reported to be 39% and 19%, respectively. For malignant tumors, local recurrences were seen in 48% and 31% of the cases after limited or standard surgery, respectively (Shikhani and Johns 1988). About 90% of the young patients with malignant tumors are diagnosed as clinically N0 (70% in adults), and occult metastases in the neck are rare (17% in the series reported by Rebours) (Rebours et al. 2017). Consequently, simultaneous neck dissection is recommended only when neck metastases are detectable.

The role of radiotherapy in salivary gland tumors remains controversial (Guzzo et al. 2006; Sessions et al. 1993; Rebours et al. 2017). The presence of high-grade malignancies, a large and aggressive tumor mass, involvement of multiple levels of cervical lymph nodes, and microscopically incomplete resection are considered the main indications for irradiation. However, in children—

given the higher risk of postirradiation complications, such as facial growth retardation, dental anomalies, and second malignant neoplasms—radiotherapy is usually recommended in highly selected cases only. Excellent outcome with only mild to moderate side effects during the treatment and no severe radiation associated late sequels are recently reported by Mao with postoperative 125I seed brachytherapy for the treatment of mucoepidermoid carcinoma (Mao et al. 2017).

There are limited clinical data to help define the role of systemic therapy in the palliative management of salivary gland cancer. Conventional cytotoxic regimens include cyclophosphamide, Adriamycin, cisplatinum, (CAP), and 5-fluorouracil (FACP) combinations. Platinum-based polychemotherapy is usually preferred for symptomatic locally recurrent or metastatic disease not amenable with further surgery or radiotherapy. The immunohistochemical and molecular profile of pediatric salivary cancer is recently investigated by Locati et al. (Locati et al. 2017) The authors concluded that they are very similar to that described in adult case with also CRTC1/MAML2 gene fusion product found in 88% of the low-grade mucoepidermoid carcinoma. Targeted therapy with cetuximab (Erbitux)—a monoclonal antibody that binds to the epidermal growth factor receptor—in combination with cisplatin has been reported to have response rate > 40% and improved overall survival in adult patients with metastatic ACC (Hitre et al. 2013).

Malignant epithelial tumors of the salivary gland in children usually have a good prognosis. The 5-year overall survival ranges from 81 to 90%, reaching 100% in some series (Guzzo et al. 2006; Zamani et al. 2019). The general good prognosis in children is probably due to the more favorable clinical presentation; however, whether age-related differences in biology exist remains unclear (Sultan et al. 2011). It is recommended that children and adolescents with salivary gland tumors are referred to specialized centers, preferably in which cooperation between pediatric oncologist, ENT surgeon, and adult experts may optimize the chances for young patients to be cured with limited morbidity (Table 14.3).

14.2.3 Very Rare Entities

Two very rare conditions shall also be mentioned. The first is sialoblastoma—a rare congenital low-grade malignant tumor with a resemblance to fetal salivary tissue. The parotid gland is affected in more than 75% of the cases. This neoplasm requires surgical treatment that is curative in about two thirds of the cases. Recurrences are common and sometimes multiple. Distant metastases are also possible. The role of chemotherapy and radiotherapy for unresectable tumors or recurrences remains to be clarified (Dalal et al. 2009; Ellis and Auclair 2008); however, more recently, chemotherapy has shown promise in selected cases (Irace et al. 2016). Another one is a tumor-like condition which can occur in HIV-infected patients. It is more common in children than in adult. Parotid gland or sometimes submandibular gland swelling may be the first clinical manifestation of HIV infection. Most of these enlargements are probably acute infections, but either lymphoid hyperplasia or lymphoepithelial cysts and lymphoepithelial lesions (salivary diffuse infiltrative lymphocytosis syndrome) can be associated. Salivary gland swelling is usually bilateral and accompanied by cervical lymph node enlargement. Medical conservative treatment with antiviral drugs has been reported to be effective in controlling parotid swelling. Repeated fine-needle aspiration and drainage, surgery, and radiation therapy have also been used (Sessions et al. 1993; Ellis and Auclair 2008; Meer 2019; Shivhare et al. 2015).

Table 14.3 A general view: practical diagnostic and therapeutic guidelines for salivary glands tumors

Physical examination	Signs and symptoms: painless glandular swelling. Parotid gland and, less frequently, submandibular gland. Rarely in the minor salivary gland of the soft and hard palate
	Anamnesis: an average duration of the symptoms of 12 months
	Children >10 years of age
Laboratory assessment	Exclude infection, acute inflammation, and lymphoma
Radiological assessment	
– First assessment	Ultrasonography
– Preop assessment	Magnetic resonance
Pathological assessment	FNAB mandatory (core biopsy preferred)
	Delay surgery when inflammatory tumors or cysts are suspected
Staging system (carcinomas of the mayor salivary glands)	TNM UICC AJCC (El Naggar et al. 2017)
	T1: tumor 2 cm or less in greatest dimension without extraparenchymal extension[a]
	T2: tumor more than 2 cm but not more than 4 cm in greatest dimension without extraparenchymal extension[a]
	T3: tumor more than 4 cm and/or tumor with extraparenchymal extension[a]
	T4a: tumor invades the skin, mandible, ear canal, and/or facial nerve
	T4b: tumor invades base of the skull and/or pterygoid plates and/or encase carotid artery
	Nx: regional lymph node metastasis cannot be assessed
	N0: no regional lymph node metastasis
	N1: metastasis in a single ipsilateral lymph node, 3 cm or less in greatest dimension
	N2: metastasis as described below
	– N2a: metastasis in a single ipsilateral lymph node, 3–6 cm
	– N2b: metastasis in multiple ipsilateral lymph nodes, <6 cm
	– N2c: metastasis in bilateral or contralateral lymph nodes, <6 cm
	N3a: metastasis in lymph node >6 cm without extranodal extension
	N3b: metastasis in lymph node >6 cm with clinical extranodal extension
	M0: no distant metastasis
	M1: distant metastasis
Stage grouping	Stage I: T1 N0 M0
	Stage II: T2 N0 M0
	Stage III: T3 N0 M0; T1, T2, T3 N1 M0
	Stage IVA: T4a, T4b N0 N1 M0; T1, T2, T3, T4a N2 M0
	Stage IVB: T4b any N M0; any T N3 M0
	Stage VIC: any T, any N M1
General treatment guidelines	Need for multidisciplinary approach
	Need for referral to primary oncology center with expert physicians professionally dedicated to the management of this cancer in adults (or strict collaboration with them)
– Surgery	Keystone of treatment
	Parotidectomy (superficial or total) is the best approach on primary
	Neck dissection is recommended only when neck metastases are clinically detected
– Radiotherapy	Recommended limiting radiation in selected patients (very rare high-grade tumors, in case of incomplete resection/irresectable tumors)
– Chemotherapy	No role

[a] Extraparenchymal extension is clinical or macroscopic evidence of invasion of soft tissue or nerve, except those listed under T4a and 4b. Microscopic evidence alone does not constitute extraparenchymal extension for classification purposes

References

Baker SR, Malone B (1985) Salivary gland malignancies in children. Cancer 55:1730–1736

Buckmiller LM (2009) Propranolol for infantile hemangiomas. Curr Opin Otolaryngol Head Neck Surg 17:458–459

Callender DL et al (1992) Salivary gland neoplasms in children. Arch Otolaryngol Head Neck Surg 118:472–476

Dalal S et al (2009) Sialoblastoma: a rare pediatric tumour of the salivary glands. Internet J Surg 2(2)

de Cassia Braga Ribeiro K et al (2002) Epithelial salivary glands neoplasms in children and adolescent: a forty-four-year experience. Med Pediatr Oncol 39: 594–600

Deng R, Huang X, Hao J, Ding J, Hu Q (2013) Salivary gland neoplasms in children. J Craniofac Surg 24(2):511–513. https://doi.org/10.1097/SCS.0b013e3182801866. PMID: 23524728

Drolet BA, Frommelt PC, Chamlin SL et al (2013) Initiation and use of propranolol for infantile hemangioma: report of a consensus conference. Pediatrics 131:128–140

El Naggar A, Chan J, Grandis J, Takata T, Slootweg P (2017) In: International Agency for Research on Cancer (IARC) (ed). Classification of head and neck tumors. 4th edn. WHO OMS, Lyon

Ellis GL, Auclair PL (2008) Tumors of the salivary glands. AFIP, Washington

Ellis GL et al (1991) Armed Force Institute of Pathology (AFIP) surgical pathology of the salivary glands. W.B. Saunders Company, Philadelphia

Ethunandan M et al (2003) Parotid neoplasms in children: experience of diagnosis and management in a district general hospital. Int J Oral Maxillofac Surg 32:373–377

Fang QG, Shi S, Li ZN, Zhang X, Liu FY, Sun CF (2013) Epithelial salivary gland tumors in children: a twenty-five-year experience of 122 patients. Int J Pediatr Otorhinolaryngol 77(8):1252–1254. https://doi.org/10.1016/j.ijporl.2013.04.034. Epub 2013 Jun 6. PMID: 23746416

Fonseca I et al (1991) Epithelial salivary gland tumors of children and adolescents in southern Portugal. Oral Surg Oral Med Oral Pathol 72:696–701

Guzzo M et al (2006) Salivary gland neoplasms in children: the experience of the Istituto Nazionale Tumori of Milan. Pediatr Blood Cancer 47(6):806–810

Hitre E, Budai B, Takacsi-Nagy Z et al (2013) Cetuximab and platinum-based chemoradio- or chemotherapy of patients with epidermal growth factor receptor expressing adenoid cystic carcinoma: a phase II trial. Br J Cancer 109:1117–1122

Ho W, Hoo C, Black C (2019) Treatment of infantile haemangioma—perspective of a regional surgical centre. Ulster Med J 88:102–104

Irace AL, Adil EA, Archer NM, Silvera VM, Perez-Atayde A, Rahbar R (2016) Pediatric sialoblastoma: evaluation and management. Int J Pediatr Otorhinolaryngol 87:44–49

Kessler A, Handler SD (1994) Salivary gland neoplasms in children: a 10-year survey at the Children's Hospital of Philadelphia. Int J Pediatr Otorhinolaryngol 29:195–202

Lack EE, Upton MP (1988) Histopathologic review of salivary gland tumors in childhood. Arch Otolaryngol Head Neck Surg 114:898–906

Laikui L, Hongwei L, Hongbing J, Zhixiu H (2008) Epithelial salivary gland tumors of children and adolescents in west China population: a clinicopathologic study of 79 cases. J Oral Pathol Med 37(4):201–205. https://doi.org/10.1111/j.1600-0714.2007.00618.x. Epub 2008 Jan 15. PMID: 18205745

Leboulanger N et al (2010) Propranolol in the therapeutic strategy of infantile laryngotracheal hemangioma: a preliminary retrospective study of French experience. Int J Pediatr Otorhinolaryngol 74:1254–1257

Leute-Labreze C et al (2008) Propranolol for severe haemangiomas of infancy. N Engl J Med 358(24):2649–2651

Liu SW, Jiang W, Zhang HQ et al (2015) Intraoperative neuromonitoring for removal of large vestibular schwannoma: facial nerve outcome and predictive factors. Clin Neurol Neurosurg 133:83–89

Locati LD, Collini P, Imbimbo M et al (2017) Immunohistochemical and molecular profile of salivary gland cancer in children. Pediatr Blood Cancer 64. https://doi.org/10.1002/pbc.26468. Epub 2017 Jan 31

Mao MH, Zheng L, Wang XM, Li H, Qin LZ, Zhang J, Han ZX, Zhang JG (2017) Surgery combined with postoperative 125 I seed brachytherapy for the treatment of mucoepidermoid carcinoma of the parotid gland in pediatric patients. Pediatr Blood Cancer 64(1):57–63. https://doi.org/10.1002/pbc.26217. Epub 2017 Aug 31. PMID: 27576792

Meer S (2019) Human immunodeficiency virus and salivary gland pathology: an update. Oral Surg Oral Med Oral Pathol Oral Radiol 128(1):52–59

Orvidas LJ et al (2000) Pediatric parotid masses. Arch Otolaryngol Head Neck Surg 126:177–184

Ramirez-Perez F, Gonzalez-Garcia R, Hernandez-Vila C, Monje-Gil F, Ruiz-Laza L (2017) Is fine-needle aspiration a reliable tool in the diagnosis of malignant salivary gland tumors? J Craniomaxillofac Surg 45:1074–1077

Rebours C, Couloigner V, Galmiche L et al (2017) Pediatric salivary gland carcinomas: diagnostic and therapeutic management. Laryngoscope 127: 140–147

Rogers DA et al (1994) Primary malignancy of the salivary gland in children. J Pediatr Surg 26:44–47

Schiestl C et al (2010) Efficacy and safety of propranolol as first-line treatment for infantile hemangiomas. Eur J Pediatr 170(4):493–501

Sessions RB et al (1993) Tumors of the salivary glands and paragangliomas. In: DeVitta V, Hellman S, Rosenberg SA (eds) Cancer: principles and practice of oncology. JB Lippincott, Philadelphia

Shikhani AH, Johns ME (1988) Tumors of the major salivary glands in children. Head Neck 10:257–263

Shivhare P, Shankarnarayan L, Jambunath U, Basavaraju SM (2015) Benign lymphoepithelial cysts of parotid and submandibular glands in a HIV-positive patient. J Oral Maxillofac Pathol 19:107

Song IH, Song JS, Sung CO et al (2015) Accuracy of core needle biopsy versus fine needle aspiration cytology for diagnosing salivary gland tumors. J Pathol Transl Med 49:136–143

Sood AJ, Houlton JJ, Nguyen SA, Gillespie MB (2015) Facial nerve monitoring during parotidectomy: a systematic review and meta-analysis. Otolaryngol Head Neck Surg 152:631–637

Sultan I et al (2011) Salivary gland carcinomas in children and adolescents population-based study, with comparison to adult cases. Head Neck 33(10):1476–1481

Thariat J, Vedrine PO, Temam S et al (2013) The role of radiation therapy in pediatric mucoepidermoid carcinomas of the salivary glands. J Pediatr 162: 839–843

Xu B, Aneja A, Ghossein R, Katabi N (2017) Salivary gland epithelial neoplasms in pediatric population: a single-institute experience with a focus on the histologic spectrum and clinical outcome. Hum Pathol 67:37–44. https://doi.org/10.1016/j.humpath.2017.07.007. Epub 2017 Jul 21. PMID: 28739497

Zamani M, Gronhoj C, Schmidt Jensen J, von Buchwald C, Charabi BW, Hjuler T (2019) Survival and characteristics of pediatric salivary gland cancer: a systematic review and meta-analysis. Pediatr Blood Cancer 66:e27543

15 Laryngeal Tumors

Roberto Bianchi, Jan Godzinski, and Marco Guzzo

Laryngeal tumors are extremely rare in children and adolescents; thus extensive experience with laryngeal neoplasms under the age of 18 is very limited, even in major head and neck cancer centers. Dyspnea, dysphonia, hoarseness, and dysphagia are symptoms which shall lead to a suspicion of laryngeal mass: in these cases flexible fiber-optic laryngoscopic examination is mandatory. Any suspicious case must be scheduled for a direct microlaryngoscopy and biopsy under general anesthesia, which allows for both establishing the local estension and taking a sample for microscopic examination (Kato et al. 1991; Sessions et al. 1993; Strong and Jako 1972). Diagnosis is frequently delayed, due to the rarity of this disease, but early detection of any malignancy located in this critical region is of greatest value, so any persistent change in a child's voice or hoarseness is an indication for prompt and adequate diagnostic workup in order to treat the disease with a conservative approach, avoiding mutilative surgery.

The clinical extension of the neoplasm must be precisely assessed. Computed tomography and MRI are useful for local–regional assessment. Distant metastasis must be searched mainly in the lungs, bones, and liver and, in case of rhabdomyosarcoma, also in bone marrow (Pransky and Kang 2003).

Among benign neoplasms, the most common is *subglottic hemangioma*: it behaves like other hemangiomas of the head and neck (see salivary gland tumors chapter for further details) with the possible additional complication of airway obstruction and/or dysphagia in the proliferative phase of a wide lesion. Subglottic hemangioma occurs in a 2:1 female to male ratio. Diagnosis is made at a mean age of 3.6 months (Bitar et al. 2005).

Infants with subglottic hemangioma and cutaneous facial hemangiomas in a "beard" distribution should be evaluated for PHACE (posterior fossa brain malformations, hemangiomas, arterial anomalies, coarctation of the aorta and cardiac defects, and eye abnormalities) syndrome (Smith et al. 2004).

The optimal treatment of subglottic hemangioma is still not defined: a wait-and-see policy, based on spontaneous regression of the lesion, is indicated in asymptomatic cases without respiratory distress. Systemic treatment includes corticosteroids, alpha-interferon, and, since 2008, propranolol, which is thought to displace other drugs in the medical cure of pediatric hemangiomas. Moreover in 2015, Elluru et al. (2015) demonstrated that the treatment with propranolol has similar effectiveness to surgical treatment modalities without major complications and should be considered as a first-line

R. Bianchi (✉) · M. Guzzo
Otolaryngology Unit, National Cancer Institute, Milan, Italy
e-mail: roberto.bianchi@istitutotumori.mi.it

J. Godzinski
Department of Pediatric Surgery, Medical University of Wroclaw, Wroclaw, Poland

D. T. Schneider et al. (eds.), *Rare Tumors in Children and Adolescents*, Pediatric Oncology,
https://doi.org/10.1007/978-3-030-92071-5_15

approach. Tracheotomy is advised to secure airway in case of extensive hemangioma.

Transoral laser resection was, in the past, the most common approach for small and circumscribed lesions, with a success rate of 88.9% using a mean of two sessions. Intralesional corticosteroid injection has been used with a success rate of 86.4%, using a mean of three injections; unfortunately, it requires general anesthesia and postoperative intubation (Bitar et al. 2005).

Open-neck surgical excision was performed in the past, but nowadays it is reserved to cases resistant to all conservative treatments (Siegel and Mehta 2015).

Other benign submucosal lesions include the exceedingly rare *nerve sheath tumors*: 10% of them are diagnosed in patients under the age of 21, and 25–40% of such lesions occur in the head and neck region. They derive from the Schwann cell of peripheral nerves and include neurilemmoma (schwannoma), which is a solitary encapsulated tumor that very rarely shows malignant change, and neurofibroma, a non-encapsulated neoplasm that can be found in multiple locations (when associated with von Recklinghausen's disease) and can undergo malignant degeneration in 10% of cases, usually into malignant peripheral nerve sheet tumor (MPNST), rarely into liposarcomas (Pulli and Coniglio 1997; Golledge et al. 1995).

The vast majority of laryngeal nerve sheath tumors are supraglottic, with the aryepiglottic fold and false vocal cord being the most common sites. They are not radio-sensitive, and thus transoral laser excision is the treatment of choice (Pulli and Coniglio 1997).

Granular cell tumors are uncommon soft tissue neoplasms that occur in 30–40% of the cases in the tongue; in pediatric population laryngeal involvement is very rare and usually subglottic. These tumors are usually benign, with slow growth; the treatment is based on a surgical approach, usually complete removal with carbon dioxide laser (Holland et al. 1998).

Inflammatory myofibroblastic tumor is an uncommon neoplasm that is usually located in the lung in pediatric population; it rarely occurs in the larynx (Coffin et al. 1995), and in this site it does not appear too aggressive as in other locations. This tumor is usually indolent, does not metastasize, and can rarely recur locally. The mainstay of treatment is wide local excision (Rodrigues et al. 2005).

Hamarthoma of the larynx is very rare; Rinaldo and colleagues reviewed 11 cases from the literature and 5 of them occurred in children. Treatment consists of local excision; recurrences are usually seen associated with incomplete removal (Rinaldo et al. 1998).

Malignant tumors of the larynx are rare in children. Two of the most extensive and recent reviews are reported by Ginhart and Ferlito in Table 15.1 (Ferlito et al. 1999; Ginhart et al. 1980).

Rhabdomyosarcoma is the most common sarcoma arising in the larynx, and the average age of the patients at the diagnosis is 9 years and 2 months (Ferlito et al. 1999). Sarcomas have well-established strategies of treatment (see Chap. 44).

The local treatment in case of laryngeal location, however, remains challenging. Radical resections are clearly mutilating, conservative surgery may not be complete, and radiotherapy is followed by well-known postirradiation complications. A limited series of laryngeal rhabdomyosarcomas from Institut Gustave Roussy, published in 1991, underlines the rarity of this location (5

Table 15.1 Summary of two reviews of malignant tumors of the larynx in children by Ginhart and Ferlito (Ferlito et al. 1999; Ginhart et al. 1980)

	Ginhart et al. (1980)	Ferlito et al. (1999)
Histotype	No. of patients (%)	No. of patients (%)
Rhabdomyosarcoma		20 (42.5)
Squamous cell carcinoma	53 (98.2)	13 (27.6)
Synovial sarcoma		3 (6.4)
Malignant fibrous histiocytoma		2 (4.3)
Non-Hodgkin's lymphoma		2 (4.3)
Chondrosarcoma		1
Ewing sarcoma		1
Fibrosarcoma		1
Malignant schwannoma		1
Mixed sarcoma		1
Mucoepidermoid carcinoma		1
Adenocarcinoma	1	
Primitive neuroectodermal tumor		1
Total	54 (100)	47 (100)

cases among 126 patients with rhabdomyosarcoma treated in that center from 1955 to 1981) and a very good survival, achieved with chemotherapy and radiotherapy, avoiding mutilative surgery (no laryngectomies in this series). Authors also emphasize on long-term important sequelae associated with radiotherapy, such as arrest in growth of irradiated structures, huskiness, hypothyroidism, abnormalities in offspring, carotid stenosis, and an increased risk of radiation-induced malignancy (Ferlito et al. 1999; Kato et al. 1991; Nikaghlagh et al. 2007).

Other malignant mesenchymal tumors located in the larynx are also reported, but taking into account the variety of the histological subtypes, the incidence of each is negligible.

Squamous cell carcinoma (SCC) is the second most frequent pediatric malignancy of the larynx. However, some authors consider this tumor more frequent than rhabdomyosarcoma (Ferlito et al. 1999; Ginhart et al. 1980; Pransky and Kang 2003; Smith 2008). SCC accounts for less than 0.1% of all head and neck malignancies in patients younger than 15 years old, with 92 cases reported in the literature since 1868 (Uloza et al. 2017). Etiology is controversial and it is not related to the well-recognized risk factors for laryngeal cancer in adults: pediatric SCC of the larynx seems to be a genetic disease in which there is an interaction between environmental, genetic, and immunological factors, such as:

- Malignant spontaneous degeneration of juvenile papilloma of the larynx (Figs. 15.1 and 15.2).
- Fanconi's anemia.
- Bloom's syndrome.
- Xeroderma pigmentosum.
- Dyskeratosis congenita.
- Chronic graft-versus-host disease.
- Epidermolysis bullosa.
- Previous radiation therapy for a benign condition, such as adenoid hypertrophy.
- Asbestos exposure.
- Secondhand smoke.
- Presence of chromosomal translocation (15;19).
- Infection with human papilloma virus (Chow et al. 2007; Ferlito et al. 1999; Joos et al. 2009(Bhanu Prasad et al. 2017)).

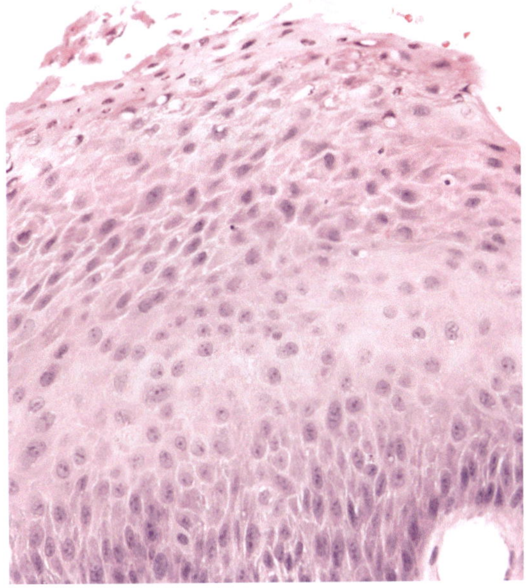

Fig. 15.1 Laryngeal papillomatosis

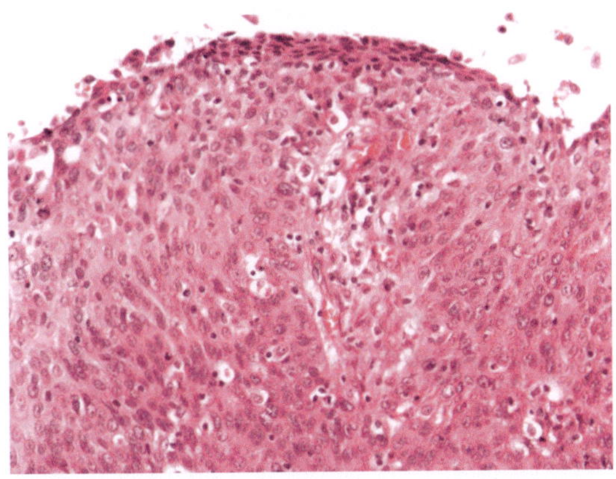

Fig. 15.2 Laryngeal papillomatosis in transformation to carcinoma

Most studies show a HPV positivity rate in head–neck SCC close to 35%; with regard to SCC of the larynx, the frequency of HPV positivity varies from 13% to 50%, and the most frequently isolated subtype is HPV-16 (Chow et al. 2007; Joos et al. 2009). In the literature there are sporadic cases of SCC of the larynx in children that are positive for HPV DNA, but recently Bayan et al. documented an increased incidence of HPV-positive glottis cancer in nonsmoker patients 30 years old or younger. The authors collected 11 of such patients, 3 of them were children and 10/11 resulted HPV-positive. Given that squamous cell papilloma (recurrent respiratory papillomatosis) is the most common benign epithelial tumor of the larynx in children associated with low-risk HPV 6–11, any effort should be done to discriminate HPV-related papillary squamous cell carcinoma that often presents with similar clinical features(Bayan et al. 2019)

In children, the average age for SCC of the larynx is 12 years, and 60% of cases affect boys, compared to adults, in whom there is a greater male predominance (Ferlito et al. 1999; Joos et al. 2009). Vocal folds are the most common site of origin followed by supraglottic and subglottic locations (Joos et al. 2009).

SCC of the children has been reported to mirror that of adults, in regard to the pattern of local spread and is usually well differentiated and keratinizing (Joos et al. 2009). This characteristic potentially offers good chance for survival, and reasonable efforts to spare good laryngeal function must be undertaken. Recently, Modh et al. reported a 5-year overall survival of 95% for laryngeal cancer and suggested that a good prognosis could be explained by early stage at presentation and different etiologic origin (high-risk HPV-16) (Modh et al. 2018). On the other hand, some reports emphasize a poorer outcome between 15 and 19 years of age (60.1% 5-year survival) than in those aged over 20 (87.7% 5-year survival) (Rutt et al. 2010). Radiotherapy and surgery are the treatment of choice and, depending on tumor extension, may be used alone or in combination (Kato et al. 1991; Pransky and Kang 2003; Preuss et al. 2009; Sessions et al. 1993; Strong and Jako 1972). Small lesions may be managed successfully with laser surgery, and by using this method only very limited sequelae were seen (Ambrosch 2007; Pransky and Kang 2003; Strong and Jako 1972; McWother and Hoffman 2005). Chemotherapy potentially applies to advanced stage laryngeal cancers and shall probably be based on the experience gained in adults (Holsinger et al. 2009; Strong and Jako 1972).

Spontaneous regression of vocal cord carcinoma has been recently described in a 10-year-old boy. The tumor, staged as cT1aN0M0 and associated with low-risk HPV type 26, did not undergo any treatment and disappeared in 2 months. The patients remained free of disease after a 12-month follow-up (Uloza et al. 2017).

NUT Carcinoma

It is a poorly differentiated carcinoma characterized by chromosomal rearrangement of the gene *NUTM1* on chromosome 15q14. The *BRD4* gene on 19q13 is the most common (70% of cases) translocation partner, resulting in a fusion oncogene, *BRD4-NUT*. This tumor is generally midline and affects the upper aerodigestive tract in 65% of the cases. The larynx involvement is very rare (Hellquist et al. 2017). Young age, female predilection, and a very poor prognosis (median overall survival of 9.8 months) (Chau et al. 2016), despite aggressive multimodal treatments, are the main features of this neoplasm (Vargas et al. 2001; Rahbar et al. 2003; French et al. 2004).

In summary, the management of children with laryngeal carcinoma (Table 15.2) remains a challenge: early diagnosis of children pre-

Table 15.2 Management of laryngeal squamous cell carcinoma in children and adolescents

Physical examination	Anamnesis: prolonged and worsening symptoms, diagnosis is frequently delayed, due to the rarity of this disease. The average age is 12 and 9 years old for SCC and sarcomas, respectively
	Signs and symptoms: persistent dysphonia or hoarseness, eventually associated with dyspnea and dysphagia; rarely cervical painless lymphadenopathy. Flexible fiber-optic laryngoscopic examination is mandatory. Any suspicious case must be scheduled for a direct microlaryngoscopy and biopsy. Vocal folds are the most common site of involvement by SCC (squamous cell carcinoma) in adolescents
Laboratory assessment	There are no specific alterations
Radiological assessment	
– First assessment	MRI or CT of the neck
– Pretreatment assessment	Metastatic workup includes CT/PET
– FU	MRI or CT, CT/PET periodically

Table 15.2 Continued

Pathological assessment	Biopsy during direct microlaryngoscopy under general anesthesia, consider tracheotomy in advanced/stenosing neoplasm, before any other treatment
Staging system (carcinomas of the larynx)	TNM UICC AJCC (Eighth ed.)
	The larynx is divided into three sites (supraglottis, glottis, and subglottis) and several subsites
	Supraglottis (suprahyoid epiglottis, aryepiglottic fold, arytenoid, infrahyoid epiglottis, and ventricular bands or false cords)
	Tis: carcinoma in situ
	T1: tumor limited to one subsite of supraglottis with normal vocal cord mobility
	T2: tumor invades mucosa of more than one adjacent subsite of supraglottis or glottis or region outside the supraglottis (e.g., base of the tongue, vallecula, and medial wall of piriform sinus) without fixation of the larynx
	T3: tumor limited to larynx with vocal cord fixation and/or invades any of the following: postcricoid area, preepiglottic space, paraglottic space, and/or inner cortex of thyroid cartilage
	T4a: tumor invades through the thyroid cartilage and/or invades tissues beyond the larynx, e.g., trachea, soft tissues of the neck including deep/extrinsic muscle of the tongue, strap muscles, thyroid, and esophagus
	T4b: tumor invades prevertebral space, encases carotid artery or mediastinal structures
	Glottis (vocal cords, anterior commissure, and posterior commissure)
	Tis: carcinoma in situ
	T1: tumor limited to vocal cord(s) (may involve anterior or posterior commissure) with normal mobility
	T1a tumor limited to one vocal cord
	T1b tumor involves both vocal cords
	T2: tumor extends to supraglottis and/or subglottis and/or with impaired vocal cord mobility
	T3: tumor limited to larynx with vocal cord fixation and/or invades paraglottic space and/or inner cortex of the thyroid cartilage
	T4a: tumor invades through the outer cortex of the thyroid cartilage and/or invades tissues beyond the larynx, e.g., trachea, soft tissues of neck including deep/extrinsic muscles of tongue, strap muscles, thyroid, and esophagus
	T4b: tumor invades prevertebral space and encases carotid artery or mediastinal structures
	Subglottis
	Tis: carcinoma in situ
	T1: tumor limited to subglottis
	T2: tumor extends to vocal cord(s) with normal or impaired mobility
	T3: tumor limited to larynx with vocal cord fixation
	T4a: tumor invades cricoid or thyroid cartilage and/or invades tissues beyond the larynx, e.g., trachea, soft tissues of neck including deep/extrinsic muscles of tongue, strap muscles, thyroid, and esophagus
	T4b: tumor invades prevertebral space, encases carotid artery or mediastinal structures
	Nx: regional lymph node metastasis cannot be assessed
	N0: no regional lymph node metastasis
	N1: metastasis in a single ipsilateral lymph node, 3 cm or less in greatest dimension without extranodal extension
	N2: metastasis as described below:
	–N2a metastasis in a single ipsilateral lymph node, more than 3 cm but not more than 6 cm in greatest dimension without extranodal extension
	–N2b metastasis in multiple ipsilateral lymph nodes, none more than 6 cm in greatest dimension without extranodal extension
	–N2c metastasis in bilateral or contralateral lymph nodes, none more than 6 cm in greatest dimension without extranodal extension
	N3a: metastasis in lymph node more than 6 cm in greatest dimension without extranodal extension
	N3b metastasis in single or multiple lymph nodes with clinical extranodal extension
	M0: no distant metastasis
	M1: distant metastasis

(continued)

Table 15.2 Continued

Stage grouping	Stage 0: Tis N0 M0
	Stage I: T1 N0 M0
	Stage II: T2 N0 M0
	Stage III: T1,T2,T3 N1 M0; T3 N0 M0
	Stage IVA: T4a N0,N1 M0; T1,T2,T3,T4a N2 M0
	Stage IVB: T4b any N M0; Any T, N3 M0
	Stage VIC: any T, Any N M1
General treatment guidelines	– Need for multidisciplinary approach
	– Need for referral to primary oncology center with expert physicians professionally dedicated to the management of this cancer in adults (or strict collaboration with them) because pediatric treatment protocols have not been well established due to the scarcity of cases; are based upon stage of the tumor
– Surgery	Conservative technique (open-neck or laser transoral surgery) is recommended when feasible; total laryngectomy is reserved in case of relapse
– Radiotherapy	Radical in early-stage disease and in sarcomas, after neoadjuvant chemotherapy; adjuvant with or without chemotherapy in high-risk patients after surgery; concomitant with chemotherapy in organ-preservation techniques. Consider long-term complications (arrest in growth of irradiated structures and radiation-induced malignancy)
– Chemotherapy	Neoadjuvant in advanced stages; concomitant with radiotherapy in organ-preservation strategies or in postoperative treatment of high-risk patients

senting with symptoms suggestive of laryngeal pathology is essential in order to secure definitive local therapy and minimize long-term complications.

A malignant hemopathy such as *non-Hodgkin's lymphoma* or, rarely, an *extramedullary plasmacytoma* could rarely affect the larynx. In these cases, histologic examination of the biopsy specimen is fundamental to address cures that are based on chemotherapy and radiotherapy (Ferlito et al. 1999; Rutherford et al. 2009).

References

Ambrosch P (2007) The role of the laser microsurgery in the treatment of laryngeal cancer. Curr Opin Otolaryngol Head Neck Surg 2(15):82–88

Bayan S, Faquin WC, Zeitels SM (2019) Glottic carcinoma in young patients. Ann Otol Rhinol Laryngol 128:25S–32S

Bhanu Prasad V, Mallick S, Upadhyay AD, Rath GK (2017) Systematic review and individual patient data analysis of pediatric head and neck squamous cell carcinoma: an analysis of 217 cases. Int J Pediatr Otorhinolaryngol 92:75–81

Bitar MA et al (2005) Management of congenital subglottic hemangioma: trends and success over the past 17 year. Otolaryngol Head Neck Surg 132:226–231

Chau NG, Hurwitz S, Mitchell CM et al (2016) Intensive treatment and survival outcomes in NUT midline carcinoma of the head and neck. Cancer 122:3632–3640

Chow CW et al (2007) Squamous cell carcinomas in children and young adults: a new wave of a very rare tumour? J Pediatr Surg 42(12):2035–2039

Coffin CM, Watterson J, Priest JR, Dehner LP (1995) Extrapulmonary inflammatory myofibroblastic tumor (inflammatory pseudotumor). A clinicopathologic and immunohistochemical study of 84 cases. Am J Surg Pathol 19:859–872

Elluru RG, Friess MR, Richter GT et al (2015) Multicenter evaluation of the effectiveness of systemic propranolol in the treatment of airway hemangiomas. Otolaryngol Head Neck Surg 153:452–460

Ferlito A et al (1999) Laryngeal malignant neoplasms in children and adolescents. Int J Pediatr Otorhinolaryngol 49:1–14

French CA et al (2004) Midline carcinoma of children and young adults with NUT rearrangement. J Clin Oncol 22:4135–4139

Ginhart TD et al (1980) Carcinoma of the larynx in childhood. Cancer 46:1683–1688

Golledge J et al (1995) Head neck liposarcoma. Cancer 76(6):1051–1058

Hellquist H, French CA, Bishop JA et al (2017) NUT midline carcinoma of the larynx: an international series and review of the literature. Histopathology 70:861–868

Holland RS et al (1998) Granular cell tumor of the larynx in a six-year-old child: case report and review of the literature. Ear Nose Throat J 77(8):652–660

Holsinger FC et al (2009) Durable long-term remission with chemotherapy alone for stage II to IV laryngeal cancer. J Clin Oncol 27:1976–1982

Joos B et al (2009) Laryngeal squamous cell carcinoma in a 13 year-old child associated with human papillomaviruses 16 and 18: a case report and review of the literature. Head Neck Pathol 3(1):37–41

Kato MA et al (1991) Rhabdomyosarcoma of the larynx in children. Med Pediatr Oncol 19(2):110–114

McWother AJ, Hoffman HT (2005) Transoral laser microsurgery for laryngeal malignancies. Curr Probl Cancer 29:180–189

Modh A, Gayar OH, Elshaikh MA, Paulino AC, Siddiqui F (2018) Pediatric head and neck squamous cell carcinoma: patient demographics, treatment trends and outcomes. Int J Pediatr Otorhinolaryngol 106:21–25

Nikaghlagh S et al (2007) Rhabdomyosarcoma of the larynx. Pak J Med Sci 23(2):280–282

Pransky SM, Kang R (2003) Tumors of the larynx, trachea and bronchi. In: Bluestone CD et al (eds) Pediatric otolaryngology. Saunders, Elsevier Science, Philadelphia

Preuss SF et al (2009) Transoral laser surgery for laryngeal cancer: outcome, complications and prognostic factors in 275 patients. Eur J Surg Oncol 35(3):235–240

Pulli R, Coniglio JU (1997) Subglottic nerve sheath tumor in a pediatric patient: case report and literature review. Head Neck 19:440–444

Rahbar R et al (2003) The role of chromosomal translocation (15;19) in the carcinoma of the upper aerodigestive tract in children. Otolaryngol Head Neck Surg 129(6):698–704

Rinaldo A et al (1998) Hamarthoma of the larynx: a critical review of the literature. Ann Otol Rhinol Laryngol 107:264–267

Rodrigues M et al (2005) Inflammatory myofibroblastic tumor of the larynx in a 2-year-old male. ORL J Otorhinolaryngol Relat Spec 67:101–105

Rutherford K et al (2009) Extramedullary plasmacytoma of the larynx in an adolescent: a case report and review of the literature. Ear Nose Throat J 88(2):E1–E7

Rutt AL et al (2010) Laryngeal cancer in patients younger than 30 years: a review of 99 cases. Ear Nose Throat J 89(4):189–192

Sessions RB et al (1993) Tumours of the larynx and hypopharynx. In: DeVitta V et al (eds) Cancer: principles and practice of oncology. JB Lippincott, Philadelphia

Siegel B, Mehta D (2015) Open airway surgery for subglottic hemangioma in the era of propranolol: is it still indicated? Int J Pediatr Otorhinolaryngol 79:1124–1127

Smith RV (2008) Merck manual for healthcare professionals. http://www.merckmanuals.com/professionals/sec08/ch093/ch093c.html

Smith DS et al (2004) Otolaryngologic manifestations of PHACE syndrome. Int J Pediatr Otorhinolaryngol 68(11):1445–1450

Strong MS, Jako GJ (1972) Laser surgery in the larynx. Early clinical experience with continuous CO_2 laser. Ann Otol Rhinol Laryngol 81:791–798

Uloza V, Ulozaite N, Vaitkus S, Sarauskas V (2017) Spontaneous regression of laryngeal carcinoma in 10 year old boy: a case report and review of literature. Int J Pediatr Otorhinolaryngol 103:10–13

Vargas SO et al (2001) Upper respiratory tract carcinoma with chromosomal translocation 15;19: evidence for a distinct disease entity of young patients with a rapidly fatal course. Cancer 92:1195–1203

Part V

Rare Tumors of the Head and Neck

16 Pathological Aspects of Mediastinal Tumors in Children and Adolescents

Alexander Marx, Claudia Spix, and Christian Vokuhl

16.1 Introduction

The mediastinum represents the space between both the lungs, the diaphragm, and the vault of the thoracic cavity. Traditionally, it has been divided in a superior, anterior (together now called prevascular), middle (visceral), and posterior (paravertebral) compartment (Carter et al. 2017), each of which harbors characteristic tumors in the pediatric and adolescent age group (Fig. 16.1). Most mediastinal, particularly thymic tumors can, however, occur in any of the mediastinal compartments due to the common occurrence of heterotopia of thymic tissue outside the anterior mediastinum (Marx et al. 2018).

16.2 Peculiarities of Mediastinal Tumors in Children and Adolescents

Epidemiology Mediastinal tumors in children and adults are rare neoplasm (incidence: 1–5 per million children and adolescence) comprising 1–1.5% of tumors in this age group, compared to

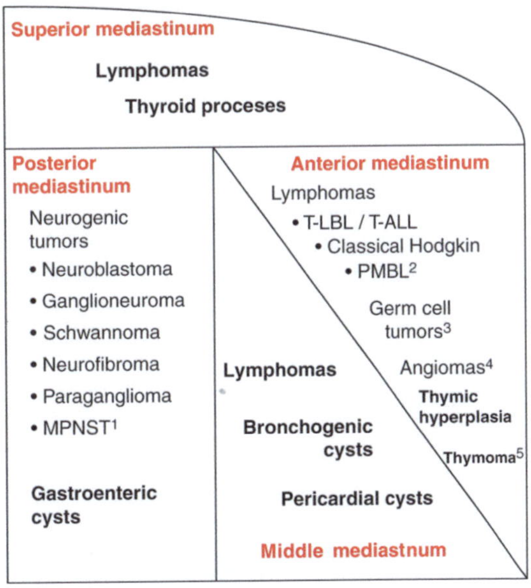

[1]Malignant peripheral nerve sheath tumor
[2]Primary mediastinal large B-cell lymphoma
[3]hemangiomas and lymphangiomas
[4]yolk sac tumors and teratomas before puberty, embyonal carcinomas, seminomas and mixed germe cell tumors after puberty
[5]thymic hyperplasia in children comprise 'true thymic hyperplasia', lymphofollicular hyperplasia and rebound hyperplasia
thymic hyperplasias comprise 'true thymic hyperplasia', lymphofollicular hyperplasia and rebound hyperplasia

Fig. 16.1 Distribution of pediatric mediastinal tumors in the prevascular (superior and anterior), visceral (middle), and paravertebral (posterior) compartments of the mediastinum. Thymomas play almost no role in children and are exceedingly rare in adolescents. For adult patients, see ref. (Roden et al. 2020)

<1% in adults (Müller-Hermelink et al. 2004). Gender plays a highly variable role in the different tumors (see below).

A. Marx (✉) · C. Spix · C. Vokuhl
University Medical Centre Mannheim,
Institute of Pathology, Heidelberg University,
Mannheim, Germany
e-mail: alexander.marx@umm.de;
Christian.Vokuhl@ukbonn.de

D. T. Schneider et al. (eds.), *Rare Tumors in Children and Adolescents*, Pediatric Oncology,
https://doi.org/10.1007/978-3-030-92071-5_16

- **Age-related spectrum of mediastinal tumors** The relative frequency of the various thymic tumors is different in children and adolescents compared to adults. While thymic epithelial tumors are the commonest mediastinal tumors in adults (Roden et al. 2020) (Fig. 16.2a), lymphomas are the commonest mediastinal and thoracic tumors in children (Marx et al. 2021a) (Fig. 16.2b, c). In data on malignant mediastinal tumors selected from the German Childhood Cancer Registry (DKKR, 2020) covering the period 2009–2018, lymphomas are commoner than malignant germ cell tumors, thymic epithelial tumors, neurogenic tumors, or sarcomas, if involvement of thoracic lymph nodes and other thoracic structures outside the mediastinum is strictly excluded (Fig. 16.2b). By contrast, if all thoracic malignancies are considered, the frequency distribution in descending order is more "conventional": lymphomas are most prevalent, being followed by neurogenic tumors, germ cell tumors, and sarcomas, while thymomas and thymic carcinomas are least common and make up only 1–2% (Marx et al. 2021a) (Fig. 16.2c). T-lymphoblastic lymphoma/T-ALL (acute lymphoblastic leukemia) is the predominant entity among pediatric/early adolescent lymphomas in the mediastinum (Burkhardt and Hermiston 2019; Minard-Colin et al. 2015), while Hodgkin lymphomas, mediastinal large B cell lymphomas, and gray zone lymphomas are most prevalent in late adolescence and adulthood (Perwein et al. 2020; Sarkozy et al. 2021). Mediastinal involvement by Burkitt lymphoma is exceptionally rare across all ages (Pillon et al. 2014). Malignant neurogenic tumors are typically encountered before the age of 5 and occur almost exclusively in the posterior mediastinum. Among germ cell tumors, yolk sac tumors and teratomas predominate before puberty with similar frequencies in boys and girls. By contrast, seminomas, embryonal carcinomas, and mixed germ cell tumors are typical mediastinal germ cell tumors after puberty with virtual restriction to male patients (Roden et al. 2021a).

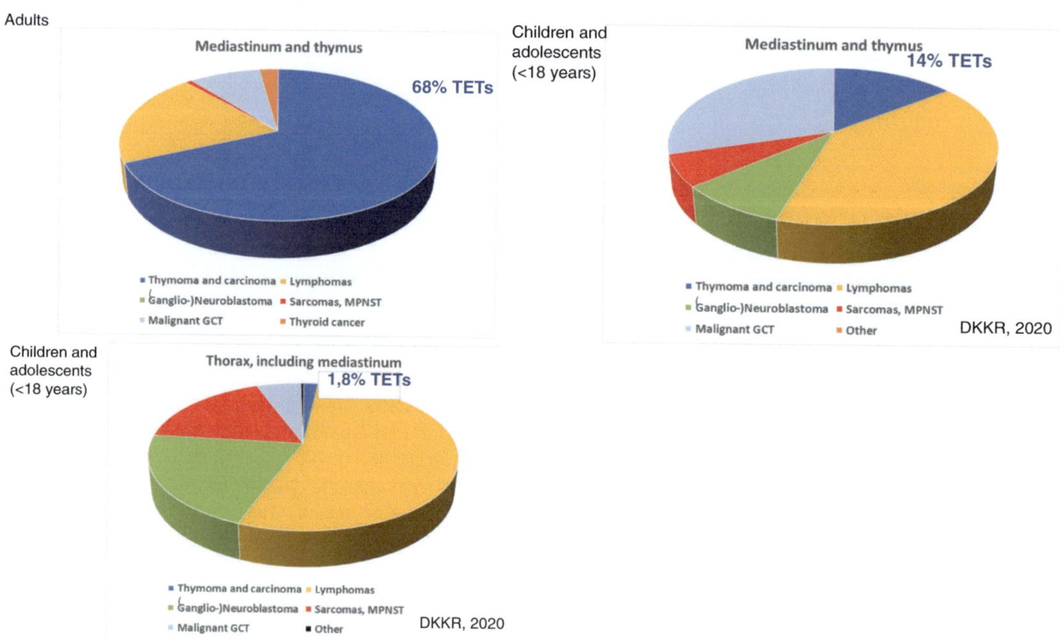

Fig. 16.2 Different proportions of the various mediastinal tumors in children and adults (Marx et al. 2021a; Müller-Hermelink et al. 2004). The adult data are from Takeda et al (2003). The children's data were selected from the German Childhood Cancer Registry (DKKR, 2020) and cover the period from 2009 to 2018. *TETs* thymic epithelial tumors (including thymomas and thymic carcinomas), *MPNST* malignant peripheral nerve sheath tumors, *GCTs* germ cell tumors

Overall, mediastinal tumors in children are more commonly malignant (in 70–95%) than in adults, and asymptomatic cases are exceptionally rare in children (Chen et al. 2019; Gun et al. 2012; Lee et al. 2020).

- **Paraneoplastic syndromes** Paraneoplastic syndromes are much less common in children and adolescents than in adults. This is due to the virtual absence of autoimmunity-prone thymomas in this age group and lower frequency of autoimmune phenomena even among pediatric thymoma patients (Fonseca et al. 2014). Therefore, thymic pathology in a child or adolescent with sero-positive myasthenia gravis (MG with autoantibodies to the acetylcholine receptor) is almost always due to lymphofollicular thymic hyperplasia. A rare pediatric paraneoplastic syndrome in conjunction with mediastinal neuroblastomas is opsomyoclonus (Simon et al. 2018).

16.3 Lymphomas and Other Hematologic Malignancies

- The most common mediastinal lymphomas in children and adolescents are T-lymphoblastic lymphomas (T-LBL) followed by classical Hodgkin lymphomas (cHL) and primary mediastinal large B cell lymphomas (PMBL) (Attias et al. 2009). Rare mediastinal hematologic malignancies that occur prior to adulthood are NK cell lymphomas and myeloid malignancies. Langerhans cell histiocytosis (LCH) is a differential diagnostic possibility particularly in cases of sclerosing mediastinitis. Mediastinal myeloid neoplasms (Kawamoto et al. 2016) including LCH may occur in isolation or as somatic malignancy associated with mediastinal germ cell tumors (Orazi et al. 2021).

16.3.1 T-Lymphoblastic Lymphoma (T-LBL)

T-LBL is a tumor composed of immature T cells mostly arising in the thymus by unknown etiological factors. By definition, the disease is called T-ALL if the percentage of blasts in the bone marrow is 25% or higher (Murphy 1980). Immature T cells may either exhibit immune phenotypes that are compatible with normal but arrested maturational stages of thymic T-cell development or show aberrant expression profiles. Furthermore, an "early thymic precursor (ETP)" subtype of T-LBL has been delineated that shares a distinct immunophenotype with ETP T-ALL (acute T-lymphoblastic leukemia of ETP-type) but may show slightly different genetic alterations (Xu et al. 2021). With current treatment protocols, the prognosis of ETP T-ALL/LBL in children (in contrast to adults) is no longer poorer than that of other T-ALLs/LBLs (Burkhardt and Hermiston 2019; Xu et al. 2021). T-LBLs comprise about 20% of lymphomas in this age group, with a major peak of incidence between late childhood and adolescence (Burkhardt and Hermiston 2019). It is the second most common pediatric NHL in children after Burkitt lymphoma (Burkhardt et al. 2005). T-LBLs affect mediastinal and other lymph nodes in about 15% of cases. Typical clinical symptoms of T-LBL are respiratory distress, superior vena cava syndrome, and pericardial and pleural effusions.

In core needle biopsies, T-LBL shows monotonous infiltrates of small- to medium-sized lymphoid blasts that commonly infiltrate beyond the thymic epithelial network and blur the normal cortico-medullary architecture of the thymus. Epithelial cell networks are typically diminished or even absent in T-LBL (Fig. 16.3). Many mediastinal T-LBLs show a regular immune phenotype corresponding to that of the major population of cortical thymocytes that is typically TdT+, CD34(−), CD1a+, CD3+, CD5+, CD4+ in addition to CD8+, with Ki67 indices of around 90%. Other T-LBL cases may show more immature (e.g., without expression of CD1a) or mature phenotypes (e.g., with isolated expression of CD4 or CD8). Finally, aberrant profiles (e.g., loss of CD5 or massive expression of CD10 and CD34) can be found as well, and their recognition is helpful for differential diagnostic purposes (see below). Most but not all T-LBL show mono-

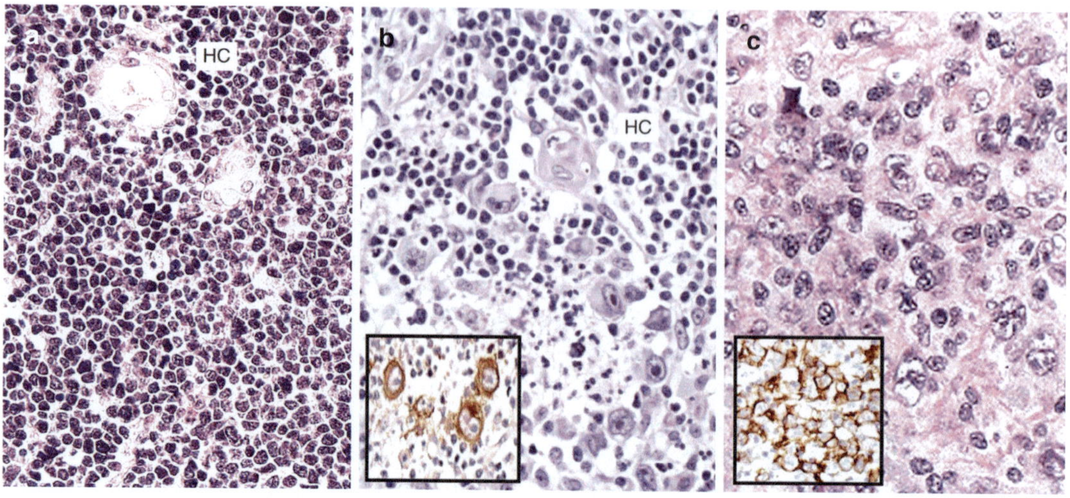

Fig. 16.3 Histology of the main lymphoma subtypes encountered in children. (**a**) T-lymphoblastic lymphoma. Monotonous medium-sized blasts infiltrating adjacent to Hassall's corpuscle (HC). (**b**) Classical Hodgkin lymphoma of the thymus, infiltrating adjacent to Hassall's corpuscle (HC). Inset: CD30 expression in Hodgkin cells. (**c**) Primary mediastinal large B-cell lymphoma. Infiltrate of pleomorphic tumor cells, some resembling Hodgkin cells. Inset: consistent strong expression of CD20 in all tumor cells

clonal rearrangements of T-cell receptor genes (Coustan-Smith et al. 2009).

16.3.2 Differential Diagnosis of T-LBL

(a) **True Thymic Hyperplasia (TTH)** is a rare proportioned enlargement of the thymus (typical weight over 100 g up to 1000 g) of unknown pathogenesis mostly in infants and young children who may suffer from respiratory and cardiac failure that may need emergency interventions (Tadiotto et al. 2019). Biopsies of sufficient size show a normal cortico-medullary architecture and normal T-cell subsets. In small biopsies the distinction between TTH and T-LBL can be difficult, particularly when the neoplastic immature T cells of T-LBL show a normal immune phenotype. Detection in most T-LBL but not TTH of reduced epithelial cells by immunohistochemistry and of monoclonal rearrangement of T-cell receptor genes can be helpful. Intrathymic bleeding is a life-threatening complication (Eifinger et al. 2007).

(b) **Rebound Hyperplasia** represents a tumor-like "over-shooting" regeneration of the thymus 2–12 months (rarely even later) after the termination of chemotherapy or steroid treatment, raising the question of local tumor recurrence or metastasis. Taking clinical history, the lack of clinical symptoms, and CT features into account, biopsies generally can be avoided or postponed (Tian et al. 2015). In equivocal cases, biopsy may clarify the situation: histology reveals normal thymic tissue and polyclonal rearrangement of T-cell receptor genes. Of note, increased tracer uptake on FDG-PET-CT is usually not helpful to distinguish tumor recurrence from rebound thymic hyperplasia (Chen et al. 2017).

(c) **Lymphoid Follicular Thymic Hyperplasia (TFH)** is an inflammatory thymic alteration (*thymitis*), due to accumulation of B-cell-rich lymphoid follicles (mostly with formation of germinal centers) in so-called perivascular spaces within the destructed thymic medulla. Thymic cortex is apparently unaltered in TFH. The triggers of TFH are unknown. TFH is the typical thymic alteration in children and adults with sero-positive "early-onset myasthenia gravis" (i.e., in patients younger than 50 years with anti-acetylcholine receptor autoantibodies). Less commonly, TFH can occur in other autoimmune states (Marx et al. 2021b; Weis et al. 2018).

(d) **Thymomas** enter the differential diagnosis of T-LBL because they also usually harbor TdT(+) immature T cells in adolescents (see below).

16.3.3 Primary Mediastinal Large B-Cell Lymphoma (PMBL)

- **PMBL** is a lymphoma of unknown etiology that typically occurs in early adulthood but rarely also in adolescents, mainly females with a mean age of 14 at first diagnosis. There is a rare familial clustering (Saarinen et al. 2013). PMBL is thought to derive from normal thymic medullary B cells. PMBL is typically located in the prevascular mediastinum and commonly elicits superior vena cava syndrome. Diagnosis usually requires (CT-guided) core biopsies. Stromal sclerosis and large, clear tumor cells are classical findings, but many morphological variants (including Hodgkin-like tumor cells) have been described. Eventual cohesive growth of tumor cells can mimic carcinomatous infiltrates (Abb.3). By immunohistochemistry, about 70% of cases show a CD20+ CD23+/− CD30+/− CD45+ CD15− CD5− HLA-DR− PDL1+ profile. There is no EBV association. Immunoglobulin genes are rearranged (Leithäuser et al. 2001). Distinction from classical Hodgkin lymphoma can be difficult (see below). Like other lymphomas, PMBL is not associated with myasthenia gravis.

16.3.4 Differential Diagnosis of PMBL

The most difficult distinction concerns classical Hodgkin lymphoma (cHL). Tumor cell of cHL can sometimes express CD20 (like PMBL) but rarely in all tumor cells and is commonly negative for CD19, CD79a, and CD45. Even more difficult is the distinction from "gray zone lymphomas," the diagnostic criteria of which await further refinement (Perwein et al. 2020; Sarkozy et al. 2020, 2021).

Rarely, diffuse large B-cell lymphomas (DLBCL) and B-lymphoblastic lymphomas/B-ALL can arise within the mediastinum but usually involve lymph nodes rather than the thymus. Also, DLBCL rarely exhibit a CD20+ CD30+ CD23+ immunophenotype and may show molecular overlap with PMBL (Duns et al. 2021). Low-grade B-cell lymphomas (e.g., MALT lymphomas) are virtually nonexistent in children. By contrast, unicentric Castleman disease (CD) is a diagnostic option in commonly asymptomatic pediatric patients with a solitary, tumor-like, hyperemic B-cell-rich mediastinal mass, while multicentric CD that is often associated with HHV8 and signs of systemic inflammation is uncommon in HIV-negative children and adolescents (idiopathic multifocal CD) (Talat and Schulte 2011; Van Rhee et al. 2018, 2020).

16.3.5 Classical Hodgkin Lymphoma (cHL)

Classical HL within the mediastinum can primarily arise from thymus (Fig. 16.3) or mediastinal lymph nodes. Nodular sclerosis predominates over mixed cellularity cHL, while "non-classical," lymphocyte-predominant HL ("paragranuloma") is virtually nonexistent in the mediastinum. Tumor cells in cHL of children and adolescents exhibit the same immune profile as in adults: CD30+ CD15+/− CD20−/+ PAX5+ (faint)/ CD45− CD23− EMA−. Expression of EBV-related LMP1 or RNA (EBER) occurs in 50% of cases (Murray and Young 2019). The differential diagnosis comprises PMBL, so-called gray zone lymphomas (Minard-Colin et al. 2015; Oschlies et al. 2011; Perwein et al. 2020; Sarkozy et al. 2019) and, rarely, cytotoxic CD30+ CD45+ EMA+ CD15− CD20− PAX5− anaplastic large

T-cell lymphoma (ALCL) that is usually Alk1(+) in children and adolescents (Ismail et al. 2019; Le Deley et al. 2008; Mussolin et al. 2020).

16.4 Germ Cell Tumors (GCTs)

In general, primary mediastinal GCT in children and adults exhibit the same histological and immunohistological features as their counterparts in adults and in testis or ovaries (Roden et al. 2021a). Metastasis of gonadal GCT to the mediastinum is rare (Böhle et al. 1986). An inconsistent but specific histological finding in mediastinal teratomas in both children and adults is a pancreatic tissue component. The various subtypes of GCT occur at significantly different frequencies before and after puberty (Table 16.1). Teratomas and yolk sac tumors are the only GCT occurring before puberty at relevant frequency (Roden et al. 2021a) (Fig. 16.4). By contrast, post-pubertal GCT resemble their counterparts in adults, including seminoma, embryonal carcinoma, and mixed GCTs. Clinically, GCTs are separated into seminomas, non-seminomatous GCTs and teratomas, and even a small non-seminomatous component in an otherwise typical seminoma results in a classification as non-seminomatous GCT. The age-related prevalence of different histotypes is mirrored by molecular features: before puberty, genetic losses (1p, 5q, 6p), and gains (1q, tetraploidy) are characteristic of non-teratomatous GCT, while presence of isochromosome 12p (in 70% of cases) and aneuploidy are typical alteration after puberty. Teratomas are subclassified as either mature or

Table 16.1 Mediastinal germ cell tumors (GCTs) in relation to puberty in children and adolescents

Age at diagnosis	Histology	Gender	Clinical course	Immune phenotype of tumor cells
Before puberty	Teratoma (immature; mature)	M = F	Usually favorable (if resectable)	Variable, dependent on composition; CK+; EMA+; CDX2+/–; Glypican-3+; SALL4+/–; OCT4–; SOX2-
	Yolk sac tumor	F > M	Malignant	CK+; EMA–; AFP+; Glypican-3+; GATA3+/– SALL4+; OCT4–; SOX2–
After puberty	Teratoma (immature; mature)	M >> > F	Usually favorable	See above
	Seminoma	M >> > F	Malignant	SALL4+; OCT4+; SOX2–; CD117+; PLAP+/–; D2–40+/–;CK+/–[a];βHCG[b];AFP–
	Yolk sac tumor	M >> > F	Malignant	See above
	Embryonal carcinoma	M >> > W	Malignant	CK+; CD30+; CD117–/+; SALL4+; OCT4+; SOX2+; HCG[b]; AFP–
	Choriocarcinoma	M >> > F	Malignant	CK+; βHCG+; CD30–; SALL4–/+; OCT4-; SOX2–
	Mixed GCT	M >> > F	Malignant	Dependent on composition
	GCT with somatic type malignancy	M >> > F	Malignant	Dependent on the type of GCT-derived carcinoma, sarcoma, or leukemia

Post-pubertal GCT is often associated with Klinefelter syndrome. For additional immunohistochemical markers (Roden et al. 2021a)

Gender (M, male; F, female); *AFP* α-Fetoprotein, *CD117* cluster of differentiation 117 (= KIT, stem cell factor receptor), *CDX2* caudal-type homeobox transcription factor 2, *CK* cytokeratin, *D2–40* podoplanin, *EMA* epithelial membrane antigen, *βHCG* human chorionic gonadotropin, *OCT4* octamer binding transcription factor 4 (=POU5F1), *PLAP* placental alkaline phosphatase, *SALL4* Sal-Like 4, *SOX2*, Sry-box 2

[a] In contrast to gonadal seminomas that are CK–

[b] In scattered syncytiotrophoblasts

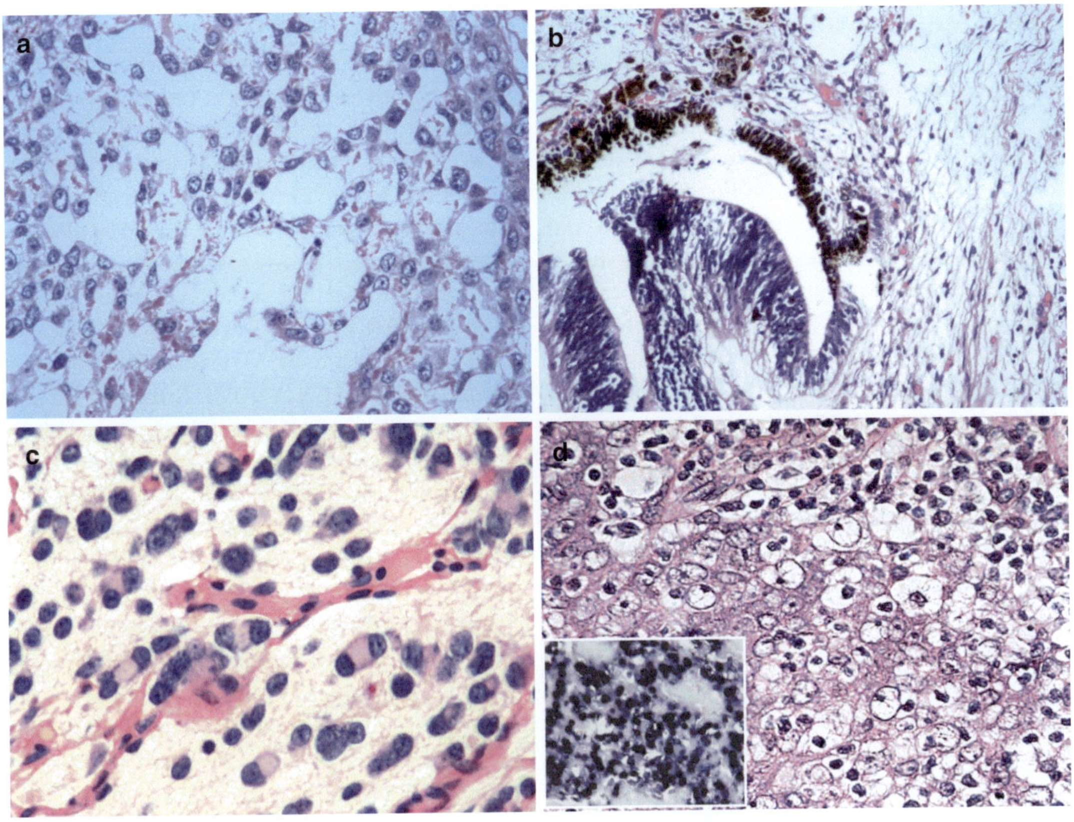

Fig. 16.4 Histology of solid mediastinal tumors occurring in children and adolescents. (**a**) Yolk sack tumor, the common non-teratomatous tumor before puberty. (**b**) Immature teratoma showing immature neuroectodermal tissue (retinal pigment epithelium). (**c**) Neuroblastoma (differentiating), a typical tumor of the posterior mediastinum in children and adolescents. (**d**) Lymphoepithelial carcinoma of the thymus (inset: EBER in situ hybridization, revealing Epstein-Barr virus RNA)

immature according to their content of immature tissue components; immature components typically represent fetal neuroectodermal structures as shown in Fig. 16.4. Recently, different modes of teratoma development have been proposed (Kao et al. 2018).

16.5 Neurogenic Tumors

Neuroblastomas (NB) are typically located in the posterior mediastinum and count among the most common mediastinal tumors in children (Fig. 16.4). Ganglioneuroblastomas and ganglioneuromas are found in slightly older children and even young adults as compared to children with neuroblastomas; they also preferentially occur in the posterior mediastinum. Rare neurogenic tumors inside the thymus occurred only in adults (Satoh 2019; Ueda et al. 2012).

A minority of benign and less commonly malignant paragangliomas ("pheochromocytomas") occur mainly in the posterior mediastinum. Occurrence of paragangliomas in children can be a hint to a variety of hereditary syndromes, such as "Carney's complex" (Stratakis and Carney 2009), due to germline mutation of the succinate dehydrogenase genes (*SDHA*, *SDHB*, *SDHC*, *SDHD*) and other genes (Bausch et al. 2017; Lazar and Cooper 2021).

16.6 Mesenchymal Tumors

Mesenchymal tumors of the mediastinum are rare in children, except for lymphangiomas and (mostly cavernous) hemangiomas/vascular malformations. Lipoma, lipoblastoma, lipoblastomatosis, well-differentiated and myxoid liposarcomas, benign and malignant nerve sheath tumors (including triton tumors in association with neurofibromatosis), hemangioendothelioma and angiosarcoma, low-grade fibromyxoid sarcoma, malignant rhabdoid tumor, rhabdomyoma, rhabdomyosarcomas of embryonal and alveolar type, chordoma, inflammatory myofibroblastic tumor (IMT), and thymolipoma have been described (Ayadi and Khabir 2010; Den Bakker et al. 2015a, b; Farber et al. 2017; Onoda et al. 2015; Schmid et al. 2018; Steiner et al. 2009; Suster and Moran 1995).

Ewing family tumors, synovial sarcomas, chondrosarcomas, and osteosarcomas in the mediastinum usually arise from the sternum or thoracic wall (Harris et al. 2020) and show the same immunohistochemical and genetic alterations as their extra-mediastinal counterparts (Fatimi et al. 2014; Mathew et al. 2019; Salah and Salem 2014; Suster and Moran 1997).

Every sarcoma in the mediastinum of a child, adolescent, or young adult should arouse suspicion of an underlying "germ cell tumor with somatic-type solid malignancy" (Faure Conter et al. 2017; Malagón et al. 2007; Roden et al. 2021b).

16.7 Thymomas, Thymic Carcinomas, and Thymic Neuroendocrine Tumors

***Thymomas** and thymic carcinomas (TCs)* are thymic epithelial tumors (TETs). Pediatric thymomas account for less than 1% of all thymomas (Rothstein et al. 2005) and for about 1% of pediatric thoracic tumors (Marx et al. 2021a). A hallmark of thymomas compared to other mediastinal tumors is the occurrence of paraneoplastic autoimmune diseases, the prevalence of which (about 25%) is, however, lower than in adults (about 50%), although the spectrum is similar (myasthenia gravis being the commonest) (Fonseca et al. 2014). Even less common is immunodeficiency associated with pediatric thymomas (Sicherer et al. 1998). In contrast to thymic carcinomas, thymomas preserve thymus-like features and almost always harbor immature, TdT+ T-cells, the bulk of which shows the immune phenotype of normal cortical thymocytes, i.e., expression of CD1a, CD3, CD5, CD4, and CD8 with lack of CD34. According to the WHO classification, they are divided into types A, AB, B1, B2, and B3 thymomas and rare others based on the morphology of neoplastic epithelial cells and the content of immature T cells (Marx et al. 2015). Most thymomas in children and adolescents are types B1, B2, and B3 that commonly behave in a clinically malignant fashion (Rod et al. 2014; Stachowicz-Stencel et al. 2015). Of note, thymomas are so rare in children and adolescents that other, more likely diagnoses need exclusion before accepting a diagnosis of pediatric thymoma, particularly when the diagnosis relies on small biopsies. If lymphadenopathy accompanies a mediastinal mass, a thymoma is even less likely. Among lymphocyte-rich TDT+ lesions, true thymic hyperplasia needs differential diagnostic consideration particularly in newborns and infants, while other thymic hyperplasias (see above) and T-LBL are much more common than thymomas in children and adolescents. Thymomas are usually distinguished from these histological mimics by an increased content of cytokeratin-positive neoplastic thymic epithelial cells. By contrast, T-LBL is the likely diagnosis, if cytologically atypical T cells, abnormal T-cell immunophenotypes, and monoclonal T-cell receptor rearrangement are encountered. However, the latter are not consistent features of T-LBL (see above). Another diagnostic pitfall in lymphocyte-poor spindle cell tumors is the interpretation of mediastinal synovial sarcoma as type A thymoma; while the former is well described in children and adolescents (Suster and Moran 2005), type A thymoma is virtually nonexistent in this age group. The prognosis of pediatric thymomas is similar to that in adults (5-year overall survival: 90%) (Stachowicz-Stencel et al. 2015).

Thymic carcinomas (TCs) account for about 50% of pediatric thymic epithelial tumors (TETs), i.e., they are relatively more common in children and adolescents than in adults (in whom TCs account for 10–20% of TETs). The epithelial cells of TCs show marked atypia and—in contrast to most thymomas—are not accompanied by significant numbers of immature, TdT+ T cells. The most common TC type in children and adolescents is lymphoepithelial TC (previously called lymphoepithelioma-like TC) that typically shows large cell features and accompanying inflammatory infiltrates of mature, TdT(−) T cells, B cells, and plasma cells and is almost always EBV-associated, as revealed by EBER in situ hybridization (Chan et al. 2021) (Fig. 16.4). Less common TC types are "conventional" squamous cell carcinomas and NUT carcinomas (which almost invariably exhibit squamous differentiation at least focally). The thorax especially the mediastinum is the preferred site of NUT carcinomas that either look like undifferentiated (small or large cell) carcinomas, poorly differentiated squamous cell carcinomas, or combinations thereof. They show translocations of the *NUTM1* gene and most commonly involve the BRD4 gene as fusion partner (Eagen and French 2021). NUT carcinomas in the thorax are almost always lethal within less than a year after the first presentation (Chau et al. 2020), while rare cases arising outside the thorax may be curable (Storck et al. 2017).

Neuroendocrine tumors (NETs) in the thymus are exceedingly rare epithelial tumors in children and adolescents (Lin et al. 1999; Soltysiak et al. 2017), but relatively common among patients with the MEN1 syndrome (multiple endocrine neoplasia type 1) (Al-Salameh et al. 2018). Morphologically, pediatric thymic NETs resemble their adult typical and atypical carcinoid counterparts (Dinter et al. 2019). In MEN1 patients, thymic NETs are highly heritable and lethal cancers due to early metastasis (Goudet et al. 2015; Kamilaris and Stratakis 2019). NETs must be distinguished from paragangliomas, i.e., non-epithelial, keratin-negative neuroendocrine neoplasms that often have a hereditary basis (see "Neurogenic Tumors" section) (Lazar and Cooper 2021).

16.8 Mediastinal Cysts

Cysts are not neoplasms but are mentioned here because they can be indicators of underlying tumors or inflammation. Among cysts, unilocular cysts are often congenital. They comprise the overall most common bronchogenic cysts (50%) that occur mainly in the middle mediastinum and show ciliated or squamous epithelial cells as inner lining. Pleural-pericardial cysts are lined by CD31−, D2–40 (podoplanin)+, and nuclear WT1+ mesothelial cells (30% of cases), while thymic cysts (15% of cases) reveal squamous or cuboidal epithelial lining cells and thymic lymphoid tissue inside or adjacent to the cyst wall. Even rarer are parathyroid and enteric cysts in the prevascular and paravertebral mediastinum, respectively (Zhang et al. 2006). In contrast to unilocular cysts, multilocular cysts are commonly acquired, covered by thymic epithelial cells and associated with thymitis, lymphadenitis (including tuberculosis), lymphomas, germ cell tumors, Langerhans cell histiocytosis, and thymic epithelial tumors (Le Pimpec-Barthes et al. 2010; Roden et al. 2020). Cysts have to be distinguished from cystic tumors, including teratomas and cystic lymphangiomas. The latter show cystic cavities lined by atypia-free, CD31+, and D2–40+ endothelial cells.

Acknowledgments The authors are grateful to Ms. Claudia Bremensdorfer of the German Childhood Cancer Registry (DKKR) for curating the childhood cancer data.

References

Al-Salameh A, Baudry C, Cohen R (2018) Update on multiple endocrine neoplasia type 1 and 2. Presse Med 47:722–731

Attias D, Hodgson D, Weitzman S (2009) Primary mediastinal B-cell lymphoma in the pediatric patient: can a rational approach to therapy be based on adult studies? Pediatr Blood Cancer 52:566–570

Ayadi L, Khabir A (2010) Pediatric angiosarcoma of soft tissue: a rare clinicopathologic entity. Arch Pathol Lab Med 134:481–485

Bausch B, Schiavi F, Ni Y et al (2017) Clinical characterization of the Pheochromocytoma and Paraganglioma susceptibility genes SDHA, TMEM127, MAX, and

SDHAF2 for gene-informed prevention. JAMA Oncol 3:1204–1212

Böhle A, Studer UE, Sonntag RW et al (1986) Primary or secondary extragonadal germ cell tumors? J Urol 135:939–943

Burkhardt B, Hermiston ML (2019) Lymphoblastic lymphoma in children and adolescents: review of current challenges and future opportunities. Br J Haematol 185:1158–1170

Burkhardt B, Zimmermann M, Oschlies I et al (2005) The impact of age and gender on biology, clinical features and treatment outcome of non-Hodgkin lymphoma in childhood and adolescence. Br J Haematol 131:39–49

Carter BW, Benveniste MF, Madan R et al (2017) ITMIG classification of mediastinal compartments and multidisciplinary approach to mediastinal masses. Radiographics 37:413–436

Chan JCK, Marx A, Detterbeck F et al (2021) Thymic carcinoma: introduction. In: Board E (ed) WHO classification of tumours editorial board. Thoracic tumours, vol 5, 5th edn. International Agency for Research on Cancer (IARC), Lyon, pp 351–353

Chau NG, Ma C, Danga K et al (2020) An anatomical site and genetic-based prognostic model for patients with nuclear protein in testis (NUT) midline carcinoma: analysis of 124 patients. JNCI Cancer Spectrum 4:pkz094

Chen CH, Hsiao CC, Chen YC et al (2017) Rebound thymic hyperplasia after chemotherapy in children with lymphoma. Pediatr Neonatol 58:151–157

Chen CH, Wu KH, Chao YH et al (2019) Clinical manifestation of pediatric mediastinal tumors, a single center experience. Medicine (Baltimore) 98:e16732

Coustan-Smith E, Mullighan CG, Onciu M et al (2009) Early T-cell precursor leukaemia: a subtype of very high-risk acute lymphoblastic leukaemia. Lancet Oncol 10:147–156

Den Bakker MA, Marx A, Mukai K et al (2015a) Mesenchymal tumours of the mediastinum—part I. Virchows Arch 467:487–500

Den Bakker MA, Marx A, Mukai K et al (2015b) Mesenchymal tumours of the mediastinum—part II. Virchows Arch 467:501–517

Dinter H, Bohnenberger H, Beck J et al (2019) Molecular classification of neuroendocrine tumors of the thymus. J Thorac Oncol 14:1472–1483

Duns G, Viganò E, Ennishi D et al (2021) Characterization of DLBCL with a PMBL gene expression signature. Blood 138:136–148

Eagen KP, French CA (2021) Supercharging BRD4 with NUT in carcinoma. Oncogene 40:1396–1408

Eifinger F, Ernestus K, Benz-Bohm G et al (2007) True thymic hyperplasia associated with severe thymic cyst bleeding in a newborn: case report and review of the literature. Ann Diagn Pathol 11:358–362

Farber BA, Shukla N, Lim I et al (2017) Prognostic factors and survival in non-central nervous system rhabdoid tumors. J Pediatr Surg 52:373–376

Fatimi SH, Khawaja RD, Majid Z (2014) Giant osteosarcoma of chest wall requiring resection and pneumonectomy. Asian Cardiovasc Thorac Ann 22:875–877

Faure Conter C, Fresneau B, Thebaud E et al (2017) Two tumors in 1: what should be the therapeutic target? Pediatric germ cell tumor with somatic malignant transformation. J Pediatr Hematol Oncol 39:388–394

Fonseca AL, Ozgediz DE, Christison-Lagay ER et al (2014) Pediatric thymomas: report of two cases and comprehensive review of the literature. Pediatr Surg Int 30:275–286

Goudet P, Dalac A, Le Bras M et al (2015) MEN1 disease occurring before 21 years old: a 160-patient cohort study from the Groupe d'étude des Tumeurs Endocrines. J Clin Endocrinol Metab 100:1568–1577

Gun F, Erginel B, Unüvar A et al (2012) Mediastinal masses in children: experience with 120 cases. Pediatr Hematol Oncol 29:141–147

Harris CJ, Helenowski I, Murphy AJ et al (2020) Implications of tumor characteristics and treatment modality on local recurrence and functional outcomes in children with Chest Wall sarcoma: a pediatric surgical oncology research collaborative study. Ann Surg

Ismail S, Haydar M, Ghanem A et al (2019) Pediatric mediastinal ALK- negative anaplastic large cell lymphoma (Hodgkin-like pattern) in a 13-year-old girl: a case report and review of literature. Oxf Med Case Reports 2019:omz077

Kamilaris CDC, Stratakis CA (2019) Multiple endocrine neoplasia type 1 (MEN1): an update and the significance of early genetic and clinical diagnosis. Front Endocrinol 10:339

Kao CS, Bangs CD, Aldrete G et al (2018) A clinicopathologic and molecular analysis of 34 mediastinal germ cell tumors suggesting different modes of teratoma development. Am J Surg Pathol 42:1662–1673

Kawamoto K, Miyoshi H, Yoshida N et al (2016) Clinicopathological, cytogenetic, and prognostic analysis of 131 myeloid sarcoma patients. Am J Surg Pathol 40:1473–1483

Lazar AJ, Cooper WA (2021) Genetic tumour syndromes involving the thorax: introduction. In: Board E (ed) WHO classification of tumours. Thoracic tumours, vol 5, 5th edn. International Agency for Research on Cancer, Lyon, pp 472–473

Le Deley MC, Reiter A, Williams D et al (2008) Prognostic factors in childhood anaplastic large cell lymphoma: results of a large European intergroup study. Blood 111:1560–1566

Le Pimpec-Barthes F, Cazes A, Bagan P et al (2010) [Mediastinal cysts: clinical approach and treatment]. Rev Pneumol Clin 66:52–62

Lee SH, Oh BL, Kimpo M et al (2020) Epidemiology of childhood malignant mediastinal masses and clinical factors associated with intensive care unit admission: a Singapore experience. J Paediatr Child Health 56:1039–1045

Leithäuser F, Bäuerle M, Huynh MQ et al (2001) Isotype-switched immunoglobulin genes with a high load of somatic hypermutation and lack of ongoing mutational activity are prevalent in mediastinal B-cell lymphoma. Blood 98:2762–2770

Lin KL, Chen CY, Hsu HH et al (1999) Ectopic ACTH syndrome due to thymic carcinoid tumor in a girl. J Pediatr Endocrinol Metab 12:573–578

Malagón HD, Valdez AM, Moran CA et al (2007) Germ cell tumors with sarcomatous components: a clinicopathologic and immunohistochemical study of 46 cases. Am J Surg Pathol 31:1356–1362

Marx A, Chan JK, Coindre JM et al (2015) The 2015 World Health Organization classification of tumors of the thymus: continuity and changes. J Thorac Oncol 10:1383–1395

Marx A, Rüdiger T, Rößner E et al (2018) [Ectopic thymic tissue and ectopic thymic tumors]. Pathologe 39:390–397

Marx A, Detterbeck F, Marom EM et al (2021a) Thymoma: introduction. In: Board E (ed) WHO classification of tumours. Thoracic tumours, vol 5, 5th edn. International Agency for Research on Cancer, Lyon, pp 320–325

Marx A, Yamada Y, Simon-Keller K et al (2021b) Thymus and autoimmunity. Semin Immunopathol 43:45–64

Mathew D, Prince DN, Mahomed N (2019) Extra-skeletal Ewing sarcoma of the chest wall in a child. SA J Radiol 23:1733

Minard-Colin V, Brugières L, Reiter A et al (2015) Non-Hodgkin lymphoma in children and adolescents: progress through effective collaboration, current knowledge, and challenges ahead. J Clin Oncol 33:2963–2974

Müller-Hermelink HK, Engel P, Kuo TT et al (2004) Tumours of the thymus: introduction. In: Travis WD, Brambilla E, Müller-Hermelink H-K, Harris CC (eds) World Health Organization classification of tumours. Pathology & genetics, tumours of the lung, pleura, thymus and heart. IARC Press, Lyon, pp 148–151

Murphy SB (1980) Classification, staging and end results of treatment of childhood non-Hodgkin's lymphomas: dissimilarities from lymphomas in adults. Semin Oncol 7:332–339

Murray PG, Young LS (2019) An etiological role for the Epstein-Barr virus in the pathogenesis of classical Hodgkin lymphoma. Blood 134:591–596

Mussolin L, Le Deley MC, Carraro E et al (2020) Prognostic factors in childhood anaplastic large cell lymphoma: long term results of the international ALCL99 trial. Cancers 12:2747

Onoda T, Meguro T, Kanno M et al (2015) Giant thymolipoma in a young child initially diagnosed as cardiomegaly. Pediatr Int 57:1051–1052

Orazi A, Moreira AL, Roden AC (2021) Mediastinal germ cell tumours with associated haematological malignancy. In: Board E (ed) WHO classification of tumors. Thoracic tumours, vol 5, 5th edn. International Agency for Research on Cancer, Lyon, pp 422–423

Oschlies I, Burkhardt B, Salaverria I et al (2011) Clinical, pathological and genetic features of primary mediastinal large B-cell lymphomas and mediastinal gray zone lymphomas in children. Haematologica 96:262–268

Perwein T, Lackner H, Ebetsberger-Dachs G et al (2020) Management of children and adolescents with gray zone lymphoma: a case series. Pediatr Blood Cancer 67:e28206

Pillon M, Aricò M, Mussolin L et al (2014) Mediastinal Burkitt lymphoma in childhood. Pediatr Blood Cancer 61:2127–2128

Rod J, Orbach D, Verité C et al (2014) Surgical management of thymic epithelial tumors in children: lessons from the French Society of Pediatric Oncology and review of the literature. Pediatr Blood Cancer 61:1910–1915

Roden AC, Fang W, Shen Y et al (2020) Distribution of mediastinal lesions across multi-institutional, international, radiology databases. J Thorac Oncol 15:568–579

Roden AC, Marom EM, Moreira AL et al (2021a) Germ cell tumours of the mediastinum: introduction. In: Board E (ed) WHO classification of tumours. Thoracic tumours, vol 5, 5th edn. International Agency for Research on Cancer, Lyon, pp 400–401

Roden AC, Ströbel P, Ulbright TM (2021b) Mediastinal germ cell tumours with somatic-type solid malignancy. In: Board WCoTE (ed) Thoracic tumours. International Agency for Research on Cancer, Lyon, pp 419–421

Rothstein DH, Voss SD, Isakoff M et al (2005) Thymoma in a child: case report and review of the literature. Pediatr Surg Int 21:548–551

Saarinen S, Kaasinen E, Karjalainen-Lindsberg ML et al (2013) Primary mediastinal large B-cell lymphoma segregating in a family: exome sequencing identifies MLL as a candidate predisposition gene. Blood 121:3428–3430

Salah S, Salem A (2014) Primary synovial sarcomas of the mediastinum: a systematic review and pooled analysis of the published literature. ISRN Oncol 2014:412527

Sarkozy C, Copie-Bergman C, Damotte D et al (2019) Gray-zone lymphoma between cHL and large B-cell lymphoma: a histopathologic series from the LYSA. Am J Surg Pathol 43:341–351

Sarkozy C, Chong L, Takata K et al (2020) Gene expression profiling of gray zone lymphoma. Blood Adv 4:2523–2535

Sarkozy C, Hung SS, Chavez EA et al (2021) Mutational landscape of gray zone lymphoma. Blood 137:1765–1776

Satoh Y (2019) A case report of a thymic neuroblastoma associated with syndrome of inappropriate secretion of antidiuretic hormone: ten-year follow-up results after surgical treatment. Int J Surg Case Rep 58:45–47

Schmid I, Klenk AK, Sparber-Sauer M et al (2018) Kaposiform hemangioendothelioma in children: a benign vascular tumor with multiple treatment options. World J Pediatr 14:322–329

Sicherer SH, Cabana MD, Perlman EJ et al (1998) Thymoma and cellular immune deficiency in an adolescent. Pediatr Allergy Immunol 9:49–52

Simon T, Cheuret E, Fiedler L et al (2018) Acute transverse myelitis following an opsoclonus-myoclonus syndrome: an unusual presentation. Eur J Paediatr Neurol 22:878–881

Soltysiak J, Ostalska-Nowicka D, Zaorska K et al (2017) Atypical thymic carcinoid manifesting with nephrotic-range proteinuria in a 7-year-old boy. Pediatr Nephrol 32:1465–1468

Stachowicz-Stencel T, Orbach D, Brecht I et al (2015) Thymoma and thymic carcinoma in children and adolescents: a report from the European cooperative study Group for Pediatric Rare Tumors (EXPeRT). Eur J Cancer 51:2444–2452

Steiner MA, Giles HW, Daley WP (2009) Massive low-grade fibromyxoid sarcoma presenting as acute respiratory distress in a 12-year-old girl. Pediatr Radiol 39:396–399

Storck S, Kennedy AL, Marcus KJ et al (2017) Pediatric NUT-midline carcinoma: therapeutic success employing a sarcoma based multimodal approach. Pediatr Hematol Oncol 34:231–237

Stratakis CA, Carney JA (2009) The triad of paragangliomas, gastric stromal tumours and pulmonary chondromas (Carney triad), and the dyad of paragangliomas and gastric stromal sarcomas (Carney-Stratakis syndrome): molecular genetics and clinical implications. J Intern Med 266:43–52

Suster S, Moran CA (1995) Chordomas of the mediastinum: clinicopathologic, immunohistochemical, and ultrastructural study of six cases presenting as posterior mediastinal masses. Hum Pathol 26:1354–1362

Suster S, Moran CA (1997) Malignant cartilaginous tumors of the mediastinum: clinicopathological study of six cases presenting as extraskeletal soft tissue masses. Hum Pathol 28:588–594

Suster S, Moran CA (2005) Primary synovial sarcomas of the mediastinum: a clinicopathologic, immunohistochemical, and ultrastructural study of 15 cases. Am J Surg Pathol 29:569–578

Tadiotto E, Clemente M, Pecoraro L et al (2019) Massive thymic hyperplasia in a 15-month-old boy: case report and literature review. Clin Case Rep 7:27–31

Takeda S, Miyoshi S, Akashi A et al (2003) Clinical spectrum of primary mediastinal tumors: a comparison of adult and pediatric populations at a single Japanese institution. J Surg Oncol 83:24–30

Talat N, Schulte KM (2011) Castleman's disease: systematic analysis of 416 patients from the literature. Oncologist 16:1316–1324

Tian L, Cai PQ, Cui CY et al (2015) Reactive thymic hyperplasia following chemotherapy for children with lymphoma: computed tomography may be able to provide valuable information to avoid over-treatment. Eur J Cardiothorac Surg 47:883–889

Ueda Y, Omasa M, Taki T et al (2012) Thymic neuroblastoma within a thymic cyst in an adult. Case Reports Oncol 5:459–463

Van Rhee F, Voorhees P, Dispenzieri A et al (2018) International, evidence-based consensus treatment guidelines for idiopathic multicentric Castleman disease. Blood 132:2115–2124

Van Rhee F, Oksenhendler E, Srkalovic G et al (2020) International evidence-based consensus diagnostic and treatment guidelines for unicentric Castleman disease. Blood Adv 4:6039–6050

Weis CA, Schalke B, Ströbel P et al (2018) Challenging the current model of early-onset myasthenia gravis pathogenesis in the light of the MGTX trial and histological heterogeneity of thymectomy specimens. Ann N Y Acad Sci 1413:82–91

Xu X, Paxton CN, Hayashi RJ et al (2021) Genomic and clinical characterization of early T-cell precursor lymphoblastic lymphoma. Blood Adv 5:2890–2900

Zhang KR, Jia HM, Pan EY et al (2006) Diagnosis and treatment of mediastinal enterogenous cysts in children. Chin Med Sci J 21:201–203

17 Mediastinal Germ Cell Tumors

Dominik T. Schneider, Giovanni Cecchetto, and Thomas A. Olson

17.1 Introduction

The general aspects of germ cell tumors common to all germ cell tumors occurring at different sites are discussed in the chapters of gonadal germ cell tumors (see Chap. 39). In the thorax, germ cell tumors almost exclusively develop in midline locations, mostly in the anterior mediastinum. Therefore, it has been debated whether such extragonadal germ cell tumors, in particular teratomas, may originate from midline somatic stem cells. On the other hand, there is molecular evidence that both gonadal and extragonadal germ cell tumors indeed originate from primordial germ cells at different stages of development. Thus, the examination of the epigenetic control of genomic imprinting reveals a methylation pattern that is characteristic of primordial germ cells during and shortly after their migration during early embryonal development (Schneider et al. 2001b; Bussey et al. 2001). In addition, this methylation pattern distinguishes germ cell tumors from other embryonal tumors with presumed stem cell origin such as nephroblastoma (Sievers et al. 2005), thus substantiating the hypothesis of their specific germ cell origin.

Some important age-dependent biologic patterns can be observed in mediastinal germ cell tumors (Schneider et al. 2002a, 2004). These are helpful for both diagnosis and prognostic assessment and therefore treatment planning. In young adults, mediastinal germ cell tumors belong to the most frequent extragonadal germ cell tumors, contributing approximately 10% to all germ cell tumors. Of note, malignant mediastinal germ cell tumors develop almost exclusively in males, while, in females, only rare teratomas are diagnosed. Individuals with a constitutional Klinefelter (47, XXY) karyotype have a significantly increased risk of developing germ cell tumors, in particular malignant nonseminomatous germ cell tumors, and they tend to develop them at a significantly younger age (Nichols et al. 1987). Accordingly, a recent report from the Children's Oncology Group found one third of pediatric patients with malignant mediastinal germ cell tumors to be affected by Klinefelter syndrome. Thus, the calculated risk of an individual with Klinefelter syndrome to develop a mediastinal germ cell tumor is 1 in 4000 (Williams et al. 2018).

In adults, malignant mediastinal germ cell tumors, in particular nonseminomatous tumors,

D. T. Schneider (✉)
Klinik für Kinder- und Jugendmedizin, Klinikum Dortmund, University Witten/Herdecke, Dortmund, Germany
e-mail: dominik.schneider@klinikumdo.de

G. Cecchetto
Department of Pediatrics, Pediatric Surgery, University of Padua, Padua, Italy

T. A. Olson
Division Pediatric Hematology/Oncology, Children's Healthcare of Atlanta at Egleston, Atlanta, GA, USA
e-mail: thomas.olson@choa.org

D. T. Schneider et al. (eds.), *Rare Tumors in Children and Adolescents*, Pediatric Oncology,
https://doi.org/10.1007/978-3-030-92071-5_17

tend to have a poor prognosis with approximately 50% long-term survival, even with intensive multimodal therapy (Hainsworth 2002; Ganjoo et al. 2000). Adult mediastinal germ cell tumors frequently include significant proportions of yolk sac tumor and/or choriocarcinoma. Although the corresponding tumor markers alpha 1-fetoprotein (AFP) and β-human chorionic gonadotropin (β-HCG) may be helpful for diagnosis, high levels of AFP and β-HCG are associated with poor prognosis (IGCCC Group 1997). In particular, mediastinal choriocarcinoma is frequently associated with widespread metastases including metastases to the central nervous system, which also bear a dismal prognosis. This finding has been confirmed for pediatric patients with malignant mediastinal germ cell tumors, too (Göbel et al. 2013).

Moreover, this unfavorable prognosis of malignant nonseminomatous germ cell tumors is also related to their ability to give rise to malignancies of non-germ cell histology such as leukemia, carcinoma, and sarcoma (Nichols et al. 1990; Motzer et al. 1998; Donadio et al. 2003; Fizazi et al. 1998; Faure Conter et al. 2017). It has been demonstrated that these secondary malignancies also display genetic aberrations that prove their origin from the malignant germ cell tumor (Chaganti et al. 1989; Oosterhuis et al. 1991; Orazi et al. 1993). In a multi-institution review, Hartmann et al. reported secondary hematologic malignancies in approximately 2% of adult patients with mediastinal nonseminomatous germ cell tumor (Hartmann et al. 2000). In contrast, such malignancies have been reported only rarely in association with gonadal tumors; in some of these cases, affected patients have been shown to have some form of XY gonadal dysgenesis (Kaplan et al. 1991; Koo et al. 1992).

Adult malignant mediastinal germ cell tumors display the characteristic genetic hallmark of adult testicular germ cell tumors, the isochromosome 12p or 12p amplification, respectively (Chaganti and Houldsworth 1998). For further details, see Chap. 39.

During childhood, the anterior mediastinum is a less frequent anatomic site of germ cell tumors, accounting for approximately 5% of all childhood germ cell tumors (Schneider et al. 2004; Billmire et al. 2001). Mediastinal germ cell tumors occurring during childhood show a clinical and biologic profile that is distinct from the corresponding tumors of adolescents and adults. During childhood, malignant germ cell tumors show a slight female preponderance and are exclusively composed of yolk sac tumor, sometimes admixed with teratoma (Schneider et al. 2002a) (Fig. 17.1). Thus, AFP is an exquisite tumor marker in tumors of the anterior mediastinum (Schneider et al. 2001a, b). If the age-related reference values are considered and disorders associated with elevated AFP levels are excluded

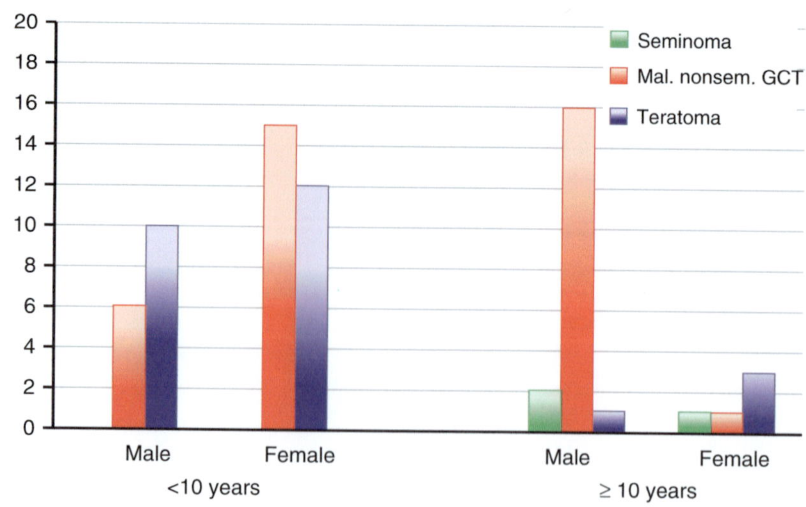

Fig. 17.1 Distribution of histologic subtypes according to age

(Blohm et al. 1998; Schneider et al. 2001a, b), an increased AFP level will prove a significant yolk sac tumor component in an anterior mediastinal tumor.

Biologically, germ cell tumors developing prior to the onset of puberty are distinct from mediastinal germ cell tumors in young men. Teratomas show no apparent chromosomal imbalances, and malignant YSTs show imbalances at 1p, 6q, and 20q, comparable to the pattern observed in gonadal germ cell tumors of this age group, while they lack 12p aberrations (Schneider et al. 2002b; Kao et al. 2018; Lee et al. 2019). Moreover, mediastinal germ cell tumors, developing in children, are not associated with secondary malignancies, and prognosis is overall favorable, comparable to that at other nongonadal sites. Accordingly, childhood germ cell tumors less frequently metastasize into the CNS, in contrast to their counterparts arising in adolescents (Göbel et al. 2013).

17.2 Clinical Diagnosis

Adolescents with germ cell tumors in the anterior mediastinum are often relatively asymptomatic, whereas infants and toddlers more often exhibit severe respiratory symptoms, including hemoptysis or upper airway obstruction (Schneider et al. 2000). Some patients may develop vena cava superior obstruction. The clinical presentation is not strictly associated with histology and biology. Thus, even "benign" teratomas may present with life-threatening complications. In such situations, the tumor markers AFP and β-HCG should be utilized immediately to guide clinical diagnosis and weigh the therapeutic options, especially whether immediate chemotherapy could be chosen to alleviate symptoms and to avoid immediate surgery with general anesthesia. The tumor markers AFP and β-HCG are also helpful in distinguishing secreting germ cell tumors from anterior mediastinal tumors with different histogenesis such as thymoma or lymphoma (Grosfeld et al. 1994).

Seminomas may be associated with elevated levels of human placenta-like alkaline phosphatase (HPLAP). However, this marker has not yet been widely studied in mediastinal seminomas. The analysis of microRNA profiles could potentially add diagnostic information in non-secreting germ cell tumors (Murray et al. 2016). Large tumors may be associated with elevated lactate dehydrogenase (LDH), which is a rather unspecific marker of tumor burden. But if LDH is significantly elevated, it may serve as an additional prognostic marker (IGCCC Group 1997; Frazier et al. 2008).

By the use of the tumor markers AFP and β-HCG, diagnostic delay by biopsy can be avoided. Considering the histologic heterogeneity of germ cell tumors, the diagnostic contribution of fine needle biopsy is mainly confirmatory and always has to be interpreted in the context of clinical tumor markers (Goel et al. 2008). It may be used in marker negative tumors, in particular if thymoma, lymphoma, or other mediastinal malignancies have to be excluded. In all other tumors that are considered assessable to complete resection based on radiographic imaging, primary complete resection should be attempted as both an initial diagnostic and therapeutic step (Table 17.1).

Radiographic imaging of mediastinal germ cell tumors commonly displays a tumor within or in close proximity to the thymus. Often invasion of the pericardium or pleura is observed, which may be associated with pericardial or pleural effusion. Teratomas tend to have cystic structures, occasional calcification, and lipid-rich tissue (Priola et al. 2006) (Fig. 17.2). Mediastinal lymph nodes may be enlarged in case of metastases, and in malignant germ cell tumors, lung metastases may be detected by CT. Choriocarcinoma has a significant tendency to metastasize into the central nervous system (Göbel et al. 2010, 2013). Therefore, a brain MRI has to be performed in every patient with elevated β-HCG or even the slightest neurological symptoms. Other metastatic sites may include the liver and rarely the bones.

During infancy and young childhood, the histologic subtypes are almost exclusively restricted to teratoma and yolk sac tumor. After the onset of puberty, histologic subtypes include most com-

Table 17.1 Specific diagnostic strategy in anterior mediastinal tumors, suspicious of germ cell tumors

Procedure	Specific questions
Clinical assessment	
Physical examination	Signs of upper airway obstruction, vena cava superior syndrome
	Pubertal status, signs of Klinefelter
	Gonadal primary
Laboratory assessment	
– AFP, β-HCG	Malignant germ cell tumor with yolk sac tumor or choriocarcinoma
– HPLAP – microRNA	Malignant seminomatous germ cell tumor If available in study setting for diagnosis and follow-up
– LDH	Unspecific marker with prognostic impact
– Catecholamines	Exclusion of neuroblastoma
– Blood count (bone marrow bx.)	Exclusion of hematologic malignancy (in adolescents and adults)
– Cytogenetics	Exclude Klinefelter syndrome (boys)
– Pregnancy test	Exclude pregnancy. If β-HCG is elevated, perform pelvic ultrasound to exclude pregnancy
Radiographic assessment	
Chest CT (alt. + chest MRI)	Site, organ of origin, cystic structures or calcification (teratoma), mediastinal metastases, lung metastases
Abdominal ultrasound	Liver metastases, lymph node metastases, testicular primary
CNS-MRI	CNS metastases (mandatory in choriocarcinoma)
Bone scan	Skeletal metastases (indicated in case of bone pain)
Histologic assessment	
H&E	Classification according to WHO
AFP	Yolk sac tumor (microfoci in teratoma)
β-HCG	Choriocarcinoma
CD-30	Embryonal carcinoma
OCT3/4	Seminoma (embryonal carcinoma)

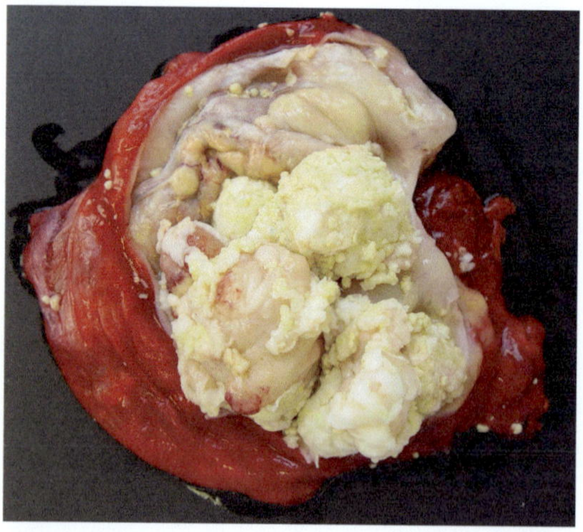

Fig. 17.2 Cystic mediastinal teratoma of a young woman

monly yolk sac tumor, germinoma, choriocarcinoma, teratoma, and immature teratoma either alone or as mixed elements (Schneider et al. 2002a). Mediastinal teratomas occasionally have sarcomatous foci-resembling rhabdomyosarcoma, angiosarcoma, or undifferentiated sarcoma. These foci are extremely aggressive, tend to overgrow the remaining teratoma, and make treatment very difficult. In adolescents and adults, malignant germ cell tumors, usually with a yolk sac tumor component, may also be associated with hematopoietic malignancies (Faure Conter et al. 2017).

17.3 Therapy

As in other sites, therapy of mediastinal germ cell tumors follows a multimodal approach. In pure teratomas, the complete resection constitutes the most important therapeutic step (Schneider et al. 2000; Billmire et al. 2001). In pure teratomas, there is no role for adjuvant chemo- or radiotherapy; only in large and irresectable tumors, an individual attempt may be made, however, with only minimal prospect of response to chemotherapy (Schneider et al. 2000). However, it should be considered that malignant germ cell tumors may include benign teratoma components. These may then respond incompletely to preoperative chemotherapy. In such situations, an attempt of delayed complete surgical resection should be taken even in bulky tumors (Billmire et al. 2001). Fortunately, compared to other nongonadal sites such as the coccygeal region, the risk of relapse after microscopically incomplete resection appears to be less, indicating yet unknown environmental factors that may influence the risk of recurrence. Nevertheless, the surgical approach in a marker negative tumor in which the radiographic assessment is suggestive of teratoma should always aim for a complete resection.

17.4 Principles of Surgical Resection of Mediastinal Germ Cell Tumors

Mediastinal germ cell tumors are mainly found in the anterior compartment, in direct contact with the thymus. The initial surgical approach depends on the likelihood of malignancy of the mass and the feasibility of a safe primary excision. A biopsy should be undertaken when a malignant germ cell tumor is suspected and if imaging investigations show an unresectable mass and if the patient is not jeopardized by the biopsy.

Biopsy technique options include open technique using the Chamberlain anterior approach (Olak 1996) or image-guided tru-cut biopsy. If the CT scan shows compression of the major airways and vena cava, an accurate assessment of the anesthetic risk is needed: actually, respiratory collapse and cardiopulmonary arrest on induction of general anesthesia are well-recognized complications also for a biopsy of an anterior mediastinal mass (Shamberger et al. 1991). Therefore, the patients must not be put at risk if the diagnosis of a malignant germ cell tumor can be established based on tumor markers and imaging.

Teratomas are also found in the pericardium, and the patient may present with cardiac tamponade. These tumors often have a stalk to the great vessels and compress the atria. Treatment requires complete resection (Gobbi et al. 2007; Schneider et al. 2000).

Initial or delayed resection of germ cell tumors can be performed by a posterolateral thoracotomy or a sternotomy depending on the extension of the disease. In some patients, partial resection of the pericardium or a partial or total thymectomy has to be performed (Schneider et al. 2000).

17.5 Multimodal Therapy in Malignant Germ Cell Tumors

In secreting tumors, diagnosis can be established based on imaging and tumor markers. By definition, secreting tumors are always malignant. Prognosis is associated with histology and age at presentation. In childhood yolk sac tumors, favorable outcome can be achieved with four cycles of platinum-based three-agent chemotherapy such as PEB, PEI, or JEB (see Table 31.6). If the lungs are compromised by mass effect, it may be prudent to use PEI, which avoids the pulmonary toxicity of bleomycin.

Ideally, chemotherapy should be given up front after establishment of the clinical diagnosis based on tumor markers. Thus, complete resection may be facilitated on delayed surgery, e.g., after three cycles of chemotherapy. In these malignant germ cell tumors, complete resection again constitutes one of the most important prognostic factors. In conclusion, initial incomplete resection at diagnosis should be avoided; if primary resection was incomplete, a second look surgery should be strongly considered. Again, the surgical approach is most often chosen via median sternotomy. Any adjacent organ such as pericardium or thymus should be resected in one piece with the tumor. In some instances, pulmonary wedge resection has to be performed in case of pulmonary metastases or pulmonary infiltration per continuitatem. On the other hand, any metastases that show complete clinical, serological (AFP), and radiographic response do not require surgical resection.

A Children's Oncology Group report has studied the impact of cisplatinum dose escalation in childhood germ cell tumors (Cushing et al. 2004). Indeed, dose escalation was associated with improved outcome, however with intolerable long-term toxicity, in particular severe ototoxicity. Nevertheless, this approach may be individually chosen in patients that are considered unfavorable risk based on clinical assessment or in relapse patients.

In postpubertal malignant nonseminomatous germ cell tumors, standard chemotherapy may not yield sufficient tumor control since with standard regimen, long-term outcome is at 50% (Bokemeyer et al. 2002; Ganjoo et al. 2000). Therefore, therapy intensification strategies, e.g., with escalated doses of ifosfamide and etoposide, have been proposed (Bokemeyer et al. 2003; Schmoll et al. 2003). Other groups have used individually intensified dose condensed regimen for selected poor prognosis patients with inappropriate marker decline (Fizazi et al. 2014). These regimens are associated with considerable toxicity and may therefore require autologous stem cell and growth factor support. However, with such strategies, long-term outcome better than 70% has been reported. Last, a recent single center study reported on the potential therapeutic impact of postchemotherapy irradiation to locally advanced mediastinal germ cell tumors, similar to strategies applied in CNS germ cell tumors (Huang et al. 2017).

In some mixed malignant germ cell tumors with teratoma elements, a specific situation termed *growing teratoma syndrome* may be observed (Logothetis et al. 1982; Afifi et al. 1997). In these patients, the serologic tumor markers show an adequate response to chemotherapy. Nevertheless, the tumor size does not decrease or may even increase. This radiographic tumor progression despite serologic response of the malignant tumor components is explained by the intrinsic resistance of teratomatous tissue to chemotherapy (Mayer et al. 2003). Therefore, continuation or even intensification of chemotherapy is obsolete. Instead, an immediate change of strategy is required, best with a surgical attempt to resect the teratoma. In tumors deemed irresectable, individual reports on alternative, e.g., antiangiogenic or immunomodulatory therapies, have been published (Calaminus et al. 2009; Postovsky et al. 2004). These will usually not induce significant tumor response but may rather induce tumor stabilization and, in ideal situations, may facilitate tumor resection.

Seminomas constitute a distinct subgroup of malignant germ cell tumors, occurring almost exclusively in male adolescent or adult patients. They are also considered malignant despite the fact that they do not secrete tumor markers. However, seminomas show an exquisite response to chemotherapy (as well as irradiation). Therefore, these tumors are currently treated with three to four cycles of platinum-based three-agent chemotherapy such as PEB, PEI, or JEB. With this standard treatment, the prognosis of these tumors is favorable and exceeds 80% long-term event-free survival. In most patients, residual tumor after chemotherapy is resected. Nevertheless, the therapeutic impact of tumor resection in highly regressive tumors is controversial. In these instances, postchemotherapy PET assessment may assist in decision-making (De et al. 2001). Any PET positive tumors should be resected irrespective of size. In contrast, PET negative tumors smaller than 1–2 cm can be followed, whereas larger tumors should also be excised, in particular in order to resect any teratoma component that cannot be distinguished by PET. In irresectable viable seminomas, irradiation constitutes a promising salvage therapy. However, it is not recommended for first-line therapy since the long-term side effects associated with mediastinal irradiations may be significant (Van den Belt-Dusebout et al. 2006).

17.6 Prognosis

More recent pediatric studies reporting outcome specifically for mediastinal subsets of children and adolescents with malignant germ cell tumors treated with platinum-based regimens suggested that although this site is considered less favorable, event-free survival of 57–88% was achieved (Schneider et al. 2000; Mann et al.

2000; Billmire et al. 2001; Cushing et al. 2004; De Pasquale et al. 2016; Depani et al. 2019). Ability to surgically resect tumor, either at onset or at postinduction surgery, improves overall survival.

Despite this encouraging data in pediatric mediastinal germ cell tumors as a whole cohort, it should always be considered that metastatic mediastinal mixed malignant germ cell tumors in adolescents (i.e., older than 8–10 years at diagnosis) and adults constitute the prognostically most unfavorable subgroup of germ cell tumors, with an overall survival hardly exceeding 50%. Therefore, a more intensive, maybe even experimental, approach is required in these patients in order to overcome the intrinsic treatment resistance in these tumors.

References

Afifi HY, Bosl GJ, Burt ME (1997) Mediastinal growing teratoma syndrome. Ann Thorac Surg 64:359–362

Billmire D, Vinocur C, Rescorla F, Colombani P, Cushing B, Hawkins E, London WB, Giller R, Lauer S (2001) Malignant mediastinal germ cell tumors: an intergroup study. J Pediatr Surg 36:18–24

Blohm ME, Vesterling-Hörner D, Calaminus G, Göbel U (1998) Alpha 1-fetoprotein (AFP) reference values in infants up to 2 years of age. Pediatr Hematol Oncol 15:135–142

Bokemeyer C, Nichols CR, Droz JP, Schmoll HJ, Horwich A, Gerl A, Fossa SD, Beyer J, Pont J, Kanz L, Einhorn L, Hartmann JT (2002) Extragonadal germ cell tumors of the mediastinum and retroperitoneum: results from an international analysis. J Clin Oncol 20:1864–1873

Bokemeyer C, Schleucher N, Metzner B, Thomas M, Rick O, Schmoll HJ, Kollmannsberger C, Boehlke I, Kanz L, Hartmann JT (2003) First-line sequential high-dose VIP chemotherapy with autologous transplantation for patients with primary mediastinal nonseminomatous germ cell tumours: a prospective trial. Br J Cancer 89:29–35

Bussey KJ, Lawce HJ, Himoe E, Shu XO, Heerema NA, Perlman EJ, Olson SB, Magenis RE (2001) SNRPN methylation patterns in germ cell tumors as a reflection of primordial germ cell development. Genes Chromosomes Cancer 32:342–352

Calaminus G, Schneider DT, Weissbach L, Schönberger S, Okpanyi V, Leuschner I, Poremba C, Göbel U (2009) Survival after an antiangiogenetic therapy and surgery in a wide spread growing teratoma originating from a testicular mixed malignant germ cell tumor. Klin Padiatr 221:136–140

Chaganti RS, Houldsworth J (1998) The cytogenetic theory of the pathogenesis of human adult male germ cell tumors. APMIS 106:80–83; discussion 83–84

Chaganti RS, Ladanyi M, Samaniego F, Offit K, Reuter VE, Jhanwar SC, Bosl GJ (1989) Leukemic differentiation of a mediastinal germ cell tumor. Genes Chromosomes Cancer 1:83–87

Cushing B, Giller R, Cullen JW, Marina NM, Lauer SJ, Olson TA, Rogers PC, Colombani P, Rescorla F, Billmire DF, Vinocur CD, Hawkins EP, Davis MM, Perlman EJ, London WB, Castleberry RP (2004) Randomized comparison of combination chemotherapy with etoposide, bleomycin, and either high-dose or standard-dose cisplatin in children and adolescents with high-risk malignant germ cell tumors: a pediatric intergroup study—Pediatric Oncology Group 9049 and Children's Cancer Group 8882. J Clin Oncol 22:2691–2700

De Pasquale MD, Crocoli A, Conte M, Indolfi P, D'Angelo P, Boldrini R, Terenziani M, Inserra A (2016) Mediastinal germ cell tumors in pediatric patients: a report from the Italian Association of Pediatric Hematology and Oncology. Pediatr Blood Cancer 63:808–812

De SM, Bokemeyer C, Becherer A, Stoiber F, Oechsle K, Kletter K, Dohmen BM, Dittrich C, Pont J (2001) Predictive impact of 2-18fluoro-2-deoxy-D-glucose positron emission tomography for residual postchemotherapy masses in patients with bulky seminoma. J Clin Oncol 19:3740–3744

Depani S, Stoneham S, Krailo M, Xia C, Nicholson J (2019) Results from the UK Children's Cancer and Leukaemia Group study of extracranial germ cell tumours in children and adolescents (GCIII). Eur J Cancer 118:49–57

Donadio AC, Motzer RJ, Bajorin DF, Kantoff PW, Sheinfeld J, Houldsworth J, Chaganti RSK, Bosl GJ (2003) Chemotherapy for teratoma with malignant transformation. J Clin Oncol 21:4285–4291

Faure Conter C, Fresneau B, Thebaud E, Bertrand A, Dijoud F, Rome A, Dumesnil C, Castex MP, Ghanem A, Orbach D (2017) Two tumors in 1: what should be the therapeutic target? Pediatric germ cell tumor with somatic malignant transformation. J Pediatr Hematol Oncol 39:388–394

Fizazi K, Culine S, Droz JP, Kramar A, Theodore C, Ruffie P, Le CT (1998) Primary mediastinal nonseminomatous germ cell tumors: results of modern therapy including cisplatin-based chemotherapy. J Clin Oncol 16:725–732

Fizazi K, Pagliaro L, Laplanche A, Fléchon A, Mardiak J, Geoffrois L, Kerbrat P, Chevreau C, Delva R, Rolland F, Theodore C, Roubaud G, Gravis G, Eymard JC, Malhaire JP, Linassier C, Habibian M, Martin AL, Journeau F, Reckova M, Logothetis C, Culine S (2014) Personalised chemotherapy based on tumour marker decline in poor prognosis germ-cell tumours (GETUG 13): a phase 3, multicentre, randomised trial. Lancet Oncol 15:1442–1450

Frazier AL, Rumcheva P, Olson T, Giller R, Cushing B, Cullen J, Marina N, London WB (2008) Application of the adult international germ cell classification system to pediatric malignant non-seminomatous germ cell tumors: a report from the Children's Oncology Group. Pediatr Blood Cancer 50:746–751

Ganjoo KN, Rieger KM, Kesler KA, Sharma M, Heilman DK, Einhorn LH (2000) Results of modern therapy for patients with mediastinal nonseminomatous germ cell tumors. Cancer 88:1051–1056

Gobbi D, Rubino M, Chiandetti L, Zanon GF, Cecchetto G (2007) Neonatal intrapericardial teratoma: a challenge for the pediatric surgeon. J Pediatr Surg 42:E3–E6

Göbel U, Schneider DT, Teske C, Schönberger S, Calaminus G (2010) Brain metastases in children and adolescents with extracranial germ cell tumor—data of the MAHO/MAKEI-registry. Klin Pädiatr 222:140–144

Göbel U, von Kries R, Teske C, Schneider DT, Beyerlein A, Bernbeck B, Calaminus G (2013) Brain metastases during follow-up of children and adolescents with extracranial malignant germ cell tumors: risk adapted management decision tree analysis based on data of the MAHO/MAKEI-registry. Pediatr Blood Cancer 60:217–223

Goel D, Prayaga AK, Sundaram C, Raghunadharao D, Rajappa SJ, Rammurti S, Rao TM, Kumar RV (2008) Utility of fine needle aspiration cytology in mediastinal lesions: a clinicopathologic study of 1617 cases from a single institution. Acta Cytol 52:404–411

Grosfeld JL, Skinner MA, Rescorla FJ, West KW, Scherer LR III (1994) Mediastinal tumors in children: experience with 196 cases. Ann Surg Oncol 1:121–127

Hainsworth JD (2002) Diagnosis, staging, and clinical characteristics of the patient with mediastinal germ cell carcinoma. Chest Surg Clin N Am 12:665–672

Hartmann JT, Nichols CR, Droz JP, Horwich A, Gerl A, Fossa SD, Beyer J, Pont J, Fizazi K, Einhorn L, Kanz L, Bokemeyer C (2000) Hematologic disorders associated with primary mediastinal nonseminomatous germ cell tumors. J Natl Cancer Inst 92:54–61

Huang J, Tan Y, Zhen Z, Lu S, Sun F, Zhu J, Wang J, Liao R, Sun X (2017) Role of post-chemotherapy radiation in the management of children and adolescents with primary advanced malignant mediastinal germ cell tumors. PLoS One 12:e0183219

IGCCC Group (1997) International germ cell consensus classification: a prognostic factor- based staging system for metastatic germ cell cancers. International Germ Cell Cancer Collaborative Group. J Clin Oncol 15:594–603

Kao CS, Bangs CD, Aldrete G, Cherry AM, Ulbright TM (2018) A clinicopathologic and molecular analysis of 34 mediastinal germ cell tumors suggesting different modes of teratoma development. Am J Surg Pathol 42:1662–1673

Kaplan SS, Bornstein SG, Christopherson WA, Surti U (1991) Associated leukemia and mixed germ cell tumor in a patient with gonadal dysgenesis. Int J Gynaecol Obstet 35:83–88

Koo CH, Reifel J, Kogut N, Cove JK, Rappaport H (1992) True histiocytic malignancy associated with a malignant teratoma in a patient with 46XY gonadal dysgenesis. Am J Surg Pathol 16:175–183

Lee T, Seo Y, Han J, Kwon GY (2019) Analysis of chromosome 12p over-representation and clinicopathological features in mediastinal teratomas. Pathology 51:62–66

Logothetis CJ, Samuels ML, Trindade A, Johnson DE (1982) The growing teratoma syndrome. Cancer 50:1629–1635

Mann JR, Raafat F, Robinson K, Imeson J, Gornall P, Sokal M, Gray E, McKeever P, Hale J, Bailey S, Oakhill A (2000) The United Kingdom Children's Cancer Study Group's second germ cell tumor study: carboplatin, etoposide, and bleomycin are effective treatment for children with malignant extracranial germ cell tumors, with acceptable toxicity. J Clin Oncol 18:3809–3818

Mayer F, Stoop H, Scheffer GL, Scheper R, Oosterhuis JW, Looijenga LH, Bokemeyer C (2003) Molecular determinants of treatment response in human germ cell tumors. Clin Cancer Res 9:767–773

Motzer RJ, Amsterdam A, Prieto V, Sheinfeld J, Murty VV, Mazumdar M, Bosl GJ, Chaganti RS, Reuter VE (1998) Teratoma with malignant transformation: diverse malignant histologies arising in men with germ cell tumors. J Urol 159:133–138

Murray MJ, Bell E, Raby KL, Rijlaarsdam MA, Gillis AJ, Looijenga LH, Brown H, Destenaves B, Nicholson JC, Coleman N (2016) A pipeline to quantify serum and cerebrospinal fluid microRNAs for diagnosis and detection of relapse in paediatric malignant germ-cell tumours. Br J Cancer 114:151–162

Nichols CR, Heerema NA, Palmer C, Loehrer PJ Sr, Williams SD, Einhorn LH (1987) Klinefelter's syndrome associated with mediastinal germ cell neoplasms. J Clin Oncol 5:1290–1294

Nichols CR, Roth BJ, Heerema N, Griep J, Tricot G (1990) Hematologic neoplasia associated with primary mediastinal germ- cell tumors. N Engl J Med 322:1425–1429

Olak J (1996) Parasternal mediastinotomy (Chamberlain procedure). Chest Surg Clin N Am 6:31–40

Oosterhuis JW, Van den Berg E, de Jong B, Timens W, Castedo SM, Rammeloo RH, Sleijfer DT (1991) Mediastinal germ cell tumor with secondary nongerm cell malignancy, and extensive hematopoietic activity. Pathology, DNA-ploidy, and karyotyping. Cancer Genet Cytogenet 54:183–195

Orazi A, Neiman RS, Ulbright TM, Heerema NA, John K, Nichols CR (1993) Hematopoietic precursor cells within the yolk sac tumor component are the source of secondary hematopoietic malignancies in patients with mediastinal germ cell tumors. Cancer 71:3873–3881

Postovsky S, Epelbaum M, Ben Itzhak O, Beck D, Ben Arush MW (2004) Growing teratoma syndrome treated by interferon alpha-2beta: case report and literature review. Pediatr Hematol Oncol 21:9–16

Priola SM, Priola AM, Cardinale L, Perotto F, Fava C (2006) The anterior mediastinum: anatomy and imaging procedures. Radiol Med 111:295–311

Schmoll HJ, Kollmannsberger C, Metzner B, Hartmann JT, Schleucher N, Schoffski P, Schleicher J, Rick O, Beyer J, Hossfeld D, Kanz L, Berdel WE, Andreesen R, Bokemeyer C (2003) Long-term results of first-line sequential high-dose etoposide, ifosfamide, and cisplatin chemotherapy plus autologous stem cell support for patients with advanced metastatic germ cell cancer: an extended phase I/II study of the German Testicular Cancer Study Group. J Clin Oncol 21:4083–4091

Schneider DT, Calaminus G, Reinhard H, Gutjahr P, Kremens B, Harms D, Göbel U (2000) Primary mediastinal germ cell tumors in children and adolescents: results of the German cooperative protocols MAKEI 83/86, 89, and 96. J Clin Oncol 18:832–839

Schneider DT, Calaminus G, Göbel U (2001a) Diagnostic value of alpha_1_-fetoprotein and human chorionic gonadotropic hormone in infancy and childhood. Pediatr Hematol Oncol 18:11–26

Schneider DT, Schuster AE, Fritsch MK, Hu J, Olson T, Lauer S, Göbel U, Perlman EJ (2001b) Multipoint imprinting analysis indicates a common precursor cell for gonadal and nongonadal pediatric germ cell tumors. Cancer Res 61:7268–7276

Schneider DT, Perlman EJ, Harms D, Fritsch MK, Calaminus G, Göbel U (2002a) Mediastinal germ cell tumors (MGCT) in children and adolescents: age correlates with histological differentiation, genetic profiles and clinical outcome. In: Harnden P, Joffe JK, Jones WG (eds) Germ cell tumours, vol 26. Springer, London, pp 127–128

Schneider DT, Schuster AE, Fritsch MK, Calaminus G, Göbel U, Harms D, Lauer S, Olson T, Perlman EJ (2002b) Genetic analysis of mediastinal nonseminomatous germ cell tumors in children and adolescents. Genes Chromosomes Cancer 34:115–125

Schneider DT, Calaminus G, Koch S, Teske C, Schmidt P, Haas RJ, Harms D, Göbel U (2004) Epidemiologic analysis of 1,442 children and adolescents registered in the German germ cell tumor protocols. Pediatr Blood Cancer 42:169–175

Shamberger RC, Holzman RS, Griscom NT, Tarbell NJ, Weinstein HJ (1991) CT quantitation of tracheal cross-sectional area as a guide to the surgical and anesthetic management of children with anterior mediastinal masses. J Pediatr Surg 26:138–142

Sievers S, Alemazkour K, Zahn S, Perlman EJ, Gillis AJ, Looijenga L, Göbel U, Schneider DT (2005) IGF2/H19 imprinting analysis with the methylation-sensitive single nucleotide primer extension method in human germ cell tumors reflects their origin from different stages of primordial germ cell development. Genes Chromosomes Cancer 44:256–264

Van den Belt-Dusebout AW, Nuver J, de Wit R, Gietema JA, ten Bokkel Huinink WW, Rodrigus PTR, Schimmel EC, Aleman BMP, van Leeuwen FE (2006) Long-term risk of cardiovascular disease in 5-year survivors of testicular cancer. J Clin Oncol 24:467–475

Williams LA, Pankratz N, Lane J, Krailo M, Roesler M, Richardson M, Frazier AL, Amatruda JF, Poynter JN (2018) Klinefelter syndrome in males with germ cell tumors: a report from the Children's Oncology Group. Cancer 124:3900–3908

18 Pleuropulmonary Blastoma

Kris Ann P. Schultz and Yoav Messinger

18.1 Background

Pleuropulmonary blastoma (PPB) is a malignant sarcoma of lung and pleura seen primarily in infants and children under age 6 years. PPB is in the family of dysembryonic developmental tumors of early childhood such as Wilms' tumor (nephroblastoma), embryonal rhabdomyosarcoma (ERMS), neuroblastoma, medulloblastoma, retinoblastoma, and others. Histopathologically, PPB recapitulates the primitive pleuropulmonary mesenchyme from which it is thought to arise (Dehner 1994; Manivel et al. 1988). Because of its rarity, PPB was recognized as a diagnostic entity only in the 1980s (Dehner 1994; Manivel et al. 1987, 1988).

Although rare, PPB is clinically significant and one of the pediatric cancers for which surveillance may be both feasible and beneficial.

18.2 Manifestations of PPB

PPB is classified into four main subtypes. The first three subtypes, type I, II, and III PPB, are most often diagnosed in very young children with 92% of type I, II, and III PPB diagnosed before 72 months of age (Messinger et al. 2015). The median ages at diagnosis for type I, type II, and type III patients are 8, 35, and 41 months, respectively (Fig. 18.1, Messinger et al. 2015).

PPB type is determined by the gross pathologic morphology augmented by radiographic and microscopic evidence (Dehner 1994; Hill et al. 2008). Type I PPB, the earliest stage of tumorigenesis, may occasionally be seen by prenatal ultrasound (Miniati et al. 2006) and typically is found in infants and toddlers with a median age at diagnosis of 8 months (Messinger et al. 2015). Radiographically and grossly, type I PPB is a relatively innocuous-appearing air-filled unilocular or multilocular cyst often located in the peripheral lung parenchyma (Fig. 18.2). The radiographic appearance of type I PPB may suggest a congenital pulmonary airway malformation (CPAM) (Priest et al. 2009; Stocker 2002). Only rarely are type I cysts fluid-filled or infected. Beneath a benign respiratory epithelium, cyst walls and septa contain a scattered, sometimes sparse, population of malignant small cells, suggesting a rhabdomyomatous lineage (Hill et al. 2008).

Type II PPB occurs generally in older children with a median age at diagnosis of 35 months (Fig. 18.1). Type II PPB has both type I cysts or cyst remnants and grossly visible thickened cyst walls or septa, solid mural nodules, or larger tumor excrescences (Fig. 18.3). The solid tume-

K. A. P. Schultz (✉) · Y. Messinger
International Pleuropulmonary Blastoma (PPB)/DICER1 Registry, Minneapolis, MN, USA

Children's Minnesota, Minneapolis, MN, USA
e-mail: krisann.schultz@childrensmn.org; yoav.messinger@childrensmn.org

D. T. Schneider et al. (eds.), *Rare Tumors in Children and Adolescents*, Pediatric Oncology,
https://doi.org/10.1007/978-3-030-92071-5_18

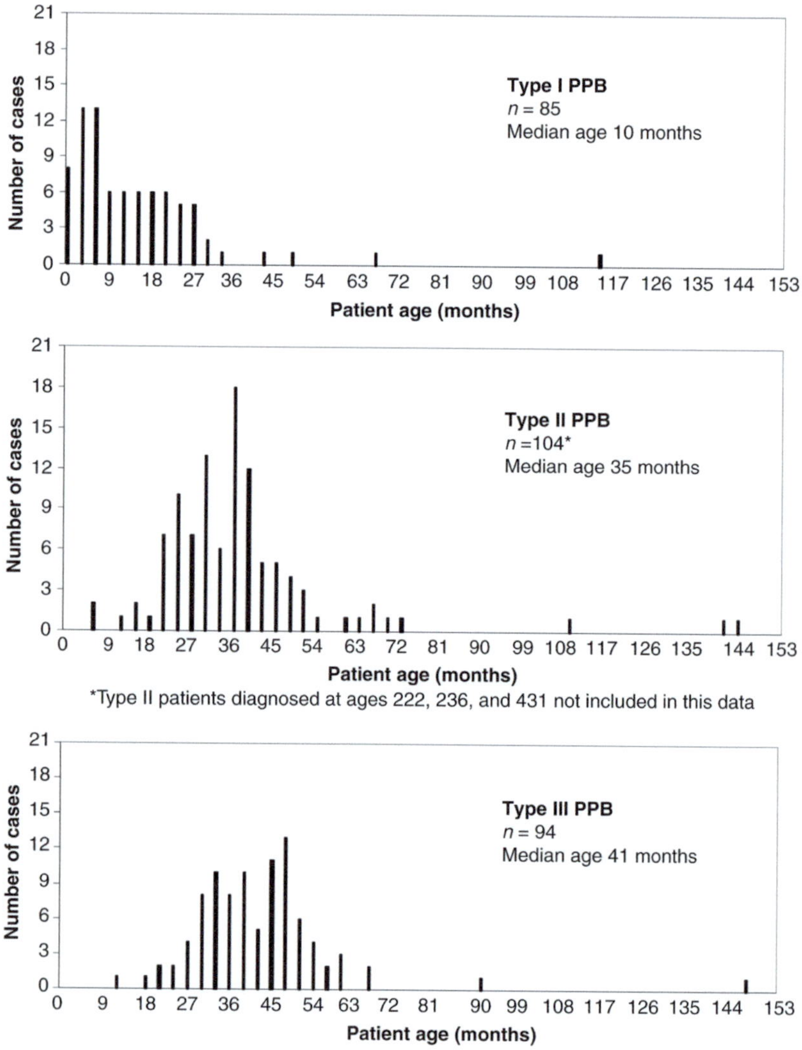

Fig. 18.1 Age at diagnosis for individuals with PPB. *PPB* pleuropulmonary blastoma. (Reprinted with permission from Messinger et al. Cancer 2015)

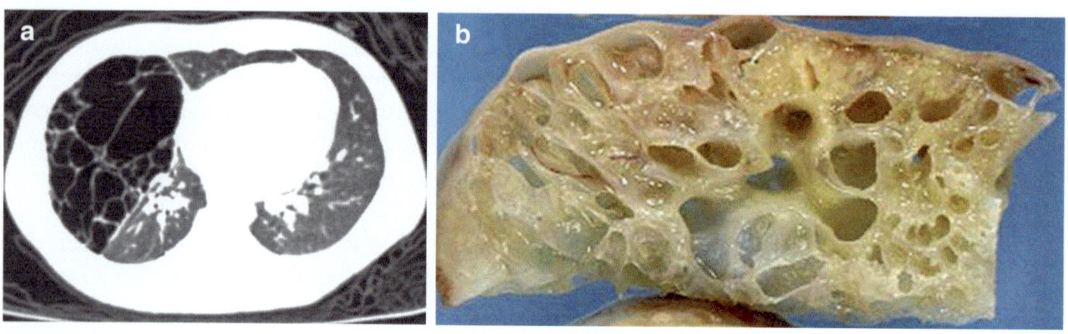

Fig. 18.2 Examples of type I PPB (different patients shown). (**a**) Axial chest CT image. Characteristic of multiloculated, air-filled cyst. CCAM may be radiographically identical. (**b**) Gross pathology (Photograph courtesy of Adrian Charles, M.D., Princess Margaret Hospital, Perth, Australia)

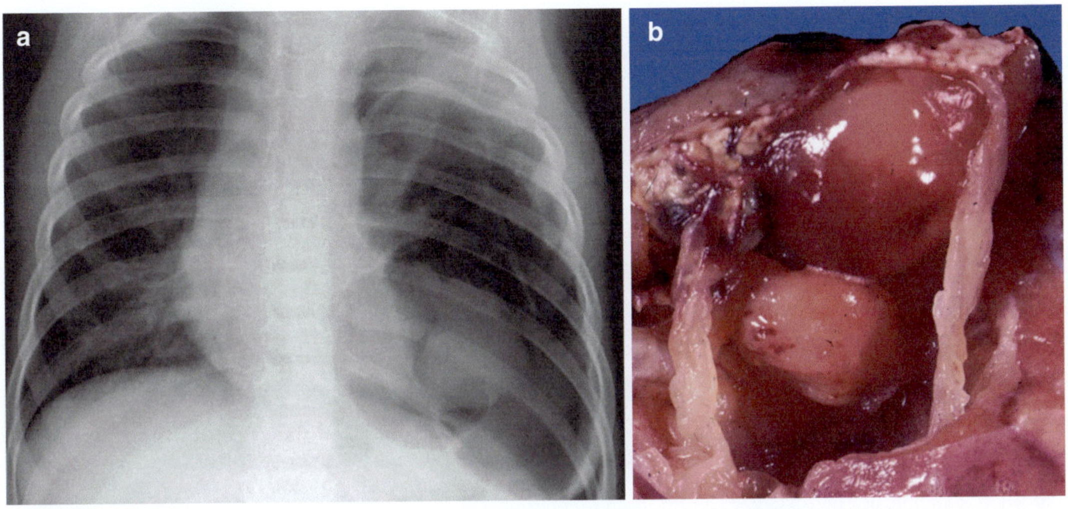

Fig. 18.3 Examples of type II PPB (different patients shown). (**a**) Chest radiograph showing solid nodules within large air-filled cyst in left hemithorax. (**b**) Gross pathology showing polypoid nodules of sarcoma botryoides inside opened pulmonary cyst (Photograph courtesy of David Kelly, M.D., Children's Health System, Birmingham, AL, USA)

factions result from sarcomatous expansion of the subepithelial malignant cells of type I PPB with overgrowth of cyst walls and septa. The solid portions clearly reveal a mixed-pattern sarcoma, indistinguishable from type III described below.

Type III PPB (Fig. 18.4a) is a completely solid mixed-pattern sarcoma diagnosed at a median age of 41 months.

Clear examples of lung cysts progressing over 6–24 months to type II or III PPB have been observed. Similarly, recurrences of type I PPB are characteristically type II or III disease (Priest et al. 2006; Messinger et al. 2015). Although progression has been documented, it is not clear if all type II or III PPBs are preceded by a purely cystic type I PPB.

In addition to *progression*, type I PPB may *regress or fail to progress* and persist without malignant potential. Residual unilocular or multiloculated cysts, termed type Ir (regressed or nonprogressed) PPB, may be diagnosed at any age. The radiographic appearance is of indistinguishable from type I PPB using current imaging modalities (Fig. 18.2a). Like type I PPB, type Ir PPB may be multifocal. Although type Ir PPBs are generally smaller than type I PPB, very large type Ir PPBs have also been seen. Regression of type II or III PPB has not been observed.

Type I PPB may present with respiratory distress related to compression or pneumothorax or may be asymptomatic and detected on chest imaging or prenatal ultrasound (Priest et al. 1997, 2009; Miniati et al. 2006). Pneumothorax, including tension pneumothorax, suggests PPB and is not common in CPAM (Priest et al. 2009; Stocker 2002). Type II PPB may also present with pneumothorax, but typically type II and III PPB may also present with cough, mild to severe respiratory distress, and nonspecific symptoms such as fever, malaise, and anorexia. Type II and III PPBs are often diagnosed as "pneumonia." Cross-sectional imaging obtained when symptoms worsen or persist shows a large mixed cystic and solid or purely solid tumor. Advanced PPBs may be very large and may grow rapidly, leading to opacification of the hemithorax and compression of mediastinal structures (Fig. 18.4a). Type II and III PPB may also extend into venous and arterial great vessels, leading to vascular symptoms and systemic embolism (Priest et al. 2011a). Type Ir PPB may also present with pneumothorax but is more commonly discovered incidentally on chest

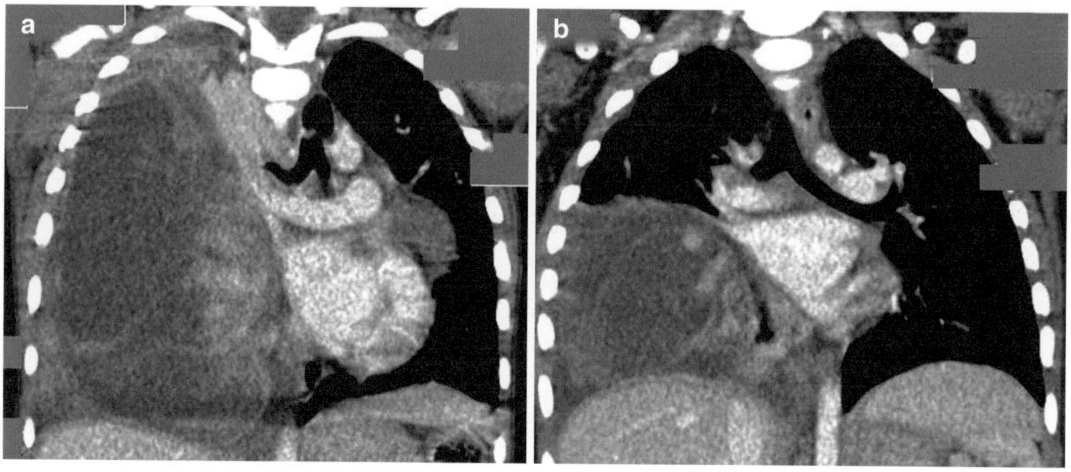

Fig. 18.4 Example of extensive type III PPB in a 33-month-old child. (**a**) Coronal CT image at carina, at diagnosis. (**b**) CT image 12 weeks later following four courses of IVADo chemotherapy

imaging during the evaluation of another condition or as a part of surveillance for known tumor predisposition.

Type I PPB has no metastatic potential; however, type II and III PPB may have metastatic disease at diagnosis, during treatment, or following completion of therapy. The central nervous system is the most common extrathoracic site of spread of PPB (Priest et al. 2007, Nakano 2019). Other metastatic sites include the pleural space, lung parenchyma, bones, and liver. Bone marrow metastases are rare but have been seen. Pleural effusion is moderately common in type II and III PPB, but cytology is rarely positive.

18.3 Pathology Overview

At gross examination, type I and Ir PPB may appear unilocular or multicystic; however, at low magnification, both demonstrate a multilocular architecture with delicate septa which are characteristic and suggest the PPB diagnosis (Hill et al. 2008). In type I PPB, a population of small primitive mesenchymal cells is found in the stroma beneath a benign respiratory epithelial lining; these cells may be a localized single focus, several foci, or a diffuse proliferation, resembling the cambium layer effect of a sarcoma botryoides. The primitive small cells may display rhabdomyoblastic differentiation, and prominent eosinophilic cytoplasm may be present. The presence of rhabdomyoblasts is not necessary for the pathologic diagnosis. Small nodules of immature cartilage are often found in the septa and are not necessarily accompanied by the small primitive cells. Because the small primitive cells or nodules of cartilage may be exquisitely focal, it may be necessary to submit an entire cyst specimen for microscopic examination. In type Ir PPB, the small cell population is not seen; there may be evidence of necrotic or hyalinized cyst walls and septa and hemosiderin-laden macrophages.

Type II PPB retains evidence of type I cysts but grossly demonstrates areas of solid tumor. The evidence for residual cysts may be clinical (pneumothorax), radiographic, or pathologic. Type III PPB is completely solid. Elsewhere in the lungs, individuals with type II or III PPB patients may have separate type I or Ir PPB. Microscopically, the solid areas of type II and III PPB reveal an aggressive, primitive mixed-pattern sarcoma: blastema, anaplasia, ERMS, chondrosarcoma, undifferentiated spindle-cell proliferations, and necrosis; rarely, other tissue types such as neuroblastoma are present. Anaplasia may be dramatic with frequent bizarre mitotic figures. Anaplasia is rare in type I PPB (~6% of cases) but is present in 77% and 90%, respectively, of type II and III PPB (Hill et al. 2008). Tumors may be extremely friable with large areas of necrosis; pseudocysts secondary to necrosis do not designate type II disease. Small biopsies of large tumors may sample a monomorphic histopathology, typically ERMS. Type III PPB may arise in and be entirely pleural based, including tumors of the parietal pleura (Fig. 18.4a). Malignant epithelium is not seen in PPB, differentiating it from "pulmonary blastoma," a biphasic tumor of adulthood, which nevertheless occurs rarely in young children (Dehner 1994).

The differential diagnosis of type I PPB includes CPAM, pulmonary interstitial emphysema, fetal lung interstitial tumor (FLIT) (Dishop et al. 2010), and cystic primary pleuropulmonary synovial sarcoma (CPPSS) (Cummings et al. 2010). FLIT is typically seen in newborns; although the histology may be reminiscent of type I PPB, the radiographic appearance of an airless opaque mass is typical of FLIT. Although CPPSS may present with pneumothorax (Belcher et al. 2007), it is a disease of teen and young adult years during which type I PPB is extraordinarily unlikely (Cummings et al. 2010). A subtle spindle-cell population in cyst walls and septa suggests type I PPB; gene fusion markers for synovial sarcoma are useful (Cummings et al. 2010).

The differential diagnosis of solid PPB includes "monomorphic" pulmonary ERMS, biphasic adult-type pulmonary blastoma, and monomorphic spindle-cell proliferations, such as monomorphic pulmonary synovial sarcoma in teens as well as malignant peripheral nerve sheath tumors and other sarcomas. Tumor-based molecular diagnostics may clarify the diagnosis (see *DICER1* pathogenic variation).

18.4 PPB Treatment

Surgical resection is the primary treatment for type I PPB. The main goal of therapy is the prevention of progression to the more advanced PPB (types II and III) that have worse prognoses. Type I PPB may be exophytic and readily removed, or it may deeply replace and distort one or more lobes, requiring lobectomy. Wedge resections are frequently performed. Negative margins may prevent the need for a subsequent surgery or other adjuvant interventions. Some type I PPBs are widely multifocal (unilateral or bilateral). In instances where surgical removal is not feasible, the largest lesion(s) should be removed for pathologic examination, and further treatment may be based on pathologic findings. A patient may have more than one type of PPB. A computed tomography (CT) scan is recommended 1 month following surgery to determine whether residual cysts remain, which may have been compressed and undetected initially. The role of chemotherapy in type I PPB is a subject of active research, and expert consultation is advised. Most children with type I PPB undergo surgery alone; however, when adjuvant chemotherapy is given, a regimen of vincristine and dactinomycin (VA) or vincristine, dactinomycin, and cyclophosphamide (VAC) is most common (Messinger et al. 2015). Chemotherapy is not generally recommended for patients with only type Ir PPB.

Type II and III PPBs require multimodal therapy. Due to tumor size and location, resection may not be feasible and biopsy is often pursued (Fig. 18.4a). Core needle biopsies may not sample diverse histologic subtypes but will probably yield a "sarcoma" diagnosis, allowing selection of neoadjuvant chemotherapy. Multiple core needle biopsies or open excisional biopsies are recommended. Fine needle aspirate and cytologic examination may fail to reveal the diagnosis. Large tumors are sometimes resected and may be encapsulated or conversely extremely friable with pre- or intraoperative rupture, gross pleural spillage, and piecemeal resection.

Type II and III PPBs are aggressive sarcomas, and chemotherapy recommendations are the same for both types. Adjuvant and neoadjuvant regimens typically follow those for other aggressive sarcomas. In Europe, VAIA (vincristine, doxorubicin [Adriamycin], ifosfamide, and dactinomycin [actinomycin D]) and IVADo (ifosfamide, vincristine, dactinomycin, and doxorubicin) have been given most commonly, and VAIA is currently included in recommendations from the EXPeRT group (Bisogno et al. 2014). The German group recently reported that

E/VAIA was effective in 23 patients (Sparber-Sauer et al. 2017). In the United States, the International PPB/*DICER1* Registry has recommended IVADo. IVADo employs four agents together for maximal early effect, especially for neoadjuvant use. Neoadjuvant responses range from approximately 40–90% three-dimensional volume reduction during 16 weeks of IVADo (Fig. 18.4b). PPB cannot be controlled by chemotherapy alone, and surgical resection by week 12 or 16 must be considered. Aggressive resections, including extrapleural pneumonectomy, may be appropriate when there is extensive involvement. Diaphragmatic resections and more rarely small chest wall resections have been done. Children appear to tolerate lobectomy or pneumonectomy. Studies of quality of life and cardiopulmonary function in PPB survivors are underway.

Type II and III PPBs are aggressive tumors, and adjunctive radiation therapy may be considered as a part of local control for residual or particularly high-risk disease. The use of thoracic radiation is limited to children with high-risk disease due to concern for toxicity in these very young children already receiving anthracycline chemotherapy. When radiation therapy is given, a sarcoma-based strategy is most often employed. Whole-lung radiation at lung tolerance doses may not be effective against this aggressive sarcoma but has not been formally evaluated.

Treatments for recurrent PPB are highly varied. Therapy for thoracic recurrence is likely to include surgery, relapse sarcoma regimens, or new agents, with or without focal radiation. For responsive disease or "consolidation" of a disease-free condition, high-dose chemotherapy with autologous stem-cell reconstitution has been used for several PPB patients who have survived.

Isolated cerebral metastases can be cured. PPB Registry data shows 11/54 individuals with PPB and CNS metastases survived (Nakano et al. 2019). Generally, CNS recurrence is treated with surgical resection followed by "sarcoma dose" radiation therapy with or without adjuvant systemic therapy (Priest et al. 2007; Nakano et al. 2019).

18.5 Prognosis

PPB type is the strongest predictor of overall survival. Children with type I PPB have an overall survival of 89%; type II, 72%; and type III, 53% (Messinger et al. 2015). Significantly, death after type I PPB occurred only after progression to type II or III. Complete resection is also correlated with improved survival (Bisogno et al. 2017, Sparber-Sauer et al. 2017). Within type II or type III, distant metastasis at diagnosis had significant detrimental prognostic effect (Messinger et al. 2015).

18.6 *DICER1* Pathogenic Variation

In 2009, germline mutations in *DICER1* were described in children with PPB and their family members with histories of PPB, lung cysts, CN, and/or ERMS (Hill et al. 2009). Subsequently, germline *DICER1* mutations have been described in more than 70% of children with PPB and in children and adults with a spectrum of neoplastic and nonneoplastic conditions (Hill et al. 2010; Slade et al. 2011; Bahubeshi et al. 2010; Rio Frio et al. 2011; Priest et al. 2011b; Brenneman et al. 2015; Hill et al. 2014). In the ovary, *DICER1* mutations are associated with Sertoli–Leydig cell tumor, gynandroblastoma, and ovarian sarcoma (Heravi-Moussavi et al. 2012; Schultz et al. 2016; Stewart et al. 2019). In the kidney, cystic nephroma is the most common *DICER1*-related manifestation with Wilms' tumor and renal sarcoma less commonly seen. Brain tumors including pineoblastoma, pituitary blastoma, and intracranial sarcoma may also be *DICER1*-related. In addition to neoplastic manifestations, thyroid nodules, macrocephaly, and renal cysts are frequently observed.

Most *DICER1*-related tumors, including PPB, have biallelic *DICER1* mutations. Generally, there is a loss of function mutation, typically germline accompanied by a second, typically tumor-specific missense mutation in the RNase IIIb domain. These missense mutations affect codons in the "hotspot" region, most commonly E1705, D1709, D1713, G1809, D1810 and E1813. These mutations alter miRNA processing via impaired cleavage of mature 5p miRNAs from the 5'end of the pre-miRNA hairpin resulting in rapid degradation of 5p miRNAs and altering downstream mRNA expression.

While "germline loss of function plus tumor-specific missense RNase IIIb mutation" is the classical pattern for PPB and many other *DICER1*-related tumors, some tumors feature biallelic somatic mutations in the absence of any apparent predisposing germline variation. Mosaicism for loss of function pathogenic variation may occur. In addition, mosaicism for an RNase IIIb hotspot mutation has been described. These individuals have an earlier age of onset and higher number of disease foci than individuals with a more typical germline loss of function variant elsewhere in the *DICER1* gene.

In individuals with a classical germline loss of function variant and somatic, tumor-specific RNase IIIb mutation, the tumor-specific RNase IIIb mutation will vary between tumor types and can thus assist in the discrimination between recurrent and metachronous tumors in situations where the clinical picture is unclear.

Germline and tumor *DICER1* testing is recommended for all individuals with *DICER1*-related conditions (Schultz et al. 2018). When a germline *DICER1* pathogenic variant is detected, genetic counseling and extension of testing to relatives is recommended. This is particularly important as many *DICER1* tumors are most curable when found in their earliest forms. In several instances, testing of children based on parental or sibling medical history has resulted in detection of PPB prior to progression to type II or II PPB. In these instances, the prognosis is favorable (Schultz et al. 2014). Likewise, most individuals with FIGO (Federation International Gynecology Oncology) Stage IA ovarian sex cord–stromal tumors will be cured with surgery alone, whereas individuals with advanced disease face intensive chemotherapy and a poorer prognosis. Other *DICER1* tumors including Wilms' tumor, renal sarcoma, and *DICER1*-related brain tumors may have better outcomes when found early.

Surveillance guidelines are now available to facilitate early detection of *DICER1*-related cancers (Schultz et al. 2018), Tables 18.1 and 18.2. Individual, family, and care provider education remains the cornerstone of the guidelines with judicious use of imaging studies at specific time points. Revision of these guidelines is expected over time as new information becomes available. All individuals with *DICER1* pathogenic varia-

Table 18.1 Indications for *DICER1* testing from Clinical Cancer Research 2018

Major:	Minor:
- Individuals with PPB (all types)	- Lung cyst(s) in adults
- Lung cyst(s) in childhood, especially if multi-septated, multiple or bilateral	- Renal cyst(s)[a]
- Thoracic ERMS[a]	- Wilms tumor
- Cystic nephroma	- Multinodular goiter or differentiated thyroid cancer
- Genitourinary sarcomas including undifferentiated sarcoma[a]	- ERMS other than thoracic or gynecologic[a]
- Ovarian SLCT	- Poorly differentiated neuroendocrine tumor
- Gynandroblastoma	- Undifferentiated sarcoma[a]
- Uterine cervical or ovarian ERMS[a]	- Macrocephaly[a]
- Genitourinary/gynecologic neuroendocrine tumors	- Consider testing for any childhood cancer in constellation with any other minor criteria
- Multinodular goiter or thyroid cancer in two or more first-degree relatives or in an index patient with a family history consistent with *DICER1* syndrome[a]	
- Childhood-onset multinodular goiter[a] or differentiated thyroid cancer[a]	
- CBME	
- NCMH	
- Pineoblastoma	
- Pituitary blastoma	

NOTE: Consider germline *DICER1* genetic testing in an individual with one major or two minor indications.
[a]Multinodular goiter, differentiated thyroid cancer (papillary or follicular carcinomas), sarcomas, Wilms tumor, neuroendocrine tumors, renal cysts, and macrocephaly may also be associated with other genetic predisposition syndromes. Consider testing for additional hereditary cancer predispositions and/or a next-generation sequencing panel that includes deletion/duplication of *DICER1* and/or other genes indicated by clinical and family history.

Table 18.2 Suggested signs and symptoms and imaging surveillance by system for individuals with *DICER1* pathogenic variation. (From Clinical Cancer Research, 2018)

System	Signs/symptoms to consider	Condition of interest	Screening: clinical and radiographic
Lung	Tachypnea, cough, fever, and pain; pneumothorax	- PPB - Lung cysts - Pulmonary blastoma	CXR at birth and every 4–6 months until 8 years of age, every 12 months 8–12 years of age; consider a CT of chest at 3–6 months of age.[a] Toddlers: if initial CT normal: repeat between 2.5 and 3 years of age.[a] If mutation detected at >12 years of age, consider baseline CXR or chest CT.
Thyroid	Visible or palpable thyroid nodule(s) Persistent cervical lymphadenopathy Hoarseness Dysphagia Neck pain Cough	- Multinodular goiter - Differentiated thyroid cancer	Baseline thyroid US by 8 years of age, then every 3 years or with symptoms/findings on physical exam. With anticipated chemotherapy or radiotherapy: baseline US and then annually for 5 years, decreasing to every 2–3 years if no nodules are detected.
Female reproductive tract	Hirsutism Virilization Abdominal distension, pain, or mass	- SLCT - Gynandroblastoma - Cervical ERMS	For females beginning at 8–10 years of age: pelvic and abdominal US every 6–12 months at least until age 40. End of interval is undetermined, but current oldest patient with *DICER1*-associated SLCT was 61 years of age. Education regarding symptoms strongly recommended.
Renal	Abdominal or flank mass and/or pain, hematuria	- Wilms tumor - Renal sarcoma - Cystic nephroma	Abdominal US every 6 months until 8 years of age, then every 12 months until 12 years of age. If mutation detected at >12 years of age, consider baseline abdominal US.
Gastrointestinal	Signs of intestinal obstruction	- Small intestine polyps	Education regarding symptoms recommended.
Central nervous system and head and neck (excluding thyroid)	Headache, emesis, diplopia, decreased ability for upward gaze, altered gait (pineoblastoma); precocious puberty; Cushing syndrome (pituitary blastoma); decreased visual acuity and leukocoria (CBME); nasal obstruction (NCMH)	- Macrocephaly - Pineoblastoma - Pituitary blastoma - CBME - NCMH	Physical exam. Annual routine dilated ophthalmologic exam (generally unsedated) with visual acuity screening from 3 years of age through at least 10 years of age. Further testing if clinically indicated. Recommend urgent MRI for any symptoms of intracranial pathology.

Abbreviation: MRI, magnetic resonance imaging.
[a]When CT is performed, techniques to minimize radiation exposure should be employed. As novel MRI techniques are developed that will eventually allow detection of small cystic lesions, transition to nonradiation containing cross-sectional imaging should be considered.

tion or *DICER1*-related cancers are encouraged to participate in ongoing research to optimize surveillance and advance knowledge regarding the best ways to diagnose and treat these rare tumors.

Acknowledgments The International PPB/*DICER1* Registry has been supported by the Pine Tree Apple Tennis Classic since 1987 and by the Theodora H. Lang Charitable Trust and Children's Minnesota Foundation. The authors are grateful for the kind assistance of Anne K. Harris CCRP in the preparation of this material and to the many children, families, and referring physicians who collaboratively support International PPB/*DICER1* Registry research.

References

Bahubeshi A, Bal N, Rio Frio T et al (2010) Germline *DICER1* mutations and familial cystic nephroma. J Med Genet 47:863–866

Belcher E, Lawson MH, Nicholson AG, Davison A, Goldstraw P (2007) Congenital cystic adenomatoid malformation presenting as in-flight systemic air embolisation. Eur Respir J 30:801–804

Bisogno G, Brennan B, Orbach D et al (2014) Treatment and prognostic factors in pleuropulmonary blastoma: an EXPeRT report. Eur J Cancer 50(1):178–184

Brenneman M, Field A, Yang J et al (2015) Temporal order of RNase IIIb and loss-of-function mutations during development determines phenoType in pleuropulmonary blastoma / *DICER1* syndrome: a unique variant of the two-hit tumor suppression model. F1000Res 4:214

Cummings NM, Desai S, Thway K et al (2010) Cystic primary pulmonary synovial sarcoma presenting as recurrent pneumothorax: report of 4 cases. Am J Surg Pathol 34:1176–1179

Dehner LP (1994) Pleuropulmonary blastoma is the pulmonary blastoma of childhood. Semin Diagn Pathol 11:144–151

Dishop MK, McKay EM, Kreiger PA et al (2010) Fetal lung interstitial tumor (FLIT): a proposed newly recognized lung tumor of infancy to be differentiated from cystic pleuropulmonary blastoma and other developmental pulmonary lesions. Am J Surg Pathol 34:1762–1772

Heravi-Moussavi A, Anglesio MS, Cheng SW et al (2012) Recurrent somatic *DICER1* mutations in nonepithelial ovarian cancers. N Engl J Med 366(3):234–242

Hill DA, Jarzembowski JA, Priest JR, Williams G, Schoettler P, Dehner LP (2008) Type I pleuropulmonary blastoma: pathology and biology study of 51 cases from the international pleuropulmonary blastoma registry. Am J Surg Pathol 32:282–295

Hill DA, Ivanovich J, Priest JR et al (2009) *DICER1* mutations in familial pleuropulmonary blastoma. Science 325:965

Hill DA, Wang JD, Schoettler P et al (2010) Germline *DICER1* mutations are common in both hereditary and presumed sporadic pleuropulmonary blastoma [abstract]. Lab Invest 90:311

Hill DA, Doros L, Schultz KA et al (2014) *DICER1*-related disorders. In: Pagon RA (ed) GeneReviews™ [Internet]. University of Washington, Seattle, Seattle. http://www.ncbi.nlm.nih.gov

Manivel C, Wick M, Dehner L (1987) Thoracopulmonary blastoma—reassessment of an embryonal neoplasm. Lab Invest 56:48

Manivel JC, Priest JR, Watterson J et al (1988) Pleuropulmonary blastoma. The so-called pulmonary blastoma of childhood. Cancer 62:1516–1526

Messinger YH, Stewart DR, Priest JR et al (2015) Pleuropulmonary blastoma: a report on 350 central pathology-confirmed pleuropulmonary blastoma cases by the International Pleuropulmonary Blastoma Registry. Cancer 121(2):276–285

Miniati DN, Chintagumpala M, Langston C et al (2006) Prenatal presentation and outcome of children with pleuropulmonary blastoma. J Pediatr Surg 41:66–71

Nakano Y, Gatell SP, Schultz KAP et al (2019) Successful treatment of metastatic cerebral recurrence of pleuropulmonary blastoma. Pediatr Blood Cancer 66(5):e27628

Priest JR, McDermott MB, Bhatia S, Watterson J, Manivel JC, Dehner LP (1997) Pleuropulmonary blastoma: a clinicopathologic study of 50 cases. Cancer 80:147–161

Priest JR, Hill DA, Williams GM et al (2006) Type I pleuropulmonary blastoma: a report from the International Pleuropulmonary Blastoma Registry. J Clin Oncol 24:4492–4498

Priest JR, Magnuson J, Williams GM et al (2007) Cerebral metastasis and other central nervous system complications of pleuropulmonary blastoma. Pediatr Blood Cancer 49:266–273

Priest JR, Williams GM, Hill DA, Dehner LP, Jaffe A (2009) Pulmonary cysts in early childhood and the risk of malignancy. Pediatr Pulmonol 44:14–30

Priest JR, Andic D, Arbuckle S, Gonzalez-Gomez I, Hill DA, Williams G (2011a) Great vessel/cardiac extension and tumor embolism in pleuropulmonary blastoma: a report from the International Pleuropulmonary Blastoma Registry. Pediatr Blood Cancer 56(4):604–609

Priest JR, Williams GM, Manera R et al (2011b) Ciliary body medulloepithelioma: four cases associated with pleuropulmonary blastoma—a report from the International Pleuropulmonary Blastoma Registry. Br J Ophthalmol 95(7):1001–1005

Rio Frio T, Bahubeshi A, Kanellopoulou C et al (2011) *DICER1* mutations in familial multinodular goiter with and without ovarian sertoli-leydig cell tumors. JAMA 305:68–77

Schultz KA, Harris A, Williams GM et al (2014) Judicious *DICER1* testing and surveillance imaging facilitates early diagnosis and cure of pleuropulmonary blastoma. Pediatr Blood Cancer 61(9):1695–1697

Schultz KA, Harris A, Messinger Y et al (2016) Ovarian tumors related to intronic mutations in *DICER1*: a report from the international ovarian and testicular stromal tumor registry. Fam Cancer. 15(1):105–110

Schultz KAP, Williams GM, Kamihara J et al (2018) *DICER1* and associated conditions: identification of at-risk individuals and recommended surveillance strategies. Clin Cancer Res 24(10):2251–2261

Slade I, Bacchelli C, Davies H et al (2011) *DICER1* syndrome—clarifying the diagnosis, clinical features and management implications of a pleiotropic tumor predisposition syndrome. J Med Genet 48(4):273–278

Sparber-Sauer M, Seitz G, Kirsch S et al (2017) The impact of local control in the treatment of type II/III pleuropulmonary blastoma. Experience of the Cooperative Weichteilsarkom Studiengruppe (CWS). J Surg Oncol 115(2):164–172

Stewart DR, Best AF, Williams GM, Harney LA, Carr AG, Harris AK, Kratz CP, Dehner LP, Messinger YH, Rosenberg PS, Hill AD, Schultz KAP (2019) Neoplasm Risk Among Individuals With a Pathogenic Germline Variant in DICER1. J Clin Oncol 37(8):668–676.

Stocker JT (2002) Congenital pulmonary airway malformation—a new name for and an expanded classification of congenital cystic adenomatoid malformation of the lung. Histopathology 41:424–431

Bronchial Carcinoids and Carcinomas

19

Dominik T. Schneider, Antje Redlich, and Peter Vorwerk

19.1 Introduction

During childhood and adolescence, lung tumors are very rare and may present with variable histological phenotype. Pleuropulmonary blastoma may contribute approximately 10% to all primary lung tumors in the pediatric cohort (Neville et al. 2009). They can arise in the context of *DICER1* genetic predisposition and may resemble characteristic patterns of embryonal tumors and sarcomas of childhood (for details, see Chap. 25). Other tumors may display neuroendocrine differentiation (neuroendocrine tumors [NET] syn. carcinoids). Bronchial NETs constitute the most frequent primary lung tumors during childhood and adolescence, accounting for half of lung tumors in this age group (Neville et al. 2009). They are rarely associated with multiple endocrine neoplasia type 1 (MEN1) (Norton et al. 2015). In contrast, classical bronchial carcinomas are rare, as they primarily constitute a tumor of adulthood and senescence, often in the context of tobacco abuse. Nevertheless, their true incidence in pediatric cohorts is largely unknown, and a significant registration gap is assumed. Only recently, they have been registered prospectively in national and international pediatric rare tumor registries. Last, the lungs present a frequent site of metastases of non-pulmonary tumors such as nephroblastoma or osteosarcoma, so that in case of lung tumors, metastasis always has to be excluded.

Bronchial NETs are tumors of the neuroendocrine system and account for 80–85% of all primary malignant lung tumors during childhood and adolescence (de Christenson et al. 1999). NETs are a group of neoplasms that histologically present with uniformly appearing cells that arise from the neuroepithelial cells within the bronchial epithelium. They may differ from each other in their biology, prognosis, and genetics. In the lungs, they are also called carcinoid. The term carcinoid was first introduced by Oberndorfer in 1907. It describes the unique feature that these tumors may show a benign clinical course despite histological features of malignancy (Oberndorfer 1907; Klöppel 2007a, b). As bronchial carcinoids were initially considered benign, they had first been classified as bronchial adenomas (Davila et al. 1993). With the increasing understanding of their biological and clinical behavior, the classification and nomenclature of these tumors has further evolved (de Christenson et al. 1999), and they are now categorized in the group of NETs. The range of morphological patterns reaches from the low-grade typical carcinoids to the intermediate-grade atypical carcinoids and high-

D. T. Schneider (✉)
Klinik für Kinder- und Jugendmedizin, Klinikum Dortmund, University Witten/Herdecke, Dortmund, Germany
e-mail: dominik.schneider@klinikumdo.de

A. Redlich · P. Vorwerk
Department of Pediatric Hematology and Oncology, University Children's Hospital, Magdeburg, Germany

D. T. Schneider et al. (eds.), *Rare Tumors in Children and Adolescents*, Pediatric Oncology,
https://doi.org/10.1007/978-3-030-92071-5_19

grade small- or large-cell neuroendocrine carcinomas (Klöppel 2007a). Thus, bronchial NETs are traditionally classified into subtypes characterized by increasing aggressiveness: typical carcinoids, atypical carcinoids, and neuroendocrine carcinomas (Pusceddu et al. 2016).

Given the rarity of bronchial NETs, it can be expected that most pediatric oncologists may encounter such a tumor once or twice in a lifetime. Cohen and Kaschula (1992) reported about eight patients in a 31-year period in a single center. In Germany, 12 children with bronchial NETs have been registered in the GPOH-MET study on malignant endocrine tumors over a period of 14 years (Redlich et al. 2013). In a recent international retrospective study of airway tumors in children, 31 of 78 tumors collected over a 15-year period were NETs, followed by inflammatory myofibroblastic tumor and mucoepidermoid carcinoma (Pio et al. 2020).

Bronchial carcinoma (i.e., classical lung cancer) is the most commonly diagnosed cancer worldwide and primarily a disease of older populations, mostly in the sixth and seventh decades of life. It is extremely rare in childhood and adolescence. Within the US SEER registry, which covers a period from 1992 to 2010 and overall includes 17,000 children and adolescents less than 20 years of age with malignant solid tumors, 47 patients with bronchial carcinoma were counted (Lit. US SEER registry (https://seer.cancer.gov), status October 2010), 31 patients in the age group from 15 to 19 years, 13 patients from 10 to 14 years, 2 patients from 5 to 9 years, and 1 patient from 0 to 4 years. In the German Rare Tumor Registry (STEP), 12 bronchial carcinomas have been registered over a 10-year period. Seven of these were mucoepidermoid carcinoma; accordingly, mucoepidermoid carcinoma was also the most common histopathological subtype in the international survey of airway tumors (Pio et al. 2020).

The low incidence of bronchial carcinoma in young patients may be explained in the light of the fact that, like almost no other tumor, the development of bronchial carcinoma is tightly correlated to toxic exogenous factor in the background of a genetic susceptibility. Thus, smoking and genetic predisposition were found as risk factors for bronchial carcinoma in young adults (under 45 years), with a predominance of adenocarcinoma (Kreuzer et al. 1998; Ramalingam et al. 1998). Bronchial carcinoma incidence trends follow the trend of prevalence of cigarette smoking, with a latency of approximately 20 years. The results of a segregation analysis suggest genetic contribution to bronchial carcinoma in the very young, particularly in nonsmokers (Kreuzer et al. 1999; Rosenberger et al. 2008).

Overall, data suggest that bronchial carcinoma is not a more aggressive disease in younger patients. In fact, most bronchial carcinoma in children or adolescents show histological differentiation with low malignancy. Therefore, all patients with lung cancer, including pediatric patients, should be managed along the same therapeutic guidelines (Ramalingam et al. 1998; Goeckenjan et al. 2010).

19.2 Clinical Diagnosis, Pretherapeutic Assessment in Lung Tumors, Staging

The detection of malignant lung tumors in children may be problematic and difficult. Children may present with unspecific respiratory complaints. The most frequent symptoms include cough in two thirds of patients, signs of pneumonia, and dyspnea (Pio et al. 2020). Moreover, hemoptysis and recurrent pneumonia (in the same lobe) may present characteristic symptoms and may be apparent for up to 1 year before diagnosis. Such symptoms may occur as isolated symptoms or in combination (Wang et al. 1993; Rizzardi et al. 2009; Srirajaskanthan et al. 2009; Pio et al. 2020). General pediatricians should be aware that wheezing localized to one lung is a characteristic finding not only of airway tumors but also of other reasons of bronchial obstruction including aspiration and always requires bronchoscopy. In addition, the presence of atelectasis, the persistence of X-ray findings after antibiotic therapy, or hemoptysis should increase awareness that further diagnostic assessment including CT and endoscopy will be required (McCahon

2006. NETs or bronchial carcinomas can also be found accidentally on chest X-rays in otherwise asymptomatic patients (Bini et al. 2008).

Neuroendocrine tumors may secrete neuroendocrine peptides, although it is extremely rare for bronchial NETs to cause a carcinoid syndrome without metastatic spread (Ward et al. 1984). However, the occurrence of Cushing's syndrome due to ectopic ACTH secretion has been reported. Typical bronchial NETs are found more frequently than atypical tumors, among which the latter are bigger in size, more peripherally located, and prognostically less favorable (Asamura et al. 2006). Local invasion and metastases are seen in 25% of children with bronchial NETs (Rizzardi et al. 2009). The propensity of the tumor to metastasize correlates with the histologic grade of atypia. The metastatic pattern includes lymph nodes, liver, and less frequently skeleton, CNS, and adrenal glands (Soga and Yakuwa 1999).

The clinical symptoms of bronchial carcinoma may also vary significantly and are undistinguishable from bronchial NETs. Because of the aggressive nature of this cancer, two thirds of patients exhibit symptoms from locally advanced or metastatic disease, such as bone pain or head swelling due to vena cava superior occlusion.

Basic preoperative diagnostic workup is comparable for NETs and carcinoma and includes clinical investigation, chest posteroanterior X-ray, CT scan of the chest (Figs. 19.1 and 19.2), and bronchoscopy with tumor biopsy. Pulmonary function tests should be performed routinely.

In NETs, somatostatin receptor scintigraphy (octreotide scan) can be used to reveal metastasis and to assess palliative treatment options, such as peptide receptor radiotargeted therapy (Hicks et al 2017). (68)Ga-DOTA use in PET/CT is the optimal tracer for NETs; however, in case of an atypical carcinoid, (18)F-DG-PET/CT is recommended (Jager et al. 2008, Caplin et al. 2015, Koopmans et al 2008).

Primary staging of the bronchial carcinoma patient includes MRI of the brain, CT or ultrasonography of the abdomen, and PET-CT scan, which may distinguish between nonmetastatic or metastatic disease (Table 19.1). In case of bone pain, bone scintigraphy is recommended. Mediastinal lymph node staging is realized by endobronchial and esophageal ultrasound. Complementary cervical mediastinoscopy or video-assisted thoracoscopy can be performed, especially in suspected N2 disease or undefined pleural effusions. The clinical and pathological staging of bronchial carcinoma is based on the TNM system.

Proof of tumor histology—with differentiation of non-small cell lung cancer vs. small cell lung cancer—has significant impact on prognosis and treatment protocols. Nowadays, analysis of molecular markers as KRAS, EGFR, and ALK mutations can indicate targeted therapeutic options individually. Nevertheless, the exceedingly rare small cell lung cancer in adolescents (with two patients reported to STEP registry over

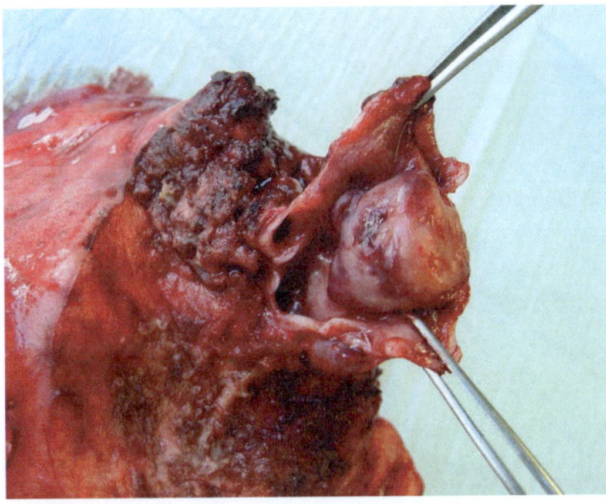

Fig. 19.1 Large lung cancer in right upper lobe (chest CT scan)

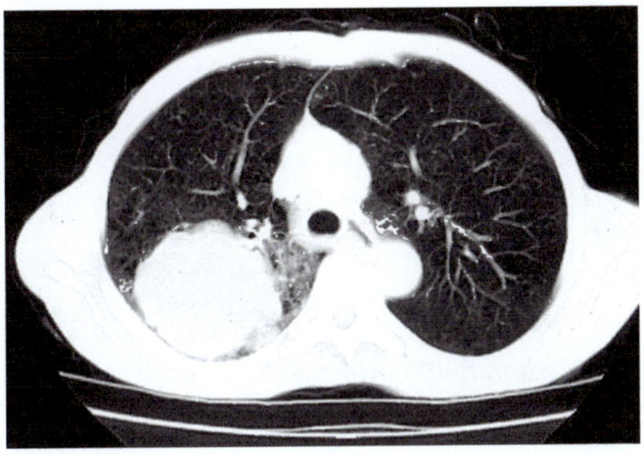

Fig. 19.2 Small cell lung cancer in right upper lobe (chest CT scan)

Table 19.1 Diagnostic assessment of bronchial carcinoids (NET) and bronchial carcinoma

Procedure	NET	Carcinoma	Specific questions
Physical examination	+	+	Airway obstruction, lymphatic metastasis, hemoptysis, wheezing, vena cava superior obstruction
Pulmonary function	+	+	Preoperative status
Laboratory assessment			
Clinical chemistry	+	+	Organ function
ChA, NSE, HIAA (urine)	+		Neuroendocrine tumor origin
ACTH, cortisone	+		Cushing?
Radiographic assessment			
Chest X-ray T	+	+	Staging
Chest CT	+	+	Local stage, lymph nodes
Abdominal ultrasound	+	+	Metastases (especially liver)
PET-CT		+	Local stage, metastases
Brain MRI	(+)	+	Brain metastases
Bone scan	(+)	(+)	Bone metastases
Octreotide scan	+		Metastases, palliative therapeutic option?
Invasive examinations			
Bronchoscopy	+	+	Preoperative staging
Endobronchial US	+	+	Local and nodal stage
Esophageal US	+	+	Local and nodal stage
Pathologic and genetic examination			
MENIN mutation	+		MEN 1?
KRAS, EGFR, ALK		+	Targeted therapy?

a 10-year period) is still a prognostically unfavorable tumor.

The pathological examination of the specimens should be performed by an experienced specialist and confirmed by reference pathologists for children. Of the NETs, 75% arise from the lobar bronchi, 10% from the mainstem bronchi, and 15% in the lung periphery (Davila et al. 1993). Small biopsies are not representative and can often be misinterpreted (Filosso et al. 2002).

Bronchial NETs can occur in 5% of patients with MEN1. Although more prevalent in older patients, an analysis of the menin gene should be performed whenever a suspicion of a genetic background exists (Sachithanandan et al. 2005).

19.3 Treatment

In experienced and skilled hands, conservative procedures are the treatment of choice for the management of pediatric bronchial NETs (Rizzardi et al. 2009). Resection is the treatment of choice for NETs in adolescents and adults (Detterbeck 2010). Lung-sparing bronchoplastic procedures and limited resections are favorable for central, most typical carcinoids (Fig. 19.3). In peripheral NETs, wedge resection is recommended for the young and lobectomy for the older adult patient. Lymphadenectomy may be beneficial, especially in N1 or N2 carcinoid tumors. In locally advanced NETs with preoperatively suspected N1 or N2 disease, mostly atypical carcinoids, neoadjuvant chemotherapy and radiation can be indicated, followed by anatomical resection.

Endobronchial resection of typical NETs is possible, but complete resection can be achieved only in half of patients. The recurrence rate is 5%, demanding subsequent surgical resection (Detterbeck 2010). Patient selection for endobronchial removal seems to be essential.

If tumors are widespread, metastatic, or unresectable, palliative and symptomatic treatment is based on surgical or endobronchial debulking, tumor embolization, and biotherapy with soma-

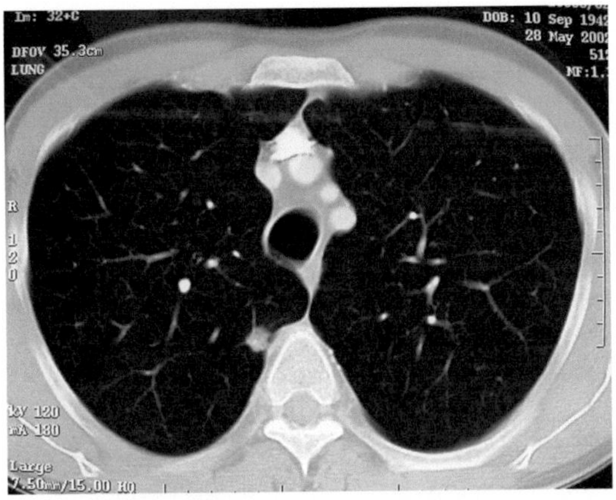

Fig. 19.3 Carcinoid tumor in central upper lobe bronchial after bronchoplastic resection (surgical specimen)

tostatin analogues. Chemotherapy and radiotherapy are usually ineffective, but novel drugs such as tyrosine kinase receptor inhibitors show promising results in phase II clinical studies (Gustafsson et al. 2008). In the international series, only one fatal outcome was reported among 31 patients (Pio et al. 2020).

Radical resection is a prerequisite of cure in bronchial carcinoma, too. Therapeutic stratification then depends on stage and histology. In adults, small cell and non-small cell carcinomas are distinguished. In children and adolescents, a specific subset of tumors with low malignant potential also has to be considered. This includes mucoepidermoid carcinomas, which have a low metastatic potential and thus primarily require radical surgical resection (Pio et al. 2020).

The therapeutic recommendations, as follows, summarize the current guidelines of the German Cancer Society in lung cancer in adults (https://www.awmf.org/uploads/tx_szleitlinien/020-007OL_l_S3_Lungenkarzinom_2018-03.pdf). After definition of tumor stage, stage-dependent treatment is indicated in the following guidelines for older adult patients. Therapy of non-small cell lung cancer is primarily surgical in stage I and II and may follow a multimodal approach in stage II–III tumors. In stage IV, systemic therapy constitutes the most validated therapeutic concept. However, on the long-term systemic therapy must be considered palliative. Anterolateral thoracotomy with anatomic lung resection (lobe or more) and lymphadenectomy is therapy of choice with best long-term survival; tumor negative resection margins (R0) are prognostically decisive. If resection is considered R1, a second look resection is recommended; if impossible, radiotherapy may be applied alternatively. In all patients, lymph node resection is required for adequate staging. After complete resection, four cycles of adjuvant (cisplatin-based, often in combination with vinorelbine) chemotherapy are recommended in pathologic N1 status (pN1 = stage II) and in stage IIIA and may improve survival (Winton and Livingston (2004). Chemotherapy can individually be considered in stage IB.

Specific recommendations apply to Pancoast tumors, with infiltration of the chest wall. In locally advanced bronchial carcinoma, mainly in stage III, extended (surgical) procedures are indicated; these are bronchoplastic or angioplastic resections; chest wall, intrapericardial, or atrial resections in T4 organ involvement; or other procedures. Stage IIIA is mainly defined by different extent of ipsilateral lymphatic metastases to the mediastinum (N2 disease), which indicate different treatment protocols (Robinson et al. 2007). Incidental N2 disease (postoperative or intraoperative diagnosis of pN2 = stage IIIA$_1$ or IIIA$_2$) should be treated with adjuvant chemotherapy and radiotherapy, sequentially. In preoperatively diagnosed N2 disease (single or several N2 = IIIA$_3$ and multilevel or bulky disease N2 = IIIA$_4$) and amenable resection, patients receive neoadjuvant chemotherapy, surgery, and radiotherapy, sequentially. Patients with tumor regression (CR, PR) or stable disease (SD) and proven resectability are operated on, with the aim of complete resection (R0). All patients with N2 disease receive adjuvant radiotherapy (50 Gy) of primary tumor lesion and mediastinum; the dose is dependent on the pathological resection status (R0 or R1/R2). Patients with tumor progression (PD) or unresectable disease receive definitive radiotherapy or combined radiochemotherapy (N3 disease).

Further adjuvant chemotherapy is chosen individually, and its choice can be influenced by the pathological tumor regression. In stage IV disease, palliative chemotherapy is state of the art and may be supplemented with targeted therapies, based on molecular stratification of ALK, BRAF, and EGFR mutation status, among others (Janne et al. 2010). Last, PD1 blockage, e.g., with durvalumab or pembrolizumab, may also provide a promising concept, however in—considering a long-term perspective—a palliative setting. Current updates on these recommendations may be found at https://www.onkopedia-guidelines.info/en/onkopedia/guidelines/lung-cancer-non-small-lung-cancer-nsclc/@@guideline/html/index.html.

For extremely rare small cell lung carcinoma (SCLC) in adolescents, the therapeutic algorithms for adult patients apply, too. Due to the high metastatic potential of SCLC, chemotherapy is also recommended in low stages and should be complemented with prophylactic brain irradiation (30 Gy) to prevent CNS metastases. Modern chemotherapy regimen of SCLC commonly includes cisplatin in combination preferably with etoposide. In this chemosensitive tumor, additional agents such as ifosfamide may yield a slight additional survival benefit. In locally advanced tumors, chemotherapy and radiotherapy should be applied simultaneously. The role of maintenance therapy following intensive radiochemotherapy is still under debate, and new targeted drugs should only be applied within clinical studies.

19.4 Results and Comment

The prognosis of bronchial NETs in children is, with 90% overall survival (OS), good (Hartman and Shochat 1983). Typical carcinoid tumors have a better outcome than atypical (60–70%) (Soga and Yakuwa 1999). A long-term follow-up including pulmonary function tests, bronchoscopy, and chest CT, if necessary, is essential, since relapses can occur even after many years. Detected in a timely manner, relapses can be successfully treated with reoperation (Rizzardi et al. 2009).

Stage-dependent survival curves of bronchial carcinomas in adults are published by Goldstraw et al. (2007). A 5-year OS (all tumor stages) is 15%. A 5-year survival following surgery was, in stage I, 73–54%; in stage II, 48–38%; in stage III, 25–19%; and, in stage IV, 21%, respectively (Goldstraw et al. 2007). For instance, in a prospective randomized phase III trial of the GLCCG for patients with stage III NSCLC, a 5-year OS could be improved to 48%, if following neoadjuvant chemotherapy or additional chemoradiotherapy and complete resection (R0), mediastinal downstaging could be achieved (Thomas et al. 2008). Induction chemotherapy has also been used to improve complete resection rate and does not appear to increase operative mortality in experienced thoracic surgeons (Fig. 19.4).

There are only little data on survival of children, adolescents, and young adults with lung cancer. In 2009, Neville et al. (2009) published data of the SEER registry from 1973 to 2004 for all patients with pulmonary tumors less than 20 years of age. They demonstrated that the incidence of pediatric lung cancer remains stable. The most common histology was endocrine tumor, followed by sarcoma and mucoepidermoid tumor. The mean age at diagnosis was 16 years. In their multivariate analysis, surgical treatment and endocrine histology were independent prognostic factors for survival.

In the Detroit SEER registry (from 1973 to 1992), overall and stage-dependent 5-year relative survival rates were significantly better in the

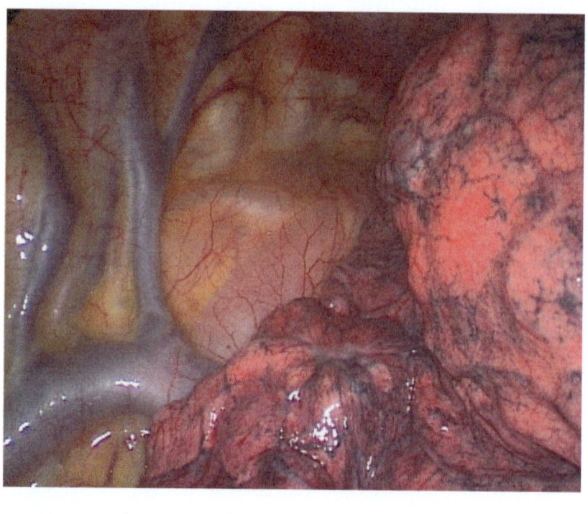

Fig. 19.4 Peripheral bronchial carcinoma in apical segment of right lower lobe (thoracoscopic view)

younger patient group (<50 years) (16.1% vs. 13.4%) (Ramalingam et al. 1998). Of 31,266 patients, 9% were under 50 years of age at diagnosis, 1.2% under 40 years, and 0.07% under 30 years. Treatment was managed in a more aggressive fashion than in older patients due to their better overall medical condition. Younger patients had a higher incidence of adenocarcinoma as histologic subtype (Ramalingam et al. 1998; Kreuzer et al. 1999).

LUCY (Lung Cancer in the Young) is an ongoing multicenter trial with 30 participating clinics all over Germany. From 2000 up to now, more than 800 young patients (<50 years) with primary lung cancer have been recruited with phenotype data. Present studies are candidate gene association studies and functional analyses of genotyping (Sauter et al. 2008). Many epidemiologic and clinical studies have indicated familial aggregation of lung cancer. Kreutzer could demonstrate a threefold increase in risk of lung cancer in patients younger than 46 years if relatives were also affected by lung cancer (Kreuzer et al. 1998). Several studies conducted in the last decades reported a preponderance of adenocarcinoma in young patients (Kreuzer et al. 1999). Although smoking is considered to be the predominant risk factor, only 10% of heavy smokers develop lung cancer. This suggests that genetic variation in sensitivity to carcinogen exposure can play an important role in the etiology of lung cancer (Sauter et al. 2008; Timofeeva et al. 2009).

Due to low incidence of lung cancer in children, adolescents and young adults will be presented in case reports or registry data, only. In future protocols, individualized and targeted therapies will be applied directed to tumor molecular markers and other tumor prognostic markers as in adult patients. Since there is no obvious evidence that histologically identical tumors differ biologically by age, these study data from young adults can be transferred to the treatment of adolescents and even children. However, data collection should be ensured, ideally to pediatric rare tumor registries that include experts from internal and surgical oncology.

References

Asamura H, Kameya T, Matsuno Y et al (2006) Neuroendocrine neoplasms of the lung: a prognostic spectrum. J Clin Oncol 24(1):70–76

Bini A, Brandolini J, Cassanelli N et al (2008) Typical and atypical pulmonary carcinoids: our institutional experience. Interact Cardiovasc Thorac Surg 7(3):415–418

Caplin ME, Baudin E, Ferolla P, Filosso P, Garcia-Yuste M, Lim E, Oberg K, Pelosi G, Perren A, Rossi RE, Travis WD (2015) Pulmonary neuroendocrine (carcinoid) tumors: European Neuroendocrine Tumor Society expert consensus and recommendations for best practice for typical and atypical pulmonary carcinoids. Ann Oncol 26(8):1604–1620

Cohen MC, Kaschula RO (1992) Primary pulmonary tumors in childhood: a review of 31 years' experience and the literature. Pediatr Pulmonol 14(4):222–232

Davila DG, Dunn WF, Tazelaar HD, Pairolero PC (1993) Bronchial carcinoid tumors. Mayo Clin Proc 68(8):795–803

de Christenson ML, Rosado AGF, Kirejczyk WM, Galvin JR, Travis WD (1999) Thoracic carcinoids: radiologic-pathologic correlation. Radiographics 19(3):707–736

Detterbeck FC (2010) Review: management of carcinoid tumours. Ann Thorac Surg 89:998–1005

Filosso PL, Rena O, Donati G et al (2002) Bronchial carcinoid tumors: surgical management and long-term outcome. J Thorac Cardiovasc Surg 123(2):303–309

Goeckenjan G, Sitter H, Thomas M et al (2010) Prevention, diagnosis, therapy, and follow-up of lung cancer. Interdisciplinary guideline of the German Respiratory Society and the German Cancer Society. Pneumologie 64(suppl 2):S23–S155

Goldstraw P, Crowley J, Chansky K et al (2007) The IASLC lung cancer staging project: proposals for the revision of the TNM stage groupings in the forthcoming (seventh) edition of the TNM classification of malignant tumours. J Thorac Oncol 2:706–720

Gustafsson BI, Kidd M, Modlin IM (2008) Neuroendocrine tumors of the diffuse neuroendocrine system. Curr Opin Oncol 20(1):1–12

Hartman GE, Shochat SJ (1983) Primary pulmonary neoplasms of childhood: a review. Ann Thorac Surg 36(1):108–119

Hicks RJ, Kwekkeboom DJ, Krenning E, Bodei L, Grozinsky-Glasberg S, Arnold R, Borbath I, Cwikla J, Toumpanakis C, Kaltsas G, Davies P, Hörsch D, Tiensuu Janson E, Ramage J (2017) ENETS consensus guidelines for the standards of care in neuroendocrine neoplasia: peptide receptor radionuclide therapy with radiolabeled somatostatin analogues. Neuroendocrinology 105(3):295–309

Jager PL, Chirakal R, Marriott CJ, Brouwers AH, Koopmans KP, Gulenchyn KY (2008) 6-L-18F-fluorodihydroxyphenylalanine PET in neuroendocrine tumors: basic aspects and emerging clinical applications. J Nucl Med 49(4):573–586

Janne PA, Wang XF, Socinski MA et al (2010) Randomized phase II trial of erlotinib (E) alone or in combination with carboplatin/paclitaxel (CP) in never or light former smokers with advanced lung adenocarcinoma: CALGB 30406 (abstract #7503). J Clin Oncol 28: 539s

Klöppel G (2007a) Oberndorfer and his successors: from carcinoid to neuroendocrine carcinoma. Endocr Pathol 18(3):141–144

Klöppel G (2007b) Tumour biology and histopathology of neuroendocrine tumours. Best Pract Res Clin Endocrinol Metab 21(1):15–31

Koopmans KP, Neels OC, Kema IP et al (2008) Improved staging of patients with carcinoid and islet cell tumors with 18F-dihydroxy-phenyl-alanine and 11C-5-hydroxy-tryptophan positron emission tomography. J Clin Oncol 26(9):1489–1495

Kreuzer M, Kreienbrock L, Gerken M et al (1998) Risk factors for lung cancer in young adults. Am J Epidemiol 147:1028–1037

Kreuzer M, Kreienbrock L, Müller K et al (1999) Histologic types of lung carcinoma and age at onset. Cancer 85:1958–1965

McCahon E (2006) Lung tumours in children. Paediatr Respir Rev 7(3):191–196

Neville H, Hogan A, Zhuge Y et al (2009) Incidence and outcomes of malignant pediatric lung neoplasms. J Surg Res 156:224–230

Norton JA, Krampitz G, Jensen RT (2015) Multiple endocrine neoplasia: genetics and clinical management. Surg Oncol Clin N Am 24(4):795–832

Oberndorfer S (1907) Karzinoide Tumoren des Dünndarms. Frankf Zschr Pathol 1:426–432

Pio L, Varela P, Eliott MJ, Couloigner V et al (2020) Pediatric airway tumors: a report from the international network of pediatric airway teams (INPAT). Laryngoscope 130:E243–E251

Pusceddu S, Lo Russo G, Macerelli M, Proto C, Vitali M, Signorelli D, Ganzinelli M, Scanagatta P, Duranti L, Trama A, Buzzoni R, Pelosi G, Pastorino U, de Braud F, Garassino MC (2016) Diagnosis and management of typical and atypical lung carcinoids. Crit Rev Oncol Hematol 2016(100):167–176

Ramalingam S, Pawlish K, Gadgeel S et al (1998) Lung cancer in young patients: analysis of a surveillance, epidemiology, and end results database. J Clin Oncol 16:651–657

Redlich A, Wechsung K, Boxberger N, Leuschner I, Vorwerk P (2013) Extra-appendiceal neuroendocrine neoplasms in children - data from the GPOH-MET 97 trial. Klin Padiatr 225(6):315–319

Rizzardi G, Marulli G, Calabrese F et al (2009) Bronchial carcinoid tumours in children: surgical treatment and outcome in a single institution. Eur J Pediatr Surg 19(4):228–231

Robinson LA, Ruckdeschel JC, Wagner H et al (2007) Treatment of stage IIIA non-small cell lung cancer. ACCP evidence-based clinical practice guidelines (2nd ed). Chest 132:243–265

Rosenberger A, Illig T, Korb K et al (2008) Do genetic factors protect for early onset lung cancer? A case control study before the age of 50 years. BMC Cancer 8:60–71

Sachithanandan N, Harle RA, Burgess JR (2005) Bronchopulmonary carcinoid in multiple endocrine neoplasia type 1. Cancer 103(3):509–515

Sauter W, Rosenberger A, Beckmann L et al (2008) Matrix metalloproteinase 1 (MMP1) is associated with early-onset lung cancer. Cancer Epidemiol Biomark Prev 17(5):1127–1135

Soga J, Yakuwa Y (1999) Bronchopulmonary carcinoids: an analysis of 1,875 reported cases with special reference to a comparison between typical carcinoids and atypical varieties. Ann Thorac Cardiovasc Surg 5(4):211–219

Srirajaskanthan R, Toumpanakis C, Karpathakis A et al (2009) Surgical management and palliative treatment in bronchial neuroendocrine tumours: a clinical study of 45 patients. Lung Cancer 65(1):68–73

Thomas M, Rübe C, Hoffknecht P et al (2008) Effect of preoperative chemoradiation in addition to preoperative chemotherapy: a randomized trial in stage III non-small-cell lung cancer. Lancet Oncol 9:636–648

Timofeeva M, Kropp S, Sauter W et al (2009) CYP450 polymorphisms as risk factors for early-onset lung cancer: gender-specific differences. Carcinogenesis 30(7):1161–1169

Wang LT, Wilkins EW Jr, Bode HH (1993) Bronchial carcinoid tumors in pediatric patients. Chest 103(5):1426–1428

Ward PS, Mott MG, Smith J, Hartog M (1984) Cushing's syndrome and bronchial carcinoid tumour. Arch Dis Child 59(4):375–377

Winton T, Livingston R (2004) A prospective randomized trial of adjuvant vinorelbine (VIN) and cisplatin (CIS) in completely resected stage I B and II non-small cell lung cancer (NSCLC): intergroup JBR 10. J Clin Oncol 22:621–626

20 Pediatric Pleural Mesothelioma

Nicolas André, Sergey K. V. V. Kashanskiy, and Abbas Agaimy

20.1 Introduction

Malignant mesothelioma is an aggressive tumor that originates from the lining cells (mesothelium) that cover the serosal surfaces of the pleural and peritoneal cavities, or more rarely the tunica vaginalis testis and the pericardium (Moore et al. 2008). Based on the stage of the disease at the time of diagnosis, mesothelioma may present as discrete multifocal nodules or as a diffuse confluent mass encasing the adjacent organs and/or obliterating the serosal cavity from which the tumor has originated.

Although, before the 1950s, the existence of adult mesothelioma was questioned by many pathologists (Moore et al. 2008), the increase in the incidence of mesothelioma, ensuing to the growing use of asbestos, definitely led to the acknowledgment of mesothelioma as a genuine clinicopathologic entity (Margery and Ruffié 2008). In children, because this is an even rarer tumor, its existence has long been debated and consequently its management neglected. Furthermore, because of the rarity of mesothelioma and the consequent difficulties in its diagnosis, a significant proportion of cases that have been diagnosed initially as pediatric mesothelioma were found to represent other entities upon a subsequent second pathological analysis (Fraire et al. 1988). Nevertheless, recent small series have been published using state-of-the-art adult diagnosis criteria (Moran et al. 2008). These recent studies have established the existence of pediatric mesothelioma and highlighted the lack of optimal strategy.

We will focus here on pleural mesothelioma and exclude peritoneal mesothelioma (see specific. Chap. 30) as well as mesothelioma of the tunica vaginalis and pericardial mesothelioma. The main challenge for pediatric oncologists remains to choose the optimal therapeutic strategy for a given patient. These options range from upfront palliative care to aggressive multimodal treatments. Meanwhile, we must increase our knowledge about this disease to codify its management (Table 20.1).

20.2 Epidemiology

In adults, it is estimated that mesothelioma represents less than 0.5% of all cancers. Among malignant mesotheliomas, pleural mesothelioma is the

N. André (✉)
Department of Pediatric Hematology, Immunology and Oncology, Children Hospital of "La Timone" AP-HM, Marseille, France
e-mail: nicolas.andre@ap-hm.fr

Sergey K. V. V. Kashanskiy
Labor Hygiene Laboratory, Yekaterinburg Medical Research Center for Prophylaxis and Health Protection in Industrial Workers, Yekaterinburg, Russian Federation

A. Agaimy
Institute of Pathology, University Hospital of Erlangen, Erlangen, Germany

D. T. Schneider et al. (eds.), *Rare Tumors in Children and Adolescents*, Pediatric Oncology,
https://doi.org/10.1007/978-3-030-92071-5_20

Table 20.1 Key points to manage a child with pleural mesothelioma

Physical examination	Signs and symptoms (cough, dyspnea, fatigue, pallor, weight loss) Anamnesis: asbestosis exposure
Laboratory assessment	None specific
Radiological assessment	
– First assessment – Local staging	Abdominal computed tomography (CT) scan
– Diagnostic workup	Chest and abdominal CT scan Positron emission tomography (PET) MRI Cardiac echography
Pathological assessment	Surgical biopsy required Always need adult's pathologist experienced with mesothelioma To get confirmation of the diagnosis of malignant mesothelioma and subtype Application of an appropriate panel of immunochemical stains
Staging systems for risk-adapted treatment strategy	None validated
General treatment guidelines	Need for multidisciplinary approach Seek for national or European group for rare tumor advice Seek advice from center with expert physician dedicated to the management of this cancer in adults
Surgery	Consider complete resection when it can be easily removable
Radiotherapy	Can be considered as part of multimodal therapy
Chemotherapy Targeted therapies Immunotherapies	First line: pemetrexed–cisplatin (bevacizumab) Second line or alternative: gemcitabine–pemetrexed Consider treatment with novel agents validated in adults Upon molecular profiling of the tumors, ALK inhibitors or others may be used Anti-PD1/L1: Consider adding as second line or as first line if high tumoral mutation burden or strong PD1/L1 staining

most common localization (Fig. 20.1). In children, pleural mesothelioma is an extremely rare disease, and no precise incidence of this disease is available. Our knowledge relies mostly on isolated case reports and rare small series. Of note, the first pediatric series was published in 1964 by Kauffman and Stout who reported five cases of both peritoneal and pleural mesotheliomas (Kauffman and Stout 1964). Based on results of autopsies, pediatric mesothelioma would represent 2–5% of all mesothelioma cases and according to epidemiologic studies would represent 0.5–1.0 case/10 millions/year (Kashanskiy and André 2010). We previously reviewed and reported epidemiologic data of 489 cases of pediatric mesothelioma; pleural mesothelioma represented approximately 60% of the cases, in line with other less extensive reviews of the literature (Fraire et al. 1988; Anderson et al. 1985).

As in adults, there is a higher frequency of pleural mesothelioma in boys (Kauffman and Stout 1964; Kashanskiy and André 2010; Brenner et al. 1981), with a sex ratio of 1.3:1 (Kashanskiy and André 2010). The mean age at presentation was 13.0 ± 0.3 years, with no difference between sexes (Kashanskiy and André 2010).

There is a strong relationship between exposure to asbestos and the subsequent development of pleural mesothelioma in adults (Moore et al. 2008). Nevertheless, in our experience, there was no such association in children. Indeed, we found only five cases with a known previous exposure to asbestos among the 110 pediatric pleural mesothelioma cases for which the exposure to asbestos was well documented (Kashanskiy and André 2010). In line with this observation, the reported pediatric cases with a prior exposure to asbestos are anecdotal. Moreover, in many countries in which the exposure to asbestos is high because of the presence of mines like in Australia, Finland, or the South African Republic, no cases have been reported. Lastly, it is generally

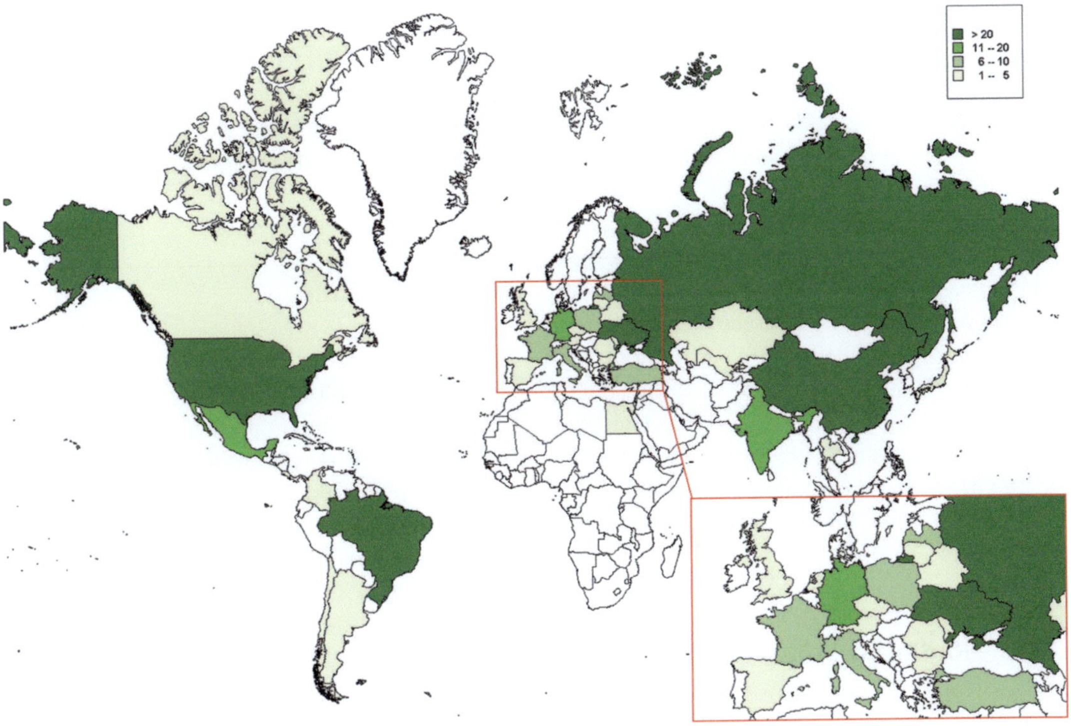

Fig. 20.1 Geographical distribution of published cases of pediatric pleural mesothelioma

accepted that it takes approximately 20–30 years after asbestos exposure to develop a mesothelioma so that it seems very unlikely that asbestosis is implicated in the genesis of mesothelioma in children. Thus, most pediatric mesotheliomas might belong to the so-called idiopathic forms of mesothelioma, which can also occur in adults with an estimated incidence of 1/million (Moore et al. 2008).

Besides asbestos exposure, other predisposing factors have been implicated in the pathogenesis of mesothelioma in children, for instance, irradiation or genetic syndromes. These suggestions rely on reported cases of pleural mesothelioma occurring after irradiation (Anderson et al. 1985; André et al. 2009; Falchero et al. 1996), as secondary malignancies especially after a Wilms' tumor or Hodgkin's disease (Anderson et al. 1985; André et al. 2009; Falchero et al. 1996; Antman et al. 1984), or in children with Proteus syndrome (Gordon et al. 1995; Malamitsi-Puchner et al. 1990). These cases suggest that in some patients, a non-identified underlying genetic background may contribute to the occurrence of a mesothelioma. Mutation of WT1 has been reported in sporadic cases of mesothelioma (Park et al. 1993) and is also frequent in patients with Wilms' tumor (Haber and Buckler 1992). However, the role of this gene in the genesis and progression of the tumor is not clear (Park et al. 1993). Some familial cases of mesothelioma have been reported with a deletion of the short arm of chromosome 9 that carries the CDKN2A gene. This gene encodes for p16^{INK4a} and p14^{ARF}. The inactivation of p16^{INK4a} has been frequently reported in mesothelioma (You et al. 2007; Ugolini et al. 2008). Nevertheless, no children have been reported to be affected in these familial series. Recently, implication of ATM has also been reported: first, in a child with ataxia telangiectasia (Rosas-Salazar et al. 2018) and in a 4-month-old child belonging to a consanguineous Bedouin family of ATM (Mijalovsky et al. 2018) who had two ATM mutations.

20.3 Clinical Presentation

Typical presenting features of children with pleural mesothelioma are chest pain, dyspnea, or both in most of the cases (Fraire et al. 1988; Kauffman and Stout 1964; Brenner et al. 1981; André et al. 2009). These symptoms develop usually quickly in a previously nonsymptomatic child. Fever is sometimes an associated symptom. Additionally, patients may very rarely present with breathlessness secondary to a pleural effusion without chest pain. A chest wall mass, weight loss, and abdominal pain and ascites due to peritoneal involvement are also common presentations. Indeed, in the SFCE series, involvement of multiple serosal cavities was seen in one third of the patients (André et al. 2009).

20.4 Radiological Presentation

Radiological imaging is critical for both the diagnosis and staging and in turn the management of mesothelioma.

20.4.1 CT

Intravenous contrast-enhanced CT is the primary imaging modality for suspected pleural malignant disease, where it can help distinguishing malignant from benign pleural disease. The most helpful CT findings suggesting a malignant pleural disease in adults are (1) a circumferential pleural rind, (2) nodular pleural thickening, (3) diffuse pleural thickening, and (4) mediastinal pleural involvement. While these features have a high positive predictive value, the absence of these signs does not reliably exclude the diagnosis of pleural malignancy (Moore et al. 2008; Wang et al. 2004).

20.4.2 MRI

In adults, MRI is not used routinely to assess malignant mesothelioma. However, it can be a valuable tool to confirm the potential surgical resectability. More specifically, using gadolinium enhancement, MRI can improve the identification of tumor extension into the diaphragm or chest wall, allowing better assessment of the individual for surgical treatment (Moore et al. 2008; Wang et al. 2004).

20.4.3 PET Scan

PET scan has been reported to have a 97% sensitivity and a 88% specificity to distinguish benign from malignant pleural disease in adults (Moore et al. 2008). Additionally, PET scanning has also increased the accuracy to diagnose mediastinal nodal metastases so that overall PET scan is useful in the staging and preoperative evaluation of mesothelioma (Moore et al. 2008; Wang et al. 2004). PET scan may also help to identify the optimal site for CT-guided pleural biopsy. Lastly, changes in the fluorodeoxyglucose (FDG) uptake within the tumor might indicate response to treatment, suggesting its role to assess the response to chemotherapy. Nevertheless, the value of PET scan to adequately stage the disease was initially controversial and recommended in adults (Pilling et al. 2010; Scherpereel et al. 2010), but it is use is. In children, very little is known regarding the use of PET scanning, but, in one case, decrease in size and uptake of FDG by a mesothelioma was documented during a treatment with pemetrexed and cisplatin (Milano et al. 2006). In another case, Abikher et al. used PET for the initial staging (Abikhzer et al. 2013).

20.5 Pathology

The pathological diagnosis of mesothelioma is acknowledged as difficult. As for adults, pathological analysis should be performed on representative biopsy specimen obtained by surgery. Given the histological heterogeneity of mesothelioma and the fact that it may mimic a variety of epithelial and mesenchymal neoplasms, needle biopsies are commonly of limited value as diagnostic tool. It is generally recommended that all cases be confirmed by a panel of pathologists including one with experience in adult mesothelioma. According to the WHO classification, malignant mesothelioma can be classified into epithelioid, sarcomatoid, or mixed (biphasic) subtypes based on tissue obtained by biopsy. The majority (almost 60%) of pediatric pleural mesotheliomas are of the epithelial subtype (Kashanskiy and André 2010).

On scanning magnification, the tumor classically displays sheets of medium-sized or large epithelioid cells with distinct cell borders arranged into well-developed tubulopapillary structures, commonly with intermixed solid areas and occasional adenomatoid pattern. At higher magnification, tumor cells have a bland cytological appearance, being polygonal in shape, with moderate amount of pale eosinophilic cytoplasm, round nuclei, and inconspicuous nucleoli (Fig. 20.2). Usually, only rare mitotic figures can be identified (<1/mm^2). In some areas, the epithelioid cells form gland-like structures and communicating cords set within abundant mucinous or myxoid stroma (Moran et al. 2008; Brenner et al. 1981; Anderson et al. 1985). The tubules occasionally contain a wispy bluish secretion that stains positive with Alcian Blue and disappears after predigestion with hyaluronidase. In contrast to adenocarcinoma, true PAS-positive mucin is usually absent in mesothelioma.

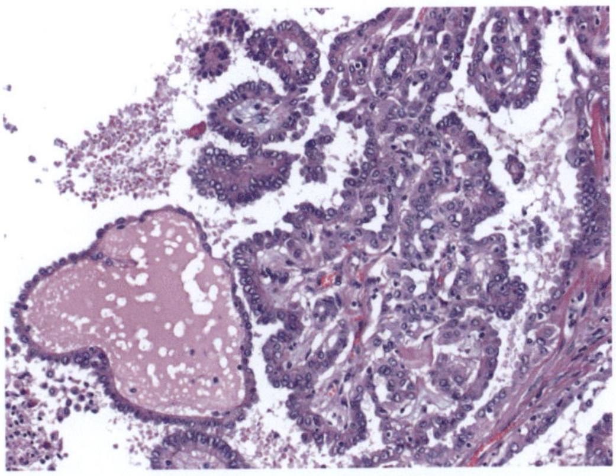

Fig. 20.2 Typical tubulopapillary pattern of mesothelioma with relatively bland-looking cuboidal cells (H&E stain, original magnification ×200)

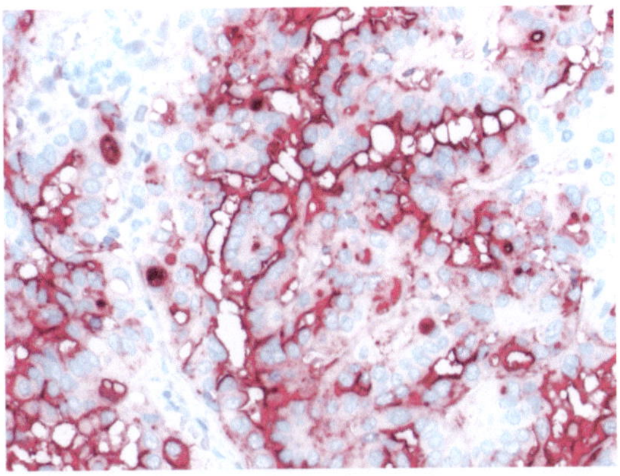

Fig. 20.3 HBME-1 showed characteristic apical (luminal) membranous staining in mesothelioma cells

Traditionally, a panel of positive and negative immunohistochemical markers is recommended to reliably diagnose mesothelioma. The tumor cells commonly express mesothelin, HBME-1 (Fig. 20.3), cytokeratin (CK) 5/6, calretinin, D2–40 (podoplanin), and vimentin. The low-molecular-weight CK (CAM5.2) is helpful in identifying less well-differentiated tumors that have lost other differentiation markers. More recently, Wilms' tumor-1 antigen (WT1) proved of value as a further marker. However, given the fair expression of this marker by serous carcinomas of the female genital tract, careful interpretation in the appropriate context is necessary. Markers that are usually absent in mesothelioma but have variable expression in carcinomas include Ber-EP4, carcinoembryonic antigen (CEA), and thyroid transcription factor 1 (TTF-1).

Interestingly, with the rapid development of molecular profiling of tumors, potential targetable mutations have been unveiled in pediatric mesothelioma. Thus, ALK translocation has been identified in pediatric patients with mesothelioma (Loharamtaweethong et al. 2016; Leal et al. 2020). In adults only a small subset (<1%) of patients demonstrate ALK or TRK rearrangements (Mian et al. 2020). Of note, unique ALK rearrangements were found in mesotheliomas lacking asbestos fibers, therapeutic radiation, and cytogenetic and molecular alterations typically found in these tumors (Hung et al. 2018).

20.6 Treatment

In adults, no standard optimal treatment strategy is currently available owing to the rarity of this tumor and the limited efficacy of treatments. Recent data and guidelines in adults suggest that multimodal (extrapleural pneumonectomy–neoadjuvant/adjuvant chemotherapy and radical hemithorax irradiation) should be proposed to patients when possible (Scherpereel et al. 2010) and within prospective randomized trials. Nothing is known about this global strategy in children; the aggressive surgery and its related mortality and morbidity, as well as radiotherapy-associated side effects, should make one highly cautious about using this strategy in children.

20.6.1 Surgery

Surgery aiming at removal of all malignant tissue is only very rarely associated with persistent durable complete remission as the disease usually has spread, at least microscopically, within the pleural cavity. Some examples can be found in pediatric literature (Flores et al. 2006). Therefore, we advocate for complete surgery only in cases of easily removable tumor. Besides, pleurectomy/decortication can be proposed but without curative intent and considered in patients to help obtaining symptom control.

20.6.2 Chemotherapy, Targeted Therapies, Immunotherapies

While the combination of pemetrexed–cisplatin is a standard first-line chemotherapy in adults with pleural mesothelioma (Vogelzang et al. 2003), there is currently no such standard chemotherapy regimen for pleural mesothelioma in children. Anyhow, these new molecules (pemetrexed, gemcitabine) indeed seem to bring clinical benefit for children with mesothelioma (Antman et al. 1984; Ugolini et al. 2008; Milano et al. 2006). Metronomic chemotherapy with oral navelbine may also allow sustained control of the disease without overt toxicities (Barlesi et al. 2017) and could be used at relapse.

Despite frequent overexpression of EGFR in mesotheliomas, TKIs and monoclonal antibodies blocking the receptor have not displayed sufficient clinical activity so far. In adult, the addition of bevacizumab to pemetrexed–cisplatin led to a significant survival advantage; this gain was only a modest 3 months (Zalcman et al. 2016). We do believe given the good tolerance in children that it shall be added as a first-line treatment in children. As mentioned above, alterations of ALK and AMT also pave the way for targeted therapies. In retrospect, these observations should not have surprised us, considering the relatively low mutational burden in mesothelioma and relative lack of oncogenic drivers. Recently, immune-checkpoint inhibitors have come into play for mesothelioma field (Scherpereel et al. 2018). In children, although the experience is very preliminary, an encouraging response has been reported recently (Geoerger et al. 2020).

20.6.3 Radiotherapy

Radiotherapy has not been demonstrated to be an effective treatment in mesothelioma in adults (Scherpereel et al. 2010), and its use is mostly restricted to try to control disease for patients receiving palliative care. As mentioned above, in adults, radical hemithorax radiotherapy has been proposed within a multimodal strategy (Scherpereel et al. 2010).

20.6.4 Outcome

Historically, the prognosis of pleural mesothelioma in children had been reported to be extremely poor. Thus, Grundy and Miller reported that death occurred within 6 months in 8 out of 12 patients with pleural mesothelioma, with the longest survival being 24 months (Grundy and Miller 1972). A more recent review only partially confirmed these findings. Indeed, the authors also reported long-term survival in two children (66 and 84 months), among whom one was treated with standard MTD chemotherapy (Brenner et al. 1981). Interestingly, Mutafoglu-Uysal et al. reported a case of relapsing malignant pleural mesothelioma that responded to the combination of VAC–ICE chemotherapy and who was alive without evidence of disease 36 months after discontinuation of the treatment (Mutafoğlu-Uysal et al. 2002). Additional cases responding to MTD chemotherapy have been reported (Kung et al. 1995). Thus, although we should be ready to face rapid progression and refractory disease, in some cases, pediatric pleural mesothelioma can respond to chemotherapy and be long-term survivors. Biologic and/or genetic differences underlying this difference of behavior must be unveiled.

20.7 Conclusion

Mesothelioma is a very rare tumor in pediatric oncology. Pediatric mesothelioma seems to be different from its adult counterpart, with less frequent primary pleural localization. Although the outcome of children with peritoneal mesothelioma is good despite frequent relapses, the outcome of pediatric pleural mesothelioma is dismal. This is in line with data obtained from adults. New therapeutic strategies with targeted therapies or immunotherapies are currently emerging and need to be properly evaluated in children within international studies, and an international registry is mandatory to increase our knowledge of this disease.

References

Abikhzer G, Gourevich K, Arkovitz M et al (2013) Role of 18F-FDG PET/CT in the staging of pediatric peritoneal mesothelioma. Clin Nucl Med 38:e331–e332

Anderson KA, Hurley WC, Hurley BT et al (1985) Malignant pleural mesothelioma following radiotherapy in a 16-year-old boy. Cancer 56:273–276

André N, Ratsimandresy R, Réguerre Y et al (2009) Paediatric malignant mesothelioma: the SFCE experience. Pediatr Blood Cancer 53:823

Antman KH, Ruxer RL Jr, Aisner J et al (1984) Mesothelioma following Wilms' tumor in childhood. Cancer 54:367–369

Barlesi F, Imbs DC, Tomasini P et al (2017) Mathematical modeling for phase I cancer trials: a study of metronomic vinorelbine for advanced non-small cell lung cancer (NSCLC) and mesothelioma patients. Oncotarget 8:47161–47166

Brenner J, Sordillo PP, Magill GB (1981) Malignant mesothelioma in children: report of seven cases and review of the literature. Med Pediatr Oncol 9:367–373

Falchero L, Coiffier B, Guibert B et al (1996) Malignant mesothelioma of the pleura following radiotherapy for Hodgkin disease. Bull Cancer 83:964–968

Flores RM, Su W, Lal D, Rusch VW, La Quaglia MP (2006) Extrapleural pneumonectomy in children. J Pediatr Surg 41:1738–1742

Fraire AE, Cooper S, Greenberg SD et al (1988) Mesothelioma of childhood. Cancer 62:838–847

Geoerger B, Kang HJ, Yalon-Oren M et al (2020) Pembrolizumab in paediatric patients with advanced melanoma or a PD-L1-positive, advanced, relapsed, or refractory solid tumour or lymphoma (KEYNOTE-051): interim analysis of an open-label, single-arm, phase 1-2 trial. Lancet Oncol 21:121–133

Gordon PL, Wilroy RS, Lasater OE et al (1995) Neoplasms in Proteus syndrome. Am J Med Genet 57:74–78

Grundy GW, Miller RW (1972) Malignant mesothelioma in childhood. Cancer 5:1216–1218

Haber DA, Buckler AJ (1992) WT1: a novel tumor suppressor gene inactivated in Wilms' tumor. New Biol 4:97–106

Hung YP, Dong F, Watkins JC et al (2018) Identification of ALK rearrangements in malignant peritoneal mesothelioma. JAMA Oncol 4:235–238

Kashanskiy SV, André N (2010) Paediatric mésothelioma: is there the such a disease? Bull Cancer 97:571–576

Kauffman SL, Stout AP (1964) Mesothelioma in children. Cancer 17:539–544

Kung FH, Desai SJ, Dickerman JD et al (1995) Ifosfamide/carboplatin/etoposide (ICE) for recurrent malignant solid tumors of childhood: a pediatric oncology group phase I/II study. J Pediatr Hematol Oncol 17: 265–269

Leal JL, Peters G, Szaumkessel M et al (2020) NTRK and ALK rearrangements in malignant pleural mesothelioma, pulmonary neuroendocrine tumours and non-small cell lung cancer. Lung Cancer 146:154–159

Loharamtaweethong K, Puripat N, Aoonjai N et al (2016) Anaplastic lymphoma kinase (ALK) translocation in paediatric malignant peritoneal mesothelioma: a case report of novel ALK-related tumour spectrum. Histopathology 68:603–607

Malamitsi-Puchner A, Dimitriadis D, Bartsocas C et al (1990) Proteus syndrome: course of a severe case. Am J Med Genet 35:283–285

Margery J, Ruffié P (2008) Environmental cancer: malignant pleural mesothelioma. Bull Cancer 95:77–86

Mian I, Abdullaev Z, Morrow B et al (2020) Anaplastic lymphoma kinase gene rearrangement in children and young adults with mesothelioma. J Thorac Oncol 15:457–461

Mijalovsky A, Halperin D, Perez Y et al (2018) Malignant peritoneal mesothelioma in an infant with familial ATM mutations. J Pediatr Hematol Oncol 40:e511–e515

Milano E, Pourroy B, Rome A, Delarue A et al (2006) Efficacy of a combination of pemetrexed and multiple redo-surgery in an 11-year-old girl with a recurrent multifocal abdominal mesothelioma. Anticancer Drugs 17:1231–1234

Moore AJ, Parker RJ, Wiggins J (2008) Malignant mesothelioma. Orphanet J Rare Dis 3:34

Moran CA, Albores-Saavedral J, Suster S (2008) Primary peritoneal mesotheliomas in children: a clinicopathological and immunohistochemical study of eight cases. Histopathology 52:824–830

Mutafoğlu-Uysal K, Kargi A, Sarialioğlu F et al (2002) Malignant pleural mesothelioma in a child: long-term survival with ICE-WAC chemotherapy regimen. Turk J Pediatr 44(3):244–247

Park S, Schalling M, Bernard A et al (1993) The Wilms tumour gene WT1 is expressed in murine mesoderm-derived tissues and mutated in a human mesothelioma. Nat Genet 4:415–420

Pilling J, Dartnell JA, Lang-Lazdunski L (2010) Integrated positron emission tomography-computed tomography does not accurately stage intrathoracic disease of patients undergoing trimodality therapy for malignant pleural mesothelioma. Thorac Cardiovasc Surg 58:215–219

Rosas-Salazar C, Gunawardena S, Spahr JE (2018) Malignant pleural mesothelioma in a child with ataxia-telangiectasia. Pediatr Pulmonol 40:e511–e515

Scherpereel A, Astoul P, Baas P et al (2010) Guidelines of the European Respiratory Society and the European Society of Thoracic Surgeons for the management of malignant pleural mesothelioma. Eur Respir J 35:479–495

Scherpereel A, Wallyn F, Albelda SM, Munck C (2018) Novel therapies for malignant pleural mesothelioma. Lancet Oncol 19:e161–e172

Ugolini D, Neri M, Ceppi M et al (2008) Genetic susceptibility to malignant mesothelioma and exposure to asbestos: the influence of the familial factor. Mutat Res 658:162–167

Vogelzang NJ, Rusthoven JJ, Symanowski J et al (2003) Phase III study of pemetrexed in combination with cisplatin versus cisplatin alone in patients with malignant pleural mesothelioma. J Clin Oncol 21:2636–2644

Wang ZJ, Reddy GP, Gotway MB, Higgins CB, Jablons DM, Ramaswamy M, Hawkins RA, Webb WR (2004) Malignant pleural mesothelioma: evaluation with CT, MR imaging, and PET. Radiographics 24:105–119

You B, Blandin S, Gérinière L et al (2007) Mésothéliomes familiaux: une composante génétique associée aux risques environnementaux? Bull Cancer 7:705–710

Zalcman G, Mazieres J, Margery J et al (2016) Bevacizumab for newly diagnosed pleural mesothelioma in the Mesothelioma Avastin cisplatin Pemetrexed Study (MAPS): a randomised, controlled, open-label, phase 3 trial. Lancet 387:1405–1414

21 Thymoma and Thymic Carcinoma in Children and Adolescents

Teresa Stachowicz-Stencel, Daniel Orbach, Jan Godzinski, and Anna Synakiewicz

21.1 Introduction

Thymomas and thymic carcinomas belong to thymic epithelial tumors (TETs) together with thymic carcinoids and thymolipoma. Primary neoplasms of the thymus constitute only 0.2–1.5% of all malignancies in adults (Girard et al. 2015), but they are the most frequent primary tumors of the thymus and apply to people between 40 and 60 years at similar rates in females and males (Safieddine et al. 2014). They are extremely rare in children's population, and need for management guideline is unprecedented (Stachowicz-Stencel et al. 2015). To date, no risk factors were found to be responsible for the development of malignancy in thymus. But strong connection with autoimmune disorders such as myasthenia gravis (MG) and paraneoplastic syndromes was observed. Autoimmune disorders are associated with favorable features but at the same time are not independent good prognostic factors for patients with TETs (Padda et al. 2018). Histology and stage of advancement are crucial for prognosis and course of the disease.

Teresa Stachowicz-Stencel and Daniel Orbach were considered as national coordinators.

T. Stachowicz-Stencel (✉) · A. Synakiewicz
Department of Pediatrics, Hematology and Oncology, Medical University, Gdansk, Poland
e-mail: tsten@gumed.edu.pl

D. Orbach
Department of Pediatrics, Insitut Curie, Paris, France

J. Godzinski
Department of Pediatric Surgery, Marciniak Hospital, Wroclaw, Poland

21.2 Symptoms

Thymic tumors, including thymoma and thymic carcinoma, may be discovered by accident in asymptomatic patients, due to symptoms resulting from mediastinal mass or due to mentioned paraneoplastic syndromes. Symptoms which are connected with anterior mediastinal mass may be as follows: shortness of breath, chest pain, dyspnea, cough, dysphagia, phrenic nerve palsy, or even vena cava superior syndrome.

21.3 Paraneoplastic Autoimmune Syndromes

Thymic tumors associate with paraneoplastic disorders concerning many areas such as hematologic disorders, pure red cell aplasia, hemolytic anemia, and pernicious anemia; neurological disorders, MG, stiff person syndrome, neuromyelitis optica, and polymyositis; dermatological disorders, pemphigus, alopecia areata, and vitiligo; and various disorders, acquired hypogammaglobulinemia, nephrotic syndrome, rheumatoid arthritis, myocarditis, hypertrophic osteoarthropathy,

D. T. Schneider et al. (eds.), *Rare Tumors in Children and Adolescents*, Pediatric Oncology,
https://doi.org/10.1007/978-3-030-92071-5_21

Addison syndrome, and thymoma-associated multiorgan autoimmunity (TAMA) (Wadhera et al. 2007). Diagnosis of these diseases depends on recognition of clinical syndromes and specific autoantibody. Management consists of tumor treatment itself and autoimmune therapy. Approximately one third of adult patients with thymoma present mainly MG which can occur up to 50% of cases, and it is particularly common in type AB, B1, and B2 thymomas and almost always associated with the presence of anti-acetylcholine receptor antibodies. As contrary among patients with MG, 20% may have a thymoma. MG is rare in thymic carcinoma (Weis et al. 2015, Evoli and Lancaster 2014). About 15% have other frequent disorders such as pure red cell aplasia (5% of cases) and hypogammaglobulinemia (Good syndrome, 5% of cases) (Evoli et al. 2007). In children, these syndromes are seldom and concern only 7% of patients (Rod et al. 2014).

21.4 Pathologic Classification and Staging

Thymic tumors are categorized according to the World Health Organization (WHO) histological classification according to their behavior from benign tumors to more aggressive ones, as thymoma with A, AB, B1, B2, and B3 subtypes and aggressive thymic carcinoma (TC; type C) defined according to adult experience and translated to pediatric tumors. TC consists about 20% of all TETs and comprises several histotypes, mostly squamous cell carcinoma with tendency to metastatic spread (Table 21.1). The Masaoka-Koga system (Table 21.2) is for determining the stages of thymic tumors. It is a postsurgical classification based on macroscopic and microscopic invasion into the tumor capsule and adjacent mediastinal fat and structures, as well as the presence of metastasis. Extrathoracic metastases of TC are rare (about 7%) and mainly occur in the lymph nodes, liver, brain, thyroid, adrenal glands, and kidney (Lewis et al. 1987). This classification is now replaced by a TNM-based system for the eighth edition of the AJCC/UICC staging

Table 21.1 WHO histologic classification of thymic epithelial tumors

Type	Histopathology
A	Tumor composed of a population of neoplastic thymic epithelial cells with spindle/oval shape. No atypia and few or no non-neoplastic lymphocytes
AB	Type A thymoma with foci of lymphocytes
B1	Plump epithelioid cells with areas resembling thymic medulla
B2	Scattered foci of atypical epithelial cells with lymphocytes
B3	Epithelial cells having a round or polygonal shape and exhibiting no or mild atypia with a minor component of lymphocytes
Thymic carcinoma (type C)	Tumor exhibiting clear-cut cytologic atypia and a set of cytoarchitectural features analogous to those seen in carcinomas of other organs

Table 21.2 Masaoka-Koga staging system for thymic malignancies

Stage	Description
I	Grossly and microscopically completely encapsulated tumor
IIa	Microscopically transcapsular invasion
b	Macroscopic invasion into thymic or surrounding fatty tissue, or grossly adherent to but not breaking through mediastinal pleura or pericardium
III	Macroscopic invasion into neighbouring organs (i.e., pericardium, great vessel, or lung)
IVa	Pleural or pericardial metastases
b	Lymphogenous or hematogenous metastasis

classification of tumors starting 2018 (Table 21.3), leading to better define the resectability of the tumor, the need of adjuvant treatment, and the harmonization of the staging of these malignancies. These classifications are mostly used for children too.

21.5 Diagnosis

21.5.1 Laboratory Studies

Complete history and physical, especially neurological, examination; laboratory tests such as complete blood count (CBC) to control anemia,

Table 21.3 Eighth TNM classification

Category	Definition		
T1			
a	Encapsulated or unencapsulated, extension into mediastinal fat present or not		
b	Mediastinal pleura extension		
T2	Pericardium involvement		
T3	Involvement of lung, brachiocephalic vein, superior vena cava, chest wall, phrenic nerve, hilar (extrapericardial) pulmonary vessels		
T4	Aorta, arch vessels, main pulmonary artery, myocardium, trachea, or esophagus		
N0	No nodal involvement		
N1	Anterior (perithymic) nodes		
N2	Deep intrathoracic or cervical nodes		
M0	No metastatic pleural, pericardial, or distant sites		
M1			
a	Separate pleural or pericardial nodule(s)		
b	Pulmonary intraparenchymal nodule or distant organ metastasis		
Stage grouping			
Stage	T	N	M
I	T1	N0	M0
II	T2	N0	M0
IIIa	T3	N0	M0
IIIb	T4	N0	M0
IVa	T any	N1	M0
	T any	N0, 1	M1a
IVb	T any	N2	M0, 1a
	T any	N any	M1b

granulocytopenia, and thrombocytopenia; and, in addition, the absence of circulating blast cells should be confirmed; immunoglobulin and immunophenotypic analysis, lactate dehydrogenase, beta-human chorionic gonadotropin, and alpha-fetoprotein help to establish diagnosis and eliminate differential diagnosis.

21.5.2 Radiological Studies

Thoracic CT scan is the imaging modality of choice. It can visualize whether anterior mediastinal tumor is more likely encapsulated or is infiltrating adjacent structures or the tumor is homogeneous (for thymoma A) or heterogeneous (for TC) or contains calcifications and necrotic areas. These features allow to suspect more likely thymoma or thymic carcinoma (Quagliano 1996). Also it may provide information about the possibility of surgical resection (Figs. 21.1 and 21.2). 18-Fluorodeoxyglucose positron emission computed tomography (PET-CT) scan is optional in suspicion aggressive histology and an advanced stage or recurrences of thymic tumors. It is often positive in carcinomas, while in thymomas it is often negative (Treglia et al. 2014). No data exist in children.

Final diagnosis should be established on the basis of histopathological examination. This is the most reliable method of mediastinal mass differentiation.

21.6 Surgical Approach to Establishing a Diagnosis

21.6.1 Biopsy

Initial biopsy is not necessary to put a diagnosis if a complete surgical resection is achievable. In this situation, pretreatment biopsy is not required. But most of the time, as other differential diagnoses are more frequent, histological confirmation before any further therapy is needed. These tumors need histology to set up precise diagnosis. It may be performed with percutaneous core-needle biopsy or incisional surgical biopsy (histology) through mediastinotomy or mini-thoracotomy. Fine-needle aspiration (cytology) is not sufficient to confirm thymic tumor. Fine-

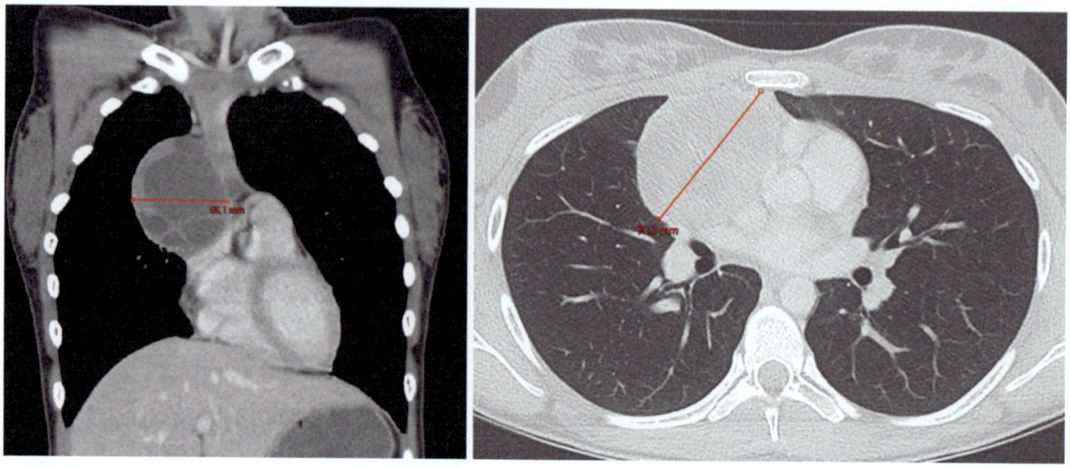

Fig. 21.1 Imaging aspect of an isolated mixed type B1/B2 thymoma treated with partial thymectomy (R1 resection), followed by an immediate re-excision (no viable cells) in a 14-year-old female. Persistent first complete remission 3 years after

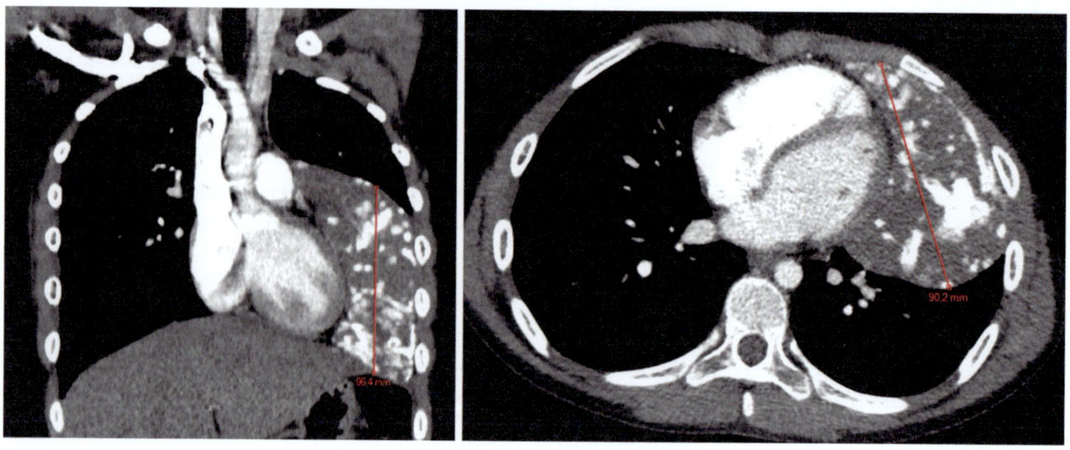

Fig. 21.2 Radiological aspect of a highly vascularized type B1 thymoma treated with incomplete thymectomy (R1 resection), in a 10-year-old female with a personal and familial history of osteochondromatosis. No adjuvant therapy. Persistent first complete remission 5 years after

needle aspiration is usually used in such mediastinal primary to eliminate malignant lymphomas. During all these diagnostic procedures, pleural spaces should be respected to avoid tumor cell seeding (Rod et al. 2014).

21.6.2 Immunochemistry

Histologic aspects define the precise subtypes (WHO classification, Table 21.1). Immunochemistry with anti-CD117/KIT and CD5 antibodies is recommended because in 80% it is present in thymic carcinomas (Asirvatham et al. 2014, Su et al. 2015). Such markers like epithelial membrane antigen, keratin, p40, p63, and PAX 8 are present both in thymoma and thymic carcinoma. Differently from TC, type A and AB thymomas may stain for CD20 (Kodama et al. 1986, Smith et al. 2016). Terminal deoxynucleotidyl transferase expression in immature T cells is observed in AB, B1, B2, and B3 thymomas (Strobel et al. 2010).

21.6.3 Molecular and Genetic Changes

Thymomas usually do not present with mutational somatic changes. General transcription factor I (*GTF2I*) mutation is seen mostly in type A and AB thymomas, followed by B1, B2, and B3 (around 80, 30, 20, and 15%, respectively) (Travis et al. 2015).

Thymic carcinogenesis can be associated with genetic changes that weaken the development of T cells and generate an increased number of self-reactive lymphocytes. It regards that PD-L1 expression is in over 90% of the normal thymic epithelial cells and correlates with clinical progression in some type of cancer because activity of PD-L1 pathway induces T cell-mediated immune suppression in the tumor microenvironment. High PD-L1 expression is correlated with advanced Masaoka staging, higher grade WHO histology, and worse clinical outcome. Apart from this high PD-L1, IDO (indoleamine 2,3-dioxygenase) expression and FOXP3 tregs are connected with high-grade histology (Yokoyama and Miyoshi 2018). IDO expression plays an immunosuppressive role in cancerogenesis and is a biomarker for poor prognosis in some cancers. Forkhead box P3 (FOXP3) is a transcriptional factor of CD4+CD25+ regulatory T cells and has an immunosuppressive function (Wei et al. 2018). Due to the rarity of this disease in children, a second advice with a pathologist expert is mandatory to confirm diagnosis and define precise subtype.

21.7 Differential Diagnosis

Hodgkin's and non-Hodgkin's lymphomas, teratomas, seminomas, and non-seminomatous germ-cell malignant tumors should be taken into consideration. Differentiating thymic malignancy from benign thymic hyperplasia may be challenging. It may be two types of hyperplasia. Thymic rebound hyperplasia may be observed after stress, injuries, chemotherapy drugs, radiotherapy, corticosteroids, or lymphoid hyperplasia in MG. There are no specific markers for thymoma and thymic carcinoma.

21.8 Treatment

Recommendations for systemic treatment of thymic carcinoma in children are only based on prospective nonrandomized studies, retrospective data, and expert opinion because of rarity of the disease and follow most of the time adults' experience. The management of thymic tumors in youths should be a strict cooperation between surgeons, pathologists, and pediatric oncologists to establish therapeutic strategy. All decisions should be taken during multi-team discussion (MTD). Treatments should also ideally be discussed with expert medical oncologists. Decisions should take into account the histological grade of the tumor (subtype), the extension of the tumor (Masaoka staging system, TNM classification), and the age of the patient.

21.9 Surgical Management

The main strategy of treatment is based on complete thymectomy including the tumor, the residual thymus gland, and perithymic fat. The standard approach is median sternotomy. In this situation, pretreatment biopsy is not required. Biopsy, such as percutaneous core-needle biopsy, incisional surgical biopsy through mediastinotomy, or mini-thoracotomy, must be done only to put diagnose if the total resection is not possible. The surgeon must evaluate pleural cavities, infiltration of perithymic and mediastinal fat, and involvement of surrounding mediastinal structures. After only partial thymectomy, the risk of local recurrence is higher (Nakagawa et al. 2014).

Exclusive thymectomy in stage I thymoma (types A to AB) is the option of treatment without further management. Subtotal resection, called "debulking resection," may be performed in thymoma but is not recommended for all other tumors, including thymic carcinoma.

21.10 Chemotherapy

Postoperative chemotherapy is not recommended in case of thymoma stages I, IIA (A, AB, B1, B2), IIIB (A, AB, B1), and any IIIB after R0 resection. In unresectable thymic tumors, where only biopsy is possible, neoadjuvant chemotherapy may be used. In metastatic thymic carcinoma, perioperative chemotherapy is also recommended associated with radiotherapy, but in metastatic thymoma chemotherapy and RTX with or without surgery is used. Cycles of chemotherapy with platinum- and etoposide-based regimens are classical options for thymic carcinomas (National Comprehensive Cancer Network 2012). Usually first-line treatment consists of CAP (cyclophosphamide, doxorubicin, and cisplatin), PE (platin, etoposide), CAP with steroids-prednisone, or ADOC (cisplatin, doxorubicin, vincristine, and cyclophosphamide). In case of failure-progression, second-line therapy with pemetrexed and octreotide may be used (Loehrer et al. 2004). Patients with primary or secondary dissemination of the disease, due to their poor prognosis, may require separate approaches, e.g., molecular targeting drugs or immunotherapy. No prospective studies even on large adult population were published so far with such new strategies, nor on children. Drugs directed against EGFR (epidermal growth factor receptor) such as cetuximab, erlotinib, or gefitinib were evaluated. In assessed patients, overexpression of EGFR was found (Yok et al. 2008, Kurup et al. 2005, Bedano et al. 2008, Palmieri et al. 2007). The number of patients is too small to propose strict recommendations. Imatinib as tyrosine kinase inhibitor is also under evaluation. CD117 expression is mandatory for use this drug. In prospective study, no benefits for patients were observed (Salter et al. 2008). Other molecular targeted substances like histone deacetylase inhibitors as belinostat or vorinostat are of interest (Giaccone et al. 2011).

21.11 Radiotherapy

Radiotherapy in thymoma and thymic carcinoma is a complementary treatment. In children, indications for radiotherapy are not clear. Panel of experts proposes in thymoma after R0 resection in stage I, IIA (A, AB, B1, B2) IIB (A, AB, B1) Masaoka-Koga: no adjuvant RT. In stages IIA (B3), IIB (B2, B3), and III, RT is advised.

In R0 thymic carcinoma, stage I and II RT is recommended but in stage III–IV chemotherapy and radiotherapy.

After R1 resection, adjuvant RT is recommended for stages I, IIA, IIB, and III–IVA for adult patients (National Comprehensive Cancer Network 2012). In children, decision about RT should also consider the patient's age, stage of disease, and the type of thymoma. After R1 resection radiotherapy in thymoma in recommended and in thymic carcinoma only in stage I, the rest stages chemotherapy and then RT.

For thymic carcinoma patients with R2 resection (macroscopic residue), adjuvant chemotherapy ± delayed surgery and radiotherapy are recommended.

Accordingly, the recommended dose of radiation for adults is 45–50 Gy in 1.8–2 Gy daily fractions over 5 weeks both to the tumor bed and surrounding mediastinum. But doses up to 60 Gy in 2 Gy daily fractions are also possible in case of microscopic or gross residual disease after R2 resection (National Comprehensive Cancer Network 2012). In children, postoperative radiotherapy (total dose of radiation proposed around 60 Gy) may be given after R2 resection especially in case of thymic carcinoma.

Proton beam radiotherapy in pediatric patients with TETs is not evaluated yet. The National Comprehensive Cancer Network (NNCN) allows its use in particular adult patients to avoid serious classical RT complications and for better local control (National Comprehensive Cancer Network 2012, Parikh et al. 2016).

21.12 Summary

Thymoma and thymic carcinomas are tumors of anterior mediastinum and belong to TETs together with thymic carcinoids and thymolipoma. Diagnosis could be established accidentally in asymptomatic patients due to performed radiological examination from other reasons or in symptomatic patients with cough, dyspnea, or vena cava syndrome. Recommended radiological diagnostic tool is CT of the chest. Additional radiological examinations are made to assess the extension of the disease. There is no biochemical marker both for thymoma and thymic carcinoma. Tests such as AFP or beta HCG serum analysis are for exclusion of other more common differential tumors in pediatric population. The only reliable method for establishing diagnosis is histopathological examination mainly after biopsy. Radical surgery when possible is the treatment of choice. Systemic therapy using classical chemotherapeutic drugs (e.g., cisplatin, cyclophosphamide, doxorubicin) is recommended for unresectable or disseminated disease. The role of radiotherapy including proton has not been established yet, although on the basis of adult experience it is also recommended in some children.

References

Asirvatham JR, Esposito MJ, Bhuiya TA (2014) Role of PAX-8, CD5,n and CD117 in distinguishing thymic carcinoma from poorly differentiated lung carcinoma. Appl Immunohistochem Mol Morphol 22(5):372

Bedano P, Perkins S, Burns M et al (2008) A phase II trial of erlotinib plus bevacizumab in patients with recurrent thymoma or thymic carcinoma. J Clin Oncol:26, 1908

Evoli A, Lancaster E (2014) Paraneoplastic disorders in thymoma patients. J Thorac Oncol 9(9 Suppl 2):S143–S147

Evoli A, Minicuci GM, Vitaliani R et al (2007) Paraneoplastic diseases associated with thymoma. J Neurol 254:756–762

Giaccone G, Rajan A, Berman A et al (2011) Phase II study of belinostat in patients with recurrent or refractory advanced thymic epithelial tumors. J Clin Oncol 29:2052–2059

Girard N, Ruffini E, Marx A, Faivre-Finn C, Peters S, ESMO Guidelines Committee (2015) Thymic epithelial tumours: ESMO clinical practice guidelines for diagnosis, treatment and follow-up. Ann Oncol 26(Suppl 5):v40–v55

Kodama T, Watanabe S, Sato Y et al (1986) An immunohistochemical study of thymic epithelial tumors. I. Epithelial component. Am J Surg Pathol 10:26–33

Kurup A, Burns M, Dropcho S et al (2005) Phase II study of gefitinib treatment in advanced thymic malignancies. J Clin Oncol 23:7068

Lewis JE, Wick MR, Scheithauer BW et al (1987) Thymoma. A clinicopathologic review. Cancer 60:2727–2743

Loehrer PJ Sr, Wang W, Johnson DH et al (2004) Octreotide alone or with prednisone in patients with advanced thymoma and thymic carcinoma: an Eastern Cooperative Oncology Group phase II trial. J Clin Oncol 22:293–299

Nakagawa K, Asamura H, Sakurai H et al (2014) Does the mode of surgical resection affect the prognosis/recurrence in patients with thymoma? J Surg Oncol 109:179–183

National Comprehensive Cancer Network guidelines. http://www.nccn.org/professionals/physician_gls/f_guidelines.asp. Accessed 17 Apr 2012

Padda SK, Yao X, Antonicelli A et al (2018) Paraneoplastic syndromes and thymic malignancies: an examination of the International Thymic Malignancy Interest Group retrospective database. J Thorac Oncol 13(3):436–446

Palmieri G, Marino M, Salvatore M et al (2007) Cetuximab is an active treatment of metastatic and chemorefractory thymoma. Front Biosci 12:757–761

Parikh RR, Rhome R, Hug E et al (2016) Adjuvant proton beam therapy in the management of thymoma: a dosimetric comparison and acute toxicities. Clin Lung Cancer 17:362–366

Rod J, Orbach D, Verité C et al (2014) Surgical management of thymic epithelial tumors in children: lessons from the French Society of Pediatric Oncology and review of the literature. Pediatr Blood Cancer 61(11):1910–1915

Quagliano PV (1996) Thymic carcinoma: case reports and review. J Thorac Imaging 11:6674

Safieddine N, Liu G, Cuningham K et al (2014) Prognostic factors for cure, recurrence and long-term survival after surgical resection of thymoma. J Thorac Oncol 9:1018–1022

Salter J, Lewis D, Yiannoutsos C et al (2008) Imatinib for the treatment of thymic carcinoma. J Clin Oncol 26:8116

Smith T, Mauri F, Naresh KN (2016) Thyroid transcription factor-1 immunostaining in World Health Organization type AB thymoma. Histopathology 68:618–619

Stachowicz-Stencel T, Orbach D, Brecht I, Schneider D, Bien E, Synakiewicz A, Rod J, Ferrari A, Cecchetto G, Bisogno G (2015 Nov) Thymoma and thymic carcinoma in children and adolescents: a report from the European Cooperative Study Group for Pediatric Rare Tumors (EXPeRT). Eur J Cancer 51(16):2444–2452

Strobel P, Hohenberger P, Marx A (2010) Thymoma and thymic carcinoma: molecular pathology and targeted therapy. J Thorac Oncol 5(10 Suppl 4):S286–S290

Su XY, Wang WY, Li JN et al (2015) Immunohistochemical differentiation between type B3 thymomas and thymic squamous cell carcinomas. Int J Clin Exp Pathol 8:5354–5362

Treglia G, Sadeghi R, Giovanella L et al (2014) Is (18) F-FDG PET useful in predicting the WHO grade of malignancy in thymic epithelial tumors? A meta-analysis. Lung Cancer 86:5–13

Wadhera A, Maverakis E, Mitsiades N et al (2007) Thymoma-associated multiorgan autoimmunity: a graft-versus-host-like disease. J Am Acad Dermatol 57:683–689

Wei YF, Chu CY, Chang CC, Lin SH, Su WC, Tseng YL, Lin CC, Yen YT (2018) Different pattern of PD-L1, IDO, and FOXP3 Tregs expression with survival in thymoma and thymic carcinoma. Lung Cancer 125:35–42

Weis CA, Yao X, Deng Y et al (2015) Contributors to the ITMIG retrospective database. The impact of thymoma histotype on prognosis in a worldwide database. J Thorac Oncol 10(2):367–372

Travyis WD, Brambilla E, Burke AP et al (eds) (2015) WHO classification of tumours of the lung, pleura, thymus, and heart, 4th edn. IARC, Lyon

Yok K, Nishiwaki Y, Ishii G et al (2008) Mutational status of EGFR and KIT in thymoma and thymic carcinoma. Lung Cancer 62:316–320

Yokoyama S, Miyoshi H (2018) Thymic tumors and immune checkpoint inhibitors. J Thorac Dis 10(Suppl 13):S1509–S1515

NUT Carcinoma

22

Christopher A. French

22.1 Definition

NC (aka NUT midline carcinoma) is a poorly differentiated carcinoma with rearrangement of the *NUTM1* (aka *NUT*) gene (French and den Bakker 2015).

22.2 Clinical Features

NC is possibly the most aggressive solid tumor known, having a median survival of 6.7–10.1 months (Bauer et al. 2012; Jung et al. 2019). The majority of tumors arise centrally near the airways in the head and neck (39%) and thorax (50%) (Bauer et al. 2012), giving the tumor's original name NUT "midline" carcinoma; however, with the increasing diagnosis of this entity, cases are being reported in a broad range of non-midline sites, including kidney (Bishop et al. 2016; Sirohi et al. 2018; Zhu et al. 2019), thyroid (Landa et al. 2016), soft tissue (Dickson et al. 2018), salivary glands (Agaimy et al. 2018; Seim et al. 2017; Vulsteke et al. 2016; Ziai et al. 2010; den Bakker et al. 2009), pancreas (Shehata et al. 2010), and bladder (French et al. 2004). In fact, non-thoracic, non-head and neck primary sites comprise ~10% of NCs (Bauer et al. 2012; Chau et al. 2019). Radiologic (CT or MRI) features are not specific, typically revealing a large, invasive, heterogenous mass that often confluently involves local lymph nodes (Polsani et al. 2012; Sholl et al. 2015) (Fig. 22.1). Metastases are common at presentation (51%) (Bauer et al. 2012), including to bone and other solid organs (Sholl et al. 2015). The early presentation of hematogenous metastases and frequent origin within the lung or mediastinum can mimic that of small cell carcinoma; however, it progresses more rapidly and often effects younger individuals.

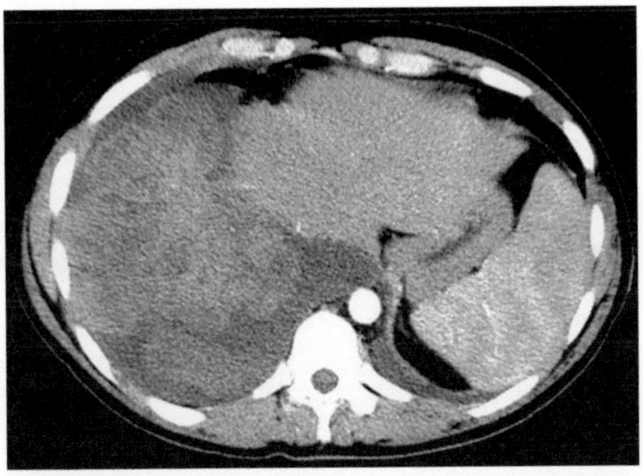

Fig. 22.1 Typical appearance of NC on thoracic CT scan reveals a large, heterogenous mass with extensive local invasion and lymph node involvement

C. A. French (✉)
Department of Pathology, Brigham and Women's Hospital/Harvard Medical School, Boston, MA, USA
e-mail: cfrench@bwh.harvard.edu

D. T. Schneider et al. (eds.), *Rare Tumors in Children and Adolescents*, Pediatric Oncology,
https://doi.org/10.1007/978-3-030-92071-5_22

22.3 Molecular Genetics

In all cases of NC, *NUTM1* is rearranged in a chromosomal translocation, most commonly (~70%) (Bauer et al. 2012; Chau et al. 2014) with *BRD4*, forming a *BRD4-NUTM1* fusion resulting from a t(15;19)(q14;p13.1). In almost every case, the breakpoint is upstream of exon 3 (transcript variant 1) of *NUTM1*, fusing this exon with the partner gene (Fig. 22.2). The most common alternative partner genes are *BRD3* (~15%) (Chau et al. 2019), which is highly homologous to *BRD4*, and *NSD3* (~6%) (Chau et al. 2019). Rare variant partners include ZNF532 and ZNF592. Interestingly, all of these encoded NUTM1 fusion partners (BRD3, BRD4, NSD3, ZNF532, ZNF592) interact with BRD4 and are critical components of the BRD4-NUT oncogenic complex (Alekseyenko et al. 2017). Thus, the fusion of any of these proteins to *NUTM1* leads to its association with BRD4 and is sufficient to recapitulate the function of the canonical BRD4-NUT oncogenic complex.

Molecular pathology utilizing next generation sequencing (NGS) has uncovered numerous novel *NUTM1*-fusions in a variety of tumors with uncertain relationship to NC. These *NUTM1*-fusion partners include *CIC* (Schaefer et al. 2018), *BCORL1* (Dickson et al. 2018), *MYXD1* (Dickson et al. 2018), *MYXD4* (Dickson et al. 2018; Tamura et al. 2018), and *MGA* (Stevens et al. 2019; Diolaiti et al. 2018) in solid tumors with various histologies, including some bearing resemblance to NC, and others with spindle cell sarcoma morphology. Remarkably, NUTM1-fusions (BRD9 (Andersson et al. 2015), *ACINI* (Andersson et al. 2015; Hormann et al. 2019; Gu et al. 2016; Liu et al. 2016), *SLC12A* (Gu et al. 2016), *ZNF618* (Gu et al. 2016), *IKZF1* (Gu et al. 2016; Lilljebjorn et al. 2016), *BPTF* (Liu et al. 2017), *CUX1*, and *IKZF1* (Hormann et al. 2019)) have also been discovered in a variety of leukemias, and CIC-NUTM1 was originally described as a variant of primitive neuroectodermal tumors (PNET) of the central nervous system (Sturm et al. 2016). The various *NUTM1*-fusions and corresponding pathology are summarized in Table 22.1.

Next-gen sequencing has also been key to characterizing exonic mutations other than the

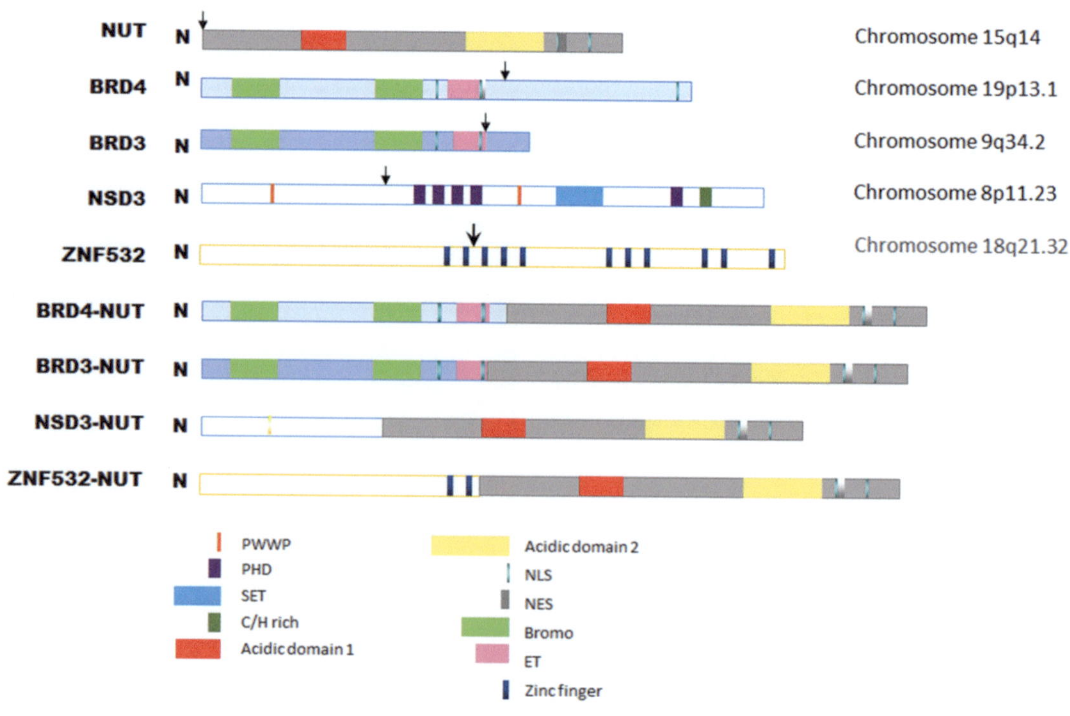

Fig. 22.2 Schematic of NUTM1 fusions reported in NC

Table 22.1 Spectrum of NUTM1-rearranged tumors

NUTM1 fusion partner	Primary site	Histology	References
BRD4	Airways, other organs	PD carcinoma	French et al. (2003); Dickson et al. (2018)
BRD3	Airways, bone and soft tissue	PD carcinoma	French et al. (2008); Dickson et al. (2018)
NSD3	Airways, bone and soft tissue	PD carcinoma	French (2014); Dickson et al. (2018)
ZNF532	Airways	PD carcinoma	Alekseyenko et al. (2017)
ZNF592	Bone and soft tissue	Undifferentiated epithelioid	Shiota et al. (2018)
CIC	CNS, bone and soft tissue	Undifferentiated epithelioid	Schaefer et al. (2018); Sturm et al. (2016)
BCOR1	Bone and soft tissue	Undifferentiated epithelioid	Dickson et al. (2018)
MYXD1	Soft tissue	Undifferentiated epithelioid	Dickson et al. (2018)
MYXD4	Colon	Undifferentiated epithelioid	Dickson et al. (2018); Tamura et al. (2018)
MGA	Lung, soft tissue, dura	Spindle cell sarcoma	Stevens et al. (2019); Diolaiti et al. (2018)
BRD9	Blood/bone marrow	Leukemia	Andersson et al. (2015)
ACINI	Blood/bone marrow	Leukemia	Andersson et al. (2015); Hormann et al. (2019); Gu et al. (2016); Liu et al. (2016)
SLC12A	Blood/bone marrow	Leukemia	Gu et al. (2016)
ZNF618	Blood/bone marrow	Leukemia	Gu et al. (2016)
IKZF1	Blood/bone marrow	Leukemia	Gu et al. (2016); Lilljebjorn et al. (2016)
BPTF	Blood/bone marrow	Leukemia	Liu et al. (2017)
CUX1	Blood/bone marrow	Leukemia	Hormann et al. (2019)
IKZF1	Blood/bone marrow	Leukemia	Hormann et al. (2019)

CNS central nervous system, *PD* poorly differentiated

NUTM1-fusion. Surprisingly, available data indicate that there are no additional oncogenic driver mutations or inactivating mutations of tumor suppressor genes, suggesting that the NUTM1 fusion may be the sole driver of NCs (Lee et al. 2017; Stathis et al. 2016).

22.4 Histology/Immunohistochemistry (IHC)

NC has a characteristic, though not diagnostic, histologic appearance. It appears as an undifferentiated, malignant neoplasm, exhibiting a sheet-like growth pattern comprised of medium-sized, round- to oval-shaped cells. Its monomorphism is distinctive (Fig. 22.3a) and distinguishes it from garden variety poorly differentiated carcinomas, which are larger and exhibit more pleomorphism (Fig. 22.3b). Another common feature is the presence of clear spaces around cells and occasional "fried egg cells" that have abundant, clear cytoplasm (Fig. 22.3a). Consistent with its rapid growth, mitoses and single-cell or geographic necrosis are characteristic. The immune infiltrate cvaries, and is either neutrophilic or lymphocytic (Fig. 22.4). As a subtype of squamous carcinoma, NC often (33–40%) (Bauer et al. 2012; Chau et al. 2019) displays morphologic squamous differentiation, which is characteristically abrupt (Fig. 22.5), rather than displaying a gradient of poorly to well-differentiated cells as seen in conventional squamous cancers. This type of abrupt squamous differentiation can also be seen in basaloid HPV-associated squamous cancers of the head and neck (Table 22.2) (Chernock et al. 2010). In keeping with its squamous lineage, NCs are typically (~75%) (Tilson and Bishop 2014) positive for p63/p40 IHC and often also stain for CK5.

Unusual cases of NC, typically arising from salivary gland (den Bakker et al. 2009) or soft tissue (Dickson et al. 2018), can display morphologic features of myoepithelial differentiation, with rhabdoid-like cells and even formation of cartilage (Fig. 22.6); however, IHC markers do not support

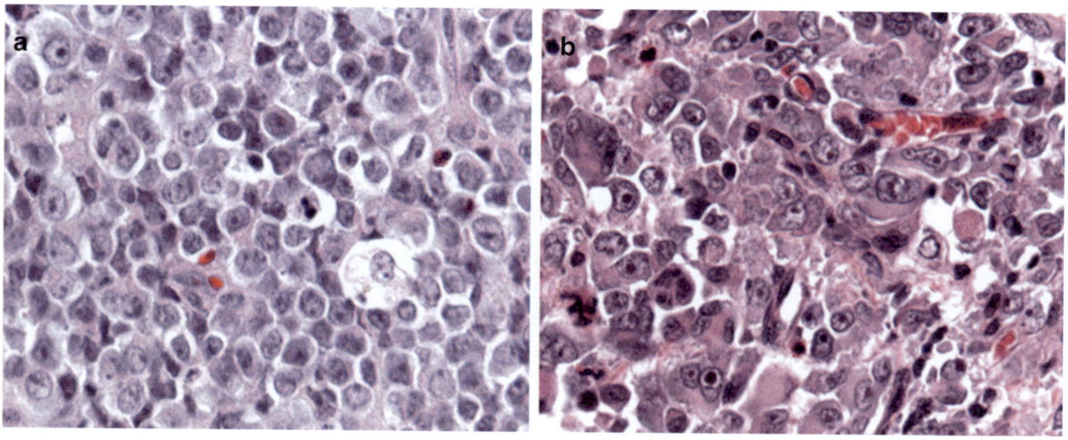

Fig. 22.3 Typical histologic appearance of (**a**) NC compared with (**b**) non-NUT poorly differentiated carcinoma. (**a**) NC is characteristically monomorphic with clear spaces separating cells and occasional "fried egg" cells. (**b**) Garden variety poorly differentiated carcinoma, by contrast, displays larger cell with greater pleomorphism. Both images are 400× magnification and H&E stained

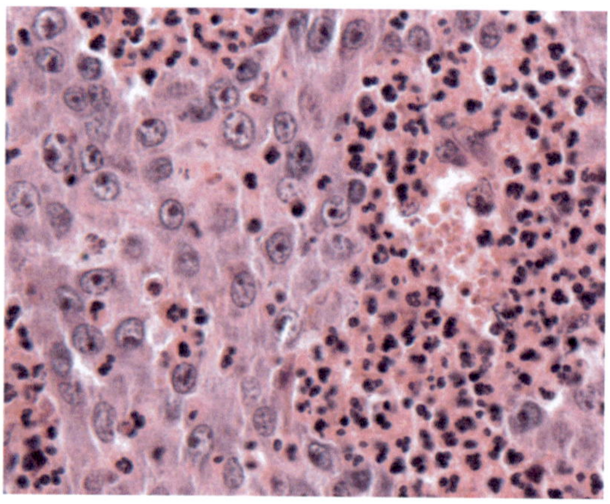

Fig. 22.4 NC showing a prominent neutrophilic infiltrate. Image is 400× magnification and H&E stained

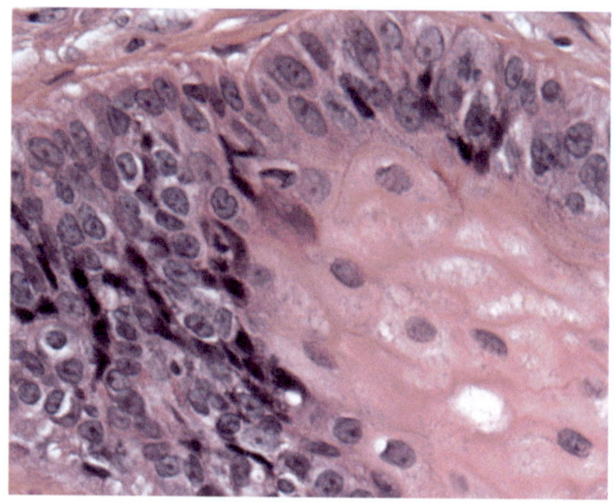

Fig. 22.5 Abrupt keratinization is a characteristic feature of NC. Image is 400× magnification and H&E stained

myoepithelial lineage; these tumors are negative for S100 and SMA and variably express p63 or GFAP (Dickson et al. 2018; Schaefer et al. 2018).

Due to the significant morphologic and immunophenotypic overlap of NC with other poorly differentiated malignancies, the diagnosis is often missed or mistaken for these other entities, including most commonly poorly differentiated carcinoma, poorly differentiated squamous carcinoma (Evans et al. 2012; Stelow et al. 2008; Stelow and French 2009; Chute and Stelow 2010), Ewing's sarcoma (Mertens et al. 2007), sino-nasal undifferentiated carcinoma (Stelow et al. 2008), and small cell carcinoma (Evans et al. 2012) (Table 22.2). Other entities that can be mistaken for NC include poorly differentiated transitional carcinoma of the genitourinary tract (Bishop et al. 2016; French et al. 2004), small-round-blue-cell tumors (blastomas) (Shehata et al. 2010), carcinoma ex pleomorphic adenoma (den Bakker et al. 2009), thymic carcinoma (Kubonishi et al. 1991; Toretsky et al. 2003; Petrini et al. 2012), and even thyroid carcinoma (Landa et al. 2016). The difficulty in distinguishing NC from these other entities by morphology alone has contributed to the vast underdiagnosis of NC (see Demographics/Prevalence, below).

The majority of NCs are carcinomas; however, a subset are so poorly differentiated that they lack

Table 22.2 Distinguishing features of tumors in the differential diagnosis of NC

Tumor	Monomorphic	Distinguishing marker	Abrupt squamous differentiation
Ewing/PNET	+		–
Extra-gonadal germ cell tumor	–	Oct3/4, CD30, β-HCG	–
Lymphoma/leukemia	+	LCA	–
Nasopharyngeal carcinoma	–	EBV	–
HPV-associated SQC	+/–	HPV	+
PD SQC	–		–
Olfactory neuroblastoma	+	S-100[a]	–
PD carcinoma	–		–
Small cell carcinoma	+	p63/p40 –	–
SNUC	+/–		–

Adapted from French CA. NUT Carcinoma: Clinicopathologic features, pathogenesis, and treatment. Pathol Int. 2018;68(11):583–595. https://doi.org/10.1111/pin.12727

EBV Epstein-Barr virus, *HMW* high molecular weight, *HPV* human papilloma virus, *LCA* leukocyte common antigen (CD45), *PNET* primitive neuroectodermal tumor, *PD* poorly differentiated, *SNUC* sino-nasal undifferentiated carcinoma, *SQC* squamous cell carcinoma

[a] Positive in sustentacular cells

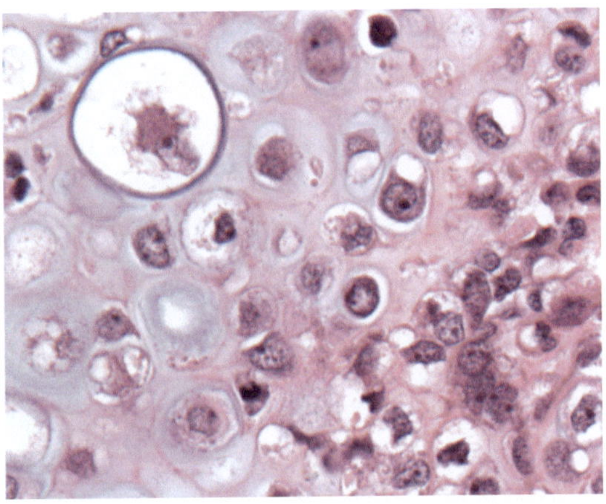

Fig. 22.6 Rare case of NC displays chondroid differentiation (left). Image is 400× magnification and H&E stained

epithelial markers (i.e., expression of keratin intermediate filaments). This has led to the misdiagnosis of leukemia or even lymphoma (unpublished observations), particularly when patient's initial biopsy is from bone marrow. Moreover, a small subset of NUTM1-rearranged malignancies, approximately 5–10% (Dickson et al. 2018; Chau et al. 2019; Stevens et al. 2019), arise from soft tissue and show variable expression of epithelial markers, raising the possibility that some of these are of different lineage from typical NC.

22.5 Diagnosis

NC is defined molecularly by *NUTM1*-rearrangement and as such historically could only be diagnosed by direct demonstration of *NUTM1* rearrangement, either by conventional cytogenetics, fluorescent in situ hybridization (FISH), or reverse-transcriptase PCR (RT-PCR). These methodologies are not widely available and thus hampered the diagnosis of NC during its early recognition. This changed in 2009 with the development of a NUT-specific antibody (Haack et al. 2009). Owing to the highly restricted expression of NUT protein to spermatids of the testis, expression of NUT is specific to NC and germ cell tumors (embryonal carcinoma, seminoma, and dysgerminoma) (Fig. 22.7); the rabbit anti-NUT monoclonal antibody clone C52B1 (Cell Signaling Technologies, Danvers, MA) exhibits a sensitivity of 87% and specificity of 100% when strict criteria are applied to interpretation: >50% of tumor nuclei positively stain (Haack et al. 2009). With this high specificity, positive NUT IHC is considered sufficient for the diagnosis of NC (French and den Bakker 2017).

Despite the high feasibility of diagnostic NUT IHC, many pathology laboratories still do not use it, due to the perceived rarity of NC; however, the

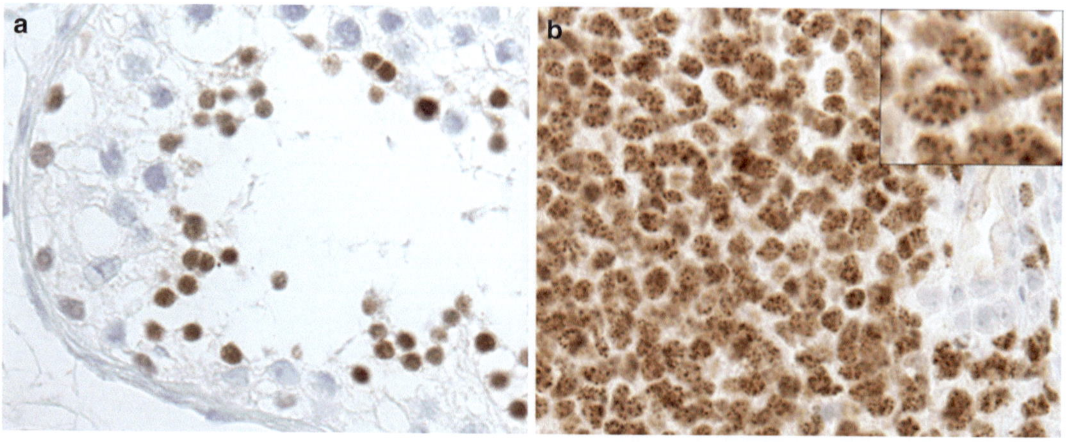

Fig. 22.7 Immunohistochemical staining of postmeiotic spermatids (**a**) and NC (**b**) nuclei using the anti-NUT, clone C52B1 antibody (Cell Signaling Technology, Inc.). The characteristic speckled nuclear staining pattern of BRD4-NUT can be seen in the inset (**b**). Images are 400× magnification

emergence of NGS is having a large impact on detecting cases not originally considered by the pathologist/oncologist. Targeted exome NGS platforms such as those provided by Foundation Medicine (Mangray et al. 2018) or Oncopanel (Stathis et al. 2016; Wagle et al. 2012) have led to the discovery of NCs, but their sensitivity is hampered by limited coverage and the large breakpoint region of *NUTM1* and *BRD4*. Rapid amplification of cDNA ends (RACE)-based NGS technology, however, is changing the landscape of *NUTM1*-rearranged tumors due to its unbiased use and high sensitivity. This test, which utilizes RNA from archival formalin-fixed paraffin-embedded material (FFPE), is able to detect the majority of *NUTM1*-rearrangements, because it can detect any fusion to *NUTM1*, including novel fusion partners, as long as the canonical exon 3 (transcript variant 1) of *NUTM1* is involved, which it is in the majority of cases (Lee et al. 2017; Thompson-Wicking et al. 2013; Stirnweiss et al. 2015, 2017; French et al. 2003; Haruki et al. 2005). Companies that offer this assay include, but are not limited to, ArcherDx (Boulder, CO) (Dickson et al. 2018; Shiota et al. 2018), Caris Life Sciences (Phoenix, AZ) (Stevens et al. 2019), and Foundation Medicine (Cambridge, MA).

22.6 When to Consider the Diagnosis of NC

Because testing and diagnosis of NC is increasing, the disease spectrum is becoming broader, with cases arising from a large variety of non-midline organs including pancreas (Shehata et al. 2010), kidney (Bishop et al. 2016), thyroid (Landa et al. 2016), bladder (French et al. 2004), salivary glands (Ziai et al. 2010; den Bakker et al. 2009; Chau et al. 2014), bone (Mertens et al. 2007), and soft tissues (Dickson et al. 2018; Stevens et al. 2019). For this reason, we recommend performing NUT IHC to rule out NC in all poorly differentiated non-cutaneous carcinomas, with or without squamous differentiation, that have a monomorphic appearance. It is important to not exclude NC on the basis of some lineage-associated markers, such as those of neuroendocrine (chromogranin or synaptophysin), pulmonary (TTF-1), or stem cell (CD34), because NCs can exhibit positive staining for any of these (French et al. 2004; Tanaka et al. 2012; Raza et al. 2015; Bishop and Westra 2012). Moreover, advanced patient age or history of smoking should not be criteria that exclude NC, because it can affect patients of all ages, including elderly patients (Bauer et al. 2012; Stelow et al. 2008), and numerous patients with a smoking history have been diagnosed.

When should one *not consider* NC? Gland-forming NCs are extremely rare, if nonexistent; thus, NC need not be considered in the differential diagnosis of adenocarcinomas. Moreover, known viral etiology, such as HPV or EBV, has never been detected in NC and can be used as a basis to exclude NC. This being said, expression of the HPV-associated marker, p16, is frequently seen in NC (Salles et al. 2014) and should not be used to exclude it.

22.7 Demographics/Prevalence

NC affects patients of all, but predominantly young, ages, with a median age of 16–22 (range 01.–81.7 years) (Bauer et al. 2012; Chau et al. 2014) and with an equal predilection for males and females (Bauer et al. 2012; Chau et al. 2019). NC is not associated with smoking, but a history of smoking is not uncommon (unpublished observations). The prevalence of NC is not precisely known; however, a recent study using the Caris RACE-NGS platform to identify *NUTM1*-fusions in a cohort of 14,107 tumors revealed 9 *NUTM1*-fusion-positive tumors, suggesting a rough incidence of ~0.06% among all tumors (Stevens et al. 2019). Extrapolating this data based on the estimated 1.7 million new cases in the USA in 2019 (American Cancer Society) would suggest an incidence of over 1000 new cases of NC in the USA per year. This estimate confirms that NC is vastly underdiagnosed and that testing must increase.

22.8 Pathogenesis (BRD4-NUT Function)

NGS indicates that BRD4-NUT is the sole oncogenic driver of NC (Lee et al. 2017; Stathis et al. 2016). The fusion protein is known to bind to acetylated histones via the dual bromodomains of BRD4 (Grayson et al. 2014), which tether NUT, an unstructured protein, to chromatin. NUT recruits the histone acetyltransferase (HAT), p300, to BRD4-NUT (Alekseyenko et al. 2017; Reynoird et al. 2010) where it is presumed to acetylate the chromatin and recruit further BRD4-NUT in an iterative process that leads to massive contiguous regions of chromatin enriched with BRD4-NUT (Alekseyenko et al. 2015). These regions are termed megadomains and function essentially to upregulate transcription of underlying coding and noncoding genes (Alekseyenko et al. 2015). A critical target of BRD4-NUT in all NCs is *MYC*, whose upregulation drives growth and arrests NC cell differentiation (Grayson et al. 2014; Alekseyenko et al. 2015). Knockdown of either MYC or BRD4-NUT results in rapid differentiation of these cells, indicating that targeting either of these proteins could be effective strategies to treat this cancer (Grayson et al. 2014; French et al. 2008).

22.9 Treatment of NC

Currently, there is no established treatment strategy for NC; however, for children, the Scandinavian Ewing SSG IX regimen has led to cure of NC in a small number ($n = 3$) of reported cases (Mertens et al. 2007; Storck et al. 2017). Thus, for pediatric patients with localized or disseminated NC, this regimen is often recommended; however, it is not effective in all patients. In addition, complete resection has been shown repeatedly to lead to significantly (p = 0.0003–0.01) improved overall survival (Bauer et al. 2012; Chau et al. 2014), and so whenever possible, surgical resection with clean margins should be performed as soon as possible after diagnosis. Often, however, the patient has disseminated or unresectable disease at the time of diagnosis, due to its rapid growth, and chemoradiation is the only available option. More often than not, chemoradiation leads to a transient response, followed by rapid progression and death; thus, there is an urgent need for novel approaches to treat NC.

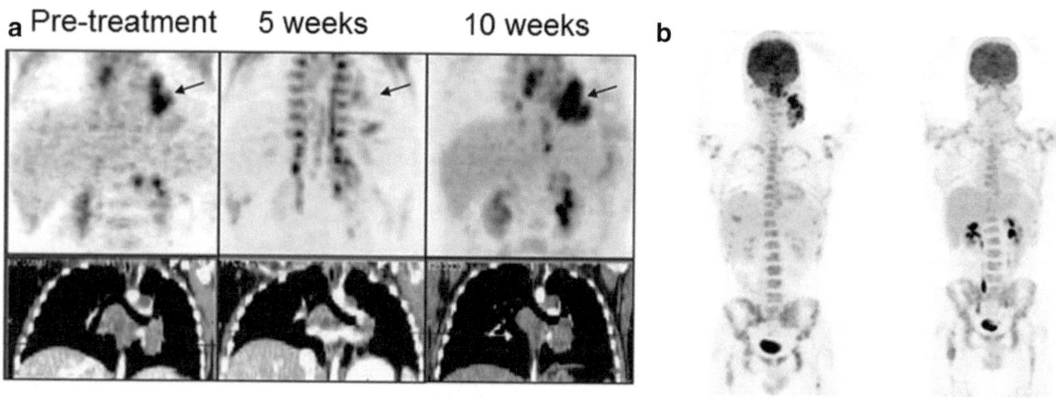

Fig. 22.8 Response of NC patients to targeted inhibitors. (**a**) PET/CT of a 10-year-old patient to single agent HDAC inhibitor, vorinostat. Recurrence at 10 weeks was due to treatment interruption secondary to gastrointestinal toxicity. (Reproduced from Schwartz BE, Hofer MD, Lemieux ME, DE, Cameron MJ, West NH, Agoston ES, Reynoird N, Khochbin S, Ince TA, Christie A, Janeway KA, Vargas SO, Perez-Atayde AR, Aster JC, Sallan SE, Kung AL, Bradner JE, French CA. Differentiation of NUT midline carcinoma by epigenomic reprogramming. Cancer Res 2011;71(7):2686–96. https://doi.org/10.1158/0008.5472.CAN-10-3513. (**b**) PET scan of patient treated with the BET inhibitor, MK-8628/OTX015 comparing baseline (left) with two cycles of treatment (right). (Reproduced from Stathis A, Zucca E, Bekradda M, Gomez-Roca C, Delord JP, de La Motte Rouge T, Uro-Coste E, de Braud F, Pelosi G, French CA. Clinical Response of Carcinomas Harboring the BRD4-NUT Oncoprotein to the Targeted Bromodomain Inhibitor OTX015/MK-8628. Cancer Discov 2016;6(5):492–500. https://doi.org/10.1158/2159-8290.CD-151335

22.10 New Treatment Strategies

NC cells are extremely sensitive to histone deacetylase (HDAC) inhibitors in cell culture experiments (Schwartz et al. 2011). The effect of HDAC inhibitors was originally ascribed to reversal of global chromatin hypoacetylation imparted by BRD4-NUT. HDAC inhibitors cause NC cells to differentiate and arrest proliferation at low doses, and activity has been seen in mouse models (Schwartz et al. 2011). Anecdotally, HDAC inhibitors, alone or in combination with chemotherapy, do show activity against NC in humans (Fig. 22.8a), though the response is transient and not curative (Schwartz et al. 2011; Maher et al. 2015).

A more precise, though still generally nonselective, approach to treating NC came about in 2010 using BET inhibitor compounds, typified by the molecule, JQ1, which are acetyl-lysine mimetic compounds that competitively inhibit the binding of BET (BRD2, BRD3, BRD4, BRDT) protein dual bromodomains to chromatin (Filippakopoulos et al. 2010; Filippakopoulos and Knapp 2012). BET inhibitors evict BET proteins, including BRD4-NUT, from chromatin, resulting in loss of function and differentiation of NC cells in vitro and in vivo (Grayson et al. 2014; Filippakopoulos et al. 2010). Multiple trials were conducted evaluating the efficacy of BET inhibitors in human cancers, including NC. On-target activity has been shown (Fig. 22.8b); however, dose-limiting toxicity has precluded cure with these drugs (Stathis et al. 2016; Lewin et al. 2018; O'Dwyer et al. 2016). Likely a combination strategy with BET and/or other targeted inhibitors will be required for the ultimate cure of this aggressive cancer. A recent CRISPR-based screen suggests that combination of BET inhibitors with a CDK4/6 inhibitor, such as palbociclib, is synergistic in inhibiting NC (Liao et al. 2018).

22.11 Conclusions

NC is a recently described predominantly pediatric and young adult cancer that remains poorly recognized and underdiagnosed. The distinctly poor prognosis and need for alternative approaches to treat NC provide a strong rationale to make the diagnosis. The longer this disease remains undiagnosed, the longer it will take to better understand it and explore novel treatment approaches.

References

Agaimy A, Fonseca I, Martins C, Thway K, Barrette R, Harrington KJ, Hartmann A, French CA, Fisher C (2018) NUT carcinoma of the salivary glands: clinicopathologic and molecular analysis of 3 cases and a survey of NUT expression in salivary gland carcinomas. Am J Surg Pathol 42(7):877–884

Alekseyenko AA, Walsh EM, Wang X, Grayson AR, Hsi PT, Kharchenko PV, Kuroda MI, French CA (2015) The oncogenic BRD4-NUT chromatin regulator drives aberrant transcription within large topological domains. Genes Dev 29(14):1507–1523

Alekseyenko AA, Walsh EM, Zee BM, Pakozdi T, Hsi P, Lemieux ME, Dal Cin P, Ince TA, Kharchenko PV, Kuroda MI, French CA (2017) Ectopic protein interactions within BRD4 chromatin complexes drive oncogenic megadomain formation in NUT midline carcinoma. Proc Natl Acad Sci U S A 114(21):E4184–E4E92

Andersson AK, Ma J, Wang J, Chen X, Gedman AL, Dang J, Nakitandwe J, Holmfeldt L, Parker M, Easton J, Huether R, Kriwacki R, Rusch M, Wu G, Li Y, Mulder H, Raimondi S, Pounds S, Kang G, Shi L, Becksfort J, Gupta P, Payne-Turner D, Vadodaria B, Boggs K et al (2015) The landscape of somatic mutations in infant MLL-rearranged acute lymphoblastic leukemias. Nat Genet 47(4):330–337

Bauer DE, Mitchell CM, Strait KM, Lathan CS, Stelow EB, Luer SC, Muhammed S, Evans AG, Sholl LM, Rosai J, Giraldi E, Oakley RP, Rodriguez-Galindo C, London WB, Sallan SE, Bradner JE, French CA (2012) Clinicopathologic features and long-term outcomes of NUT midline carcinoma. Clin Cancer Res 18(20):5773–5779

Bishop JA, Westra WH (2012) NUT midline carcinomas of the sinonasal tract. Am J Surg Pathol 36(8):1216–1221

Bishop JA, French CA, Ali SZ (2016) Cytopathologic features of NUT midline carcinoma: a series of 26 specimens from 13 patients. Cancer Cytopathol 124(12):901–908

Chau NG, Mitchell CM, Aserlind A, Grunfeld N, Kaplan L, Bauer DE, Lathan CS, Rodriguez-Galindo C, Hurwitz S, Tishler RB, Haddad RI, Sallan SE, Bradner JE, French CA (2014) Aggressive treatment and survival outcomes in NUT midline carcinoma (NMC) of the head and neck (HN). J Clin Oncol, 2014 ASCO Annual Meeting Abstracts 32(15_suppl)

Chau NG, Ma C, Danga K, Al-Sayegh H, Nardi V, Barrette R, Lathan CS, DuBois SG, Haddad RI, Shapiro GI, Sallan SE, Dhar A, Nelson JJ, French CA (2019) An anatomical site and genetic-based prognostic model for patients with nuclear protein in testis (NUT) midline carcinoma: analysis of 124 patients. JNCI Cancer Spectr 4(2):pkz094. https://doi.org/10.1093/jncics/pkz094. PMID: 32328562; PMCID: PMC7165803

Chernock RD, Lewis JS Jr, Zhang Q, El-Mofty SK (2010) Human papillomavirus-positive basaloid squamous cell carcinomas of the upper aerodigestive tract: a distinct clinicopathologic and molecular subtype of basaloid squamous cell carcinoma. Hum Pathol 41(7):1016–1023

Chute DJ, Stelow EB (2010) Cytology of head and neck squamous cell carcinoma variants. Diagn Cytopathol 38(1):65–80

den Bakker MA, Beverloo BH, van den Heuvel-Eibrink MM, Meeuwis CA, Tan LM, Johnson LA, French CA, van Leenders GJ (2009) NUT midline carcinoma of the parotid gland with mesenchymal differentiation. Am J Surg Pathol 33(8):1253–1258

Dickson BC, Sung YS, Rosenblum MK, Reuter VE, Harb M, Wunder JS, Swanson D, Antonescu CR (2018) NUTM1 gene fusions characterize a subset of undifferentiated soft tissue and visceral tumors. Am J Surg Pathol 42(5):636–645

Diolaiti D, Dela Cruz FS, Gundem G, Bouvier N, Boulad M, Zhang Y, Chou AJ, Dunkel IJ, Sanghvi R, Shah M, Geiger H, Rahman S, Felice V, Wrzeszczynski KO, Darnell RB, Antonescu CR, French CA, Papaemmanuil E, Kung AL, Shukla N (2018) A recurrent novel MGA-NUTM1 fusion identifies a new subtype of high-grade spindle cell sarcoma. Cold Spring Harb Mol Case Stud 4(6):a003194

Evans AG, French CA, Cameron MJ, Fletcher CD, Jackman DM, Lathan CS, Sholl LM (2012) Pathologic characteristics of NUT midline carcinoma arising in the mediastinum. Am J Surg Pathol 36(8): 1222–1227

Filippakopoulos P, Knapp S (2012) The bromodomain interaction module. FEBS Lett 586(17):2692–2704

Filippakopoulos P, Qi J, Picaud S, Shen Y, Smith WB, Fedorov O, Morse EM, Keates T, Hickman TT, Felletar I, Philpott M, Munro S, McKeown MR, Wang Y, Christie AL, West N, Cameron MJ, Schwartz B, Heightman TD, La Thangue N, French CA, Wiest O, Kung AL, Knapp S, Bradner JE (2010) Selective inhibition of BET bromodomains. Nature 468(7327):1067–1073

French CA, Rahman S, Walsh EM, Kühnle S, Grayson AR, Lemieux ME, Grunfeld N, Rubin BP, Antonescu CR, Zhang S, Venkatramani R, Dal Cin P, Howley PM (2014) NSD3-NUT fusion oncoprotein in NUT midline carcinoma: implications for a novel oncogenic mechanism. Cancer Discov 4(8):928–941. https://doi.org/10.1158/2159-8290. CD-14-0014. Epub 2014 May 29. PMID: 24875858; PMCID: PMC4125436

French CA, den Bakker MA (2015) In: Travis WD, Brambilla E, Burke AP, Marx A, Nicholson AG (eds)

NUT carcinoma, 4th edn. International Agency for Research on Cancer (IARC), Lyon, pp 229–230
French CA, den Bakker MA (2017) In: El-Naggar A, Chan JKC, Grandis JR, Takata T, Slootweg P (eds) WHO classification of head and neck tumours, 4th edn. International Agency for Research on Cancer (IARC), Lyon, pp 20–21
French CA, Miyoshi I, Kubonishi I, Grier HE, Perez-Atayde AR, Fletcher JA (2003) BRD4-NUT fusion oncogene: a novel mechanism in aggressive carcinoma. Cancer Res 63(2):304–307
French CA, Kutok JL, Faquin WC, Toretsky JA, Antonescu CR, Griffin CA, Nose V, Vargas SO, Moschovi M, Tzortzatou-Stathopoulou F, Miyoshi I, Perez-Atayde AR, Aster JC, Fletcher JA (2004) Midline carcinoma of children and young adults with NUT rearrangement. J Clin Oncol 22(20):4135–4139
French CA, Ramirez CL, Kolmakova J, Hickman TT, Cameron MJ, Thyne ME, Kutok JL, Toretsky JA, Tadavarthy AK, Kees UR, Fletcher JA, Aster JC (2008) BRD-NUT oncoproteins: a family of closely related nuclear proteins that block epithelial differentiation and maintain the growth of carcinoma cells. Oncogene 27(15):2237–2242
Grayson AR, Walsh EM, Cameron MJ, Godec J, Ashworth T, Ambrose JM, Aserlind AB, Wang H, Evan GI, Kluk MJ, Bradner JE, Aster JC, French CA (2014) MYC, a downstream target of BRD-NUT, is necessary and sufficient for the blockade of differentiation in NUT midline carcinoma. Oncogene 33(13):1736–1742
Gu Z, Churchman M, Roberts K, Li Y, Liu Y, Harvey RC, McCastlain K, Reshmi SC, Payne-Turner D, Iacobucci I, Shao Y, Chen IM, Valentine M, Pei D, Mungall KL, Mungall AJ, Ma Y, Moore R, Marra M, Stonerock E, Gastier-Foster JM, Devidas M, Dai Y, Wood B, Borowitz M et al (2016) Genomic analyses identify recurrent MEF2D fusions in acute lymphoblastic leukaemia. Nat Commun 7:13331
Haack H, Johnson LA, Fry CJ, Crosby K, Polakiewicz RD, Stelow EB, Hong SM, Schwartz BE, Cameron MJ, Rubin MA, Chang MC, Aster JC, French CA (2009) Diagnosis of NUT midline carcinoma using a NUT-specific monoclonal antibody. Am J Surg Pathol 33(7):984–991
Haruki N, Kawaguchi KS, Eichenberger S, Massion PP, Gonzalez A, Gazdar AF, Minna JD, Carbone DP, Dang TP (2005) Cloned fusion product from a rare t(15;19)(q13.2;p13.1) inhibit S phase in vitro. J Med Genet 42(7):558–564
Hormann FM, Hoogkamer AQ, Beverloo HB, Boeree A, Dingjan I, Wattel MM, Stam RW, Escherich G, Pieters R, den Boer ML, Boer JM (2019) NUTM1 is a recurrent fusion gene partner in B cell precursor acute lymphoblastic leukemia associated with increased expression of genes on chromosome band 10p12.31-12.2. Haematologica 104(10):e455–e459. https://doi.org/10.3324/haematol.2018.20696
Jung M, Kim S, Lee JK, Yoon SO, Park HS, Hong SW, Park WS, Kim JE, Kim J, Keam B, Kim HJ, Kang HJ, Kim DW, Jung KC, Kim YT, Heo DS, Kim TM, Jeon YK (2019) Clinicopathological and preclinical findings of NUT carcinoma: a multicenter study. Oncologist 24(8):e740–e748
Kubonishi I, Takehara N, Iwata J, Sonobe H, Ohtsuki Y, Abe T, Miyoshi I (1991) Novel t(15;19)(q15;p13) chromosome abnormality in a thymic carcinoma. Cancer Res 51(12):3327–3328
Landa I, Ibrahimpasic T, Boucai L, Sinha R, Knauf JA, Shah RH, Dogan S, Ricarte-Filho JC, Krishnamoorthy GP, Xu B, Schultz N, Berger MF, Sander C, Taylor BS, Ghossein R, Ganly I, Fagin JA (2016) Genomic and transcriptomic hallmarks of poorly differentiated and anaplastic thyroid cancers. J Clin Invest 126(3):1052–1066
Lee JK, Louzada S, An Y, Kim SY, Kim S, Youk J, Park S, Koo SH, Keam B, Jeon YK, Ku JL, Yang F, Kim TM, Ju YS (2017) Complex chromosomal rearrangements by single catastrophic pathogenesis in NUT midline carcinoma. Ann Oncol 28(4):890–897
Lewin J, Soria JC, Stathis A, Delord JP, Peters S, Awada A, Aftimos PG, Bekradda M, Rezai K, Zeng Z, Hussain A, Perez S, Siu LL, Massard C (2018) Phase Ib trial with Birabresib, a small-molecule inhibitor of bromodomain and extraterminal proteins, in patients with selected advanced solid tumors. J Clin Oncol 36(30):3007–3014
Liao S, Maertens O, Cichowski K, Elledge SJ (2018) Genetic modifiers of the BRD4-NUT dependency of NUT midline carcinoma uncovers a synergism between BETis and CDK4/6is. Genes Dev 32(17–18):1188–1200
Lilljebjorn H, Henningsson R, Hyrenius-Wittsten A, Olsson L, Orsmark-Pietras C, von Palffy S, Askmyr M, Rissler M, Schrappe M, Cario G, Castor A, Pronk CJ, Behrendtz M, Mitelman F, Johansson B, Paulsson K, Andersson AK, Fontes M, Fioretos T (2016) Identification of ETV6-RUNX1-like and DUX4-rearranged subtypes in paediatric B-cell precursor acute lymphoblastic leukaemia. Nat Commun 7:11790
Liu YF, Wang BY, Zhang WN, Huang JY, Li BS, Zhang M, Jiang L, Li JF, Wang MJ, Dai YJ, Zhang ZG, Wang Q, Kong J, Chen B, Zhu YM, Weng XQ, Shen ZX, Li JM, Wang J, Yan XJ, Li Y, Liang YM, Liu L, Chen XQ, Zhang WG et al (2016) Genomic profiling of adult and pediatric B-cell acute lymphoblastic leukemia. EBioMedicine 8:173–183
Liu Y, Easton J, Shao Y, Maciaszek J, Wang Z, Wilkinson MR, McCastlain K, Edmonson M, Pounds SB, Shi L, Zhou X, Ma X, Sioson E, Li Y, Rusch M, Gupta P, Pei D, Cheng C, Smith MA, Auvil JG, Gerhard DS, Relling MV, Winick NJ, Carroll AJ, Heerema NA et al (2017) The genomic landscape of pediatric and young adult T-lineage acute lymphoblastic leukemia. Nat Genet 49(8):1211–1218
Maher OM, Christensen AM, Yedururi S, Bell D, Tarek N (2015) Histone deacetylase inhibitor for NUT midline carcinoma. Pediatr Blood Cancer 62(4):715–717
Mangray S, Kelly DR, LeGuellec S, Fridman E, Aggarwal S, Shago M, Matoso A, Madison R, Pramanik S, Zhong S, Li R, Lombardo KA, Cramer S, Pressey

J, Ross JS, Corona RJ, Bratslavsky G, Argani P, Coindre JM, Somers GR, Ali SM, Yakirevich E (2018) Clinicopathologic features of a series of primary renal CIC-rearranged sarcomas with comprehensive molecular analysis. Am J Surg Pathol 42(10):1360–1369

Mertens F, Wiebe T, Adlercreutz C, Mandahl N, French CA (2007) Successful treatment of a child with t(15;19)-positive tumor. Pediatr Blood Cancer 49(7):1015–1017

O'Dwyer PJ, Piha-Paul SA, French CA, Harward S, Ferron-Brady G, Wu Y, Barbash O, Wyce A, Annan M, Horner T, Parr NJ, Prinjha RK, Carpenter C, Shapiro G, Dhar A, Hann C (2016) Abstract CT014: GSK525762, a selective bromodomain (BRD) and extra terminal protein (BET) inhibitor: results from part 1 of a phase I/II open-label single-agent study in patients with NUT midline carcinoma (NMC) and other cancers. Cancer Res 76(14 supplement):CT014

Petrini P, French CA, Rajan A, Cameron MJ, Jaffe ES, Zucali PA, Xie J, Wang Y, Giaccone G (2012) NUT rearrangement is uncommon in human thymic epithelial tumors. J Thorac Oncol 7(4):744–750

Polsani A, Braithwaite KA, Alazraki AL, Abramowsky C, Shehata BM (2012) NUT midline carcinoma: an imaging case series and review of literature. Pediatr Radiol 42(2):205–210

Raza A, Cao H, Conrad R, Cobb C, Castelino-Prabhu S, Mirshahidi S, Shiraz P, Mirshahidi HR (2015) Nuclear protein in testis midline carcinoma with unusual elevation of alpha-fetoprotein and synaptophysin positivity: a case report and review of the literature. Expert Rev Anticancer Ther 15(10):1199–1213

Reynoird N, Schwartz BE, Delvecchio M, Sadoul K, Meyers D, Mukherjee C, Caron C, Kimura H, Rousseaux S, Cole PA, Panne D, French CA, Khochbin S (2010) Oncogenesis by sequestration of CBP/p300 in transcriptionally inactive hyperacetylated chromatin domains. EMBO J 29(17):2943–2952

Salles PG, Moura Rde D, Menezes LM, Bacchi CE (2014) Expression of P16 in NUT carcinomas with no association with human papillomavirus (HPV). Appl Immunohistochem Mol Morphol 22(4):262–265

Schaefer IM, Dal Cin P, Fletcher CDM, Hanna GJ, French CA (2018) CIC-NUTM1 fusion: a case which expands the spectrum of NUT-rearranged epithelioid malignancies. Genes Chromosomes Cancer 57(9):446–451

Schwartz BE, Hofer MD, Lemieux ME, Bauer DE, Cameron MJ, West NH, Agoston ES, Reynoird N, Khochbin S, Ince TA, Christie A, Janeway KA, Vargas SO, Perez-Atayde AR, Aster JC, Sallan SE, Kung AL, Bradner JE, French CA (2011) Differentiation of NUT midline carcinoma by epigenomic reprogramming. Cancer Res 71(7):2686–2696

Seim NB, Philips RHW, Schoenfield L, Teknos TN, Rocco JW, Agrawal A, Ozer E, Carrau RL, Kang SY, Old MO (2017) NUT midline carcinoma of the sublingual gland: clinical presentation and review. Head Neck Pathol 11(4):460–468

Shehata BM, Steelman CK, Abramowsky CR, Olson TA, French CA, Saxe DF, Ricketts RR, Katzenstein HM (2010) NUT midline carcinoma in a newborn with multiorgan disseminated tumor and a 2-year-old with a pancreatic/hepatic primary. Pediatr Dev Pathol 13(6):481–485

Shiota H, Elya JE, Alekseyenko A, Chou PM, Gorman SA, Barbash O, Becht K, Danga K, Kuroda MI, Nardi V, French CA (2018) 'Z4' complex member fusions in NUT carcinoma: implications for a novel oncogenic mechanism. Mol Cancer Res 16(12):1826–1833

Sholl LM, Nishino M, Pokharel S, Mino-Kenudson M, French CA, Janne PA, Lathan C (2015) Primary pulmonary NUT midline carcinoma: clinical, radiographic, and pathologic characterizations. J Thorac Oncol 10(6):951–959

Sirohi D, Garg K, Simko JP, Grenert JP (2018) Renal NUT carcinoma: a case report. Histopathology 72(3):528–530

Stathis A, Zucca E, Bekradda M, Gomez-Roca C, Delord JP, de La Motte Rouge T, Uro-Coste E, de Braud F, Pelosi G, French CA (2016) Clinical response of carcinomas harboring the BRD4-NUT oncoprotein to the targeted bromodomain inhibitor OTX015/MK-8628. Cancer Discov 6(5):492–500

Stelow EB, French CA (2009) Carcinomas of the upper aerodigestive tract with rearrangement of the nuclear protein of the testis (NUT) gene (NUT midline carcinomas). Adv Anat Pathol 16(2):92–96

Stelow EB, Bellizzi AM, Taneja K, Mills SE, Legallo RD, Kutok JL, Aster JC, French CA (2008) NUT rearrangement in undifferentiated carcinomas of the upper aerodigestive tract. Am J Surg Pathol 32(6): 828–834

Stevens TM, Morlote D, Xiu J, Swensen J, Brandwein-Weber M, Miettinen MM, Gatalica Z, Bridge JA (2019) NUTM1-rearranged neoplasia: a multi-institution experience yields novel fusion partners and expands the histologic spectrum. Modern Pathol 32:764–773. https://doi.org/10.1038/s41379-019-0206

Stirnweiss A, McCarthy K, Oommen J, Crook ML, Hardy K, Kees UR, Wilton SD, Anazodo A, Beesley AH (2015) A novel BRD4-NUT fusion in an undifferentiated sinonasal tumor highlights alternative splicing as a contributing oncogenic factor in NUT midline carcinoma. Oncogenesis 4:e174

Stirnweiss A, Oommen J, Kotecha RS, Kees UR, Beesley AH (2017) Molecular-genetic profiling and high-throughput in vitro drug screening in NUT midline carcinoma-an aggressive and fatal disease. Oncotarget 8(68):112313–112329

Storck S, Kennedy AL, Marcus KJ, Teot L, Vaughn J, Gnekow AK, Markl B, Leuschner I, DuBois SG, French CA, Fruhwald MC (2017) Pediatric NUT-midline carcinoma: therapeutic success employing a sarcoma based multimodal approach. Pediatr Hematol Oncol 34(4):231–237

Sturm D, Orr BA, Toprak UH, Hovestadt V, Jones DTW, Capper D, Sill M, Buchhalter I, Northcott PA, Leis I, Ryzhova M, Koelsche C, Pfaff E, Allen SJ, Balasubramanian G, Worst BC, Pajtler KW, Brabetz S, Johann PD, Sahm F, Reimand J, Mackay A, Carvalho

DM, Remke M, Phillips JJ et al (2016) New brain tumor entities emerge from molecular classification of CNS-PNETs. Cell 164(5):1060–1072

Tamura R, Nakaoka H, Yoshihara K, Mori Y, Yachida N, Nishikawa N, Motoyama T, Okuda S, Inoue I, Enomoto T (2018) Novel MXD4-NUTM1 fusion transcript identified in primary ovarian undifferentiated small round cell sarcoma. Genes Chromosomes Cancer 57(11):557–563

Tanaka M, Kato K, Gomi K, Yoshida M, Niwa T, Aida N, Kigasawa H, Ohama Y, Tanaka Y (2012) NUT midline carcinoma: report of 2 cases suggestive of pulmonary origin. Am J Surg Pathol 36(3):381–388

Thompson-Wicking K, Francis RW, Stirnweiss A, Ferrari E, Welch MD, Baker E, Murch AR, Gout AM, Carter KW, Charles AK, Phillips MB, Kees UR, Beesley AH (2013) Novel BRD4-NUT fusion isoforms increase the pathogenic complexity in NUT midline carcinoma. Oncogene 32(39):4664–4674

Tilson MP, Bishop JA (2014) Utility of p40 in the differential diagnosis of small round blue cell tumors of the sinonasal tract. Head Neck Pathol 8(2):141–145

Toretsky JA, Jenson J, Sun CC, Eskenazi AE, Campbell A, Hunger SP, Caires A, Frantz C, Hill JL, Stamberg J (2003) Translocation (11;15;19): a highly specific chromosome rearrangement associated with poorly differentiated thymic carcinoma in young patients. Am J Clin Oncol 26(3):300–306

Vulsteke C, Lurquin E, Debiec-Rychter M, Gheysens O, Nuyts S, Schoenaers J, Politis C, Mebis J, Hauben E, Clement PM (2016) First evidence of treatment efficacy in metastatic carcinoma of the parotid gland with BRD4/NUT translocation. J Chemother 28(3):242–246

Wagle N, Berger MF, Davis MJ, Blumenstiel B, Defelice M, Pochanard P, Ducar M, Van Hummelen P, Macconaill LE, Hahn WC, Meyerson M, Gabriel SB, Garraway LA (2012) High-throughput detection of actionable genomic alterations in clinical tumor samples by targeted, massively parallel sequencing. Cancer Discov 2(1):82–93

Zhu Y, Liu YF, Zhao J, Yu YW (2019) [BRD4-NUT fusion oncogene carcinoma in the kidney]. Zhonghua Bing Li Xue Za Zhi 48(3):237–9

Ziai J, French CA, Zambrano E (2010) NUT gene rearrangement in a poorly-differentiated carcinoma of the submandibular gland. Head Neck Pathol 4(2):163–168

Part VI

Rare Tumors of the Gastrointestinal Tract

Pathology and Differential Diagnosis

23

Bahig M. Shehata and Sarah S. Kappa

23.1 Gastrointestinal Stromal Tumor (GIST)

23.1.1 Introduction

GISTs are the most common mesenchymal tumor of the gastrointestinal tract (Figs. 23.1, 23.2, 23.3, 23.4, and 23.5). They primarily affect middle-aged or older adults, and they occur only rarely in children and adolescents. It has been proposed that GIST arises from the interstitial cells of Cajal (Liegl-Atzwanger et al. 2010; Benesch et al. 2009; Kaemmer et al. 2009; Machairas et al. 2010; Shimomura et al. 2010). Besides GIST, the family of mesenchymal tumors includes plexosarcomas, leiomyoblastomas, leiomyosarcomas (LMS), gastrointestinal autonomic nerve tumors (GANT), and gastrointestinal pacemaker cell tumors (GIPACT). While extensive research has been done on adult GIST by the National Comprehensive Cancer Network, the European Society of Medical Oncology, and others, standard practice and guidelines for children affected by GIST have not yet been established (Benesch et al. 2009) (Table 23.1).

B. M. Shehata
Department of Pathology, Wayne State University School of Medicine, Detroit, MI, USA
e-mail: bshehat@emory.edu

S. S. Kappa (✉)
Cancer and Hematology Center, Texas Children's Hospital, Houston, TX, USA
e-mail: sskappa@texaschildrens.org

23.1.2 Presentation

Pediatric GIST is most commonly found in the stomach (typically in the antrum), although cases have been identified in the small intestine, colon/rectum, omentum, and abdominal wall (Benesch et al. 2009; Shimomura et al. 2010). The average size of the tumor is 5.7 cm in greatest dimension with a range of 1.5–35 cm. Some patients, even unaffected by an associated tumor syndrome, present with multiple tumors or tumors with numerous satellite lesions. Metastasis is not uncommon, and it typically presents in the liver (Fig. 23.2), lymph nodes, peritoneum, and mesentery. These lesions, however, rarely present at diagnosis (Benesch et al. 2009).

23.2 Pathology/Molecular Biological Findings

Pediatric gastric GISTs are most commonly epithelioid cell tumors (Fig. 23.3) or mixed spindle and epithelioid cell tumors, whereas, in adults, spindle cell tumors are the most frequent Shimomura et al. 2010). Two genes have been implicated in the pathogenesis of GIST: *KIT* and *PDGFRA* (4q11–q12). Both genes encode for

D. T. Schneider et al. (eds.), *Rare Tumors in Children and Adolescents*, Pediatric Oncology,
https://doi.org/10.1007/978-3-030-92071-5_23

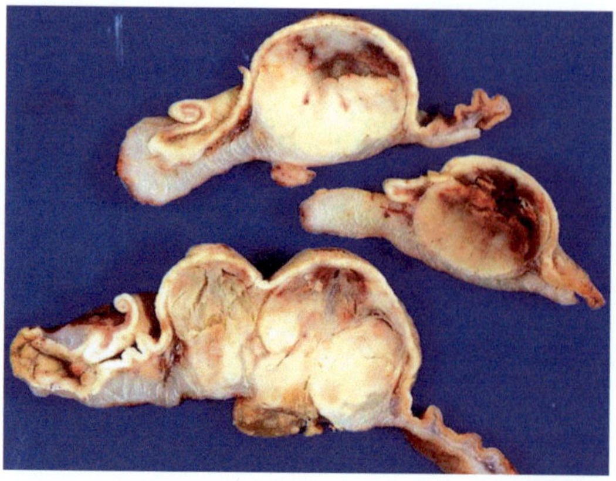

Fig. 23.1 Gastrointestinal stroma tumor: multiple submucosal nodules showing gray–tan myxoid cut surface

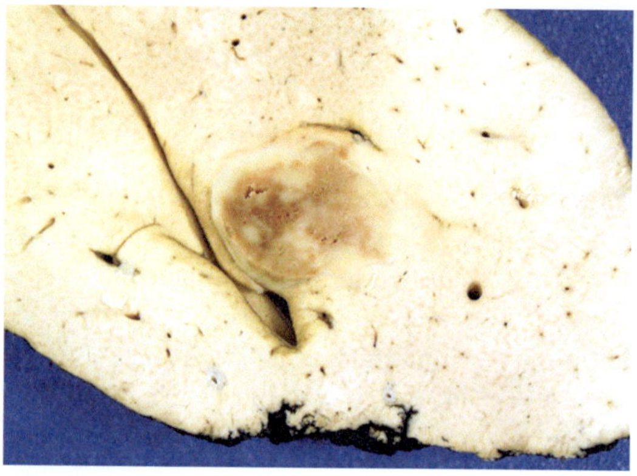

Fig. 23.2 Gastrointestinal stroma tumor: liver metastasis from partial hepatectomy

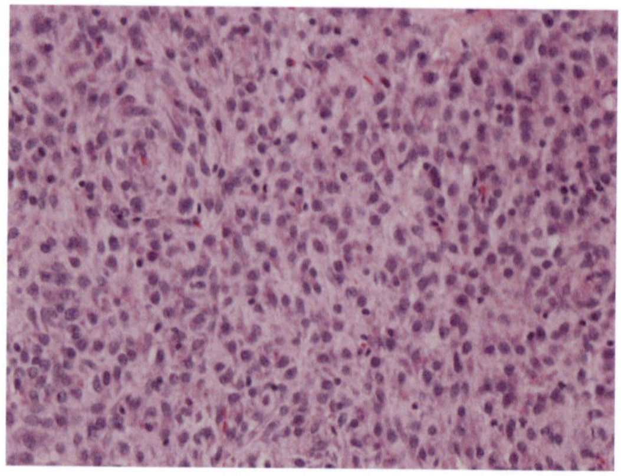

Fig. 23.3 Gastrointestinal stroma tumor: sheets of epithelioid cells with neuroendocrine differentiation (400×)

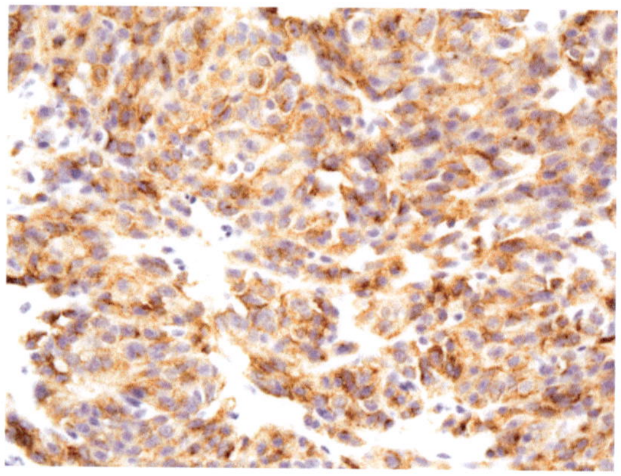

Fig. 23.4 Gastrointestinal stroma tumor: strong positive c-kit immunohistochemical stain

transmembrane growth factor receptors which exhibit tyrosine kinase activity. The expression of these genes leads to the activation of several pathways which regulate cell proliferation, adhesion, motility, and differentiation. These pathways include MEK-MAPK, STAT5, RAS, JAK2, and PI3-AKT (Liegl-Atzwanger et al. 2010; Machairas et al. 2010). Both mutations are early events in the development of GIST. Researchers have found that these mutations are not involved in the malignant transformation of this tumor, only in the development and proliferation. In approximately 66% of mutated GISTs, monosomy 14 or partial loss of 14q is identified, and in approximately 50%, loss of 22q is identified. The latter is associated with the progression of GIST to a borderline or malignant lesion. Losses on chromosomes 1p, 9q, 11p, and 17q and gains on chromosomes 8q and 17q have also been identified, albeit their occurrence is rare. These mutations are also linked with malignancy. Both adult and pediatric GISTs without *KIT* or *PDGFRA* mutations display a much lower level of cytogenetic progression than mutant GISTs (Liegl-Atzwanger et al. 2010).

Expression of *KIT* is integral for the growth and preservation of cell types including germ cells, hematopoietic cells, mast cells, melanocytes, interstitial cells of Cajal, and intestinal pacemaker cells. Along with GIST, mutations in *KIT* have been identified in mast cell tumors, myelofibrosis, chronic myelogenous leukemia, and germ cell tumors. Mutations in the c-kit proto-oncogene have also been associated with

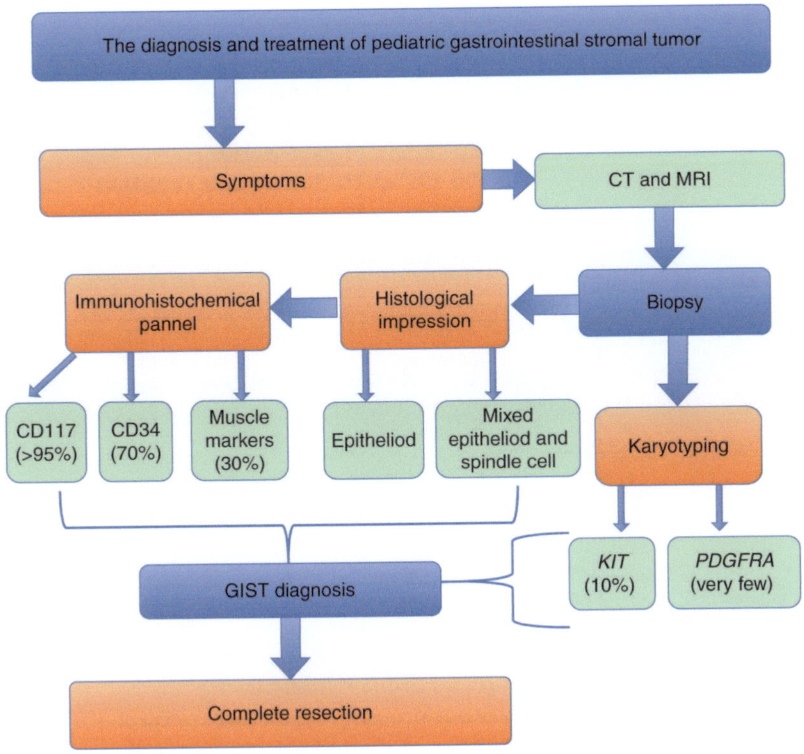

Fig. 23.5 Road map outlining the diagnosis and treatment of pediatric GIST

the activation of the *KIT* receptor, leading to constant proliferation (Machairas et al. 2010). Mutations in *KIT* exist on exon 11 (68%), exon 9 (11%), and exons 13 and 17 (0.6–4%) (Liegl-Atzwanger et al. 2010; Kaemmer et al. 2009; Machairas et al. 2010).

When a *KIT* mutation is not identified in GIST, typically a *PDGFRA* mutation is present (Liegl-Atzwanger et al. 2010; Kaemmer et al. 2009). *PDGFRA* mutations occur on either exon 18 or exon 14 (7%) and rarely on exon 12 (<1%). In adults, characteristics of *PDGFRA* mutated GISTs include presentation in the stomach and omentum, the appearance of epithelioid morphology, and an association with a benign clinical course (Liegl-Atzwanger et al. 2010).

No more than 10% of pediatric GIST patients display an oncogenic *KIT* mutation, and only two patients have displayed a *PDGFRA* mutation to date. The upregulation of fibroblast growth factor 4 (FGF 4), brain and acute leukemia, cytoplasmic (BAALC), and insulin-like growth factor 1 (IGFR1), among others, has been reported in pediatric GIST (Benesch et al. 2009).

The immunohistochemical pattern of pediatric GIST is similar to that of adult GIST as it stains positive for CD117 (c-kit) (>95%) (Fig. 23.4); CD34 (70%); muscle markers including smooth muscle actin, calponin, and caldesmon (30%); and very rarely desmin and S100 (Benesch et al. 2009; Kaemmer et al. 2009; Machairas et al. 2010). Cytokeratins 8 and 18 are expressed in only a small percentage of GISTs, while nestin, which is found in other mesenchymal tumors and schwannomas, is expressed in the majority of GISTs (Machairas et al. 2010). A road map pertaining to the diagnosis and treatment of GIST is presented in Fig. 23.5.

23.3 GANT

GANT is a recently described variant of GIST. Required for the diagnosis of GANT is the absence of myogenic, Schwann, and epithelial features (Kerr et al. 1999). They are also differentiated from GIST by showing neural differentiation using electron microscopy. While only a few

Table 23.1 Overview of rare pediatric abdominal tumors

Tumor type	Adrenocortical tumors	Gastric tumors	Pancreatic tumors
Classification	• Adenoma • Carcinoma	• Epithelioid leiomyoma • Leiomyosarcoma • Carcinoid • Non-Hodgkin lymphoma	• Papillary–cystic carcinoma • Pancreatoblastoma • Acinic cell carcinoma • Malignant insulinoma • Glucagonoma • Gastrinoma • PNET • Lymphoma
Associated syndrome	• Li–Fraumeni syndrome • Beckwith–Wiedemann syndrome • Hemihypertrophy	• Epithelioid leiomyoma and LMS: Carney's triad	• Pancreatoblastoma: Beckwith–Wiedemann syndrome and Cushing's syndrome
Metastasis	• Lymph node • Kidney • Lung • Bone • Brain	N/A	• Direct invasion of liver
Treatment	• Surgical removal • Hormone therapy • Chemotherapy	• Surgical removal • Radiation therapy • Chemotherapy	• Surgical removal: partial or complete pancreatectomy • Chemotherapy
Prognosis	• Excellent: small resectable tumors • Fair: large primary tumors or metastatic disease at diagnosis	• Dependent on extent of disease and treatment success; no comprehensive studies	• Good: complete surgical resection • Poor: pancreatoblastoma

Rare tumors of the liver such as undifferentiated embryonal sarcoma are not included in this table as they are mentioned in the liver chapter
PNET primitive neuroectodermal tumor

cases of pediatric GANT have been reported, a slight predilection for females has been noted (Kerr et al. 1999; Benesch et al. 2009). In comparison to adult GANT, pediatric GANT tends to be smaller in size, is most commonly found in the stomach, and has a better prognosis. Pediatric GANT is typically treated using surgical resection (Kerr et al. 1999).

23.4 Colorectal Adenocarcinoma (CRAC)

CRAC is the third most common malignancy in the adult population, surpassed by only lung and breast cancers (Sultan et al. 2010). An annual average of 9.4% of adult cancer cases and 7.9% of adult cancer deaths are attributed to CRAC, and, therefore, it has been widely studied in this population. Pediatric CRAC, however, has not been extensively studied due to its rarity. Only one to two cases of CRAC per million children are reported annually (Sultan et al. 2010). The incidence of colorectal carcinoma in patients under 20 is on the rise (O'Connell et al. 2003). Sultan's investigation of the Surveillance, Epidemiology, and End Results database between 1986 and 1995 yielded 34 cases of colorectal carcinoma in patients <20 years of age; this figure nearly tripled to 94 between 1996 and 2005 (Sultan et al. 2010).

In adults, there is a slight predilection for males; however, this trend has not been reported in pediatric CRAC (Saab and Furman 2008). Patients, including those in younger age groups, typically present with abdominal pain, hematochezia, altered bowel habits, weight loss, and anemia. Pediatric patients often also complain of nausea, vomiting, abdominal distention, and abdominal mass. Acute abdominal conditions such as acute obstruction, perforation, or severe pain mimicking appendicitis are also more common in children than in adults. The common occurrence of these symptoms in children may be attributed to their misdiagnosis until the mass reaches a large size. In children, the time from onset of symptoms to diagnoses is on average 3 months. This delay in diagnosis might be due to a combination of the rarity of CRAC in children and the symptomatic overlap with more common benign pediatric abdominal conditions (Saab and Furman 2008).

The pathology of CRAC is that of a malignant adenocarcinoma which often arise from polyps which undergo malignant degeneration (Fig. 23.6). In comparison to adults, where only 10–15% of tumors are of mucinous histology, pediatric CRACs have a high preponderance of mucinous lesions. More than 40% of tumors are signet cell carcinomas and poorly differentiated lesions (Figs. 23.7 and 23.8). The presence of this histology in adult CRAC is typically associated with an unfavorable outcome, yet due to the rarity of these tumors in children, the histological significance in this age group is unknown (Saab and Furman 2008).

A prognostic factor in adults, E-cadherin expression has not been studied in children with CRAC. Researchers have found that a decrease in E-cadherin expression in adults is an adverse prognostic indicator in several carcinomas, including esophageal, endometrial, ovarian, thyroid, and gastric (Lin et al. 2004; Mell et al. 2004; Brecelj et al. 2005; Faleiro-Rodrigues et al. 2005; Kim et al. 2009). Additionally, loss of E-cadherin is a characteristic of signet ring cell carcinoma, and it is surmised that this is an indicator for the more aggressive nature of such less differentiated colorectal carcinomas (Fig. 23.9) (Kim et al. 2002; Khoursheed et al. 2003; Borger et al. 2007). The author's present study shows no correlation between E-cadherin expression and the prognosis/staging of CRAC in children.

Adult CRAC staging guidelines based on surgery and pathology are typically used for children. The current staging system, developed by the American Joint Committee on Cancer, is based on the tumor pathology, lymph node involvement, margin infiltration, and occurrence of metastasis. Histologically, low-grade lesions (grades 1 and 2), which have no angiolymphatic invasion and no marginal involvement, are classified as favorable histology. If invasion is documented, total colonoscopy, complete blood count, blood chemistry panel with liver enzymes, and the carcinoembryonic antigen (CEA) level should be completed. While the CEA level in adults can help in the prediction of recurrence, the usefulness of this antigen in children remains unclear (Saab and Furman 2008). A road map pertaining

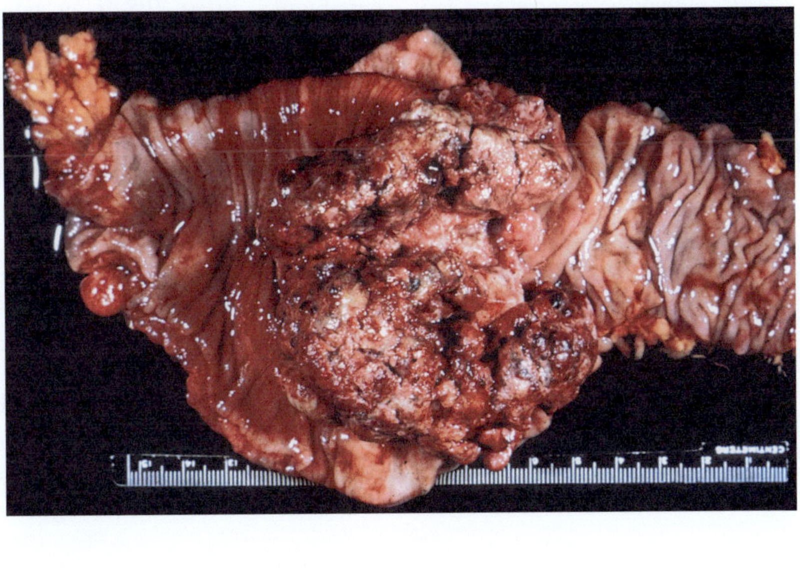

Fig. 23.6 Colon with invasive adenocarcinoma

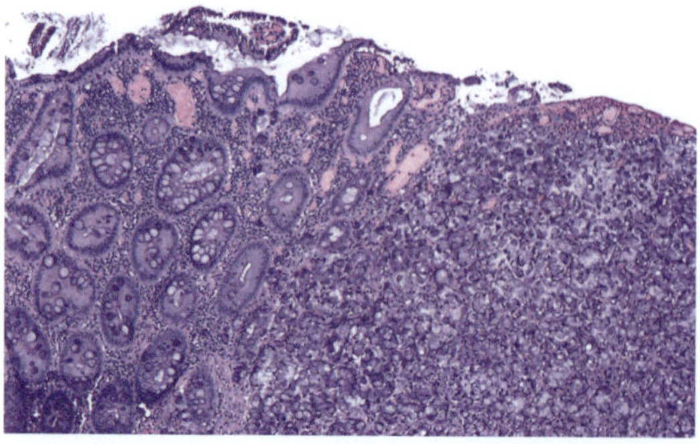

Fig. 23.7 Microscopic picture showing the transition from normal colonic mucosa to signet ring adenocarcinoma (100×)

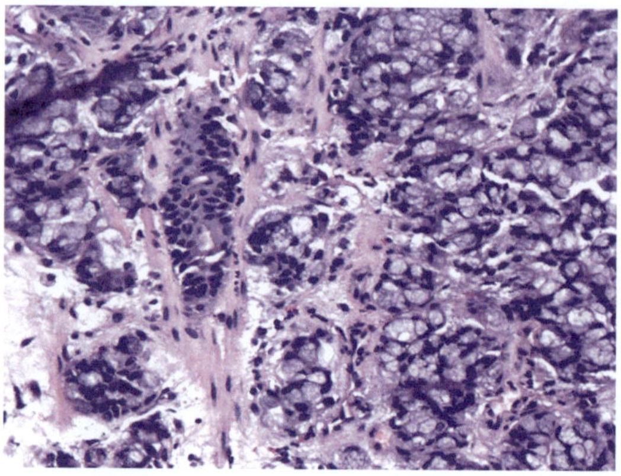

Fig. 23.8 Higher magnification of signet ring adenocarcinoma (400×)

to the diagnosis and treatment of CRAC is presented in Fig. 23.10.

There are three broad categories of pediatric CRAC: polyposis-associated CRAC, hereditary nonpolyposis colorectal cancer (HNPCC), and adenocarcinoma resulting from malignant degeneration of ulcerative colitis (UC). Polyposis-associated CRAC is linked with multiple familial polyposis syndromes, including familial adenomatous polyposis (FAP), MUTYH-associated polyposis syndrome (MAP), Peutz–Jeghers syndrome (PJS), juvenile polyposis syndrome (JPS), and juvenile hyperplastic polyposis syndrome (HPP) (Saab and Furman 2008). Peutz–Jeghers syndrome has not been reported in the pediatric population so it will not be further discussed.

FAP is an autosomal dominant disorder with a 100% incidence rate of CRAC. Indicated in the

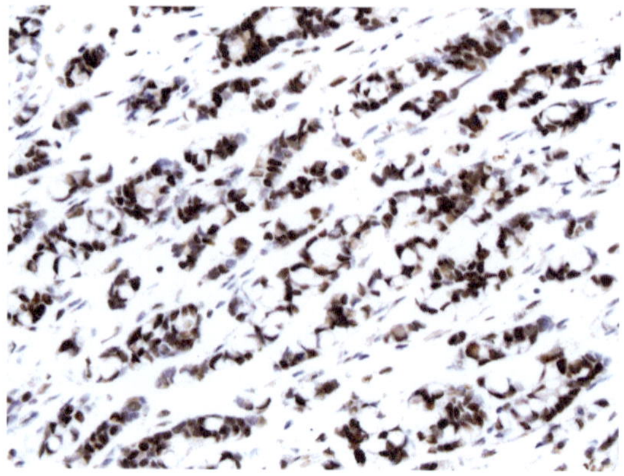

Fig. 23.9 Positive E-cadherin immunostain in signet ring adenocarcinoma

etiology of this disorder is an inactivating germline mutation in 5q21, the adenomatous polyposis coli (*APC*) tumor suppressor gene. Acquired mutations of this gene are found in most sporadic cases of CRACs, and the youngest reported patient with FAB-associated CRAC was 5 years of age (Durno and Gallinger 2006; Saab and Furman 2008; Jasperson et al. 2010). MUTYH-associated polyposis syndrome, an autosomal recessive disorder, stems from a biallelic mutation in the *MUTYH* gene. According to Durno et al., only one pediatric patient (21 years of age) has had MAP-associated CRAC; however, they note that testing for this genetic mutation has not widely been performed in the pediatric population (Durno and Gallinger 2006; Jasperson et al. 2010). JPS is an autosomal dominant disorder with suggested germline inactivation mutations in *SMAD4* and *BMPR1A*. In patients under 35 years of age with JPS, there is a 15% incidence of CRAC (Saab and Furman 2008; Jasperson et al. 2010). Finally, the etiology of HPP is unknown (Jasperson et al. 2010).

An autosomal dominant condition, HNPCC or Lynch syndrome, accounts for roughly 3% of CRACs (Lynch et al. 2009). Patients with Lynch syndrome have an increased risk of developing extracolonic cancers including those of the endometrium (~40%), stomach (~15%), ovary (~10%), hepatobiliary tract and pancreas (~5%), urinary tract (~4%), small bowel (~3%), and CNS (~2%) (Lagerstedt Robinson et al. 2007;

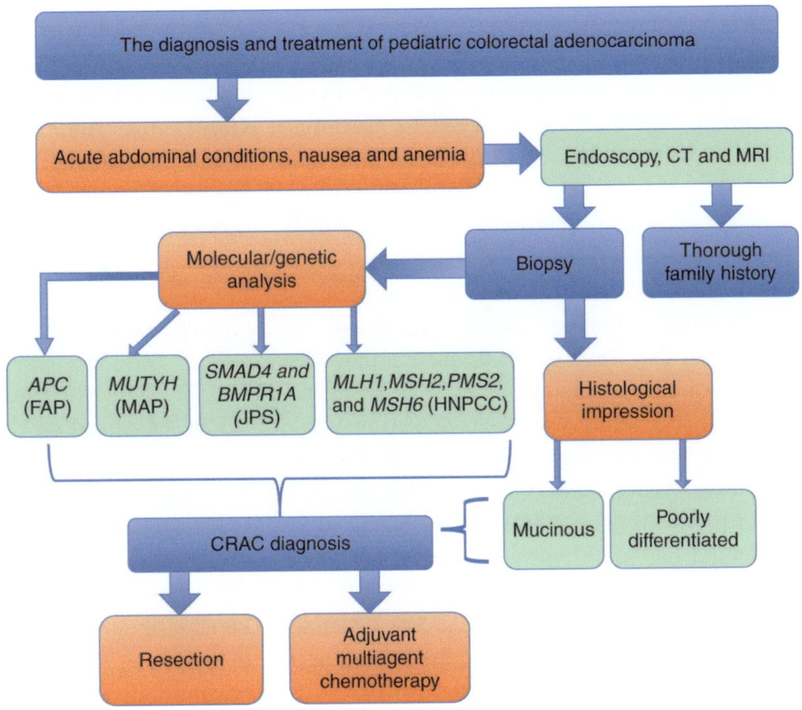

Fig. 23.10 Road map outlining the diagnosis and treatment of pediatric CRAC

Jang and Chung 2010). In comparison to patients with sporadic CRAC, those with HNPCC-related CRAC are often present at a lower stage, have lower incidence of metastases, and have more favorable prognosis (Saab and Furman 2008).

The biological basis of Lynch syndrome has been widely studied. Heterozygous germline mutations in four specific DNA mismatch repair (MMR) genes, *MLH1*, *MSH2*, *PMS2*, and *MSH6*, have been linked with this disorder (5, 6). These genes are responsible for fixing sequencing errors that arise during DNA replication; therefore, if they become impaired, genetic errors may accumulate and, ultimately, carcinoma may occur. The accumulation of errors during DNA replication can occasionally lead to microsatellite instability (MSI), which is defined as erroneously lengthened or shortened repetitive DNA sequences. Most Lynch syndrome patients display MSI; however, it can also occur in up to 15% of CRACs unrelated to Lynch syndrome. In non-HNPCC patients, MSI is typically due to acquired hypermethylation of the *MLH1* gene promoter (Lagerstedt Robinson et al. 2007; Boland and Goel 2010; Jang and Chung 2010; Gonzalez et al. 2012). *MLH1* and *MSH2* gene mutations are seen in up to 90% of Lynch syndrome patients, while *MSH6* and *PMS2* gene mutations constitute the remaining 10% of cases (Jasperson et al. 2010). The biallelic mutations of one of the MMR genes lead to a distinct phenotype that includes multiple adenomatous polyps and café au lait skin macules (Poley et al. 2007; Durno et al. 2010).

To ensure early diagnosis of this rare disease, strict diagnostic criteria (the Amsterdam criteria) were created in 1990 with the hopes of improving morbidity and mortality rates. Since its inception, modifications have been made to include other HNPCC-related cancers (Amsterdam II criteria). The diagnostic criteria of HNPCC require the patient to have (1) three or more family members with colorectal carcinoma where one is a first-degree relative of another, (2) two successive affected generations, and (3) the diagnosis of an HNPCC-related cancer relative before 50 years of age (Lynch et al. 2009).

Due to the rarity of CRAC in the pediatric population, routine workup should include a thorough family history and pending results, genetic testing performed (Davidson 2007;

Jasperson et al. 2010). While FAP, JPS, and Peutz–Jeghers syndrome predispose patients to the formation of multiple polyps, Lynch syndrome—the most common genetic abnormalities associated with CRAC—does not, and, therefore, patients with this syndrome require a higher level of clinical suspicion (Jasperson et al. 2010). If a patient is suspected of having HNPCC, genetic tests for MMR genes and immunohistochemical stains that demonstrate the absence of the protein that corresponds to the aberrant gene are available (Lynch et al. 2009). Immunohistochemical staining for MSI may also be performed in cases suspicious for HNPCC with excessive mucin or poorly differentiated signet ring cells (Jass 2007).

Behind FAP and Lynch syndrome, UC is the third highest condition at risk for CRAC. The development of CRAC in UC patients is mainly related to long-standing chronic inflammation of the bowel, and the longer symptoms of UC persist, the greater the chances that CRAC will occur. One study found that the presence of UC increases the risk of CRAC by 19-fold compared to the general population. When associated with UC, CRAC develops in the affected mucosa and in areas proximal to gross colitis. When UC is found in the pediatric population, the risk of CRAC is heightened (Saab and Furman 2008; Kulaylat and Dayton 2010). One report noted that children who have UC for more than 5 years are more prone to develop CRAC, whereas in the adult population, this risk does not increase until after 10 years (Saab and Furman 2008). The subtypes most often observed of UC-associated CRAC are mucinous or signet cell, and multiple lesions are typically found. Surveillance measures include regular colonoscopies as well as random serial biopsies (Kulaylat and Dayton 2010).

23.4.1 Cancer of the Stomach

Adenocarcinomas account for 95% of gastric cancers. They are extremely rare in children and adolescents (Schwartz and Sgaglione 1984). Gastric adenocarcinoma and MALT lymphoma are associated with *Helicobacter pylori*, chronic carrier (Blosse and Lehours 2019; Correa and Blanca Piazuelo 2011). Another relatively common tumor is GIST, which can be associated with Carney triad. Additionally, Carney–Stratakis syndrome is characterized by GIST, chondromas of the lung, and paragangliomas caused by germline mutations of the SDHB, SDHC, and SDHD genes (Falcone 2012) (Fig. 23.1). Additionally, rare tumors can be seen in this age group including squamous cell carcinomas, carcinoids, and LMS.

23.4.2 Cancer of the Pancreas

Pancreatic cancer is a frequent cause of death from cancer in adults. Pancreatic tumors are extremely rare in children and adolescents (Dall'igna et al. 2010; Chung et al. 2006). Pancreatic cancers present variable histologies that include papillary–cystic carcinomas, adenocarcinomas, squamous cell carcinomas, acinic cell carcinomas, liposarcomas, pancreatoblastomas, glucagonomas, gastrinomas, and malignant insulinomas (Vossen et al. 1998; Shorter et al. 2002; Raffel et al. 2004). Primitive neuroectodermal tumors and lymphomas have also been reported (Movahedi-Lankarani et al. 2002). Many of these tumors do not produce hormones. Pancreatic carcinoma and pancreatoblastoma can produce hormones and may be associated with wasting and pain (Murakami et al. 1996; Schwartz 1997; Imamura et al. 1998). Pancreatoblastoma has been associated with Cushing's syndrome and Beckwith–Wiedemann syndrome (Muguerza et al. 2005). Complete resection is the mainstay of treatment. Solid pseudopapillary neoplasm of the pancreas has been reported in children. It has been called a "borderline" malignancy. It is also treated with surgical excision. AFP elevation has also been reported in pancreatoblastoma (Dhebri et al. 2004).

23.4.3 Carcinoid Tumor

Carcinoid tumors are rare in children but may be located in the esophagus and bronchi in the thorax.

In the abdomen, they occur in the pancreas and small and large bowel, including the appendix. Many are found after appendectomy. Tumors of appendix are usually benign. Tumors contain argentaffin granules which are thought to arise from small intestine Kulchitsky cells. These cells may secrete proteins, such as somatostatin, leading to the clinical symptoms of carcinoid syndrome.

23.4.4 Cancer of the Bladder, Cervix, and Vagina

Bladder carcinomas are extremely rare in children. Most pediatric bladder carcinomas are low grade, in contrast to similar tumors in adults. Papillary urothelial neoplasm of low malignant potential (PUNLUP) may be the most common entity in children (Alanee and Shukla 2010). Most of these tumors are superficial and easily treated with surgery. Squamous cell carcinomas do occur in children (Sung and Koyle 2000; Lezama-del Valle et al. 2004). In pediatric cancer survivors, there is an association between the development of bladder carcinoma and treatment with alkylating agents, such as cyclophosphamide (Johansson and Cohen 1997). Adenocarcinomas of cervix and vagina are extremely rare in children and adolescents (McNall et al. 2004). The median age of presentation is 15 years, and two-thirds are associated with exposure to diethylstilbestrol in utero. These tumors tend to present at higher stage III or IV in these adolescents. This may be because this population is not routinely examined with routine PAP smears.

References

Alanee S, Shukla AR (2010) Bladder malignancies in children aged <18 years: results from the Surveillance, Epidemiology and End Results database. BJU Int 106(4):557–560

Benesch M, Wardelmann E et al (2009) Gastrointestinal stromal tumors (GIST) in children and adolescents: a comprehensive review of the current literature. Pediatr Blood Cancer 53(7):1171–1179

Blosse A, Lehours P (2019) Deregulation of miRNA in Helicobacter pylori-induced gastric MALT lymphoma. J Clin Med 8(6):845

Boland CR, Goel A (2010) Microsatellite instability in colorectal cancer. Gastroenterology 138(6):2073–2087.e3

Borger ME, Gosens MJ et al (2007) Signet ring cell differentiation in mucinous colorectal carcinoma. J Pathol 212(3):278–286

Brecelj E, Frkovic Grazio S et al (2005) Prognostic value of E-cadherin expression in thyroid follicular carcinoma. Eur J Surg Oncol 31(5):544–548

Chung EM, Travis MD et al (2006) Pancreatic tumors in children: radiologic-pathologic correlation. Radiographics 26(4):1211–1238

Correa P, Blanca Piazuelo M (2011) Helicobacter pylori infection and gastric adenocarcinoma. US Gastroenterol Hepatol 7(1):59–64

Dall'igna P, Cecchetto G et al (2010) Pancreatic tumors in children and adolescents: the Italian TREP project experience. Pediatr Blood Cancer 54(5):675–680

Davidson NO (2007) Genetic testing in colorectal cancer: who, when, how and why. Keio J Med 56(1):14–20

Dhebri AR, Connor S et al (2004) Diagnosis, treatment and outcome of pancreatoblastoma. Pancreatology 4(5):441–451; discussion 452–453

Durno CA, Gallinger S (2006) Genetic predisposition to colorectal cancer: new pieces in the pediatric puzzle. J Pediatr Gastroenterol Nutr 43(1):5–15

Durno CA, Holter S et al (2010) The gastrointestinal phenotype of germline biallelic mismatch repair gene mutations. Am J Gastroenterol 105(11):2449–2456

Falcone ME (2012) Pediatric gastrointestinal tumors. J Diagn Med Sonography 28(3):131–134

Faleiro-Rodrigues C, Macedo-Pinto IM et al (2005) Biological relevance of E-cadherin-catenin complex proteins in primary epithelial ovarian tumours. Gynecol Obstet Invest 60(2):75–83

Gonzalez RS, Shulman SC et al (2012) Colorectal adenocarcinoma: a pediatric case review with a focus on mismatch repair gene mutations and E-cadherin expression. Pediatr Dev Pathol 15:192–198

Imamura A, Nakagawa A et al (1998) Pancreatoblastoma in an adolescent girl: case report and review of 26 Japanese cases. Eur J Surg 164(4):309–312

Jang E, Chung DC (2010) Hereditary colon cancer: lynch syndrome. Gut Liver 4(2):151–160

Jasperson KW, Tuohy TM et al (2010) Hereditary and familial colon cancer. Gastroenterology 138(6):2044–2058

Jass JR (2007) Classification of colorectal cancer based on correlation of clinical, morphological and molecular features. Histopathology 50(1):113–130

Johansson SL, Cohen SM (1997) Epidemiology and etiology of bladder cancer. Semin Surg Oncol 13(5):291–298

Kaemmer DA, Otto J et al (2009) The Gist of literature on pediatric GIST: review of clinical presentation. J Pediatr Hematol Oncol 31(2):108–112

Kerr JZ, Hicks MJ et al (1999) Gastrointestinal autonomic nerve tumors in the pediatric population: a report of four cases and a review of the literature. Cancer 85(1):220–230

Khoursheed MA, Mathew TC et al (2003) Expression of E-cadherin in human colorectal cancer. Surgeon 1(2):86–91

Kim HC, Kim HJ et al (2002) Reduced E-cadherin expression as a cause of distinctive signet-ring cell variant in colorectal carcinoma. J Korean Med Sci 17(1):23–28

Kim MA, Lee HS et al (2009) Prognostic importance of epithelial-mesenchymal transition-related protein expression in gastric carcinoma. Histopathology 54(4):442–451

Kulaylat MN, Dayton MT (2010) Ulcerative colitis and cancer. J Surg Oncol 101(8):706–712

Lagerstedt Robinson K, Liu T et al (2007) Lynch syndrome (hereditary nonpolyposis colorectal cancer) diagnostics. J Natl Cancer Inst 99(4):291–299

Lezama-del Valle P, Jerkins GR et al (2004) Aggressive bladder carcinoma in a child. Pediatr Blood Cancer 43(3):285–288

Liegl-Atzwanger B, Fletcher JA et al (2010) Gastrointestinal stromal tumors. Virchows Arch 456(2):111–127

Lin YC, Wu MY et al (2004) Prognostic and clinicopathological features of E-cadherin, alpha-catenin, beta-catenin, gamma-catenin and cyclin D1 expression in human esophageal squamous cell carcinoma. World J Gastroenterol 10(22):3235–3239

Lynch HT, Lynch PM et al (2009) Review of the Lynch syndrome: history, molecular genetics, screening, differential diagnosis, and medicolegal ramifications. Clin Genet 76(1):1–18

Machairas A, Karamitopoulou E et al (2010) Gastrointestinal stromal tumors (GISTs): an updated experience. Dig Dis Sci 55(12):3315–3327

McNall RY, Nowicki PD et al (2004) Adenocarcinoma of the cervix and vagina in pediatric patients. Pediatr Blood Cancer 43(3):289–294

Mell LK, Meyer JJ et al (2004) Prognostic significance of E-cadherin protein expression in pathological stage I–III endometrial cancer. Clin Cancer Res 10(16):5546–5553

Movahedi-Lankarani S, Hruban RH et al (2002) Primitive neuroectodermal tumors of the pancreas: a report of seven cases of a rare neoplasm. Am J Surg Pathol 26(8):1040–1047

Muguerza R, Rodriguez A et al (2005) Pancreatoblastoma associated with incomplete Beckwith-Wiedemann syndrome: case report and review of the literature. J Pediatr Surg 40(8):1341–1344

Murakami T, Ueki K et al (1996) Pancreatoblastoma: case report and review of treatment in the literature. Med Pediatr Oncol 27(3):193–197

O'Connell JB, Maggard MA et al (2003) Rates of colon and rectal cancers are increasing in young adults. Am Surg 69(10):866–872

Poley JW, Wagner A et al (2007) Biallelic germline mutations of mismatch-repair genes: a possible cause for multiple pediatric malignancies. Cancer 109(11):2349–2356

Raffel A, Cupisti K et al (2004) Therapeutic strategy of papillary cystic and solid neoplasm (PCSN): a rare non-endocrine tumor of the pancreas in children. Surg Oncol 13(1):1–6

Saab R, Furman WL (2008) Epidemiology and management options for colorectal cancer in children. Paediatr Drugs 10(3):177–192

Schwartz MZ (1997) Unusual peptide-secreting tumors in adolescents and children. Semin Pediatr Surg 6(3):141–146

Schwartz MG, Sgaglione NA (1984) Gastric carcinoma in the young: overview of the literature. Mt Sinai J Med 51(6):720–723

Shimomura M, Ikeda S et al (2010) Gastrointestinal stromal tumors of the small intestine in pediatric populations: a case report and literature review. Pediatr Surg Int 26(6):649–654

Shorter NA, Glick RD et al (2002) Malignant pancreatic tumors in childhood and adolescence: the Memorial Sloan-Kettering experience, 1967 to present. J Pediatr Surg 37(6):887–892

Sultan I, Rodriguez-Galindo C et al (2010) Distinct features of colorectal cancer in children and adolescents: a population-based study of 159 cases. Cancer 116(3):758–765

Sung JD, Koyle MA (2000) Squamous cell carcinoma of the bladder in a pediatric patient. J Pediatr Surg 35(12):1838–1839

Vossen S, Goretzki PE et al (1998) Therapeutic management of rare malignant pancreatic tumors in children. World J Surg 22(8):879–882

24 Tumors of the Esophagus and the Stomach

Dietrich von Schweinitz

24.1 Tumors of the Esophagus

In contrast to adults, neoplastic tumors of the esophagus are exceedingly rare during childhood and adolescence (Rodriguez-Galindo and Furman 2016). As primary tumors of other parts of the gastrointestinal tract, also those of the esophagus almost never affect infants and toddlers but rather school-age children and adolescents (Ladd and Grosfeld 2006). In the SEER registry of 1992–2007, a rate of < 0.02 per one million children was documented. But also in this age group, carcinomas are the most frequent neoplasms, and both adenocarcinomas and squamous cell carcinomas can occur (Rodriguez-Galindo and Furman 2016). Esophageal carcinomas may be more frequent in Asia than in Europe or North America proposedly both on the basis of environmental and on genetic factors (Khushed et al. 2007). Adenocarcinomas of the esophagus in adults are usually associated with Barrett's esophagus because of chronic gastroesophageal reflux, and there have been reports on this association also in children. Esophageal carcinomas can occur during childhood in the context of cancer predisposing syndromes and are more frequent in boys than in girls. According to reports on single patients, other malignant neoplasms as leiomyosarcomas and undifferentiated mesenchymal tumors and also benign tumors as leiomyomas, hamartomas, lipomas, and fibromatosis can be found in children (Heij 2008). Also inflammatory myofibroblastic tumors can be encountered in the esophagus of children (Doussek et al. 2015).

D. von Schweinitz (✉)
Kinderchirurgische Klinik und Poliklinik, Dr. von Haunersches Kinderspital, Munich, Germany
e-mail: dietrich_schweinitz@hotmail.de

D. T. Schneider et al. (eds.), *Rare Tumors in Children and Adolescents*, Pediatric Oncology,
https://doi.org/10.1007/978-3-030-92071-5_24

SEER data 1992–2007															
Males and females				0–14 years		0–19 years		0–4 years		5–9 years		10–14 years		15–19 years	
ICCC code	ICCC	SRCode	Site recode	Rate	Count	Rate	Count	Rate	Count	Rate	Count	Rate	Count	Rate	Count
42	IX(d.1) Ewing tumor and Askin tumor of soft tissue	10	Esophagus	0	0	0.01	1	0	0	0	0	0	0	0.02	1
89	XI(f.10) Carcinomas of other specified sites	10	Esophagus	0.02	3	0.02	4	0	0	0.02	1	0.04	2	0.02	1
			Sum	**0.02**	**3**	**0.03**	**5**	**0**	**0**	**0.02**	**1**	**0.04**	**2**	**0.04**	**2**
38	IX(b.1) Fibroblastic and myofibroblastic tumors	11	Stomach	0.01	1	0.01	1	0	0	0	0	0.02	1	0	0
39	IX(b.2) Nerve sheath tumors	11	Stomach	0	0	0.01	1	0	0	0	0	0	0	0.02	1
47	IX(d.6) Leiomyosarcomas	11	Stomach	0.02	3	0.03	5	0	0	0.07	3	0	0	0.05	2
53	IX(e) Unspecified soft tissue sarcomas	11	Stomach	0.01	1	0.01	1	0	0	0	0	0.02	1	0	0
61	X(b.2) Malignant teratomas: extracranial/extragonadal	11	Stomach	0.01	1	0.01	1	0.02	1	0	0	0	0	0	0
89	XI(f.10) Carcinomas of other specified sites	11	Stomach	0.01	2	0.1	19	0	0	0	0	0.04	2	0.4	17
91	XII(a.1) Gastrointestinal stromal tumor	11	Stomach	0.02	3	0.03	5	0	0	0.02	1	0.04	2	0.05	2
97	XII(b) Other unspecified malignant tumors	11	Stomach	0.01	1	0.01	2	0.02	1	0	0	0	0	0.02	1
			Sum	**0.09**	**12**	**0.21**	**35**	**0.04**	**2**	**0.09**	**4**	**0.12**	**6**	**0.54**	**23**

Patients with an esophageal tumor usually present with dysphagia and weight loss. Other typical symptoms are vomiting, cough, regurgitation and hematemesis, and retrosternal pain. In patients with these symptoms, other more frequent causes as foreign body impactation, inflammatory diseases of the esophagus, and malformations as bronchogenic cysts and esophageal duplications have to be ruled out. The diagnostic procedure should include conventional radiology with contrast medium, a CT or MRI scan, and an esophagoscopy with biopsies. Early-stage tumors are asymptomatic and may be found incidentally during endoscopy for other reasons. A histological confirmation of the diagnosis is mandatory. In case of malignancy, other diagnostic procedures as thoracic CT, bone scan, FDG-PET scan, and cerebral MRI become necessary for identification of metastases and staging. Esophageal carcinomas are staged according to the TNM system (Table 24.1; UICC 2017).

The mainstay of treatment of esophageal tumors is a complete surgical resection. Depending on tumor extension, this can be accomplished by a local excision or by a removal of the esophagus with a replacement by either a gastric or a colonic interposition. In case of a malignant tumor, especially a carcinoma, it is important to perform a thorough lymph node dissection. Adjuvant chemotherapy and/or radiation may be administered for malignant neoplasms. In carcinomas, these are of very little to no effect, while in sarcomas they can be cytotoxic in a regime according to the existing different national and international soft tissue sarcoma trials (Rodriguez-Galindo and Furman 2016).

The prognosis of children with a benign tumor is good; however, depending of the extension of the tumor, long-term functional problems may be a result of surgical treatment. In case of mesenchymal neoplasms, the patients' chance for survival will be similar to that of the same entities (i.e., leiomyosarcoma, undifferentiated mesenchymal tumor) at other locations and the tumor extension. Other factors for survival are completeness of resection and response of the tumor to chemotherapy and radiation. The prognosis of children with esophagus carcinoma has been dismal in the very few reported cases. This may be due to an advanced stage of disease at diagnosis but possibly also of an increased aggressiveness of carcinomas in young patients in comparison to adults (Heij 2008).

Table 24.1 TNM clinical classification of esophageal cancer

T—primary tumor	
TX	Primary tumor cannot be assessed
T0	No evidence of primary tumor
Tis	Carcinoma in situ/high-grade dysplasia
T1	Tumor invades lamina propria, muscularis mucosae, or submucosa
T1a	Tumor invades lamina propria or muscularis mucosae
T1b	Tumor invades submucosa
T2	Tumor invades muscularis propria
T3	Tumor invades adventitia
T4	Tumor invades adjacent structures
T4a	Tumor invades pleura, pericardium, or diaphragm
T4b	Tumor invades other adjacent structures such as aorta, vertebral body, or trachea
N—regional lymph nodes	
NX	Regional lymph nodes cannot be assessed
N0	No regional lymph node metastasis
N1	Metastasis in one to two regional lymph nodes
N2	Metastasis in three to six regional lymph nodes
N3	Metastasis in seven or more regional lymph nodes
M—distant metastasis	
M0	No distant metastasis
M1	Distant metastasis

24.2 Tumors of the Stomach

Although not as exceedingly rare in childhood and adolescence as esophageal neoplasms, primary tumors of the stomach occur only sporadically in the pediatric age group; thus, only 0.05% of all gastric cancers are found in children (Rodriguez-Galindo and Furman 2016), and the SEER registry for 1992–2007 documented a rate of 0.21 per one million population <20 years of age. In contrast to adults, carcinomas do not comprise the vast majority of all gastric neoplasms of the young age. As primary benign tumors of the stomach, teratomas, hamartomas, lipomas, and inflammatory myoblastic tumors, as well as leiomyomas and leiomyomatosis, have been described in children. Soft tissue sarcomas, mostly leiomyosarcomas, and lymphomas are the most common malignant tumors of the stomach in children; also gastrointestinal stromal tumors (GIST) are found (Heij 2008; Curtis et al. 2008). Adenocarcinomas comprise only 5% of all gastric tumors in this age group (Rodriguez-Galindo and Furman 2016). While as in adults the carcinomas seem to be associated with *Helicobacter pylori* infection, this was also proposed for lymphomas in childhood (Imrie et al. 2001). Gastric neoplasms may also be associated with tumor predisposing syndromes in children. A combination of GIST with extra-adrenal paraganglioma and pulmonary chondroma in children has been called Carney's triad.

Over 100 cases of gastric teratomas have been described in the literature (Heij 2008). These usually occur in early childhood and behave like teratomas of other localizations. Thus, they usually are benign but with increasing age become malignant. Therefore, a complete excision is important at an early stage. Inflammatory myoblastic tumors occur rarely in the gastrointestinal tract. Here they are found mostly in the stomach. They are benign, grow slowly, and do not metastasize but often demonstrate local infiltration and a relatively high rate of local recurrences after surgery. Leiomyomas can grow in the stomach mainly in young children. As they are essentially benign tumors, surgical resection usually leads to cure.

Also malignant leiomyosarcomas are mostly found in children of young age; a number of these occur during the newborn period (Ladd and Grosfeld 2006). Other cases have been described in patients with a depression of the immune system, e.g., after organ transplantation or HIV infection. These tumors are highly malignant with a frequent development of metastases (Heij 2008). Some lymphomas are thought to develop from atopically arising mucosa-associated lymphatic tissue (MALT) after a *Helicobacter pylori* infection, which then can develop into a low malignant lymphoma. These MALT lymphomas are usually locally spreading and seldomly disseminate. In a longer course of disease, however, they can transform into highly malignant lymphomas, which takes place in 20% of the cases (Imrie et al. 2001). However, also typical Burkitt lymphomas of the stomach have been found in some pediatric cases.

GIST is a malignant mesenchymal tumor arising from primitive precursor cells which are related to the interstitial cells of Cajal. The majority (88%) of GISTs occurring in children are located in the stomach and are diagnosed in school-age girls (Miettinen et al. 2005). The biological and histological characteristics of GISTs are described in detail in a separate chapter of this book. Some GISTs of the stomach metastasize at local lymph nodes and the liver. The response rate of GISTs in children to imatinib mesylate is estimated to be approximately 50%.

The very rare carcinomas of the stomach in school-age children and adolescents do not seem to differ very much from those in adults concerning histopathology and biological behavior. Thus, they grow locally aggressive and spread via lymphatic and blood vessels as well as by peritoneal seeding. Therefore, they can involve adjacent organs such as esophagus, duodenum, pancreas, colon, and liver. Distant metastases can affect the liver, lungs, bones, and skin (Rodriguez-Galindo and Furman 2016). The tumor status and the extension of disease can best be classified with the TNM system (Table 24.2; UICC 2017).

The clinical symptoms of gastric tumors are quite uniform. The patients have epigastric discomfort or pain, nausea and vomiting, and sometimes anorexia and weight loss. Also hematemesis and anemia as well as occult blood in the stool may appear. Often the tumor is palpable in the upper abdomen at the time of diagnosis. For differential diagnosis, mainly space-occupying malformations of the stomach, especially a gastric duplication, have to be taken into account but also extragastric tumors such as tumors of the pancreas, the liver, and the retroperitoneum.

Table 24.2 TNM clinical classification of gastric cancer

T—primary tumor	
TX	Primary tumor cannot be assessed
T0	No evidence of primary tumor
Tis	Carcinoma in situ: intraepithelial tumor without invasion of the lamina propria, high-grade dysplasia
T1	Tumor invades lamina propria, muscularis mucosae, or submucosa
T1a	Tumor invades lamina propria or muscularis mucosae
T1b	Tumor invades submucosa
T2	Tumor invades muscularis propria
T3	Tumor invades subserosa
T4	Tumor perforates serosa or invades adjacent structures[a–c]
T4a	Tumor perforates serosa
T4b	Tumor invades other adjacent structures[a–c]
N—regional lymph nodes	
NX	Regional lymph nodes cannot be assessed
N0	No regional lymph node metastasis
N1	Metastasis in one to two regional lymph nodes
N2	Metastasis in three to six regional lymph nodes
N3	Metastasis in seven or more regional lymph nodes
N3a	Metastasis in 7–15 regional lymph nodes
N3b	Metastasis in 16 or more regional lymph nodes
M—distant metastasis	
M0	No distant metastasis
M1	Distant metastasis

[a]The adjacent structures of the stomach are the spleen, transverse colon, liver, diaphragm, pancreas, abdominal wall, adrenal gland, kidney, small intestine, and retroperitoneum
[b]Intramural extension of the duodenum or esophagus is classified by the depth of greatest invasion in any of these sites, including stomach
[c]Tumor that extends into gastrocolic or gastrohepatic ligaments or into greater or lesser omentum, without perforation of visceral peritoneum, is T3

Therefore, besides a laboratory workup, the diagnostic procedures should include abdominal ultrasound, radiology with an upper gastrointestinal contrast medium passage, a CT and/or MRI scan, and a gastroscopy. During this procedure, the essential biopsies can be taken. In case of malignancy, investigations for staging with thoracic CT, bone scan, and eventually a FDG-PET scan should follow. In patients with a suspected gastric lymphoma, it is important to gain tumor material through a biopsy or from other materials as ascites, pleural effusion, or bone marrow before planning of treatment.

The best therapy for most gastric tumors is a primary complete resection (Heij 2008). Obviously, this has to be more extensive in malignant than in benign tumors. Therefore, if the diagnosis is not established by a biopsy beforehand, intraoperative frozen sections should be performed by the pathologist. In benign tumors, a local excision usually with preservation of some parts of the stomach is sufficient. In contrast to malignant tumors, a resection with wide margins and excision of regional lymph nodes is the procedure of choice. For pediatric GIST and sarcomas but also for gastric carcinomas, it is not clear whether a limited lymph node dissection with a low rate of surgical complication or an extended dissection with a high risk of complications is the better procedure. In relatively extended tumors, complete gastrectomies can be performed also in children without taking a risk for acute complications and long-term sequelae which would be higher than in adults.

Only for gastric lymphomas as for non-Hodgkin's lymphomas of other sites, the treatment of choice is primary chemotherapy according to the schemes of non-Hodgkin's lymphoma trials. In most cases, this is very effective, and the tumors show an extensive decrease of size. In some patients in whom this diagnosis has been established before start of treatment, surgery is not necessary any more after a complete regression of the tumor (Rodriguez-Galindo and Furman 2016).

Adjuvant therapy is indicated in many cases with another malignant tumor. In sarcomas, chemotherapy according to the different soft tissue sarcoma protocols often has at least some effect, and, in cases of GIST, adjuvant therapy should mainly contain imatinib mesylate. Although gastric carcinomas mostly show a very poor response to chemotherapy, different cytotoxic agents such as 5-FU, doxorubicin, cisplatin, etoposide, mitomycin, and irinotecan have been administered adjuvantly. Sarcomas and some carcinomas are responsive to radiation which may preferably be administered in addition to chemotherapy, especially after marginal resections. Patients with unresectable or metastasized malignant tumors should receive neoadjuvant treatment. For sarcomas, the chemotherapy regimens shown to be effective in soft tissue sarcomas of other localizations should be applied. For GIST, imatinib mesylate should be administered while the effect of conventional chemotherapy is not clear especially in children. In extended unresectable and/or metastasized carcinomas, pre- or intraoperative radiation but also chemotherapy can be tried (Rodriguez-Galindo and Furman 2016).

The prognosis of gastric tumors depends on the dignity, the histological diagnosis, the extension of disease, surgical resectability, and the response to chemotherapy and radiation. Benign tumors usually have a very good prognosis. This also accounts for gastric lymphomas, while the prognosis for sarcomas is dependent on resectability and sensitivity to chemotherapy and radiation. For GIST, it seems that children have a slightly poorer outcome than adults; approximately two thirds of the pediatric patients could be cured in the recent years (Cypriano et al. 2004). The prognosis of gastric carcinoma in childhood is very poor; only very few survivors have been reported (Rodriguez-Galindo and Furman 2016; Heij 2008).

References

Curtis JL, Burns RC, Wang L et al (2008) Primary gastric tumors of infancy and childhood: 54-year experience at a single institution. J Pediatr Surg 43:1487–1493

Cypriano MS, Jenkins JJ, Pappo AS et al (2004) Pediatric gastrointestinal stromal tumors and leiomyosarcoma. Cancer 101:29–50

Doussek R, Tuma J, Planka L et al (2015) Inflammatory myofibroblastic tumor of the esophagus in childhood: a case report and a review of the literature. J Pediatr Hematol Oncol 37:121–124

Heij HA (2008) Rare tumors. In: Carachi R, Grosfeld JL, Azy AF (eds) The surgery of childhood tumors, 2nd edn. Springer, Heidelberg

Imrie C, Rowland M, Bourke B et al (2001) Is *Helicobacter pylori* infection in childhood a risk factor for gastric cancer? Pediatrics 107:373–380

Khushed A, Ahmed R, Bhurgri Y (2007) Primary gastrointestinal malignancies in childhood and adolescents—an Asian perspective. Asian Pac J Cancer Prev 8:613–617

Ladd AP, Grosfeld JL (2006) Gastrointestinal tumors in children and adolescents. Semin Pediatr Surg 15:37–47

Miettinen M, Lasota J, Sobin LH (2005) Gastrointestinal stromal tumors of the stomach in children and young adults: a clinicopathologic, immunohistochemical and molecular genetic study of 44 cases with long-term follow-up and review of the literature. Am J Pathol 29:1373–1381

Rodriguez-Galindo C, Furman WL (2016) Rare pediatric tumors. In: Pizzo PA, Poplack DG (eds) Principles and practice of pediatric oncology, 7th edn. Lippincott Williams & Wilkins, Philadelphia, pp 946–966

SEER Registry 1992–2007. www.seer.cancer.gov

UICC (2017) TNM classification of malignant tumours, 8th edn. Wiley Blackwell, New York

Tumors of the Small Intestine, Colon, and Rectum

25

Stefano Signoroni, Maria Di Bartolomeo, and Andrea Ferrari

25.1 Epidemiology

Carcinomas of the small intestine, colon, and rectum are malignant epithelial tumors, originating from glandular epithelium of the intestinal mucosa. They represent one of the leading malignancies among adults worldwide. While adenocarcinoma of the small bowel (duodenum, jejunum, and ileum) is less frequent, colorectal carcinoma (CRC) is the third most common malignancy in adults worldwide after lung and breast cancers, with 945.000 new cases a year (9.4% of the world total) and 492.000 deaths (7.9% of the total) (Parkin 2001). However, these tumors are extremely rare among children, particularly before puberty (Fig. 25.1). In the Survival Epidemiology and End Result (SEER) public-access database, only 31 cases younger than 15 years old and 143 aged from 15 to 19 years old were collected between 1973 and 2006, as compared to 584.427 adult cases (Ferrari et al. 2010). Age-adjusted incidence rates calculated from the SEER database in children/adolescents and adults were reported to be 0.38 and 802 per million, respectively (Sultan et al. 2010). Therefore, pediatric oncologists and pediatric surgeons only occasionally encounter these tumors in their clinical activity. When this happens, their limited experience and the scanty data available in the literature make the management of these patients a real challenge, also because the clinical appearance, the anatomical sites involved, and the tumor's clinical course but also the related risk stratification, the applicable staging systems, and recommended investigations, as well as the therapeutic procedures, are generally very different from what pediatric oncologists have learned from years of experience in managing typical childhood embryonal tumors.

25.2 Gastrointestinal Cancer Predisposition Syndromes

Bowel cancer has been defined as the most frequent form of hereditary neoplasia (Fearon 1997), and approximately 10–20% of CRCs occur in familial aggregations (Saab and Furman 2008a, b).

The two best characterized familial syndromes, Lynch syndrome and familial adenomatous polyposis (FAP), are autosomal dominant inherited disorders accounting for

S. Signoroni (✉)
Unit of Hereditary Digestive Tract Tumours, Fondazione IRCCS Istituto Nazionale Tumori, Milano, Italy
e-mail: stefano.signoroni@istitutotumori.mi.it

M. Di Bartolomeo
Medical Oncology, Fondazione IRCCS Istituto Nazionale Tumori, Milano, Italy

A. Ferrari
Pediatric Oncology Unit, Fondazione IRCCS Istituto Nazionale Tumori, Milano, Italy

D. T. Schneider et al. (eds.), *Rare Tumors in Children and Adolescents*, Pediatric Oncology,
https://doi.org/10.1007/978-3-030-92071-5_25

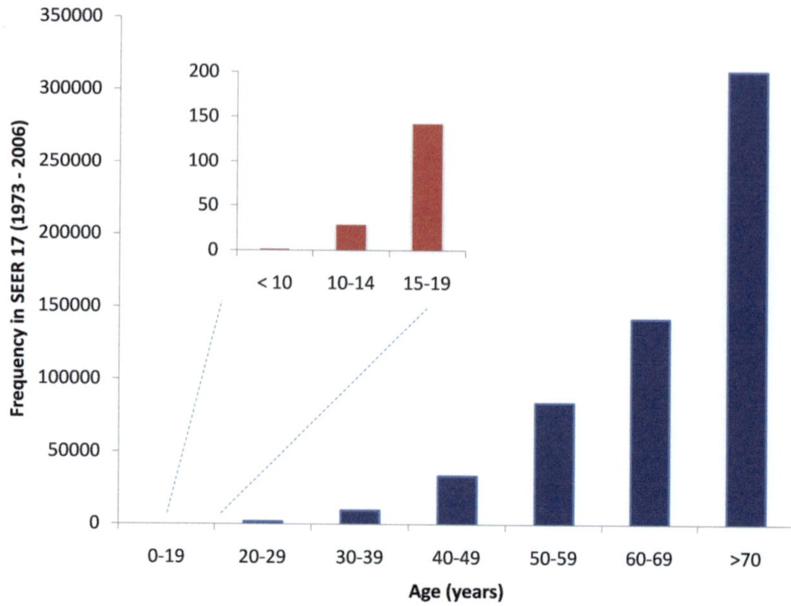

Fig. 25.1 Colorectal cancer by age from the SEER public-access database (1973–2007) (www.seer.cancer.gov) (courtesy dr. Iyad Sultan, King Hussein Cancer Center, Amman, Jordan)

approximately 2% and 0.1–1% of all adult cases of CRCs, respectively. Other polyposis syndromes affect children: Peutz-Jeghers syndrome (PJS) and juvenile polyposis coli. All the syndromes cited rarely cause malignant colorectal tumours in young carriers; however, extracolonic manifestations and preneoplastic lesions must be considered and often occur in pediatric patients.

25.2.1 Adenomatous Polyposis Syndrome (FAP)

FAP (OMIM N175100) is a dominantly inherited colorectal cancer predisposition syndrome in which hundreds to thousands of precancerous colonic polyps (adenomas) and extracolonic manifestations and/or neoplasms (tumours) are variably present.

FAP is generally caused by germline inactivating mutations in the adenomatous polyposis coli (APC) gene at 5q21, which encodes a protein of 2843 amino acids (Vasen et al. 2008). APC is a tumor suppressor gene, member of the WNT pathway. Normally, the WNT pathway leads to changes in gene expression profile; in fact, APC is able to form a multiprotein complex with glycogen synthesis kinase-3ß and axin and to bind ß-catenin, which in turn is phosphorylated by glycogen synthase kinase-3ß and subsequently degraded by the proteasome. If APC is mutated, the multiprotein complex could not be formed, and, therefore, ß-catenin accumulates into the cytoplasm and then translocates to the nucleus, where it activates the T-cell factor, which in turn causes transcription of target genes, influencing different cellular processes such as cell migration, cell cycle control, differentiation, and apoptosis (Kundu et al. 2006).

APC gene is considered at high penetrance activity, so patients carrying a germline mutation have theoretically the 100% of risk to develop at early age a colorectal cancer if not adequately treated.

The standard prophylactic approach is still surgical. Generally, a total colectomy (extended to the rectum in specific pathological conditions) is required to interrupt the sequence from adenoma to cancer, and the frequent endoscopic screening of the individuals at risk is mandatory from the age of 10–14 years. However, it is imperative to have the best risk estimation and to submit to endoscopy only individuals that with high probability could develop colorectal lesions (Vasen et al. 2008).

A specific experience in pediatric setting has been reported by the Istituto Nazionale Tumori, Milan, describing 16 patients aged 13–18 years who underwent prophylactic total colectomy with a laparoscopic approach (Vitellaro et al. 2012). The laparoscopic surgery (less invasive as compared to open surgery) may have various advantages: it may require short hospital stay with acceptable postsurgical outcomes, and therefore it can be appealing for young patients. It is important to remember that the decision-making for prophylactic surgery for FAP may be an intricate process, in particular for very young individuals (depending on family experience, emotional stage, support, compliance). Laparoscopy can help in the anticipation of the prophylactic operation from the third to fifth decades of life (as was in the past) to the second decade: it can support the decision-making for prophylactic surgery in adolescent patients, thus reducing the risk of cancer. In addition, laparoscopy may reduce the risk of future occurrence of desmoid tumors (Vitellaro et al. 2012).

Similarly, wireless capsule endoscopy may be seen as a feasible and well-tolerated first screening examination in adolescent patients and can increase early adherence to a surveillance program (Cavallo et al. 2016).

FAP affects about 1 in 7000 individuals. Two types of FAP exist, and a relationship between the location of mutations in the gene and the phenotypic expression of FAP has been established (Vasen et al. 2008; Signoroni et al. 2010): the sparse or attenuated type (generally defined as AFAP) is characterized by hundreds of polyps, and the profuse type presents with thousands of polyps (Fig. 25.2). In general, adenomas tend to develop near puberty, although early childhood presentations can occur.

Another polyposis-causing gene was detected on chromosome 1p33-34, the MUTYH gene (OMIM n. 608456). Mutations in this gene have been found to be associated with milder form of polyposis named MAP. MUTYH germline mutations are related to an attenuated phenotype and have been reported in 10–30% of patients without an APC mutation. For these reasons, it could be considered another important biomarker in identifying polyposis and in particular attenuated phenotype patients. Recent studies have also demonstrated that germline MUTYH mutations predispose to colorectal cancer with an autosomal recessive pattern, accounting for up to 1% of these neoplasms. In this setting, biallelic MUTYH mutations have been found to be associated with a 93-fold excess risk of colorectal cancer, with almost complete penetrance by 60 years of age. Interestingly, in up to one third of these patients, no associated adenoma was found (Vasen et al. 2008; Kundu et al. 2006; Signoroni et al. 2010; Al-Sukhni et al. 2008). In contrast, the influence of monoallelic MYH mutations on colorectal risk remains controversial, although recent studies suggest a modest effect (Jenkins et al. 2006). The MUTYH gene encodes a member of the base excision repair system. This system is composed of three enzymes (MYH, OGG1, and MTH1) that contribute to protect cells against the mutagenic effects of aerobic metabolism. MUTYH is a DNA glycosylase, which acts at a third level of defense, and is responsible for the removal of adenines mispaired with 8-oxoguanine, one of the most mutagenic DNA products of oxidative DNA damage. Failure to correct these mispairs leads to somatic G:C→T:A transversions in target genes, namely, APC and KRAS. Somatic G:C→T:A transversions in the APC gene were described, and, in addition, G:C→T:A transversions in the KRAS gene were also observed in adenomas from AFAP patients (David et al. 2007).

Although MAP patients have milder disease, starting later in life, it should be considered that colorectal cancer was frequently found in these subjects and so they need strict surveillance programs like classical FAP patients, to reduce risk of developing cancer. Some reports have identified cases of upper gastrointestinal adenomas/polyps also in MAP patients, so also upper gastrointestinal tract needs controls (Bouguen et al. 2007).

The gastrointestinal tract is also affected in FAP: duodenal, particularly water papilla, and gastric polyps seem to be an important and typical manifestation of FAP patients but generally related to an adult age.

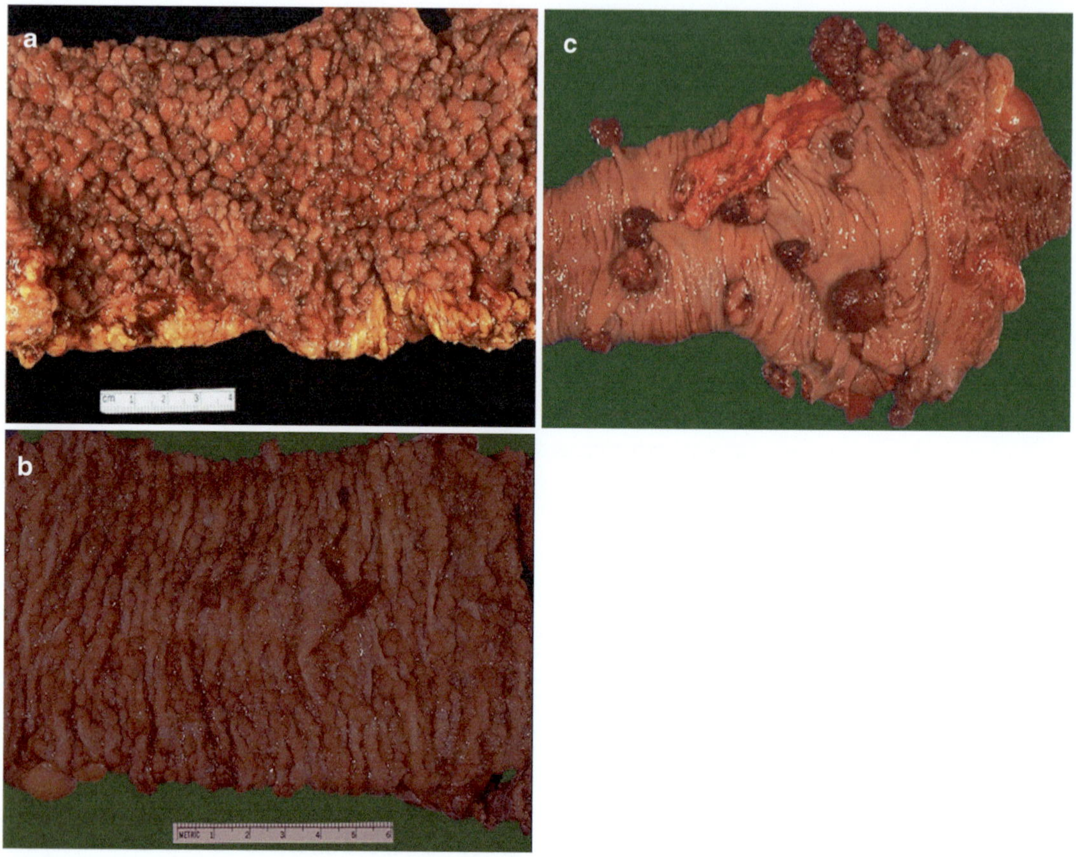

Fig. 25.2 The variability of FAP phenotype: (**a**) severe polyposis, (**b**) classical polyposis, (**c**) attenuated polyposis (see from previous edition, Fig. 30.1)

FAP is also associated with the development of extracolonic malignancies including thyroid carcinoma and hepatoblastoma. Clinical phenotype, including the presence of extracolonic abnormalities, appears to vary according to the site of the APC gene mutation and the presentation of modifying genes. After a diagnosis is made, annual sigmoidoscopy is recommended starting about 10 years of age (Table 25.1). As soon as polyps are identified, prophylactic colectomy can be considered at 15 years of age unless suspicious lesions are found earlier (Signoroni et al. 2010).

Two variants of FAP, with the same propensity to progress to CRC and extraintestinal disease manifestations, must be considered. One is Gardner syndrome in which FAP is associated with desmoid tumors, epidermoid cysts, fibromas, osteomas, and congenital hypertrophy of the retinal pigment epithelium. Patients with Gardner syndrome are at high risk to develop a desmoids of the abdominal wall and mesentery after colectomy, which can then be a leading cause of morbidity and mortality (Saab and Furman 2008a, b; Vasen et al. 2008; Signoroni et al. 2010).

Table 25.1 Colorectal surveillance protocol in family member at risk for (A) FAP

	Type of investigation	Lower age limit	Interval
Classical FAP	Sigmoidoscopy[a]	10–12 years	2 years[a]
AFAP	Colonoscopy	18–20 years	2 years[a]

From Vasen et al. (2008)
(A)FAP (attenuated) familial adenomatous polyposis
[a]Once adenomas are detected annual colonoscopy should be performed until colectomy is planned

Turcot syndrome is another FAP variant that includes multiple pediatric brain tumours (medulloblastoma, glioma, and ependymoma) in conjunction with FAP (Saab and Furman 2008a, b; Vasen et al. 2008; Signoroni et al. 2010).

25.2.2 Hamartomatous Polyposis Syndromes

Hamartomatous polyposis syndromes are a rare group of hereditary autosomal dominant disorders that comprise less than 1% of all hereditary colorectal cancers (Manfredi 2010). Hamartomatous polyps, in and of themselves, are benign entities; however, these hamartomatous polyposis syndromes have a malignant potential for the development of colorectal cancer as well as extracolonic cancers. Early detection and proper surveillance are vital to minimizing the risk of carcinoma.

The hamartomatous polyposis syndromes include juvenile polyposis syndrome (JPS); PTEN hamartoma tumor syndrome, which includes Cowden syndrome (CS) and Bannayan-Riley-Ruvalcaba syndrome (BRRS); and PJS (Manfredi 2010).

25.2.3 Peutz-Jeghers Syndrome

PJS, as with the other hamartomatous syndromes, is an autosomal dominant syndrome that is typified by its characteristic mucocutaneous pigmentation and intestinal hamartomatous polyps. The incidence of PJS is reported to be 1 in 150.000–200.000 individuals (Boardman 2002; Kutscher et al. 1960). Pigmentation is seen around the vermilion border of the lips in over 95% of cases, with the buccal mucosa being the second most common site (80%) (Utsunomiya et al. 1975) (Fig. 25.2). Other areas of pigmentation include the hands, feet, genitals, and around the nose and eyes. Pigmentation typically presents in early childhood and starts to fade with age usually after the start of puberty (Giardiello and Trimbath 2006).

Hamartomatous polyps in PJS are commonly found in the small intestine; however, they are also found in the stomach and colon. The number of polyps in the intestine may range from 1 to a complete carpeting of the gastrointestinal tract (Utsunomiya et al. 1975; Westerman and Wilson 1999). The most common presentation of PJS is abdominal pain secondary to intussusception. Other clinical presentations include anemia, melena, hematochezia, hematemesis, and obstruction. Approximately one third of PJS patients present in the first decade of life, with up to 60% presenting by the second or third decade (Giardiello and Trimbath 2006; Brosens et al. 2007).

The diagnosis of PJS is clinically established on the presence of histologic tissue that is consistent with hamartomatous polyps and two of the following criteria (Giardiello et al. 1987): a family history of PJS, the presence of mucocutaneous pigmentation (Fig. 25.3), and the presence of small bowel polyps.

PJS, as with the other hamartomatous syndromes, has an autosomal dominant pattern of inheritance with both familial and sporadic transmission. The gene associated with PJS is a serine-threonine kinase that is located on chromosome 19p13.3 (Hemminki et al. 1997). Hemminki and coworkers and Jenne and associates independently identified the gene in this region as *LKB1/STK11* (Hemminki et al. 1998; Jenne et al. 1998). This gene has been reported in 80% of patients with PJS. Common mutations are frameshift and nonsense mutations in exons 1–6; however, large

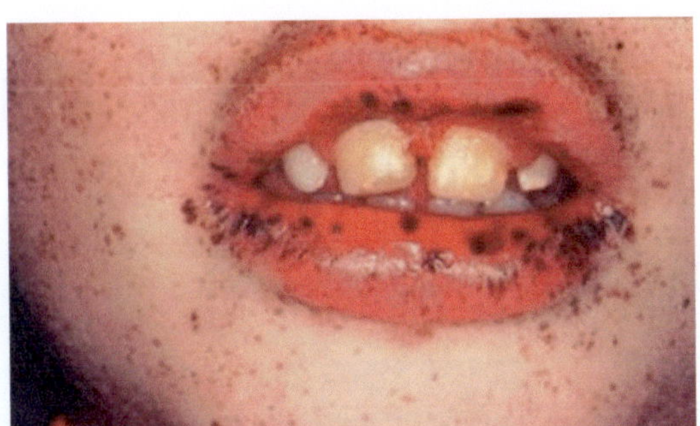

Fig. 25.3 Mucocutaneous pigmentation around lips in PJS

deletion mutations missed by direct sequencing have been recently described using multiple ligation probes (Volikos et al. 2006).

LKB1/STK11 is a tumor suppressor gene that encodes a serine-threonine kinase that phosphorylates and activates members of the AMPK-related subfamily of protein kinases (Forcet et al. 2005). LKB1/STK11 has an essential role in G1 cell cycle arrest, cell polarity, p53-dependent apoptosis, and cellular energy levels (Forcet and Billaud. 2007, Marignani 2005). *LKB1* (+/−) mice develop gastrointestinal polyps with histologic characteristics resembling those of human PJS polyps (Miyoshi et al. 2002).

Individuals with PJS are at risk for the development of colorectal, gastric, small intestinal, esophageal, and pancreatic cancers but generally not in pediatric age. PJS patients are also at risk for extraintestinal cancer such as lung, breast, ovarian, testicular, and endometrial cancers (Saab and Furman 2008a, b; Zbuk and Eng 2007; Giardiello and Trimbath 2006). A meta-analysis showed that the risk of developing any type of cancer by 64 years of age was 93% (relative risk of 15) (Giardiello et al. 2000).

25.2.4 PTEN Hamartoma Tumor Syndrome: Cowden Syndrome and Bannayan-Riley-Ruvalcaba Syndrome

CS is a rare autosomal dominant syndrome, with a reported incidence of 1 in 200.000 individuals (Nelen et al. 1997). This syndrome is characterized by macrocephaly, mucocutaneous lesions (such as facial trichilemmoma), acral keratosis, and papillomatous papules. It is also associated with thyroid, breast, and endometrial manifestations, including cancer in all of these areas (Zbuk and Eng 2007; Calva and Howe 2008; Starink et al. 1986). CS has been linked to Lhermitte-Duclos disease, which is characterized by hamartomas of the cerebellum (Albrecht et al. 1992). Hamartomatous polyps throughout the gastrointestinal tract are associated with this syndrome but are not as common as the extraintestinal findings associated with the syndrome. The incidence of gastrointestinal polyps in CS varies in the literature, ranging anywhere from 30% (Starink et al. 1986). It is generally thought that the incidence of gastrointestinal polyps in CS is less than that of BRRS, though this belief is debated in the literature (Eng 2000). Another gastrointestinal manifestation of CS is glycogenic acanthosis of the esophagus, which involves large benign glycogen-filled epithelial cells that are gray to white in color (McGarrity et al. 2003).

The BRRS is characterized by macrocephaly, developmental delays, pigmented speckling of the penis, lipomas, and hamartomatous polyps of the intestine. The incidence of gastrointestinal polyps in BRRS has been reported to be 45% (Gorlin et al. 1992).

CS and BRRS have an autosomal dominant inheritance pattern with variable penetrance. Both syndromes have been associated with the *PTEN* gene, which is located on chromosome 10q22-23.

The *PTEN* gene is a tumor suppressor gene that is also a tyrosine phosphatase that dephosphorylates tyrosine, serine, and threonine (Suzuki et al. 1998). PTEN is a negative regulator of the Akt/PKB signaling pathway (Suzuki et al. 1998; Waite and Eng 2002), which controls the levels of phosphoinositol triphosphate. PTEN is also involved in regulating cell cycle, apoptosis, and angiogenesis (Waite and Eng 2002; Chow and Baker 2006).

Individuals with CS are at risk for developing breast, thyroid, and endometrial cancers. The risk of adenocarcinoma of the breast has been reported to range from 30% to 50% in women with CS (Zbuk and Eng 2007; Starink et al. 1986; Eng 2000). In addition, there are reports of breast cancer in men with CS (Fackenthal et al. 2001). Individuals with CS are also subject to benign conditions of the breast such as fibrocystic disease (Starink et al. 1986). Thyroid abnormalities such as multinodular goiter and thyroglossal duct cysts are associated with this syndrome, as well as a 10% risk of thyroid cancer. CS patients also have a risk of leiomyomas, as well as an up to 10% risk of endometrial cancer; renal cell cancer has also been associated with CS (Starink et al. 1986). The risk of developing gastrointestinal carcinoma in CS is unclear at this point. It has been reported by some studies that there is no increased risk of gastrointestinal cancer; however, there are multiple case reports of gastric and colorectal cancer (Starink et al. 1986; Carlson et al. 1984).

In BRRS, the cancer risk is unclear. The limited number of patients with this disease makes it difficult to determine the risk; however, there have been case reports of breast and endometrial cancer (Marsh et al. 1999, Longy et al. 1998). With additional evidence supporting the idea that CS and BRRS are variable phenotypic expressions in the *PTEN* gene, it is therefore recommended that individuals with BRRS be considered at risk for malignancy, as with CS.

25.2.5 Juvenile Polyposis Syndrome

Juvenile polyps are the most common type of pediatric gastrointestinal polyps. Solitary juvenile polyps can develop at any age, though they appear most frequently in preschool children and have an incidence of 2% in children under 10 years of age. Solitary polyps are generally located in the rectosigmoid area and are usually considered to be a separate entity from JPS, which has an incidence of 1 in 100.000–160.000 individuals (Chow and Macrae 2005). A family history of juvenile polyps is found in 20–50% of patients with JPS, with an autosomal dominant inheritance pattern of variable penetrance (Chow and Macrae 2005; Attard and Young 2006).

The diagnosis of JPS is clinically established based on the presence of at least one of the following criteria (Jass et al. 1988; Giardiello et al. 1991): at least three to ten polyps detected on colonoscopy, polyps located outside of the colon, and any number of polyps in a patient with a family history of juvenile polyps (Table 25.2).

The gross appearance of a juvenile polyp is spherical to slightly lobular in shape, and most are pedunculated with long stalks (Horrilleno et al. 1957). In patients with JPS, polyps may have a multilobulated appearance of a villiform or papillary shape (Desai et al. 1995). Jass and colleagues reported that approximately 20% of polyps have the latter appearance (Jass et al. 1988). Polyp size can range from several millimeters to 3 cm. These polyps are typically very vascular, with a smooth and glistening appearance on the surface; however, they may also have an ulcerated surface from auto-infarction.

Table 25.2 Juvenile[a] polyposis syndrome (JPS) is diagnosed if at least one of the following clinical criteria is present

Criteria
More than five juvenile polyps of the colorectum
Multiple juvenile polyps of the upper and lower GI tract
Any number of juvenile polyps and a family history of juvenile polyps

[a]The term "juvenile" refers to the type of polyp not the age of onset of polyps. Juvenile polyps are hamartomas that develop from an abnormal collection of tissue elements normally present at this site

A family history of JPS is found in 20–50% of patients with JPS, with an autosomal dominant inheritance pattern of variable penetrance (Jass et al. 1988; Coburn et al. 1995). Three genes have been associated with JPS: *SMAD4*, *BMPR1A*, and *ENG*, all of which are part of the transforming growth factor-b (TGF-b) superfamily of proteins. The *PTEN* gene mutation in patients with juvenile polyposis is a controversial topic. It is generally thought that patients with the *PTEN* gene mutation likely represent CS or BRRS patients who have not yet expressed the extraintestinal clinical features of these conditions (Zbuk and Eng 2007).

Individuals with JPS are at risk for the development of colorectal, gastric, small intestinal, and pancreatic cancers. The risk of developing colorectal cancer from solitary juvenile polyps is thought to be negligible or nonexistent. However, individuals with JPS are at risk for developing adenomatous change and carcinoma. The incidence of colorectal cancer has been reported by Jass and associates to be 20.7%, with a mean age of 34 years (age range, 15–59 years) and an estimated cumulative colorectal cancer risk of 68% by 60 years of age (Jass et al. 1988).

25.2.6 Serrated Polyposis Syndrome (SPS)

The SPS is a heterogeneous disease (generally in adult age) defined by the presence of multiple serrated polyps throughout the colon, causing an increased risk (16%) of CRC (Carballal et al. 2016). The clinical definition of SPS is based on the fulfillment of one of the revised World Health Organization (WHO) criteria: (i) at least five serrated polyps proximal to the sigmoid colon, two of them larger than 10 mm; (ii) any number of serrated polyps proximal to the sigmoid colon in an individual with one first-degree relative with SPS; or (iii) more than 20 serrated polyps distributed throughout the colon (Rex et al. 2012). Patients with SPS are at high risk of developing colorectal cancer and need expert and intensive surveillance.

Being this entity mostly sporadic, generally not associated with family history, diagnosed between 50 and 60 years of age, and believed to be strongly associated with environmental factors (IJspeert et al. 2017), it has been suggested that, overall, SPS is not an inherited genetic syndrome but rather behaves as a complex disorder consequence of the interaction of genetic susceptibility and environment.

However, evidence indicates that a small proportion of cases may be due to an inherited genetic syndrome. In 2014, by performing WES in 20 SPS families, Gala et al. identified in two independent families a germline deleterious variant, c.337C>T (p.Arg113*), in the RING-type E3 *ubiquitin ligase RNF43* – inhibitor of the Wnt pathway (Gala et al. 2014). To date, a total of 13 carriers (seven families) of *RNF43* (likely) pathogenic variants have been reported, 12 of whom are affected with serrated polyposis and/or CRC (mean age at diagnosis, 44; range, 18–65). Moreover, knockout of *RNF43* contributes to an intestinal polyposis phenotype in mice (Koo et al. 2012).

25.3 Polymerase Proofreading-Associated Polyposis (PPAP)

POLE and POLD1 belong to the B family of replicative and repair DNA polymerases. In DNA replication, they act as the major catalytic and proofreading subunits of the POL epsilon and POL delta complexes, respectively, synthesizing the leading and lagging DNA strands (Nick McElhinny et al. 2008). They have a proofreading function, performed by their exonuclease domain, which detects and removes misincorporated bases in the daughter strand through failed complementary pairing with the parental strand (Miyabe et al. 2011). Germline pathogenic variants in human *POLE* and *POLD1* exonuclease domains have recently been reported to predispose to PPAP. This disease is characterized by multiple colorectal adenomas and carcinomas following an autosomal dominant pattern of inheritance and suspected high penetrance. Regarding associated phenotypes, pathogenic germline variants in *POLE* and *POLD1*were initially implicated in genetic predisposition to multiple polyposis and CRC (Palles et al. 2013). Later on, the phenotypic spectrum broadened to include other neoplasms such as endometrial cancer (Church et al. 2013), ovarian and brain tumors (Rohlin et al. 2014), pancreatic and small intestine cancer (Hansen et al. 2015), melanoma (Aoude et al. 2015), or a clinical phenotype suggestive of constitutional MMR deficiency (CMMRD) (Wimmer et al. 2017). In 2018, Buchanan et al., after estimating CRC risks for POLE mutation carriers, recommended annual colonoscopy screening and clinical management guidelines comparable to those currently recommended for Lynch syndrome or FAP (Buchanan et al. 2018).

25.4 Other Polyposes

25.4.1 *NTHL1*-Associated Polyposis

A recent whole-exome sequencing (WES) study, in which a stringently selected cohort of 51 cases who developed multiple adenomatous polyps at an early age in life were investigated, led to the identification of *NTHL1*, another base excision repair gene, as a predisposing gene for polyposis and CRC (Weren et al. 2015). Generally, carriers of biallelic *NTHL1* pathogenic variants may develop multiple adenomas in the colon and also tumors, including CRC and endometrial cancer.

25.4.2 *MSH3*-Associated Polyposis

Biallelic pathogenic variants of MSH3 gene, a mismatch repair gene, is not associated with Lynch syndrome but generally is associated with the presence of colorectal adenomatous polyposis. The phenotype observed in *MSH3* biallelic carriers largely resembles that of attenuated FAP, although still conserving some features of CMMRD occurring at more advanced age (not in the childhood) (Adam et al. 2016).

25.5 Lynch Syndrome

Lynch syndrome (once hereditary nonpolyposis colorectal cancer) is a rare hereditary disease that accounts for about 1–5% of all colorectal cancers (Gryfe 2009). It is an autosomal dominant condition caused by the mutation of one of several DNA mismatch repair (MMR) genes: MLH1, MSH2, MSH6, and PMS2, leading to microsatellite instability (MSI). The average age of colorectal cancer diagnosis in Lynch syndrome mutation carriers is 44 years, compared with 64 years in sporadic colorectal cancer. Individuals with a Lynch syndrome gene mutation have an estimated 80% lifetime risk of developing colorectal cancer. The identification of Lynch syndrome patients is fundamental to address them to correct intensive surveillance programs and to the right therapeutic strategies (Gryfe 2009).

The research criteria for defining Lynch syndrome were established by the International Collaborative Group (ICG) meeting in Amsterdam in 1990 and are known as the Amsterdam criteria. However, these criteria are not considered comprehensive; a number of families who do not meet these criteria, but have germline MMR gene mutations, have been reported. For this reason, another set of clinical criteria that can be used to identify Lynch syndrome families is the revised Bethesda guidelines. These criteria are less stringent for identifying families with MSI and germline mutations in one of the MMR genes (Mukherjee et al. 2010).

It is difficult to precisely determine the prevalence of HNPCC in children and adolescents with CRC. Case series reporting children and adolescents with colorectal cancer have not focused on the underlying genetic aspects of the tumor or genetic susceptibility of the families (Bethel et al. 1997; Vastyan et al. 2001a, b; Kam et al. 2004a, b). Single case reports describe adolescents with CRC with HNPCC, one 13-year-old with an MSH2 mutation (Madlensky et al. 1997), another 13-year-old with a PMS2 mutation (Hamilton et al. 1995), and a 14-year-old with an MLH1 mutation (Huang et al. 2001).

Extremely rarely MMR gene mutations can occur in homozygosis or compound heterozygous. This condition is known as CMMRD (constitutional mismatch repair deficiency) and generally brings to the development of hematologic malignancies, brain tumours, or both in their first decade of life (Durno and Gallinger 2006).

25.6 Multigene Panel

Recent advances in technology and research are rapidly changing the diagnostic approach to hereditary gastrointestinal cancer syndromes. Although the practice of clinical genetics is currently transitioning from targeted criteria-based testing to multigene panels, important challenges remain to be addressed.

The advent of next-generation sequencing (NGS) and the application to "whole-exome analysis" brought to the discovery of a lot of variants in human genome, but it is not easy to give them a significance of clinical impact. Moreover, NGS has enabled the massively parallel testing of multiple genes (panel-based testing). A wide range of multigene panels has been developed, and their use for the diagnosis of hereditary cancer has increased dramatically over the past 5 years (Fecteau et al. 2014; Gonzaga-Jauregui et al. 2012; Lapunzina et al. 2014). Although multigene testing has been proven to be an efficient approach for comprehensive, cost-effective, and time-saving evaluation of multiple genes

(Frey et al. 2015; Gallego et al. 2015; Hansen et al. 2017), its introduction into routine practice raises many concerns about its impact on result interpretation as well as patient counseling and management (Bombard et al. 2013; Maga et al. 2017).

Therefore, the introduction of panel-based testing in routine clinical practice will necessitate implementing novel genetic counseling models to ensure adequate pretest and posttest information provision and to better prepare patients for the possibility of results of uncertain clinical impact (Ricci et al. 2019).

25.6.1 Pediatric Series on Intestinal Carcinoma: Peculiarities of Disease When Arising in Children

Intestinal cancer is extremely rare in children and adolescents, and there is a limited list of published series, as shown in Table 25.3. Various reports have been published on a series of CRC in young people, but most of these studies included patients up to the age of 30 or more, treated over lengthy periods of time. As a matter of fact, the real number of prepubertal cases (or under 18-year-olds at least) is only a few dozen (Andersson and Bergdahl 1976; Rao et al. 1985; Lamego and Torloni 1989a, b; Taguchi et al. 1991a, b; Bhatia et al. 1999; Brown et al. 1992; Chantada et al. 2005; Chen et al. 2001; Chung et al. 1998; Cozart et al. 1993; Durno et al. 2005; Ferrari et al. 2008; Hill et al. 2007, Kam et al. 2004a, b; Karnak et al. 1999; Kravarusic et al. 2007; Lamego and Torloni 1989a, b; LaQuaglia et al. 1992; Lee et al. 1994; Minardi Jr et al. 1998; Pratt et al. 1999; Radhakrishnan and Bruce 2003; Rao et al. 1985; Rodriguez-Bigas et al. 1996; Salas-Valverde et al. 2009; Sebbag et al. 1997; Shahrudin and Noori 1997; Stones and McGill 2003; Sule and Mandong 1999; Taguchi et al. 1991a, b; Vastyan et al. 2001a, b; Singer and Hoellwarth 2012; Kim et al. 2013; Kaplan et al. 2013; Al-Tonbary et al. 2013; Rahman et al. 2014; Poles et al. 2016; Indini et al. 2017; Weber et al. 2016; Attard and Lawson 2019). The largest hospital-based series included 77 children and adolescents (up to 19 years of age) referring to the St. Jude Children's Research Hospital over a period of 40 years (Hill et al. 2007). A comprehensive literature review (Saab and Furman 2008a, b) and a population-based study using the SEER data (Sultan et al. 2010) were also published. The latter, in particular, compared the clinical features and outcomes of 159 patients less than 20 years old (only 12 cases were under 12 years old) with those of a large cohort of over 550.000 adult cases.

A relative small prospective nationwide cooperative pediatric series has been published in 2016 by the Italian TREP Project (period 2000–2015) (Indini et al. 2017). The study included 15 patients less than 18 years of age, treated at six pediatric oncology centers and prospectively registered in the TREP database. Twelve were CRC, two patients had small bowel cancer, and one had gastric carcinoma. That report described also the annual number of cases of GI tract carcinomas to be expected in Italy in the population aged 0–17 years according to Italian epidemiology data (AIRTum—Associazione Italiana Registri Tumori, the Italian network of population-based cancer registries), i.e., 1.75/year. The annual number of cases actually registered in the TREP database was 0.93, giving a ratio of observed to expected cases of 0.53 (Indini et al. 2017). The Italian study supported clinical findings already published by others. In fact, despite the limited sources, all the published experiences were consistent in drawing a similar picture, suggesting that CRC in children may behave differently when they occur in adults. Hallmarks of this tumor in the younger age groups are (1) a higher incidence of unfavorable aggressive histotypes, (2) an advanced clinical stage at onset (in many cases with peritoneal carcinomatosis), and (3) a worse survival rate for pediatric cases than for adults.

As for the first of these features, all the publications report frequently finding poorly differentiated or signet-ring or mucinous adenocarcinoma subtypes in children and adolescents. On the contrary, most tumors in adults are moderately or well differentiated. This may suggest that CRC in

Table 25.3 Published series on colorectal carcinoma of children and adolescents

Author	Main features
Rao (1985)	St. Jude Children's Research Hospital, Memphis; review of 30 pts < 25 years, in a 20-year period; inadequate rate of complete resection
Lamego and Torloni (1989a, b)	Review of 11 pts < 15 yrs; delayed diagnosis, advanced stage
Taguchi et al. (1991a, b)	Case report and review of 40 cases aged < 15 years reported in the Japanese literature; unfavorable prognosis (delayed diagnosis)
LaQuaglia et al. (1992)	Memorial Sloan-Kettering Cancer Center, New York; review of 29 pts < 21 yrs, in a 40-year period; poor outcome, high incidence of high-grade histologies
Brown (1992)	7 pts < 15 yrs, in a 28-year period, all 7 pts died of disease
Cozart (1993)	55 pts < 30 yrs from 24 different centers (Southwestern Surgical Congress Unusual Case Registry)
Rodriguez-Bigas (1996)	Retrospective review of 68 pts < 30 yrs (median age 27 yrs), in a 25-year period; poor prognosis
Shahrudin and Noori (1997)	Retrospective review of 4 pts < 20 yrs (out of 21 < 30 yrs), in a 5-year period
Sebbag (1997)	Case report of three adolescent patients
Chung (1998)	23 pts < 29 yrs (out of 110 < 40 yrs), in a 9-year period
Karnak (1999)	Retrospective review of 20 pts < 16 yrs, in a 25-year period
Pratt (1999)	St. Jude: 13 patients 11–23 years of age; 5-Fluorouracil, leucovorin, α-interferon for advanced disease
Bhatia (1999)	St. Jude: 53 pts < 21 years, seen from 1960 to 1998; increased risk of colorectal cancer in relatives
Sule and Mandong (1999)	35 cases < 30 yrs (median age 25 yrs)
Vastyan et al. (2001a, b)	7 cases < 15 yrs, in a 16-year period
Chen (2001)	Retrospective review of 28 cases < 20 yrs
Stones and McGill (2003)	3 cases <15 yrs, in a 5-year period
Radhakrishnan and Bruce (2003)	Record of 8 pts < 16 yrs; all died of tumor
Durno (2005)	Retrospective analysis of 16 cases <24 years; genetic analysis: inherited predisposition for early-onset cases
Chantada (2005)	Retrospective evaluation of 14 pts < 20 yrs
Kravarusic (2007)	7 children ≤ 18 yrs (1980–2004)
Hill (2007)	St. Jude: review of 77 children and adolescents (aged 7–19 years), from 1964 to 2003; high frequency of mucinous histology, poor outcomes
Ferrari (2008)	Istituto Nazionale Tumori, Milan, Italy: retrospective report of 7 children (<18 yrs), compared to 20 young adults (<30 yrs) and 2.340 older adults; young adults similar to older adult series
Salas-Valverde (2009)	Retrospective review of 11 children (7–17 years)
Sultan et al. (2010)	SEER (Surveillance, Epidemiology, and End Results) database; 159 children/adolescents (aged 4–20 years); high-risk features and worse outcome than adults
Singer and Hoellwarth (2012)	3 cases (12–16 years)
Kim (2013)	4 cases (11–14 years)
Kaplan (2013)	Retrospective review of 76 pts (<25 years) from 2003 to 2010
Al-Tonbary (2013)	3 cases (aged 12–13 years)
Rahman (2014)	7 cases
Poles et al. (2016)	Epidemiology series (US National Cancer Database); analysis of the subgroup of pts (n = 918) aged ≤ 21 years (1998–2011)
Indini (2017)	TREP Italian project: prospective cooperative nationwide series; 15 children/adolescents (<18 yrs); aggressive histology, advanced stage, poor outcomes
Weber (2016)	31 patients aged ≤ 18 years (1990–2012); a high percentage of pediatric CRC patients presented with a tumor predisposition syndrome and showed an especially favorable OS
Attard and Lawson (2019)	Epidemiology data on hospital admission (AHRQ online resource HCUPnet/KID database)

pediatric age is biologically more aggressive. The reasons for this situation remain substantially unclear. In addition to this high incidence of unfavorable histotypes, a particular MSI has also been reported in younger patients (Kim et al. 2003). New studies are needed to clarify speculative hypotheses on the tumorigenesis of childhood CRC differing from the well-known multistep process occurring in adults (which is assumed to take around 10 years) and probably taking an alternative, shorter path (Durno et al. 2005; Fearon 1997). The rarity of the tumor in childhood and the fact that tissue collections are unavailable make biological studies on the disease's pathogenesis extremely difficult.

The second peculiarity of CRC in children is the advanced stage at onset: in the SEER review, only 19% of children/adolescents had localized disease, while their chances of having distant spread were twice as high as in adults (Sultan et al. 2010). Clearly, the possible different biological aggressiveness of CRC in pediatric age may have a relevant role in determining the initial spread of the disease. However, some studies suggested that diagnostic delays may have a role as well (Karnak et al. 1999; Lamego and Torloni 1989a, b; Rao et al. 1985; Salas-Valverde et al. 2009): long symptom intervals have been reported on various occasions for children with CRC, e.g., in a recent Argentina series, the median time elapsing between the first symptoms and diagnosis was reportedly 3 months for patients less than 20 years old, as opposed to 1 month for those over 20 (Chantada et al. 2005). This finding may be related to the scarce awareness (not only of young people but also of their parents and physicians) that CRC can occur in this age group. It is assumed that adolescents do not get cancer, and particularly not this type, so little clinical attention is paid to telltale signs, and the rather vague and nonspecific symptoms (mild abdominal pain, constipation or diarrhea, hematochezia, weight loss) are often underestimated. Moreover, even when the disease is suspected, its diagnosis by means of a fiber-optic exam may be more difficult in children, and rectosigmoidoscopy may fail to identify the tumor, because of the relatively high frequency of right-sided lesions (while in most adult cases of colonic cancer, the tumor is usually located within 25 cm of the anus) (Ferrari et al. 2008).

Finally, pediatric CRC cases are characterized by a worse survival than adults. The study on the SEER series showed survival estimates at 5 and 10 years of 40% and 31% for children/adolescents and 60% and 54% for adults (Sultan et al. 2010); furthermore, no improvement in survival rates seemed to be between 1973 and 2005 for the children/adolescents included in the SEER database. The poor prognosis for pediatric CRC may be related to various factors. Above all, these tumors usually present in an advanced stage and with aggressive histological features. An advanced stage at diagnosis is a variable that affects survival not only in itself but also because it strongly reduces the chances of adequate surgery: CRC remains a primarily "surgical disease," and the rate of complete resection in children is reportedly suboptimal, to say the least (Rao et al. 1985). Whether the rarity of the tumor and the inexperience of pediatric oncologists and surgeons contribute to the poor outcome for children with CRC is hard to say, but it may be of interest to recall that some adult studies have identified the surgeon's experience and level of specialization as a prognostic variable (Simons et al. 1997; Porter et al. 1998).

It remains to be clarified whether and why GI carcinomas developing in pediatric age may have a different pathogenesis and more aggressive biological features, as compared to adult counterpart. In the model of adult colorectal carcinogenesis, cell transformation is the result of a slow, multistep process that includes many genetic changes, each contributing to the acquisition of an invasive phenotype (Tariq and Ghias 2016). This long process results in many cases in well- or moderately differentiated histology. Though it is still unclear, it is possible to hypothesize that the epithelial transformation process in pediatric age might follow different ways, with no age-related cell degeneration or association to environmental exposure to carcinogens.

25.6.2 Diagnosis

Initial signs and symptoms may be aspecific. Local symptoms include changes in bowel habit (new-onset constipation or diarrhea in the absence of another cause), rectal tenesmus and reduction in diameter of stool, bleeding, or increased presence of mucus. In advanced cases, bowel obstruction may occur (Fig. 25.4). In case of chronic occult bleeding, iron-deficiency anemia with fatigue, palpitations, and pallor may be the initial sign. Weight loss is a frequent constitutional symptom.

In case of suspected signs or symptoms, first-level investigations may be digital rectal exam, fecal occult blood test, abdominal ultrasound, and colonoscopy, with eventual biopsy. Tumor stage is based on surgery and histopathological diagnosis. Computed tomography (CT) scan and positron emission tomography (PET) are required for the detection of metastases. The level of carcinoembryonic antigen (CEA) in the blood and, less significantly, CA19-9 and CA 242 are markers of the disease (especially for adenocarcinoma). CEA may be used to monitor and assess response to treatment in patients with metastatic disease and can also be used to monitor recurrence.

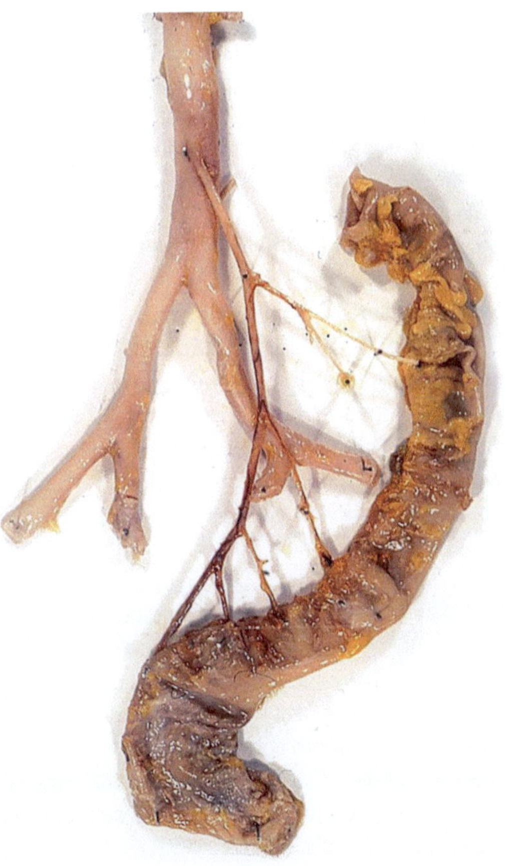

Fig. 25.4 From an autopsy: advanced rectal tumor (courtesy Dr. Gianfranco Gallino, Colorectal Cancer Surgery Unit, Fondazione IRCCS Istituto Nazionale Tumori, Milano, Italy)

The most common staging system is the TNM (for tumors/nodes/metastases) system, from the American Joint Committee on Cancer (AJCC), based on the level of the invasion of the primary tumor (mucosa, submucosa, muscularis propria, sierosa, or beyond) and the number of lymph node metastases (Fig. 25.5). Other previously used staging classifications are the Dukes and the Astler-Coller classifications.

25.7 Systemic Treatment

Since the rarity of the tumor prevents the feasibility of clinical trials dedicated to pediatric CRC, then the therapeutic recommendations should stay the same as for adults, i.e., a multimodality treatment guided by precise staging and histopathology (Gustafsson et al. 2019). In children with known polyposis syndromes, the presence of cancer early onset within a polyp can be cured with a polypectomy during a colonoscopy.

In other cases, the surgical approach is the standard care of localized CRC and must be timely adequate and radical. The resection of the colon with sufficient margins, en bloc with mesentery and lymph nodes (radical colectomy), is necessary. Laparoscopic-assisted colectomy may be used in some cases to reduce surgical morbidity. Since surgery remains the most reliable way to cure patients with CRC, early diagnosis is crucial: it is important for pediatricians to be aware that CRC does occur in children, so that they can refer suspect cases to a prime oncology center with expert physicians professionally dedicated to the management of this cancer in adults. Close cooperation with adult surgeons and medi-

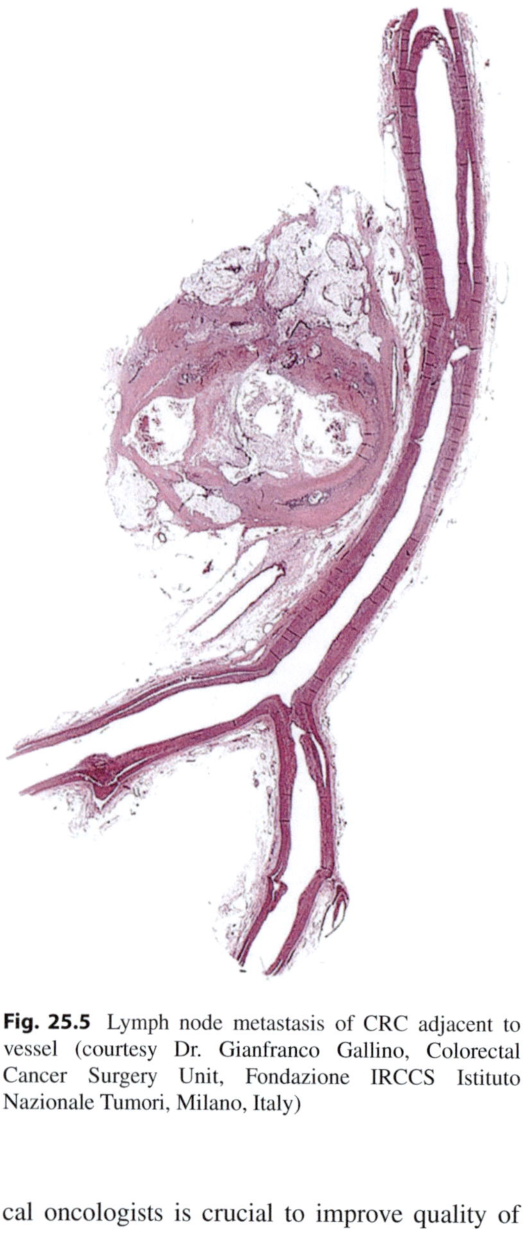

Fig. 25.5 Lymph node metastasis of CRC adjacent to vessel (courtesy Dr. Gianfranco Gallino, Colorectal Cancer Surgery Unit, Fondazione IRCCS Istituto Nazionale Tumori, Milano, Italy)

cal oncologists is crucial to improve quality of cure for children and adolescents with CRC.

25.7.1 Adjuvant Therapy

The indication for adjuvant treatment depends on the individual patient's staging and, again, should follow the recommendations in the guidelines for adult CRC. Survival for early stage tumors (TNM stage pT1-2, pN0, M0) is over 90% at 5 years: in this case, surgery may be the only treatment (Schmoll et al. 2012).

In patients with resected CRC stage II, the adjuvant therapy with 5-fluorouracil/folinic acid (5-FU/LV) or oral fluoropyrimidine is recommended only if one of the following risk factors is documented: pT4 tumor, tumor perforation, grade 3, and fewer than 12 lymph nodes resected (Benson 3rd et al. 2004; Shi et al. 2013). Data available about the use of an oral fluoropyrimidine/oxaliplatin (CAPOX scheme) combination were not able to show a significant survival benefit for the combination treatment when compared with fluoropyrimidine single agent. For all stage II tumors, the absolute benefit is about 2% in 3-year DFS, and there is very small benefit in overall survival, so adjuvant treatment is not recommended (André et al. 2009). Patients without high-risk features who have MSI-unstable (MSI-H/dMMR) tumor have a favorable prognosis and are not likely to derive significant benefit from adjuvant fluoropyrimidine-based therapy. It is suggested observation alone for these patients (Hong et al. 2012).

For patients with lymph node involvement (stage III), standard adjuvant chemotherapy is based on a combination of 5-FU/LV and oxaliplatin (FOLFOX-4 regimen) or CAPOX for a duration of 6 months, as defined by the pivotal MOSAIC and NSABP C-07 trials (André et al. 2009, 2015; Kuebler et al. 2007). Based on oxaliplatin neuropathy that depends on the duration of oxaliplatin treatment, it was conducted a pooled data from eight clinical adjuvant trials (the IDEA collaboration) to answer the question of whether 3 months of adjuvant therapy is as effective as 6 months of treatment with regard to 3-year DFS. With more than 12.800 patients pooled, the trial was not able to establish the non-inferiority for 3 months of treatment compared with 6 months of treatment. On the other hand, toxicities especially neuropathy were significantly less frequent in the 3-month cohort. However, a subgroup analysis showed that a higher risk recurrence (T4 or N2 stage) group 3 months of treatment was inferior to 6 months (Shi et al. 2018a, b).

Surgical resection is the cornerstone of curative therapy for patients with early stage rectal cancer (Kikuchi et al. 1995). Superficially invasive, small cancers may be effectively managed with limited surgery (such as local excision)

(Clancy et al. 2015). However, in the presence of deeply invasive tumors, a low anterior resection or abdominoperineal resection is required. For T3/T4 and/or clinically node-positive T1/T2 tumor, the addition of neoadjuvant chemoradiotherapy can enhance local control and cure rates and enhance the ability to preserve the anal sphincter (Sebag-montefiore et al. 2009; Bosset et al. 2006). Moreover, such therapy is characterized by more favorable long-term toxicity profile compared with postoperative treatment. Whereas a neoadjuvant chemoradiotherapy is a standard approach in order to prevent local recurrence, the postoperative chemotherapy after surgery remains important for the control of distant metastasis (Bosset et al. 2014; Sauer et al. 2004).

25.7.2 Metastatic Disease and Molecular Features

The treatment of metastatic colorectal cancer in pediatric patients has the same standard recommendation for IV stage in adults. A large cohort of pediatric CRC patients, from the National Cancer Data Base from 1998 to 2011, documented a more aggressive tumor histology and behavior in children, particularly in rectal cancer. Despite standard oncologic treatment, age ≤21 was a significant predictor of mortality. This is likely owing to worse tumor biology rather than treatment disparities and may signal the need for different therapeutic strategies (Poles et al. 2016).

Clinical evaluation of patients including performance status, comorbidities, history of cancer, and previous treatments is a strong prognostic and predictive factor for chemotherapy. Nevertheless, biological data including MSI status, RAS mutation, BRAF mutation, and tumor sidedness are critical in the choice of treatment. Colorectal cancers in younger patients often lack *KRAS* mutations and other cytogenetic anomalies seen in older patients. In a genomic study that used exome and RNA sequencing to identify mutational differences in CRCs of adults ($n = 30$), adolescents and young adults ($n = 30$), and children ($n = 2$), five genes (*MYCBP2*, *BRCA2*, *PHLPP1*, *TOPORS*, and *ATR*) were identified that were more frequently mutated in adolescents and young adult patients. These genes contained a damaging mutation and were identified through whole-exome sequencing and RNA sequencing. In addition, higher mutational rates in DNA mismatch and DNA repair pathways, such as *MSH2*, *BRCA2*, and *RAD9B*, were more prevalent in adolescent and young adult samples, but the results were not validated by RNA sequencing (Tricoli et al. 2018).

The optimal management of metastatic CRC needs the involvement of an expert multidisciplinary team, including medical oncologist, colorectal surgeon, a specialist hepatobiliary and/or lung surgeon, a diagnostic radiologist, and a radiation oncologist.

A recent review of nine clinical trials comprising 138 patients younger than 40 years demonstrated that the use of combination chemotherapy improved PFS and OS in these patients. Furthermore, OS and response rates to chemotherapy were similar to those observed in older patients (Blanke et al. 2011).

An active agent used in adults includes oxaliplatin, bevacizumab, panitumumab, cetuximab, aflibercept, and regorafenib (Saltz et al. 2008; Heinemann et al. 2014; Van Cutsem et al. 2012; Pratt et al. 1999).

Immunotherapy with ipilimumab and nivolumab demonstrated high response rates in pediatric patients aged 12 years and older with MSI-high or mismatch repair-deficient metastatic colorectal cancer who had disease progression after treatment with a fluoropyrimidine, oxaliplatin, and irinotecan (Overman et al. 2018).

In patients with oligometastatic disease, surgical resection may be an important therapeutic option with or without perioperative chemotherapy. In patients with unresectable metastases, a conversion therapy strategy including chemotherapy followed by surgical resection provided improved resection rate and a good long-term disease control.

Nevertheless, the systemic therapy, including cytotoxic agents and targeted agents, plays a dominant role in metastatic disease. The typical first-line chemotherapy backbone comprises a fluoropyrimidine (intravenous 5-FU or oral capecitabine) used in various combinations and schedules with irinotecan or oxaliplatin. In the last year, several studies have shown an increased activity and a better survivor of the monoclonal antibody bevacizumab in association with chemotherapy. The combination of FOLFOXIRI and bevacizumab has shown a better survivor respect to the doublet FOLFIRI plus bevacizumab (Cremolini et al. 2015). This combination is the paradigm of systemic therapy in patients with BRAF mutation (Loupakis et al. 2014).

The EGFR antibody agents cetuximab and panitumumab, in combination with cytotoxic agents, must be considered only in patients not harboring RAS mutation (Douillard et al. 2014; Tejpar et al. 2017).

Second- and third-line chemotherapy may be proposed on patients with good performance status and adequate organ function, and in patients in whom the initial chemotherapy backbone has failed, the chemotherapy backbone should be changed.

Regorafenib and trifluridine/tipiracil are recommended in patients pre-treated with fluoropyrimidines, oxaliplatin, irinotecan, and bevacizumab and in *RAS* wild-type patients with EGFR antibodies.

25.7.3 Risk Factors

Most of the risk factors related to lifestyle that have been described for adult CRC (smoking, diet high in red meat and low in fresh fruit and vegetables, alcohol, physical inactivity) are most unlikely to play a role in the pathogenesis of CRC in children. If prevention based on improving lifestyle is not feasible in children, focus should be directed to early diagnosis and increased surveillance in the case of familiarity.

Bowel cancer has been defined as the most frequent form of hereditary neoplasia (Fearon 1997), and approximately 10–20% of CRCs occur in familial aggregations, in particular in FAP and hereditary nonpolyposis colorectal cancer (HNPCC). Genetic counseling is mandatory for young people with CRC. However, the association of these inherited autosomal dominant conditions with early-onset tumors seems to be more common in young adults than in children (Durno et al. 2005; Ferrari et al. 2008; Losi et al. 2005; Leppert et al. 1987; Pinto et al. 2006), and it is still debated whether a family history of bowel cancer increases the risk of CRC in pediatric age, i.e., the tumorigenesis of childhood CRC may differ from the well-described multistep process of adult CRC (which usually takes around 10 years).

References

Adam R, Spier I, Zhao B, Kloth M, Marquez J, Hinrichsen I, Kirfel J, Tafazzoli A, Horpaopan S, Uhlhaas S, Stienen D, Friedrichs N, Altmüller J, Laner A, Holzapfel S, Peters S, Kayser K, Thiele H, Holinski-Feder E, Marra G, Kristiansen G, Nöthen MM, Büttner R, Möslein G, Betz RC, Brieger A, Lifton RP, Aretz S (2016) Exome sequencing identifies biallelic MSH3 germline mutations as a recessive subtype of colorectal adenomatous polyposis. Am J Hum Genet 99(2):337–351

Albrecht S, Haber RM, Goodman JC, Duvic M (1992) Cowden syndrome and Lhermitte-Duclos disease. Cancer 70:869–876

Al-Sukhni W, Aronson M, Gallinger S (2008) Hereditary colorectal cancer syndromes: familial adenomatous polyposis and lynch syndrome. Surg Clin North Am 88:819–844

Al-Tonbary Y, Darwish A, El-Hussein A, Fouda A (2013) Adenocarcinoma of the colon in children: case series and mini-review of the literature. Hematol Oncol Stem Cell Ther 6(1):29–33

Andersson A, Bergdahl L (1976) Carcinoma of the colon in children: a report of six new cases and a review of the literature. J Pediatr Surg 11:967–971

André T, Boni C, Navarro M, Tabernero J, Hickish T, Topham C, Bonetti A, Clingan P, Bridgewater J, Rivera F, de Gramont A (2009) Improved overall survival with oxaliplatin, fluorouracil, and leucovorin as adjuvant treatment in stage II or III colon cancer in the MOSAIC trial. J Clin Oncol 27(19):3109–3116

André T, de Gramont A, Vernerey D, Chibaudel B, Bonnetain F, Tijeras-Raballand A, Scriva A, Hickish T, Tabernero J, Van Laethem JL, Banzi M, Maartense E, Shmueli E, Carlsson GU, Scheithauer W, Papamichael D, Möehler M, Landolfi S, Demetter P, Colote S, Tournigand C, Louvet C, Duval A, Fléjou JF, de Gramont A (2015) Adjuvant fluorouracil, leucovorin, and oxaliplatin in stage II to III colon cancer: updated 10-year survival and outcomes according to BRAF mutation and mismatch repair status of the MOSAIC study. J Clin Oncol 33(35):4176–4187

Aoude LG, Heitzer E, Johansson P, Gartside M, Wadt K, Pritchard AL, Palmer JM, Symmons J, Gerdes AM,

Montgomery GW, Martin NG, Tomlinson I, Kearsey S, Hayward NK (2015) POLE mutations in families predisposed to cutaneous melanoma. Fam Cancer 14:621–628

Attard TM, Lawson CE (2019 Feb) Comparison of the demographic characteristics of pediatric and adult colorectal cancer patients: a national inpatient sample based analysis. World J Pediatr 15(1):37–41

Attard TM, Young RJ (2006) Diagnosis and management of gastrointestinal polyps: pediatric considerations. Gastroenterol Nurs 29:16–22

Benson AB 3rd, Schrag D, Somerfield MR, Cohen AM, Figueredo AT, Flynn PJ, Krzyzanowska MK, Maroun J, McAllister P, Van Cutsem E, Brouwers M, Charette M, Haller DG (2004) American Society of Clinical Oncology recommendations on adjuvant chemotherapy for stage II colon cancer. J Clin Oncol 22(16):3408–3419. Review

Bethel CA, Bhattacharyya N, Hutchinson C, Ruymann F, Cooney DR (1997) Alimentary tract malignancies in children. J Pediatr Surg 32:1004–1008. discussion 1008–1009

Bhatia S, Pratt CB, Sharp GB, Robison LL (1999) Family history of cancer in children and young adults with colorectal cancer. Med Pediatr Oncol 33:470–475

Blanke CD, Bot BM, Thomas DM et al (2011) Impact of young age on treatment efficacy and safety in advanced colorectal cancer: a pooled analysis of patients from nine first-line phase III chemotherapy trials. J Clin Oncol 29:2781–2786

Boardman LA (2002) Heritable colorectal cancer syndromes: recognition and preventive management. Gastroenterol Clin N Am 31:1107–1131

Bombard Y, Bach PB, Offit K (2013) Translating genomics in cancer care. J Natl Compr Canc Netw 11:1343–1353

Bosset JF, Collette L, Calais G, Mineur L, Maingon P, Radosevic-Jelic L, Daban A, Bardet E, Beny A, Ollier JC, EORTC Radiotherapy Group Trial 22921 (2006) Chemotherapy with preoperative radiotherapy in rectal cancer. N Engl J Med 355(11):1114–1123. Erratum in: N Engl J Med. 2007 Aug 16;357(7):728

Bosset JF, Calais G, Mineur L, Maingon P, Stojanovic-Rundic S, Bensadoun RJ, Bardet E, Beny A, Ollier JC, Bolla M, Marchal D, Van Laethem JL, Klein V, Giralt J, Clavère P, Glanzmann C, Cellier P, Collette L, EORTC Radiation Oncology Group (2014) Fluorouracil-based adjuvant chemotherapy after preoperative chemoradiotherapy in rectal cancer: long-term results of the EORTC 22921 randomised study. Lancet Oncol 15(2):184–190

Bouguen G, Manfredi S, Blayau M, Dugast C, Buecher B, Bonneau D, Siproudhis L, David V, Bretagne JF (2007) Colorectal adenomatous polyposis aAssociated with MYH mutations: genotype and phenotype characteristics. Dis Colon Rectum 50:1612–1617

Brosens LA, van Hattem WA, Jansen M, de Leng WW, Giardiello FM, Offerhaus GJ (2007) Gastrointestinal polyposis syndromes. Curr Mol Med 7:29–46

Brown RA, Rode H, Millar AJ et al (1992) Colorectal carcinoma in children. J Pediatr Surg 27:919–921

Buchanan DD, Stewart JR, Clendenning M, Rosty C, Mahmood K, Pope BJ, Jenkins MA, Hopper JL, Southey MC, Macrae FA, Winship IM, Win AK (2018) Risk of colorectal cancer for carriers of a germ-line mutation in POLE or POLD1. Genet Med 20:890–895

Calva D, Howe JR (2008) Hamartomatous polyposis syndromes. Surg Clin North Am 88:779–817

Carballal S, Rodríguez-Alcalde D, Moreira L, Hernández L, Rodríguez L, Rodríguez-Moranta F, Gonzalo V, Bujanda L, Bessa X, Poves C, Cubiella J, Castro I, González M, Moya E, Oquiñena S, Clofent J, Quintero E, Esteban P, Piñol V, Fernández FJ, Jover R, Cid L, López-Cerón M, Cuatrecasas M, López-Vicente J, Leoz ML, Rivero-Sánchez L, Castells A, Pellisé M, Balaguer F, Gastrointestinal Oncology Group of the Spanish Gastroenterological Association (2016) Colorectal cancer risk factors in patients with serrated polyposis syndrome: a large multicentre study. Gut. 65:1829–1837

Carlson GJ, Nivatvongs S, Snover DC (1984) Colorectal polyps in Cowden's disease (multiple hamartoma syndrome). Am J Surg Pathol 8:763–770

Cavallo D, Ballardini G, Ferrari A, Delconte G, Signoroni S, Sala P, Chiaravalli S, Massimino M, Bertario L, Vitellaro M (2016) Wireless capsule endoscopy in adolescents with familial adenomatous polyposis. Tumori J 102(1):40–44

Chantada GL, Perelli VB, Lombardi MG et al (2005) Colorectal carcinoma in children, adolescents, and young adults. J Pediatr Hematol Oncol 27:39–41

Chen LK, Hwang SJ, Li AF et al (2001) Colorectal cancer in patients 20 years old or less in Taiwan. South Med J 94:1202–1205

Chow LM, Baker SJ (2006) PTEN function in normal and neoplastic growth. Cancer Lett 241:184–196

Chow E, Macrae F (2005) A review of juvenile polyposis syndrome. J Gastroenterol Hepatol 20:1634–1640

Chung YF, Eu KW, Machin D et al (1998) Young age is not a poor prognostic marker in colorectal cancer. Br J Surg 85:1255–1259

Church DN, Briggs SE, Palles C, Domingo E, Kearsey SJ, Grimes JM, Gorman M, Martin L, Howarth KM, Hodgson SV, NSECG Collaborators, Kaur K, Taylor J, Tomlinson IP (2013) DNA polymerase ε and δ exonuclease domain mutations in endometrial cancer. Hum Mol Genet 22(14):2820–2828

Clancy C, Burke JP, Albert MR, O'Connell PR, Winter DC (2015) Transanal endoscopic microsurgery versus standard transanal excision for the removal of rectal neoplasms: a systematic review and meta-analysis. Dis Colon Rectum 58(2):254–261

Coburn MC, Pricolo VE, DeLuca FG, Bland KI (1995) Malignant potential in intestinal juvenile polyposis syndromes. Ann Surg Oncol 2:386–391

Cozart DT, Lang NP, Hauer-Jensen M (1993) Colorectal cancer in patients under 30 years of age. Contributors to the Southwestern Surgical Congress Unusual Case Registry. Am J Surg 166:764–767

Cremolini C, Loupakis F, Antoniotti C, Lupi C, Sensi E, Lonardi S, Mezi S, Tomasello G, Ronzoni M, Zaniboni A, Tonini G, Carlomagno C, Allegrini G, Chiara S, D'Amico M, Granetto C, Cazzaniga M, Boni L, Fontanini G, Falcone A (2015) FOLFOXIRI plus bevacizumab versus FOLFIRI plus bevacizumab as first-line treatment of patients with metastatic colorectal cancer: updated overall survival and molecular subgroup analyses of the open-label, phase 3 TRIBE study. Lancet Oncol 16(13):1306–1315

David SS, O'Shea VL, Kundu S (2007) Base-excision repair of oxidative DNA damage. Nature 447:941–950

Desai DC, Neale KF, Talbot IC, Hodgson SV, Phillips RK (1995) Juvenile polyposis. Br J Surg 82:14–17

Douillard JY, Siena S, Cassidy J, Tabernero J, Burkes R, Barugel M, Humblet Y, Bodoky G, Cunningham D, Jassem J, Rivera F, Kocákova I, Ruff P, Błasińska-Morawiec M, Smakal M, Canon JL, Rother M, Oliner KS, Tian Y, Xu F, Sidhu R (2014) Final results from PRIME: randomized phase III study of panitumumab with FOLFOX4 for first-line treatment of metastatic colorectal cancer. Ann Oncol 25(7):1346–1355

Durno CA, Gallinger S (2006) Genetic predisposition to colorectal cancer: new pieces in the pediatric puzzle. J Pediatr Gastroenterol Nutr 43:5–15. Review

Durno C, Aronson M, Bapat B et al (2005) Family history and molecular features of children, adolescents, and young adults with colorectal carcinoma. GUT 54:1146–1150

Fackenthal JD, Marsh DJ, Richardson AL, Cummings SA, Eng C et al (2001) Male breast cancer in Cowden syndrome patients with germline PTEN mutations. J Med Genet 38:159–164

Fearon ER (1997) Human cancer syndromes: clues to the origin and nature of cancer. Science 278:1043–1050

Fecteau H, Vogel KJ, Hanson K, Morrill-Cornelius S (2014) The evolution of cancer risk assessment in the era of next generation sequencing. J Genet Couns 23:633–639

Ferrari A, Rognone A, Casanova M et al (2008) Colorectal carcinoma in children and adolescents: the experience of the Istituto Nazionale Tumori of Milan, Italy. Pediatr Blood Cancer 50:588–593

Ferrari A, Casanova M, Massimino M, Sultan I (2010) Peculiar features and tailored management of adult cancers occurring in pediatric age. Expert Rev Anticancer Ther 10:1837–1851

Forcet C, Billaud M (2007) Dialogue between LKB1 and AMPK: a hot topic at the cellular pole. Sci STKE 2007(404):pe51

Forcet C, Etienne-Manneville S, Gaude H, Fournier L, Debilly S et al (2005) Functional analysis of Peutz-Jeghers mutations reveals that the LKB1 C-terminal region exerts a crucial role in regulating both the AMPK pathway and the cell polarity. Hum Mol Genet 14:1283–1292

Frey MK, Kim SH, Bassett RY, Martineau J, Dalton E, Chern JY, Blank SV (2015) Rescreening for genetic mutations using multi-gene panel testing in patients who previously underwent non-informative genetic screening. Gynecol Oncol 139:211–215

Gala MK, Mizukami Y, Le LP, Moriichi K, Austin T, Yamamoto M, Lauwers GY, Bardeesy N, Chung DC (2014) Germline mutations in oncogene-induced senescence pathways are associated with multiple sessile serrated adenomas. Gastroenterology 146:520–529

Gallego CJ, Shirts BH, Bennette CS, Guzauskas G, Amendola LM, Horike-Pyne M, Hisama FM, Pritchard CC, Grady WM, Burke W, Jarvik GP, Veenstra DL (2015) Next-generation sequencing panels for the diagnosis of colorectal cancer and polyposis syndromes: a cost-effectiveness analysis. J Clin Oncol 33:2084–2091

Giardiello FM, Trimbath JD (2006) Peutz-Jeghers syndrome and management recommendations. Clin Gastroenterol Hepatol 4:408–415

Giardiello FM, Welsh SB, Hamilton SR, Offerhaus GJ, Gittelsohn AM et al (1987) Increased risk of cancer in the Peutz-Jeghers syndrome. N Engl J Med 316:1511–1514

Giardiello FM, Hamilton SR, Kern SE, Offerhaus GJ, Green PA et al (1991) Colorectal neoplasia in juvenile polyposis or juvenile polyps. Arch Dis Child 66:971–975

Giardiello FM, Brensinger JD, Tersmette AC, Goodman SN, Petersen GM et al (2000) Very high risk of cancer in familial Peutz-Jeghers syndrome. Gastroenterology 119:1447–1453

Gonzaga-Jauregui C, Lupski JR, Gibbs RA (2012) Human genome sequencing in health and disease. Annu Rev Med 63:35–61

Gorlin RJ, Cohen MM Jr, Condon LM, Burke BA (1992) Bannayan-Riley-Ruval-caba syndrome. Am J Med Genet 44:307–314

Gryfe R (2009) Inherited colorectal cancer syndromes. Clin Colon Rectal Surg 22:198–208

Gustafsson UO, Scott MJ, Hubner M, Nygren J, Demartines N, Francis N, Rockall TA, Young-Fadok TM, Hill AG, Soop M, de Boer HD, Urman RD, Chang GJ, Fichera A, Kessler H, Grass F, Whang EE, Fawcett WJ, Carli F, Lobo DN, Rollins KE, Balfour A, Baldini G, Riedel B, Ljungqvist O (2019) Guidelines for perioperative care in elective colorectal surgery: Enhanced Recovery After Surgery (ERAS®) society recommendations: 2018. World J Surg 43(3):659–695

Hamilton SR, Liu B, Parsons RE, Papadopoulos N, Jen J, Powell SM, Krush AJ, Berk T, Cohen Z, Tetu B et al (1995) The molecular basis of Turcot's syndrome. N Engl J Med 332:839–847

Hansen MF, Johansen J, Bjørnevoll I, Sylvander AE, Steinsbekk KS, Sætrom P, Sandvik AK, Drabløs F, Sjursen W (2015) A novel POLE mutation associated with cancers of colon, pancreas, ovaries and small intestine. Fam Cancer 14:437–448

Hansen MF, Johansen J, Sylvander AE, Bjørnevoll I, Talseth-Palmer BA, Lavik LAS, Xavier A, Engebretsen LF, Scott RJ, Drabløs F, Sjursen W (2017) Use of multigene-panel identifies pathogenic variants in several CRC-predisposing genes in patients previously tested for Lynch Syndrome. Clin Genet 92:405–414

Heinemann V, von Weikersthal LF, Decker T et al (2014) FOLFIRI plus cetuximab versus FOLFIRI plus bevacizumab as first-line treatment for patients with metastatic colorectal cancer (FIRE-3): a randomised, open-label, phase 3 trial. Lancet Oncol 15:1065–1075

Hemminki A, Tomlinson I, Markie D, Järvinen H, Sistonen P et al (1997) Localization of a susceptibility locus for Peutz-Jeghers syndrome to 19p using comparative genomic hybridization and targeted linkage analysis. Nat Genet 15:87–90

Hemminki A, Markie D, Tomlinson I, Avizienyte E, Roth S et al (1998) A serine/threonine kinase gene defective in Peutz-Jeghers syndrome. Nature 391:184–187

Hill DA, Furman WL, Billups CA et al (2007) Colorectal carcinoma in childhood and adolescence: a clinicopathologic review. J Clin Oncol 25:5808–5814

Hong SP, Min BS, Kim TI, Cheon JH, Kim NK, Kim H, Kim WH (2012) The differential impact of microsatellite instability as a marker of prognosis and tumour response between colon cancer and rectal cancer. Eur J Cancer 48(8):1235–1243

Horrilleno EG, Eckert C, Ackerman LV (1957) Polyps of the rectum and colon in children. Cancer 10:1210–1220

Huang SC, Lavine JE, Boland PS, Newbury RO, Kolodner R, Pham TT, Arnold CN, Boland CR, Carethers JM (2001) Germline characterization of early-aged onset of hereditary non-polyposis colorectal cancer. J Pediatr 138:629–635

IJspeert JE, Rana SA, Atkinson NS, van Herwaarden YJ, Bastiaansen BA, van Leerdam ME, Sanduleanu S, Bisseling TM, Spaander MC, Clark SK, Meijer GA, van Lelyveld N, Koornstra JJ, Nagtegaal ID, East JE, Latchford A, Dekker E, Dutch Workgroup Serrated Polyps & Polyposis (WASP) (2017) Clinical risk factors of colorectal cancer in patients with serrated polyposis syndrome: a multicentre cohort analysis. Gut 66:278–284

Indini A, Bisogno G, Cecchetto G et al (2017) Gastrointestinal tract carcinoma in pediatric and adolescent age: the Italian TREP project experience. Pediatr Blood Cancer 64(12):e26658

Jass JR, Williams CB, Bussey HJ, Morson BC (1988) Juvenile polyposis—a precancerous condition. Histopathology 13:619–630

Jenkins MA, Croitoru ME, Monga N, Cleary SP, Cotterchio M, Hopper JL, Gallinger S (2006) Risk of colorectal cancer in monoallelic and biallelic carriers of MYH mutations: a population-based case-family study. Cancer Epidemiol Biomark Prev 15:312–314

Jenne DE, Reimann H, Nezu J, Friedel W, Loff S et al (1998) Peutz-Jeghers syndrome is caused by mutations in a novel serine threonine kinase. Nat Genet 18:38–43

Kam MH, Eu KW, Barben CP et al (2004a) Colorectal cancer in the young: a 12 year review of patients 30 years or less. Colorectal Dis 6:191–194

Kam MH, Eu KW, Barben CP, Seow-Choen F (2004b) Colorectal cancer in the young: a 12-year review of patients 30 years or less. Colorectal Dis 6:191–194

Kaplan MA, Isikdogan A, Gumus M, Arslan UY, Geredeli C, Ozdemir N et al (2013) Childhood, adolescents, and young adults (≤25 y) colorectal cancer: study of Anatolian Society of Medical Oncology. J Pediatr Hematol Oncol 35(2):83–89

Karnak I, Ciftci AO, Senocak ME et al (1999) Colorectal carcinoma in children. J Pediatr Surg 34:1499–1504

Kikuchi R, Takano M, Takagi K, Fujimoto N, Nozaki R, Fujiyoshi T, Uchida Y (1995) Management of early invasive colorectal cancer. Risk of recurrence and clinical guidelines. Dis Colon Rectum 38(12):1286–1295

Kim HC, Kim CN, Yu CS et al (2003) Methylation of the hMLH1 and hMSH2 promoter in early-onset sporadic colorectal carcinomas with microsatellite instability. Int J Colorectal Dis 18:196–202

Kim G, Baik SH, Lee KY, Hur H, Min BS, Lyu CJ et al (2013) Colon carcinoma in childhood: review of the literature with four case reports. Int J Colorectal Dis 28:157–164

Koo BK, Spit M, Jordens I, Low TY, Stange DE, van de Wetering M, van Es JH, Mohammed S, Heck AJ, Maurice MM, Clevers H (2012) Tumour suppressor RNF43 is a stem-cell E3 ligase that induces endocytosis of Wnt receptors. Nature 30(488):665–669

Kravarusic D, Feigin E, Dlugy E et al (2007) Colorectal carcinoma in childhood: a retrospective multicenter study. J Pediatr Gastroenterol Nutr 44:209–211

Kuebler JP, Wieand HS, O'Connell MJ, Smith RE, Colangelo LH, Yothers G, Petrelli NJ, Findlay MP, Seay TE, Atkins JN, Zapas JL, Goodwin JW, Fehrenbacher L, Ramanathan RK, Conley BA, Flynn PJ, Soori G, Colman LK, Levine EA, Lanier KS, Wolmark N (2007) Oxaliplatin combined with weekly bolus fluorouracil and leucovorin as surgical adjuvant chemotherapy for stage II and III colon cancer: results from NSABP C-07. J Clin Oncol 25(16):2198–2204

Kundu JK, Choi KY, Surh YJ (2006) beta-Catenin-mediated signaling: a novel molecular target for chemoprevention with anti-inflammatory substances. Biochim Biophys Acta 1765:14–24

Kutscher AH, Zegarelli EV, Rankow RM, Slaughter TW (1960) Incidence of Peutz-Jeghers syndrome. Am J Dig Dis 5:576–577

Lamego CM, Torloni H (1989a) Colorectal adenocarcinoma in childhood and adolescence. Report of 11 cases and review of the literature. Pediatr Radiol 19:504–508

Lamego CM, Torloni H (1989b) Colorectal adenocarcinoma in childhood and adolescent. Report of 11 cases and review of the literature. Pediatr Radiol 19:504–508

Lapunzina P, López RO, Rodríguez-Laguna L, García-Miguel P, Martínez AR, Martínez-Glez V (2014) Impact of NGS in the medical sciences: genetic syndromes with an increased risk of developing cancer as an example of the use of new technologies. Genet Mol Biol 37:241–249

LaQuaglia MP, Heller G, Filippa DA et al (1992) Prognostic factors and outcome in patients 21 years and under with colorectal carcinoma. J Pediatr Surg 27:1085–1089

Lee PY, Fletcher WS, Sullivan ES et al (1994) Colorectal cancer in young patients: characteristics and outcome. Am Surg 60:607–612

Leppert M, Dobbs M, Scambler P et al (1987) The gene for familial polyposis coli maps to the long arm of chromosome 5. Science 238:1411–1413

Longy M, Coulon V, Duboue B, David A, Larrègue M et al (1998) Mutations of PTEN in patients with Bannayan-Riley-Ruvalcaba phenotype. J Med Genet 35:886–889

Losi L, Di Gregorio C, Pedroni M et al (2005) Molecular genetic alterations and clinical features in early-onset colorectal carcinomas and their role for the recognition of hereditary cancer syndromes. Am J Gastroenterol 100:2280–2287

Loupakis F, Cremolini C, Salvatore L, Masi G, Sensi E, Schirripa M, Michelucci A, Pfanner E, Brunetti I, Lupi C, Antoniotti C, Bergamo F, Lonardi S, Zagonel V, Simi P, Fontanini G, Falcone A (2014) FOLFOXIRI plus bevacizumab as first-line treatment in BRAF mutant metastatic colorectal cancer. Eur J Cancer 50(1):57–63

Madlensky L, Bapat B, Redston M, Pearl R, Gallinger S, Cohen Z (1997) Using genetic information to make surgical decisions: report of a case of a 13-year-old boy with colon cancer. Dis Colon Rectum 40:240–243

Maga T, Balay L, Jung B (2017) Advantages and some remaining challenges in hereditary gastrointestinal cancer panel testing. Clin Transl Gastroenterol 8(5):e92

Manfredi M (2010) Hereditary hamartomatous polyposis syndromes. Gastroenterol Hepatol 6:185–196

Marignani PA (2005) LKB1, the multitasking tumour suppressor kinase. J Clin Pathol 58:15–19

Marsh DJ, Kum JB, Lunetta KL, Bennett MJ, Gorlin RJ et al (1999) PTEN mutation spectrum and genotype-phenotype correlations in Bannayan-Riley-Ruvalcaba syndrome suggest a single entity with Cowden syndrome. Hum Mol Genet 8:1461–1472

McGarrity TJ, Wagner Baker MJ, Ruggiero FM, Thiboutot DM, Hampel H et al (2003) GI polyposis and glycogenic acanthosis of the esophagus associated with PTEN mutation positive Cowden syndrome in the absence of cutaneous manifestations. Am J Gastroenterol 98:1429–1434

Minardi AJ Jr, Sittig KM, Zibari GB et al (1998) Colorectal cancer in the young patients. Am Surg 64:849–853

Miyabe I, Kunkel TA, Carr AM (2011) The major roles of DNA polymerases epsilon and delta at the eukaryotic replication fork are evolutionarily conserved. PLoS Genet 7(12):e1002407

Miyoshi H, Nakau M, Ishikawa TO, Seldin MF, Oshima M, Taketo MM (2002) Gastrointestinal hamartomatous polyposis in Lkb1 heterozygous knockout mice. Cancer Res 62:2261–2266

Mukherjee A, McGarrity TJ, Ruggiero F, Koltun W, McKenna K, Poritz L, Baker MJ (2010) The revised Bethesda guidelines: extent of utilization in a university hospital medical center with a cancer genetics program. Hered Cancer Clin Pract 22(8):9

Nelen MR, van Staveren WC, Peeters EA, Hassel MB, Gorlin RJ et al (1997) Germline mutations in the PTEN/MMAC1 gene in patients with Cowden disease. Hum Mol Genet 6:1383–1387

Nick McElhinny SA, Gordenin DA, Stith CM, Burgers PM, Kunkel TA (2008) Division of labor at the eukaryotic replication fork. Mol Cell 30:137–144

Overman MJ, Lonardi S, Wong KYM et al (2018) Durable clinical benefit with Nivolumab Plus Ipilimumab in DNA Mismatch repair-deficient/microsatellite instability-high metastatic colorectal cancer. J Clin Oncol 36:773–779

Palles C, Cazier JB, Howarth KM, Domingo E, Jones AM, Broderick P, Kemp Z, Spain SL, Guarino E, Salguero I, Sherborne A, Chubb D, Carvajal-Carmona LG, Ma Y, Kaur K, Dobbins S, Barclay E, Gorman M, Martin L, Kovac MB, Humphray S, CORGI Consortium, WGS500 Consortium, Lucassen A, Holmes CC, Bentley D, Donnelly P, Taylor J, Petridis C, Roylance R, Sawyer EJ, Kerr DJ, Clark S, Grimes J, Kearsey SE, Thomas HJ, McVean G, Houlston RS, Tomlinson I (2013) Germline mutations affecting the proofreading domains of POLE and POLD1 predispose to colorectal adenomas and carcinomas. Nat Genet 45:136–144

Parkin DM (2001) Global cancer statistics in the year 2000. Lancet Oncol **2**:533–543

Pinto C, Veiga I, Pinheiro M et al (2006) MSH6 germline mutations in early-onset colorectal cancer patients without family history of the disease. Br J Cancer 95:752–756

Poles GC, Clark DE, Mayo SW, Beierle EA, Goldfarb M, Gow KW et al (2016) Colorectal carcinoma in pediatric patients: a comparison with adult tumors, treatment and outcomes from the National Cancer Database. J Pediatr Surg 51(7):1061–1066

Porter GA, Soskolne CL, Yakimets WW, Newman SC (1998) Surgeon-related factors and outcome in rectal cancer. Ann Surg 227:157–167

Pratt CB, Rao BN, Merchant TE et al (1999) Treatment of colorectal carcinoma in adolescents and young adults with surgery, 5-fluorouracil/leucovorin/interferon-alpha 2a and radiation therapy. Med Pediatr Oncol 32:459–460

Radhakrishnan CN, Bruce J (2003) Colorectal cancers in children without any predisposing factors. A report of eight cases and review of the literature. Eur J Pediatr Surg 13:66–68

Rahman MA, Chowdhury TK, Bhuiyan MA, Al Farooq MA, Sajid MM, Banu T (2014) Colorectal carcinoma in first decade of life: our experience. Pediatr Surg Int 30:847–851

Rao BN, Pratt CB, Fleming ID et al (1985) Colon carcinoma in children and adolescents. A review of 30 cases. Cancer 55:1322–1326

Rex DK, Ahnen DJ, Baron JA, Batts KP, Burke CA, Burt RW, Goldblum JR, Guillem JG, Kahi CJ, Kalady MF, O'Brien MJ, Odze RD, Ogino S, Parry S, Snover DC, Torlakovic EE, Wise PE, Young J, Church J (2012) Serrated lesions of the colorectum: review and recommendations from an expert panel. Am J Gastroenterol 107:1315–1329. quiz 1314, 1330

Ricci MT, Volorio S, Signoroni S, Mariani P, Mariette F, Sardella D, Pensotti V, Vitellaro M (2019) Development, technical validation, and clinical application of a multigene panel for hereditary gastrointestinal cancer and polyposis. Tumori J 8:300891619847085

Rodriguez-Bigas MA, Mahoney MC, Weber TK et al (1996) Colorectal cancer in patients aged 30 years or younger. Surg Oncol 5:189–194

Rohlin A, Zagoras T, Nilsson S, Lundstam U, Wahlström J, Hultén L, Martinsson T, Karlsson GB, Nordling M (2014) A mutation in POLE predisposing to a multitumour phenotype. Int J Oncol 45:77–81

Saab R, Furman WL (2008a) Epidemiology and management options for colorectal cancer in children. Paediatr Drugs 10:177–192

Saab R, Furman WL (2008b) Epidemiology and management options for colorectal cancer in children. Pediatr Drugs 10:177–192

Salas-Valverde S, Lizano A, Gamboa Y et al (2009) Colon carcinoma in children and adolescents: prognostic factors and outcome—a review of 11 cases. Pediatr Surg Int 25:1073–1076

Saltz LB, Clarke S, Díaz-Rubio E et al (2008) Bevacizumab in combination with oxaliplatin-based chemotherapy as first-line therapy in metastatic colorectal cancer: a randomized phase III study. J Clin Oncol 26:2013–2019

Sauer R, Becker H, Hohenberger W, Rödel C, Wittekind C, Fietkau R, Martus P, Tschmelitsch J, Hager E, Hess CF, Karstens JH, Liersch T, Schmidberger H, Raab R, German Rectal Cancer Study Group (2004) Preoperative versus postoperative chemoradiotherapy for rectal cancer. N Engl J Med 351(17):1731–1740

Schmoll HJ, Van Cutsem E, Stein A, Valentini V, Glimelius B, Haustermans K, Nordlinger B, van de Velde CJ, Balmana J, Regula J, Nagtegaal ID, Beets-Tan RG, Arnold D, Ciardiello F, Hoff P, Kerr D, Köhne CH, Labianca R, Price T, Scheithauer W, Sobrero A, Tabernero J, Aderka D, Barroso S, Bodoky G, Douillard JY, El Ghazaly H, Gallardo J, Garin A, Glynne-Jones R, Jordan K, Meshcheryakov A, Papamichail D, Pfeiffer P, Souglakos I, Turhal S, Cervantes A (2012) ESMO Consensus Guidelines for management of patients with colon and rectal cancer. a personalized approach to clinical decision making. Ann Oncol 23(10):2479–2516

Sebag-Montefiore D, Stephens RJ, Steele R, Monson J, Grieve R, Khanna S, Quirke P, Couture J, de Metz C, Myint AS, Bessell E, Griffiths G, Thompson LC, Parmar M (2009) Preoperative radiotherapy versus selective postoperative chemoradiotherapy in patients with rectal cancer (MRC CR07 and NCIC-CTG C016): a multicentre, randomised trial. Lancet 373(9666):811–820

Sebbag G, Lantsberg L, Arish A et al (1997) Colon carcinoma in the adolescent. Pediatr Surg Int 12:446–448

Shahrudin MD, Noori SM (1997) Cancer of the colon and rectum in the first three decades of life. Hepatogastroenterology 44:441–444

Shi Q, Andre T, Grothey A, Yothers G, Hamilton SR, Bot BM, Haller DG, Van Cutsem E, Twelves C, Benedetti JK, O'Connell MJ, Sargent DJ (2013) Comparison of outcomes after fluorouracil-based adjuvant therapy for stages II and III colon cancer between 1978 to 1995 and 1996 to 2007: evidence of stage migration from the ACCENT database. J Clin Oncol 31(29):3656–3663

Shi Q, Paul J, Grothey A (2018a) Duration of adjuvant chemotherapy for stage III colon cancer. N Engl J Med 379(4):396–397

Shi Q, Paul J, Grothey A (2018b) Duration of adjuvant chemotherapy for stage III colon cancer. N Engl J Med 378(13):1177–1188

Signoroni S, Vitellaro M, Sala P, Bertario L (2010) Biomarkers in familial adenomatous polyposis: role and significance. Front Biosci (Schol Ed) 2:413–421. Review

Simons AJ, Ker R, Groshen S et al (1997) Variations in treatment of rectal cancer: the influence of hospital type and caseload. Dis Colon Rectum 40:641–646

Singer G, Hoellwarth ME (2012) Colorectal carcinomas in children: an institutional experience. Pediatr Surg Int 28(6):591–595

Starink TM, van der Veen JP, Arwert F, de Waal LP, de Lange GG et al (1986) The Cowden syndrome: a clinical and genetic study in 21 patients. Clin Genet 29:222–233

Stones DK, McGill N (2003) Colon carcinoma in African children. Med Pediatr Oncol 40:410–411

Sule AZ, Mandong BM (1999) Malignant colorectal tumours in patients 30 years and below: a review of 35 cases. Cent Afr J Med 45:209–212

Sultan I, Rodriguez-Galindo C, El-Tani H et al (2010) Colorectal cancer in children and adolescents: a population based study of 159 cases with comparison to adult cases. Cancer 116:758–765

Suzuki A, de la Pompa JL, Stambolic V, Elia AJ, Sasaki T et al (1998) High cancer susceptibility and embryonic lethality associated with mutation of the PTEN tumor suppressor gene in mice. Curr Biol 8:1169–1178

Taguchi T, Suita S, Hirata Y et al (1991a) Carcinoma of the colon in children: a case report and review of 41 Japanese cases. J Pediatr Gastroenterol Nutr 12:394–399

Taguchi T, Suita S, Hirata Y, Ishii E, Ueda K (1991b) Carcinoma of the colon in children: a case report and review of 41 Japanese cases. J PediatrGastroenterol Nutr 12:394–399

Tariq K, Ghias K (2016) Colorectal cancer carcinogenesis: a review of mechanisms. Cancer Biol Med 13:120–135

Tejpar S, Stintzing S, Ciardiello F, Tabernero J, Van Cutsem E, Beier F, Esser R, Lenz HJ, Heinemann

V (2017) Prognostic and predictive relevance of primary tumor location in patients with RAS wild-type metastatic colorectal cancer: retrospective analyses of the CRYSTAL and FIRE-3 trials. JAMA Oncol 3(2):194–201

Tricoli JV, Boardman LA, Patidar R et al (2018) A mutational comparison of adult and adolescent and young adult (AYA) colon cancer. Cancer 124:1070–1082

Utsunomiya J, Gocho H, Miyanaga T, Hamaguchi E, Kashimure A (1975) Peutz-Jeghers syndrome: its natural course and management. Johns Hopkins Med J 136:71–82

Van Cutsem E, Tabernero J, Lakomy R et al (2012) Addition of aflibercept to fluorouracil, leucovorin, and irinotecan improves survival in a phase III randomized trial in patients with metastatic colorectal cancer previously treated with an oxaliplatin-based regimen. J Clin Oncol 30:3499–3506

Vasen HF, Möslein G, Alonso A, Aretz S, Bernstein I, Bertario L, Blanco I, Bülow S, Burn J, Capella G, Colas C, Engel C, Frayling I, Friedl W, Hes FJ, Hodgson S, Järvinen H, Mecklin JP, Møller P, Myrhøi T, Nagengast FM, Parc Y, Phillips R, Clark SK, de Leon MP, Renkonen-Sinisalo L, Sampson JR, Stormorken A, Tejpar S, Thomas HJ, Wijnen J (2008) Guidelines for the clinical management of familial adenomatous polyposis (FAP). Gut 57:704–713

Vastyan AM, Walker J, Pinter AB et al (2001a) Colorectal carcinoma in children and adolescents-a report of seven cases. Eur J Pediatr Surg 11:338–341

Vastyan AM, Walker J, Pintér AB, Gerrard M, Kajtar P (2001b) Colorectal carcinoma in children and adolescents--a report of seven cases. Eur J Pediatr Surg 11:338–341

Vitellaro M, Ferrari A, Trencheva K, Sala P, Massimino M, Piva L, Bertario L (2012) Is laparoscopic surgery an option to support prophylactic colectomy in adolescent patients with Familial Adenomatous Polyposis (FAP)? Pediatr Blood Cancer 59(7):1223–1228

Volikos E, Robinson J, Aittomäki K, Mecklin JP, Järvinen H et al (2006) LKB1 exonic and whole gene deletions are a common cause of Peutz-Jeghers syndrome. *J Med Genet* 43:e18

Waite KA, Eng C (2002) Protean PTEN: form and function. Am J Hum Genet 70:829–844

Weber ML, Schneider DT, Offenmüller S et al (2016) Pediatric colorectal carcinoma is associated with excellent outcome in the context of cancer predisposition syndromes. Pediatr Blood Cancer 63(4):611–617

Weren RD, Ligtenberg MJ, Kets CM, de Voer RM, Verwiel ET, Spruijt L, van Zelst-Stams WA, Jongmans MC, Gilissen C, Hehir-Kwa JY, Hoischen A, Shendure J, Boyle EA, Kamping EJ, Nagtegaal ID, Tops BB, Nagengast FM, Geurts van Kessel A, van Krieken JH, Kuiper RP, Hoogerbrugge N (2015) A germline homozygous mutation in the base-excision repair gene NTHL1 causes adenomatous polyposis and colorectal cancer. Nat Genet 47:668–671

Westerman AM, Wilson JH (1999) Peutz-Jeghers syndrome: risks of a hereditary condition. Scand J Gastroenterol 230:64–70

Wimmer K, Beilken A, Nustede R, Ripperger T, Lamottke B, Ure B, Steinmann D, Reineke-Plaass T, Lehmann U, Zschocke J, Valle L, Fauth C, Kratz CP (2017) A novel germline POLE mutation causes an early onset cancer prone syndrome mimicking constitutional mismatch repair deficiency. Fam Cancer 16:67–71

Zbuk KM, Eng C (2007) Hamartomatous polyposis syndromes. Nat Clin Pract Gastroenterol Hepatol 4:492–502

Neuroendocrine Tumors (Carcinoids) of the Appendix

26

A. Redlich, M. Kuhlen, and P. Vorwerk

Although rare, NET of the appendix are the most common tumors of the gastrointestinal tract in children, accounting for 0.3% of all histologically evaluated appendiceal specimens (Njere et al. 2018; Parkes et al. 1993). The term "carcinoid" was first introduced at the beginning of the last century indicating a rather benign behavior compared to adenocarcinoma (Oberndorfer 1907; Stinner and Rothmund 2005). Appendiceal NET need to be distinguished from very rare, rather malignant tumors such as goblet cell carcinoids (Kim et al. 2017).

NET of the appendix are usually asymptomatic and diagnosed incidentally following appendectomy for acute appendicitis. Carcinoid syndrome may only be present in patients with retroperitoneal or liver metastases. In about 10% of patients, a yellowish tumor is discovered during surgery (Njere et al. 2018). The majority of appendiceal NET, however, are initially diagnosed postoperatively by histopathological evaluation. About two-thirds of the NET occur in the tip of the appendix, and less than 8% are found at the base of the organ.

Tumor size is the most important predictor of metastatic disease. Other potential risk factors including infiltration of the mesoappendix, Ki-67 proliferation index, invasion of blood or lymph vessels, infiltration of the appendiceal wall, and presence of mucin-producing cells are still under evaluation (Thirlby et al. 1984; Böger and Leuschner 2009). In tumors >15 mm, the rate of metastatic disease to regional lymph nodes is up to 35% (Boxberger et al. 2013). A meta-analysis including 958 children with appendiceal carcinoids reports a 28-fold increased risk of positive lymph nodes in tumors >20 mm compared to tumors ≤20 mm (Njere et al. 2018). The clinical significance of micrometastases, however, is not clear yet. An increased likelihood of coexisting neoplasms is reported (Sandor and Modlin 1998; Spunt et al. 2000).

The management of appendiceal NET, particularly the need of extended surgery including locoregional lymph nodes, is still a matter of debate. Second surgical interventions aim at removing tumor cells within lymph nodes and lymphatic drainage of the appendix. In a systematic review and meta-analysis, Daskalakis et al. determined the risk of lymph node metastases and their impact on survival in children with NET of the appendix (Daskalakis et al. 2020). In 77 children, morphological parameters did not predict lymph node metastases. Even more

A. Redlich · P. Vorwerk (✉)
Department Pediatric Oncology, Otto-von-Guericke University Magdeburg, Magdeburg, Germany
e-mail: antje.redlich@med.ovgu.de; Peter.Vorwerk@med.ovgu.de

M. Kuhlen
Swabian Children's Cancer Center, University Children's Hospital Augsburg, Augsburg, Germany
e-mail: michaela.kuhlen@med.ovgu.de

D. T. Schneider et al. (eds.), *Rare Tumors in Children and Adolescents*, Pediatric Oncology,
https://doi.org/10.1007/978-3-030-92071-5_26

importantly, the 10-year disease-specific survival was 100% irrespective of the extent of surgery. The authors concluded that there is a need of longitudinal studies to determine the real impact of lymph node metastases on survival.

In adults, the European Neuroendocrine Tumor Society (ENETS) guidelines recommend simple appendectomy for well-differentiated NET of the appendix ≤20 mm and right hemicolectomy for tumors >20 mm. If positive surgical margins and/or deep mesoappendiceal invasion is observed, right hemicolectomy is indicated (Plockinger et al. 2008). As opposed to this, a review by Bamboat et al. concludes that tumors >20 mm can be managed effectively with simple appendectomy (Bamboat and Berger 2006).

In children, no consensus guideline for the management of these tumors exists. The Italian Tumori Rari in Etá Pediatrica (TREP) project considers simple appendectomy for most patients (Virgone et al. 2014). In case of incomplete tumor resection, they recommend a more extended surgical approach. A French multicenter study in 114 children concludes that appendectomy alone is curative independent of tumor size and local invasion status (de Lambert et al. 2016).

The Malignant Endocrine Tumors registry of the Society for German Paediatric Oncology and Haematology (GPOH-MET) recommends a second surgery in children with tumors >15 mm and/or incomplete resection considering the long life expectancy of children, the potential risk of late recurrences, and the unclear significance of micrometastases (Table 26.1) (Boxberger et al. 2013). Since NET of the appendix are slow growing tumors, re-surgery can electively be planned after recovering from acute appendicitis and obtaining informed consent from the patient and her/his legal guardians.

NET-specific imaging is not required for children with appendiceal NET. Biochemical testing should be performed to establish baseline measures for future surveillance and disease monitoring. Appendiceal NET, however, are not commonly biochemically active. The most common metabolites produced by appendiceal NET include chromogranin A (evaluated with serum) and 5-hydroxyindoleacetic acid (5-HIAA, evaluated with 24-h urine collection).

Table 26.1 German recommendations for therapy and follow-up of appendiceal NET in children (Boxberger et al. 2013)

Therapy	
Tumor size	
≤ 15 mm, R0 resection	No further surgical therapy
≤ 15 mm, R1 resection	Local revision with lymph node sampling
> 15 mm, R0/1 resection	Right hemicolectomy

Follow-up		
Year after diagnosis	Interval	
1	Quarterly	Physical examination, abdominal ultrasound, serum chromogranin, 5-HIAA in urine
2	Biannual	
3 to >10	Annual	

Long-term follow-up for children and adolescents with appendiceal NET is necessary enabling evidence-based reduction of surgical procedures (Boxberger et al. 2013; Prommegger et al. 2002). Enlarged lymph nodes in routinely performed ultrasound scans (mesenterial lymphadenitis) are very common in children with various gastrointestinal viral infections. Therefore, these findings should be interpreted carefully during follow-up.

References

Bamboat ZM, Berger DL (2006) Is right hemicolectomy for 2.0-cm appendiceal carcinoids justified? Arch Surg 141(4):349–352

Böger CV, Leuschner I (2009) Clinicopathological investigation of carcinoid tumors of the appendix in children and adolescents: is extended resection necessary? Eur J Pediatr 168:375–386

Boxberger N, Redlich A, Boger C et al (2013) Neuroendocrine tumors of the appendix in children and adolescents. PediatrBlood Cancer 60(1):65–70

Daskalakis K, Alexandraki K, Kassi E et al (2020) The risk of lymph node metastases and their impact on survival in patients with appendiceal neuroendocrine neoplasms: a systematic review and meta-analysis of adult and paediatric patients. Endocrine 67(1):20–34

de Lambert G, Lardy H, Martelli H, Orbach D, Gauthier F, Guerin F (2016) Surgical Management of Neuroendocrine Tumors of the Appendix in Children and Adolescents: A Retrospective French

Multicenter Study of 114 Cases. Pediatr Blood Cancer 63(4):598–603

Kim JY, Hong SM, Ro JY (2017) Recent updates on grading and classification of neuroendocrine tumors. Ann Diagn Pathol 29:11–16

Njere I, Smith LL, Thurairasa D et al (2018) Systematic review and meta-analysis of appendiceal carcinoid tumors in children. Pediatr Blood Cancer 65(8):e27069

Oberndorfer S (1907) Karzinoide tumoren des dunndarms. FrankfZschrPathol 1:426–432

Parkes SE, Muir KR, Al Sheyyab M et al (1993) Carcinoid tumours of the appendix in children 1957–1986: incidence, treatment and outcome. Br J Surg 80(4):502–504

Plockinger U, Couvelard A, Falconi M et al (2008) Consensus guidelines for the management of patients with digestive neuroendocrine tumours: well-differentiated tumour/carcinoma of the appendix and goblet cell carcinoma. Neuroendocrinology 87(1):20–30

Prommegger R, Obrist P, Ensinger C, Profanter C, Mittermair R, Hager J (2002) Retrospective evaluation of carcinoid tumors of the appendix in children. World J Surg 26(12):1489–1492

Sandor A, Modlin IM (1998) A retrospective analysis of 1570 appendiceal carcinoids. Am J Gastroenterol 93(3):422–428

Spunt SL, Pratt CB, Rao BN et al (2000) Childhood carcinoid tumors: the St Jude Children's Research Hospital experience. JPediatrSurg 35(9):1282–1286

Stinner B, Rothmund M (2005) Neuroendocrine tumours (carcinoids) of the appendix. BestPractResClinGastroenterol 19(5):729–738

Thirlby RC, Kasper CS, Jones RC (1984) Metastatic carcinoid tumor of the appendix. Report of a case and review of the literature. DisColon Rectum 27(1):42–46

Virgone C, Cecchetto G, Alaggio R et al (2014) Appendiceal neuroendocrine tumours in childhood: Italian TREP project. JPediatrGastroenterolNutr 58(3):333–338

27 Gastrointestinal Stromal Tumors in Children and Adolescents

M. Benesch and P. Reichardt

27.1 Introduction

Gastrointestinal stromal tumors (GIST) are the most common mesenchymal tumors of the gastrointestinal tract in adults but are very uncommon in children and adolescents. The exact incidence of GIST in this population has not been determined. In the three largest GIST series to date, the percentage of patients below the age of 21 ranged from 0.5% to 2.7%. There is a reported annual incidence of 6.5–14.5 per million cases of GIST overall, while the UK National Registry of Childhood Tumors has reported an annual incidence of 0.02 per million cases of GIST in children below the age of 14 years (Stiller 2007). In children and adolescents, GIST are most commonly found in the stomach and predominantly in females. In contrast to adult GIST cases, lymph node metastases are frequent in pediatric GIST.

M. Benesch (✉)
Division of Pediatric Hemato-Oncology, Pediatric Palliative Care Team, Medical University of Graz, Graz, Austria
e-mail: martin.benesch@medunigraz.at; martin.benesch@klinikum-graz.at

P. Reichardt
Oncology and Palliative Care, Helios Klinikum Berlin-Buch, Berlin, Germany
e-mail: peter.reichardt@helios-gesundheit.de

27.2 Pathology and Biology

Until the 1980s, these tumors were classified as gastrointestinal leiomyomas, or leiomyosarcomas. In 1983, Mazur and Clark proposed to term these neoplasms stromal tumors (Mazur and Clark 1983). Three morphological variants (epithelioid, spindle cell, and mixed cell) are distinguished (Corless and Heinrich 2008). Ultrastructural and immunophenotypic studies showed that GIST share many morphological features with the interstitial cell of Cajal (ICC), a gastrointestinal pacemaker cell (Kindblom et al. 1998). In addition, ICC and the majority of GIST stain positive for both CD34 and CD117 (KIT) (Corless and Heinrich 2008; Hirota et al. 1998). Expression of the cell surface transmembrane receptor KIT and to a lesser extent of the platelet-derived growth factor receptor alpha (PDGFRA) makes GIST amenable to treatment with receptor tyrosine kinase inhibitors (RTKI) such as imatinib, sunitinib, or regorafenib. Among adult cases, 95% and 70% of GIST are positive for CD117 and CD34, and 60–80% carry gain-of-function mutations of the *KIT* gene leading to its oncogenic activation (Corless and Heinrich 2008; Hirota et al. 1998).

Pediatric GIST are mostly of epithelioid or mixed type morphology, and, in contrast to adult cases, only about 0–10% of pediatric GIST have an oncogenic *KIT* mutation (Miettinen et al. 2005; Agaram et al. 2008; Janeway et al. 2007).

D. T. Schneider et al. (eds.), *Rare Tumors in Children and Adolescents*, Pediatric Oncology,
https://doi.org/10.1007/978-3-030-92071-5_27

Only two pediatric patients were reported with a mutation of the *PDGFRA* gene to date (Kuroiwa et al. 2005; Benesch et al. 2009). The majority, however, show a loss of succinate dehydrogenase (SDH) and therefore lack SDH expression by immunohistochemistry (Miettinen and Lasota 2014). This has led to the category of "SDH-deficient GIST." Approximately half of the patients with SDH deficiency carry a germline mutation of the SDH complex, mostly involving SDHA. Rare cases show SDHC promoter hypermethylation resulting in gene silencing (Killian et al. 2014). A significant expression of the insulin-like growth factor 1 receptor (IGF1R) in GIST was also reported (Agaram et al. 2008; Tarn et al. 2008). Recently, FGFR1 and NTRK3 actionable alterations have been identified in cases without activating *KIT* or *PDGFR* mutations, opening personalized additional treatment options for these patients (Shi et al. 2016).

27.3 Syndromic/Inherited GIST

GIST occur either sporadically or rarely in association with other tumor syndromes (e.g., neurofibromatosis type 1 (NF1)) (Nannini et al. 2013). The familial occurrence of GIST has also been reported (Nishida et al. 1998). Phenotypic characteristics associated with familial GIST include mastocytosis, dysphagia, cutaneous hyperpigmentation, multiple lesions, location in the small intestine, and/or urticaria pigmentosa (Benesch et al. 2009). The nonhereditary association of gastric leiomyosarcoma, extra-adrenal paraganglioma, and pulmonary chondroma is termed Carney triad (CT) (Carney et al. 1977). An inherited tumor syndrome comprising GIST and paragangliomas ("Carney-Stratakis syndrome" [CSS] or "Carney-Stratakis dyad") has to be separated from the "classic" CT (Carney and Stratakis 2002). Recently, germline mutations encoding the SDH subunits B, C, and D have been identified in patients with CSS (McWhinney et al. 2007). Both CT- and CSS-associated GIST belong to the category of SDH-deficient GIST. The term familial GIST was originally used to refer to germline *KIT* mutations. Since GIST are heritable in the case of either germline KIT or germline SDH mutations, these two forms of heritable GIST have to be distinguished. The occurrence of familial GIST has not been reported in pediatric patients; however, an 18-year-old who had surgery for a jejunum tumor eventually developed familial recurrent GIST later in life (Benesch et al. 2009).

27.4 Symptoms

Although GIST have been observed in newborns, most cases are diagnosed at the end of the first or during the second decade of life (Benesch et al. 2009). The average age of pediatric patients is 13 years, and there is a predilection for females of 2.5:1 (Benesch et al. 2009). Hypochromic, microcytic anemia and anemia-related symptoms resulting from upper gastrointestinal bleeding are commonly observed at presentation. Nonspecific symptoms include loss of appetite, abdominal pain, nausea, vomiting, constipation, and diarrhea. The majority of pediatric GIST are located in the stomach (typically in the antrum), although GIST are occasionally found in the small intestine, colon/rectum, omentum, and abdominal wall with the tumor size ranging widely (1.5–35 cm) (Benesch et al. 2009). Multiple tumors or tumors with numerous satellite lesions are found in a considerable number of patients. Metastasis is not uncommon, and it typically occurs in the liver, lymph nodes, peritoneum, and mesentery; these lesions, however, rarely present at diagnosis (Benesch et al. 2009).

27.5 Diagnosis

Pediatric patients suspected of having GIST are worked up using the following: conventional abdominal radiographs, upper gastrointestinal contrast series, ultrasound, upper and lower endoscopy, computed tomography (CT), magnetic resonance imaging (MRI), flurodeoxyglucose-positron emission tomography (FDG-PET), angiography, fecal occult blood test, and labeled red cell scans. GIST often present as either single or multiple well-circumscribed solid nodular masses. CT or

MRI is mandatory both in the diagnostic workup and follow-up of patients with GIST (Benesch et al. 2009). To keep radiation exposure as low as possible, MRI is strongly preferred over CT imaging. FDG-PET is useful to detect occult metastatic disease and particularly to monitor treatment response. Endoscopy is done in some patients, particularly in case of upper gastrointestinal bleeding, but endoscopic biopsies are often nondiagnostic. The final diagnosis is based on histology and immunohistochemistry. Tissue samples can be obtained either by biopsy or resection of the tumor. A tumor biopsy is unnecessary, if the tumor is localized and resectable.

27.6 Treatment

Management guidelines for adult patients with GIST have been presented by different groups (e.g., the GIST Task Force of the NCCN, ESMO) (Demetri et al. 2007; Casali et al. 2018) but are not available for children. Thus far surgery is the mainstay of treatment aiming at local excision, ideally with microscopically free margins (Demetri et al. 2007; Casali et al. 2018). However, a report from the National Institutes of Health Pediatric and Wildtype GIST Clinic has shown that, in addition to a high rate of progression, resection margin status did not affect event-free survival (Weldon et al. 2017). Removal of liver metastases may be indicated in selected cases. Since GIST do not respond to conventional cytotoxic chemotherapy, its use is not recommended. Although RTKI are increasingly used in the pediatric age group, the total number of reports on patients receiving imatinib and/or sunitinib for GIST is still low (Agaram et al. 2008; Benesch et al. 2009). Children with GIST who present with activating *KIT* or *PDGFR* mutations should be treated according to recommendations in adult GIST (i.e., with imatinib, sunitinib, and regorafenib). For the majority of patients with no activating *KIT* or *PDGFR* mutation, especially those with SDH deficiency, imatinib treatment is not recommended. Given the much broader spectrum of kinase inhibition, sunitinib, and also regorafenib, has been shown to be more active in these cases (Demetri et al. 2013). If available, patients should be included into clinical trials. In agreement with the guidelines for adult patients (Demetri et al. 2007; Casali et al. 2018), treatment with RTKI is recommended only in children and adolescents with extensive GIST (i.e., metastatic or initial R0 resection not feasible). There are currently insufficient data to recommend adjuvant RTKI treatment in R0 resected pediatric GIST. Risk stratification in adult patients with GIST is based on tumor size, mitotic index, and location of the primary tumor (Demetri et al. 2007; Casali et al. 2018). The risk stratification system has not been evaluated systematically in pediatric GIST. The majority of patients with GIST can be cured with complete surgical resection alone. In view of the mostly indolent course of pediatric GIST, all treatment should be indicated carefully, avoiding extensive mutilating or repetitive surgery on the one hand and withholding systemic treatment until proven progression leading to symptoms.

27.7 Prognosis

Prognosis is dismal, if the tumor and/or metastatic lesions are not completely resectable (Benesch et al. 2009). However, even with extensive disease, some pediatric patients may have a prolonged and slowly progressing clinical course. Current evidence suggests that GIST in the pediatric and adolescent population behave differently from those in adults. In adults, prognosis is determined by tumor size, mitotic activity, and location of the primary lesion. In the pediatric population, these three factors do not seem to be predictive of outcome. In general, pediatric GIST tend to be less aggressive in nature, and despite recurrence of metastases, the clinical course is quite favorable in comparison to adults (Benesch et al. 2009).

27.8 Conclusion

Data on the pathogenesis, clinical course, and prognosis of these tumors in this pediatric population are currently insufficient. In order to prospectively collect more data from children and adolescents with GIST, these patients should be included into national (rare tumor or soft tissue sarcoma) registries and clinical trials.

References

Agaram NP, Laquaglia MP, Ustun B (2008) Molecular characterization of pediatric gastrointestinal stromal tumors. Clin Cancer Res 14:3204–3215

Benesch M, Wardelmann E, Ferrari A et al (2009) Gastrointestinal stromal tumors (GIST) in children and adolescents: a comprehensive review of the current literature. Pediatr Blood Cancer 53:1171–1179

Carney JA, Stratakis CA (2002) Familial paraganglioma and gastric stromal sarcoma: a new syndrome distinct from the Carney triad. Am J Med Genet 108:132–139

Carney JA, Sheps SG, Go VL et al (1977) The triad of gastric leiomyosarcoma, functioning extra-adrenal paraganglioma and pulmonary chondroma. N Engl J Med 296:1517–1518

Casali PG, Abecassis N, Aro HT et al (2018) Gastrointestinal stromal tumours: ESMO-EURACAN Clinical Practice Guidelines for diagnosis, treatment and follow-up. Ann Oncol 29(Suppl. 4):iv267

Corless CL, Heinrich MC (2008) Molecular pathobiology of gastrointestinal stromal sarcomas. Annu Rev Pathol Mech Dis 3:557–586

Demetri GD, Benjamin RS, Blanke CD et al (2007) NCCN Task Force report: optimal management of patients with gastrointestinal stromal tumors (GIST)–update of the NCCN clinical practice guidelines. J Natl Compr Cancer Netw 5(Suppl. 2):S1–S29

Demetri GD, Reichardt P, Kang YK et al (2013) Efficacy and safety of regorafenib for advanced gastrointestinal stromal tumours after failure of imatinib and sunitinib (GRID): an international, multicentre, randomised, placebo-controlled, phase 3 trial. Lancet 381(9863):295–302

Hirota S, Isozaki K, Moriyama Y et al (1998) Gain-of-function mutations of c-kit in human gastrointestinal stromal tumors. Science 279(5350):577–580

Janeway KA, Liegl B, Harlow B (2007) Pediatric KIT–wild-type and platelet-derived growth factor receptor alpha–wild-type gastrointestinal stromal tumors share KIT activation but not mechanisms of genetic progression with adult gastrointestinal stromal tumors. Cancer Res 67:9084–9088

Killian JK, Miettinen M, Walker RL et al (2014) Recurrent epimutation of SDHC in gastrointestinal stromal tumors. Sci Transl Med 6(268):268ra177

Kindblom LG, Remotti HE, Aldenborg F et al (1998) Gastrointestinal pacemaker cell tumor (GIPACT): gastrointestinal stromal tumors show phenotypic characteristics of the interstitial cells of Cajal. Am J Pathol 152:1259–1269

Kuroiwa M, Hiwatari M, Hirato J (2005) Advanced-stage gastrointestinal stromal tumor treated with imatinib in a 12-year-old girl with a unique mutation of PDGFRA. J Pediatr Surg 40:1798–1801

Mazur MT, Clark HB (1983) Gastric stromal tumors. Reappraisal of histogenesis. Am J Surg Pathol 7:507–519

McWhinney SR, Pasini B, Stratakis CA (2007) Familial gastrointestinal stromal tumors and germ-line mutations. New Engl J Med 357:1054–1056

Miettinen M, Lasota J (2014) Succinate dehydrogenase deficient gastrointestinal stromal tumors (GISTs)—a review. Int J Biochem Cell Biol 53:514–519

Miettinen M, Lasota J, Sobin LH (2005) Gastrointestinal stromal tumors of the stomach in children and young adults: a clinicopathologic, immunohistochemical, and molecular genetic study of 44 cases with long-term follow-up and review of the literature. Am J Surg Pathol 29:1373–1381

Nannini M, Biasco G, Astolfi A, Pantaleo MA (2013) An overview on molecular biology of KIT/PDGFRA wild type (WT) gastrointestinal stromal tumours (GIST). J Med Genet 50:653–661

Nishida T, Hirota S, Taniguchi M et al (1998) Familial gastrointestinal stromal tumours with germline mutation of the KIT gene. Nat Genet 19:323–324

Shi E, Chmielecki J, Tang CM et al (2016) NTRK3 actionable alterations in "Wild-Type" gastrointestinal stromal tumors. J Transl Med 14:339

Stiller C (2007) Childhood cancer in Britain: incidence, survival and mortality. Oxford University Press Inc, New York

Tarn C, Rink L, Merkel E et al (2008) Insulin-like growth factor 1 receptor is a potential therapeutic target for gastrointestinal stromal tumors. Proc Natl Acad Sci U S A 105:8387–8392

Weldon CB, Madenci AL, Boikos SA et al (2017) Surgical management of wild-type gastrointestinal stromal tumors: a report From the National Institutes of Health Pediatric and Wildtype GIST Clinic. J Clin Oncol 35:523–528

28 Pancreatic Tumors

Ewa Bien, Winfried Barthlen, Ines B. Brecht, and Bence Sipos

28.1 Introduction

Pancreatic tumors in infancy and childhood are extremely rare. Even larger institutions can report only few cases over a time period of 20 and more years (Yu et al. 2009). Perez et al. identified 58 patients under the age of 20 years with malignant pancreatic tumors within the US Surveillance, Epidemiology, and End Results registry (SEER, 1973–2004), accounting for an age-population-adjusted incidence of around 0.018 cases/100,000 in the United States (Perez et al. 2009). In the UK National Registry, 41 pancreatic tumors have been counted in 30 years (Brennan et al. 2004); the Italian TREP project identified 21 patients under the age of 18 years with malignant pancreatic tumors within a 10-year period (Dall'igna et al. 2010). Recently, Mylonas et al. reported an updated analysis of 114 patients with malignant pancreatic tumors within the SEER registry and performed a comprehensive systematic review of 32 studies reporting on 489 children with pancreatic tumors (Mylonas et al. 2018a, b).

28.2 Differential Diagnosis

The differential diagnosis for malignant pancreatic tumors includes benign tumors, as hemangiomas, cystic lesions, like enterogenous cysts, pseudocysts, and abscesses. Also, tumors from adjacent organs like neuroblastoma, Wilms' tumor, and hepatoblastoma, as well as involvement of the pancreas in case of leukemia, lymphoma, or lymphoproliferative disorders, are more common than primary pancreatic tumors (Rebhandl et al. 2001). In case of a primary pancreatic tumor, pancreatoblastoma has to be considered especially in a child under the age of 10 years, while a solid-pseudo-papillary neoplasm (SPN) - rather in a female adolescent (Mylonas et al. 2018b). Because of similar morphology, SPN might easily be confused with neuroendocrine tumors. The pathology and clinical behavior of pancreatoblastoma and acinar cell

E. Bien (✉)
Department of Pediatrics, Hematology and Oncology, Medical University of Gdansk, Gdansk, Poland
e-mail: ewa.bien@gumed.edu.pl

W. Barthlen
Pediatric Surgery, University Medicine Greifswald, Greifswald, Germany

I. B. Brecht
Department of Pediatric Hematology/Oncology, University Children's Hospital Tuebingen, Tuebingen, Germany
e-mail: ines.brecht@med.uni-tuebingen.de

B. Sipos
Department of Pediatric Hematology/Oncology, University Children's Hospital Tuebingen, Tuebingen, Germany

Internal Medicine VIII, University Hospital Tuebingen, Tuebingen, Germany
e-mail: Bence.Sipos@med.uni-tuebingen.de; bence.sipos@pathologie-stuttgart.de

D. T. Schneider et al. (eds.), *Rare Tumors in Children and Adolescents*, Pediatric Oncology,
https://doi.org/10.1007/978-3-030-92071-5_28

Table 28.1 Differential diagnosis of pancreatic tumors in children and adolescents

Group	Entity
Malignant pancreatic tumors	Pancreatoblastoma
	Acinar cell carcinoma
	Ductal adenocarcinoma
Tumors with low malignant potential	Solid-pseudopapillary neoplasm
	Mucinous cystic neoplasm
	Inflammatory myofibroblastic tumor
Gastroenteropancreatic neuroendocrine tumors (GEP-NETs)	Insulinoma Gastrinoma
	Others (VIP) oma, glucagonoma, somatostatinoma)
Benign tumors	Hemangioma
	Teratoma (see Chap. 39)
Tumor-like lesions	Cyst Local fibrous focus
	Pseudocyst
Congenital hyperinsulinism	
Secondary tumor manifestations	Lymphoma
	Rhabdomyosarcoma
	Primitive neuroectodermal tumor
	Neuroblastoma
	Hepatoblastoma
	Wilms' tumor

carcinoma (ACC) are very similar, and differentiation between the two can be difficult (Shorter et al. 2002). Anyway, ACC as well as ductal adenocarcinoma are extremely rarely seen in children (Luttges et al. 2004; Perez et al. 2009; Mylonas et al. 2018a) (Table 28.1).

Differential diagnosis of pediatric pancreatic neoplasms should be very cautious both in terms of radiologic findings and pathologic decisions. In the series reported by Ellerkamp et al., initial radiological images led to an incorrect tentative diagnosis in nearly 70% of cases. There were also up to 50% of false initial histopathological diagnoses regarding SPT and pancreatic carcinoma (Ellerkamp et al. 2012). Therefore, the necessity of involving reference pathology and reference radiology in a diagnostic workup of all cases of pediatric pancreatic tumors should be underlined.

28.3 Biology, Pathology, and Tumor Characteristics

28.3.1 Pancreatoblastoma

Pancreatoblastoma is the most common pancreatic tumor in children in the first decade of life, accounting for approximately 25% of cases (Shorter et al. 2002). A joint analysis of the European Pediatric Rare Tumor Group (EXPeRT) collected 20 cases treated between 2000 and 2009 (Bien et al. 2011). It is a malignant tumor, which mainly occurs in children under the age of 10 years and is rarely reported in neonates (an incidence peak between second and third years of life, mean age 5 years) (Klimstra et al. 1995; Defachelles et al. 2001; Shorter et al. 2002; Mylonas et al. 2018a). Pancreatoblastomas have a bimodal age distribution: two-thirds of the cases occur in children and one-third in adults. This embryonal neoplasm has many similarities with hepatoblastoma concerning age group, genetic alterations, and the response to chemotherapy. It shows alterations of the APC/β-catenin pathway and a loss of heterozygosity on chromosome 11p15.5 (Abraham et al. 2001; Isobe et al. 2017). Pancreatoblastoma can be associated with Wilms' tumor, Beckwith–Wiedemann syndrome, and familiar adenomatous polyposis (Kerr et al. 2002; Antonello et al. 2009; Mylonas et al. 2018a). The association with Beckwith–Wiedemann syndrome is significantly higher in patients with congenital and infantile PBLs (50%) than in the whole group of patients with PBL (4.5%) (Chisholm et al. 2012).

The tumor is frequently found in the pancreatic head or tail, well defined, and surrounded by a fibrous capsule (Dhebri et al. 2004). It is composed of cells showing predominantly acinar differentiation divided by septa. Neonatal pancreatoblastomas associated with Beckwith–Wiedemann syndrome are cystic (Kerr et al. 2002). Necrotic areas with calcifications are typical. The most important criterion for the histological diagnosis is the presence of squamoid nests (Fig. 28.1). Pancreatoblastomas may exhibit partially endocrine and ductal differentiation or even contain primitive compo-

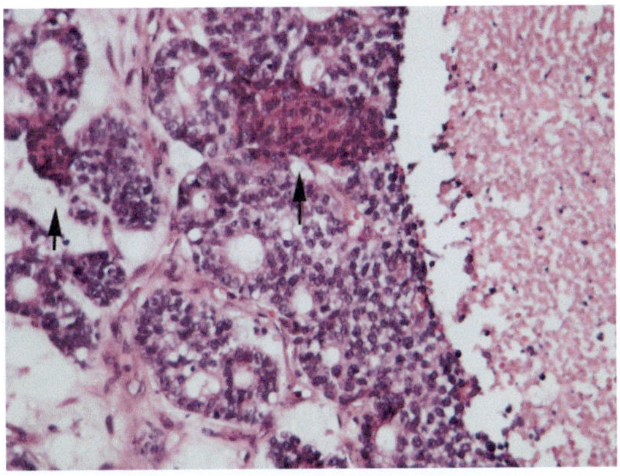

Fig. 28.1 Pancreatoblastoma with acinar-glandular features and with squamoid nests (*arrows*, H & E, ×400)

nents, somehow recapitulating the embryonic features of pancreas. The proliferative activity is between <1 and 42 mitoses/high power field (HPF). Nuclear polymorphism is low, and tumor cell invasion in perineural space and vessels is rare. The frequency of metastases in regional lymph nodes and liver has been reported to vary between 17% and 50% (Dhebri et al. 2004; Perez et al. 2009). In most cases, expression and secretion of AFP can be observed, and serum AFP level may serve as tumor marker to follow the response to the therapy (Saif 2007; Antonello et al. 2009; Belletrutti et al. 2013; Mylonas et al. 2018a).

28.3.2 Solid-Pseudopapillary Neoplasm (SPN)

SPNs are rare tumors of the pancreas of low malignant potential (Casamassima et al. 2016; Lubezky et al. 2017; Mylonas et al. 2018a), occurring mainly in young females (10:1, mean age 22 years) (Papavramidis and Papavramidis 2005; Laje et al. 2013; Morita et al. 2014). SPNs were also known as "solid and papillary tumor," "solid-cystic tumor," "papillary cystic tumor," "solid and pseudopapillary epithelial neoplasm," "solid and cystic acinar cell neoplasm," and "Frantz tumor" (Kloppel et al. 1996; Papavramidis and Papavramidis 2005; Chung et al. 2006a, b; Shet et al. 2014). Not seldom they were misdiagnosed as nonfunctioning islet cell tumors, adenocarcinomas, cystadenocarcinomas, or pseudocysts (Todani et al. 1988; Sclafani et al. 1991; Kloppel et al. 1996; Papavramidis and Papavramidis 2005; Chung et al. 2006a, b). Recently, the tumor has been more recognized and therefore more often diagnosed, accounting for approximately 6% of all exocrine pancreatic tumors in all age groups (Papavramidis and Papavramidis 2005). In children, they account for 8–17% of all cases of pancreatic tumors (Grosfeld et al. 1990; Jaksic et al. 1992).

Solid-pseudopapillary neoplasms are enigmatic tumors, with regard to their cell of origin and phenotype. SPNs are composed of unique cells which may exhibit epithelial, mesenchymal, and neuroendocrine features. SPNs do not express major transcription factors involved in pancreatic development and differentiation, which does not allow for precise identification of the pancreatic lineage of the tumor cells (Calvani et al. 2019). During fetal development, there is a close relationship between the left genital ridge and the pancreatic anlage. It is speculated, therefore, that SPNs arise from pluripotent precursor cells from this area (Kosmahl et al. 2000). This would explain the female preponderance of >90%. In 95% of the cases, SPNs show an alteration of the APC/β-catenin signaling pathway and LOH on chromosome 5q22.1 (Antonello et al. 2009). In one-third of the SPNs, Fli-1 is overexpressed without exhibiting EWS/Fli-1 translocation, which is observed in pediatric tumors, mostly in Ewing sarcomas. The tumor localization is equally distributed in the pancreas (Rebhandl et al. 2001; Papavramidis and Papavramidis 2005). SPNs are often large tumors with a mean diameter of 6 cm (0.5–34.5 cm). The tumor consistency is soft with friable necrotic gray-hemorrhagic material in the center. Smaller tumors may be completely solid, mimicking neuroendocrine neoplasms. Usually, the tumor is well demarcated and surrounded by a pseudocapsule, which can be infiltrated by tumor cells (Fig. 28.2). This feature, however, is not an established sign of malignancy in SPNs (Fig. 28.3). Histologically, the eponymous pseudopapillary appearance is found around the lacunae. Monomorphous polygonal tumor cells form solid

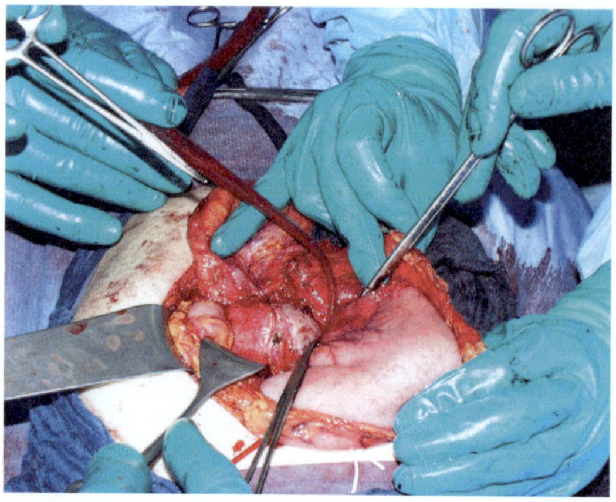

Fig. 28.2 Intraoperative view of an SPN in the head of the pancreas in a 14-year-old female

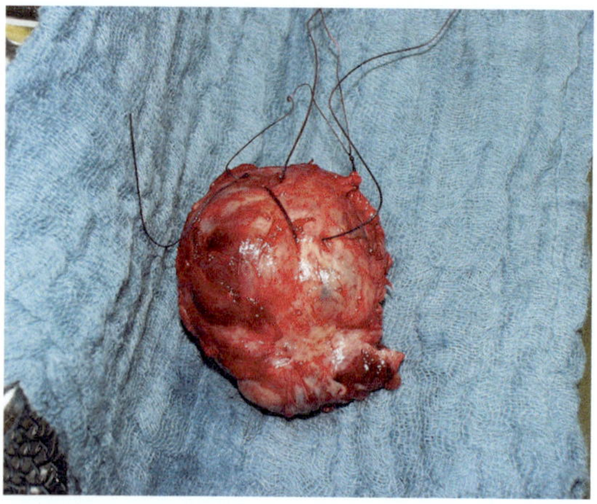

Fig. 28.3 Specimen of the SPN with free margins. Neither the pancreatic nor the choledochal duct has been touched

areas or are arranged in pseudo-rosettes. The stromal component is often imperceptible, but it can be myxoid or sclerotic. The proliferation rate is very low (Rebhandl et al. 2001; Kosmahl et al. 2004). SPNs display a characteristic immunohistochemical pattern with expression of nuclear β-catenin, cyclin D, vimentin, CD56, synaptophysin, and progesterone receptor (Fig. 28.4). Calcifications were revealed in approximately one-third of cases (Shet et al. 2014). SPNs have no specific tumor markers; however, elevated AFP, carcinoembryonic antigen (CEA), cancer antigen 19-9 (CA 19-9), and cancer antigen 125 (CA 125) in some patients with SPT were reported (Morita et al. 2014; Bender et al. 2018).

Most SPNs (>90%) behave in a benign fashion. A possible malignant potential of the remaining small proportion of SPNs cannot be easily predicted by radiologic preoperative findings and immunohistochemical stainings, apart from cases with evident presence of infiltration of surrounding tissues and distant metastases. In other cases, possible malignancy of SPN may be suggested when CT or MRI reveals a large tumor with high rate of solid component (Hwang et al. 2014), focal lobulated margins and incomplete capsule (Chung et al. 2009), or exophytic growth pattern (Ye et al. 2012). Additionally, most authors used the WHO-defined criteria for classification of SPNs, such as angioinvasion, perineural invasion, or deep infiltration of the pancreatic parenchyma to confirm the diagnosis of malignant SPN (Hwang et al. 2014).

28.3.3 Gastroenteropancreatic Neuroendocrine Tumors (GEP-NETs) and Congenital Hyperinsulinism

Neuroendocrine tumors (NETs) are a heterogeneous group of malignancies, characterized by production of hormones and vasoactive peptides. Currently, the term "NETs" encompasses carcinoid tumors, islet cell tumors, and amine precursor uptake and decarboxylation (APUD) tumors. Although these tumors can produce distinct clinical syndromes, their diagnosis in children remains challenging due to wide variations in presentation and slow onset of symptoms (Hsieh and Burjonrappa 2016; Broaddus et al. 2003). Gastroenteropancreatic NETs (GEP-NETs) are significantly rising in incidence due to advances in anatomic imaging and incorporation of metabolic imaging techniques which enable improved detection of these tumors. GEP-NETs have currently the highest prevalence among upper gastrointestinal tumors with one-third of GEP-NETS found in the pancreas (Hsieh and Burjonrappa 2016). They constitute 1–2% of all tumors of

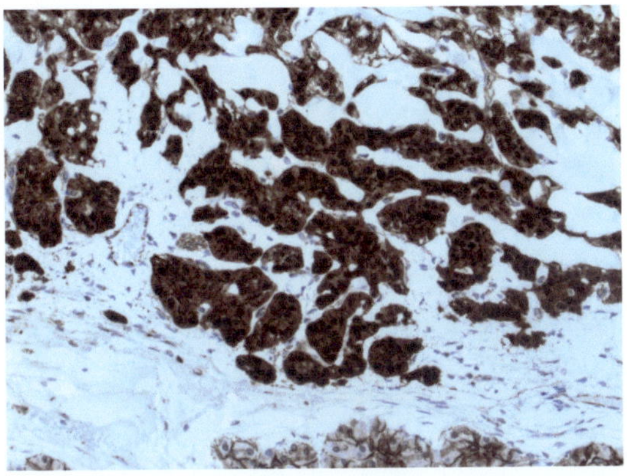

Fig. 28.4 Nuclear *β*-catenin expression in SPN. At the bottom, normal pancreatic acini with membrane-bound staining (×400)

pancreas and can be associated with familial syndromes, such as multiple endocrine neoplasia (MEN) 1/2, von Hippel–Lindau (VHL), and tuberous sclerosis (Shorter et al. 2002).

The prognostic stratification of GEP-NETs is based on tumor size, proliferation rate, angioinvasion, and infiltration of surrounding tissue (Hamilton and Aaltonen 2000) (Table 28.2). The WHO classification from 2010 provided a more simplified system for risk stratification (Bosman et al. 2010) (Table 28.3).

The islet cell tumors derive from any of the cell types of the islets and may be benign (adenomas) or malignant (carcinomas) and occur equally often in male and female (Chung et al. 2006a, b). They account for 1–2% of all pancreatic neoplasms at all age groups, but the prevalence is estimated to be much higher – around 1/100,000. Insulinomas and gastrinomas arise either sporadically, or, as in most pediatric cases, they are associated with MEN 1 (Nasher et al. 2015). Importantly, most MEN 1-associated GEP-NETs are nonfunctioning and frequently multifocal. Monohormonal endocrine cell clusters and microadenomas are well-defined precursor lesions of MEN-associated NETs. Up to the fourth decade, gastrinomas develop in about 40% and insulinomas in 10% of all MEN 1 carriers. Additionally, adenomas are observed in the para-

Table 28.2 Classification of pancreatic GEP-NETs (Solcia et al. 2000; Hamilton and Aaltonen 2000)

Well-differentiated endocrine tumor
Functioning
Insulin-producing (insulinoma)
Glucagon-producing (glucagonoma)
Somatostatin-producing (somatostatinoma)
Gastrin-producing (gastrinoma)
VIP-producing (VIPoma)
Others
Nonfunctioning
Microadenoma (<0.5 cm)
Others
Well-differentiated endocrine carcinoma
Functioning
Insulin-producing (insulinoma)
Glucagon-producing (glucagonoma)
Somatostatin-producing (somatostatinoma)
Gastrin-producing (gastrinoma)
VIP-producing (VIPoma)
Serotonin-producing with carcinoid syndrome
ACTH-producing with Cushing syndrome
Nonfunctioning
Poorly differentiated endocrine carcinoma—small-cell carcinoma
Mixed exocrine–endocrine carcinoma
VIP, vasoactive intestinal peptide; ACTH, adrenocorticotropic hormone

Table 28.3 Recent classification of neuroendocrine neoplasms of the gastrointestinal tract including pancreas (Bosman et al. 2010)

Nomenclature	Features
1. Neuroendocrine Tumor Grade 1 (carcinoid)	Well-differentiated, Ki-67 Index <2%, <2 mitoses/10 HPF
2. Neuroendocrine Tumor Grade 2	Well-differentiated, Ki-67 Index <20%, <20 mitoses/10 HPF
3. Neuroendocrine carcinoma	Poorly differentiated, small or large cell, Ki-67 Index >20%, >20 mitoses/10 HPF
4. Mixed adenoneuroendocrine carcinoma (MANEC)	Epithelial and neuroendocrine components, at least 30% of either
5. Hyperplastic and preneoplastic lesions	

thyroid gland in 90% and in the pituitary gland in 29% of the cases (Brandi et al. 2001). Other functionally active tumors like glucagonoma, VIPoma, and somatostatinoma, are extremely rare in children. In contrast to adults, pediatric vasoactive intestinal peptide (VIP)-producing tumors are more frequently associated with non-pancreatic tumors (e.g., neuroblastoma) (Nasher et al. 2015). Hybrid tumors with characteristics of both insulinoma and gastrinoma have been described (Lodish et al. 2008).

Insulinomas are the most common type of GEP-NETs found in children. They are solid, well-circumscribed tumors, approximately 1–3 cm in size (Bartsch et al. 2000). In contrast to the foci in congenital hyperinsulinism, they can be well distinguished macroscopically from normal pancreatic tissue (Figs. 28.5–28.9). Insulin and proinsulin expressions can be shown by immunohistochemistry.

In childhood, >90% of insulinomas are benign (Fig. 28.10). Malignant behavior of insulinoma is proven by metastases which arise in the regional lymph nodes and in the liver (Padidela et al. 2014). In contrast, gastrinomas developing as a component of the MEN 1 usually demonstrate a malignant potential, and more than half of them have metastasized at the time of diagnosis (Brandi et al. 2001). Alike insulinomas, they are solid, well-defined encapsulated tumors (Fig. 28.11). Because of their malignant behavior, small size,

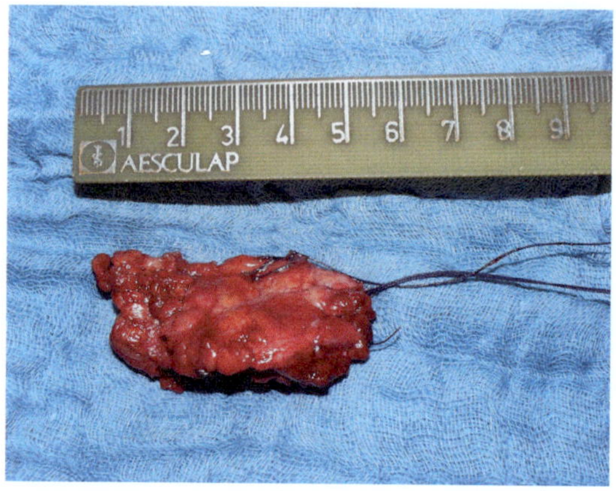

Fig. 28.6 Gross specimen of an insulinoma with free margins

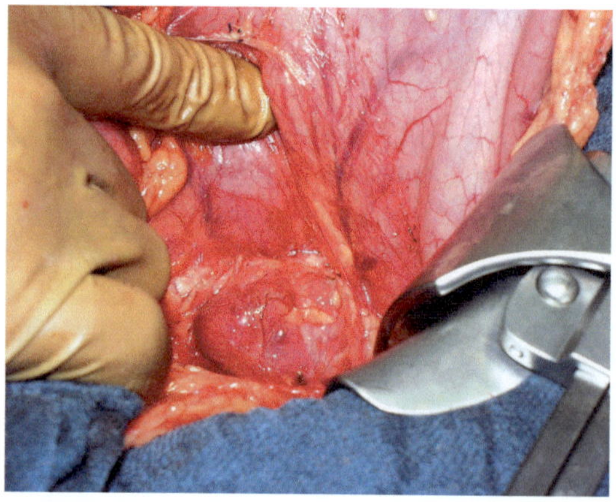

Fig. 28.7 Intraoperative view of an insulinoma in the middle of the pancreas in a 17-year-old female with the MEN 1 syndrome

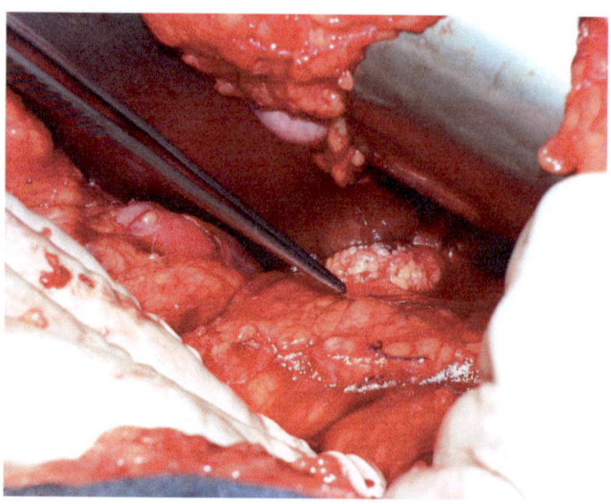

Fig. 28.5 Intraoperative view of an insulinoma (forceps tip) in the middle of the pancreas in a 16-year-old male with the MEN 1 syndrome

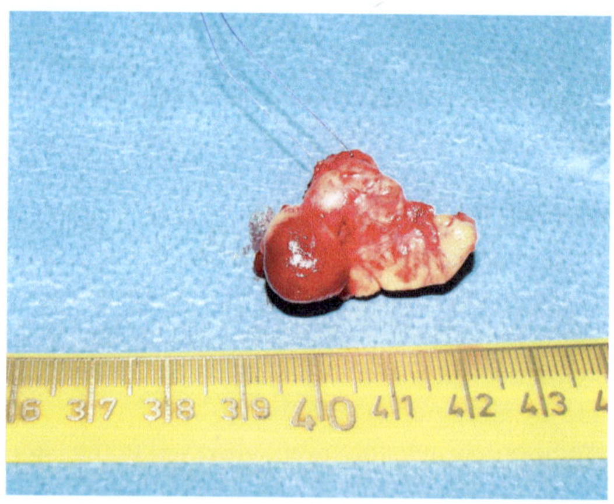

Fig. 28.8 Specimen of an insulinoma of a 14-year-old male with the MEN 1 syndrome

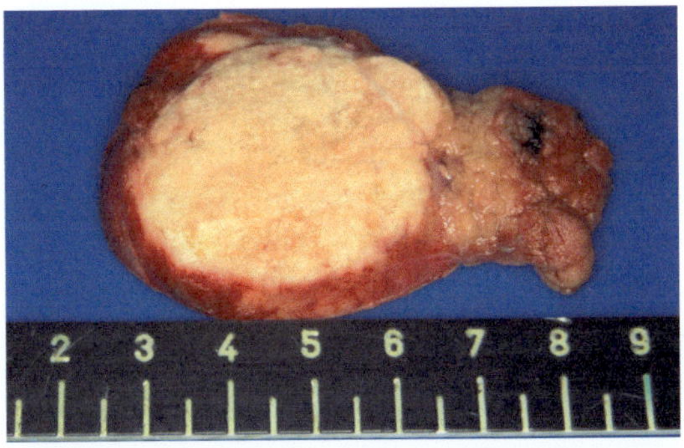

Fig. 28.9 Gross features of pancreatic NET: well-circumscribed, *white-yellow* nodule without necrosis

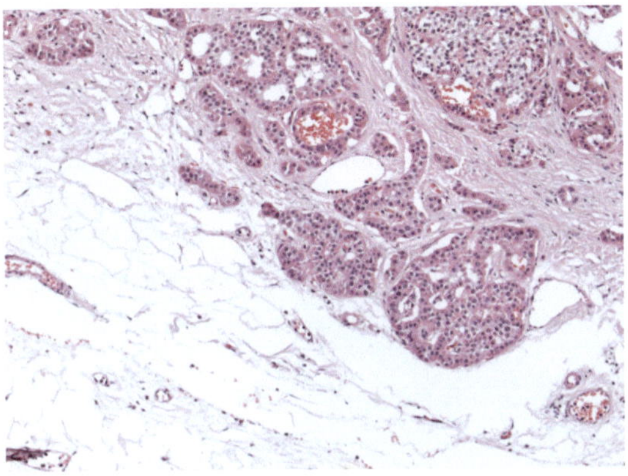

Fig. 28.10 Well-differentiated NET composed of monomorphous round/oval cells arranged in nests (HE, ×200)

multiplicity, and frequent localization in the duodenum, MEN-1-associated gastrinomas represent a diagnostic and therapeutic challenge (Norton et al. 2001).

28.3.3.1 Congenital Hyperinsulinism

Congenital hyperinsulinism – formerly called nesidioblastosis—is defined by morphologic changes in the endocrine pancreas causing hyperinsulinemic hypoglycemia in the absence of an insulinoma. Congenital hyperinsulinism occurs more commonly in infancy with the annual incidence 1 in 50,000 births in sporadic forms and 1 in 2500 births in familial disease (Padidela et al. 2014). Focal congenital hyperinsulinism is not a neoplastic lesion and represents the most important differential diagnosis of insulinoma.

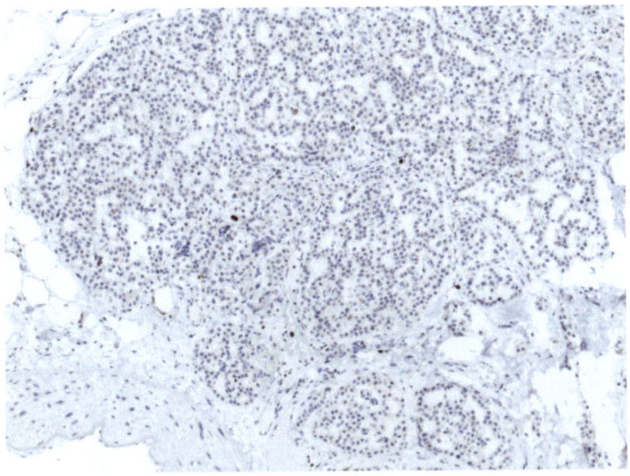

Fig. 28.11 Low proliferation rate in a well-differentiated neuroendocrine tumor (Ki-67 immunostaining, ×200)

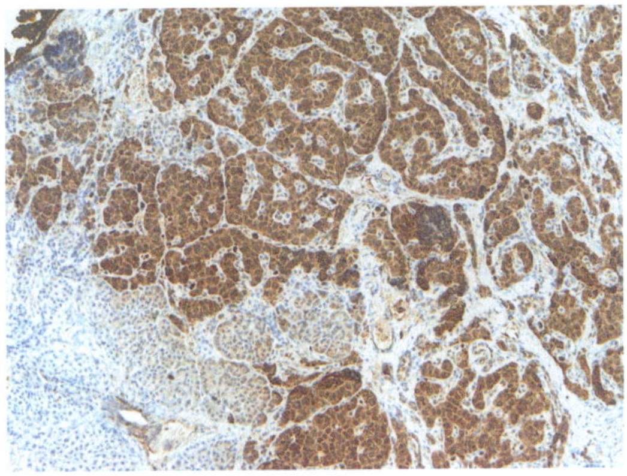

Fig. 28.12 Congenital hyperinsulinism (ancient name: nesidioblastosis) (IHC proinsulin)

Congenital hyperinsulinism is caused by impaired control of insulin secretion from functionally defective pancreatic beta cells. The defect of the beta cells resides in the glucose recognition system. In most cases of focal congenital hyperinsulinism, there is a general paternal mutation of the K_{ATP} channels on the cellular level and a maternal loss of heterozygosity only in the cells of the focal lesion (de Lonlay et al. 2006; Shet et al. 2014). Morphologically, there is a diffuse (75%) or focal hypertrophy of beta cells (Anlauf et al. 2005a, b; Shet et al. 2014) that are macroscopically not recognizable. The histological diagnosis is based on immunohistochemical detection of insulin in the hypertrophic Langerhans islets (Fig. 28.12).

28.3.4 Acinar Cell Carcinoma (ACC)

ACCs arise from the exocrine acinar cells secreting the pancreatic enzymes. They show similarity to pancreatoblastomas harboring LOH on chromosome 11p in 50% of cases and alterations of the APC/β-catenin signaling pathway in 24% (Abraham et al. 2002; Al-Hader et al. 2017). ACCs are large tumors at presentation, averaging 10 cm in diameter. Most ACCs are subdivided by large fibrotic septa and show pushing borders. Frequently, there is a nodular infiltration in the surrounding tissues and vessels. Necrotic areas are typical. Histologically, ACCs are solid but may exhibit a wide range of cell types: acinar, monotonous endocrine-like, trabecular, cystic, or even hepatoid differentiation (Sipos and Kloppel 2005). The mitotic activity is usually high (>50/10 HPF) (Abraham et al. 2002). Immunohistochemically, pancreatic enzymes such as trypsin, chymotrypsin, and amylase are expressed in ACCs (Chaudhary 2015).

28.3.5 Ductal Adenocarcinoma

Ductal adenocarcinoma is the most frequent malignant pancreatic tumor in the adult age group but is extremely rare in childhood (Grosfeld et al. 1990; Perez et al. 2009; Mylonas et al. 2018b). Most cases date to the pre-immunohistochemical era and are usually not well documented. It has been speculated that in ancient reports, some SPNs or pancreatoblastomas had been misinterpreted as pediatric ductal adenocarcinomas (Shorter et al. 2002; Luttges et al. 2004). Nevertheless, according to the SEER registry, ductal adenocarcinomas of the childhood were associated with adverse outcome, exhibiting a 15-year survival rate of 23% (Perez et al. 2009).

28.3.6 Benign Tumors

28.3.6.1 Inflammatory Myofibroblastic Tumor (IMT)

IMTs of pancreas are extremely rare in children, with only 12 cases reported in the literature (summarized by Liu et al. 2017). IMTs, known also as inflammatory pseudotumors or plasma cell granulomas, affect more commonly girls than boys (Shet et al. 2014). These enigmatic tumors represent a range from truly mesenchymal tumors to reactive-inflammatory lesions. They consist of myofibroblastic spindle cells admixed with inflammatory cells, predominantly with plasma cells, lymphocytes, and eosinophils. The clinical symptoms of pancreatic IMTs are nonspecific, including pain, jaundice, and a palpable mass. In US examination, IMT presents as a solid isoechoic or hypoechoic, well-defined mass. In CT, the tumor enhances comparably to the remainder of the pancreas (Chung et al. 2006a, b). Unlike in adults, the literature review did not show the predomination of the location of pediatric IMT in the head of pancreas (Liu et al. 2017). The proliferation rate of IMT of the pancreas is low. It does not show a malignant behavior but is able to grow by infiltration (McClain et al. 2000). After incomplete resection, the rate of local recurrences is high (Mizukami et al. 2006).

28.3.6.2 Teratoma

Like in other locations, teratomas in the pancreas show components of all three germinal sheets (Mester et al. 1990). Most of the cases published so far have been dermoid cysts (Kela et al. 2008). Please also refer to Chap. 39 ("Germ Cell Tumors").

28.3.6.3 Mucinous Cystic Neoplasm (MCN)

MCN is very rare in childhood. In adults, virtually all tumors arise in women and are located in the pancreatic body and tail. By imaging, it is difficult to distinguish MCN from pseudocysts or other cystic tumors (Fukushima and Fukayama 2007). MCNs have no connection to pancreatic ducts. Microscopically, the solitary or multiple cysts are lined by tall, columnar epithelium with mucin secretion. The intra-cystic connective tissue resembles ovarian stroma by conventional histopathology and also by immunohistochemistry, exhibiting expression of estrogen and progesterone receptors as well as α-inhibin. In MCNs, the classical sequence from dysplasia and adenoma to carcinoma is well known. This is associated with a loss of tumor suppressor genes Smad4 and p53 and an increasing frequency of K-ras oncogene mutations (Fukushima and Fukayama 2007; Garcea et al. 2008). In children, no malignant transformation has been reported to date.

28.3.6.4 Fibrous Focus

Chronic pancreatitis can result in circumscribed fibrotic indurations in the pancreas which may mimic a tumor. Pancreatitis in childhood can originate from cholelithiasis, choledochal cysts, pancreas divisum, medications, metabolic diseases, hemolytic–uremic syndrome, viral diseases (predominantly mumps and coxsackie), and hereditary chronic pancreatitis of childhood with mutations in the PRSS1 gene (Chung et al. 2006a, b; Rebours et al. 2009). Hereditary pancreatitis is frequently associated with an adenocarcinoma of the pancreas occurring later in life.

28.3.6.5 Pancreatic Pseudocysts

Pancreatic pseudocysts are by far the most common cystic lesions in the pediatric pancreas. In most cases, they originate from blunt abdominal trauma, rarely from chronic pancreatitis.

28.4 Diagnosis of Pancreatic Tumors

28.4.1 Clinical Presentation

Pancreatic tumors in children normally present with a palpable mass, abdominal pain, or general symptoms like weight loss, fatigue, and mild gastrointestinal problems (Lack et al. 1983; Klimstra et al. 1995; Shorter et al. 2002, Nasher et al. 2015). As tumors can arise at any site within the pancreas and origin from the ductal epithelium is rare, jaundice is less often seen in children than in adults (Lack 1989; Shorter et al. 2002; Nasher et al. 2015). Many cystic tumors are incidentally discovered, some after blunt abdominal trauma (Rebhandl et al. 2001; van den Akker et al. 2012). Most children with pancreatic malignancies present with advanced tumors. In case of a tumor arising from the head of the pancreas, the patient might present with mechanical obstruction of the duodenum and gastric outlet, jaundice, and gastrointestinal bleeding. However, these symptoms are rare in childhood, most likely due to the soft consistency of the tumors. Varices, hemorrhage, and ascites, possibly resulting from hepatic failure, may be seen due to venous obstruction (Pappo and Furman 2006). In case of ACC, painful, subcutaneous nodules and polyarthritis might be seen, which is caused by elevated lipase secretion by the tumor (Klimstra et al. 1992).

Functioning GEP-NETs may produce hormones which lead to specific symptoms. In case of insulinoma, hypoglycemic symptoms, which might manifest as weakness, fatigue, sweating, change in behavior, confusion, seizures, or coma, are seen (Field 1993). Blood glucose levels under 50 mg/dl, hypoglycemia in case of fasting, and immediate disappearance of symptoms with intravenous administration of glucose are typical symptoms (Whipple's triad). The diagnosis of insulinoma is frequently delayed, particularly in younger children <10 years of age. Some children with insulinoma were initially diagnosed and treated for seizure disorders (Peranteau et al. 2013). Serum insulin levels are elevated with a higher proportion of proinsulin (Field 1993). Gastrinoma causes the Zollinger–Ellison syndrome with gastric hyperacidity, multiple and recurrent peptic ulcers in uncommon locations, gastroesophageal reflux, and diarrhea (Zollinger 1987; Nasher et al. 2015). Another functioning islet cell tumor exceedingly rarely seen in children is the VIPoma causing Verner–Morrison syndrome (massive watery diarrhea, hypokalemia, and achlorhydria, WDHA syndrome) (Grosfeld et al. 1990; Chung et al. 2006a, b). In children, however, VIP-secreting tumors are more often of neurogenic than islet cell origin (Shet et al. 2014) (Table 28.4).

28.4.2 Laboratory

In pancreatic tumors in childhood, the routine laboratory tests are of little value. Often there are no abnormal laboratory findings, no evidence of pancreatic insufficiency, cholestasis, impaired liver function, or endocrine syndrome. Even lactate dehydrogenase in the serum is rarely elevated.

Table 28.4 Diagnostic strategy in pediatric pancreatic tumors

Procedure	Specific questions
Clinical assessment	
Physical examination	Mostly mild and unspecific (gastrointestinal) symptoms but also signs of obstruction of duodenum, gastric outlet, biliary tract or venous obstruction, and palpable mass
Laboratory assessment	
– Hepatic function: Bil (dir. + indir.), AP, γ-GT, GOT, GPT, total protein, and albumin	Elevated in case of obstructive jaundice
– Calcium, parathormone, prolactin, chromogranin A, and a hormone profile including insulin, proinsulin, VIP, gastrin, somatostatin, and glucagon	In case of suspected endocrine active tumor
– LDH, amylase, lipase	Unspecific marker
– AFP	Pancreatoblastoma, suitable to differentiate among pancreatic tumors, may be used to monitor the response to chemotherapy and completeness of surgery and to detect cancer recurrence. Sporadically elevated in ACC, pancreatic ductal adenocarcinoma
– NSE	Sporadically elevated in SPN
– CA 19.9	Pancreatic ductal adenocarcinoma, sporadically elevated in SPN; not suitable to detect early stages, may be used to monitor for cancer recurrence; also elevated in chronic pancreatitis, benign obstructive jaundice, and cystic lesions
– CEA	Assists with evaluating pancreatic cysts as benign or malignant
– CA 125	Pancreatic ductal adenocarcinoma
– Pancreatic oncofetal antigen	Pancreatic ductal adenocarcinoma
– Catecholamines	Exclusion of neuroblastoma, sporadically elevated in SPN
– Blood count	Exclusion of hematologic malignancy
Radiographic assessment	
Abdominal ultrasound and MRI	Tumor size, localization and tumor borders, consistency, presence of cystic and solid components, necrosis, calcification, hemorrhage, dilatation of the pancreatic and bile duct, local and vascular infiltration, ascites, lymphadenopathy, and liver metastases
Abdominal CT and MRI	Site, tumor size, organ of origin, cystic structures or calcification, ascites, obstruction, or invasion of other organs
Chest CT	Lung metastases
CNS MRI	CNS metastases
Bone scan	Skeletal metastases
Histologic assessment	
See above for details	Classification according to WHO
Genetics	
MEN 1	Gastrinoma
KRAS2 gene	Ductal adenocarcinoma
PRSS1 gene	Familial chronic pancreatitis
Other assessments	
Secretin test	In case of suspected gastrinoma
Fasting blood glucose	In case of endocrine active tumor
Screening methods	
Screening tests	Not available, currently ongoing research, e.g., Johns Hopkins Medicine http://pathology.jhu.edu/pc/BasicScreening.php?area=ba

Anyway, alpha-fetoprotein (AFP) is increased in about 50–70% of cases of pancreatoblastoma and can serve as a tumor marker. However, AFP was also reported to be elevated in epithelial exocrine carcinomas, particularly in ACC; therefore, in cases with increased AFP, careful differential diagnosis is required (Ellerkamp et al. 2012; Mylonas et al. 2018a). However, an increased AFP value may help to distinguish between PBL and ACC on the one hand and SPT on the other hand. Ectopic secretion of ACTH causing Cushing syndrome was detected in sporadic cases of PBL, islet cell tumors, and ACC (Hinnie et al. 2000; Ilyes et al. 2007; Kletter et al. 2007; Matarazzo et al. 2011). In SPN, elevated serum levels of neuron-specific enolase (NSE) and CA 19.9 and elevation of urinary vanillylmandelic and homovanillic acids have been reported in sporadic cases (Casanova et al. 2003).

If cystic lesions are present, the differential diagnosis between pseudocysts, true cysts (von Hippel–Lindau, cystic fibrosis, and lymphoepithelial cyst), and cystic tumors (SPN, cystic pancreatoblastoma, and cystic teratoma) can be very difficult (Correa-Gallego et al. 2010; Farrell 2007). Pseudocysts are the most frequent cystic lesions encountered (70%) (Singhal et al. 2006). A cystic tumor can be suspected if there is no history of pancreatitis or blunt abdominal trauma; if the cyst has thick walls, septa, and lobuli; if there is no connection to the pancreatic duct; and if cystic fluid shows low level of amylase (Chung et al. 2006a, b). The detection of elevated tumor markers like CEA and CA 19.9 in the cystic fluid shows low sensitivity and high specificity.

If an endocrine active tumor is suspected, fasting blood glucose and MEN-1-associated parameters, calcium, parathormone, prolactin, chromogranin A, and a hormone profile, including insulin, proinsulin, VIP, gastrin, somatostatin, and glucagon, should be assessed. In suspected gastrinoma, a secretin test is performed.

28.4.3 Imaging

The first-line tool is ultrasonography on suspicion of a pancreatic mass. Tumor size, localization and tumor borders, consistency, presence of cystic and solid components, necrosis, hemorrhage, dilatation of the pancreatic and bile ducts, local and vascular infiltration, lymphadenopathy, and liver metastases can be demonstrated (Montemarano et al. 2000). The value of sonography, however, largely depends on the personal experience of the examiner and is often impaired by air superposition in the bowel. Additionally, defining the exact margins of the tumors of pancreas may be problematic due to the heterogeneous echogenicity of pancreatic lesions, so that CT or MRI may be of assistance regarding localization, extension of the lesion, and presence of metastases (Hammond et al. 2012; Shet et al. 2014). In the case of suspected pancreatoblastoma, CT or MRI is mandatory for precise staging. Also for precise detection of insulinoma, MRI should be used as a first-line imaging with or without endoscopic ultrasound (Peranteau et al. 2013). However, lymph node metastasis or duodenal or vascular infiltration by the tumor may be missed even using up-to-date imaging methods (Montemarano et al. 2000; Chung et al. 2006a, b). A preoperative ERCP or MRCP is indicated if there is a dilatation of the bile or pancreatic ducts.

In the adult age group, the ^{18}fluorodeoxyglucose (^{18}FDG)-PET-CT was able to distinguish between malignant and benign pancreatic lesions (Herrmann et al. 2008). The utility of ^{18}FDG-PET-CT/MRI scanning in differential diagnosis of pancreatic tumors in children is not yet completely determined. However, primary pancreatic tumors as well as PBL metastasis to retroperitoneal lymph nodes have been recently reported to display elevated ^{18}FDG uptake in FDG-PET-CT scans (Corrias et al. 2017; Bohl et al. 2018). In case of insulinoma not identified on MRI, the PET-CT/MRI scans may successfully identify the location of the tumor (Padidela et al. 2014). If neuroendocrine tumors are clinically suspected, PET-CT with new, innovative tracers (^{18}F-L-DOPA, ^{68}Ga-DOTATOC, and ^{11}C-5-hydroxytryptophane) has been giving promising results (Orlefors et al. 2005; Kauhanen et al. 2007; Tessonnier et al. 2010). If congenital hyperinsulinism is suspected, an ^{18}F-L-DOPA-PET-CT is able to distinguish between diffuse and focal forms and in the latter case to localize the focus exactly (Barthlen et al. 2016).

Table 28.5 Imaging characteristics of pancreatoblastoma and SPN

Pancreatoblastoma	SPN
– Child <10 years	– Young female adolescent
– Well-defined, solitary lesion in the pancreas of considerable size	– Usually large, well circumscribed
– Half of the cases occurring in the head of the pancreas	– Equally distributed over the pancreas
– Heterogeneous tumor with septa and few calcifications, hemorrhagic and necrotic areas, simultaneous solid and cystic areas	– Heterogeneous tumor with simultaneous occurrence of solid, cystic, hemorrhagic, and necrotic areas in the tumor; calcification in the tumor capsule
– Metastasis in regional lymph nodes and liver (up to 50%)	– No metastasis
– Well-vascularized tumor without hemorrhage	– Well-vascularized tumor with hemorrhage
– Rare dilatation of the choledochal duct	– Very rare dilatation of the choledochal duct
– Fibrous capsule	– Thick, fibrous tumor capsule
– Often compressing nearby organs without invading them	– Compression of adjacent structures is more often seen than invasion

Skeletal scintigraphy is indicated for pancreatoblastoma to look for bone metastasis. If a neuroendocrine tumor is suspected, a somatostatin receptor scintigraphy (^{111}In-DTPA-DPhe-octreotide) can aid to establish the diagnosis and localize the tumor. Especially for gastrinomas which are often small, multiple, and submucous in the duodenal wall, the somatostatin receptor scintigraphy became an important diagnostic tool (Norton et al. 2001; Yeung and Pasieka 2009). Functional localization of gastrinomas, measuring gastrin gradients, is performed by hepatic venous sampling after the selective intra-arterial injection of secretin (Norton et al. 2004) (Table 28.5).

28.4.4 Biopsy

In most pancreatic tumors in childhood, it will be impossible to establish a diagnosis from imaging alone. There have been cases of pancreatoblastoma which have been misinterpreted as intraperitoneal cysts prenatally (Sugai et al. 2006). In principle, a tumor biopsy would be advantageous before making a decision for therapy. This biopsy could be done by fine-needle aspiration (Nadler et al. 2002), by laparoscopy (Metzelder et al. 2007), or by open incision. In fine-needle aspiration, however, the amount of tissue obtained is often very small. A definitive diagnosis is difficult to establish, especially concerning the heterogeneity of most pancreatic tumors in childhood. Biopsy by laparoscopy for diagnostic purposes is a well-accepted strategy in pediatric surgery (Metzelder et al. 2007). However, the assessment of resectability of a pancreatic tumor by laparoscopy is by far more difficult than by the open approach. The risk of misinterpretation, therefore, is increased, and the chance of a complete healing in the first step is decreased. Additionally, there is the possibility of tumor cell spillage by the CO_2 insufflation. A tight closure of the tumor capsule after the biopsy by laparoscopy is technically demanding. Several cases of local or disseminated peritoneal recurrences of an SPN after laparoscopic biopsy have been reported, even in case of clear margins in initial resection (Fais et al. 2009). Therefore, and with the exception of small, localized tumors in the pancreatic tail which can be resected by laparoscopy, a primary open approach for the definite diagnosis and treatment of pancreatic tumors in childhood and adolescence of unknown biological behavior is strongly recommended.

28.4.5 Staging

The TNM staging system is not specific and thus not used for the very heterogeneous group of pediatric pancreatic and neuroendocrine tumors, and currently no other staging system is in common use. Anyway, for NETs, the WHO classification combines different clinical prognostic factors to differentiate between well-differentiated NETs with benign or uncertain behavior, well-differentiated neuroendocrine carcinoma, and poorly differentiated neuroendocrine carcinoma (see Table 28.3). In most cases, they are hormonally active, though with more advanced diagnostic and surgical methods, the percentage of nonfunctioning islet cell tumors has risen in the last decades (Anlauf et al. 2005a, b; Hsieh and Burjonrappa 2016). The active polypeptide can produce clinical symptoms (functioning or hyperfunctioning islet cell tumors) or not (nonfunctioning or clinically silent tumors). Functioning islet cell tumors are further classified into insulinomas, glucagonomas, somatostatinomas, gastrinomas, and VIPomas according to the hormone they produce (see also Table 28.4). In case of production of more than one hormonally active peptide, clinical symptoms are related to one hormone being predominant. Under all types of functioning islet cell tumors, insulinoma (47%) and gastrinoma (30%) are most often seen (Chung et al. 2006a, b). Microadenomas are tumor nodules with a diameter of less than 0.5 cm, which is the minimum size required for gross detection.

28.5 Treatment of Pancreatic Tumors

Though treatment strategies for pancreatic tumors in children mainly have to be derived from experience in adults, more and more experience is available to understand specific treatment approaches for children and adolescents. The treatment mainly relies on complete resection as most tumors are considered to be not or little radio- or chemosensitive (Pappo and Furman 2006). An exception seems to be pancreatoblastomas that proved to be sensitive to chemotherapy (Klimstra et al. 1995; Murakami et al. 1996; Chun et al. 1997; Defachelles et al. 2001; Bien et al. 2011). Anyway, metastases might occur in several entities, and systemic therapy therefore has to be considered.

28.5.1 Surgical Therapy

With the rare exception of unequivocally proven unresectability and metastasis, all pancreatic tumors must be treated surgically in curative intention. The surgical procedure depends on the malignancy of the tumor and the location. In case of a tumor of the tail or body, a distal pancreatic tail resection with preservation of the spleen can be performed. This can be done conveniently by a laparoscopic approach. The standard surgical procedure for tumors of the head of the pancreas is the Whipple procedure (partial pancreatoduodenectomy), although a less radical resection like pylorus-sparing partial pancreatoduodenectomy (PPPD/Traverso–Longmire), partial pancreatic resection, or even enucleation might be more adequate in some cases. Some patients also seem to profit from tumor debulking in case of unresectability (Scandavini et al. 2018; Varshney et al. 2018).

28.5.1.1 Surgical Approach

After a transverse laparotomy, the omental bursa is opened, and the situation is evaluated:

- Is an enucleation or a local resection of the tumor possible?
- Is there evidence of peritoneal infiltration or of local or liver metastasis?
- Is there evidence of an infiltration of the duodenum, the choledochal duct, the porta hepatis, the caval vein, or the superior mesenteric vessels?

If the tumor seems to be resectable, it should be removed totally even without knowledge of the histological diagnosis (Perez et al. 2009; Snajdauf et al. 2009). Open biopsy should only be performed in all cases that would necessitate extended surgery (e.g., partial duodenopancreatectomy) for complete resection. The final histopathological diagnosis should be awaited. Frozen sections are valuable for detection of residual tumor cells in the resection margins. However, final diagnosis may not be achieved in all cases because of the necessity of additional immunohistochemical examination in certain tumors

(SPN vs. endocrine; pancreatoblastoma/ACC vs. endocrine). Intraoperative tumor cell spillage, however, must be strictly avoided. The tumor capsule must be closed carefully after the biopsy.

28.5.2 Therapy and Prognosis of Specific Entities

28.5.2.1 Pancreatoblastoma

Patients with pancreatoblastoma have good chances for cure, if radical resection of all vital tumor tissue is performed (Brennan et al. 2004; Saif 2007; Perez et al. 2009; Yu et al. 2009). In most cases, the tumor is located ventrally in the pancreatic head, surrounded by a capsule, and has no connections to the duct system. Therefore, a local resection without mutilating surgery is possible in many cases (Dhebri et al. 2004). However, achieving safe tumor-free margins is crucial since relapses are likely to occur after enucleation of the tumor, in spite of adjuvant chemotherapy (Ellerkamp et al. 2012).

There are no sufficient data about the extent of lymphadenectomy in PBL. However, lymph node metastasis occurs in up to 30% of patients at diagnosis (Mylonas et al. 2018a, b). Since the prognosis is significantly worse in patients with involved lymph nodes and when lymph node metastasis develops after tumor resection (Dhebri et al. 2004), an extended and radical lymphadenectomy should be performed in every case. Both enlarged, PET-CT/MRI positive and normal lymph nodes should be removed and checked for the presence of PBL metastasis histologically.

The pylorus-preserving strategy of Traverso–Longmire has been preferred in adult oncology because the quality of life of patients was regarded significantly better than that after a classical Whipple operation. However, recent systematic review has shown that pancreatic insufficiency occurred significantly more often in children following PPPD (45.7%) than Whipple surgery (2.9%). Also, the local relapse rates were higher in patients treated with PPPD than in those treated with Whipple surgery (14.3% vs. 5.7%). The surgery-associated morbidity was comparable between the two modalities (Mylonas et al. 2018a). These new observations need to be analyzed more cautiously; however, it should be underlined that the surgical intervention in children with PBL should be performed only by experienced surgeons who are familiar with the technique of partial duodenopancreatectomy as well.

Though the mainstay of treatment is complete surgical resection, patients often present with metastases and/or unresectable tumor at the time of diagnosis. Therefore, preoperative chemotherapy might be needed and in fact has led to marked tumor reduction in several cases (Defachelles et al. 2001; Bien et al. 2011; Belletrutti et al. 2013; Ghaffarian et al. 2018). Anyway, the most effective chemotherapy for pancreatoblastoma is not known, and a variety of different regimes have been used so far (Dhebri et al. 2004). The PLADO regime (cisplatin and doxorubicin), as recommended for hepatoblastoma in the SIOPEL study, is the most widely used protocol for PBL (Ogawa et al. 2000; Perilongo et al. 2000). It was reported to be efficient in the EXPeRT series, where 73% of patients with initially unresectable PBL responded to primary PLADO chemotherapy (Bien et al. 2011). Different regimes other than PLADO, including usually cisplatin and/or doxorubicin but also other chemotherapeutics, such as cyclophosphamide, etoposide, vincristine, dactinomycin, gemcitabine, ifosfamide, carboplatin, 5-fluorouracil, vinblastine, and irinotecan, have also been successfully used and might be considered for treatment (Chun et al. 1997; Vossen et al. 1998; Defachelles et al. 2001; Dhebri et al. 2004; Dall'Igna et al. 2010; Belletrutti et al. 2013; Dhamne and Herzog 2015). In single cases of highly advanced and/or metastatic PBL, the high-dose chemotherapy with autologous hematopoietic transplantation has been successfully used to diminish the extent of the disease preoperatively (Ibuka et al. 2017) (Fig. 28.13).

So far, it is not known whether adjuvant postoperative chemotherapy results in improved survival rates, especially in cases feasible to primary complete resection (Shorter et al.

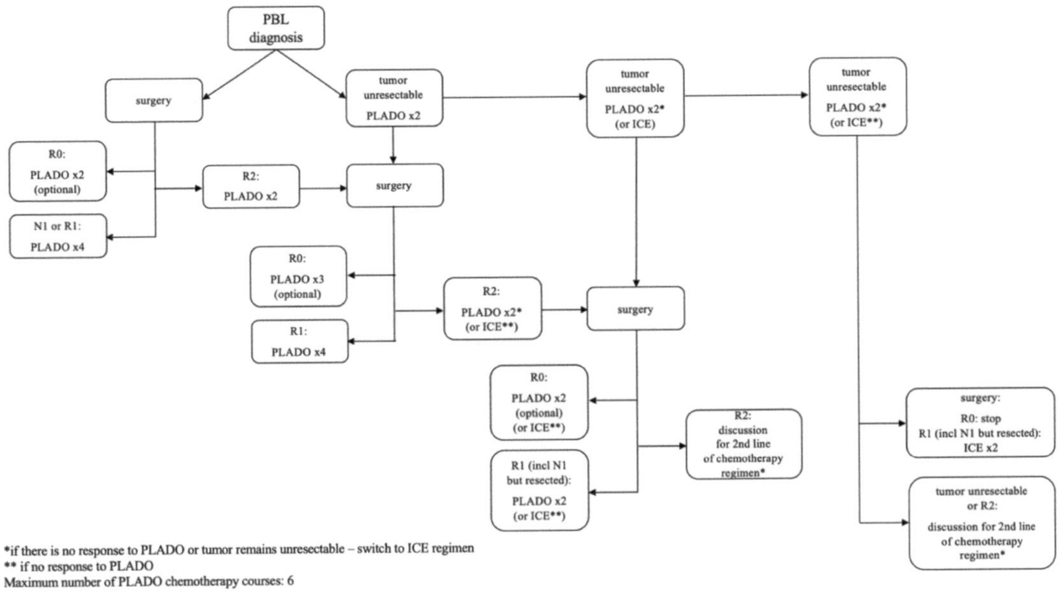

Fig. 28.13 The strategy of management of pediatric pancreatoblastoma, recommended by the European Cooperative Study on Pediatric Rare Tumors (EXPeRT). *ICE* ifosfamide carboplatin and etoposide, *N1* involved lymph nodes, *PLADO* platinum + doxorubicin chemotherapy, R0 complete excision, R1 microscopic residues, R2 macroscopic residues (Bien E et al. 2021)

2002). Also, the role of radiotherapy remains unclear though response to irradiation in case of recurrent or incompletely resected pancreatoblastoma has been reported (Griffin et al. 1987; Murakami et al. 1996; Defachelles et al. 2001; Ellerkamp et al. 2012). Surgical resection of liver metastases should be considered (Grosfeld et al. 1990; Murakami et al. 1996, Belletrutti et al. 2013). The long-term survival has been achieved in PBL metastatic to the liver treated with neoadjuvant chemotherapy followed by pancreatectomy, total hepatectomy, and liver transplant (Ghaffarian et al. 2018).

28.5.2.2 Prognosis

Approximately one-third of the reported PBL cases of all age groups present with metastases to the liver and abdominal lymph nodes and less commonly to the lung, brain, and peritoneum (Klimstra et al. 1995; Imamura et al. 1998; Gupta et al. 2000; Montemarano et al. 2000; Mylonas et al. 2018b). While in adults pancreatoblastoma is reported to be fatal, especially in case of metastases and unresectability (Dhebri et al. 2004; Bassarova et al. 2015; Zouros et al. 2015), the tumor seems to behave less aggressively in pediatric patients, showing a better outcome (Kohda et al. 2000; Defachelles et al. 2001; Saif 2007). Congenital and infantile PBLs are associated with particularly favorable prognosis (Chisholm et al. 2012). The analysis of the EXPeRT group on 20 children with PBL reported a 5-year event-free survival and OS of 58.8% and 79.4%, respectively. Outcome did not correlate with tumor site and size but was strongly influenced by the tumor stage and by the feasibility of complete resection. All patients who underwent complete resection at the time of initial laparotomy survived at the end of the review period. Also initially inoperable and/or metastatic cases that responded well to neoadjuvant chemotherapy and became feasible to subsequent complete delayed surgery had good prognosis (Bien et al. 2011). The response rate to chemotherapy was 73% (Bien et al. 2011). Long-term survival after response to radiation and chemotherapy in case of metastatic disease was reported (Griffin et al. 1987; Vannier et al. 1991; Klimstra et al. 1995; Murakami et al. 1996; Vossen et al. 1998; Ogawa et al. 2000; Dhebri et al. 2004). Anyway, recurrence may occur even after complete surgery, though based on meta-analysis by Mylonas et al., it is now regarded much less frequent than reported earlier in small series of patients with PBL (14.7% vs. 60%) (Shorter et al. 2002; Mylonas et al. 2018a). Nevertheless, close follow-up is necessary.

28.5.2.3 SPN

Specific treatment experience for children with SPN does not exist. Because of the low grade of malignancy of SPNs and the existence of a fibrous pseudo-capsule, an enucleation of the tumor might be sufficient, especially in pediatric cases (Grosfeld et al. 1990; Matsunou and Konishi 1990; Jaksic et al. 1992; Wunsch et al. 1997). But as metastatic and local recurrences do occur in case of incomplete resection or enucleation, complete resection with safe margins should be the aim (Todani et al. 1988; Sclafani et al. 1991; Klimstra et al. 2000; Zhou et al. 2001; Papavramidis and Papavramidis 2005). It is particularly important because even well-circumscribed tumors seen on imaging, may have incomplete tumor capsule with local infiltration into surrounding parenchyma, pancreatic duct and vascular or perineural invasion, revealed by pathologic studies (Namgoong et al. 2014). Papavramidis et al. reported that complete resection of SPN was achieved by local excision in 22%, by pancreatic tail resection in 40%, by a Whipple resection in 22%, and by a Traverso–Longmire partial duodenopancreatectomy in 4% of the cases (Papavramidis and Papavramidis 2005). Anyway, radical local approaches or extensive lymphatic dissection is not necessary, and tumor size, recurrence, and limited metastases as well as local invasion (e.g., into the portal vein or superior mesenteric artery) should not lead to the conclusion of unresectability (Jeng et al. 1993; Martin et al. 2002). Even highly locally advanced and metastatic SPNs can have a very indolent course and are often amenable to complete surgical resection (Lubezky et al. 2017). Some of these patients can survive more than 10 years after surgery (Kaufman et al. 1986; Nishihara et al. 1993a; Mao et al. 1995; Papavramidis and Papavramidis 2005; Farrell 2007).

If the tumor is not excised completely, the rate of local recurrence is very high (73%), and the almost 100% survival rate after R0 resection decreases dramatically (Campanile et al. 2011; Namgoong et al. 2014). Apart from positive surgical margins, an important risk factor for recurrence was patients' age less than 13.5 years at diagnosis (Irtan et al. 2016).

If a central pancreatic resection has to be performed, the drainage of the tail must be accomplished by a Roux-en-Y jejunal loop or a pancreaticogastrostomy (Fisher et al. 2007). If the portal vein, the mesenteric vein, or the venous confluens are infiltrated, a bypass can be constructed using jugular vein graft or a Goretex graft (Goh et al. 2007; Sperti et al. 2008). The spleen should be preserved in any case of childhood SPN to avoid the overwhelming postsplenectomy infection (OPSI) syndrome.

Laparoscopic tumor biopsy is not recommended in suspected SPN because of the risk of tumor cell spillage (Fais et al. 2009). However, laparoscopic central pancreatectomy with distal pancreaticogastrostomy and laparoscopic distal pancreatectomy with preservation of the spleen have been proven to be safe and efficient in the tumors of the body and tail of the pancreas, respectively (Nasher et al. 2015; Stewart et al. 2016). For isolated tumors in the body or tail of the pancreas, primary laparoscopic excision appears to be the optimal treatment resulting in cure and improved quality of life in the majority of cases (Nasher et al. 2015).

Surgical treatment for metastases should be considered, especially in case of single liver metastases (Nishihara et al. 1993b; Ogawa et al. 1993; Panieri et al. 1998; Klimstra et al. 2000; Saiura et al. 2000; Martin et al. 2002). Patients profit from debulking if complete resection is not possible (Todani et al. 1988; Sclafani et al. 1991; Nishihara et al. 1993a; Mao et al. 1995; Wang et al. 1998; Papavramidis and Papavramidis 2005). In case of a local recurrence of SPN, even multiple resections may be of value because the overall prognosis of this slowly growing tumor is excellent (Tipton et al. 2006; Goh et al. 2007; Perez et al. 2009; Irtan et al. 2016). There is no consensus regarding the value of lymphadenectomy for SPNs. Generally, the routine lymphadenectomy is not indicated since the incidence of lymph node involvement in SPN is very low (Tipton et al. 2006). However, some authors advocate for the lymph node dissection in patients with tumors >5 cm due to their potentially malignant behavior.

The role of chemotherapy and radiotherapy in SPT is not clear (Mylonas et al. 2018a). In a recent review of the literature by Bender et al., only 3.8% of children with SPN received adjuvant therapy, including chemotherapy in 12 and radiotherapy in 6 out of 523 evaluable patients (Bender et al. 2018). Rebhandl et al. report successful postoperative treatment of a pediatric patient with metastasized SPN with ifosfamide, cisplatin, and VP16 (Rebhandl et al. 2001). Gemcitabine (Maffuz et al. 2005) and a combination of cisplatin and 5-fluorouracil (Strauss et al. 1993) have been successfully used as preoperative chemotherapy regimes in two adult patients with unresectable SPN. Neoadjuvant chemotherapy with cisplatinum, ifosfamide, etoposide, and vincristine followed by intraoperative radiofrequency ablation of metastatic liver lesions was proven successful in a child with inoperable SPN (Hah et al. 2007). Also, radiotherapy might be of value in cases of unresectable tumors (Fried et al. 1985; Matsunou and Konishi 1990; Rebhandl et al. 2001). It was also shown that peritoneal carcinomatosis can be successfully treated with complete cytoreductive and hyperthermic intraperitoneal chemotherapy (HIPEC) with irinotecan and oxaliplatin (Honore et al. 2012). Multiple liver metastasis from SPN can be effectively treated with trans-arterial chemoembolization (TACE) with gemcitabine and lipoidal followed by Gelfoam embolization (Prasad et al. 2017).

As diagnosis might not be established until intraoperative frozen section biopsy, the surgeon and pathologist should be aware of this entity as correct diagnosis might lead to a different surgical approach in case of SPT.

28.5.2.4 Prognosis

Unlike other malignant pancreatic tumors occurring in children, SPNs show a slow-growing, low malignant behavior and therefore have an excellent prognosis with surgery alone. Approximately 85% of the patients present with local disease (Mao et al. 1995; Wang et al. 1998; Klimstra et al. 2000), and 95% of these patients can be cured by complete surgical excision (Kaufman et al. 1986; Mao et al. 1995; Papavramidis and Papavramidis 2005). Despite low malignant potential of SPN, the possibility of aggressive behavior exists in approximately 15–20% of patients. According to Hwang et al., malignant SPNs are usually bigger than benign (median diameter 10 cm vs. 5 cm, respectively), and the proportion of solid component within the tumor in CT imagings is higher (median 88.5% vs. 41.5%) (Hwang et al. 2014).

In the case of recurrence (up to 10%), the tumor spread to liver or peritoneum and more rarely to lymph nodes, lung, and skin is seen (Rebhandl et al. 2001; Papavramidis and Papavramidis 2005; Morita et al. 2014). The risk of relapse is higher in patients with pancreas parenchyma infiltration and incomplete tumor capsule (Marchegiani et al. 2016; Song et al. 2017). In single cases, repeated surgeries for local recurrence and metastasis have proven to be of value (Rebhandl et al. 2001). Metastases occur late (average disease-free survival of 8.5 years) (Gonzalez-Campora et al. 1995; Lam et al. 1999) and are seen more often in older women (Todani et al. 1988; Matsunou and Konishi 1990; Nishihara et al. 1993a; Wang et al. 1998; Zhou et al. 2001). It was reported that clinical presentation and survival outcomes are similar in SPN of children and adults, suggesting that the management approaches in adult SPN may be appropriate for children (Leraas et al. 2018).

28.5.2.5 GEP-NETs

A multidisciplinary approach is crucial in appropriate management of the diverse group of GEP-NETs. Currently available therapeutic options for GEP-NETs include surgery, long-acting somatostatin analogues (e.g., octreotide), targeted agents (everolimus, sunitinib), peptide receptor radionuclide therapy (PRRT), and chemotherapy. Despite promising results from recent trials, the challenge is to establish the optimal sequencing of therapies to optimize outcome and preserve the quality of life (Khanna et al. 2008).

The short-term therapy of insulinoma is to prevent severe hypoglycemia including administration of high-dose glucose i.v. and glucagon and octreotide s.c. It may allow for symptomatic control during preoperative evaluation to localize the tumor (Esposito et al. 2015).

In case of gastrinoma, conservative therapy to alleviate symptoms consists of oral PPI. The best long-term survival has been seen in case of complete surgical resection, absence of liver metastases, or aggressive treatment of them, if present (Chu et al. 2002); 90% of insulinomas and most gastrinomas present as solitary mass and therefore can be cured by complete resection alone (Service et al. 1991). Usually, insulinomas are well circumscribed and can be enucleated without touching the pancreatic duct (Peranteau et al. 2013). To decrease the risk of formation of postoperative pancreatic fistulas, the tissue sealants and mattress sutures are used to reinforce the site of enucleation. If there is a concern for ductal involvement, partial pancreatectomy is preferred (Peranteau et al. 2013). If an insulinoma is located in the pancreatic tail, a spleen-preserving resection is indicated. It can be completed, if necessary, by enucleation of additional tumors in the pancreatic corpus or head (Bartsch et al. 2000; Padidela et al. 2014). If insulinoma cannot be localized, intraoperative ultrasound should be performed (Peranteau et al. 2013).

In case of MEN 1, therapy is complicated by often multiple pancreatic NETs (Service et al. 1991; Mergo et al. 1997). Therefore, during surgery, the pancreas must be carefully scrutinized with inspection, bimanual palpation, and intraoperative sonography from the uncinate process to the tip of the tail in order to find and resect all existing tumors. A systematic lymphadenectomy, however, is not routinely recommended in insulinoma. Management of metastatic insulinoma remains challenging and includes multimodal therapies, including chemotherapy, radiofrequency ablation, chemoembolization, and somatostatin analogues. Liver transplantation has also been used in cases with multifocal metastases limited to the liver (Casamassima et al. 2016).

As most of the gastrinomas occur in the so-called gastrinoma triangle around the head of the pancreas, resection for gastrinoma has to involve this area (Machado et al. 2001). As long as additional gastrinomas in the duodenum are excluded, a duodenopancreatectomy is not necessary in most cases (Bartsch et al. 2000; Brandi et al. 2001). A duodenotomy, however, is performed as a routine since duodenal gastrinomas frequently escape preoperative imaging (Norton et al. 2004). MEN-1-associated gastrinomas present as multiple, small nodules in the duodenum. Therefore, duodenotomy with transillumination is mandatory (Norton et al. 2004). However, the role of surgery is controversial in MEN-1-associated gastrinoma because complete cure by surgery is extremely rare.

Lymph node metastases are frequent (ca. 70%). An extended lymphadenectomy, therefore, must be performed in all cases of MEN-1-associated gastrinoma. Following these rules, young adults with advanced disease without disseminated distant metastases, who underwent surgical resection, showed comparable 15-year survival rates (89–100%) to those with limited disease or without an identifiable tumor (Norton et al. 2001). Hypergastrinemia, however, persists in most cases.

Debulking and metastasectomy can diminish the associated endocrine syndrome and might therefore be appropriate. Also, antihormonal pharmacologic therapy (e.g., pantoprazole in the ulcer-producing Zollinger–Ellison syndrome) has to be considered in these cases (Shorter et al. 2002). The role of chemotherapy and radiotherapy, though, is not clear.

28.5.2.6 Prognosis

In childhood, over 90% of insulinomas show a benign biological behavior; therefore, the prognosis is very good (Nasher et al. 2015). However, benign course is the case for only 40% of gastrinomas and 20–30% of glucagonomas (Grosfeld et al. 1990). Large tumors might have metastasized at the time of diagnosis, and metastases may also occur many years after diagnosis (Buetow et al. 1995). Different parameters for prediction of biological behavior and outcome have been found: tumors larger than 2–3 cm, tumor necrosis, well-differentiated tumors, vascular and perineural invasion, high mitotic count, high proliferation, and tumor biology (insulinoma vs. non-insulinoma) have been strongly correlated with malignant behavior (Donow et al. 1990; La Rosa et al. 1996; Hochwald et al. 2002). As insulinoma is slow-growing, these patients might show long survival, which is seen in only 20–30% in cases of sporadic gastrinoma (Norton et al. 2004). The prognosis of metastatic insulinoma remains relatively poor with a median survival period of approximately 2 years (Casamassima et al. 2016). Careful long-lasting postoperative follow-up is necessary, especially for patients with MEN-1, in whom the risk of recurrence is higher at 10 years than in individuals without MEN-1 (21% vs. 5%) (Padidela et al. 2014; Peranteau et al. 2013).

28.5.2.7 Other Rare Malignant and Low-Malignancy Pancreatic Tumors

The ACC probably grows less aggressively in childrenhood than in adults (Klimstra et al. 1992; Shorter et al. 2002). The prognosis of the rare pediatric ductal adenocarcinoma is as bad as that in the adult age group (Ivy et al. 1990). In general, a 5-year survival in epithelial exocrine carcinomas in children does not exceed 50% (Luttges et al. 2004; Perez et al. 2009; Ellerkamp et al. 2012; Mylonas et al. 2018a). Of utmost importance is the complete surgical resection. Since exocrine carcinomas develop most often in the head of pancreas, pancreaticoduodenectomy is the most commonly used surgical procedure. The impact of chemo- and radiotherapy is not clear (Shorter et al. 2002).

The IMT has a high tendency for local recurrence. A radical surgical resection, therefore, is of vital importance (Mizukami et al. 2006; Liu et al. 2017). Since anaplastic lymphoma kinase (ALK) and p80 expression as well as chromosomal rearrangements involving 2p23 have been reported to be related to IMT (Coffin et al. 2001; Nikitakis et al. 2004), a successful treatment using steroids and ALK inhibitors has been described in single cases (Dagash et al. 2009; Mosse et al. 2017).

28.5.2.8 Benign Tumors

The mucinous cystic adenoma is a benign tumor with the potential of malignant transformation and must be totally resected (Grosfeld et al. 1990; Farrell 2007). For hemangioma, there is an anecdotal report about a spontaneous regression after the biopsy (England et al. 2006). Teratoma must be totally resected. A circumscribed fibrotic focus associated with pediatric pancreatitis may mimic a neoplastic process (Adsay et al. 2004). This is one more reason why a mutilating resection of a pancreatic lesion should not be performed without knowing the final histological diagnosis.

Pancreatic pseudocysts have a high spontaneous healing rate. Initially, therefore, a wait-and-see policy is indicated. However, such factors as patient's comorbidity, age, and quality of life should be carefully considered based on the results of CT, MR, and endoscopic ultrasound imagings with cyst fluid analysis while at the same time balancing the risks of both surveillance and surgical intervention (Farrell 2007). If the size of the cyst does not decrease and symptoms persist, however, a drainage is necessary. This can be achieved by stent insertion directly into the cyst either percutaneously under sonographic or CT control imaging (Cannon et al. 2009) or endoscopically via ERCP or through the gastric wall (Sharma and Maharshi 2008; Maharshi 2008). If this fails, an open or laparoscopic cystogastrostomy or cystojejunostomy can be performed (Seitz et al. 2006; Yoder et al. 2009). A cystic pancreatic tumor, however, must be excluded before the drainage (Cannon et al. 2009). If the history or the diagnostic findings are equivocal, there is the rule: better resect a cyst than drain a tumor!

28.5.2.9 Focal Congenital Hyperinsulinism

If the existence and location of a focal congenital hyperinsulinism have been confirmed by

^{18}F-DOPA-PET-CT/MRI, surgical resection is indicated. Initially, three small biopsies are taken from unaffected areas and examined as frozen sections to exclude diffuse congenital hyperinsulinism. Then, the focal lesion is excised by atypical excision under frozen section monitoring. If the lesion is located in the pancreatic tail, a left resection is indicated which can be done by laparoscopy. Care is taken to preserve as much pancreatic tissue as possible. The excision is finished if all resection margins of the remaining pancreas are clear. If the pancreatic duct is involved, it must be drained by a Roux-en-Y pancreaticojejunostomy (Barthlen et al. 2016).

28.5.2.10 Laparoscopy

In adults, the number of minimally invasive pancreatic surgeries (MIPS) performed is increasing, and, in some centers, MIPS tend to replace traditional open approach. If performed by experienced laparoscopic surgeons, the outcomes are comparable to laparotomic surgeries (Umemura et al. 2018). There are numerous reports with reasonable patient numbers about laparoscopic pancreatic resections of both benign and malignant diseases (Palanivelu et al. 2007; Senthilnathan et al. 2015). In a study including 103 patients, the conversion rate was only 7% (Fernandez-Esparrach et al. 2007).

In children, laparoscopy has been also reported to be successfully used in the treatment of benign pancreatic tumors and SNP (Senthilnathan et al. 2014; Stewart et al. 2016; Esposito et al. 2015). For malignant solid tumors in childhood, however, the favorable results obtained in the adult group have not been reproducible (Warmann et al. 2003). The development of metastasis on the trocar sites seems to be quite rare. But even highly experienced centers report about high conversion rates in abdominal tumors (up to 42%) because a satisfying overview cannot be achieved (Metzelder et al. 2007). As outlined before, therefore, the laparoscopic approach for pediatric tumors in the pancreatic head and body is not recommended, neither for the biopsy (Fais et al. 2009) nor for the resection with curative intention (Spurbeck et al. 2004). An exception are small, delimited tumors in the pancreatic body or tail, which can be removed by pancreatic tail resection (Sokolov et al. 2009). Possible complications of pancreatic surgery are shown in Table 28.6. They are rare and do not seem to have significant impact on further child's growth (Sugito et al. 2012; Scandavini et al. 2018).

Table 28.6 Possible complications of pancreatic surgery (Adham et al. 2008; Mylonas et al. 2018a)

Complications	
Postoperative bleeding	From the remaining pancreas, small vessels to the splenic vein, bleeding from the splenic vein, portal vein, and superior mesenteric vein
	CAVE! Dangerous are erosion bleedings after leaking of the suture line or septic complications
Thrombosis or ischemia	Of the splenic artery, splenic vein, portal vein, mesenterial vessels, choledochal duct (after close preparation with stricture)
Loss of the spleen	Due to bleeding or thrombosis with risk of OPSI
Insufficiency Ileus Postoperative diabetes mellitus	Stump insufficiency of the pancreas after tail resection, insufficiency of the suture line of a pancreatojejunostomy with secretion of digestive juices, abscess, and pseudocyst Endocrine insufficiency due to resection of significant part of pancreas

28.6 Summary and Conclusions

In case of unspecific pain or a palpable mass in the upper abdomen, a pancreatic tumor should be considered, especially in adolescent females. Ultrasound examination in combination with MR/CT is mandatory. Because imaging alone is not able to assure proper diagnosis, the tumor should be exposed by an open approach, and the possibility of a primary complete resection without extensive surgery should be evaluated. Laparoscopy is indicated in tumors confined to the pancreatic body and tail, which can be resected without touching the tumor itself. If a complete resection does not seem feasible, biopsy should be performed only. Extensive resections of the pancreas and adjacent organs in childhood are justified only if they are beneficial for the child in knowledge of the histopathology and the staging. The surgical resection of local recurrences and metastases in childhood is always justified, even multiple times. The role of chemotherapy has been confirmed as a neoadjuvant treatment for initially inoperable and/or metastatic pancreatoblastoma; high rate of responses to chemotherapy allows for delayed complete surgeries, which improve the outcome. The role of radiotherapy in pediatric pancreatic tumors currently is hard to define because only single-case reports have been published.

Endocrine tumors are characterized by their hormone profile, imaging, and scintigraphy. Insulinomas must be treated by surgery, whereas the cure rate of gastrinomas by surgery alone is very low, especially in MEN 1 patients.

Children with pancreatic tumors show generally better prognosis than adults, mainly because of a different histologic pattern of the tumors occurring in that age group, but even in the few cases of pediatric pancreatic carcinomas, better results have been observed. Underlying reasons for a different prognosis, e.g., differences in biology and/or genetic makeup over age groups, are still to be investigated.

References

Abraham SC, Wu TT et al (2001) Distinctive molecular genetic alterations in sporadic and familial adenomatous polyposis-associated pancreatoblastomas: frequent alterations in the APC/beta-catenin pathway and chromosome 11p. Am J Pathol 159(5):1619–1627

Abraham SC, Wu TT et al (2002) Genetic and immunohistochemical analysis of pancreatic acinar cell carcinoma: frequent allelic loss on chromosome 11p and alterations in the APC/beta-catenin pathway. Am J Pathol 160(3):953–962

Adham M, Giunippero A et al (2008) Central pancreatectomy: single-center experience of 50 cases. Arch Surg 143(2):175–180. discussion 180–171

Adsay NV, Basturk O et al (2004) Pancreatic pseudotumors: non-neoplastic solid lesions of the pancreas that clinically mimic pancreas cancer. Semin Diagn Pathol 21(4):260–267

Al-Hader A, Al-Rohil RN et al (2017) Pancreatic acinar cell carcinoma: a review on molecular profiling of patient tumors. World J Gastroenterol 23(45):7945–7951

Anlauf M, Sipos B et al (2005a) Tumors of the endocrine pancreas. Pathologe 26(1):46–51

Anlauf M, Wieben D et al (2005b) Persistent hyperinsulinemic hypoglycemia in 15 adults with diffuse nesidioblastosis: diagnostic criteria, incidence, and characterization of beta-cell changes. Am J Surg Pathol 29(4):524–533

Antonello D, Gobbo S et al (2009) Update on the molecular pathogenesis of pancreatic tumors other than common ductal adenocarcinoma. Pancreatology 9(1–2):25–33

Barthlen W, Varol E et al (2016) Surgery in Focal Congenital Hyperinsulinism (CHI)—the "Hyperinsulinism Germany International" experience in 30 children. Pediatr Endocrinol Rev 14(2):129–137

Bartsch DK, Kersting M et al (2000) Low frequency of p16(INK4a) alterations in insulinomas. Digestion 62(2–3):171–177

Bassarova A, Sedloev T et al (2015) Pancreatoblastoma in an adult patient with late recurrence. J Cytol Histol 6(4):338

Belletrutti MJ, Bigam D et al (2013) Use of gemcitabine with multi-stage surgical resection as successful second-line treatment of metastatic pancreatoblastoma. J Pediatr Hematol Oncol 35(1):e7–e10

Bender AM, Thompson ED et al (2018) Solid pseudopapillary neoplasm of the pancreas in a young pediatric patient. A case report and systematic review of the literature. Pancreas 47(10):1364–1368

Bien E, Godzinski J, Dall'igna P et al (2011) Pancreatoblastoma: a report from the European cooperative study group for paediatric rare tumours (EXPeRT). Eur J Cancer 47(15):2347–2352. Epub 2011 Jun 21

Bien E, Roganovic J et al (2021) Pancreatoblastoma in children: EXPeRT/PARTNER diagnostic and therapeutic recommendations. Pediatr Blood Cancer 68(Suppl. 4):e29112. https://doi.org/10.1002/pbc.29112

Bohl CE, Federico SM et al (2018) FDG-PET CT in the evaluation of primary and secondary pancreatic malignancies. Pediatr Blood Cancer 65(10):e27115

Bosman FT, Carneiro F, Hruban RH, Theise ND (eds) (2010) WHO classification of tumours of the digestive system. World Health Organization, Lyon

Brandi ML, Gagel RF et al (2001) Guidelines for diagnosis and therapy of MEN type 1 and type 2. J Clin Endocrinol Metab 86(12):5658–5671. Review

Brennan MF, Kattan MW et al (2004) Prognostic nomogram for patients undergoing resection for adenocarcinoma of the pancreas. Ann Surg 240(2):293–298

Broaddus RR, Herzog CE, Hicks MJ (2003) Neuroendocrine tumors (carcinoid and neuroendocrine carcinoma) presenting at extra-appendiceal sites in childhood and adolescence. Arch Pathol Lab Med 127:1200–1203

Buetow PC, Parrino TV et al (1995) Islet cell tumors of the pancreas: pathologic-imaging correlation among size, necrosis and cysts, calcification, malignant behavior, and functional status. AJR Am J Roentgenol 165(5):1175–1179

Calvani J, Lopez P et al (2019) Solid pseudopapillary neoplasms of the pancreas do not express major pancreatic markers in pediatric patients. Hum Pathol 83:29–35

Campanile M, Nicolas A et al (2011) Frantz's tumor: is mutilating surgery always justified in young patients? Surg Oncol 20(2):121–125

Cannon JW, Callery MP et al (2009) Diagnosis and management of pancreatic pseudocysts: what is the evidence? J Am Coll Surg 209(3):385–393

Casamassima MGS, Gause CD et al (2016) Pancreatic surgery for tumors in children and adolescents. Pediatr Surg Int 32(8):779–788

Casanova M, Collini P et al (2003) Solid-pseudopapillary tumor of the pancreas (Frantz tumor) in children. Med Pediatr Oncol 41(1):74–76

Chaudhary P (2015) Acinar Cell Carcinoma Of The Pancreas: A Literature Review And Update. Indian Journal of Surgery 77(3):226–231

Chisholm KM, Hsu CH et al (2012) Congenital Pancreatoblastoma. J Pediatr Hematol Oncol 34(4):310–315

Chu QD, Hill HC et al (2002) Predictive factors associated with long-term survival in patients with neuroendocrine tumors of the pancreas. Ann Surg Oncol 9(9):855–862

Chun Y, Kim W et al (1997) Pancreatoblastoma. J Pediatr Surg 32(11):1612–1615

Chung EM, Travis MD et al (2006a) Pancreatic tumors in children: radiologic-pathologic correlation. Radiographics 26(4):1211–1238

Chung EM, Travis MD, Conran RM (2006b) Pancreatic tumors in children: radiologic-pathologic correlation. Radiographics 26:1211–1238

Chung YE, Kim MJ et al (2009) Differentiation of benign and malignant solid pseudopapillary neoplasms of the pancreas. J Comput Assist Tomogr 33(5):689–694

Coffin CM, Patel A et al (2001) ALK1 and p80 expression and chromosomal rearrangements involving 2p23 in inflammatory myofibroblastic tumor. Mod Pathol 14(6):569–576

Correa-Gallego C, Ferrone CR et al (2010) Incidental pancreatic cysts: do we really know what we are watching? Pancreatology 10(2–3):144–150

Corrias G, Ragucci M et al (2017) Pancreatoblastoma with metastatic retroperitoneal lymph node and PET/CT. Clin Nucl Med 42(11):e482–e483

Dagash H, Koh C et al (2009) Inflammatory myofibroblastic tumor of the pancreas: a case report of 2 pediatric cases–steroids or surgery? J Pediatr Surg 44(9):1839–1841

Dall'igna P, Cecchetto G et al (2010) Pancreatic tumors in children and adolescents: the Italian TREP project experience. Pediatr Blood Cancer 54(5):675–680

de Lonlay P, Simon-Carre A et al (2006) Congenital hyperinsulinism: pancreatic [18F]fluoro-L-dihydroxyphenylalanine (DOPA) positron emission tomography and immunohistochemistry study of DOPA decarboxylase and insulin secretion. J Clin Endocrinol Metab 91(3):933–940

Defachelles AS, Martin De Lassalle E et al (2001) Pancreatoblastoma in childhood: clinical course and therapeutic management of seven patients. Med Pediatr Oncol 37(1):47–52

Dhamne C, Herzog CE (2015) Response of relapsed pancreatoblastoma to a combination of vinorelbine and oral cyclophosphamide. J Pediatr Hematol Oncol 37(6):e378–e380

Dhebri AR, Connor S et al (2004) Diagnosis, treatment and outcome of pancreatoblastoma. Pancreatology 4(5):441–451. discussion 452–443

Donow C, Pipeleers-Marichal M et al (1990) The pathology of insulinoma and gastrinoma. The location, size, multicentricity, association with multiple endocrine type-I neoplasms and malignancy. Dtsch Med Wochenschr 115(37):1386–1391

Ellerkamp V, Warmann SW et al (2012) Exocrine pancreatic tumors in childhood in Germany. Pediatr Blood Cancer 58(3):366–371

England RJ, Woodley H et al (2006) Pediatric pancreatic hemangioma: a case report and literature review. JOP 7(5):496–501

Esposito I, Segler A, Steiger K, et al (2015) Pathology, genetics and precursors of human and experimental pancreatic neoplasms: An update. Pancreatology 15(6):598–610. https://doi.org/10.1016/j.pan.2015.08.007, indexed in Pubmed: 26365060

Fais PO, Carricaburu E et al (2009) Is laparoscopic management suitable for solid pseudo-papillary tumors of the pancreas? Pediatr Surg Int 25(7):617–621

Farrell J (2007) Pancreatic cysts and guidelines. Dig Dis Sci 62(7):1827–1839

Fernandez-Esparrach G, Gines A et al (2007) Comparison of endoscopic ultrasonography and magnetic resonance cholangiopancreatography in the diagnosis of pancreatobiliary diseases: a prospective study. Am J Gastroenterol 102(8):1632–1639

Field JB (1993) Insulinoma. In: Mazzaferri EL, Samaan NA (eds) Endocrine tumors. Blackwell Scientific Publications, Boston, pp 497–530

Fisher JC, Kuenzler KA et al (2007) Central pancreatectomy with pancreaticogastrostomy in children. J Pediatr Surg 42(4):740–746

Fried P, Cooper J et al (1985) A role for radiotherapy in the treatment of solid and papillary neoplasms of the pancreas. Cancer 56(12):2783–2785

Fukushima N, Fukayama M (2007) Mucinous cystic neoplasms of the pancreas: pathology and molecular genetics. J Hepato-Biliary-Pancreat Surg 14(3):238–242

Garcea G, Ong SL et al (2008) Cystic lesions of the pancreas. A diagnostic and management dilemma. Pancreatology 8(3):236–251

Ghaffarian AA, Book L et al (2018) Liver transplant for metastatic pancreatoblastoma: 7-year event-free survival after chemotherapy, pancreatectomy, complete hepatectomy, and liver transplant. Pediatr Transplant 22(1):e13098

Goh BK, Tan YM et al (2007) Solid pseudopapillary neoplasms of the pancreas: an updated experience. J Surg Oncol 95(8):640–644

Gonzalez-Campora R, Rios Martin JJ et al (1995) Papillary cystic neoplasm of the pancreas with liver metastasis coexisting with thyroid papillary carcinoma. Arch Pathol Lab Med 119(3):268–273

Griffin BR, Wisbeck WM et al (1987) Radiotherapy for locally recurrent infantile pancreatic carcinoma (pancreatoblastoma). Cancer 60(8):1734–1736

Grosfeld JL, Vane DW et al (1990) Pancreatic tumors in childhood: analysis of 13 cases. J Pediatr Surg 25(10):1057–1062

Gupta AK, Mitra DK et al (2000) Sonography and CT of pancreatoblastoma in children. AJR Am J Roentgenol 174(6):1639–1641

Hah JO, Park WK et al (2007) Preoperative chemotherapy and intraoperative radiofrequency ablation for unresectable solid pseudopapillary tumor of the pancreas. J Pediatr Hematol Oncol 29(12):851–853

Hamilton SR, Aaltonen LA (eds) (2000) World Health Organization classification of tumours. Pathology and genetics of tumours of the digestive system. IARC Press, Lyon

Hammond NA, Miller FH et al (2012) Imaging features of the less common pancreatic masses. Abdom Imaging 38(3):561–572

Herrmann KA, Helmberger T et al (2008) Solid pseudopapillary pancreas tumors–often neglected. Radiologe 48(8):764–769

Hinnie J, Gray CE et al (2000) Cushing's syndrome in a 16 year old girl due to ectopic ACTH precursor production from a pancreatic tumour. Clin Endocrinol 53(4):539–540

Hochwald SN, Zee S et al (2002) Prognostic factors in pancreatic endocrine neoplasms: an analysis of 136 cases with a proposal for low-grade and intermediate-grade groups. J Clin Oncol 20(11):2633–2642

Honore C, Goere D et al (2012) Peritoneal carcinomatosis from solid pseudopapillary neoplasm (Frantz's tumour) of the pancreas treated with HIPEC. Anticancer Res 32(3):1069–1073

Hsieh L, Burjonrappa S (2016) Pediatric pancreatic tumors: a review of current concepts JOP. J Pancreas (Online) 17(3):257–262

Hwang J, Kim DY et al (2014) Solid-pseudopapillary neoplasm of the pancreas in children: can we predict malignancy? J Pediatr Surg 49(12):1730–1733

Ibuka S, Uehara S et al (2017) Complete resection of pancreatoblastoma with portal vein obstruction after high-dose chemotherapy. J Pediatr Hematol Oncol 39(5):e275–e278

Ilyes G, Luzcay A et al (2007) Cushing's syndrome in a child with pancreatic acinar cell carcinoma. Endocr Pathol 18:95–102

Imamura A, Nakagawa A et al (1998) Pancreatoblastoma in an adolescent girl: case report and review of 26 Japanese cases. Eur J Surg 164(4):309–312

Irtan S, Galmiche-Rolland L et al (2016) Recurrence of solid pseudopapillary neoplasms of the pancreas: results of a Nationwide Study of Risk Factors and Treatment Modalities. Pediatr Blood Cancer 63(9):1515–1521

Isobe T, Seki M et al (2017) Integrated molecular characterization of the lethal pediatric cancer pancreatoblastoma. Cancer Res 78(4):865–876

Ivy EJ, Sarr MG et al (1990) Nonendocrine cancer of the pancreas in patients under age forty years. Surgery 108(3):481–487

Jaksic T, Yaman M et al (1992) A 20-year review of pediatric pancreatic tumors. J Pediatr Surg 27(10):1315–1317

Jeng LB, Chen MF et al (1993) Solid and papillary neoplasm of the pancreas. Emphasis on surgical treatment. Arch Surg 128(4):433–436

Kaufman SL, Reddick RL et al (1986) Papillary cystic neoplasm of the pancreas: a curable pancreatic tumor. World J Surg 10(5):851–859

Kauhanen S, Seppanen M et al (2007) Fluorine-18-L-dihydroxyphenylalanine (18F-DOPA) positron emission tomography as a tool to localize an insulinoma or beta-cell hyperplasia in adult patients. J Clin Endocrinol Metab 92(4):1237–1244

Kela M, Singh S, Lahoti B (2008) Immature cystic teratoma of head of pancreas. J Indian Assoc Pediatr Surg 13(2):85–87

Kerr NJ, Chun YH et al (2002) Pancreatoblastoma is associated with chromosome 11p loss of heterozygosity and IGF2 overexpression. Med Pediatr Oncol 39(1):52–54

Khanna G, O'Dorisio SM, Menda Y et al (2008) Gastroenteropancreatic neuroendocrine tumors in children and young adults. Pediatr Radiol 38: 251–259

Kletter GB, Sweetser DA et al (2007) Adrenocorticotropin-secreting pancreatoblastoma. J Pediatr Endocrinol Metab 20(5):639–642

Klimstra DS, Heffess CS et al (1992) Acinar cell carcinoma of the pancreas. A clinicopathologic study of 28 cases. Am J Surg Pathol 16(9):815–837

Klimstra DS, Wenig BM et al (1995) Pancreatoblastoma. A clinicopathologic study and review of the literature. Am J Surg Pathol 19(12):1371–1389

Klimstra DS, Wenig BM et al (2000) Solid-pseudopapillary tumor of the pancreas: a typically cystic carcinoma of low malignant potential. Semin Diagn Pathol 17(1):66–80

Kloppel G, Solcia E et al (1996) Histological typing of tumors of the exocrine pancreas. WHO international histological classification of tumors, 2nd edn. Springer, Berlin/Heidelberg/New York

Kohda E, Iseki M et al (2000) Pancreatoblastoma. Three original cases and review of the literature. Acta Radiol 41(4):334–337

Kosmahl M, Seada LS et al (2000) Solid-pseudopapillary tumor of the pancreas: its origin revisited. Virchows Arch 436(5):473–480

Kosmahl M, Pauser U et al (2004) Cystic neoplasms of the pancreas and tumor-like lesions with cystic features: a review of 418 cases and a classification proposal. Virchows Arch 445(2):168–178

La Rosa S, Sessa F et al (1996) Prognostic criteria in nonfunctioning pancreatic endocrine tumours. Virchows Arch 429(6):323–333

Lack EE (1989) Primary tumors of the exocrine pancreas. Classification, overview, and recent contributions by immunohistochemistry and electron microscopy. Am J Surg Pathol 13(Suppl. 1):66–88

Lack EE, Cassady JR et al (1983) Tumors of the exocrine pancreas in children and adolescents. A clinical and pathologic study of eight cases. Am J Surg Pathol 7(4):319–327

Laje P, Bhatti TR et al (2013) Solid pseudopapillary neoplasm of the pancreas in children: a 15-year experience and the identification of a unique immunohistochemical marker. J Pediatr Surg 48(10):2054–2060

Lam KY, Lo CY et al (1999) Pancreatic solid-cystic-papillary tumor: clinicopathologic features in eight patients from Hong Kong and review of the literature. World J Surg 23(10):1045–1050

Leraas HJ, Kim J et al (2018) Solid pseudopapillary neoplasm of the pancreas in children and adults. J Pediatr Hematol Oncol 40(4):233–236

Liu HK, Lin YC et al (2017) Inflammatory myofibroblastic tumors of the pancreas in children. Medicine 96(2):2–5

Lodish MB, Powell AC et al (2008) Insulinoma and gastrinoma syndromes from a single intrapancreatic neuroendocrine tumor. J Clin Endocrinol Metab 93(4):1123–1128

Lubezky N, Papoulas M et al (2017) Solid pseudopapillary neoplasm of the pancreas: Management and long-term outcome. Eur J Surg Oncol 43(6):1056–1060

Luttges J, Stigge C et al (2004) Rare ductal adenocarcinoma of the pancreas in patients younger than age 40 years. Cancer 100(1):173–182

Machado MC, da Cunha JE et al (2001) Insulinoma: diagnostic strategies and surgical treatment. A 22-year experience. Hepato-Gastroenterology 48(39):854–858

Maffuz A, Bustamante Fde T et al (2005) Preoperative gemcitabine for unresectable, solid pseudopapillary tumour of the pancreas. Lancet Oncol 6(3):185–186

Mao C, Guvendi M et al (1995) Papillary cystic and solid tumors of the pancreas: a pancreatic embryonic tumor? Studies of three cases and cumulative review of the world's literature. Surgery 118(5):821–828

Marchegiani G, Andrianello S et al (2016) Solid pseudopapillary tumors of the pancreas: specific pathological features predict the likelihood of postoperative recurrence. J Surg Oncol 114(5):597–601

Martin RC, Klimstra DS et al (2002) Solid-pseudopapillary tumor of the pancreas: a surgical enigma? Ann Surg Oncol 9(1):35–40

Matarazzo P, Tuli G et al (2011) Cushing syndrome due to ectopic adrenocorticotropic hormone secretion in a 3-year-old child. J Pediatr Endocrinol Metab 24(3–4):219–222

Matsunou H, Konishi F (1990) Papillary-cystic neoplasm of the pancreas. A clinicopathologic study concerning the tumor aging and malignancy of nine cases. Cancer 65(2):283–291

McClain MB, Burton EM et al (2000) Pancreatic pseudotumor in an 11-year-old child: imaging findings. Pediatr Radiol 30(9):610–613

Mergo PJ, Helmberger TK et al (1997) Pancreatic neoplasms: MR imaging and pathologic correlation. Radiographics 17(2):281–301

Mester M, Trajber et al (1990) Cystic teratomas of the pancreas. Arch Surg 125(9):1215–1258

Metzelder ML, Kuebler JF et al (2007) Role of diagnostic and ablative minimally invasive surgery for pediatric malignancies. Cancer 109(11):2343–2348

Mizukami H, Yajima N et al (2006) Pancreatic malignant fibrous histiocytoma, inflammatory myofibroblastic tumor, and inflammatory pseudotumor related to autoimmune pancreatitis: characterization and differential diagnosis. Virchows Arch 448(5):552–560

Montemarano H, Lonergan GJ et al (2000) Pancreatoblastoma: imaging findings in 10 patients and review of the literature. Radiology 214(2): 476–482

Morita K, Urushihara N et al (2014) Solid pseudopapillary tumor of the pancreas in children: surgical intervention strategies based on pathological findings. Pediatr Surg Int 30:253–257

Mosse YP, Voss SD et al (2017) Targeting ALK with crizotinib in pediatric anaplastic large cell lymphoma and inflammatory myofibroblastic tumor: a Children's Oncology Group Study. J Clin Oncol 35(28):3215–3221

Murakami T, Ueki K et al (1996) Pancreatoblastoma: case report and review of treatment in the literature. Med Pediatr Oncol 27(3):193–197

Mylonas KS, Doulamis IP et al (2018a) Solid pseudopapillary and malignant pancreatic tumors in childhood: a systematic review and evidence quality assessment. Pediatr Blood Cancer 65(10):1–9

Mylonas KS, Nasioudis D et al (2018b) A population-based analysis of a rare oncologic entity: malignant pancreatic tumors in children. J Pediatr Surg 53(4):647–652

Nadler EP, Novikov A et al (2002) The use of endoscopic ultrasound in the diagnosis of solid pseudopapillary tumors of the pancreas in children. J Pediatr Surg 37(9):1370–1373

Namgoong JM, Kim DY et al (2014) Laparoscopic distal pancreatectomy to treat solid pseudopapillary tumors in children: transition from open to laparoscopic approaches in suitable cases. Pediatr Surg Int 30(3):259–266

Nasher O, Hall NJ et al (2015) Pancreatic tumours in children: diagnosis, treatment and outcome. Pediatr Surg Int 31(9):831–835

Nikitakis NG, Brooks JK et al (2004) Inflammatory myofibroblastic tumour of oral cavity: review of literature and presentation of an ALK positive case. Oral Surg Oral Med Oral Pathol Oral Radiol Endod 98: 197–198

Nishihara K, Nagoshi M et al (1993a) Papillary cystic tumors of the pancreas. Cancer 71(1):82–92

Nishihara K, Tsuneyoshi M et al (1993b) Papillary cystic tumor of the pancreas. Is it a hormone-dependent neoplasm? Pathol Res Pract 189(5):521–526

Norton JA, Alexander HR et al (2001) Comparison of surgical results in patients with advanced and limited disease with multiple endocrine neoplasia type 1 and Zollinger-Ellison syndrome. Ann Surg 234(4):495–505. discussion 505–496

Norton JA, Alexander HR et al (2004) Does the use of routine duodenotomy (DUODX) affect rate of cure, development of liver metastases, or survival in patients with Zollinger-Ellison syndrome? Ann Surg 239(5):617–625; discussion 626

Ogawa T, Isaji S et al (1993) A case of radical resection for solid cystic tumor of the pancreas with widespread metastases in the liver and greater omentum. Am J Gastroenterol 88(9):1436–1439

Ogawa B, Okinaga K et al (2000) Pancreatoblastoma treated by delayed operation after effective chemotherapy. J Pediatr Surg 35(11):1663–1665

Orlefors H, Sundin A et al (2005) Whole-body (11)C-5-hydroxytryptophan positron emission tomography as a universal imaging technique for neuroendocrine tumors: comparison with somatostatin receptor scintigraphy and computed tomography. J Clin Endocrinol Metab 90(6):3392–3400

Padidela R, Fiest M et al (2014) Insulinoma in childhood: clinical, radiological, molecular and histological aspects of nine patients. Eur J Endocrinol 170(5):741–747

Palanivelu C, Jani K et al (2007) Laparoscopic pancreaticoduodenectomy: technique and outcomes. J Am Coll Surg 205(2):222–230

Panieri E, Krige JE et al (1998) Operative management of papillary cystic neoplasms of the pancreas. J Am Coll Surg 186(3):319–324

Papavramidis T, Papavramidis S (2005) Solid pseudopapillary tumors of the pancreas: review of 718 patients reported in English literature. J Am Coll Surg 200(6):965–972

Pappo AS, Furman WL (2006) Management of infrequent cancers in childhood. In: Pizzo PA, Poplack DC (eds) Principles and practice of pediatric oncology, 5th edn. Lippincott Williams & Wilkins, Philadelphia, pp 1180–1182

Peranteau WH, Palladino AA et al (2013) The surgical management of insulinomas in children. J Pediatr Surg 48(12):2517–2524

Perez EA, Gutierrez JC et al (2009) Malignant pancreatic tumors: incidence and outcome in 58 pediatric patients. J Pediatr Surg 44(1):197–203

Perilongo G, Brown J et al (2000) Hepatoblastoma presenting with lung metastases: treatment results of the first cooperative, prospective study of the International Society of Paediatric Oncology on childhood liver tumors. Cancer 89(8):1845–1853

Prasad T, Madhusudhan K et al (2017) Transarterial chemoembolization for liver metastases from solid pseudopapillary epithelial neoplasm of pancreas: a case report. World J Radiol 7(3):61

Rebhandl W, Felberbauer FX et al (2001) Solid-pseudopapillary tumor of the pancreas (Frantz tumor) in children: report of four cases and review of the literature. J Surg Oncol 76(4):289–296

Rebours V, Boutron-Ruault MC et al (2009) The natural history of hereditary pancreatitis: a national series. Gut 58(1):97–103

Saif MW (2007) Pancreatoblastoma. JOP 8(1):55–63

Saiura A, Umekita N et al (2000) Successful surgical resection of solid cystic tumor of the pancreas with multiple liver metastases and a tumor thrombus in the portal vein. Hepato-Gastroenterology 47(33):887–889

Scandavini C, Valente R et al (2018) Pancreatectomies for pancreatic neoplasms in pediatric and adolescent age: a single institution experience. Pancreatology 18(2):204–207

Sclafani LM, Reuter VE et al (1991) The malignant nature of papillary and cystic neoplasm of the pancreas. Cancer 68(1):153–158

Seitz G, Warmann SW et al (2006) Laparoscopic cystojejunostomy as a treatment option for pancreatic pseudocysts in children—a case report. J Pediatr Surg 41(12):e33–e35

Senthilnathan P, Patel N et al (2014) Laparoscopic pylorus preserving pancreaticoduodenectomy in paediatric age for solid pseudopapillary neoplasm of head of the pancreas—case report. Pancreatology 14(6):550–552

Senthilnathan P, Srivatsan Gurumurthy S et al (2015) Long-term results of laparoscopic pancreaticoduodenectomy for pancreatic and periampullary cancer—experience of 130 cases from a tertiary-care center in South India. J Laparoendosc Adv Surg Tech 25(4):295–300

Service FJ, McMahon MM et al (1991) Functioning insulinoma–incidence, recurrence, and long-term survival of patients: a 60-year study. Mayo Clin Proc 66(7):711–719

Sharma SS, Maharshi S (2008) Endoscopic management of pancreatic pseudocyst in children-a long-term follow-up. J Pediatr Surg 43(9):1636–1639

Shet NS, Cole BL et al (2014) Imaging of pediatric pancreatic neoplasms with radiologic-histopathologic correlation. Am J Roentgenol 202(6):1337–1348

Shorter NA, Glick RD et al (2002) Malignant pancreatic tumors in childhood and adolescence: the Memorial Sloan-Kettering experience, 1967 to present. J Pediatr Surg 37(6):887–892

Singhal D, Kakodkar R et al (2006) Issues in management of pancreatic pseudocysts. JOP 7(5):502–507

Sipos B, Kloppel G (2005) Acinar cell carcinomas and pancreatoblastomas: related but not the same. Pathologe 26(1):37–40

Snajdauf J, Rygl M et al (2009) Duodenum-sparing technique of head resection in solid pseudopapillary tumor of the pancreas in children. Eur J Pediatr Surg 19(6):354–357

Sokolov YY, Stonogin SV et al (2009) Laparoscopic pancreatic resections for solid pseudopapillary tumor in children. Eur J Pediatr Surg 19(6):399–401

Solcia E, Klöppel G et al (2000) Histological typing of endocrine tumours. WHO international histological classification of tumours, 2nd edn. Springer, Berlin

Song H, Dong M et al (2017) Solid pseudopapillary neoplasm of the pancreas: clinicopathologic feature, risk factors of malignancy, and survival analysis of 53 cases from a single center. Biomed Res Int 2017: 1–7

Sperti C, Berselli M et al (2008) Aggressive behaviour of solid-pseudopapillary tumor of the pancreas in adults: a case report and review of the literature. World J Gastroenterol 14(6):960–965

Spurbeck WW, Davidoff AM et al (2004) Minimally invasive surgery in pediatric cancer patients. Ann Surg Oncol 11(3):340–343

Stewart CL, Meguid C et al (2016) Evolving trends towards minimally invasive surgery for solid-pseudopapillary neoplasms. Ann Surg Oncol 23(13):4165–4168

Strauss JF, Hirsch VJ et al (1993) Resection of a solid and papillary epithelial neoplasm of the pancreas following treatment with cis-platinum and 5-fluorouracil: a case report. Med Pediatr Oncol 21(5): 365–367

Sugai M, Kimura N et al (2006) A case of pancreatoblastoma prenatally diagnosed as intraperitoneal cyst. Pediatr Surg Int 22(10):845–847

Sugito K, Furuya T et al (2012) Long-term follow-up of nutritional status, pancreatic function, and morphological changes of the pancreatic remnant after pancreatic tumor resection in children. Pancreas 41(4):554–559

Tessonnier L, Sebag F et al (2010) Limited value of 18F-F-DOPA PET to localize pancreatic insulin-secreting tumors in adults with hyperinsulinemic hypoglycemia. J Clin Endocrinol Metab 95(1):303–307

Tipton SG, Smyrk TC et al (2006) Malignant potential of solid pseudopapillary neoplasm of the pancreas. Br J Surg 93(6):733–737

Todani T, Shimada K et al (1988) Frantz's tumor: a papillary and cystic tumor of the pancreas in girls. J Pediatr Surg 23(2):116–121

Umemura A, Nitta H et al (2018) Current status of laparoscopic pancreaticoduodenectomy and pancreatectomy. Asian J Surg 41(2):106–114

Van Den Akker M, Angelini P et al (2012) Malignant pancreatic tumors in children: a single-institution series. J Pediatr Surg 47(4):681–687

Vannier JP, Flamant F et al (1991) Pancreatoblastoma: response to chemotherapy. Med Pediatr Oncol 19(3):187–191

Varshney A, Dhua A et al (2018) Whipple's pancreaticoduodenectomy in pediatric patients: an experience from a tertiary care center. J Indian Assoc Pediatr Surg 23(4):212

Vossen S, Goretzki PE et al (1998) Therapeutic management of rare malignant pancreatic tumors in children. World J Surg 22(8):879–882

Wang KS, Albanese C et al (1998) Papillary cystic neoplasm of the pancreas: a report of three pediatric cases and literature review. J Pediatr Surg 33(6):842–845

Warmann S, Fuchs J et al (2003) A prospective study of minimally invasive techniques in pediatric surgical oncology: preliminary report. Med Pediatr Oncol 40(3):155–157

Wunsch LP, Flemming P et al (1997) Diagnosis and treatment of papillary cystic tumor of the pancreas in children. Eur J Pediatr Surg 7(1):45–47

Ye J, Ma M et al (2012) Solid-pseudopapillary tumor of the pancreas: clinical features, pathological characteristics, and origin. J Surg Oncol 106(6):728–735

Yeung MJ, Pasieka JL (2009) Gastrinomas: a historical perspective. J Surg Oncol 100(5):425–433

Yoder SM, Rothenberg S et al (2009) Laparoscopic treatment of pancreatic pseudocysts in children. J Laparoendosc Adv Surg Tech A 19(Suppl. 1):S37–S40

Yu DC, Kozakewich HP et al (2009) Childhood pancreatic tumors: a single institution experience. J Pediatr Surg 44(12):2267–2272

Zhou H, Cheng W et al (2001) Solid-cystic papillary tumor of the pancreas in children. Pediatr Surg Int 17(8):614–620

Zollinger RM (1987) Gastrinoma: the Zollinger-Ellison syndrome. Semin Oncol 14(3):247–252

Zouros E, Manatakis DK et al (2015) Adult pancreatoblastoma: a case report and review of the literature. Oncol Lett 9(5):2293–2298

29 Liver Tumors

Howard M. Katzenstein and Michela Casanova

29.1 Genetics and Etiology

The underlying etiology of most pediatric liver tumors remains largely unknown; however, several genetic syndromes have been observed to be associated with liver tumors. Beckwith-Wiedemann syndrome (BWS) is an overgrowth syndrome linked to chromosome 11p and is present in approximately 2% of patients with hepatoblastoma. Patients with BWS are at increased risk for the development of several cancers including hepatoblastoma, Wilms' tumor, neuroblastoma, and adrenocortical carcinoma. A BWS registry has observed that hepatoblastoma is the most common tumor that occurs in BWS and that the risk for the development of hepatoblastoma in children with BWS is over 2000-fold higher than normal (DeBaun and Tucker 1998). Accordingly, it is recommended that BWS children be routinely screened with abdominal ultrasounds and serum alpha-fetoprotein levels every 3 months during the first decade of life to facilitate early detection (Clericuzio et al. 2003). Importantly, BWS patients can develop multiple primary tumors over the first decade of life, and so screening needs to continue even after the diagnosis of an initial malignancy.

Familial adenomatous polyposis (FAP) is an autosomal dominant disorder in which colonic polyp growth develops during adolescence and, without medical intervention, leads to colon cancer. FAP is also associated with a high risk of hepatoblastoma (Clericuzio et al. 2003). Mutations in the adenomatous polyposis coli (APC) gene on chromosome 5q can be detected in children with hepatoblastoma who have a family history of early occurrence of colon cancer. While it is unclear what the risk of this cancer predisposition is in children with hepatoblastoma without a history of FAP, it has been recommended that all children with hepatoblastoma should be evaluated for APC mutations and that asymptomatic children from FAP kindreds be screened to detect the presence of the mutation. If APC mutations are observed, then accordingly periodic screening for hepatoblastoma is also warranted (Hirschman et al. 2005) with abdominal ultrasounds and serum alpha-fetoprotein levels every 3 months.

Several other syndromes have been reported in association with hepatoblastoma including Simpson-Golabi-Behmel syndrome and trisomy of chromosome 8. A range of rare genetic disorders with underlying liver disease can be seen and may be linked to the development hepatocellular carcinoma (HCC), including progressive familial intrahepatic cholestasis, Alagille syn-

H. M. Katzenstein (✉) · M. Casanova
Division of Hematology/Oncology and BMT, Department of Pediatrics, Nemours Children's Specialty Care, Wolfson Children's Hospital, Jacksonville, FL, USA
e-mail: howard.katzenstein@nemours.org

D. T. Schneider et al. (eds.), *Rare Tumors in Children and Adolescents*, Pediatric Oncology,
https://doi.org/10.1007/978-3-030-92071-5_29

drome, hereditary tyrosinemia, and glycogen storage disease. HCC has also been described to occur in children with Fanconi's anemia who receive treatment with androgenic steroids.

The strongest risk factor associated with the development of HCC is hepatitis B or C infection. This is rare in North America, while in endemic areas of Southeast Asia, where hepatitis B and C infection rates are high, HCC is associated with the preponderance of malignant pediatric liver cancers (Chang et al. 1997). The utilization of hepatitis B vaccine has significantly diminished the incidence of HCC. In children, hepatocellular carcinoma can develop without any previous viral infections, and tumor development may be associated with congenital hepatic disorders (Czauderna 2002; Czauderna et al. 2002).

Epidemiologic studies have observed an increased risk of hepatoblastoma in children with fetal alcohol syndrome, with maternal use of oral contraceptives, and in parents who smoke. Surveys of exposures related to parental occupations in children with hepatoblastoma have shown a higher incidence of exposure to metals, welding, petroleum products, paints, and pigments (Buckley et al. 1989).

An increased risk of hepatoblastoma has been observed in children born prematurely, and this risk is inversely related to birth weight (Spector et al. 2004). The improved survival of low-birth-weight infants over recent decades may be an important contributing factor to the increased incidence of liver tumors observed over the past 20 years (Spector et al. 2004). Studies have yet to ascertain the etiology behind this phenomenon, which may be related to environmental exposures within newborn nurseries, enhanced sensitivity of the premature liver, interference in prenatal developmental pathways, or a multifactorial combination of such events.

29.2 Pathology and Cellular Classification

An international effort has been made over the last decade to unify the language of liver tumor pathology. This is important going forward and also in considering prior results where the terminology used to define liver tumor variants may have been different. Hepatoblastoma is the most common malignant liver tumor in children. Hepatoblastoma arises from hepatic precursors and may present with varying histology. Histology, typical for hepatoblastoma, is shown in Fig. 29.1. The tumors often contain a mixture

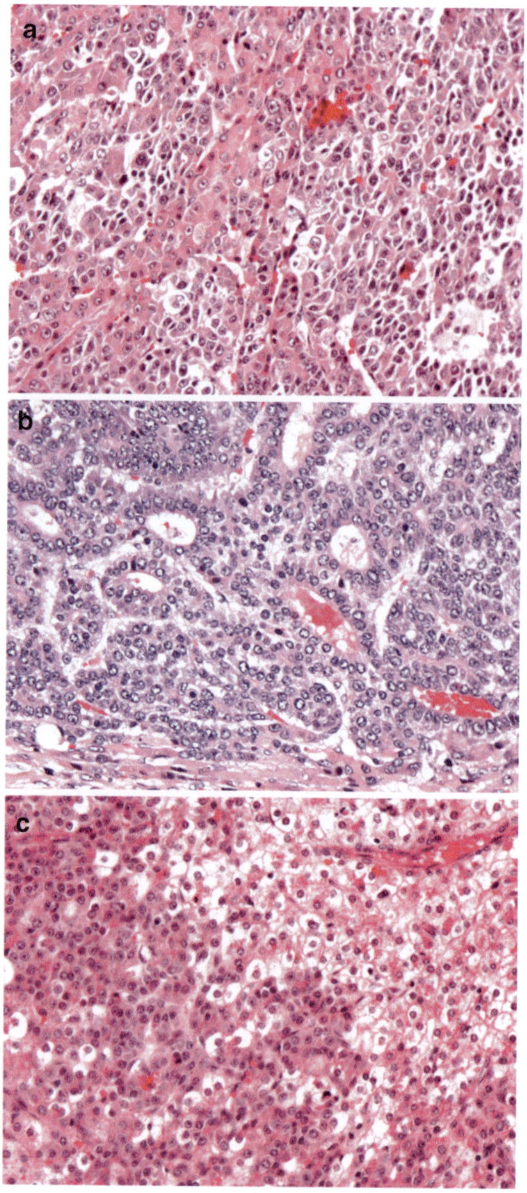

Fig. 29.1 (**a**) Hepatoblastoma, epithelial mixed type (embryonal and fetal). (**b**) Hepatoblastoma, pure embryonal type. (**c**) Hepatoblastoma, pure fetal type showing light and dark pattern

of epithelial hepatocytic precursors or pure hepatic embryonal cells. Two important variants may have clinical relevance: 100% pure fetal histology (throughout the entire tumor) and foci of small undifferentiated cells. In the USA, the treatment strategy has favored surgical resection at diagnosis, if the surgeon is confident that complete resection can be obtained. Again over the last decade, surgical guidelines have been created to try to provide objective criteria using the pretreatment extent of disease (PRETEXT) staging system and incorporated annotation factors. Patients whose tumors have pure fetal histology and undergo complete resection at diagnosis have a better prognosis (Ortega et al. 2000; Malogolowkin et al. 2011) and are treated with surgery alone. Confirmation of this pathologic finding by central expert review is essential as discrepancies between local and central review may happen more than 20% of the time. The presence of all pure fetal histology at a delayed resection is not prognostic as it is unclear what pathology cell types were present at diagnosis. Small cell undifferentiated hepatoblastoma is uncommon and is often seen under 1 year of age (Haas et al. 2001; Rowland 2002; Trobaugh-Lotrario et al. 2009), and the AFP is often low. Histologically, small cell undifferentiated hepatoblastoma presents with a diffuse population of small cells with scant cytoplasm. However, low AFP tumors with small cells may actually be rhabdoid tumors. The current use of INI1 staining and the detection of mutations in the hSNF5/INI1 gene (SMARCB1) on chromosome 22q functions, which functions as a tumor suppressor gene, can now be used to make an accurate pathologic diagnosis of rhabdoid tumors.

29.2.1 HCC

HCC can be seen in children, and the histology has predominately epithelial features (Fig. 29.2). They may form sinusoidal-like vascular channels with trabeculations. A distinct variant, fibrolamellar carcinoma has been described in older children and young adults (Katzenstein et al. 2003b). While sometimes considered to have a more favorable diagnosis, the long outcome of HCC of any pathologic subtype is dismal unless all disease is resectable and has recently been identified to have a specific genetic alteration resulting in a DNAJBI-PRKACA chimeric transcript. Transitional liver cell tumors/hepatocellular neoplasm, not otherwise specified, have been recently identified in older children and adolescents (Prokurat et al. 2002). They usually present as a solitary large mass (often in right lobe of liver). Cells are described as intermediate between hepatoblasts and mature hepatocytes.

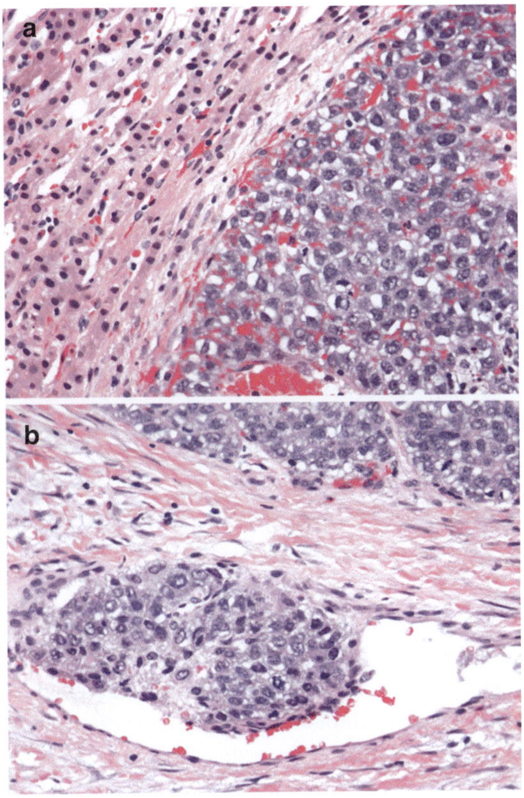

Fig. 29.2 (**a**) HCC, showing normal liver on left and tumor on right. (**b**) HCC, showing angiolymphatic invasion

29.2.2 Sarcomas and Undifferentiated Embryonal Sarcoma of the Liver

Various sarcomas have been identified in the liver including biliary rhabdomyosarcoma, angiosarcoma, and undifferentiated embryonal sarcoma of the liver which is a unique entity. Histologically, intracellular hyaline globules and marked anaplasia are seen in a mesenchymal background. Infantile choriocarcinoma of the liver are identified by closely packed cells with clear cytoplasm and multinucleated syncytia formation.

29.3 Clinical Diagnosis

Liver tumors in children have a wide constellation of presenting symptoms but do not have a pathognomonic presentation. Most patients present with an asymptomatic lesion or with an incidentally detected right upper quadrant mass in patients with other complaints such as abdominal pain, nausea, vomiting, weight loss, and fever. Systemic symptoms may indicate tumor rupture. At diagnosis, most children will not have any evidence of underlying liver disease such as ascites, jaundice, or abnormal tests of liver function. Hepatoblastoma is high in the differential diagnosis of patients with predisposing conditions such as a history of prematurity, hemihypertrophy, BWS, a family history of early colon cancers, or precocious puberty. HCC usually occurs in an otherwise asymptomatic patient but may arise in patients with antecedent conditions producing underlying liver disease such as cirrhosis, galactosemia, tyrosinemia, α-1 antitrypsin deficiency, or glycogen storage disease. As noted, hepatitis B and C are rarely detected as the cause of hepatocellular carcinoma in North America. The rarest of malignant pediatric liver tumors, sarcomas and rhabdoid tumors, are usually not considered as a diagnosis until review of tissue biopsies or in patients with characteristic radiographic findings. Metastatic involvement of the liver from neuroblastoma, Wilms' tumor, lymphoma, leukemia, and Langerhans cell histiocytosis are more common than most primary liver malignancies and may be identifiable within the characteristic presentations of such oncologic processes.

Benign tumors are also often asymptomatic at diagnosis. Hemangiomas and hemangioendotheliomas usually occur early in life and may present as part of the Kasabach-Merritt syndrome with high-output cardiac failure or consumptive coagulopathy. In adolescent girls with a history of using oral contraceptive, adenomas should be considered.

29.3.1 Diagnosis and Evaluation

Serum alpha-fetoprotein (AFP) is an extremely helpful tumor marker in the diagnosis and follow-up of liver tumor patients and should be evaluated in all patients at presentation. AFP elevation is almost always a sign of malignant disease, especially when it is >100 ng/ml. Rarely, tests for AFP can be falsely low in what is referred to as the "hook effect" if the assay is not sensitive enough to detect a very high level (Jassam et al. 2006). Normal AFP levels in suspected malignancies should have serial dilutions performed to ascertain whether or not the hook effect is present and also to get an accurate level at diagnosis (to follow response to therapy) if there is an upper limit of the AFP detected by the test. In the first year of life, and especially in the first 6 months, interpretation of AFP levels can be difficult and must be evaluated within the context of age appropriate normal values (Wu et al. 1981; Blohm et al. 1998). AFP levels are elevated at diagnosis in the majority of hepatoblastoma patients but in only about half of HCC patients. A normal AFP level should question the diagnosis of hepatoblastoma, and in such cases other pathologic liver tumor variants should be strongly considered as a normal AFP level is usually found in cases of fibrolamellar HCC, undifferentiated sarcomas, rhabdoid tumors, and metastatic disease. The decline of the AFP in response to chemotherapy is a useful marker of tumor response. Failure of the AFP level to decline or AFP increases during both therapy and follow-up can signify resistant or recurrent disease. Minimal elevations can be seen following surgery, as a result of tumor necrosis following the initiation of therapy. Recurrent disease as suggested by elevations of AFP should be confirmed by imaging studies although occasional small rises (<100 ng/ml) can be seen and serial AFP levels will typically give an answer. However, it is sometimes difficult to find recurrent lesions when the AFP has just started to increase, and it is generally recommended to wait to reinitiate therapy until the recurrent disease can be identified in this "surgical" disease. In fibrolamellar HCC, elevated levels of vitamin B12-binding protein can sometimes be used to monitor disease (Lin et al. 2010).

Thrombocytosis and anemia can sometimes be observed at diagnosis. In most instances, liver function tests are usually normal, except in the setting of underlying liver disease.

Abdominal ultrasound is typically the first radiologic exam performed in patients with newly identified liver lesions. Computed tomography (CT) and/or magnetic resonance imaging of the abdomen provides definitive tumor imaging. As the lungs are the primary site of metastatic disease, a CT scan of the chest should be performed preoperatively in all patients suspected of malignancy. Angiographic studies which delineate tumor vascularity and blood supply are often extremely helpful in guiding decisions about tumor resectability. The utility of positron emission tomography (PET) imaging in pediatric liver tumors is not established at this time but is sometimes utilized without defined utility when looking for occult recurrent disease.

Metastatic disease to sites other than lung is extremely rare but has been described to occur in the bone, bone marrow, and brain. Imaging of these sites should only be considered if the clinical scenario suggests the presence of such disease.

29.4 Tumor Staging

The Children's Oncology Group has used a surgical staging system (Table 29.1). Stages I and II are grossly resected tumors with and without microscopic residual, respectively. The majority of tumors are stage III with gross residual disease but no extrahepatic spread. Stage IV patients have distant metastasis. In contrast, the International Childhood Liver Tumor Strategy Group (SIOPEL) has established the PRETEXT system (Fig. 29.3) which uses the radiologic appearance of the tumor to determine tumor involvement of four different sectors and the eight different Couinaud segments (Aronson et al. 2005). This system guides resectability and is linked to outcome. Some initial studies suggested significant over-staging using this system as well as questionable interobserver reliability (Aronson et al. 2005). This system is now being used as the standard staging system on international trials but still requires further validation for prognostic significance (Lopez-Terrada et al. 2014).

Table 29.1 Children's Oncology Group: surgical staging of primary tumor at time of initial surgery

Stage	Description
Stage I:	Completely resected tumors
	All stage I tumors require rapid pathology review
Stage II:	Grossly resected tumors with evidence of microscopic residual
	Resected tumors with microscopic positive margins or preoperative (intraoperative) rupture
Stage III:	Unresectable tumors
	Partially resected tumors with measurable tumor left behind or patients with abdominal lymph node involvement
Stage IV:	Metastatic disease to lungs, other organs, or sites distant from the abdomen

29.5 Prognostic Factors

The surgical resectability of the tumor and the absence of metastatic disease are the most important prognostic factors in pediatric liver tumors. The PRETEXT system can predict outcome. More recent evidence has revealed that tumor pathology can also predict outcome. Patients with 100% pure fetal histology hepatoblastoma tumors that are completely resected at diagnosis have a superb outcome (Malogolowkin et al. 2011). Patients with fibrolamellar HCC subtype, though previously described to be associated

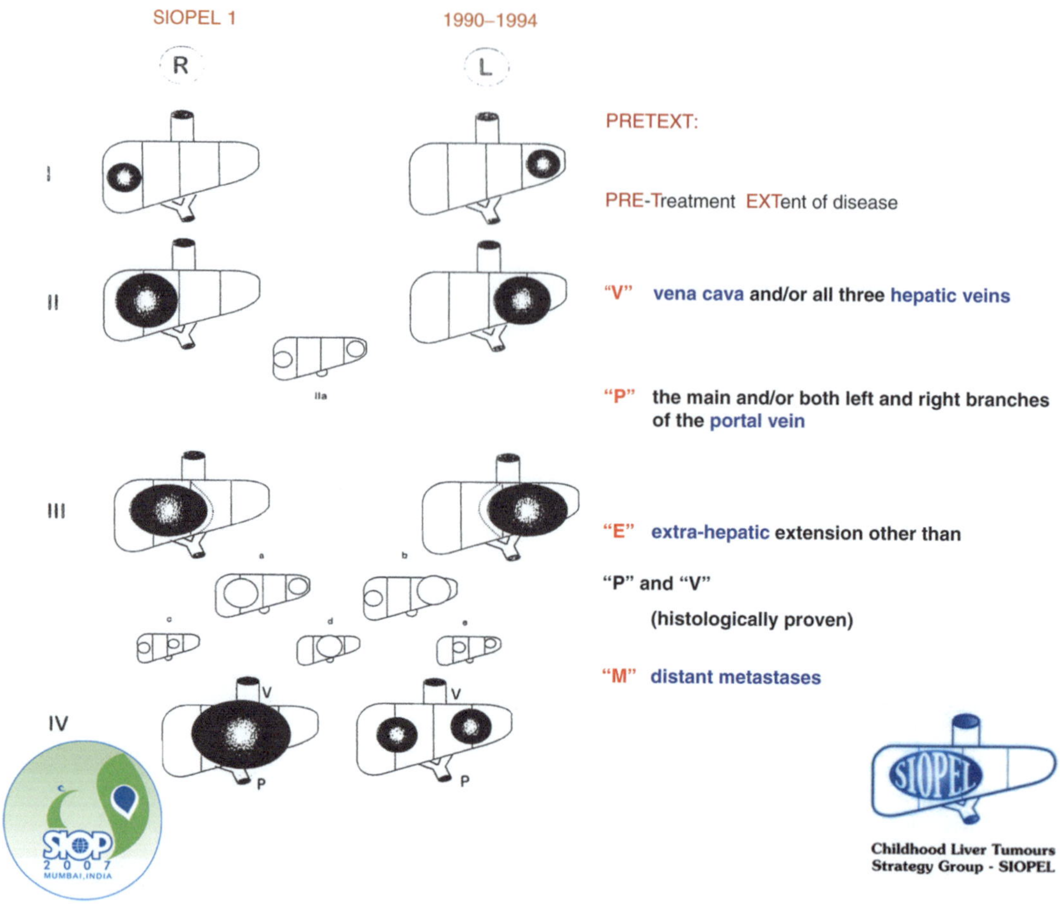

Fig. 29.3 PRETEXT classification of liver tumors

with a survival advantage, have a similar overall outcome as other HCC patients (Katzenstein et al. 2003b). The total overall decline of AFP levels is another prognostic variable, as patients with hepatoblastoma, who have a >1 log decline over the entire course of therapy, do better (Van Tornout et al. 1997). However, the rate of AFP decline during therapy has not been shown to predict outcome and should not be used to guide therapeutic decisions. Undifferentiated embryonal sarcoma of the liver and rhabdoid tumor of the liver are considered more aggressive but do have reasonable outcomes if all disease can be surgically removed.

The Children's Hepatic Tumors International Collaboration (CHIC) developed a novel risk stratification system. Definitions were standardized. This enabled the comparison of data from studies conducted by different national groups (Meyers et al. 2017). Analysis of combined data allowed for the identification of prognostic factors Czauderna et al. 2016). These factors were based on PRETEXT stage, AFP level, presence of metastatic disease, and annotation factors.

29.6 Treatment

Surgical resection is the foundation of curative treatment for both hepatoblastoma and HCC. Recent data suggest that patients who undergo upfront resection require limited postoperative chemotherapy and achieve an excellent outcome. This data suggests that patients who undergo earlier resection may require less overall therapy. Liver transplantation, as potential curative therapy, is an important alternative for achieving surgical resection (Otte et al. 2004). Patients who undergo liver transplantation have an outcome similar to those who undergo conventional resection. There is no data in children with liver tumors that demonstrates the use of immune suppression makes a patient more likely to relapse. Extrahepatic disease is an absolute contraindication to liver transplantation. However, if metastatic disease is eradicated in full, then liver transplantation becomes an immediate therapeutic option as there is no evidence-based data that suggests that such patients should be observed for any specific period of time. Therefore, strong consideration should be given to the aggressive early removal of metastatic foci to make a patient a viable candidate for liver transplant. The scarcity of liver tumors makes it crucial to consider early referral to centers with experience and expertise in performing liver transplantation for any patient who has unresectable disease at diagnosis. Ultimately, novel therapies are needed to improve the response to induction chemotherapy and decrease the need for liver transplantation. Most importantly, patients who undergo a liver transplant for recurrent disease have an inferior outcome. Therefore, it is critical that the correct initial surgery (resection vs transplant) be performed for every patient. Typically, less than half of children with hepatoblastoma and one third of patients with HCC have resectable disease at diagnosis. Patients who do not undergo upfront resection usually receive a more prolonged course of chemotherapy treatment with potential for an increased amount of late effects. While hepatoblastoma is considered a surgical disease, the importance and role of surgical resection of metastatic sites remain unclear (Meyers et al. 2007). It requires a prospective study to determine whether there is a difference in outcome for patients who have chemotherapeutic eradication of metastatic disease compared with those who undergo surgical metastasectomy.

Over the last two decades, chemotherapy has been demonstrated to be effective in improving the survival of patients with hepatoblastoma by making tumors surgically resectable. Treatment approaches in North American cooperative group trials have differed somewhat from international treatment regimens (Perilongo et al. 2004; Katzenstein et al. 2019; Zsíros et al. 2013). Cisplatin and doxorubicin are considered to be the most effective agents. The combination of cisplatin, 5-flourouracil, and vincristine (C5V) has demonstrated excellent survival in the approximately one third of patients with low-risk disease who are able to undergo resection at diagnosis (Ortega et al. 2000). The role of doxorubicin has been debated but is used in the majority of patients with high-risk disease that is either unresectable or metastatic (Pritchard et al. 2000; Malogolowkin et al. 2008). Carboplatin, ifosfamide, and etoposide have been used in treatment regimens, but there are no single agent data establishing the effectiveness of these drugs (von Schweinitz et al. 1997). Due to the low numbers of cases of pediatric liver tumors, it has been challenging to identify active new compounds in phase I and II trials. Irinotecan is a newer agent which has shown some efficacy and is being studied in current trials (Katzenstein et al. 2017; Qayed et al. 2010). Contrastingly, the novel platin compound oxaliplatin had disappointing phase II results against liver tumors (Beaty et al. 2010). SIOPEL-4 was a multinational feasibility trial of dose-dense cisplatin/doxorubicin chemotherapy and radical surgery for a group of children with high-risk hepatoblastoma. Neoadjuvant chemotherapy (three cycles) was administered followed, in patients with a response, by surgical removal (which may include liver transplantation). Patients with no response received additional two cycles (Zsiros et al. 2013).

The chemotherapy drugs used for the treatment of hepatoblastoma have also been utilized in combined trials for HCC but with much different results. Patients with resected HCC have received chemotherapy post-resection with excellent results. It is unclear if these patients were cured with surgery alone or if there was any contributing role for chemotherapy (Katzenstein et al. 2002). This remains a study question for future trials. On the other hand, for patients with unresectable or metastatic disease, chemotherapy is largely ineffective in rendering a tumor resectable or in eliminating metastatic disease. Interferon has been used in adult trials without much success. Sorafenib has shown some efficacy in prolonging survival in adult trials and is now widely considered as standard of care (Llovet et al. 2008; Abou-Alfa et al. 2010). This agent has been used in pediatric phase I and II studies but has yet to be formally evaluated in a pediatric liver tumor trial. Because of the lack of chemotherapeutic efficacy, earlier consideration should be given to children with HCC for liver transplantation so that tumor does not spread during the administration of chemotherapy that is likely to cause toxicity with little to no therapeutic effect. Pediatric HCC should not be evaluated and treated in the same manner as adult HCC because these tumors arise in different settings. It is unknown if the biology of pediatric tumors are the same as or different from the lesions that occur in adults. Lesions from other malignancies that arise in both pediatric and adult populations suggest there is likely to be different biology requiring distinct therapeutic strategies for both groups. Therefore, in HCC it would seem that separate transplant criteria need to be established for pediatric patients to offer them the optimal chance at survival.

Radioembolization, chemoembolization, radiofrequency ablation, and cryosurgery are alternative methods that have been used in adult trials and have demonstrated the ability to cause decrease in liver tumor size. There are rare reports on the use of these techniques in pediatric patients (Malogolowkin et al. 2000). The identification of effective therapies against HCC is essential to improving the dismal outcomes for these patients.

Rhabdoid tumor of the liver has a poor prognosis unless resected. Different chemotherapy regimens have been used, and there has been evidence of chemosensitivity, with ifosfamide being potentially recognized as the most active agent (Katzenstein et al. 2003a). However, there is no established chemotherapeutic regimen that is effective in producing long-term survival for these patients. Undifferentiated sarcoma of the liver is usually treated with a sarcoma-based approach with surgery and chemotherapy (Baron et al. 2007) and has reasonable survival if resected.

Radiation therapy has no definitive role in the treatment of primary malignant liver tumors or metastatic liver lesions and has been mostly used in palliative care settings (Habrand et al. 1992).

29.7 Outcome

Surgical resection is critical to survival in patients with pediatric liver tumors. Patients with hepatoblastoma or HCC that are resected have excellent survival, while those that are unable to undergo surgical eradication of disease do poorly. Chemotherapy can result in tumor shrinkage that can often make resection feasible in children with hepatoblastoma, while this is rarely achievable in patients with HCC. Metastatic disease remains an adverse prognostic factor and predicts a poor outcome in all affected patients.

29.8 Practical Strategy for Liver Tumors

This discussion has centered on the diagnosis and treatment of malignant liver tumors. However, there are many benign tumors that present in childhood and adolescent. Many are only seen in infants and toddlers. Both malignant and benign liver tumors may be age specific (Table 29.2). A practical strategy for diagnosis of liver tumors is described. Many benign tumors have

Table 29.2 Common liver tumors

Benign tumors	Age at presentation
Mesenchymal hamartoma	<5 years (usually infancy)
Teratoma	<5 years (usually infancy)
Hemangioma Kaposiform hemangioendothelioma Hepatic adenoma	Infancy Infancy Older children and adolescents
Focal nodular hyperplasia	Older children and adolescents
Malignant tumors	
Hepatoblastoma	<5 years (usually infancy)
Hepatocellular carcinoma	Older children and adolescents
Sarcomas Malignant rhabdoid tumor Germ cell tumor Nested epithelial stromal tumor	Older children and adolescents Any age Any age Older children and adolescents
Metastatic disease	Any age

characteristic imaging findings. Biopsy is not always needed and may be detrimental, especially given a highly vascular lesion. Careful observation may be appropriate. A careful understanding of the natural history of the more common benign hepatic tumors of childhood is warranted (Table 29.3). A more complex issue is the treatment strategy for hepatoblastoma. In the USA (COG), an attempt is made to perform initial resection at diagnosis for PRETEXT I and II tumors. Some patients will not need chemotherapy, for example, stage I with pure fetal histology (Malogolowkin et al. 2011). Others would need only two cycles. In the SIOPEL strategy, neoadjuvant chemotherapy is administered to the vast majority of patients (Perilongo et al. 2009). This may improve event-free survival, but all patients receive increased cisplatin and are at risk for late toxicity. COG, SIOPEL, and the Japanese Liver Tumor Group (JPLT) are now working together on an international trial. In addition, the Children's Hepatic tumors International Collaboration (CHIC) includes data from the above groups as well as the German Pediatric Oncology Group (GPOH) and has helped establish prognostic variables now being used for risk stratification on treatment protocols. This collaboration is extremely important to produce timely results in this rare disease as well as unified criteria for pathologic and radiologic evaluation as well as surgical interventions. The collection of tumor samples for all of these primary liver lesions is vital as biological studies may greatly inform investigators on which patients are most likely to relapse and may need more or less therapy.

Table 29.3 Management of benign liver tumors

Tumor	Diagnosis	Treatment
Infantile hepatic hemangioma	• Most common benign tumor in infancy	• Can have spontaneous remission
	• Contrast-enhanced CT findings—diagnostic	• Steroids, IFN
	• May be able to avoid biopsy	• Surgery should be reserved for life-threatening cases
Kaposiform hemangioendothelioma	• Rare, benign but behaves aggressively, may have true Kasabach-Merritt with platelet and factor consumption	• IFN • Multidrug regimens with vincristine, cyclophosphamide, actinomycin D, and methotrexate
Mesenchymal hamartoma	• Abdominal mass in healthy child	• Surgery may be the only option
	• Right lobe most affected	• Medical treatment—debatable
	• CT shows multiple cysts, rare solid	
	• AFP may be slightly elevated	
Focal nodular hyperplasia	• Any age, but usually 2–5 years	• Surgical treatment
	• Associated with syndromes such as Klinefelter's	• Questionable role for arterial embolization
	• Associated with past chemotherapy treatment	
	• CT angiography/MRI—well demarcated, hyperechoic, homogeneous	

References

Abou-Alfa GK, Johnson P et al (2010) Doxorubicin plus sorafenib vs. doxorubicin alone in patients with advanced hepatocellular carcinoma: a randomized trial. JAMA 304(19):2154–2160

Aronson DC, Schnater JM et al (2005) Predictive value of the pretreatment extent of disease system in hepatoblastoma: results from the International Society of Pediatric Oncology Liver Tumor Study Group SIOPEL-1 study. J Clin Oncol 23(6):1245–1252

Baron PW, Majlessipour F et al (2007) Undifferentiated embryonal sarcoma of the liver successfully treated with chemotherapy and liver resection. J Gastrointest Surg 11(1):73–75

Beaty O 3rd, Berg S et al (2010) A phase II trial and pharmacokinetic study of oxaliplatin in children with refractory solid tumors: a Children's Oncology Group study. Pediatr Blood Cancer 55(3):440–445

Blohm ME, Vesterling-Horner D et al (1998) Alpha 1-fetoprotein (AFP) reference values in infants up to 2 years of age. Pediatr Hematol Oncol 15(2):135–142

Buckley JD, Sather H et al (1989) A case-control study of risk factors for hepatoblastoma. A report from the Children's Cancer Study Group. Cancer 64(5):1169–1176

Chang MH, Chen CJ et al (1997) Universal hepatitis B vaccination in Taiwan and the incidence of hepatocellular carcinoma in children. Taiwan Childhood Hepatoma Study Group. N Engl J Med 336(26):1855–1859

Clericuzio CL, Chen E et al (2003) Serum alpha-fetoprotein screening for hepatoblastoma in children with Beckwith-Wiedemann syndrome or isolated hemihyperplasia. J Pediatr 143(2):270–272

Czauderna P (2002) Adult type vs. Childhood hepatocellular carcinoma—are they the same or different lesions? Biology, natural history, prognosis, and treatment. Med Pediatr Oncol 39(5):519–523

Czauderna P, Mackinlay G et al (2002) Hepatocellular carcinoma in children: results of the first prospective study of the International Society of Pediatric Oncology group. J Clin Oncol 20(12):2798–2804

Czauderna P, Haeberle B, Hiyama E et al (2016) The Children's Hepatic tumors International Collaboration (CHIC): Novel global rare tumor database yields new prognostic factors in hepatoblastoma and becomes a research model. Eur J Cancer 52:92–101

DeBaun MR, Tucker MA (1998) Risk of cancer during the first four years of life in children from The Beckwith-Wiedemann Syndrome Registry. J Pediatr 132(3 Pt 1):398–400

Haas JE, Feusner JH et al (2001) Small cell undifferentiated histology in hepatoblastoma may be unfavorable. Cancer 92(12):3130–3134

Habrand JL, Nehme D et al (1992) Is there a place for radiation therapy in the management of hepatoblastomas and hepatocellular carcinomas in children? Int J Radiat Oncol Biol Phys 23(3):525–531

Hirschman BA, Pollock BH et al (2005) The spectrum of APC mutations in children with hepatoblastoma from familial adenomatous polyposis kindreds. J Pediatr 147(2):263–266

Jassam N, Jones CM et al (2006) The hook effect: a need for constant vigilance. Ann Clin Biochem 43(Pt 4):314–317

Katzenstein HM, Krailo MD et al (2002) Hepatocellular carcinoma in children and adolescents: results from the Pediatric Oncology Group and the Children's Cancer Group intergroup study. J Clin Oncol 20(12):2789–2797

Katzenstein HM, Kletzel M et al (2003a) Metastatic malignant rhabdoid tumor of the liver treated with tandem high-dose therapy and autologous peripheral blood stem cell rescue. Med Pediatr Oncol 40(3):199–201

Katzenstein HM, Krailo MD et al (2003b) Fibrolamellar hepatocellular carcinoma in children and adolescents. Cancer 97(8):2006–2012

Katzenstein HM, Furman WL, Malogolowkin MH et al (2017) Upfront window vincristine/irinotecan treatment of high-risk hepatoblastoma: a report from the Children's Oncology Group AHEP0731 study committee. Cancer 123(12):2360–2367

Katzenstein HM, Langham MR, Malogolowkin MH et al (2019) Minimal adjuvant chemotherapy for children with hepatoblastoma resected at diagnosis (AHEP0731): a Children's Oncology Group, multicentre, phase 3 trial. Lancet Oncology

Lin CY, Kuo CS et al (2010) Elevated serum vitamin B(12) levels in association with tumor markers as the prognostic factors predictive for poor survival in patients with hepatocellular carcinoma. Nutr Cancer 62(2):190–197

Llovet JM, Ricci S et al (2008) SHARP Investigators Study Group. Sorafenib in advanced hepatocellular carcinoma. N Engl J Med 359(4):378–390

Lopez-Terrada D et al (2014) Towards an international pediatric liver tumor consensus classification: proceedings of the Los Angeles COG liver tumors symposium. Mod Pathol 27(3):472–491

Malogolowkin MH, Stanley P et al (2000) Feasibility and toxicity of chemoembolization for children with liver tumors. J Clin Oncol 18(6):1279–1284

Malogolowkin MH, Katzenstein HM et al (2008) Redefining the role of doxorubicin for the treatment of children with hepatoblastoma. J Clin Oncol 26(14):2379–2383

Malogolowkin MH, Katzenstein HM, Krailo M, Rowland J, Haas J, Meyers RL, Finegold M (2011) Complete surgical resection is curative for children with hepatoblastoma with pure fetal histology. J Clin Oncol 29(24):3301–3306

Meyers RL, Katzenstein HM et al (2007) Surgical resection of pulmonary metastatic lesions in children with hepatoblastoma. J Pediatr Surg 42(12):2050–2056

Meyers RL, Maibach R, Hiyama E et al (2017) Risk-stratified staging in paediatric hepatoblastoma:

a unified analysis from the Children's Hepatic tumors International Collaboration. Lancet Oncol. 18(1):122–131

Ortega JA, Douglass EC et al (2000) Randomized comparison of cisplatin/vincristine/fluorouracil and cisplatin/continuous infusion doxorubicin for treatment of pediatric hepatoblastoma: a report from the Children's Cancer Group and the Pediatric Oncology Group. J Clin Oncol 18(14):2665–2675

Otte JB, Pritchard J et al (2004) Liver transplantation for hepatoblastoma: results from the International Society of Pediatric Oncology (SIOP) study SIOPEL-1 and review of the world experience. Pediatr Blood Cancer 42(1):74–83

Perilongo G, Shafford E et al (2004) Risk-adapted treatment for childhood hepatoblastoma. Final report of the second study of the International Society of Paediatric Oncology–SIOPEL 2. International Society of Paediatric Oncology-SIOPEL 2. Eur J Cancer 40(3):411–421

Perilongo G, Maibach R et al (2009) Cisplatin versus cisplatin plus doxorubicin for standard-risk hepatoblastoma. N Engl J Med 361(17):1662–1670

Pritchard J, Brown J et al (2000) Cisplatin, doxorubicin, and delayed surgery for childhood hepatoblastoma: a successful approach—results of the first prospective study of the International Society of Pediatric Oncology. J Clin Oncol 18(22):3819–3828

Prokurat A, Kluge P et al (2002) Transitional liver cell tumors (TLCT) in older children and adolescents: a novel group of aggressive hepatic tumors expressing beta-catenin. Med Pediatr Oncol 39(5):510–518

Qayed M, Powell C et al (2010) Irinotecan as maintenance therapy in high-risk hepatoblastoma. Pediatr Blood Cancer 54(5):761–763

Rowland JM (2002) Hepatoblastoma: assessment of criteria for histologic classification. Med Pediatr Oncol 39(5):478–483

Spector LG, Feusner JH et al (2004) Hepatoblastoma and low birth weight. Pediatr Blood Cancer 43(6):706

Trobaugh-Lotrario AD, Tomlinson GE et al (2009) Small cell undifferentiated variant of hepatoblastoma: adverse clinical and molecular features similar to rhabdoid tumors. Pediatr Blood Cancer 52(3):328–334

Van Tornout JM, Buckley JD et al (1997) Timing and magnitude of decline in alpha-fetoprotein levels in treated children with unresectable or metastatic hepatoblastoma are predictors of outcome: a report from the Children's Cancer Group. J Clin Oncol 15(3):1190–1197

von Schweinitz D, Byrd DJ et al (1997) Efficiency and toxicity of ifosfamide, cisplatin and doxorubicin in the treatment of childhood hepatoblastoma. Study Committee of the Cooperative Paediatric Liver Tumour Study HB89 of the German Society for Paediatric Oncology and Haematology. Eur J Cancer 33(8):1243–1249

Wu JT, Book L et al (1981) Serum alpha fetoprotein (AFP) levels in normal infants. Pediatr Res 15(1):50–52

Zsiros J, Brugieres L, Brock P et al (2013) Dose-dense cisplatin-based chemotherapy and surgery for children with high-risk hepatoblastoma (SIOPEL-4): a prospective, single-arm, feasibility study. Lancet Oncol 14(9):834–842

30 Paediatric Peritoneal Mesothelioma

Nicolas André and Abbas Agaimy

30.1 Introduction

Malignant mesothelioma is an aggressive tumour that originates from the surface mesothelial layer which covers the serosal surfaces, such as the pleura, the peritoneum or more rarely the tunica vaginalis testis and the pericardium (Moore et al. 2008). Before the 1950s, the existence of adults' mesothelioma was questioned by many pathologists (Moore et al. 2008). Nevertheless, the increase in the incidence of mesothelioma, following the growing use of asbestos, definitely established mesothelioma as a real disease (Margery and Ruffié 2008). In children, because this is an extremely rare tumour, some paediatric oncologists still doubt its existence. Moreover, the diagnosis is appreciated as being difficult, and many cases that were reported as paediatric mesothelioma were not confirmed by recent second pathological analysis (Antman et al. 1984). Nevertheless, recently, small series have been published with the use of state-of-the-art adults' diagnosis criteria (Husain et al. 2017; Moran et al. 2008).

We will focus here on peritoneal mesothelioma and exclude pleural mesothelioma (which is presented in a separate chapter (Chap. 20); we also exclude mesothelioma of the tunica vaginalis testis and precardial mesothelioma).

To decide on the optimal treatment for individual patients and to try to increase our knowledge on this disease to understand its biological basis still represent great challenges for those involved with patient care, particularly paediatric oncologists.

30.2 Epidemiology

Peritoneal mesothelioma is an extremely rare disease in children, and no precise epidemiologic data on the incidence of this disease are available. Our knowledge is mainly based on case reports and on small series of cases. The first paediatric series was published in 1964 (Kauffman and Stout 1964). According to autopsies' results, paediatric mesothelioma should represent 2–5% of all mesothelioma cases and according to epidemiologic studies would represent 0.5–1.0 case/10 millions/year (Kashanskiy and André 2010). We previously reviewed and reported epidemiologic data of 489 cases of paediatric mesothelioma, and peritoneal mesothelioma accounted for one-fourth among these cases, in line with another

N. André (✉)
Department of Pediatric Hematology, Immunology and Oncology, Children Hospital "la Timone"AP-HM, Marseille, France
e-mail: nicolas.andre@ap-hm.fr

A. Agaimy
Institute of Pathology, University Hospital of Erlangen, Erlangen, Germany
e-mail: abbas.agaimy@uk-erlangen.de

D. T. Schneider et al. (eds.), *Rare Tumors in Children and Adolescents*, Pediatric Oncology,
https://doi.org/10.1007/978-3-030-92071-5_30

less extensive previous review of the literature (Kauffman and Stout 1964). As in adults, there is a higher frequency of peritoneal mesothelioma in girls (Kauffman and Stout 1964) with a female/male ratio of 2:1 (Kashanskiy and André 2010). The mean age at presentation was 11.9 ± 0.6 years with no difference between sexes (Kashanskiy and André 2010). An unusual case of peritoneal mesothelioma occurred in a 6-week-old girl (Silberstein et al. 1983).

Although a strong link with prior exposure to asbestosis and mesothelioma is well known and generally accepted (Moore et al. 2008), in our experience, there was no association with asbestos exposure in children. Only four children had a confirmed previous exposure to asbestos among the 50 cases for which the exposure to asbestos was documented (Kashanskiy and André 2010). Similarly, the reported paediatric cases with a prior exposure to asbestos are anecdotal, and in many countries in which the exposure to asbestos is high because of the presence of mines like in Australia, no cases have been reported. Moreover, as it usually takes 20 years or longer after asbestos exposure to develop mesothelioma, it seems very unlikely that asbestosis is implicated in the pathogenesis of mesothelioma in children and more specifically for peritoneal mesothelioma. Thus, most paediatric mesothelioma cases might be idiopathic forms of mesothelioma, which can also occur in adults with an incidence of one per million (Moore et al. 2008).

Furthermore, other predisposing factors have been proposed for childhood mesothelioma such as irradiation and genetic syndromes. These hypotheses are based on reported cases of paediatric mesothelioma developing after irradiation (Stock et al. 1979; Anderson et al. 1985; André et al. 2009), as secondary malignancies especially after Wilms' tumour and Hodgkin disease (Anderson et al. 1985; André et al. 2009; Falchero et al. 1996; Antman et al. 1984) or in children with Proteus syndrome (Gordon et al. 1995; Malamitsi-Puchner et al. 1990). Indeed, these cases suggest that an underlying genetic background may contribute to the occurrence of a mesothelioma in these affected patients. Mutation of WT1 has been reported in sporadic cases of mesothelioma, but the role of this gene in the genesis and progression of the tumour is not clear yet (Park et al. 1993). Some familial cases of mesothelioma have been reported with a deletion of the short arm of chromosome 9 that carry the CDKN2A gene. This gene encodes for $p16^{INK4a}$ and $p14^{ARF}$, and inactivation of these oncoproteins has been frequently reported in mesothelioma (You et al. 2007; Ugolini et al. 2008). Nevertheless, no children have been reported to be affected in these familial series. More recently, functional mutations were detected in EGFR in 31% of peritoneal mesothelioma. All mutations are clustered near the ATP-binding cleft of the tyrosine kinase domain. However, it still remains to be determined if these mutations represent gatekeeper events in the development of peritoneal mesothelioma or are a mere secondary event occurring during later progression of the disease (Foster et al. 2010).

Bap-1 deletion has over the last decade been identified as an important feature of peritoneal mesothelioma. Indeed, BAP1 encodes an enzyme that catalyses the removal of ubiquitin from protein substrates. Germline mutations of BAP1 are responsible for a novel cancer syndrome with high incidence of malignant mesothelioma (Testa et al. 2013). In children, Taylor et al. reported an adolescent with peritoneal mesothelioma with a cytoplasmic BAP1 staining associated with a 3p deletion detected by conventional cytogenetics (Taylor et al. 2015). Elsewhere, the rapid development of molecular profiling of tumours has led to the identification of potential targetable mutations in paediatric mesothelioma. Thus, ALK translocation has been identified in paediatric patients with mesothelioma (Loharamtaweethong et al. 2016; Leal et al. 2020). Of note, unique ALK rearrangements were found in mesotheliomas lacking asbestos fibres, therapeutic radiation and cytogenetic and molecular alterations typically found in these tumours (Hung et al. 2018).

Recently, implication of ATM has also been reported: first, in a child with ataxia telangiectasia (Rosas-Salazar et al. 2018) and in a 4-month-old child belonging to a consanguineous Bedouin family of ATM (Mijalovsky et al. 2018) who had two ATM mutations.

30.3 Clinical Presentation

A long delay is usually observed between the appearance of the first clinical signs and diagnosis. Peritoneal mesothelioma typically presents with non-specific symptoms such as weight loss, abdominal distension and ascites in which ascites represented the most common initial clinical finding (Antman et al. 1984; Moran et al. 2008; Kauffman and Stout 1964; André et al. 2009; Fraire et al. 1988). As tumours grow, pain and extension to other serosal surfaces may be seen. In a paediatric series, 3 out of 12 patients displayed involvement of more than one serosal surface (André et al. 2009).

30.4 Radiological Presentation

Malignant peritoneal mesothelioma tends to spread in sheets of tissue over the parietal and visceral peritoneal surfaces and to become confluent, thereby encasing the abdominal organs. In such cases, extensive lesions may be accompanied by ascites. The CT features of malignant peritoneal mesotheliomas range from a "dry" appearance, consisting of peritoneum-based masses, to a "wet" appearance, consisting of ascites, irregular or nodular peritoneal thickening and one or several omental masses. The latter is the most frequent presentation in children (Silberstein et al. 1983; Terry and Fowler 2009; Milano et al. 2006). Scalloping or direct invasion of adjacent abdominal organs can also be seen (Milano et al. 2006). Frequently, CT appears as a multilocular cystic mass. Cystic mesothelioma typically consists of multiple grape-like clusters of mesothelium-lined cysts. In our experience, the bulky tumour may be more extensive in the pelvic peritoneum, thereby extending into the ovaries. This may, in part, result in the under-recognition of peritoneal mesothelioma in females and its misinterpretation as advanced ovarian cancer.

Although FDG-PET is not reliable in detecting non-bulky tumour growth in the peritoneum, it is a useful modality to explore a peritoneal mesothelioma in children. It can also show metabolic active components (Abikhzer et al. 2013) even within cystic lesions (Milano et al. 2006).

30.5 Pathology

The pathological diagnosis of mesothelioma is recognised as difficult. As for adults, pathologic analysis should be performed on specimens obtained by surgery and not on limited needle biopsies or cytology material. All cases should also be confirmed by a panel of pathologists including one with experience in adult mesothelioma and the application of an appropriate panel of immunohistochemical stains. Grossly, the tumours showed multiple, diffuse or confluent peritoneal nodules or larger masses. Histologically, in a series of eight cases (Moran et al. 2008), most cases corresponded to epithelioid mesotheliomas, and one case displayed biphasic (epithelioid and spindle) cellular pattern. In our review, we also found that a majority of peritoneal mesotheliomas were of the epithelioid type regardless of age and sex (Kashanskiy and André 2010) (Figs. 30.1–30.4, Table 30.1).

On scanning magnification, the tumour classically displays sheets of medium-sized or large epithelioid cells with well-developed tubulopapillary structures. At higher magnification, the tumour cells display bland cytological appearance composed of polygonal cells with moderate amount of pale eosinophilic frequently vacuolated cytoplasm, round nuclei and inconspicuous nucleoli. Usually, only rare mitotic figures can be identified ($<1/mm^2$). In some areas, the epithelioid cells could be seen within an abundant mucinous or myxoid stroma (Moran et al. 2008; Silberstein et al. 1983). A few scattered psammoma bodies are frequently seen, particularly in tumours with prominent papillary pattern. This feature together with others represents a pitfall in the diagnosis of peritoneal mesothelioma in women and girls and probably suggests misinterpretation of some cases as serous carcinomas of the ovaries (Fig. 30.3). Accordingly, we suspect that peritoneal mesotheliomas in children and young women might be under-diagnosed by gen-

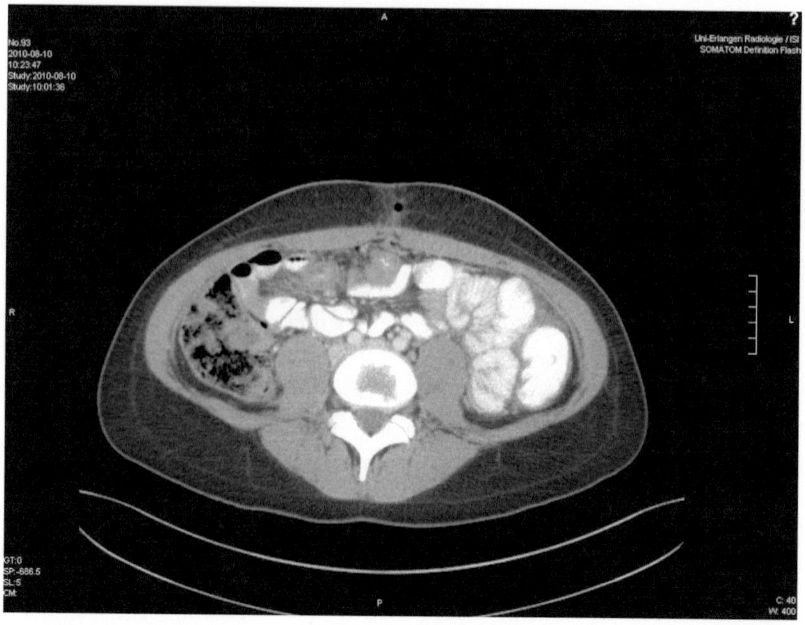

Fig. 30.1 CT scan of a 16-year-old girl with peritoneal mesothelioma. Solid and cystic tumourous masses occupying the pelvic cavity seem to involve the ovaries. There is accumulation of ascitic fluid between the liver and the diaphragm and in the precardial and the ileocecal region. Note also some prominent mesenteric lymph nodes

eral pathologists who are unfamiliar with the histology of adult mesothelioma.

The International Mesothelioma Interest Group recommends analysis of calretinin, cytokeratins 5/6, WT1 and D2–40 as positive mesothelial markers and ACE and MOC-31 as positive carcinoma markers to differentiate malignant mesotheliomas from adenocarcinoma, ovarian carcinoma or renal carcinoma (Churg et al. 2015). Classical immunohistochemical studies for cytokeratin (CK) 5/6 and low molecular weight CK (CAM5.2) show strong cytoplasmic positivity in the neoplastic cells. In addition, peritoneal mesothelioma expresses vimentin, calretinin, podoplanin (D2–40), mesothelin, HMBE-1 and WT1 (Fig. 30.4). It is noteworthy that WT1, CK7 and CA12.5 are regularly expressed both in mesothelioma and serous carcinoma and are thus of no value in their distinction. PAX8 is a recent marker that is expressed in the nuclei of serous carcinomas but not in mesothelioma. Similarly, some keratin markers, Ber-EP4 and carcinoembryonic antigen (CEA), are regularly negative in mesothelioma. The value of BAP1 immunohistochemistry as a potential adjunct for mesothelioma diagnosis in children has not been explored.

Besides, one should be aware of an even rarer entity called multicystic mesothelioma of the peritoneum. This rare benign or indolent tumour commonly occurs in young to middle-aged women and also may affect children. The classic signs and symptoms are abdominal pain, tenderness or distension with an abdominal or pelvic mass. The lesion is composed of fluid-filled thin-walled cystic spaces lined by flat cuboidal mesothelial cells that may confluent to a large multicystic mass or even spread along the peritoneal surface. Multiple recurrences can occur (Terry and Fowler 2009) as well as malignant degeneration (Milano et al. 2006). Accordingly, surgical removal of this rare tumour should be attempted and the patient carefully monitored. Multicystic mesothelioma should therefore be distinguished from focal cystic areas within malignant peritoneal mesothelioma.

30.6 Treatment and Outcome

In adults, no standard treatment strategy is currently available owing to the rarity of this tumour, which is even rarer in young children.

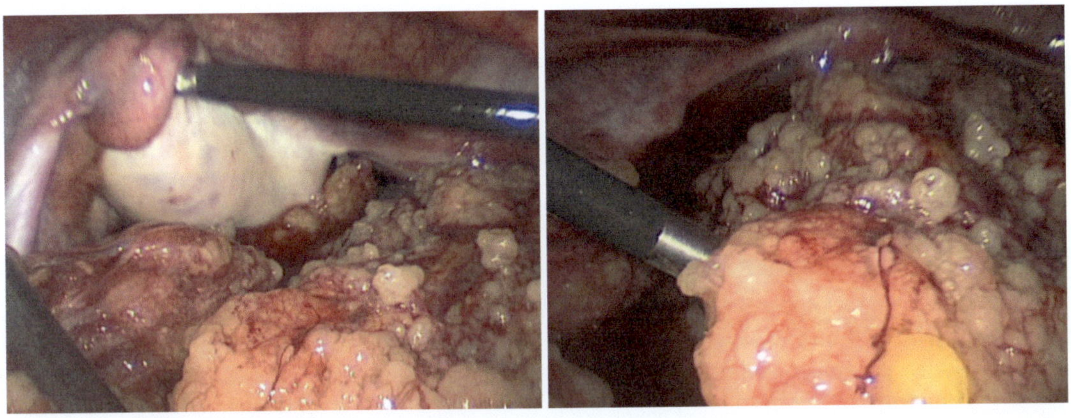

Fig. 30.2 Intraoperative laparoscopic view: confluent nodular masses involve the whole greater omentum and both ovaries. In the right lower abdomen, thickened cysts with evidence of torsion, bleeding and partial rupture are seen

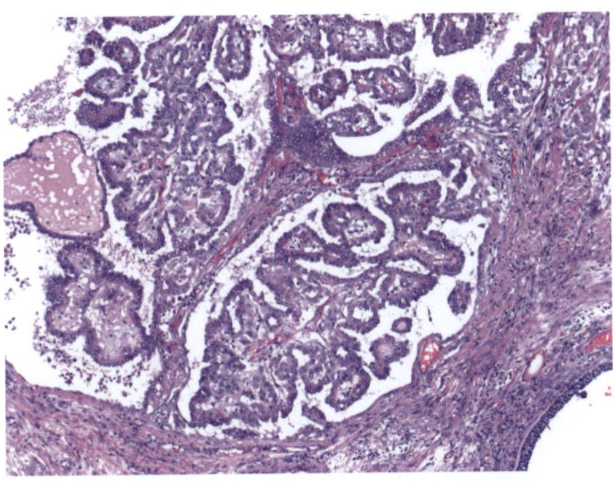

Fig. 30.3 Histological features: mesothelioma tissue composed of characteristic tubulopapillary structures is seen within the ovary adjacent to a follicle cyst (*lower right*). This finding closely mimics serous ovarian cancer and may be misdiagnosed if mesothelioma is not thought of

Recent data (Moran et al. 2008; André et al. 2009; Milano et al. 2006; Cioffredi et al. 2009) suggest that the prognosis of these patients is far better than what was generally believed with mesothelioma. Using multimodal approach, in the SFCE series of paediatric mesothelioma, all eight patients with peritoneal mesothelioma were alive with a mean follow-up of 61 months, following multimodal therapy and often several lines of chemotherapy (André et al. 2009).

Similar findings have been reported elsewhere (Cioffredi et al. 2009). Nevertheless, paediatric peritoneal mesotheliomas have an unpredictable biologic behaviour, requiring individual treatment strategies.

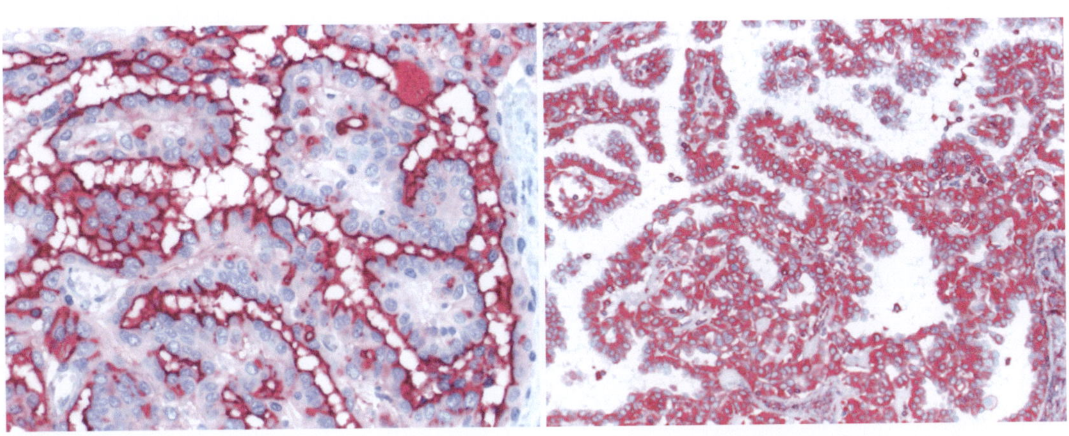

Fig. 30.4 In addition to expression of typical immunohistochemical mesothelioma markers (D2–40, *left* image), detection of the mesenchymal marker vimentin (*right* image) in a papillary ovarian neoplasm strongly suggests mesothelioma

Table 30.1 Key points to manage a child with peritoneal mesothelioma

Physical examination	Signs and symptoms: constipation/diarrhoea, tenesmus, bowel obstruction, fatigue, weight loss
	Clinical history: personal cancerin the last section regarding treatment
Laboratory assessment	Immunotherapies
Radiological assessment	
– First assessment	Abdominal ultrasound
– Local staging	Abdominal computed tomography (CT) scan
	Surgical staging
Diagnostic work	Chest and abdominal CT scan, positron emission tomography (PET)
Pathological assessment	– Surgical biopsy required
	– Confirmation of diagnosis by pathologist(s) with experience in adult's mesothelioma always necessary
	– Confirm the diagnosis of malignant mesothelioma and subtype
	– Application of an appropriate panel of immunohistochemical stains
Staging systems for risk-adapted treatment strategy	None validated
General treatment guidelines	– Need for multidisciplinary approach
	– Seek advice from national and/or European group for rare tumours
	– Seek advice from centre with expert physicians professionally dedicated to the management of this cancer in adults
– Surgery	– Keystone of treatment
	– Consider multivisceral resections, peritonectomy or procedures as hyperthermic intraperitoneal chemoperfusion (HIPEC)
– Radiotherapy	None
– Chemotherapy – Targeted therapies – Immunotherapies	– First line: pemetrexed–cisplatin- (bevacizumab)
	– Second line or alternative: gemcitabine–pemetrexed
	– Consider chemotherapy with novel agents for advanced disease validated in adults Upon molecular profiling of the tumours, ALK inhibitors or others may be used Anti-PD1/L1: consider adding as second-line or as first-line therapy, if high tumoural mutation burden or strong PD1/L1 staining

30.6.1 Surgery

Surgery aiming at removal of all malignant tissue is only very rarely associated with persistent durable complete remission as the disease is usually, at least microscopically, spread within the peritoneal cavity. Therefore, we advocate for complete surgery only in cases of easily removable tumour. If complete remission cannot be achieved without sequelae, debulking surgery is another option and should be then followed by chemotherapy. An interesting alternative is cytoreductive surgery and hyperthermic intraperitoneal chemotherapy which is gaining interest in adults (Yan et al. 2009) and can yield sustained remissions in children (André et al. 2009). Indeed, recently, in a retrospective analysis of 14 paediatric cases, ten patients were treated with cytoreductive surgery followed by hyperthermic intraperitoneal chemotherapy. In eight cases, the procedure was performed after induction chemotherapy and as an upfront treatment in two cases. Intraperitoneal chemotherapy was cisplatin/mitomycin for four patients, oxaliplatin/irinotecan for two patients and cisplatin/doxorubicin for one patient (missing data for one patient) (Vermersch et al. 2020).

30.6.2 Chemotherapy

While the combination of pemetrexed–cisplatin is a standard in adults with pleural mesothelioma (Vogelzang et al. 2003), there is currently no standard chemotherapy regimen for peritoneal mesothelioma. Nevertheless, a combination of gemcitabine and pemetrexed has recently been reported to have an interesting efficacy in adults with peritoneal mesotheliomas (Simon et al. 2008) and could be used for children, too. Moreover, these new molecules (pemetrexed, gemcitabine) indeed seem to bring clinical benefit to children with mesothelioma (André et al. 2009; Milano et al. 2006; Cioffredi et al. 2009). In adults, the addition of bevacizumab to pemetrexed/cisplatin led to a significant survival advantage (Zalcman et al. 2016). Though this gain of survival was only a modest 3 months, we do believe—given the good tolerance in children—that bevacizumab shall be added as a first-line treatment in children.

30.6.3 Radiotherapy

Radiotherapy has not been demonstrated to be an effective treatment in mesothelioma, and its use is limited to the control of the disease in a palliative setting.

30.6.4 Targeted Therapy

As to date, there is no specific therapy that targets molecular pathways in malignant mesothelioma. This is because, despite recent progress, the major molecular mechanisms involved in the initiation, development and progression of mesothelioma are still largely unknown. A recent study has demonstrated the occurrence of novel oncogenic mutations in the tyrosine kinase domain of the epidermal growth factor receptor (EGFR) in 31% of cases of peritoneal mesothelioma investigated (Foster et al. 2010). Anyhow, despite frequent overexpression of EGFR in mesotheliomas, TKIs and monoclonal antibodies blocking the receptor have not displayed sufficient clinical activity so far. As mentioned above, alterations of ALK and AMT also pave the way for targeted therapies.

30.6.5 Immunotherapy

Recently, immune-checkpoint inhibitors have come into play for mesothelioma (Scherpereel et al. 2018). In children, although the experience is very preliminary, an encouraging response has been reported (Geoerger et al. 2020). This new observation might open a new option as part of multi-agent therapy for affected patients including children, but this remains to be confirmed in larger controlled clinical studies.

30.7 Conclusion

Mesothelioma is a very rare tumour in paediatric oncology. Paediatric mesothelioma seems to be different from its adult counterpart with less frequent primary pleural localisation. The outcome of children with peritoneal mesothelioma is good despite frequent relapses by using effective treatment (multimodal therapy, the use of recent cytotoxic agents, hyperthermic intraperitoneal chemotherapy). These strategies need to be properly evaluated in children, and an international registry is mandatory to increase our knowledge of this disease. Thus, we encourage reporting cases of mesothelioma in children to national registries for rare paediatric tumours and choosing an interdisciplinary and international approach in the management of these extremely rare entities.

References

Abikhzer G, Gourevich K, Arkovitz M, Postovsky S, Keidar Z (2013) Role of 18F-FDG PET/CT in the staging of pediatric peritoneal mesothelioma. Clin Nucl Med 38:e331–e332

Anderson KA, Hurley WC, Hurley BT et al (1985) Malignant pleural mesothelioma following radiotherapy in a 16-year-old boy. Cancer 56:273–276

André N, Ratsimandresy R, Réguerre Y et al (2009) Paediatric malignant mesothelioma: the SFCE experience. Pediatr Blood Cancer 53:823

Antman KH, Ruxer RL Jr, Aisner J et al (1984) Mesothelioma following Wilms' tumor in childhood. Cancer 54:367–369

Churg A, Sheffield BS, Galateau-Salle F (2015) New markers for separating benign from malignant mesothelial proliferations: are we there yet? Arch Pathol Lab Med 140:318–321
Cioffredi LA, Jänne P, Jackman D (2009) Treatment of peritoneal mesothelioma in pediatric patients. Pediatr Blood Cancer 1:127–129
Falchero L, Coiffier B, Guibert B et al (1996) Malignant mesothelioma of the pleura following radiotherapy for Hodgkin disease. Bull Cancer 83:964–968
Foster JM, Radhakrishna U, Govindarajan V et al (2010) Clinical implications of novel activating EGFR mutations in malignant peritoneal mesothelioma. World J Surg Oncol 8:88
Fraire AE, Cooper S, Greenberg SD et al (1988) Mesothelioma of childhood. Cancer 62:838–847
Geoerger B, Kang HJ, Yalon-Oren M et al (2020) Pembrolizumab in paediatric patients with advanced melanoma or a PD-L1-positive, advanced, relapsed, or refractory solid tumour or lymphoma (KEYNOTE-051): interim analysis of an open-label, single-arm, phase 1-2 trial. Lancet Oncol 21:121–133
Gordon PL, Wilroy RS, Lasater OE et al (1995) Neoplasms in Proteus syndrome. Am J Med Genet 57:74–78
Hung YP, Dong F, Watkins JC et al (2018) Identification of ALK rearrangements in malignant peritoneal mesothelioma. JAMA Oncol 4:235–238
Husain AN, Colby TV, Ordóñez NG, Guidelines for Pathologic Diagnosis of Malignant Mesothelioma et al (2017) Update of the consensus statement from the International Mesothelioma Interest Group. Arch Pathol Lab Med 142:89–108
Kashanskiy SV, André N (2010) Paediatric mésothelioma: is there such a disease? Bull Cancer 97:571–576
Kauffman SL, Stout AP (1964) Mesothelioma in children. Cancer 17:539–544
Leal JL, Peters G, Szaumkessel M et al (2020) NTRK and ALK rearrangements in malignant pleural mesothelioma, pulmonary neuroendocrine tumours and non-small cell lung cancer. Lung Cancer 146:154–159
Loharamtaweethong K, Puripat N, Aoonjai N et al (2016) Anaplastic lymphoma kinase (ALK) translocation in paediatric malignant peritoneal mesothelioma: a case report of novel ALK-related tumour spectrum. Histopathology 68:603–607
Malamitsi-Puchner A, Dimitriadis D, Bartsocas C et al (1990) Proteus syndrome: course of a severe case. Am J Med Genet 35:283–285
Margery J, Ruffié P (2008) Environmental cancer: malignant pleural mesothelioma. Bull Cancer 95:77–86
Mijalovsky A, Halperin D, Perez Y et al (2018) Malignant peritoneal mesothelioma in an infant with familial ATM mutations. J Pediatr Hematol Oncol 40:e511–e515
Milano E, Pourroy B, Rome A, Delarue A, Coze C, Gorincour G, Bouvier C, Braguer D, André N (2006) Efficacy of a combination of pemetrexed and multiple redo-surgery in an 11-year-old girl with a recurrent multifocal abdominal mesothelioma. Anti-Cancer Drugs 17:1231–1234
Moore AJ, Parker RJ, Wiggins J (2008) Malignant mesothelioma. Orphanet J Rare Dis 3:34
Moran CA, Albores-Saavedra JI, Suster S (2008) Primary peritoneal mesotheliomas in children: a clinicopathological and immunohistochemical study of eight cases. Histopathology 52:824–830
Park S, Schalling M, Bernard A, Maheswaran S, Shipley GC, Roberts D, Fletcher J, Shipman R, Rheinwald J, Demetri G et al (1993) The Wilms tumour gene WT1 is expressed in murine mesoderm-derived tissues and mutated in a human mesothelioma. Nat Genet 4:415–420
Rosas-Salazar C, Gunawardena S, Spahr JE (2018) Malignant pleural mesothelioma in a child with Ataxia-Telangiectasia. Pediatr Pulmonol 40:e511–e515
Scherpereel A, Wallyn F, Albelda SM, Munck C (2018) Novel therapies for malignant pleural mesothelioma. Lancet Oncol 19:e161–e172
Silberstein MJ, Lewis JE, Blair JD, Graviss ER, Brodeur AE (1983) Congenital peritoneal mesothelioma. J Pediatr Surg 18:243–245
Simon GR, Verschraegen CF, Jänne PA et al (2008) Pemetrexed plus gemcitabine as first-line chemotherapy for patients with peritoneal mesothelioma: final report of a phase II trial. J Clin Oncol 26:3567–3572
Stock RJ, Fu YS, Carter JR (1979) Malignant peritoneal mesothelioma following radiotherapy for seminoma of the testis. Cancer 44:914–919
Taylor S, Carpentieri D, Williams J et al (2015) Malignant peritoneal mesothelioma in an adolescent male with BAP1 deletion. J Pediatr Hematol Oncol 37:e323–e327
Terry NE, Fowler CL (2009) Benign cystic mesothelioma in a child. J Pediatr Surg 44:e9–e11
Testa JE, Malkin D, Schiffman JD (2013) Connecting molecular pathways to hereditary cancer risk syndromes. Am Soc Clin Oncol Educ Book:81–90
Ugolini D, Neri M, Ceppi M et al (2008) Genetic susceptibility to malignant mesothelioma and exposure to asbestos: the influence of the familial factor. Mutat Res 658:162–167
Vermersch S, Arnauld A, Orbach D et al (2020) Multicystic and diffuse malignant peritoneal mesothelioma in children. Pediatr Blood Cancer 67:e28286
Vogelzang NJ, Rusthoven JJ, Symanowski J et al (2003) Phase III study of pemetrexed in combination with cisplatin versus cisplatin alone in patients with malignant pleural mesothelioma. J Clin Oncol 21:2636–2644
Yan TD, Deraco M, Baratti D et al (2009) Cytoreductive surgery and hyperthermic intraperitoneal chemotherapy for malignant peritoneal mesothelioma: multi-institutional experience. J Clin Oncol 27:6237–6242
You B, Blandin S, Gérinière L et al (2007) Mésothéliomes familiaux: une composante génétique associée aux risques environnementaux ? Bull Cancer 7:705–710
Zalcman G, Mazieres J, Margery J et al (2016) Bevacizumab for newly diagnosed pleural mesothelioma in the Mesothelioma Avastin Cisplatin Pemetrexed Study (MAPS): a randomised, controlled, open-label, phase 3 trial. Lancet 387:1405–1414

Part VII

Germ Cell Tumors and Genitourinary Tumors

Gonadal and Extragonadal Germ Cell Tumors, Sex Cord Stromal and Rare Gonadal Tumors

31

Dominik T. Schneider, Monica Terenziani, Giovanni Cecchetto, and Thomas A. Olson

31.1 Overview on Epidemiology, Biology, Histology, and Clinic

Dominik T. Schneider

Monica Terenziani, and Thomas A. Olson

Germ cell tumors include a group of tumors that are highly heterogeneous regarding their clinical and histologic appearance. Altogether they comprise approximately 2–3% of cancers diagnosed in children and adolescents younger than 15 years (Ries et al. 1999a; Kaatsch 2004a; Kaatsch et al. 2015). During childhood and adolescence, approximately half of all germ cell tumors develop at extragonadal midline sites. Sacrococcygeal germ cell tumors constitute the most frequent tumor in neonates, and extracranial germ cell tumors account for 14% of all cancers in adolescents of the 15–19 age group. An epidemiological analysis of patients reported to the German germ cell tumor trials from 1981 to 2000 showed a bimodal age distribution with a small peak during infancy and a larger peak after puberty, to be continued among adults, among which germ cell tumors constitute the most common cancer in young men (Schneider et al. 2004a). During the first year of life, teratomas predominate, with a slight female preponderance (Fig. 31.1a, b). After the first 6 months of life, yolk sac tumors are the most frequent histologic subtype. This histology is slightly more often seen in boys than in girls. Tumors with germinoma histology (syn. seminoma or dysgerminoma) are first observed in girls at 5 years of age and show a gradually increasing incidence during adolescence. Seminomas are not seen in boys, until they reach puberty. The same accounts for other nongerminomatous histologies such as embryonal carcinoma and choriocarcinoma, which are mainly seen during and after puberty, in most cases as components of mixed malignant germ cell tumors (Fig. 31.1c) (Schneider et al. 2004a).

D. T. Schneider (✉)
Klinik für Kinder- und Jugendmedizin, Klinikum Dortmund, University Witten/Herdecke, Dortmund, Germany
e-mail: dominik.schneider@klinikumdo.de

M. Terenziani
Pediatric Oncology Fondazione IRCCS Istituto Nazionale deiTumori, Milan, Italy

G. Cecchetto
Department of Pediatrics, Pediatric Surgery, University of Padua, Padua, Italy

T. A. Olson
Division Pediatric Hematology/Oncology, Children's Healthcare of Atlanta at Egleston, Atlanta, GA, USA
e-mail: thomas.olson@choa.org

D. T. Schneider et al. (eds.), *Rare Tumors in Children and Adolescents*, Pediatric Oncology,
https://doi.org/10.1007/978-3-030-92071-5_31

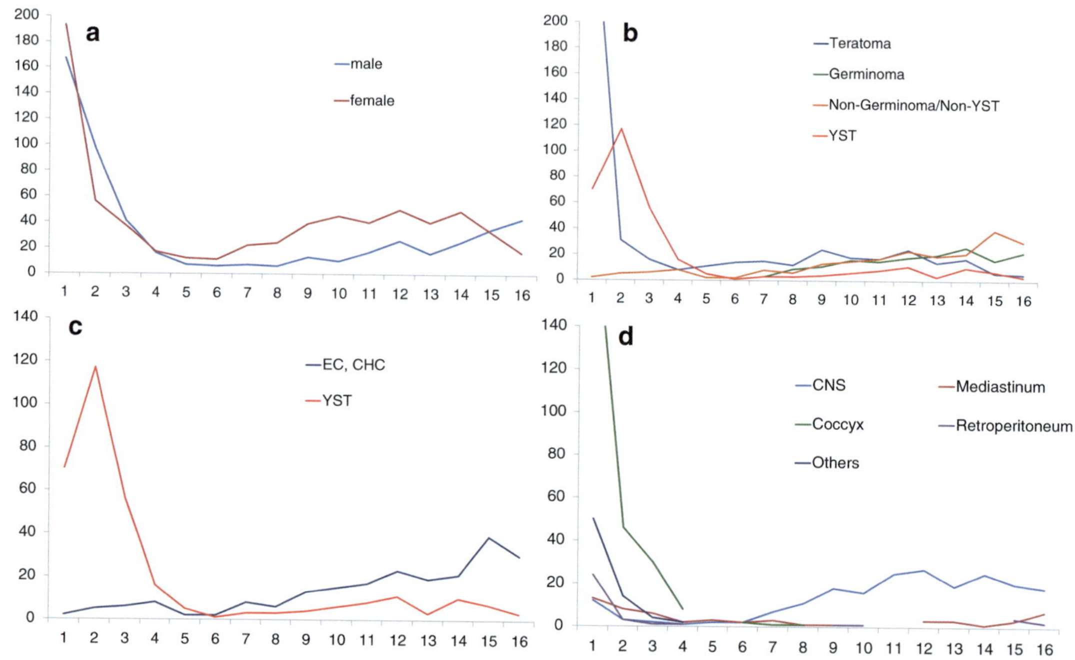

Fig. 31.1 (**a**) Age distribution of germ cell tumors by age and sex. (**b**) Age distribution of germ cell tumors by histology—teratomas. (**c**) Age distribution of germ cell tumors by histology—nongerminomatous. (**d**) Age distribution of germ cell tumors by site

This bimodal age distribution is also demonstrated by the Surveillance Epidemiology and End Results Registry (SEER). For adult patients with germ cell tumors, the SEER data also demonstrated higher incidence rates among Caucasian compared to African American males. Of note, there appears to be a significant increase of the incidence in specific subgroups such as adolescent boys and prepubertal girls (Poynter et al. 2010). This study suggests that the biology of germ cell tumors may differ between different populations and clinical subgroups. The overall incidence of germ cell tumors has been increasing at a global level (being higher in Europe, Australia, and the USA), especially for testicular tumors (de Angelis et al. 2014). The rising incidence is in part explained by western lifestyle habits, including the developmental exposure to endocrine disruptors (Kaushik and Bhartiya 2018).

Separate groups are marked by distinct clinical and molecular features. The distribution of gonadal and extragonadal tumor sites by age is shown in Fig. 31.1d. This figure illustrates that for some specific tumor sites such as the testis and the mediastinum, a bimodal age distribution can be recognized, with a subgroup occurring during infancy and a separate group developing after the onset of puberty (Schneider et al. 2002a). In contrast, no separate epidemiological groups can be appreciated in CNS and ovarian germ cell tumors, which only show an incidence peak after the onset of puberty. Lastly, some germ cell tumors such as vaginal and sacrococcygeal germ cell tumors only develop during infancy and childhood but not after the onset of puberty (Fig. 31.2) (Schneider et al. 2004a).

The survival of children with pediatric germ cell tumors has greatly improved with the application of lessons from adult germ cell tumors. For some patients with germ cell tumors, a reduction in therapy may be warranted. However, there is still a small population for which more intensive or adaptive therapy is warranted. The paucity of such events suggests that international collaborations and advances in molecular understanding of germ cell tumor may be crucial.

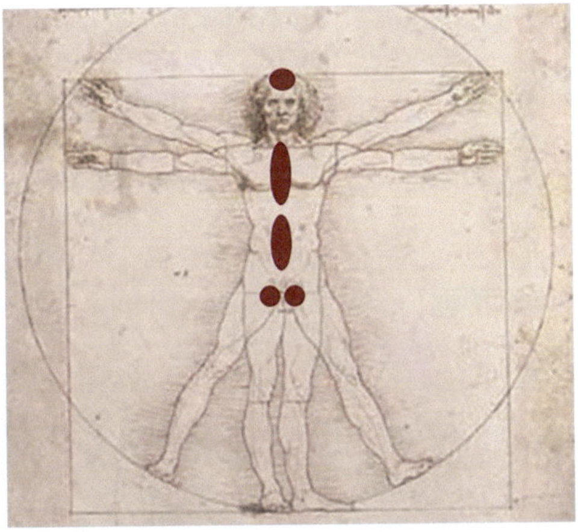

	<10	>10 years
CNS	10%	35%
Ovary	15%	45%
Testis	25%	10%
Coccyx	35%	0%
Others	15%	10%

1442 patients from the MAHO/MAKEI/SIOP registry

Fig. 31.2 Distribution of germ cell tumors by site and age

31.1.1 Histogenesis and Biology of Extragonadal Germ Cell Tumors

As we investigate molecular differences in germ cell tumor from children and adolescents, it should be recognized that few pediatric tumors have been studied (Palmer et al. 2007). When addressing tumor-specific genetic changes, the heterogeneity of the pediatric germ cell tumors is evident also in studies investigating their genetic and molecular properties. Biologically distinct subcategories have been described in the pediatric population (Bussey et al. 1999a; Perlman et al. 2000; Schneider et al. 2006; Palmer et al. 2007).

31.1.2 Sex-Chromosomal Abnormalities in Germ Cell Tumors

Sex-chromosomal abnormalities have been associated with the development of germ cell tumors. The most recognized association is the one of ovarian germ cell tumors with Turner syndrome, in particular, in patients with microscopic residues of Y-chromosomal sequences. In these patients, dysgerminomas may develop within gonadoblastomas, which therefore constitutes a precursor lesion of invasive germ cell tumors (Cools et al. 2006). Moreover, testicular feminization and Swyer syndrome, a disorder characterized by a female appearance but with gonadal dysgenesis, i.e., hypoplastic streak gonads in a cytogenetically male patient, are also associated with the development of gonadoblastoma and overt germ cell tumor over time. Therefore, prophylactic oophorectomy is recommended in these patients.

Moreover, some extragonadal germ cell tumors are also associated with sex-chromosomal aberrations. Thus, mediastinal germ cell tumor have been associated with Klinefelter's syndrome (47,XXY) (Nichols et al. 1987a). Approximately 50% of adolescents with mediastinal germ cell tumors have cytogenetic changes consistent with Klinefelter's syndrome (Schneider et al. 2002a) (see Chap. 24). In addition, a high frequency of numeric aberrations of sex chromosomes has been demonstrated in germ cell tumors of the central nervous system (Yu et al. 1995).

31.1.3 The Primordial Germ Cell Hypothesis of Extragonadal Germ Cell Tumors

More than 35 years ago, Teilum postulated that all different histologic entities of germ cell tumors develop from an omnipotent primordial germ cell that is capable of differentiation along the germ line and into embryonic and extraembryonic tissues (Teilum et al. 1975a) (Fig. 31.3). This so-called holistic concept of the histogenesis of germ cell tumors remains fascinating since it provides a very instructive theory that is able to explain both the apparent heterogeneity of germ cell tumors and the observation of tumors with mixed histology. Moreover, patients who at relapse present with a histology different from that at initial diagnosis can be explained based on this theory. Lastly, if the holistic concept is considered in the light of the knowledge of primordial germ cell migration during early embryonal development, even the development of seminomatous and nonseminomatous germ cell tumors at extragonadal sites can be explained. However, several aspects still remain elusive. For instance, it is unclear why the histologic differentiation of germ cell tumors is restricted to specific subtypes at specific sites, while it is not at others. For instance, at the sacrococcygeal region, teratomas and yolk sac tumors can be found, while vaginal germ cell tumors always present as pure yolk sac tumors. Therefore, it can be assumed that the microenvironment may play a substantial role in modulating tumor development and differentiation.

There has been considerable debate as to whether the heterogeneous germ cell tumors, in particular extragonadal teratomas, may originate from midline somatic stem cells (Kaushik and Bhartiya 2018). This debate has been fostered by the experimental observation that teratoma-like tumors may develop at the injection site of cultured embryonal stem cells (Thomson et al. 1998). Moreover, the development of an

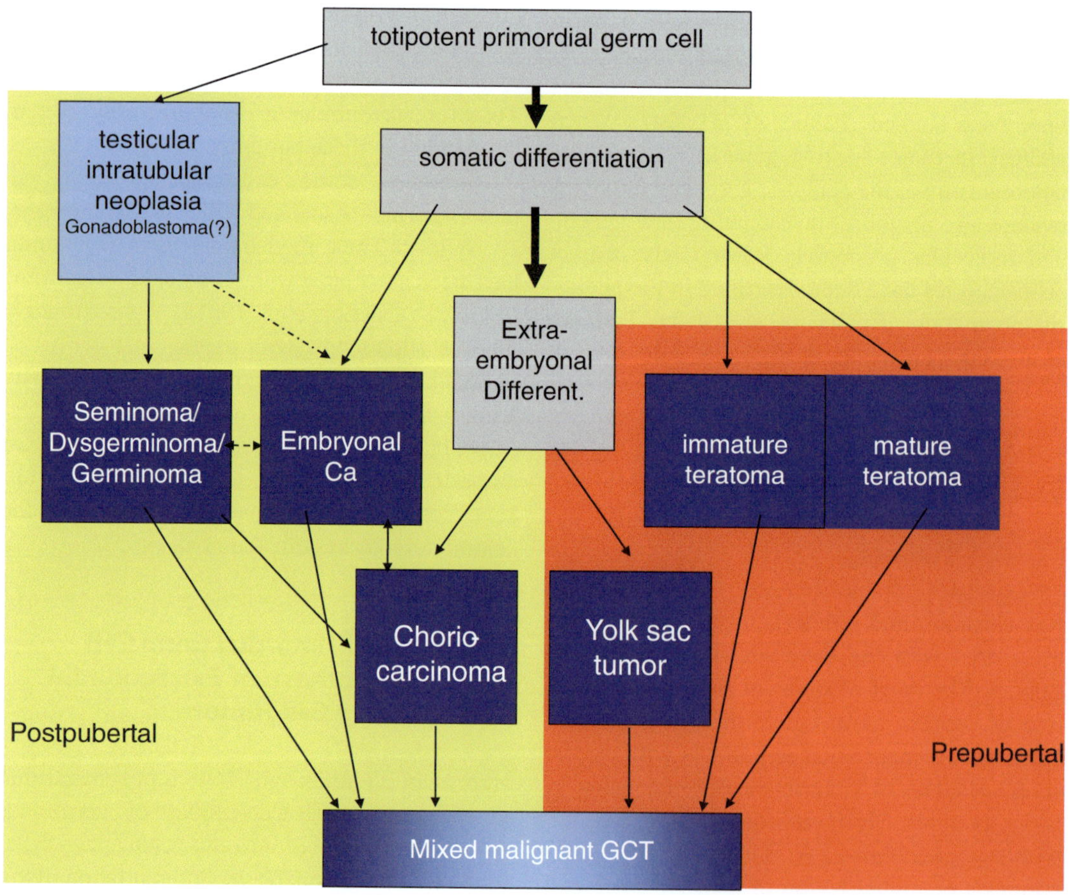

Fig. 31.3 Primordial germ cell hypothesis of extragonadal germ cell tumor development

isochromosome 12p, the pathognomic marker of germ cell tumors in young men, has been described in long-term culture of embryonal stem cells (Draper et al. 2004).

On the other hand, there is biological evidence that both gonadal and extragonadal germ cell tumors originate from primordial germ cells at different stages of development (Honecker et al. 2004). Thus, the examination of the epigenetic control of genomic imprinting reveals a methylation pattern that is characteristic of primordial germ cells during and shortly after their migration during early embryonal development (Bussey et al. 1999a; Schneider et al. 2001a). Moreover, the tumors cells retain a specific embryonal stem-cell-like expression pattern, characteristic of primordial germ cells (Hoei-Hansen et al. 2006). However, this hypothesis has recently been challenged by the observation that neural stem cells may also show loss of the methylation imprint, e.g., of SNRPN, making these cells alternative candidates from which CNS germ cell tumors may be derived (Lee et al. 2010). For testicular germ cell tumors, embryonal stem cells have been proposed as alternative sources of type 2 germ cell tumors (Kaushik and Bhartiya 2018). The loss of methylation pattern of other genes such as IGF-2 however distinguishes germ cell tumors from other embryonal tumors with presumed stem cell origin such as nephroblastoma (Sievers et al. 2005a). This observation, as well as modern findings on the role of the microenvironment for the development of extragonadal germ cell tumors, still supports the hypothesis of a specific germ cell origin of these tumors (Oosterhuis et al. 2007).

The primordial germ cells first become evident in the extraembryonic yolk sac by the fourth week of gestation. By the fifth week, the germ cells migrate through the mesentery to the gonadal ridge. This migration appears to be mediated by the c-kit receptor and its ligand, stem-cell factor, or steel factor. Primordial germ cells express c-kit. Stem-cell factor is expressed with an increasing gradient from yolk sac to gonadal ridge, guiding germ cells to the gonadal ridge. In animal models, primordial germ cells not expressing c-kit are unable either to migrate to the gonad or to proliferate during this migration (Godin et al. 1991; Dolci et al. 1993; Orth et al. 1997).

The association of c-kit mutations (codon 816) with bilateral or familial germ cell tumors underlines the importance of this gene during germ cell development (Looijenga et al. 2003; Rapley et al. 2004). In addition, c-kit mutations or c-kit amplifications have also been reported in 27% of unilateral ovarian dysgerminomas (Cheng et al. 2010).

Germ cell migration is also controlled by additional mediators such as the chemokine soluble derived factor 1 (SDF-1) and its receptor CXCR-4 (Doitsidou et al. 2002). Germ cells express CXCR-4, and their migration is directed by the expression and secretion of SDF-1 (CXCL-12) in the mesenchyme of the gonadal ridges. Mice that lack either SDF-1 or CXCR-4 also fail to populate the gonadal ridges and may persist at extragonadal sites. Moreover, aberrant migration of germ cells can be induced by aberrant expression of SDF-1 (Molyneaux et al. 2003). Of note, expression analysis of SDF-1 and CXCR-4 has demonstrated aberrant expression of CXCR-4 in extragonadal germ cell tumors, which typically locate at sites known to express SDF-1 (Gilbert et al. 2009). These data from embryological and tumor genetic studies support the hypothesis that extragonadal germ cell tumors may indeed arise from germ cells that have migrated aberrantly, and in which expression of growth factors aberrantly persists beyond the embryonal period. While no mutations of CXCR-4 have been reported in extragonadal germ cell tumors to date (D.T.S. unpublished data), recently changes of miRNA expression, e.g., by environmental factors have been detected, which may affect expression of CXCR4 and other factors that direct PGC migration (McIver et al. 2013). Thus, perturbances in the SDF-1 and CXCR-4 axis may be involved in the development of extragonadal germ cell tumors.

31.1.4 Complex Correlation of Biology, Site, and Histology

It should be noted that apart from the predominance of midline sites and the histologic similarity to the histologic spectrum of gonadal germ cell tumors, there are pronounced biologic and histologic differences between germ cell tumors at different anatomical sites.

Thus, during childhood the histologic appearance of germ cell tumors is almost exclusively restricted to teratoma and yolk sac tumor, and the sacrococcygeal region is the most frequent tumor site during infancy (Table 31.1). Tumors at other sites such as vaginal germ cell tumors only present as yolk sac tumors. Both sacrococcygeal and vaginal germ cell tumors are not seen during adolescence. After the onset of puberty, mediastinal and central nervous system germ cell tumors predominate among extragonadal germ cell tumors. These tumors present with the whole spectrum of adult germ cell tumors, including seminomas, nonseminomas, and teratomas. Of note, mediastinal germ cell tumors may present with both patterns, one consisting of teratomas and yolk sac tumors during childhood and one with seminomas, nonseminomas, and teratomas during adolescence. These two groups are distinguished by different genetic profiles, both corresponding to the genetic aberrations seen in germ cell tumors at other anatomical sites during the corresponding age group (Schneider et al. 2002a).

Thus, genetic studies have substantially helped in categorizing the different distinct clinical entities of germ cell tumors and in defining childhood germ cell tumors at a distinct site, despite their heterogeneous clinical presentation at different anatomical sites. Genetic studies have also provided information regarding the pathogenesis of pediatric germ cell tumors including information on constitutional genetic changes that may lead to increased susceptibility and tumor-specific genetic changes. However, little is still known regarding the former, particularly with regard to infantile germ cell tumors. Nevertheless, it has become clear that with the onset of puberty, the spectrum of genetic changes seen in germ cell tumors changes and so does tumor biology.

31.1.5 Genetics of Prepubertal Germ Cell Tumors

In children younger than 10 years, germ cell tumors arising in gonadal and extragonadal sites are similar in clinical presentation, histology, and genetics (Table 31.2). Most teratomas in this age group are diploid, have normal karyotypes, and, if completely resected, behave in a benign fashion regardless of degree of immaturity and site of origin (Kaplan et al. 1979a; Silver et al. 1994; Bussey et al. 1999a; Schneider et al. 2001b, c; Harms et al. 2006a). Malignant germ cell tumors in these young children are almost exclusively yolk sac tumors, may arise from a preexisting teratoma, and most often are diploid or tetraploid (Perlman et al. 1994a; Silver et al. 1994; Bussey et al. 1999a). Recurrent cytogenetic

Table 31.1 Histology and genetics

Group	Histology	Epigenetics	Genetics
GCTs of infancy and childhood	Teratoma	Premeiotic	Normal
	Yolk sac tumor	Loss of imprinting	$-1p, +1p, -6p, +20$
GCTs of adolescence and adulthood	Teratoma	Meiosis I	+12p
	Seminoma	Loss of imprinting	
	Mal. nonseminoma		
Spermatocytic seminoma (testis)		Meiosis II	+9
		Gamete specific imprinting	
Cystic teratoma (ovary)		Meiosis II	(23,X) × 2
		Gamete specific imprinting	

Table 31.2 Histology and markers

Histology	AFP	β-HCG	Immunohisto-marker	Prepubertal	Postpubertal
Teratoma, mature	–	–	–	+	+
Teratoma, immature	(+)	–	–	+	+
Teratoma with mal.	(+)	–	–	–	+
Transformation, e.g., carcinoma					
Germinoma (syn. seminoma, dysgerminoma)	–	(+)	OCT3/4, c-kit	–	+
Embryonal			CD30		
Carcinoma	–	–	OCT3/4	–	+
Choriocarcinoma	–	+++	β-HCG	(+)	+
Yolk sac tumor	+++	–	AFP	+	+
			CD34		
Mixed malignant				TER + YST	
GCT	–/+	–/+	As above		All comb.
Gonadoblastoma	–	–	OCT3/4	–	+
Polyembryoma	–	–	–	–	–

abnormalities involve chromosomes 1, 6, and 20 among others, but only rarely the 12p (Bussey et al. 1999a; Perlman et al. 1994a, 2000; Mostert et al. 2000; Schneider et al. 2001b, c, 2006; Palmer et al. 2007).

In situ hybridization and loss of heterozygosity studies have demonstrated deletion of 1p36 in 80–100% of infantile malignant germ cell tumors arising from testicular and extragonadal sites (Jenderny et al. 1995; Bussey et al. 2001; (Zahn et al. 2006; Perlman et al. 1996). Genetic surveys of regions of gain or loss in these infantile yolk sac tumors document recurrent loss of 6q24-qter, gain of 20q and 1q, and loss of 1p. A small number of tumors show evidence for c-myc or n-myc amplification (Schneider et al. 2002a, Germ Cell Tumours V, 127–128). The clinical significance for these markers is however entirely unknown.

Expression studies of mRNAs and micro-RNAs in childhood germ cell tumors have revealed recurrent mRNA and micro-RNA profiles that segregate tumors primarily according to histology (Palmer et al. 2008, 2010). Furthermore, expression profiles distinguished between childhood and adult germ cell tumors. Of note, within a distinct histology, the yolk sac tumor, tumors had different expression profiles for different ages. As miRNAs are also detectable in bodily fluids, these may potentially serve as additional serum tumor markers (Murray et al. 2017). In contrast, no site-specific differences were reported within a given histology and age group. Gene expression studies have also yielded insights into the molecular biology of childhood germ cell tumors. Thus, in pediatric yolk sac tumors, genes associated with activation of the canonical WNT pathway were expressed at high levels (Fritsch et al. 2006; Palmer et al. 2008). Additional studies have shown that this pattern is associated primarily with epigenetic dysregulation of WNT control genes among others, the adenomatosis poliposis gene and cell surface regulators of *wnt* signaling (unpublished data).

Figures 31.4 and 31.5 demonstrate a summary of CGH profiles of 116 malignant germ cell tumors and 32 pure teratomas, respectively. The results are separated by age, demonstrating frequent chromosomal imbalances of chromosomes 1p, 6q, and 20q in prepubertal tumors, irrespective of tumor site. Postpubertal tumors show recurrent gain of 12p and other less recurrent imbalances. Of note, all pure teratomas prior to puberty are balanced, while postpubertal teratomas may show recurrent imbalances, resembling a pattern seen in malignant germ cell tumors of the same age group. However, the number of

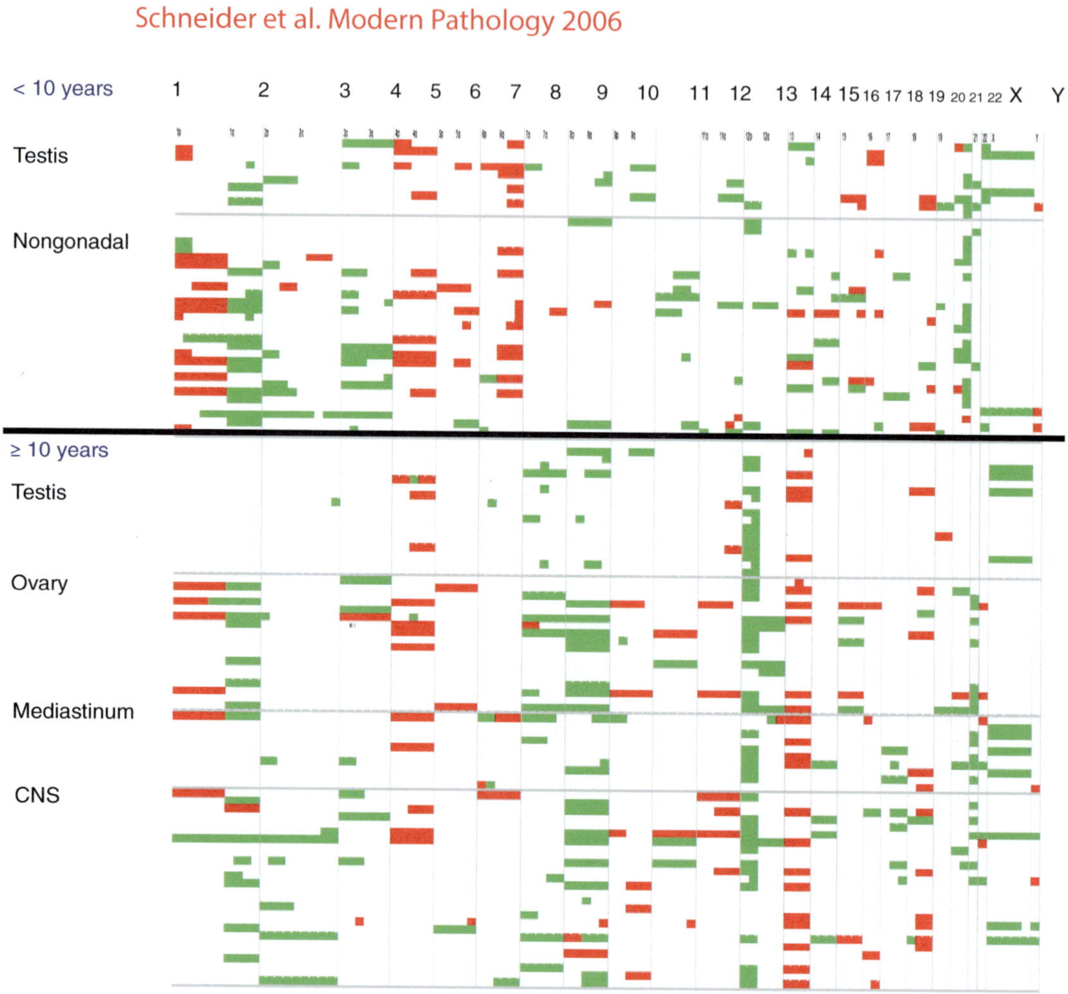

Fig. 31.4 CGH profiles of 116 malignant germ cell tumors (Schneider et al. 2006)

Fig. 31.5 CGH profiles of pure teratomas (Schneider et al. 2006)

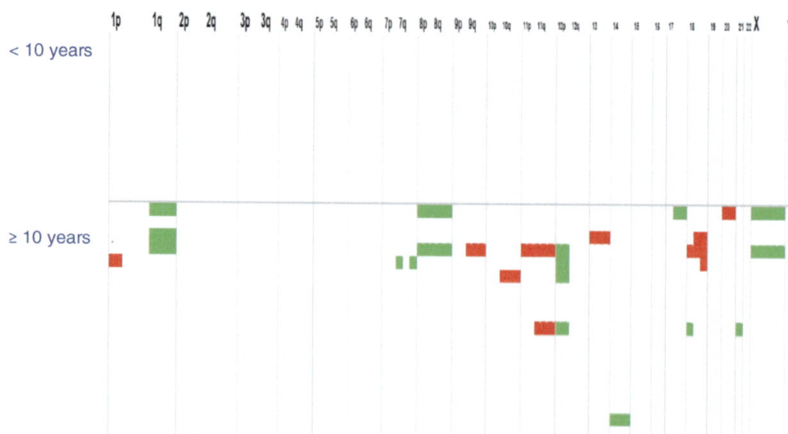

chromosomal imbalances is smaller than in corresponding malignant tumors (Schneider et al. 2006).

In conclusion, tumors in children younger than 10 years of age are biologically distinct from those tumors that develop in adolescents and adults. This is true, even if the histology, e.g., yolk sac tumor, is microscopically undistinguishable.

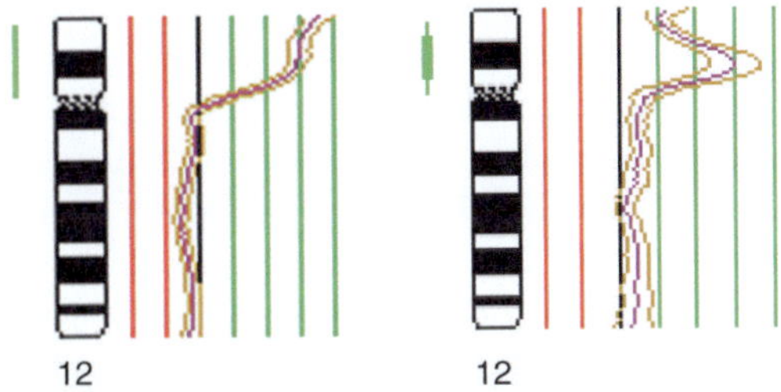

Fig. 31.6 CGH of CNS germ cell tumor with amplification at 12p22 (isochromosome 12p)

31.1.6 Genetics of Postpubertal Germ Cell Tumors

Testicular germ cell tumors of the young adult constitute the best studied entity of germ cell tumors. These tumors appear to arise from a precursor lesion, which is histologically defined as testicular intratubular neoplasia (TIN). TIN may grow within the seminiferous tubules. Tumor cells express specific transcription factors such as c-kit and OCT3/4, indicating their origin from immature pluripotent gonocytes (Oosterhuis and Looijenga 2005a). Obviously, the progression of TIN to invasive germ cell cancer is associated with the development of additional cytogenetic events, including aberrations of chromosome 12p. Bilateral testicular (2–5%) and familial (2%) cases have been reported. Thus, family members with malignant germ cell tumors are associated with higher risk of developing testicular germ cell tumor. Having a brother or father with testicular GCT increases the risk 8–10 and 4–6 times, respectively; in twins (monozygotic and dizygotic) the risk is also increased 76 and 35 times, respectively.

The isochromosome 12p constitutes the biologic hallmark of testicular and extragonadal germ cell tumors in adults (Atkin and Baker 1982; Rodriguez et al. 1992). It is formed by centromeric fusion of two short arms of chromosome 12, with loss of the long arms. The isochromosome 12p can be detected in approximately 80% of adult malignant germ cell tumors. In addition, in adults, even pure teratomas may display 12p aberrations. In those cases with no isochromosome 12p, amplification of 12p chromosomal material can be detected with molecular techniques such as fluorescence in situ hybridization or comparative genomic hybridization (Samaniego et al. 1990; Schneider et al. 2006). Figure 31.6 demonstrates a comparative genomic hybridization of a central nervous system germ cell tumor with an amplicon at 12p22. The region from 12p11 to 12p12 has been defined as the region most commonly involved in amplification. Chromosomal amplification is cytogenetically recognizable as double minutes or homogeneously staining region, e.g., on marker chromosomes. In this chromosomal region, several candidate proto-oncogenes Cyclin D2, SOX5, and KRAS are located. However, their etiopathogenetic role remains unclear. In addition, this region harbors stem cell genes such as *STELLAR* and *NANOG* (Oosterhuis and Looijenga 2005a).

The development of adult testicular germ cell tumors is associated with cryptorchidism and testicular dysgenesis together with hypospadia, testicular atrophy, inguinal hernia, and impaired spermatogenesis, leaving a proportion of patients infertile (Skakkebaek et al. 2003; Skakkebaek 2004). In the context of a testicular dysgenesis syndrome, TIN and invasive germ cell tumors may be detected “accidentally” during medical evaluation of infertility. Recently, it has been discussed, to what extent exposure to endocrine disruptors during early germ cell development may increase the risk of germ cell tumor development in the context of genetic predisposition (Nettersheim et al. 2016; Skakkebaek 2016) For general pediatricians and pediatric surgeons, question arises whether medical or surgical treatment of cryptorchidism may influence the risk of germ cell tumor development in the cryptorchid testis. The lifetime risk of later development of germ cell tumors in cryptorchid children is estimated to 2–18% (Buetow 1995). In this context, the biologic association between cryptorchidism and germ cell tumor is still elusive. It remains unclear if the risk of later germ cell tumor development can be reduced by early orchidopexy (and at what age) or whether it is inherent to an underlying testicular dysgenesis and maturation disorder. Other risk factors are related to fetal exposure to estrogens and anti-androgens, resulting in dysregulation of prenatal hormone signaling (e.g., low-high birth weight, decreased GA, maternal bleeding). External risk factors to be considered include diet (including synthetic hormones), sedentary lifestyle, occupational exposure, and recently marijuana smoking.

While ovarian germ cell tumors are associated with testicular feminization, constitutional loss of one X chromosome, and presence of aberrant Y chromosomal genetic material, no such association has been reported in girls with extragonadal germ cell tumors. However, mediastinal germ cell tumors are associated with constitutional Klinefelter's syndrome (Nichols et al. 1987a). Compared to patients with normal constitutional karyotype, these tumors tend to occur at a younger age and predominantly with malignant nonseminomatous histology. Of note, the risk of germ cell tumors at other anatomical sites including the testis does not appear to be significantly increased in Klinefelter's syndrome (Hasle et al. 1995), although some single patients with CNS germ cell tumors and Klinefelter's syndrome have been reported (Prall et al. 1995).

The two most common sites for extragonadal germ cell tumors in adolescents and adults are mediastinum and brain. Cytogenetic analysis of central nervous system teratoma has shown a high frequency of sex-chromosome abnormalities, most commonly increased copies of the X chromosome (Yu et al. 1995). The i (12p) has been described in some, but not all, pineal germinomas, but it has not been seen in pineal teratoma (Schneider et al. 2006). Ploidy analyses of mediastinal germ cell tumors suggest that most are diploid or tetraploid (Oosterhuis et al. 1990), and those that are malignant contain the i (12p) and the other genetic changes seen in adolescent testicular germ cell tumors (Dal Cin et al. 1989; Schneider et al. 2002a). The extragonadal germ cell tumors (almost exclusively, nonseminomatous mediastinal tumors) in adolescents and adults are associated with hematopoietic malignancies of various cell lineages that present soon after the initial presentation of the germ cell tumors. The most common presentation is acute megakaryocytic leukemia, and the malignant hematopoietic clone commonly demonstrates i (12p). This differs from hematopoietic malignancies that arise secondary to therapy (Chaganti et al. 1994; Hartmann et al. 2000).

31.1.6.1 Pathology

Germ cell tumors comprise numerous histologic subtypes; however, the microscopic morphology of a distinct histologic subentity is undistinguishable regardless of age at diagnosis, tumor site, and genetic background (Hawkins and Perlman 1996a). Thus, tissue from ovarian cystic teratoma, a tumor arising from premeiotic cells, is undistinguishable from mature cystic teratoma of the sacrococcygeal region or the CNS.

Currently, germ cell tumors are most commonly classified according to the World Health Organization classification for testicular, ovarian, and central nervous system tumors, latest revision in 2016. Still, there are some inconsistencies in the site-specific classification, in that different terms are used for histologically and biologically identical tumors, i.e., seminomas of the testis, dysgerminomas of the ovary, and germinoma of the CNS. These inconsistencies are mainly explained by the historical development of the site-specific classifications. However, in all classification systems, the approach to mixed malignant germ cell tumors composed of different histologic components is comparable. Thus, it is highly recommended that all different histologic entities present in each single tumor should be listed separately so that a specific description is provided that may assist in the optimal planning of the multimodal therapy. For instance, in a mixed malignant germ cell tumor with germinoma and teratoma, a 2-cm tumor residue after chemotherapy should be interpreted differently from a 2-cm residue of a pure germinoma; the

Table 31.3 Pediatric germ cell tumor—histology

– Teratoma
Mature teratoma
Immature teratoma (grades 1–3)
– Germinoma (seminoma and dysgerminoma)
– Embryonal carcinoma
– Choriocarcinoma
– Polyembryoma
– Mixed malignant germ cell tumor
Teratoma or immature teratoma with malignant GCT elements
Teratoma with other malignant elements (e.g., squamous cell carcinoma)

first could represent residual teratoma requiring resection, whereas a residue of pure germinoma may be pure scar to be followed only.

The histologic classification of these tumors is shown in Table 31.3. The pathologic features of each histologic subtype are discussed separately.

31.1.6.2 Mature Teratoma

Teratomas are the most common histologic subtype of childhood germ cell tumors (Dehner 1983a; Harms and Janig 1986; Hawkins 1990; Young and Scully 1990a). They can arise in the gonads and virtually all extragonadal locations. In fact, sacrococcygeal teratoma constitutes the most common tumor in neonates. Mature teratomas of the gonads are encapsulated and present as multicystic or solid tumors. Extragonadal teratomas differ from their gonadal counterparts in that they commonly lack a clearly defined external capsule, which interferes with surgical preparation and hence complete tumor resection. In sacrococcygeal teratoma, this characteristic requires the coccyx to be removed during surgery to reduce the risk of recurrence (Göbel et al. 1997a, 1998a). A simple enucleation of a mature teratoma may be possible in skilled surgical hands.

The mature teratoma is composed of mature tissues from one or up to all three germ cell layers: ectoderm, mesoderm, and endoderm (Fig. 31.7a). Although any tissue type may be seen, the most commonly found are skin and skin appendages, adipose tissue, mature brain, intestinal epithelium, and cystic structures lined by squamous, cuboidal, or flattened epithelium. Some tissue types are site-specific. For example, hematopoietic, pancreatic, or pituitary tissues are frequently found in mediastinal tumors and rarely in teratoma at other sites. Components of the mature teratoma occasionally may be biologically active, with secretion of enzymes or hormones, including insulin, growth hormone, prolactin, and vasopressin.

31.1.6.3 Immature Teratoma

Pediatric immature teratomas primarily occur in extragonadal sites in children and in the ovaries of girls near puberty (Göbel et al. 1998a; Marina et al. 1999a). Immature teratomas have a gross appearance similar to mature teratoma and are composed of representative tissues from all three germ layers. Unique to these tumors is the presence of various immature tissues, usually neuroepithelium, although immature ectodermal, mesodermal, and endodermal elements also may be observed (Fig. 31.7b). A number of grading systems have been established for immature teratoma, all of which are variations of the system originally devised by Thurlbeck and Scully (1960). All currently used grading systems, such as the one proposed by Gonzalez-Crussi (Gonzalez-Crussi et al. 1978), quantify the degree of immaturity in the lesion. Grade 0 contains only mature tissue, while grade 3 contains more than three areas of immature tissue per low power slide. This grading system to pediatric germ cell tumors has not consistently been applied. Only, within the German MAKEI studies, a consistent reference pathologic evaluation of mature and immature teratomas has been implemented, allowing for evaluating the clinical impact of immaturity and the detection of microfoci of yolk sac tumor within teratomas.

The prognostic impact of grading of immature elements in childhood immature teratoma is not clear. High immaturity itself does not confer a poor prognosis if the tumor is completely resected. However, the risk of incomplete resection is obviously higher in very immature teratomas that tend to show more infiltrative growth in the absence of a clearly distinguished tumor capsule (Göbel et al. 1997a, 1998a).

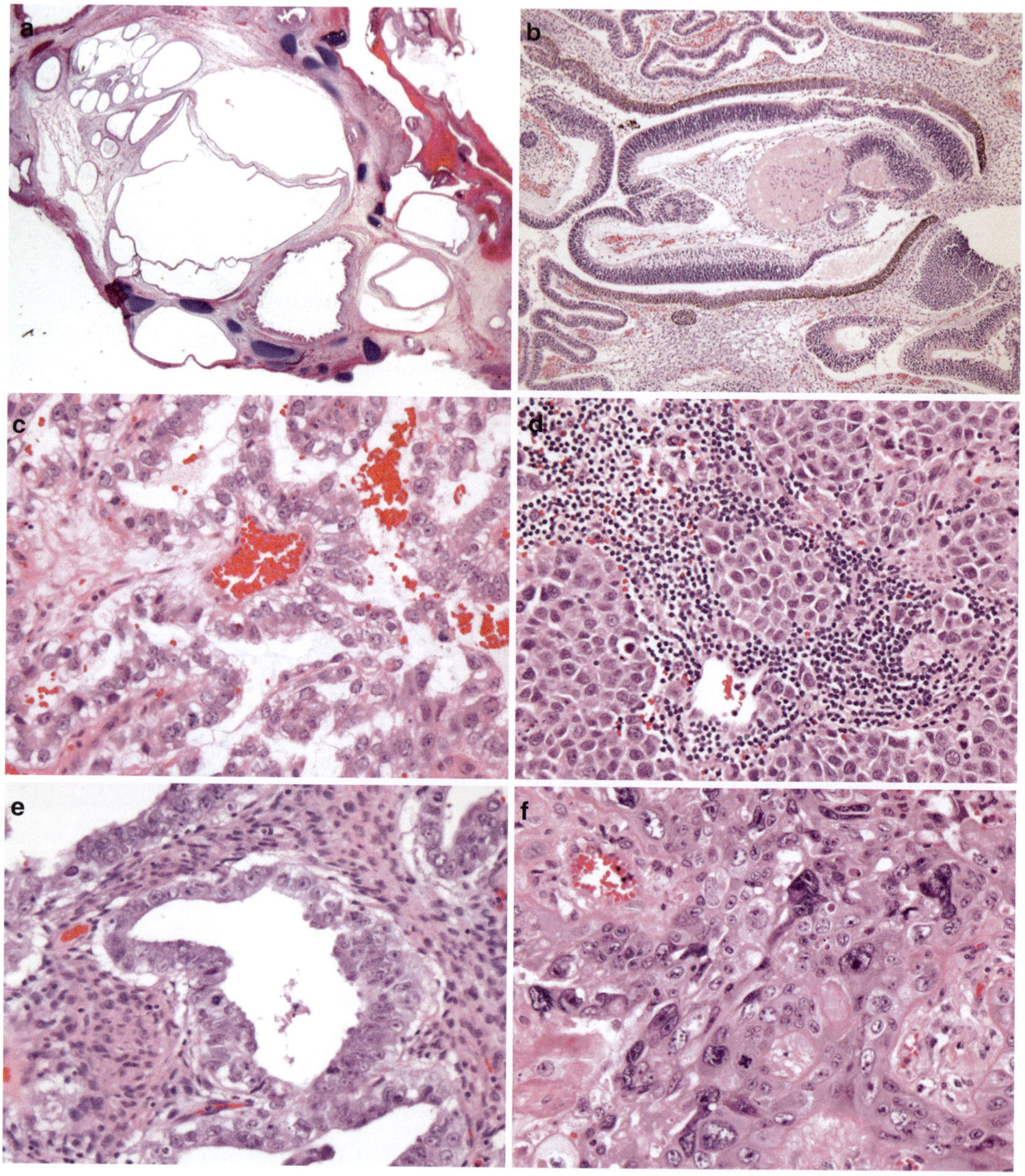

Fig. 31.7 (**a**) Teratoma—encapsulated cystic structure with ectoderm, mesoderm, and endoderm. In this area, cartilage and skin tissue is apparent. (**b**) Immature teratoma—myxoid background with large areas of immature neuroepithelium. (**c**) Yolk sac tumor showing Schiller-Duval body with central blood vessel surrounded by tumor cells and a space before next layer of tumor cells. (**d**) Germinoma showing monomorphic cells with abundant clear cytoplasm surrounded by lymphocytic infiltrate. (**e**) Embryonal carcinoma showing large overlapping nuclei with eosinophilic cytoplasm. (**f**) Choriocarcinoma showing small cells associated with large giant syncytiotrophoblasts

Immature teratomas in children behave in a malignant fashion only if foci of malignant germ cell elements (usually yolk sac tumor) or malignant transformed cells from epithelial or mesenchymal origin are present, and if they are resected incompletely. Clusters of yolk sac tumor can be easily overlooked because they may be very small. Since these may not stain for AFP by immunohistochemistry, the experience of the pathologist is of crucial importance. Tumors containing such foci likely are responsible for the reports that immature teratoma may metastasize. Surgical resection is not always possible, and in some cases, a "benign" immature teratoma proves fatal.

31.1.6.4 Yolk Sac Tumor

Yolk sac tumors are the most common pure malignant germ cell tumor in young children (Young and Scully 1990a). Apart from very few exceptions, it is the only malignant germ cell tumor type occurring during infancy. Yolk sac tumors rarely occur in pure form in adolescents, but more frequently, they are a component of the mixed malignant germ cell tumors occurring in these locations. Grossly, these tumors consist of friable, pale-gray, mucoid tissue with variable amounts of hemorrhage and necrosis. The microscopic features are also wide and have been characterized fully only in the last two decades. Four general patterns and a number of variations have been recognized. These patterns are useful in the recognition of yolk sac tumor, but their clinical relevance is currently unknown.

The pseudopapillary or festoon pattern and the microcystic or reticular patterns are the most common and widely recognized. Both contain Schiller-Duval bodies (Fig. 31.7c). The microcystic or reticular pattern is associated most often with eosinophilic globules and strands that only occasionally stain positively for AFP or α_1-antitrypsin. The pseudopapillary and parietal patterns often are observed after chemotherapy (Ulbright et al. 1990). The solid pattern usually is found only focally and may mimic embryonal carcinoma. A variant of the solid pattern is the hepatoid pattern, which closely resembles fetal liver (Nakashima et al. 1987). A fourth pattern is the polyvesicular vitelline pattern, characterized by small, empty cystic structures lined by a single layer of malignant cells that merge from cuboidal to flat. The cells often are embedded in a loose, frequently myxoid stroma. Two other patterns have been described. The enteric pattern resembles the fetal human gastrointestinal tract and typically stains positively for AFP and chorionic embryonic antigen (Clement et al. 1987; Cohen et al. 1987; Ulbright and Roth 1987). The mesenchyme-like pattern stains positively for cytokeratin and vimentin but not for AFP and has been implicated as the source of the sarcomas that occasionally occur in patients who have had a yolk sac tumor (Nakashima et al. 1987).

In general, AFP is the characteristic immunohistochemical (and clinical) marker of yolk sac tumors. Remarkably, it may not consistently stain all tumor cells but may rather show a spotty staining pattern, so that a negative AFP staining of yolk sac tumor microfoci may not exclude the presence of yolk sac tumor. Therefore, the measurement of AFP in the serum (and cerebrospinal fluid in case of a CNS tumor) is complementary to immunohistochemistry.

31.1.6.5 Germinoma

Germinomas, also termed dysgerminomas (ovary) or seminomas (testis), are the most common pure malignant germ cell tumors that occur in the ovary and central nervous system in adolescents (Talerman 1987; Ho and Liu 1992). Pure seminomas are unusual in men younger than 20 years and rarely occur prior to the onset of puberty. The exception is in patients with sex-chromosomal abnormalities or cryptorchidism, where tumors often present at an earlier age.

On gross pathology, germinomas are encapsulated, solid, gray-pink tumors with a rubbery consistency and occasional small foci of hemorrhage and necrosis. Microscopically, the tumor cells are arranged in nests separated by bands of fibrous tissue in which variable numbers of lymphocytes are identified (Fig. 31.7d). The cells are large, with clear cytoplasm, distinct cell membranes, and large round nuclei having one or two prominent nucleoli. Granulomas with giant cells frequently are present.

Syncytiotrophoblasts also may be present, but they do not alter the prognosis of the tumor unless they are associated with cytotrophoblasts in foci of choriocarcinoma. These tumors are then termed mixed malignant germ cell tumors. Immunohistochemically, the germinoma cells have strong staining for the stem cell marker OCT3/4, placental alkaline phosphatase (PLAP), and c-kit, whereas the syncytiotrophoblasts may stain for human chorionic gonadotropin beta-subunit (β-HCG). In such tumors, a slight elevation of β-HCG may be found in the serum or the cerebrospinal fluid ion case of CNS tumors.

31.1.6.6 Embryonal Carcinoma

Embryonal carcinoma rarely occurs in a pure form in children and is more often a component of a mixed malignant germ cell tumor of adolescents (Young and Scully 1990a; Hawkins and Perlman 1996a). This component is commonly seen in adult testicular germ cell tumor. They are characterized by large cells with large, overlapping nuclei and very large, round nucleoli. The major pattern is epithelial and consists of large nests of cells with varying amounts of central necrosis (Fig. 31.7e). Pseudotubular and papillary patterns that may be confused with those of yolk sac tumor are frequent, but the cells are AFP-negative, and the tumors typically lack the eosinophilic hyaline globules characteristic of yolk sac tumors. Unlike other germ cell tumors, embryonal carcinoma is consistently positive for CD30 by immunohistochemical staining. In addition, they stain positive for OCT3/4 (Looijenga et al. 2003).

31.1.6.7 Choriocarcinoma

Choriocarcinoma rarely occurs outside the context of malignant mixed germ cell tumors in adolescents (Young and Scully 1990a; Hawkins and Perlman 1996a). The rare case of pure choriocarcinoma detected in infants almost always represents metastasis from maternal or placental gestational trophoblastic primary tumor (Belchis et al. 1993). These tumors characteristically are very hemorrhagic and friable. Microscopically, two types of cells must be present to confirm the diagnosis: cytotrophoblasts, which classically appear as closely packed nests of relatively uniform, medium-sized cells having clear cytoplasm, distinct cell margins, and vesicular nuclei, and syncytiotrophoblasts, which represent multinucleate syncytial trophoblastic cells (Fig. 31.7f). The syncytiotrophoblastic elements stain positively for β-HCG, accounting for the associated high concentrations of serum β-HCG in these patients. If choriocarcinoma arises in the CNS, β-HCG may be detected both in the cerebrospinal fluid and the serum, sometimes with discrepant findings in the two compartments. Clinically, choriocarcinoma is associated with widespread hematogenic metastases including CNS metastases, which may be complicated by CNS hemorrhage.

31.1.7 Serum Tumor Markers

Due to their crucial importance for the categorization of childhood germ cell tumors, the serological markers α_1-fetoprotein (AFP) and β-human chorionic gonadotropin (β-HCG) are discussed in detail. AFP, an α_1-globulin, is the earliest and predominant serum-binding protein in the fetus, reaching its peak concentration at 12–14 weeks' gestation and gradually falling to reach an adult normal level of less than 10 ng per dL at approximately age 1 year (Gitlin et al. 1972) (Table 31.4). In some patients, adult AFP normal serum levels of AFP are reached only at the end of the second year of life (Blohm et al. 1998). As AFP levels begin to decline in fetal development, albumin becomes the principal serum-binding protein. In early embryogenesis, AFP is produced in the yolk sac and later by hepatocytes and the gastrointestinal tract. Since AFP may cross the placenta, AFP of pregnant mothers may be significantly elevated.

In 1974, the association between serum elevation of AFP and the natural history of adult germ cell tumors was described. Elevated serum levels or positive immunohistochemical staining of germ cell tumors for AFP indicates the presence

Table 31.4 Serum AFP levels in first year of life for preterm and term infants

Age	Preterm (<37 weeks)	Term
Birth	31,261–799,834	9120–190,546
1 week	6039–311,889	1480–58,887
1 month	389–79,433	16–1995
3–4 months	9–18,620	3–417
6–24 months	0–372	0.8–87

Adapted from report by Blohm et al. (1998)
AFP levels (ng/ml) reported as 95.5% intervals

of malignant components, specifically yolk sac or embryonal carcinoma (Table 31.2). The serum half-life ($t_{1/2}$) of AFP is 5–7 days, but may be longer in particular at lower levels, e.g., during the second half of the first year of life (Blohm et al. 1998). Because of the wide variation in levels at birth, especially with infants of less than 40 weeks' gestational age, and the wide variability in $t_{1/2}$ at different ages within the first year of life, difficulties arise in interpreting decay of serum AFP as an indication of residual or recurrent germ cell tumor in infants younger than 12 months (Blohm et al. 1998; Schneider et al. 2001a).

Increasing levels of serum AFP, however, are not necessarily indicative of tumor progression. Abrupt rise in serum AFP can occur after chemotherapy-induced tumor lysis (Schneider et al. 2001a). Spurious persistence of elevated serum AFP may reflect an alteration in hepatic function from such conditions as viral hepatitis (hepatitis B, hepatitis C, and human immunodeficiency virus–associated hepatitis), cholestasis secondary to anesthesia, metabolic disease (e.g., tyrosinemia type I), or exposure to phenytoin or methotrexate. Other neoplastic conditions associated with elevated serum AFP include hepatoblastoma, hepatocellular carcinoma, pancreaticoblastoma, and pancreatic, gastrointestinal, or bronchial adenocarcinomas (Schneider et al. 2001a). AFP is not only helpful in detecting significant yolk sac tumor components but may also assist in prognostic assessment. During and after treatment, an elevation in AFP identifies progression or recurrence before tumor can be identified by imaging. In a large cooperative analysis of adult germ cell tumors, high AFP and/or β-HCG levels indicated poor prognosis (Group 1997a). In the British childhood cancer studies, high AFP levels above 1000 μg/L were associated with unfavorable outcome (Mann et al. 1989a). In the international collaborative study (MAGIC), high AFP levels above 10,000 μg/L were again associated with worse outcome (Frazier et al. 2015) Furthermore, an inadequate decline of AFP that does not follow its half time of 5–7 days indicates pure response to chemo or tumor progression after tumor resection (Schneider et al. 2005a).

Human chorionic gonadotropin (HCG) is a glycoprotein comprised of α- and β-peptide subunits and normally is synthesized during pregnancy by syncytiotrophoblasts of the placenta to maintain viability of the corpus luteum. The α-subunit is similar to α-peptides of other hormones, such as luteinizing hormone, follicle-stimulating hormone, and thyroid-stimulating hormone. The β-subunit is antigenically distinct, serving as the basis for the method of serum assay. Minute amounts, less than 5 mIU per mL, are detected in serum of healthy adults; serum $t_{1/2}$ of β-HCG is 24–36 h.

The most frequent cause of significant rise of β-HCG is pregnancy. Therefore, in case of suspected germ cell tumor and elevated β-HCG, pregnancy must be excluded with other techniques, e.g., ultrasound.

Elevation of serum β-HCG in patients with germ cell tumors implies the presence of clones of syncytiotrophoblasts, such as choriocarcinoma, or of syncytiotrophoblastic giant cells, found frequently in germinomas (pure seminomas or dysgerminomas) and occasionally in adult embryonal carcinoma.

Like serum AFP, sudden elevation of serum β-HCG may occur after cell lysis secondary to chemotherapy (Vogelzang et al. 1982). Iatrogenic hypogonadism secondary to bilateral orchiectomy, oophorectomy, or chemotherapy also may be associated with rising levels of serum β-HCG because of an increase in luteinizing hormone that results in immunologic cross-reactivity. Other conditions in which modest elevations of serum β-HCG have been reported include multiple myeloma and other malignancies of the liver, pancreas, gastrointestinal tract, breast, lung, and bladder. Simultaneous elevation of serum AFP and β-HCG has been described in ovarian embryonal carcinoma in an 11-year-old and in patients with polyembryoma.

31.1.7.1 Other Markers

Because some germ cell tumors with identifiable malignant elements do not produce measurable amounts of serum AFP or β-HCG, other markers with potential prognostic value have been investigated. Serum LDH, a glycolytic enzyme that appears to correlate with growth and regression of various solid neoplasms, has not shown specificity for a specific histologic subtype of germ cell tumors. In patients with dysgerminoma, serum levels of the LDH isoenzyme 1, the gene which resides on 12p, correlate with the tumor burden and aid in the planning and assessment of surgical management (Schwartz and Morris 1988). Elevated serum LDH levels have not been prognostic in germ cell tumors of prepubertal children.

Human placenta like alkaline phosphatase (PLAP) is a fetal isoenzyme of alkaline phosphatase that is elevated in the sera of up to 30% of patients with stage I disease and of almost 100% of cases with advanced seminoma (Koshida et al. 1991). As with AFP and β-HCG, immunohistochemical staining for PLAP sometimes is useful in determining the origin of histologically undifferentiated tumors.

Although elevated serum levels of carcinoembryonic antigen (CEA) are reported in patients with ovarian tumors, the usefulness of this antigen has been hampered by lack of tumor specificity and correlation to disease natural history.

The carbohydrate antigen CA-125, which is related to the tissues of the coelomic epithelium and müllerian ducts, has been assessed in ovarian cancers of germ cell and epithelial origin. CA125 may be elevated as a result of peritoneal irritation. It has been reported to have some correlation with other tumor markers and to be of value in monitoring patients with ovarian tumors of germ cell, epithelial, and stromal origin (Altaras et al. 1986), although its utility in these patients remains to be defined because of the limited numbers of patients studied to date.

Recently, miRNA profiles have been evaluated as specific serum tumor markers of malignant germ cell tumors (Murray et al. 2017). However, these await further evaluation in diagnostic studies to validate their differential diagnostic accuracy and sensitivity for monitoring during therapy and follow-up.

31.1.8 Treatment Overview

The treatment of benign and malignant germ cell tumors requires a coordinated multimodality approach. The strategy is chosen based on data on site, staging, biology, histology, and marker levels (Table 31.5). The development of effective chemotherapy regimens has allowed a more adaptive surgical approach that is specific to anatomic site of germ cell tumors. These specifics will be discussed in sections that follow on testicular, ovarian, and extragonadal germ cell tumors. A few guiding principles can be outlined.

31.1.9 Surgical Treatment of Germ Cell Tumors in the Context of Multimodal Therapy

Surgery is a mainstay in the treatment of germ cell tumors. Complete surgical resection is the standard treatment for benign tumors, such as teratomas. In pure teratoma, there is no evidence that chemotherapy has any significant therapeutic effects (Göbel et al. 1998a; Marina et al. 1999a; Pashankar et al. 2016). Considering the possibility of late relapse, a prolonged follow-up especially after immature teratoma resection is recommended.

Table 31.5 Sensitivity to treatment

	Histologic grading	Sensitivity to chemo	Sensitivity to radiation
Seminoma/germinoma	Malignant	+++	>24 Gy
Embryonal carcinoma	Malignant	+++	>45 Gy
Yolk sac tumor	Malignant	+++	>45 Gy
Choriocarcinoma	Malignant	+++	>45 Gy
Teratoma, mature/immature	Benign/potential for malignant development	?	?

The complete surgical removal of malignant lesions is also indicated, if possible. However, the surgical approach to malignant germ cell tumors may be influenced by effective neoadjuvant chemotherapy. In this situation, biopsy followed by delayed resection (following neo-adjuvant chemotherapy) may be appropriate.

It must be emphasized that surgical recommendations may differ significantly for children and adolescents and for gonadal and extragonadal germ cell tumors. In general, gonadal tumors are more assessable to complete tumor resection, since most present with a clearly defined tumor capsule often in combination with the organ capsule of the gonad. Therefore, most gonadal tumors are resected completely and the local relapse rate is low. In contrast, extragonadal tumors more often show infiltrating growth and a poorly defined pseudocapsule. These tumors present with considerable size and often develop in anatomically problematic regions such as the brain, mediastinum, or the pelvic floor. Therefore, complete resection with free margins of extragonadal germ cell tumors is often impossible. In this situation, neoadjuvant chemotherapy may substantially facilitate complete resection on delayed surgery.

The question "is a biopsy needed prior to neoadjuvant chemotherapy?" is approached differently by various groups. Most physicians are more comfortable treating with chemotherapy when a pathologic diagnosis is confirmed. In addition, material for molecular studies of germ cell tumor may be crucial to future treatments. However, in patients with secreting tumors, it may be in the patient's interest not to biopsy, for example, in the presence of respiratory distress due to mediastinal disease or if an intracavitary tumor spread is possible during the procedure.

Malignant germ cell tumors may respond dramatically to neoadjuvant chemotherapy, allowing a less aggressive surgical approach at specific sites such as vaginal yolk sac tumors (Mauz-Körholz et al. 2000a, b). Therefore, resection should not be undertaken to the point of sacrificing vital structures. Chemotherapy may thus allow a patient to be spared mutilating surgery. In many large extragonadal malignant germ cell tumors, neoadjuvant chemotherapy may increase the chance of complete resection. Eventual complete resection (post-chemotherapy) is the goal if cure of an extragonadal germ cell tumor is to be achieved (Schneider et al. 2000a; Göbel et al. 2001a). Stable radiologic disease with marker normalization may not always suggest resistant disease. In this case, however, a removal of residual disease after chemotherapy is recommended whenever feasible. Thus, surgical resection plays a final therapeutic role and provides information with regard to the histologic composition of residual disease. Lastly, surgery also plays a significant role in relapsed germ cell tumors.

31.1.9.1 Radiotherapy

Radiotherapy has been used to effectively treat germ cell tumors of germinomatous origin including germinoma (CNS), seminoma (testis), and dysgerminoma (ovarian). Radiation sensitivity correlates with histology (Table 31.5). However, the role of radiation in seminoma and dysgerminoma has been reduced by the advent of platinum-based chemotherapy. Nevertheless, radiation therapy, applied as craniospinal irradiation, remains standard treatment for CNS germinoma. However, currently new strategies have been developed that combine chemotherapy with irradiation to reduced fields and with reduced doses, in order to reduce the risk of long-term radiotherapy-associated sequelae. Radiation therapy may also play a role in the treatment of recurrent germ cell tumors, in particular, if tumors still cannot be resected completely after up-front salvage chemotherapy.

31.1.10 Chemotherapy

The prognosis of germ cell tumors has improved significantly with the development of cisplatin-based therapy in adult testicular germ cell tumor patients (DFS 68–92%) (Einhorn and Donohue 1977a; Logothetis et al. 1985; Bosl et al. 1988; Einhorn et al. 1989a). Prior to this effective chemotherapy, children with extracranial malignant germ cell tumors had 3-year survival rates of 15–20% with surgery and radiation therapy

(Kurman and Norris 1976a; Billmire and Grosfeld 1986). However, boys with localized testicular tumors did well with surgical resection (Hawkins et al. 1986). Prognosis and appropriate treatment depend on factors such as histology (e.g., seminomatous vs. nonseminomatous), age (young children vs. adolescents), stage of disease, and primary site (Baranzelli et al. 1999a; Marina et al. 2006a). Cisplatin-based chemotherapy has dramatically improved the outcome for children with extracranial germ cell tumor, with 5-year overall survival rates of more than 90% (Göbel et al. 2001a; Cushing et al. 2004a; Rogers et al. 2004a). Table 31.6 describes successful regimens developed by various national pediatric groups. In general, the clinical outcome is comparable with the different protocols; however, the toxicity profile may vary. To develop an optimal consensus treatment strategy, an international meta-analysis would be beneficial. However, such a project is still problematic due to several issues such as different staging systems, different histopathologic classification systems, as well as considerable differences in risk stratification. Current international initiatives evaluate whether the efficacy of cisplatin-based chemotherapy can further be enhanced by time condensed regimen (Lawrence et al. 2018). Moreover, based on the MAGIC risk stratification, a first retrospective and now prospective comparison between cis- and carboplatin-based regimen for intermediate-risk germ cell tumors has been launched (Shaikh et al. 2013). The background of this initiative is that in all adult randomized clinical trials, cisplatin has proven superior to carboplatin, while the outcome of the British protocol that used carboplatin-based regimen at a dose of 6 AUC was favorable (Mann et al. 2000). Moreover, there are considerable concerns about potential late effects of cisplatin in children.

In general, substantial reduction of cumulative chemotherapy has become possible with the optimization of multimodal therapeutic strategies, including optimal timing of surgical resection in locally advanced tumors. Thus, acute and long-term side effects can be minimized while maintaining excellent survival. This goal can only be achieved through ongoing cooperative group studies. Advances in molecular understanding of these rare pediatric tumors may additionally help in the development of risk-adapted strategies. Site-specific details will be discussed in the following chapters.

31.1.11 Salvage Therapy

The treatment of recurrent germ cell tumors in children has mostly not been studied systematically. Recurrent disease must be categorized based on histology (benign or malignant) and extent (local or distant). In addition, the first-line treatment has a substantial impact on both the choice of salvage treatment and prognosis. Thus, tumors that progress after surgery and watch-and-wait strategy commonly have a favorable prognosis with standard platin-based chemotherapy. In contrast, malignant tumors that relapse after first-line treatment are often resistant to further therapy, and prognosis is poor. Recurrent benign tumors (mature teratomas and most immature teratomas) must be treated with surgery. Chemotherapy has not yielded significant improvement in these benign tumors. One example that demonstrates this phenomenon is the "growing teratoma syndrome." A mixed tumor with teratoma and yolk sac tumor continues to grow despite normalization of markers. At surgery, only viable mature teratoma persists (Afifi et al. 1997). Of note, these growing teratomas retain the cytogenetic aberrations also present in malignant germ cell tumors (van Echten et al. 1997a, b). It may be concluded that in these tumors, terminal differentiation presents a way to evade cytotoxic treatment and to induce resistance to chemotherapy (Mayer et al. 2003a). For these tumors, alternative strategies with either immunomodulation (interferon) (van der Gaast et al. 1991) or antiangiogenetic therapy (Calaminus et al. 2009) have been applied with some success. Nevertheless, definitive therapy always requires complete surgical resection, even if intermittent stable disease can be achieved with such strategies. In 3–6% of adult cases, somatic transformation is evident.

Table 31.6 Pediatric treatment strategies

Drug	Doses	No. of cycles
US Children's Oncology Group: PEB (9048/8891;9049/8890)		
Cisplatin	20 mg/m², day 1, 2, 3, 4, 5	3–4 cycles
	or 33 mg/m², day 1, 2, 3	
Etoposide	100 mg/m², day 1, 2, 3, 4, 5	
	or 167 mg/m², day 1, 2, 3	
Bleomycin	15 U/m², day 1	
German MAKEI study group: PE and PEI (MAKEI 96)/SIOP CNS GCT I-II		
Cisplatin	20 mg/m², day 1,2,3,4,5	2–4 cycles
Etoposide	100 mg/m², day 1,2,3	
Ifosfamide	1500 mg/m², day 1,2,3,4,5	
French TGC study group: PVB and VIP (TGM 2011)		
Cisplatin	20 mg/m², day 1,2,3,4,5	Up to 3 cycles
Vinblastin	3 mg/m², day 1,2	
Bleomycin	15 U/m², day 1	
Cisplatin	20 mg/m², day 1,2,3,4,5	Up to 4 cycles
Etoposide	75 mg/m², day 1,2,3,4,5	
Ifosfamide	3000 mg/m², day 1,2	
*Italian GCT study group (PEB) (*Terenziani et al. 2017, 2018*)*		
Cisplatin	25 mg/m², day 1,2,3,4	Up to 4 cycles
Etoposide	100 mg/m², day 1,2,3,4	
Bleomycin	15 mg/m², day 2	
*Brazilian TCG [PE (high-dose PE), IVB] (*Lopes et al. 2009, b*)*		
Cisplatin	20 mg/m², day 1,2,3,4,5	5 cycles
Etoposide	100 mg/m², day 1,2,3,4,5	
HD-Cisplatin	30 mg/m², day 1,2,3,4,5	5 cycles
HD-Etoposide	120 mg/m², day 1,2,3,4,5	
Ifosfamide	1500 mg/m², day 1,2,3	3 cycles
Velban	3 mg/m², day 1	
Bleomycin	15 mg/m², day 1	
SIOP central nervous system germ cell tumor protocol (SIOP CNS GCT) (HD-PEI) (Schmoll et al. 2003a, b)		
Cisplatin	100 mg/m², day 1,2,3,4,5	3 cycles (after one initial cycle of conventional PEI)
Etoposide	300 mg/m², day 1,2,3,4,5	
Ifosfamide	2000 mg/m², day 1,2,3,4,5	
Plus autologous stem cell support plus G-CSF at day 7		
SIOP central nervous system germ cell tumor protocol (SIOP CNS GCT) (Carbo-PEI)		
Carboplatin	600 mg/m², day 1	2 cycles
Etoposide	100 mg/m², day 1,2,3,22,23,24	
Ifosfamide	1800 mg/m², day 22,23,24,25,26	
*UK CCLG (*Mann et al. 2000*)*		
Carboplatin	600 mg/m², day 2	Until remission + 2 cycles
Etoposide	120 mg/m², day 1,2,3	
Bleomycin	15 mg/m², day 3	

During cisplatin therapy, intensive infusion therapy with 3 L/m²/day accompanied by mannitol forced diuresis is mandatory. During ifosfamide, uroprotection with mesna is recommended

The prospective assessment of salvage therapies in recurrent or refractory malignant pediatric germ cell tumors is limited by the small numbers of patients.

The treatment of recurrent malignant pediatric germ cell tumors is anecdotal. In contrast to adult patients, many children have local relapses, and treatment may include intensive chemotherapy and local therapy (Schneider et al. 2001d). For these purposes a strategy that utilizes up-front chemotherapy followed by delayed tumor resection has proven effective. In selected patients, locoregional control can be supported by the combination of cisplatin chemotherapy and regional deep hyperthermia (Wessalowski et al. 1997a, 2003a, 2013). In addition, it is certainly helpful to concentrate surgical therapy of patients with recurrent malignant germ cell tumors in specific national surgical centers. This provides the opportunity to centralize experience in these often delicate surgical procedures and to advance scientific research on salvage surgery.

Radiation therapy with at least 45 Gy for nonseminomatous germ cell tumors (Table 31.5) may also be considered to improve local control, in particular, in tumors not assessable to complete resection (Schneider et al. 2001d).

A multimodal strategy that combines chemotherapy, surgery, and possibly radiotherapy is necessary for recurrent malignant tumors. Trials in adult patients with recurrent or persistent malignant germ cell tumors have provided potential strategies for salvage chemotherapy. Complete responses from 50 to 77% have been obtained in patients, who relapsed after cisplatin therapy (Motzer et al. 2000). Combinations of paclitaxel, ifosfamide, and cisplatin; vinblastine, ifosfamide, and cisplatin; or vincristine, bleomycin, and cisplatin, and more recently paclitaxel, gemcitabine, and oxaliplatin have been used. To date, no molecular targeted agent has shown reasonable activity (Oing et al. 2017). Autologous marrow transplantation has also been used to treat these adult patients (Einhorn et al. 2007). However, in particular, for extragonadal germ cell tumors, the therapeutic impact of high-dose chemotherapy is limited, if no local control can be achieved (Schneider et al. 2001d; Faure-Conter et al. 2014). However, in a prospective protocol using thermochemotherapy in combination with surgical resection (and irradiation of unresectable tumors) for 44 patients with refractory or recurrent malignant germ cell tumors, a 5-year event-free survival of 62% and overall survival of 72% were achieved (Wessalowski et al. 2013).

Retroperitoneal lymph node dissection (RPLND) has not been part of standard pediatric germ cell tumor treatment. Post-chemotherapy followed by RPLND may be an integral part of treatment in adolescent and adult males. These tumors may progress in the retroperitoneal lymph nodes, and residual teratoma may dedifferentiate into malignant germ cell tumor or somatic malignant differentiation (Carver et al. 2007a, b, c). Site-specific salvage therapies will be discussed with anatomic sites.

31.1.12 Late Effects

In the study of late effects of therapy, attention must be paid to those late effects from tumor and local therapy and those effects secondary to systemic therapy (Table 31.7).

Among the various possible late effects of germ cell tumors, local sequelae after surgery and/or radiotherapy must be distinguished from systemic late effects as a consequence of chemotherapy. Local effects can be caused both by tumor and by local treatment. For instance, teratomas of the head and neck can involve the thy-

Table 31.7 Potential late treatment effects

I. Late effects from tumor and local therapy
– CNS
Diabetes insipidus, GH, and other endocrine deficiencies
Hemianopsia, cranial nerve palsies, bone growth
– Head and neck tumors—hypothyroid, tracheal malacia
– SCT—incontinence
– Gonadal—sterility, lack of function
– Polyembryoma
– Mixed malignant germ cell tumor
Teratoma or immature teratoma with malignant GCT elements
Teratoma with other malignant elements (e.g., squamous cell carcinoma)
II. Late effects from systemic therapy
– Cisplatin—ototoxicity and renal toxicity, secondary malignancy
– Bleomycin—pulmonary dysfunction and cutaneous toxicity
– Etoposide—secondary leukemia
– Ifosfamide—renal toxicity

roid gland, which must then be removed with the tumor. As a consequence a proportion of children with cervical teratoma may suffer from insufficiency of the thyroid or parathyroid glands (Bernbeck et al. 2009a). Chronic endocrine insufficiency is also characteristic of hypophyseal germ cell tumors. In these tumors, diabetes insipidus may be the key symptom of the tumor. Diabetes insipidus will usually persist even after successful treatment of the germ cell tumors. Hypophyseal insufficiency may also result in other hormone deficiencies such as growth hormone deficiency.

Sacrococcygeal teratomas are often very large at presentation. They may distort the anatomic situation of the pelvic floor so that the muscles of the pelvic floor have to be reconstructed during tumor resection. However, still some patients may develop palsy of the pelvic floor, in particular, if a malignant tumor infiltrates the nerves of the sacral plexus. As a result, these patients may be incontinent for stool and/or urine, or they may suffer from chronic obstipation (Güler et al. 2018; Shalaby et al. 2014). The risk of recurrent urinary infections is also increased. Since many germ cell tumors grow to a considerable size, a broad surgical approach is required, thus giving rise to scars at considerable size. Nevertheless, as presented in the respective chapters, most patients even with gross tumors grow up with a good quality of life and without mutilation. To achieve this goal, the possibility to apply up-front chemotherapy prior to surgery should be considered in all malignant germ cell tumors.

The issue of chemotherapy-related late effects is multifactorial and varies with the different chemotherapy combinations applied according to the different protocols.

Cisplatin era has greatly improved survival in children with malignant germ cell tumors. However, significant toxicity and late effects have occurred. Hearing impairment, in particular, high tone loss, was noted in a substantial proportion of pediatric patients treated with high-dose cisplatin (Cushing et al. 2004a). However, individual audiograms have already documented significant hearing loss with both standard- and high-dose cisplatin (Li et al. 2004). Amifostine, as a protectant, did not lessen ototoxicity (Marina et al. 2003). Young children are particularly sensitive to toxic effects of cisplatin. Importantly, ototoxicity in a young child may significantly impair speech, academic, and social development (Knight et al. 2005). A Dutch study reported on a frequency of ototoxicity of 45% for cisplatin, 17% for carboplatin, and 75% for the combination of both drugs. With the cumulative dose of cisplatin of 300 mg/mq or more, a fivefold increase of ototoxicity is observed, and the concomitant use of carboplatin, furosemide, aminoglycoside, brain radiotherapy, and CSF shunts increases the risk (for details see Chaps. 3 and 9 in clinical and genetic determinants of ototoxicity after childhood cancer. 2019 Eva Clemes ed.)

A study in adults suggests that cisplatin ototoxicity may be associated with specific glutathione S-transferase genotypes (Oldenburg et al. 2007). In addition, genetic polymorphism of the megalin gene (Riedemann et al. 2008) may eventually provide a diagnostic tool to assessing the risk of ototoxicity prospectively. Genetic susceptibility associations have not been consistent or replicated for children, to date, and thus, evidence-based recommendations cannot be made with regard to the risk hearing impairment. Genetic susceptibility associations are not consistent or not replicated, and to date, no evidence-based recommendations can be made for prophylaxis of hearing impairment (Chap. 4 in clinical and genetic determinants of ototoxicity after childhood cancer. 2019 Eva Clemes ed.) A recent randomized trial of thiosulfate prior to the infusion of cisplatin for children with hepatoblastoma demonstrated a significant otoprotective effect with no adverse tumor-related outcome (Brock et al. 2018).

Nephrotoxicity may be enhanced when cisplatin and ifosfamide are used concurrently. In particular, children may develop tubulopathy with loss of electrolytes and glucose (secondary Fanconi syndrome). Therefore, renal function and urinary excretion of electrolytes should be monitored during follow-up in order to prevent renal osteopathy.

The risk of pulmonary toxicity of bleomycin in toddlers and infants is controversial. In adult germ cell tumors, there are reports on an increased risk of cardiovascular disease, including atherosclerosis and coronary heart disease. However, there are no comparable long-term follow-up data available for patients treated for a germ cell tumor during childhood. In the German MAKEI registry, two patients are documented, who developed lethal pulmonary fibrosis and pulmonary failure after bleomycin and anesthesia required for tumor resection (Göbel et al. 2000a). In adults, the risk of lethal pulmonary toxicity is estimated to be approximately 1% (Osanto et al. 1992). Most adult patients develop some gradual impairment of pulmonary function during bleomycin chemotherapy. However, these changes are mostly intermittent and resolve after cessation of chemotherapy. Nevertheless, since an increased pulmonary sensitivity is suspected for children and since pulmonary function cannot be monitored in infants, most pediatric protocols have either reduced bleomycin doses (15 mg/m^2 per cycle), reduced chemotherapy to a two-agent regimen, or replaced bleomycin with ifosfamide, even if ifosfamide is more myelo- and gonadotoxic.

The risk of secondary neoplasms such as therapy-related acute myelogenous leukemias has been debated intensively, both for adult and pediatric patients treated with etoposide. According to the MAKEI series, the 10-year cumulative risk of secondary leukemia can be estimated to be approximately 1% in patients treated with chemotherapy alone and 4.2% in patients treated with both radio- and chemotherapy (Schneider et al. 1999). In the US pediatric intergroup study, there were four cases of acute myelocytic leukemia. None were associated with 11q23 abnormality, supporting that the regimen commonly prescribed for childhood germ cell tumors only has a low leukemogenic potential.

In this context, it should also be noted that some malignant germ cell tumors, in particular, malignant mediastinal nonseminomatous germ cell tumors, may be associated with concurrent or metachronous leukemia. However, this leukemic clone is intrinsic to the germ cell tumor and presents a somatic malignant transformation within the germ cell tumor. This is proven by the observation that the isochromosome 12p, which is pathognomic of the germ cell tumor, is also detectable in the leukemic cell (Orazi et al. 1993).

In adult patients, chemotherapy for malignant germ cell tumors is associated with a significant long-time risk of cardiovascular disease. Thus, the risk of myocardial infarction, angina pectoris, and heart failure is increased compared to healthy adults of the same age group (Gietema et al. 1992; Bokemeyer et al. 1996; van den Belt-Dusebout et al. 2006). Compared to adults, no comprehensive data on long-term cardiovascular risk for children treated with chemotherapy is currently available. However, considerable research activities are currently focusing on the issue of cancer survivorship. This data may then assist in evaluating different therapeutic strategies for childhood germ cell tumors that take both the therapeutic efficacy and long-term sequelae of therapy into account. The quality of semen is very poor in adults, even in those patients not treated with chemotherapy. This has not been well investigated in adults who were treated for germ cell tumors as children. Any efforts should be done to reduce the gonadotoxic treatments and to adopt preventive strategies for preserving fertility.

31.2 Extragonadal Germ Cell Tumors

Dominik T. Schneider

Giovanni Cecchetto, and Thomas A. Olson

Germ cell tumors include a group of tumors that is highly heterogeneous regarding their clinical and histologic appearance. During childhood and adolescence, approximately half of all germ cell tumors develop at extragonadal midline sites.

Sacrococcygeal germ cell tumors constitute the most frequent tumor in neonates, and extracranial germ cell tumors account for 14% of all cancers in adolescents of the 15–19 age group. Accordingly, an epidemiological analysis of patients reported to the German germ cell tumor trials from 1981 to 2000 showed a bimodal age distribution with a small peak during infancy and a larger peak after puberty (Schneider et al. 2004b). These separate groups were marked by distinct clinical and molecular features. The distribution of extragonadal tumor sites by age is shown in Figs. 31.1 and 31.2 of Sect. 31.1.1.

Experience gained in the successful chemotherapy of testicular germ cell tumors in adults has successfully been translated to the treatment of childhood extragonadal germ cell tumors. Several prospective trials of different national study groups have demonstrated that cis- or carboplatin-based combination chemotherapy is effective in extragonadal germ cell tumors, too (Kapoor et al. 1995; Cushing et al. 2004b; Göbel et al. 2000b; Lopes et al. 2009; Mann et al. 2000a). In addition, substantial reduction of cumulative chemotherapy has become possible with the optimization of multimodal therapeutic strategies, including optimal timing of surgical resection in locally advanced tumors. Thus, acute and long-term side effects can be minimized, while maintaining excellent survival. This goal can only be achieved through ongoing cooperative group studies. Advances in molecular understanding of these rare pediatric tumors may additionally help in the development of risk-adapted strategies (Oosterhuis and Looijenga 2005b).

31.2.1 Histogenesis, Biology, and Histology of Extragonadal Germ Cell Tumors

These aspects are extensively discussed in Sect. 31.1. In summary, the histologic appearance of extragonadal germ cell tumors is undistinguishable from that of their gonadal counterparts. Moreover, within the corresponding age groups, they share the same genetic aberrations such as the isochromosome 12p or deletion of 1p and 6q. At the epigenetic level, both gonadal and extragonadal germ cell tumors show erasure of genomic imprinting, substantiating the holistic concept of Teilum that all germ cell tumors arise from primordial germ cells (Teilum et al. 1975b).

Nevertheless, some peculiar and site-specific features have to be considered. Thus, the histologic differentiation may be restricted to specific subtypes such as teratoma and yolk sac tumor in the coccygeal region (Göbel et al. 2001a, b; Harms and Jänig 1986) and yolk sac tumor in the vagina (Mauz-Körholz et al. 2000a, b). At these sites, no germinomatous tumors can be observed.

In addition, the development of germ cell tumors may be restricted to specific age groups. Sacrococcygeal or vaginal germ cell tumors only develop in prepubertal children, while ovarian and central nervous system germ cell tumors mainly develop during and after puberty (Schneider et al. 2004b). Lastly, some extragonadal germ cell tumors may be associated with specific genetic aberrations such as Klinefelter's syndrome in mediastinal germ cell tumors, while this constellation is not observed at other sites (Nichols et al. 1987b; Schneider et al. 2002b). These clinical observations illustrate that some yet unknown site-specific environmental factors significantly modulate the development as well as histologic and clinical appearance of extragonadal germ cell tumors. In how far such factors also impact on therapy is currently speculative.

31.2.2 Pathology

Germ cell tumors show numerous histologic subtypes; however, the microscopic morphology of a distinct histologic subentity is undistinguishable regardless of age at diagnosis, tumor site, and genetic background (Dehner 1983b). Thus, tissue from ovarian cystic teratoma, a tumor arising from premeiotic cells, is undistinguishable from mature cystic teratoma of the sacrococcygeal region or the central nervous system. Currently, germ cell tumors are most commonly classified according to the World Health Organization revised classification for testicular, ovarian, and central nervous system tumors (Young 2005a; Kleihues et al. 1993; Mostofi and Sobin 1993; Serov and Scully 1973; Williamson et al. 2016; Meinhold-Heerlein et al. 2016). Still, there are some inconsistencies in the site-specific classification, in that different terms are used for histologically and biologically identical tumors, i.e., seminomas of the testis, dysgerminomas of the ovary, and germinoma of the CNS. These inconsistencies are mainly explained by the historical development of the site-specific classifications. However, in all classification systems, the approach to mixed malignant germ cell tumors composed of different histologic components is comparable. Thus, all different histologic entities present in each single tumor are listed separately so that a specific description is provided that may assist in the optimal planning of the multimodal therapy. For instance, in a mixed malignant germ cell tumor with germinoma and teratoma, a 2-cm tumor residue after chemotherapy should be interpreted different from a 2-cm residue of a pure germinoma; the first could represent residual teratoma, whereas a residue of pure germinoma may be pure scar tissue.

The histologic classification of these tumors is shown in Table 31.3 of Sect. 31.1.1. The pathologic features of each histologic subtype are discussed separately in Sect. 31.1.1 too.

31.2.3 Clinical Diagnosis

31.2.3.1 Clinical Symptoms

The diagnosis of extragonadal germ cell tumors primarily depends on the clinical and radiographic assessment as well as the evaluation of the "specific" tumor markers AFP and β-HCG. In most patients, germ cell tumors present as considerably large indolent tumors. In contrast, childhood testicular germ cell tumors are mainly diagnosed at a comparably small size, since in young infants these tumors are detected by the parents while the diapers are changed. In analogy, vaginal yolk sac tumors are mostly diagnosed at comparable moderate size, because these may become apparent after vaginal bleeding.

Regardless of benign or malignant histology, large tumors may result in significant local complications. Thus, head and neck teratomas may result in acute life-threatening airway obstruction, requiring an anticipating and qualified perinatal management [Fig. 19.1 in Chap. 19 (Head and Neck Teratomas)]. Sacrococcygeal teratomas may cause tumor bleeding if extrapelvic cysts rupture during vaginal delivery (Fig. 31.8). On

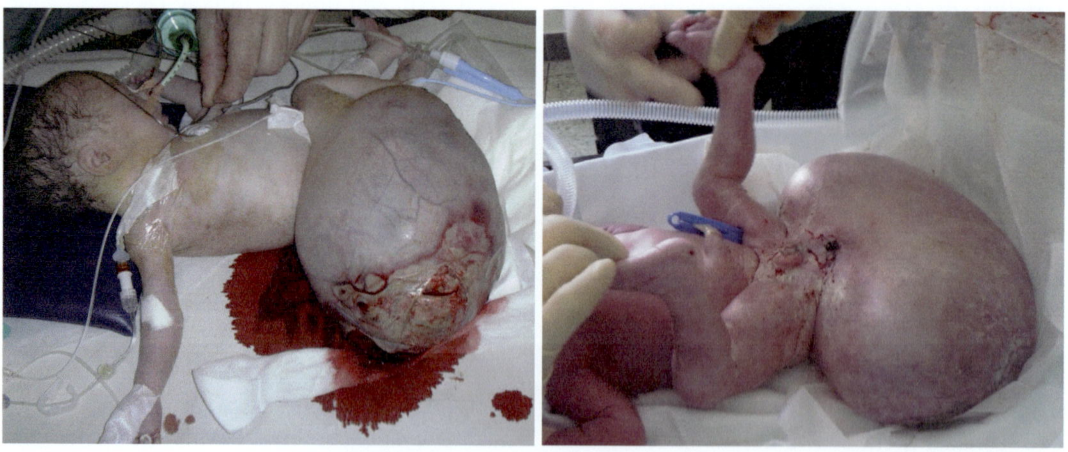

Fig. 31.8 Clinical presentation of neonatal sacrococcygeal teratomas. The tumor shown to the left is incompletely covered with skin and ruptured during delivery (cesarean section), leading to hemorrhagic shock

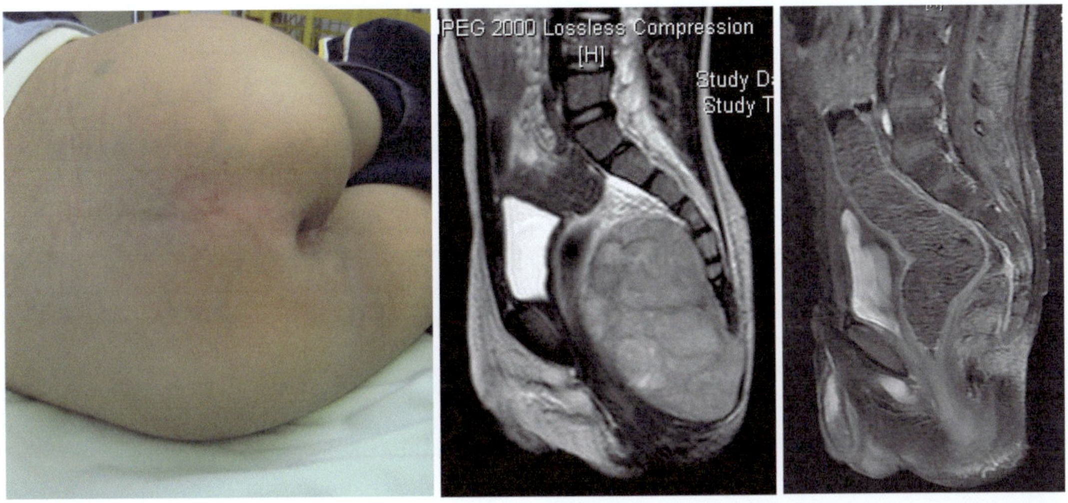

Fig. 31.9 Sacrococcygeal yolk sac tumor (Altman III/IV) in a 3-year-old boy: clinical presentation and MRI prior to (*left*) and after (*right*) chemotherapy with three cycles of cisplatin, etoposide, and etoposide

the other hand, sacrococcygeal germ cell tumors may lead to chronic obstipation if they show predominantly intrapelvic extension (Fig. 31.9). Some sacrococcygeal yolk sac tumors may lead to skeletal metastases including the vertebral columns (Fig. 31.10). Spinal invasion may then lead to acute paralysis. Vaginal yolk sac tumors may lead to vaginal bleeding.

At other sites, the diagnosis even of small tumors is also guided by local symptoms and complications. Thus, CNS germ cell tumors of the hypophyseal region frequently present with diabetes insipidus, or pineal tumors may result in symptoms resulting from increased intracranial pressure or in vertical ocular paralysis (Parinaud's syndrome) (Fig. 31.11) (Cho et al. 1998; Diez et al. 1999; Hieda and Fukui 2008). Apart from this, unspecific personality changes have also been reported. Rarely, differentiated elements within teratomas may result in endocrinological perturbances, e.g., by inadequate hormone secretion (Esik et al. 1994; Lam and Cheung 1996; Yassa et al. 2008). Lastly, due to their specific location at very sensible midline sites, CNS germ cell tumors often lead to obstructive hydrocephalus, as it is demonstrated in Fig. 31.12, showing an infant with a huge teratoma (Fig. 31.13).

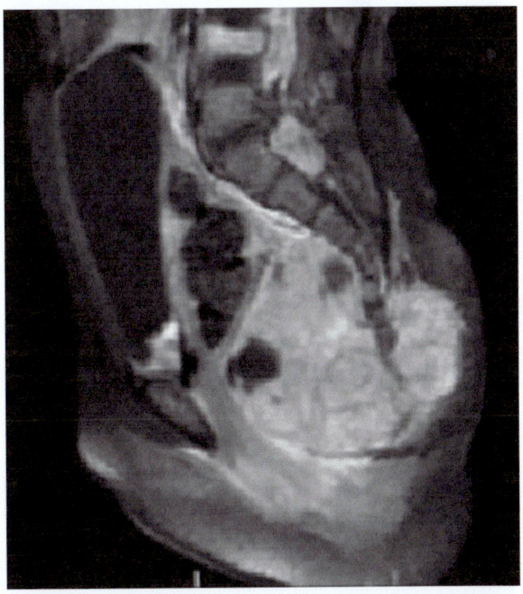

Fig. 31.10 Sacrococcygeal yolk sac tumor (Altman III) of a 2-year-old girl with bone metastasis in lumbar spine

31.2.4 Diagnostic Assessment

The diagnostic assessment is also outlined for sacrococcygeal, retroperitoneal, and central nervous system germ cell tumors in Tables 31.8, 31.9, and 31.10. The medical history and physical examinations should consider signs of congenital malformations such as anal atresia (Currarino et al. 1981) or sex-chromosomal aberrations such as Ullrich-Turner and Klinefelter's syndrome, which may be associated with specific subtypes of germ cell tumors. In each child, the pubertal status has to be documented. Both testes have to be palpated. Rarely, a retroperitoneal teratoma may interfere with testicular descensus, so that a "retroperitoneal" tumor may arise in an undescended testis (Schwabe et al. 2000).

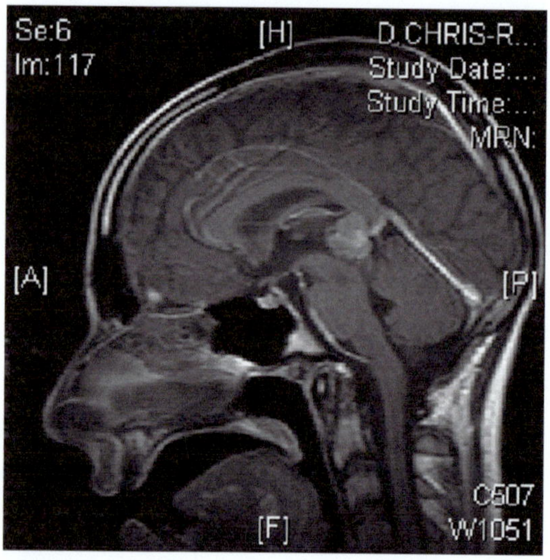

Fig. 31.11 Pineal mixed malignant germ cell tumor in a 15-year-old male

In sacrococcygeal tumors (Table 31.8), a rectal examination should be performed to palpate for intrapelvic tumor extension and to consider a potential proximity to or infiltration of the rectum. The anal sphincter tone should also be documented preoperatively, since in some rare patients, paralysis of the pelvic floor may develop following surgery. These examinations should also be performed during follow-up investigations.

The first radiographic assessment is usually made by ultrasound, which should always include the draining lymph nodes. Sonography is the most commonly applied initial imaging technique and is usually followed by magnetic resonance imaging, which should always depict the tumor in all three dimensions. For sacrococcygeal tumors, the intrapelvic anatomy, i.e., the association to the rectum, has to be carefully considered, since this may have important implications for surgical therapy. In addition, any extension into the spinal canal should be excluded

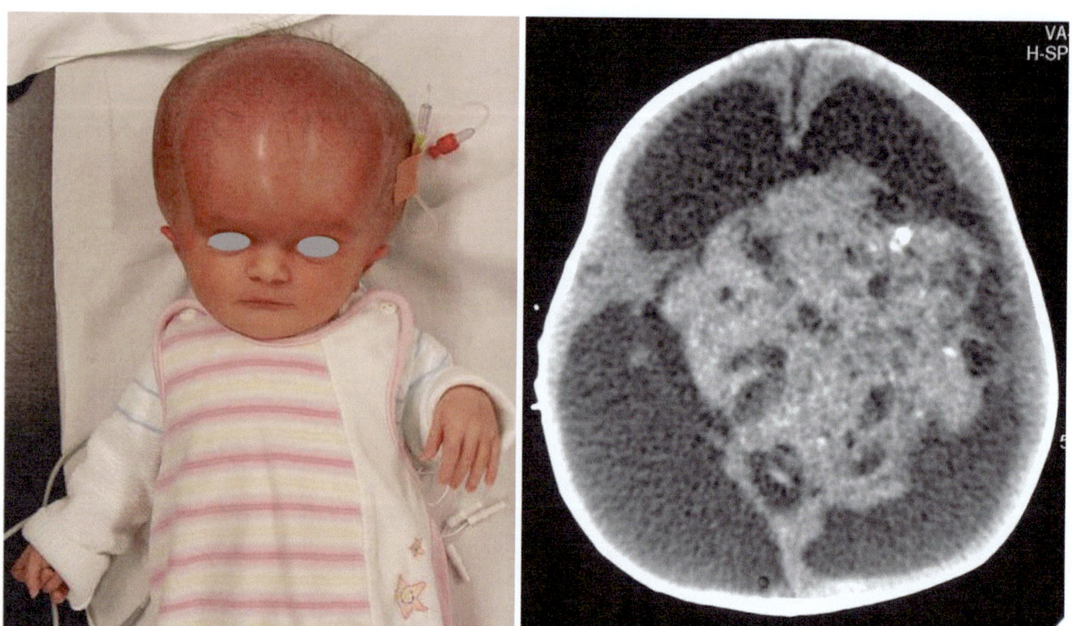

Fig. 31.12 One-month-old infant with an unresectable intracranial teratoma

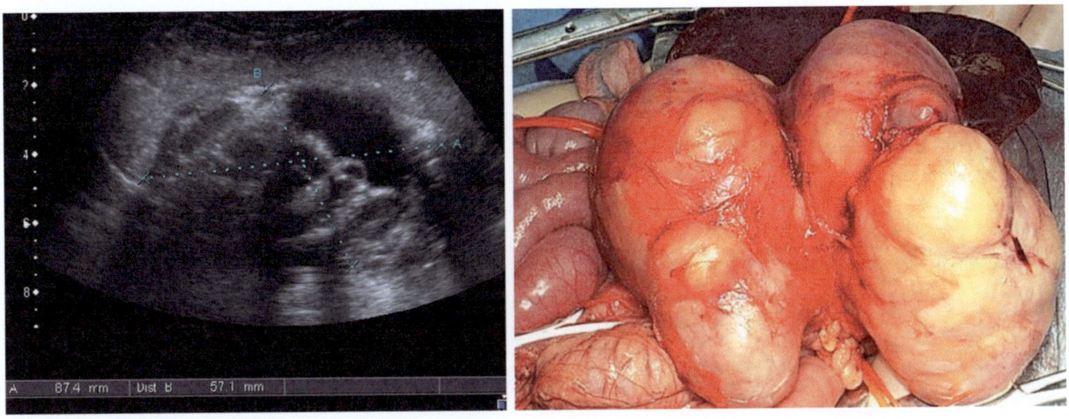

Fig. 31.13 Retroperitoneal teratoma in a 1-year-old girl: ultrasound and operative situs

Table 31.8 Specific diagnostic strategy in sacrococcygeal germ cell tumors

Procedure	Specific questions
Clinical assessment	
Medical history	Obstipation? Continence? Urinary retention? Anal atresia/malformation?
Phys. examination	Rectal examination: intrapelvic tumor component/relation to rectum. Anal sphincter tone?
Audiometry	Sensorineural hearing loss?
Laboratory assessment	
– Creatinine clearance/cystatin c	Assessment of renal function
– AFP	Malignant GCT with yolk sac tumor (consider age-related reference values)
– LDH	Unspecific marker with prognostic impact
Radiographic assessment	
Ultrasound	Tumor size and extension in 3 dimensions, anatomical relation to rectum, extension into spinal canal, lymph node, or liver metastases
Abdominal and pelvic MRI	Tumor size and extension in 3 dimensions, anatomical relation to rectum, extension into spinal canal, lymph node metastases, vertebral metastases
Chest X-ray	Lung metastases
Chest CT	Lung (micro-) metastases
Brain MRI	CNS metastases (indicated in case of pulmonary or visceral metastases and/or neurological symptoms)
Bone scan	Skeletal metastases (indicated in case of pulmonary or visceral metastases and/or bone pain)
Histologic assessment	
H&E	Classification according to WHO, in teratoma grading of immaturity according to Gonzalez-Crussi or Skullbeck
AFP	Yolk sac tumor (microfoci in teratoma)

with MRI (Jelin et al. 2009; Ribeiro et al. 1999). Rarely intrapelvic teratomas may develop as a manifestation of the Currarino triad, which describes the association of anal atresia, sacral hemiagenesis, and intrapelvic masses such as dermoid cyst or teratoma (Currarino et al. 1981).

Due to their crucial importance for the categorization of childhood germ cell tumors, the serological markers alpha$_1$-fetoprotein (AFP) and β-human chorionic gonadotropin (β-HCG) are discussed in detail in Sect. 31.1.1. Because of the wide variation in levels at birth, especially with

Table 31.9 Specific diagnostic strategy in retroperitoneal germ cell tumors

Procedure	Specific questions
Clinical assessment	
Medical history	Obstipation? Klinefelter's syndrome? Maldescensus testis? Ullrich-Turner syndrome? Gynecological anamnesis?
Phys. examination	Tumor size, pubertal status, testicular palpation
Audiometry	Sensorineural hearing loss?
Laboratory assessment	
– Creatinine clearance/cystatin c	Assessment of renal function
– AFP	Malignant GCT with yolk sac tumor (consider age-related reference values)
– β-HCG	Malignant GCT with choriocarcinoma
– LDH	Unspecific marker with prognostic impact
Radiographic assessment	
Ultrasound	Tumor size and extension in 3 dimensions, anatomical relation to the intestine, lymph node, or liver metastases
Abdominal and pelvic MRI	Tumor size and extension in 3 dimensions, anatomical relation to the intestine, lymph node metastases
Chest X-ray	Lung metastases
Chest CT	Lung (micro-) metastases
Brain MRI	CNS metastases (indicated in case of choriocarcinoma and/or pulmonary or visceral metastases and/or neurological symptoms)
Bone scan	Skeletal metastases (indicated in case of pulmonary or visceral metastases and/or bone pain)
Histologic assessment	
H&E	Classification according to WHO, in teratoma grading of immaturity according to Gonzalez-Crussi or Skullbeck
AFP	Yolk sac tumor (microfoci in teratoma)
β-HCG	Choriocarcinoma
HPLAP, OCT3/4	Seminoma
CD30	Embryonal carcinoma

infants of less than 40 weeks' gestational age, and the wide variability in $t_{1/2}$ at different ages within the first year of life, difficulties arise in interpreting decay of serum AFP as an indication of residual or recurrent germ cell tumor in infants younger than 12 months (Schneider et al. 2001f; Blohm et al. 1998).

Slightly increasing levels of serum AFP, however, are not necessarily indicative of tumor progression. Abrupt escalation in serum AFP can occur after chemotherapy-induced tumor lysis (Schneider et al. 2001f). Otherwise, the decline of AFP during chemotherapy of yolk sac tumor strongly indicates a favorable response to therapy and thus favorable prognosis (Calaminus et al. 1991). Spurious persistence of elevated serum AFP may reflect an alteration in hepatic function from such conditions as viral hepatitis (hepatitis B, hepatitis C, and human immunodeficiency virus–associated hepatitis), cholestasis secondary to anesthesia, metabolic disease (e.g., tyrosinemia type I), or exposure to phenytoin or methotrexate. Other neoplastic conditions associated with elevated serum AFP include hepatoblastoma, hepatocellular carcinoma, pancreaticoblastoma, pancreatic, gastrointestinal, and bronchial adenocarcinomas (Schneider et al. 2001f).

AFP is not only helpful in detecting significant yolk sac tumor components but may also assist in prognostic assessment. In a large cooperative analysis of adult germ cell tumors, high AFP and/or β-HCG levels indicated poor prognosis (International-Germ-Cell-Cancer-Collaborative-Group 1997). In the British childhood cancer studies, high AFP levels above 1000 μg/L were associated with unfavorable outcome (Mann et al. 1989b). In an international

Table 31.10 Specific diagnostic strategy in central nervous system germ cell tumors

Procedure	Specific questions
Clinical assessment	
Medical history	Signs of intracranial hypertension? Signs of diabetes insipidus. Pubertal development
Phys. examination	Complete neurological assessment: cerebral palsy? Parinaud's phenomenon? Klinefelter's syndrome? Pubertal status? Testicular palpation
Ophthalmology including perimetry	Intracranial hypertension? Hemianopsia?
Audiometry	Sensorineural hearing loss?
Phys. examination	Complete neurological assessment: cerebral palsy? Parinaud's phenomenon? Klinefelter's syndrome? Pubertal status? Testicular palpation
Laboratory assessment	
– Serum and urine osmolarity	Diabetes insipidus
– Serum sodium	Diabetes insipidus
– Creatinine clearance	Assessment of renal function
– AFP (serum + CSF)	Malignant GCT with yolk sac tumor (cutoff 25 μg/L)
– β-HCG (serum + CSF)	Malignant GCT with choriocarcinoma (cutoff 50 U/μL)
– HPLAP	Malignant GCT with germinoma
– LDH	Unspecific marker with prognostic impact
– CSF cytology	Detection of (micro-) metastatic spread
Radiographic assessment	
Brain MRI	Tumor extension, uni- or bifocal disease, ventricular or brain metastases
Spinal MRI	Spinal metastases
Chest X-ray	Lung metastases
Abdominal ultrasound	Liver metastases, exclusion of renal disease
Bone scan	Skeletal metastases (indicated in case of pulmonary or visceral metastases and/or bone pain)
Histologic assessment	
H&E	Classification according to WHO
AFP	Yolk sac tumor (microfoci in teratoma)

meta-analysis, the prognostic cutoff was reported at 10,000/μL (Frazier et al. 2015). Furthermore, an inadequate decline of AFP that does not follow its half time of 5–7 days indicates pure response to chemo or tumor progression after tumor resection (Calaminus et al. 1991).

The most frequent cause of significant rise of β-HCG is pregnancy. Therefore, in case of suspected germ cell tumor and elevated β-HCG, pregnancy must be excluded with other techniques, e.g., ultrasound. Elevation of serum β-HCG in patients with germ cell tumors implies the presence of clones of syncytiotrophoblasts, such as choriocarcinoma, or of syncytiotrophoblastic giant cells, found frequently in germinomas (pure seminomas or dysgerminomas) and occasionally in adult embryonal carcinoma. Immunoperoxidase staining of tumor for β-HCG detects these hormone-containing elements.

31.2.5 Staging of Extracranial Extragonadal Germ Cell Tumors

Pure teratomas of childhood do not metastasize. However, since they may include microscopic foci of malignant yolk sac tumor, the draining lymph nodes should be examined with ultrasound or MRI, and an initial chest X-ray can be performed in order to document absence of metastases. It should be noted that teratomatous tumors arising after puberty may sometimes be associated with metastatic spread. Thus, clinical staging with ultrasound, MRI, and chest X-ray is certainly justified. If absence of metastases is documented, the follow-up of childhood teratomas should primarily focus on the primary tumor site, since relapses most commonly develop locally.

Malignant yolk sac tumors of childhood show a tendency to metastasize into the locoregional lymph nodes and into the lungs, justifying a limited staging assessment focusing on these sites. Currently, there is no prospectively proven evidence as to whether pulmonary micrometastases detected with CT scans of the lungs are therapeutically and prognostically relevant. In fact, pulmonary metastases of childhood yolk sac tumor commonly show a favorable response to platin-based chemotherapy and rarely require surgical treatment. However, germ cell tumors with pulmonary micrometastases are certainly eligible to intensive chemotherapy with four cycles of chemotherapy so that CT scans are commonly used and currently recommended in order to increase the accuracy of clinical staging.

Rarely, metastases at other sites such as the liver, the bones, or the CNS are noted. However, these metastases almost never present in the absence of lung metastases or site-specific symptoms such as bone pain (Calaminus et al. 2003). Therefore, clinical staging should be expanded to bone scan and MRI of the brain if lung metastases are diagnosed or if specific symptoms such as bone pain are reported. In fact, the highest risk of CNS metastases was observed in mediastinal malignant germ cell tumors with other extracranial metastases (Göbel et al. 2013a, b).

The use of PET scan for staging of childhood germ cell tumors is still awaiting evaluation in clinical trials. Currently, it cannot be considered routine. In fact, PET scan may misinterpret teratomatous components in mixed malignant germ cell tumors and may also be unable to distinguish necrosis from residual teratoma in postchemotherapeutic masses.

31.2.6 Clinical Staging Systems for Extracranial Extragonadal Germ Cell Tumors

Different staging systems are used for extragonadal malignant germ cell tumors, which all have several advantages and disadvantages. The main problem is that extragonadal germ cell tumors may arise at different anatomical sizes, which of course cannot be considered in a general staging system. Therefore, the currently applied staging systems reflect general characteristics such as infiltration into neighboring organs and metastatic spread into the lymph nodes or the lungs or other visceral organs. The German MAKEI group is currently applying a modified TNM staging system for soft tissue sarcomas, according to which tumor size (<5 cm vs. >5 cm diameter) and local infiltration are considered for T-staging. Lymph node and distant metastases are counted separately as either negative or positive (Table 31.11). For therapy stratification, the completeness of resection is considered as a separate variable.

In contrast, the staging system according to the US COG also integrates information on resection status as well as the initial surgical procedure. Thus, all patients who undergo a biopsy prior to the start of chemotherapy are considered stage III (Table 31.12). A main advantage of this

Table 31.11 Staging system for extragonadal germ cell tumors adapted from the TNM staging system for soft tissue sarcomas

Category		Parameters	
Local stage			
T	1a	No infiltration of neighboring organs	<5 cm
	1b		>5 cm
	2a	Infiltration of neighboring organs	<5 cm
	2b		>5 cm
N	0	No lymphatic metastases	
	1	Lymphatic metastases	
M	0	No distant metastases	
	1	Distant metastases	

Table 31.12 US COG staging system for gonadal and extragonadal germ cell tumors

Children's Oncology Group staging of extragonadal germ cell tumors	
I	Complete resection at any site, coccygectomy for sacrococcygeal site, negative tumor margins. No evidence of metastases. Appropriate marker decline
II	Microscopic residual; lymph nodes negative
III	Gross residual disease or biopsy only; lymph node involvement with metastatic disease; retroperitoneal nodes positive or negative
IV	Metastatic disease including liver

staging system is that it is similarly applied to gonadal germ cell tumors, facilitating comparison of prognostic and therapeutic data regardless of site. However in contrast to the TNM system, biopsy procedures will always upstage tumors to stage III, irrespective of anatomical stage.

31.2.7 Germ Cell Tumors of the Central Nervous System

Since CNS germ cell tumors are described extensively in this series' book on CNS tumors, only a brief description of the general diagnostic and therapeutic strategies is provided in this chapter.

Primary intracranial germ cell tumors primarily develop during adolescence and young adulthood. They may be located in the pineal gland (62%) or suprasellar region (31%), or they may span both areas (7%) (Balmaceda and Finlay 2004; Bamberg et al. 1999; Calaminus et al. 2005). Symptomatology depends on site, growth pattern, and histology of the tumor and may include personality changes, visual disturbances, diabetes insipidus, hypopituitarism, Parinaud's syndrome (convergence nystagmus), anorexia, and precocious puberty. Histologically, two thirds of the tumors are germinomas, and the rest are nongerminomatous, some mixed with yolk sac tumor, choriocarcinoma, or teratocarcinoma.

The clinical assessment of central nervous system germ cell tumors is outlined in Table 31.10. Since hypophyseal germ cell tumors may induce diabetes insipidus, specific attention should be paid to the serum electrolytes as well as serum and urine osmolarity. The presence of diabetes insipidus would have significant impact on infusion therapy during chemotherapy, since severe electrolyte imbalances may develop during intensive infusion therapy required during platin chemotherapy (Bryant et al. 1994).

It is important to note that CNS germ cell tumors show a marked tendency to metastasize through the cerebrospinal fluid. Thus, metastases within the ventricular system as well as drop metastases to the spine may occur (Alapetite et al. 2002, 2010; Calaminus et al. 2002). Extracranial spread to lung and bones has also been reported, however very rarely. Considering their tendency to spread within the cerebrospinal fluid, cytological evaluation after lumbar tap or of cerebrospinal fluid collected during surgery is absolutely mandatory for initial staging. If cytological examination is not performed perioperatively, tumors should be considered potentially metastatic, with a significant impact on local treatment, i.e., radiotherapy (Calaminus et al. 1997a).

There is no specific staging system for central nervous system germ cell tumors. Thus, they are staged in analogy to other CNS tumors such as medulloblastoma (Chang et al. 1969). Mainly, the presence of tumor cells in the cerebrospinal fluid as well as metastases to different sites of the CNS is considered. Local radiotherapy is planned according to this initial staging, with inclusion of craniospinal irradiation in micrometastases and an additional boost to any visible metastases apparent on MRI.

AFP and β-HCG should be measured both in the serum and the cerebrospinal fluid, because they indicate secreting malignant nonseminomatous germ cell tumors. Of note, discrepant levels between serum and cerebrospinal fluid may be detected in some patients. There is considerable debate regarding the appropriate cut-off levels for AFP and β-HCG, since in some rare patients histologically pure germinoma may be associated with significant β-HCG secretion. However, in the current international SIOP study on CNS germ cell tumors, cutoff levels of AFP, 25 μg/L, and β-HCG, 50 IU/μL, have been defined (Calaminus et al. 1994, 2002, 2005). Tumors associated with higher levels either in the serum or the cerebrospinal fluid are considered secreting tumors and selected for more intensive chemotherapy with cisplatin instead of carboplatin and higher irradiation doses (Calaminus et al. 2017). Of note, these tumor markers also assist in establishing a clinical diagnosis in that a significant elevation is considered sufficient for the clinical diagnosis of a malignant germ cell tumor even without biopsy. Lastly, high AFP levels above 1000 µg/L may be used for therapy stratification in the current SIOP protocol.

31.2.8 Treatment Overview

For all extragonadal germ cell tumors, an individualized multimodal treatment plan has to be chosen that takes histology, the site of origin, and stage into account. The treatment of teratoma is surgical; apart from single-case reports (Garre et al. 1996), there is no evidence of significant therapeutic effects of chemotherapy in pure teratomas (Göbel et al. 1997a, b, 1998a; Marina et al. 1999b). In malignant germ cell tumors, surgical resection is also of vital importance for successful treatment, since extragonadal germ cell tumors show a high tendency to relapse at the site of origin. Therefore, complete resection constitutes the mainstay of treatment (Göbel et al. 2001a, b; Schneider et al. 2000b). In rare, circumscribed, and nonmetastatic malignant germ cell tumors, patients may not require additional chemotherapy following complete surgical resection. However, in most extragonadal germ cell tumors, chemotherapy is indicated to consolidate remission after initial resection. Alternatively, up-front chemotherapy may be applied to facilitate complete resection on delayed surgery. Radiotherapy is rarely applied in extragonadal germ cell tumors. In contrast, it is commonly applied in central nervous system germ cell tumors, in which it may partly replace surgical resection as a measure to achieve local tumor control (Bamberg et al. 1999; Calaminus et al. 2005, 2013, 2017).

Chemotherapy is given according to the regimens also administered for gonadal germ cell tumors (see Table 31.4 in Sect. 31.1.1).

31.2.9 Principles of Surgery of Extragonadal Extracranial Germ Cell Tumors

Surgical resection is the therapy of choice in benign tumors, such as teratomas. With malignant lesions, removal is indicated, if possible. However, given the availability of effective chemotherapy, resection should not be undertaken to the point of sacrificing vital structures. In this situation, biopsy may be appropriate. Biopsy will not only support, confirm, and specify clinical diagnosis but also opens perspectives for genetic analysis and molecular research.

It must be emphasized that surgical recommendations may differ significantly for children and adolescents. After initial chemotherapy, second-look surgery serves to assist in achieving complete response in selected patients. Specific surgical strategies for specific extragonadal germ cell tumors of the mediastinum and the head and neck region are described in Chap. 19 and below for sacrococcygeal germ cell tumors.

31.2.10 Principles of Chemotherapy for Extragonadal Germ Cell Tumors

Substantial improvements in the cure rates for pediatric germ cell tumors have occurred, stemming in large part from the evolution of effective chemotherapeutic strategies, most developed for the larger adult population with these neoplasms. Most pediatric germ cell tumor trials are limited by the small numbers of tumors at each site of origin with specific histology and stage.

Most chemotherapeutic studies have been conducted in patients with testicular and extragonadal tumors, primarily with advanced or disseminated disease. These data indicated that extragonadal germ cell tumors show a similar response to cisplatin-based combination chemotherapy as gonadal germ cell tumors do (Mann et al. 2000a; Göbel et al. 2000a, b). However, mediastinal germ cell tumors constitute the largest subgroup of extragonadal germ cell tumors in adults, and they commonly have an unfavorable prognosis (Ganjoo et al. 2000). Therefore, strategies for chemotherapy intensification have been proposed that incorporate dose-escalated chemotherapy as well as high-dose chemotherapy with autologous stem cell transplantation (Bokemeyer et al. 2003; Schmoll et al. 2003a, b).

Pediatric studies have mirrored the adult experience. Combination chemotherapy has been found to be superior to single or dual agents, and the addition of cisplatin has increased the efficacy of these regimens (Billmire et al. 2003; Billmire et al. 2004a; Cushing et al. 2004b; Rogers et al. 2004b; Lopes et al. 2008, 2009; Göbel et al. 2000a, b). In the intergroup study conducted by the Pediatric Oncology Group (POG) and the Children's Cancer Group (CCG), PEB, as standard treatment, was compared to a combination of high-dose cisplatin plus etoposide and bleomycin (Cushing et al. 2004b). This regimen did differ from adult PEB treatments because bleomycin was not administered weekly. Patients with localized gonadal germ cell tumors were treated with standard PEB. All other gonadal and all extragonadal germ cell tumors were randomized to standard PEB or a regimen with high-dose cisplatin (200 mg/m^2). Although tumor control was better in high-risk patients who received high-dose cisplatin, significant toxicity appeared to limit its use.

Studies conducted by the United Kingdom Children's Cancer Study Group suggest the superiority of carboplatin over standard-dose cisplatin in reducing permanent toxicity. Comparison was not made, however, to high-dose cisplatin (Mann et al. 1998; Mann et al. 2000a).

The Brazilian pediatric germ cell tumor group applied a response-based strategy. Bleomycin was omitted for both intermediate- and high-risk patients (Lopes et al. 2008, 2009). Cisplatin, at 30 mg/m^2/day for 5 days, was administered to high-risk patients. After three cycles patients from both risk categories, who did not achieve CR, were switched to ifosfamide, vinblastine, and bleomycin. Though the study was limited by small sample size, some patients were treated successfully without bleomycin. In addition, a rationale for response-based treatment was suggested (Lopes et al. 2009). Marrow-ablative doses of carboplatin and etoposide followed by autologous marrow reinfusion may provide a method of salvaging patients who experience relapse or whose disease proves refractory to treatment.

The French group has utilized both carboplatin- and cisplatin-based regimen. In the late 1980s and 1990s, carboplatin-based regimen have been applied, with doses of carboplatin at 400 mg/m^2/cycle (Baranzelli et al. 1999b, 2000a), which is considerably lower than in the British studies. In this study, inferior response rates have been reported, in particular, for extragonadal germ cell tumors (Baranzelli et al. 1999b). However, patients could be salvaged with second-line cisplatin-based regimen. In the current studies, a combination of cisplatin, etoposide, and ifosfamide is applied, using a response-based strategy. Thus, patients receive two additional cycles after complete response, summing up to a median of three cycles in intermediate-risk patients and five cycles in high-risk patients.

In the German MAKEI protocols, therapy is stratified according to site, stage, and completeness of tumor resection (Göbel et al. 1999, 2000a, b). In locally advanced and metastatic tumors, up-front chemotherapy after clinical diagnosis based on markers or biopsy is strongly advocated. In completely resected, low-stage tumors, a watch-and-wait strategy is chosen, or patients are treated with two to three cycles of a two-agent regimen including cisplatin and etoposide. In all other tumors, cisplatin and etoposide are combined with ifosfamide. In previous studies, bleomycin has substituted for ifosfamide. However, after two lethal pulmonary toxicities occurred in young infants, ifosfamide was chosen but is withheld in young toddlers (Göbel et al. 2000a, b). Up to four cycles of PEI are administered to high-risk patients. For patients with unresectable tumors that respond inadequately to up-front chemotherapy or relapse, a local therapy intensification with locoregional hyperthermia and thermochemotherapy is recommended (Wessalowski et al. 2003b, 2013).

One difficulty of establishing clear recommendations for treatment of pediatric germ cell tumors is the inability to define risk groups. Most trials are small and have been conducted by individual national groups. Most pediatric trials combine different sites of origin, staging, and histology to the same stratum for therapy to achieve adequate statistical power. In contrast, for adult germ cell tumors, a large international meta-analysis has led to the introduction of a risk categorization that is currently used for the development and comparison of therapeutic trials (International-Germ-Cell-Cancer-Collaborative--Group 1997). A recent analysis of the US Children's Oncology Group has shown that this prognostic staging system, when adopted to a pediatric cohort, leads to a different stratification (Frazier et al. 2008). This is mainly explained by the different biology of germ cell tumors, in particular, during early childhood. Thus, the impact of high AFP levels has to be evaluated critically and under the consideration of yolk sac tumor being the only malignant histology in childhood.

Based on this consideration, an international attempt with a combined analysis of the US and British study registries has been taken to develop a new prognostic stratification system (Frazier et al. 2015). This analysis shows that a highly unfavorable risk group is defined for extragonadal, in particular, mediastinal and metastatic germ cell tumors in adolescents. In fact, age emerges as a prognostic factor for extragonadal germ cell tumors. In line with the previous report from the German MAKEI study and the molecular genetic study (Schneider et al. 2002b; Frazier et al. 2015). Thus, mediastinal nonseminomatous germ cell tumors of adolescents older than 10 years of age are prognostically unfavorable, whereas the corresponding tumors in young infants are not (Hale et al. 2010).

Specific recommendations for incorporating chemotherapy into the management of pediatric extragonadal germ cell tumors are discussed separately for each tumor. The dosages and methods of administration of current regimens employed in pediatric germ cell tumors [cisplatin, vinblastine, and bleomycin (PVB); cisplatin, etoposide, and bleomycin (PEB); and carboplatin, etoposide, and bleomycin (JEB)] are shown in Table 31.4 in Sect. 31.1.1.

It should be noted that complete initial resection with wide margins is rarely achieved in malignant extragonadal germ cell tumors. Therefore, apart from teratoma, only rare extragonadal malignant tumors are eligible for a watch-and-wait strategy. Patients with moderate-risk gonadal tumors or progression of disease in untreated tumors may be managed adequately with three to four cycles of a platinum-containing regimen. For higher-risk patients (higher-stage extragonadal tumors), four (to six) cycles of a platinum-based or dose-intensified chemotherapeutic regimen is indicated, and currently the evaluation of an accelerated cisplatin-based strategy is under evaluation (Lawrence et al. 2018).

31.2.11 Treatment of Sacrococcygeal Germ Cell Tumors

31.2.11.1 Sacrococcygeal Tumors

Sacrococcygeal germ cell tumors constitute the most frequent germ cell tumors during childhood and adolescence. In fact, sacrococcygeal teratoma is the overall most frequent neonatal tumor. The risk of malignancy increases with age. The surgical approach strongly depends on the anatomical site according to the Altman classification (Altman et al. 1974a). This classification categorizes tumors with regard to the extrapelvic (dorsal to the coccyx) and intrapelvic extension of the tumor. It is hypothesized that malignant tumors show a higher tendency to grow inside the pelvis. Although this classification is not consistently used, the basic consideration to evaluate preoperatively for intra- and extrapelvic tumor extension has a significant impact on surgical access and strategy.

31.2.11.2 Resection of Neonatal Sacrococcygeal Teratomas

Most neonatal teratomas, both immature and mature, present as large exophytic tumors that may be as large as the rest of the neonate. Moreover, during pregnancy large and fast growing tumors can cause cardiac failure, fetal hydrops, and intrauterine death. Attempts of minimally invasive fetal therapy have been described (Van Mieghem et al. 2014). If the tumor is diagnosed with prenatal ultrasound, the child should not be delivered through vaginal delivery, since tumor rupture and severe hemorrhage may develop (Fig. 31.8). If the tumor is intact, there is no need for immediate resection, and preoperative imaging can be completed.

If the tumor has ruptured, then a pressure bandage may diminish the blood loss for a limited period of time. Prior to surgical resection, the degree of abdominal extension should be accurately evaluated if possible with US and MRI, to plan the approach.

The patient is usually positioned in the prone position, with a roll under the hips. Surgical principles that lead to a complete removal include a posterior approach with an inverted V shape to allow for excision of the tumor and to facilitate an eventually satisfactory cosmetic closure. This approach affords the surgeon excellent exposure for most neonatal sacrococcygeal germ cell tumors and may obviate the need for intra-abdominal exposures. The incision should be placed as to preserve as much normal skin as possible: Excess skin can always be trimmed later if necessary.

Immature lesions are more vascular with significantly greater blood loss during surgery, and it is often necessary to perform blood transfusions (Altman et al. 1974a). The tumor is dissected from gluteus muscles, the coccyx is dissected at the sacrococcygeal joint, and the middle sacral vessels are controlled to minimize intraoperative hemorrhage. Failure to resect the complete coccyx is associated with increased risk of local recurrence (Göbel et al. 1997a, b, 1998a).

The presacral extent of the tumor can compress the perineal structures forward; since the tumor may be adherent to the rectum, sharp dissection can be directed by placing a finger or a Hegar dilator in the rectum. The mass should be mobilized close to its pseudocapsule and removed, without spillage, en bloc with the coccyx. Then the anorectal and the retrorectal muscles are reconstructed. Closed suction drainage is adopted to evacuate fluid, and the wound is closed in layers.

If the tumor extends deeply through the bony pelvis into the retroperitoneum, an abdominal approach allows the mobilization of the mass and the control of the sacral artery. In some patients, a combined posterior and abdominal approach has to be chosen.

The tumor is eventually removed from the perineum. Hemorrhagic mortality of neonates with sacrococcygeal teratoma is relatively high (3.8%) representing almost 70% of the overall mortality in the neonatal period. If the tumor has been ruptured or if a bleeding is possible, primary abdominal exploration is required to control the aorta and the arterial blood supply of the tumor before resection (Angel et al. 1998). The aim is to find and ligate the middle sacral vessels; if this is not possible, an occlusive sling is placed across the aorta below the origin of the inferior mesenteric artery (Lindahl 1988). The ligation of the median sacral artery before posterior resection has been described also using a laparoscopic approach. Alternatively, preoperative successful embolization of the middle sacral and other feeding arteries with angiographic procedure has been reported (Rossi et al. 2013).

Intraoperative hemorrhage and postoperative wound infections constitute the most frequent complications of excision of sacrococcygeal teratoma. The major cause of mortality is hemorrhagic shock, since an unsuspected teratoma may rupture during delivery. Neonatal teratomas need accurate clinical follow-up since local recurrences are observed in 4–20% of cases, in particular, if the coccyx is not removed. Of note, 50% of relapses are malignant (Fig. 31.14) (Göbel et al. 1998a). The infant should be followed up with visits (including rectal examination), ultrasound, and AFP at 3-month intervals for at least 3 years and then annually. Recurrences rarely develop after the age of 2 years. The development of a malignant recurrence may be the result of an incomplete resection or a pathologic sampling error.

In a study from the UK, the 5-year event-free survival for both mature and immature sacrococcygeal teratomas was approximately 75% (Mann

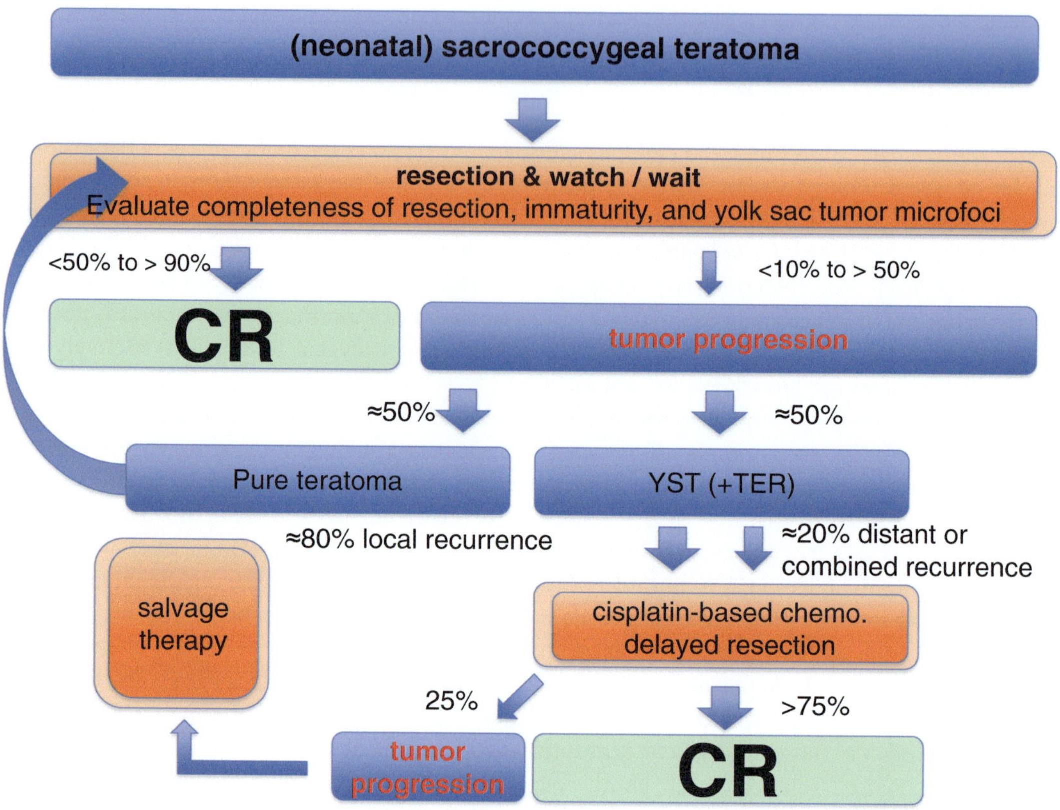

Fig. 31.14 Therapeutic algorithm in sacrococcygeal teratomas

et al. 2008a). Accordingly, the recurrence rate was 23% in 132 patients reported to the German MAKEI studies. Of note, the risk of malignant relapse with yolk sac tumor was minimized when postoperative chemotherapy was administered to patients with incomplete initial resection. However, the overall relapse rate was not reduced by chemotherapy (Göbel et al. 1998a). In a study from Italy, the 5-year event-free survival for both mature and immature sacrococcygeal teratomas was 88.9%, treated with surgery only (Terenziani et al. 2015). Cautious monitoring of such patients is required, because malignant germ cell tumors are well recognized to recur either from unnoticed malignant elements in the original tumor or from malignant transformation in residual tissue. Until recently, only a 10% salvage rate for malignant lesions was expected. In a study from Italy, the 5-year event-free survival for both mature and immature sacrococcygeal teratomas was 88.9%, treated with surgery only (Terenziani et al. 2015).

31.2.11.3 Resection of Malignant Sacrococcygeal Germ Cell Tumors in Toddlers

At the sacrococcygeal region, the risk of malignant germ cell tumor increases with age. However, even in neonates, malignant components may be detected histologically, the so-called yolk sac tumor microfoci (Harms and Jänig 1986). Therefore, accurate preoperative evaluation of the tumor markers and radiographic staging are necessary. Nevertheless, in case of complete resection, the risk of recurrence is not elevated even in the presence of malignant yolk sac tumor microfoci; in fact, also sacrococcygeal mixed malignant germ cell tumors stages I–II could potentially be treated with surgery alone

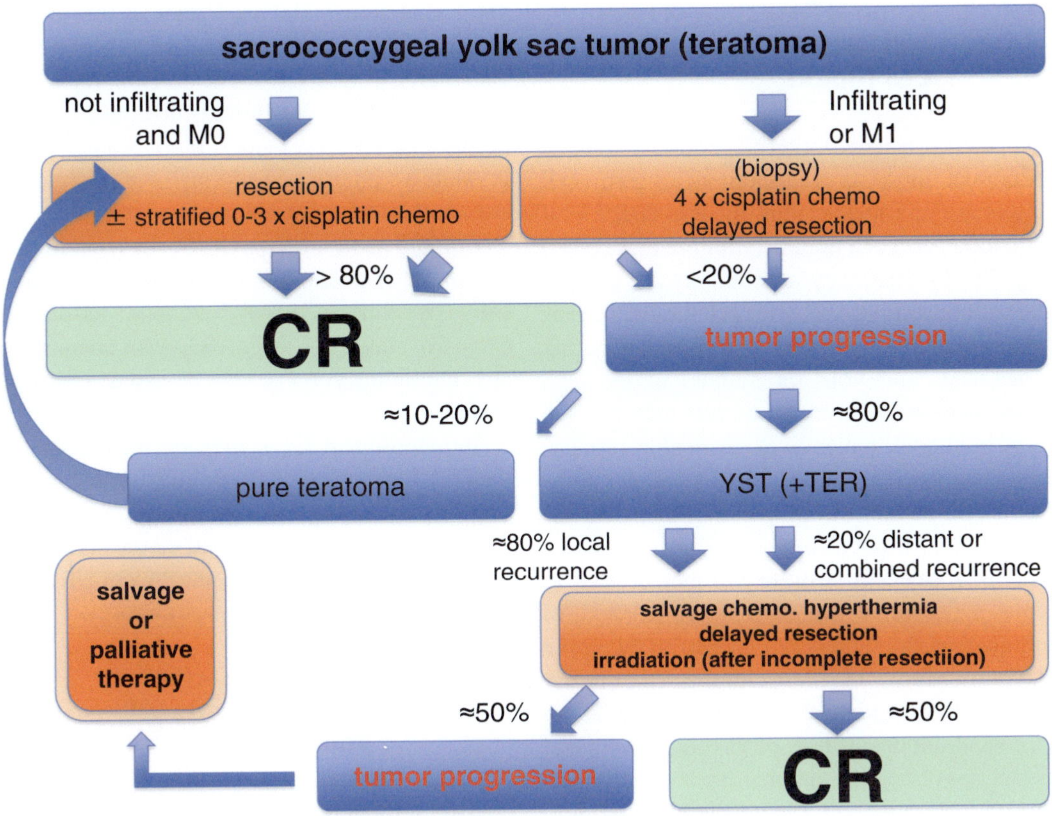

Fig. 31.15 Therapeutic algorithm in malignant sacrococcygeal yolk sac tumors

(Göbel et al. 1998a, b, c, d; Egler et al. 2017). The strategy for postoperative follow-up or adjuvant treatment and estimated prognosis is illustrated in Fig. 31.15.

Tumors are frequently non-capsulated and may develop in close proximity to the rectum. When invasion of the pelvic structures and/or extension into the spine are found or uncertain, the mass should be considered unresectable, and a primary excision is discouraged. In these patients, an initial biopsy followed by neoadjuvant chemotherapy is the best choice (Göbel et al. 2000a, b). Tumor shrinkage from platinum-based chemotherapy is highly successful and increases the achievement of complete resection with negative margins (Göbel et al. 2001a, b).

Primary or delayed excision can be performed with posterior or combined (abdominal plus posterior) approach, depending on the site and extension of the tumor [according to Altman classification (Altman et al. 1974a)], and the surgical principles are the same, adopted for neonatal germ cell tumors, taking into consideration the crucial importance of a microscopically complete resection in patients with malignant lesions. The mass is removed with the coccyx, and multiple biopsies on the tumor bed should be performed to verify the completeness of the excision. Biopsy of suspected regional nodes (pelvic or inguinal) is recommended. If no residual disease is visible at imaging after neoadjuvant chemotherapy, coccygectomy is still required.

Surgery for extragonadal malignant germ cell tumors may be difficult due to the invasiveness of the tumor and the involvement of pelvic structures. Temporary colostomies may be required if rectal damages are caused during the resection. Neuropathic bladder or bowel disorders are reported in up to 30% of cases after major procedures (Rescorla 2008; Shalaby et al. 2014).

31.2.12 Surgical Resection of Intra- and Retroperitoneal Germ Cell Tumors

Compared to sacrococcygeal germ cell tumors, abdominal intra- or retroperitoneal germ cell tumors are rare and account for less than 5% of childhood germ cell tumors (Billmire et al. 2003) (Fig. 31.16). Histology and biology are comparable to other childhood germ cell tumors such as mediastinal tumors, with teratoma predominating in neonates and yolk sac tumors in toddlers. Mixed malignant germ cell tumors are observed in postpubertal patients. A testicular primary should always be excluded by clinical and ultrasound examination. In prepubertal patients, testicular biopsy is not recommended. However, it is often performed in postpubertal patients and in adults. Differential diagnosis is problematic, in particular, if the tumors are located in the upper retroperitoneum. In these tumors, the tumor marker AFP is equivocal, since other upper retroperitoneal tumors such as pancreatic tumors and metastases of hepatic tumors may also be associated with elevated AFP (Schneider et al. 2001e).

As for germ cell tumors arising at other sites, retroperitoneal germ cell tumors should also be resected in one piece and without spillage. In order to facilitate complete resection, a median laparotomy is chosen based on the anatomical situation of the tumor, alternatively a large transverse laparatomy. Benign teratomas are usually well capsulated and not attached to retroperitoneal organs (Fig. 31.13). The excision represents the only therapy, and usually it is not difficult because they have a modest blood supply which is simply interrupted during the dissection. Adjacent lymph node should be sampled.

For large and invasive GCTs, the most important initial step is to establish the diagnosis clinically or with a biopsy, without performing extensive surgery. After neoadjuvant chemotherapy, mutilating surgery may be avoided in most cases.

Intraperitoneal GCT may be located in the liver or attached to the stomach or omentum. Gastric teratomas require the removal of a part of the gastric wall, which depend on the size of the tumor and the depth of the attachment (Billmire et al. 2003).

31.2.12.1 Surgical Resection of Vaginal Germ Cell Tumors

Although vaginal germ cell tumors are extraordinarily rare, they constitute a specific subgroup that is characterized by its limitation to yolk sac tumor histology in the absence of teratoma (Mauz-Körholz et al. 2000a, b; Lopes et al. 1999). Moreover, these tumors show a low incidence of metastases. In the pre-platinum era, these tumors have been considered

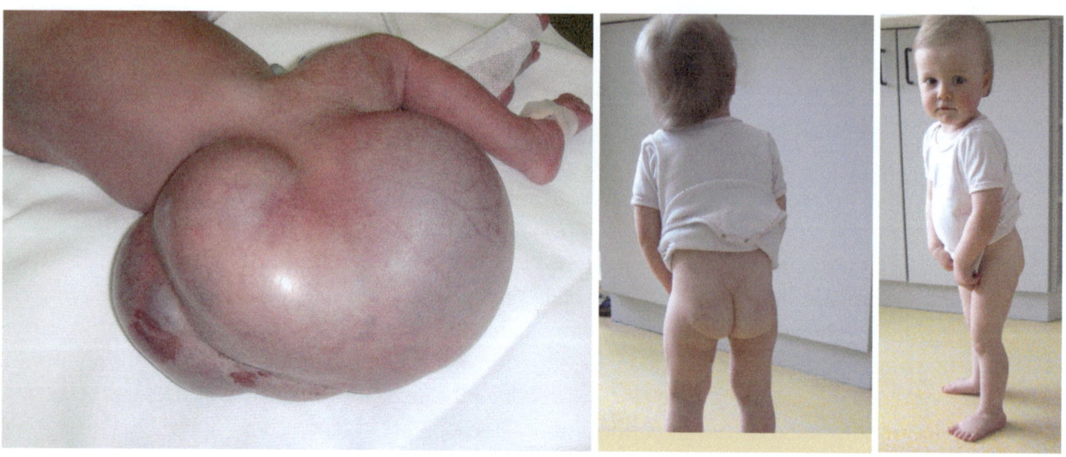

Fig. 31.16 Clinical presentation of a neonatal sacrococcygeal teratoma in a preterm girl delivered in the 32th week of pregnancy. The girl has become continent for both urine and stool at the age of 2 years

prognostically unfavorable, and extensive surgical resection including hysterectomy has been advocated. With the development of intensive platin-based combination chemotherapy, prognosis has dramatically improved. In fact, vaginal yolk sac tumors belong to the most curable subtypes of childhood germ cell tumors with a low relapse rate and excellent overall survival (Mauz-Körholz et al. 2000b). The prerequisite of this success has been the implementation of up-front chemotherapy, which usually induces excellent tumor response, thus allowing for only limited resection on delayed surgery.

In most patients, enucleation of the pretreated tumor, often in combination with partial vaginectomy, is performed. In contrast to sacrococcygeal germ cell tumors, in which microscopically incomplete resection is associated with a high rate of local recurrences, microscopic residues obviously do not bear a dismal prognostic impact in vaginal yolk sac tumors.

Lastly, germ cell tumors may also rarely arise at other urogenital sites such as the penis or the prostate. In these tumors, complete surgical resection is considered a prerequisite of cure. In order to avoid mutilating surgery, a preoperative chemotherapy is recommended after initial diagnostic biopsy. The surgical strategy follows the general guidelines for oncologic surgery at the specific site.

31.2.12.2 Germ Cell Tumors of the Central Nervous System

Since CNS germ cell tumors are described extensively in this series' book on CNS tumors, only a brief description of the general therapeutic strategies is provided in this chapter.

As CNS germ cell tumors may develop at different, mostly midline sites, they may pose a significant challenge to the neurosurgeon (Figs. 31.11 and 31.12). In fact, large neonatal midline teratomas may be completely inassessable to treatment (Fig. 31.12). On the other hand, malignant germ cell tumors show a favorable response to chemotherapy and radiotherapy, in particular, in case of germinoma. Therefore, an initial surgical procedure should not be performed at the risk of provoking neurological damage or of sacrificing structures of vital importance such as vessels (Nicholson et al. 2002). Moreover, venous plexus may be in close neighborhood to, e.g., larger pineal tumors, so that surgery may be complicated by hemorrhage. Lastly, surgical resection of hypophyseal tumors will lead to hypophyseal insufficiency with a lifelong need of hormone replacement.

In addition, it should always be considered in brain tumors that secreting germ cell tumors may easily be diagnosed based on serum and CSF tumor markers AFP and β-HCG. In patients with unequivocally elevated tumor markers, the clinical diagnosis may be established on markers and imaging even without surgical procedure and histologic confirmation. As a consequence, only a subset with marker of negative tumors requires histologic confirmation. The neurosurgical resection should be limited to initial (stereotactic, endoscopic, or open) biopsy. In patients with significant intracranial hypertension, biopsy may be combined with insertion of a ventricular-peritoneal drainage, or ventricular drainage can ideally be combined with biopsy during endoscopic surgery. There is no convincing evidence that aggressive surgical resection at diagnoses improves patients' oncologic prognosis, but there is considerably a concern that it may be associated with significant sequelae. Thus, many patients can be spared major brain surgery and can be cured with chemo- and/or radiotherapy.

The adjuvant chemo- and radiotherapy treatment heavily depends on histology and stage. Evidence of secreting tumor (AFP 25 μg/L and β-HCG 50 IU/μL) will lead to more intensive chemotherapy and higher radiotherapy doses. Evidence of (micro-) metastases on the cerebrospinal fluid will justify extended radiation fields including the cerebrospinal axis or at least the ventricular field. Therefore, complete initial diagnostic assessment and staging constitutes the mainstay of treatment stratification. Moreover, the presence of diabetes insipidus has significant impact on infusion therapy during chemotherapy, since severe electrolyte imbalances may develop during hyperhydration required during platin chemotherapy.

Germinomas have traditionally been treated with radiotherapy, consisting of craniospinal irradiation with a tumor boost to 36 Gy (Bamberg et al. 1999). More recently, several studies from the USA and Europe reported that both germinomas and secreting germ cell tumors can be successfully managed with a carboplatin-based chemotherapeutic regimen (Balmaceda et al. 1996; da Silva et al. 2010; Kellie et al. 2004; Khatua et al. 2010; Alapetite et al. 2002). However, omitting radiotherapy is associated with an increased risk of local recurrence. In analogy, the omission of craniospinal irradiation in patients receiving radiochemotherapy including focal irradiation is associated with an increased risk of ventricular recurrences (Alapetite et al. 2010). Therefore, the current international SIOP protocol proposes ventricular irradiation after carboplatin-based combination chemotherapy, in order to minimize this risk of ventricular relapse. For metastatic germinomas, craniospinal irradiation is proposed, with excellent outcome (Calaminus et al. 2013). The prognostic impact of residual tumor following chemo- and radiotherapy has to be considered carefully and in the context of the histology, in particular, the presence of additional teratomatous components.

For secreting tumors, a combination of four cycles of cisplatin-based chemotherapy (PEI) supplemented by local (localized tumor) or craniospinal (metastatic tumors) irradiation with 45 Gy is recommended. In tumors with high AFP levels, chemotherapy is intensified with dose escalation of ifosfamide and etoposide (Calaminus et al. 2017).

31.2.13 Salvage Strategies

Therapy of malignant extragonadal germ cell tumors depends on histology at diagnosis and at relapse, site of recurrence, and first-line treatment (Figs. 31.14 and 31.15). In general, extragonadal germ cell tumors tend to recur at the primary tumor site. Nevertheless, prognosis of malignant extragonadal germ cell tumors that recur after platin-based chemotherapy is poor. This is primarily related to the fact that these tumors may develop resistance to chemotherapy (Mayer et al. 2003b). Second, the (surgical) chances to obtain a complete local control are usually significantly impaired at second-look surgery. Thus, scarring and changes in the normal anatomy after first surgery may impair surgical access to the recurrent tumor. Therefore, salvage strategy must always take both the local surgical situation and the general oncologic situation (metastases) into account. In general, salvage strategy must be planned and performed following an interdisciplinary approach.

The chances to successfully treat a malignant recurrence of a neonatal sacrococcygeal teratoma are good, in particular, if recurrence is detected at an early stage during regular follow-up. These tumors are usually treated with up-front cisplatin-based chemotherapy, followed by delayed tumor resection, which should be reserved to experienced pediatric surgeons (Fig. 31.14). If complete resection is obtained, the prognosis is comparable to that of primary sacrococcygeal yolk sac tumor.

In contrast, the outlook of recurrence after first-line chemotherapy is impaired. A switch, ideally an intensification of chemotherapy, is indicated in case of recurrence after first-line chemotherapy. In case of carboplatin-based first-line therapy, carboplatin can be replaced with cisplatin, and studies have shown that a substantial proportion of patients can be salvaged after the introduction of cisplatin (Baranzelli et al. 1999a, b, c). Otherwise, salvage chemotherapy regimens in children including high-dose chemotherapy strategies are commonly derived from studies performed in adult patients. This experience is extensively reviewed in Sect. 31.1.1.

Ideally, a strategy should be developed that allows both to overcome resistance of tumor cells to chemotherapy and to facilitate local tumor control (Fig. 31.15). In this context, regional deep hyperthermia may provide promising aspects. Wessalowski and colleagues have treated children and adolescents with recurrent gonadal but mostly extragonadal germ cell tumors with cisplatin, etoposide, and ifosfamide in combination with regional deep hyperthermia

(Wessalowski et al. 1997b, 2003b, 2013). The majority of patients were suffering from recurrent malignant sacrococcygeal germ cell tumors. Therapy was administered in a neoadjuvant strategy, with a delayed resection usually performed after the third or fourth cycles of thermochemotherapy. Of note, surgical resection was centralized to few experienced pediatric surgical centers, and in case of still incomplete resection, a proportion of patients additionally received local radiotherapy (Schneider et al. 2001e). With this approach, response to thermochemotherapy was favorable, as demonstrated by reduction of tumor size and decline of tumor markers. In addition, complete resection could be obtained in a proportion of patients, and in those not assessable to complete resection, radiotherapy appeared to enhance local tumor control additionally. With this strategy, a salvage rate almost comparable to that in first-line treatment was obtained—however, such favorable outcome was only achieved in patients referred to thermochemotherapy at first relapse (Wessalowski et al. 2013). In later relapses, thermochemotherapy strategies are not as promising. This indicates that in case of relapse, early treatment intensification and stringent multimodal treatment strategies are an absolute prerequisite of cure (Schneider et al. 2001e). Unfortunately, thermochemotherapy is available only in few pediatric oncologic centers. Even more, any salvage strategy should nevertheless aim for the best possible tumor control. For this purpose, careful planning of surgical resection and, if required, radiotherapy is essential.

These considerations can be transferred to recurrent extragonadal germ cell tumors at any other site, including retroperitoneal, mediastinal, and vaginal germ cell tumors. For intracranial germ cell tumors, the same biologic and clinical observations can be made. They only rarely metastasize outside of the central nervous system. However, metastases within the ventricular system are not infrequent (Alapetite et al. 2010). In addition, local recurrences can be observed, in particular, in nonseminomatous germ cell tumors. Unfortunately, the chances to intensify local and systemic tumor control in recurrent central nervous system germ cell tumors are very restricted. Thus, most patients have been treated with intensive first-line chemotherapy. Only in case of carboplatin-based chemotherapy, a switch to cisplatin regimen opens the perspective to intensive chemotherapy significantly. If tumors recur outside of the radiation field, irradiation can be administered to these areas. However, it should be considered that usually such tumors present as metastatic tumors, thus requiring consolidating irradiation of the whole craniospinal axis.

If high cumulative doses are required, toxicity may thus interfere with this approach. Thus, alternative strategies including intraventricular chemotherapy can also be administered, however, with currently only limited experience. Unfortunately, the outcome especially of recurrent secreting CNS germ cell tumors is unfavorable, using current salvage strategies (Murray et al. 2017). Therefore, any salvage strategy in recurrent central nervous system germ cell tumors should be discussed with the respective study coordinator. Ideally, clinical data should be collected centrally in order to support the development of standardized and effective strategies including new irradiation techniques (e.g., protons), alternative chemotherapy strategies (e.g., high-dose chemotherapy), and alternative drugs (e.g., kinase inhibitors or antiangiogenetic drugs).

31.2.14 Prognosis and Late Effects

The prognosis of extragonadal teratomas is excellent if complete tumor resection is obtained. If tumor resection is incomplete, the risk of recurrence correlates with the grade of immaturity. Lastly, the recurrence risk also correlates with site, with incompletely resected sacrococcygeal teratomas being at the highest risk. Of note, half of recurrences present with malignant histology so that monitoring of AFP during follow-up is helpful in detecting these malignant relapses (Göbel et al. 1998a, b). It should be considered that despite the "benign" histology, teratomas are potentially lethal tumors. In a large series of 270 extracranial non-testicular teratomas, relapse rates of mature and immature teratoma were 10% and 18%, respectively. 25% of patients with tumor recurrence died, and almost half of the survivors underwent mutilating surgery with long-term sequelae such as palsy of the pelvic floor and incontinence (Göbel et al. 1998a). In contrast, the long-term outcome of patients who were successfully operated at initial diagnosis is favorable. Only a minority of patients with sacrococcygeal teratoma suffer from neurologic sequelae related to the tumor infiltrating the spinal canal, such as weakness of the lower limbs or incontinence, illustrated by the little girl of Fig. 31.16, who presented with a giant neonatal teratoma and was continent at the age of 2 years. Nevertheless, a proportion of patients may describe episodal or chronic constipation, which may rarely be significant (Draper et al. 2009).

The prognosis of teratomas at other extragonadal sites is comparably favorable and clearly exceeds 90% long-term survival (Göbel et al. 1998a; Marina et al. 1999b). Fortunately, the surgery-associated risks are tolerable, too. In head and neck teratomas, secondary hypothyroidism or parahypothyroidism has been reported (Bernbeck et al. 2009b).

A comparably favorable outcome has been reported for patients with malignant extragonadal yolk sac tumors. Certainly, vaginal yolk sac tumors appear to have the best overall prognosis with a cure rate exceeding 95%. This therapeutic success is the result of the exquisite chemotherapy sensitivity of these tumors so that even less-radical surgical procedures such as partial vaginectomy can be performed that may potentially lead to less long-term functional deficits (Lopes et al. 1999; Mauz-Körholz et al. 2000a, b). In contrast, the prognosis of sacrococcygeal yolk sac tumors heavily depends on a radical surgical therapy with microscopically complete resection. If resection is incomplete, long-term outcome falls below 50%, whereas cure rates above 85% can be achieved after complete resection (Göbel et al. 2001a, b). Accordingly, outcome is more favorable even in high-stage tumors if a neoadjuvant strategy with up-front chemotherapy and delayed resection is chosen, since at delayed resection a higher chance of complete resection can be obtained. Even if published experience is limited, there is no evidence that the cosmetic and functional outcome of malignant sacrococcygeal germ cell tumors is significantly different from that of sacrococcygeal teratomas. The most adverse indicator is invasion of the spinal canal and the sacral nerve plexus by the tumor, which may lead to pelvic palsy be it by the tumor or the surgeon (Draper et al. 2009).

Long-term toxicity related to chemotherapy is extensively discussed in Sect. 31.1.1. The same considerations can be taken into account for gonadal and extragonadal germ cell tumors.

31.3 Testicular Germ Cell Tumors

31.3.1 Introduction

Gonadal and extragonadal germ cell tumors (GCT) comprise approximately 2–3% of cancers diagnosed in children and adolescents younger than 15 years (Ries et al. 1999b; Kaatsch 2004b). The survival of boys with testicular germ cell tumors has greatly improved with the application of lessons from adult GCT trials. However, significant differences exist between germ cell tumors in prepubertal boys compared to those in adolescents and young adults. Long-term toxicity may be a significant problem especially following chemotherapy as a young child. We will explore the molecular basis of testicular germ cell tumor and risk-adaptive strategies that may be applicable to young boys and adolescents with malignant testicular germ cell tumors.

31.3.1.1 Testicular Germ Cell Tumors of Young Children: Genetics

In children younger than 4 years, germ cell tumors arising in gonadal and extragonadal sites are histologically, clinically, and genetically similar (for more details see Sect. 31.1.1). Most teratomas in this age group are diploid, have normal karyotypes, and, if completely resected, behave in a benign fashion regardless of degree of immaturity and site of origin (Kaplan et al. 1979b; Bussey et al. 1999b; Harms et al. 2006b; Göbel et al. 1998a, b, c, d). Malignant germ cell tumors in prepubertal children are almost exclusively yolk sac tumors (Perlman et al. 1994b).

Cytogenetic abnormalities involving chromosomes 1, 3, and 6 have been reported (Oosterhuis et al. 1988; Bussey et al. 1999b, Schneider et al. 2001a, b, c, d, e, f, g, h). In situ hybridization and loss of heterozygosity studies have demonstrated deletion of 1p36 in 80–100% of infantile malignant germ cell tumors arising from testicular and extragonadal sites (Stock et al. 1994; Sievers et al. 2005b).

31.3.1.2 Testicular Tumors in Adolescents and Adults: Genetics

Adolescent testicular germ cell tumors most commonly become clinically evident several years after puberty, suggesting that a critical genetic event occurs with, or is unmasked at, puberty. Germ cell tumors of the adolescent and adult testis demonstrate homogeneous genetic patterns including aneuploid DNA content and the isochromosome 12p or i (12p) (Oosterhuis et al. 1989; Atkin and Baker 1992; el-Naggar et al. 1992). Postpubertal testicular teratomas may have cytogenetic evidence of i (12p) and spread as a malignant GCT (Harms et al. 2006b).

The i (12p) can be found in 80% of postpubertal germ cell tumors and is comprised of two copies of the short arm of chromosome 12, fused at the centromere (Fig. 31.6 from gonadal chapter). Testicular tumors lacking i (12p) often show gain of 12p material within marker chromosomes (Rodriguez et al. 1993). The i (12p) has been documented by fluorescent in situ hybridization. This finding of i (12p) in intratubular germ cell neoplasia, a precursor lesion of testicular germ cell tumors, suggests that this genetic alteration occurs early in germ cell tumor pathogenesis (Looijenga et al. 1993). Testicular germ cell tumors also have exhibited loss of chromosome 13 (38%), gain of chromosome 21 (45%), gain of chromosome 8 (45%), gain of chromosome 1q (36%), and high-level gain of 12p11.2–12.1 (Mostert et al. 1996). Other less frequent genetic changes have been noted. Adolescent testicular germ cell tumors, like normal embryonic germ cells, demonstrate biallelic expression of multiple imprinted genes including H19 and insulin-like growth factor-2 (van Gurp et al. 1994) and loss of DNA methylation within imprinting control regions (Schneider et al. 2001a, b, c, d, e, f, g, h; Sievers et al. 2005a, b).

31.3.1.3 Pathology

Germ cell tumors comprise several histologic subtypes. The histologic features of each subtype are independent of presenting clinical characteristics. Both tumor biology and clinical behavior vary with site of origin, stage, and age of the patient (Altman et al. 1974b; Hawkins and Perlman 1996b). In contrast to mature teratomas which are almost always benign and diploid in infants or located in the ovary, the same histologic features are aneuploid and potentially malignant in the adult testis (Young and Scully 1990b). The histologic and pathologic classifications and descriptions have been previously described in Table 31.3 and Fig. 31.7 from gonadal chapter.

There are several points that are particular to testicular germ cell tumors. Teratomas and yolk sac tumors are the predominant histology prior to puberty. After puberty, other elements, seminoma, choriocarcinoma, and embryonal carcinoma are demonstrated. Pediatric immature teratomas primarily occur in extragonadal sites in children and in the ovaries of girls near puberty (Marina et al. 1999c). They are only rarely present in the male testis. Yolk sac tumors (YST) are the most common pure malignant germ cell tumor in young children and are the most common germ cell tumor, benign or malignant, in the testes of infants and young boys (Young and Scully 1990b). Pure seminomas represent the most common malignant germ cell tumor in men older than 20 years. However, pure seminomas are unusual in men younger than 20 years. Embryonal carcinoma rarely occurs in a pure form in children and is more often a component of a mixed malignant germ cell tumor (Young and Scully 1990b; Hawkins and Perlman 1996b). This component is seen in adolescent testicular germ cell tumor (Fig. 31.7e, Sect. 31.1.1).

31.3.2 Clinical Diagnosis

The signs and symptoms of germ cell tumors are dependent on the site of origin of the tumor (Table 31.13). The typical finding in testicular germ cell tumor—as for other testicular tumors—is a non-painful enlarging mass. Pain especially may be associated with testicular torsion (Giwercman et al. 1987). The absence of other clinical findings often delays the diagnosis. Testicular GCTs present in two peaks during childhood and adolescence. The first peak is usually under age 4 years. Parents generally note these lesions, and patients may be brought to the attention of primary care physician in timely fashion (Fig. 31.17, left and 31.18). Postpubertal males usually identify a mass but often delay reporting to their family or physician so that tumors are often diagnosed at considerable size (Fig. 31.17, right). Perhaps this may also increase the risk for metastases. Diagnostic strategies specific for testicular germ cell tumors are described in Table 31.14. A crucial point in the diagnosis and treatment of testicular GCT is referral to an appropriate surgeon. Testicular GCTs, in particular, in prepubertal children, can often be treated with surgery and observation. If the wrong surgical approach is taken, the patient may require chemotherapy. This will be discussed further in treatment section.

Table 31.13 Testicular germ cell tumor—Group presentation

– Teratoma	– Enlarging non-painful scrotal mass, surgery alone
– Yolk sac tumor	– Most common pediatric malignant germ cell tumor histology, enlarging non-painful scrotal mass
– Embryonal carcinoma	– More common in adolescents, may require more extensive surgery including retroperitoneal lymph node resection, similar presentation to above
– Mixed	– Less common in young males, combination of yolk sac tumor, embryonal carcinoma, and teratoma in postpubertal males
– Gonadoblastoma	– Bilateral 30%, poor sexual development
– Choriocarcinoma	– Rare, most often seen in mixed tumors, in adolescents, findings consistent with Klinefelter's

31.3.3 Staging

Staging of testicular germ cell tumors is closely linked to treatment. An improper diagnostic procedure, for example, a trans-scrotal biopsy with contamination, will upstage a patient. This patient will then require chemotherapy. Table 31.15 shows the clinical surgical staging system as defined by intergroup pediatric trials from the USA. Ideally, patients with testicular masses should have appropriate imaging and marker studies prior to diagnostic biopsy or orchiectomy.

Several features must be considered in stage I testicular germ cell tumor. The surgical approach may determine stage and need for further treatment. An inguinal approach with high ligation of spermatic cord and vessels may ensure complete resection and classification of stage I disease. An additional feature is marker decay. Most prepubertal males have yolk sac tumor with elevated AFP as the predominant histology. An appropriate AFP decline (half-life, 5–7 days) would confirm stage I disease during follow-up. An AFP that does not return to normal or rises would suggest stage II disease even in the absence of positive imaging. This patient would need to be treated with chemotherapy. The prognosis is excellent for stage I with more than 70% of patients requiring no chemotherapy. The remaining patients can usually be salvaged with standard cisplatin chemotherapy. The treatment of postpubertal males must be informed by adult germ cell tumor studies, which will incorporate histology (embryonal carcinoma associated with a worse prognosis) and vascular invasion. Testicular germ cell tumors have a propensity to metastasize to retroperitoneal lymph nodes. Postpubertal males, in particular, often have residual teratomatous material that has the potential to dedifferentiate later into malignant disease. For this reason, many physicians, treating adult patients with germ cell tumors, recommend

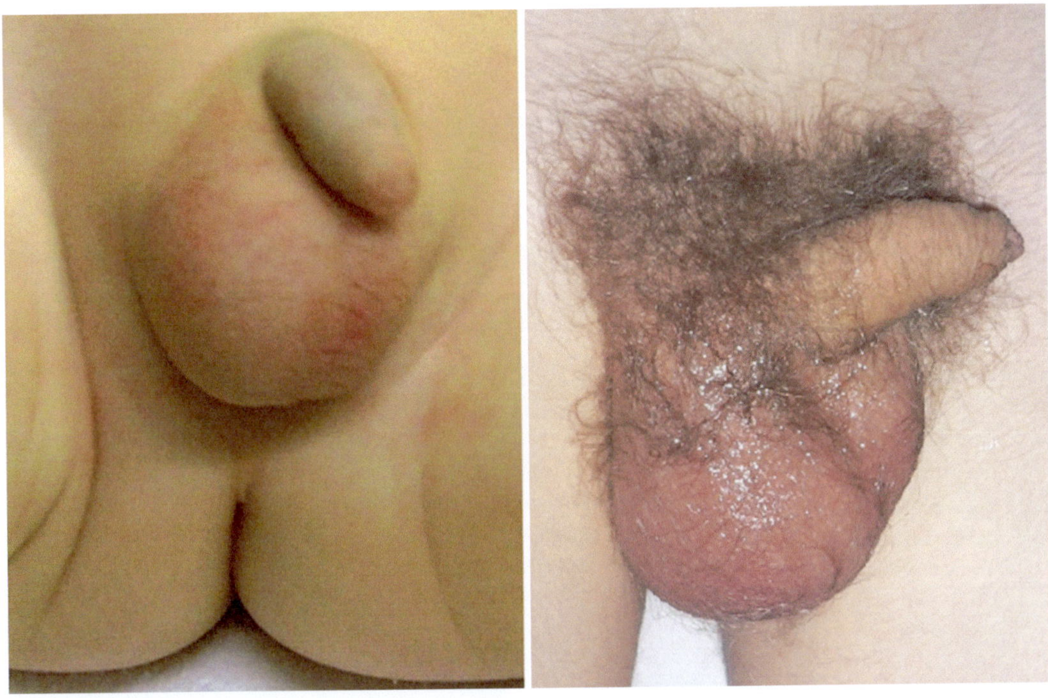

Fig. 31.17 Clinical presentation of testicular germ cell tumor in an infant (6 months old, immature teratoma + yolk sac tumor) and adolescent boy (15 years old, mixed malignant germ cell tumor with nodal metastases)

removal of residual tissue. Figure 31.19 demonstrates the full extent of nodal metastases from an initial testicular primary. A mixed YST and embryonal carcinoma spread to retroperitoneal nodes, posterior mediastinal nodes, and eventually to left supraclavicular nodes. The last finding brought patient to medical attention, as the testicular primary was small.

The question of retroperitoneal lymph node dissection (RPLND) for accurate staging of testicular germ cell tumors has been long standing and complex. In boys less than 4 years of age, there are no data to suggest that this surgical approach is warranted. The outcome, even in stage IV, is excellent, and residual teratoma is not usually present. In adolescent males, this is still an important question. Figure 31.19 shows recurrence of seminoma in an adolescent who did not have RPLND or return for observational studies.

31.3.4 Therapy

An individualized, multimodality treatment plan is necessary due to the heterogeneity of pediatric germ cell tumors relative to site of origin, age, histology, and stage. Different subsets have been described for childhood and adolescent germ cell tumors (Schneider et al. 2004c). Most patients are referred after orchiectomy, and treatment will be directed based on staging. In the USA, the Children's Oncology Group staging for testicular germ cell tumors reflects other pediatric tumors. The advent of effective chemotherapy may mitigate the need for initial extensive surgery. Figure 31.20 details practical options in the treatment of testicular germ cell tumors.

Surgery represents the cornerstone of the management of testicular germ cell tumors. Generally, a primary complete excision is feasible. Protocols recommend an inguinal approach with vascular control before mobilization of the testis (Schmidt et al. 2002a; Lo Curto et al. 2003). If a malignant germ cell tumor is confirmed by frozen section examination of the mass, en bloc resection of testis and spermatic structures with ligation of the cord at the inguinal ring is required (Schlatter et al. 2003). Patients with scrotal skin involvement and those operated or biopsied through a scrotal

Table 31.14 Specific diagnostic strategy in testicular GCT

Procedure	Specific questions
Clinical assessment	
Phys. examination	Non-tender testicular mass, suspected torsion of testis, undescended testis, Klinefelter's syndrome
Laboratory assessment	
– AFP (+β-HCG)	Malignant GCT with yolk sac tumor—consider age-related reference range (or choriocarcinoma)
– LDH	May be prognostic in older males
Radiographic assessment	
Chest—CT, abdomen, pelvis—MRI	Most common sites of metastatic spread from testis are retroperitoneal lymph nodes and lungs
Testicular ultrasound	Examine both testes (bilateral cases possible)
Bone scan	Not usually required in young boys but may need evaluation in older males
Histologic assessment	
H&E	Classification according to WHO
AFP	Yolk sac tumor (microfoci in teratoma)
β-HCG	Exclusion of choriocarcinoma
(CD-30)	Exclusion of embryonal carcinoma
(OCT3/4)	Exclusion of seminoma (embryonal carcinoma)

Table 31.15 Testicular germ cell tumor—Childrens Oncology Group staging

I	Complete resection. Disease limited to testis. Surgical approach—high inguinal ligation or trans-scrotal (with no spillage). No evidence of metastases. Appropriate marker decline
II	Microscopic disease in scrotum or spermatic cord (≤5 cm from proximal end). Transscrotal biopsy/resection with spillage
III	Retroperitoneal involvement (>2 cm sized nodes) or biopsy positive
IV	Metastatic

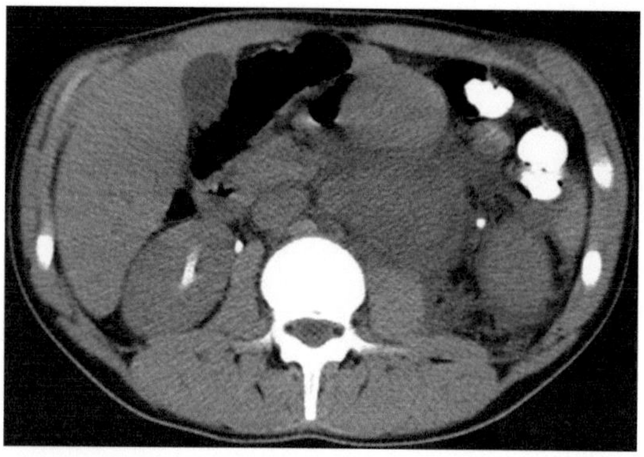

Fig. 31.18 Recurrent retroperitoneal seminoma, 4 years after surgery for stage I seminoma Testicular germ cell tumor with yolk sac tumor and embryonal carcinoma histology metastatic throughout retroperitoneal and posterior mediastinal lymph nodes to supraclavicular nodes

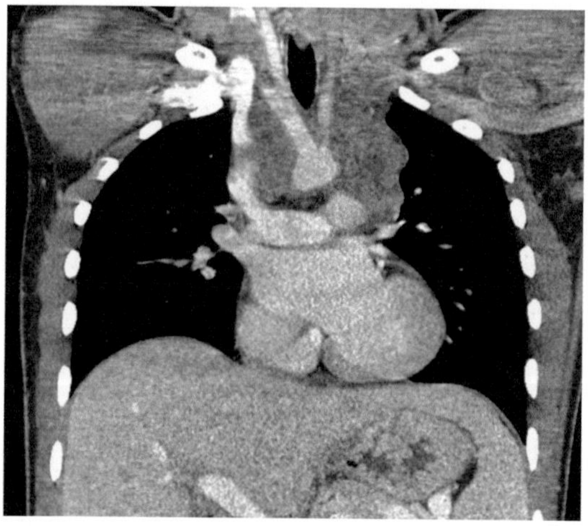

Fig. 31.19 Testicular germ cell tumor with yolk sac tumor and embryonal carcinoma histology metastatic throughout retroperitoneal and posterior mediastinal lymph nodes to supraclavicular nodes

approach should undergo a hemiscrotectomy to ensure local control. Some authors state that this procedure can be avoided if patient is upstaged from stage I to stage II and receives chemotherapy (Billmire 2006a). However, a recent study reported favorable outcome after watch-and-wait strategy following a non-study compliant transscrotal, however only for infants

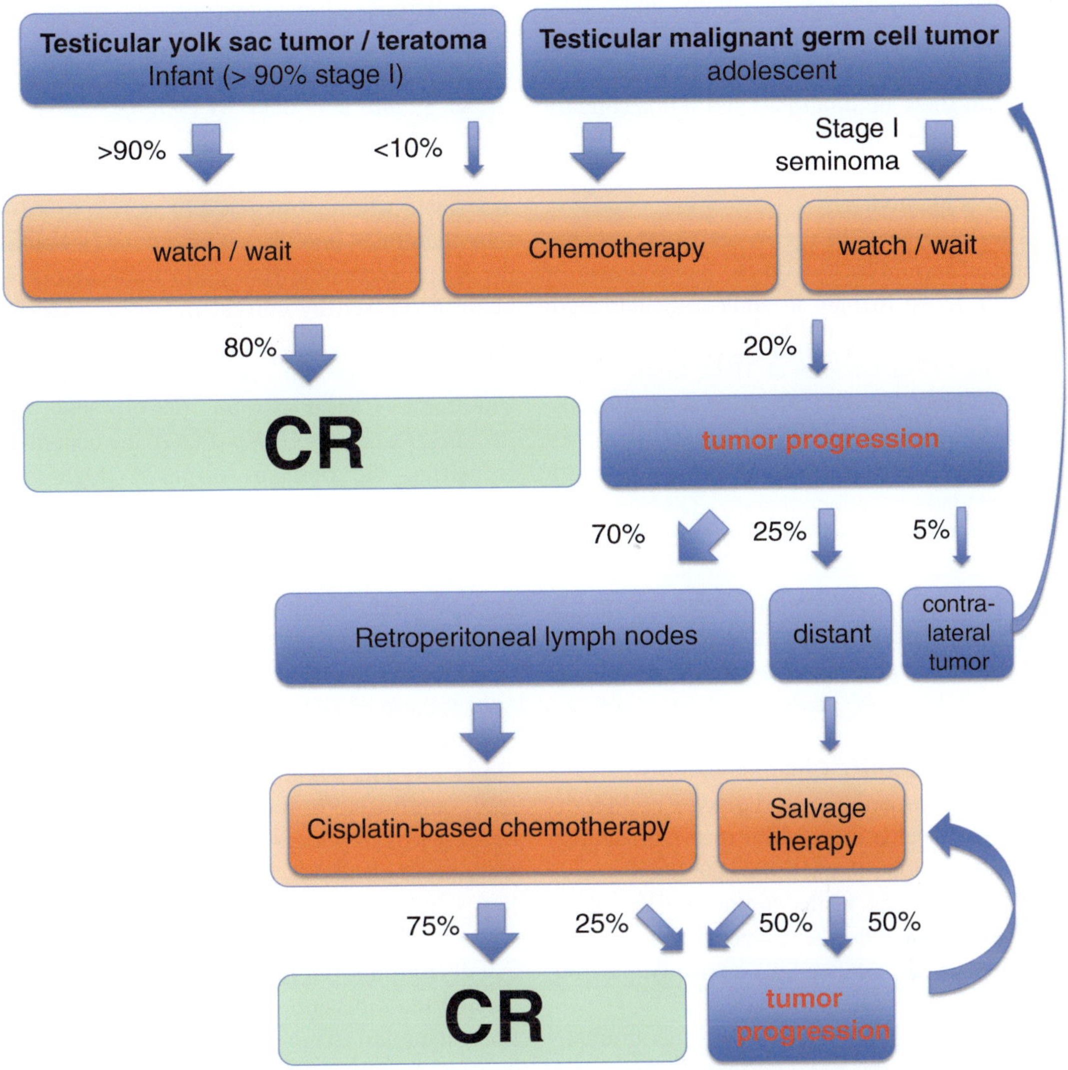

Fig. 31.20 Treatment algorithm for malignant testicular germ cell tumors

(Göbel et al. 2013a, b). Primary retroperitoneal lymph node dissection (RPLND) is not indicated in prepubertal boys, since malignant germ cell tumors are highly responsive to chemotherapy (Haas et al. 1999; Göbel et al. 2013a, b). Limited biopsy may be necessary to define staging when the involvement of retroperitoneal lymph nodes is uncertain after imaging. However, open or laparoscopic RPLND may be necessary when enlarged nodes remain after chemotherapy. Inguinal node exploration is indicated only in patients with scrotal involvement.

Patients with completely resected testicular germ cell tumors do not require chemotherapy. The "watch-and-wait" approach requires scheduled serial physical examination, tumor marker determination, and primary tumor imaging to ensure that a recurrent tumor is detected without delay. A discussion of tumor marker is warranted, especially in testicular stage I germ cell tumor. Tumor markers, especially AFP in prepubertal male, must fall according to AFP half-life. While it is usually 5–7 days, some patients will have longer half-life. The failure to normalize or any significant rise in AFP suggests the presence of residual tumor, and patient should receive chemotherapy even without imaging or biopsy confirmation. In a few cases AFP can show minimal rise and fall secondary to other causes. Many investigators agree that in this population, five times the upper limit or normal is too high.

The prognosis of germ cell tumors has improved significantly with the development of cisplatin-based therapy in adult testicular germ cell tumor patients (DFS 68–92%) (Einhorn and Donohue 1977b; Ozols et al. 1988; Einhorn et al. 1989b). Prior to this effective chemotherapy, children with extracranial malignant germ cell tumors had 3-year survival rates of 15–20% with surgery and radiation therapy (Kurman and Norris 1976b). However, boys with localized testicular tumors do well with surgical resection (Schlatter et al. 2003). Prognosis and appropriate treatment depend on factors such as histology (e.g., seminomatous vs. nonseminomatous), age (young children vs. adolescents), stage of disease, and primary site (Baranzelli et al. 1999c; Marina et al. 2006b). Children with extracranial malignant germ cell tumors should be cared for at pediatric cancer centers with experience treating these rare tumors, to maximize the likelihood of long-term survival while minimizing the likelihood of treatment-related long-term sequelae (e.g., secondary leukemias, infertility, hearing loss, renal dysfunction).

Cisplatin-based chemotherapy has dramatically improved the outcome for children with extracranial germ cell tumors, with 5-year survival rates of more than 90% (Mann et al. 2000b; Göbel et al. 2002a; Cushing et al. 2004c; Rogers et al. 2004c). Chemotherapy strategies developed by various international pediatric germ cell tumor committees were previously described in Table 31.6 (gonadal chapter). The standard chemotherapy regimen for both adults and children with malignant nonseminomatous GCT includes cisplatin, etoposide, and bleomycin (PEB), though children receive fewer doses of bleomycin than adults. The combination of carboplatin, etoposide, and bleomycin (JEB) has undergone clinical investigation in the UK in children younger than 16 years and is reported to have a similar event-free survival (EFS) by site and stage as PEB (Mann et al. 2000b). It must be noted that these were not randomized trials. The use of JEB appears to be associated with less ototoxicity and nephrotoxicity than PEB, and the use of cis- or carboplatin for intermediate-risk germ cell tumors is being addressed by current initiatives (Shaikh et al. 2013).

In an intergroup study conducted by the Children's Cancer Group (CCG) and the Pediatric Oncology Group (POG), the benefit of increasing the dose of cisplatin [high-dose (HD)-PEB: 200 mg/m^2 vs. PEB: 100 mg/m^2 of cisplatin] was studied in a randomized manner in patients with extragonadal and advanced gonadal germ cell tumors (Cushing et al. 2004c). Intensification of cisplatin in the HD-PEB regimen provided some improvement in EFS; however, the use of HD-PEB was associated with a significantly higher incidence and severity of ototoxicity and nephrotoxicity. In a subsequent study, amifostine was not effective in preventing hearing loss in patients who received HD-PEB (Marina et al. 2005). Moreover, semen collection should be considered in pubertal patients, whenever feasible.

Other groups (Germany, Brazil, France) have studied the omission of bleomycin from frontline therapies. The Italian group have still applied bleomyin but reduced the dose of Etoposide to 400 mg/m2 per cycle, without negative impact on outcome (Terenziani et al. 2018). Regimens without bleomycin were developed for favorable-risk germ cell tumors. Excellent outcomes were maintained, too. In the most recent analysis of the German consecutive protocols, all of 128 prepubertal children with testicular germ cell tumors survived, including 82 malignant germ cell tumors. Among the latter, 68 were followed with a watch-and-wait strategy, with five tumor progressions in this group. These 5 and additional 14 stage II or higher tumors were successfully treated with chemotherapy (Göbel et al. 2013a, b).

The treatment of testicular germ cell tumors in adolescents and adults has been analyzed by a large meta-analysis study. Postpubertal males with testicular GCT should be treated according to these guidelines (Group 1997b). In fact, it should be considered that in this age group, there is a considerable group of patients with advanced and metastatic tumors, which require intensive chemotherapy (Göbel et al. 2014).

There are several points that should be made concerning treatment approaches in patients with testicular germ cell tumors containing specific benign or malignant elements.

31.3.4.1 Teratoma

Immature teratomas are rarely found in the prepubertal testis. Teratomas, in prepubertal males, almost always take a favorable clinical course. Surgery is the treatment for these patients with such benign teratomas. Inguinal orchiectomy is usually required for mature and immature germ cell tumors (Mann et al. 2008b). However, testis-sparing procedure through the inguinal canal may be considered when markers and investigations suggest a benign process. The feasibility of a conservative resection (tumorectomy) depends on the location of the mass and on the frozen section pathology results. The tumor size cutoff at 2 cm does not appear to accurately predict the final pathology as it happens in adults. Re-excision may be necessary for residual tumor or in the case of malignancy at definitive histology. Inguinal orchiectomy may be required for mature and immature germ cell tumors (Mann et al. 2008b). The postpubertal adolescent patient with a germ cell tumor presents additional challenges. Residual teratomatous material has been associated with significant malignant germ cell tumor recurrence within 10 years. Therefore, several institutions advocate resection of all residual material in postpubertal males. This may include retroperitoneal lymph node resection (RPLND) (Carver et al. 2005, 2007d).

31.3.4.2 Seminoma

Seminomas of the testis are almost exclusive to the postpubertal male. Seminomas display an outstanding response to treatment, both chemotherapy and radiation therapy. In most patients, residual tumor after chemotherapy is resected. Nevertheless, the therapeutic impact of tumor resection in highly regressive tumors is controversial. In these instances, post-chemotherapy PET assessment may assist in decision-making. Any PET positive tumors should be resected irrespective of size. In contrast, PET negative tumors smaller than 1–2 cm can be followed, whereas larger tumors should also be excised. In unresectable viable seminomas, irradiation constitutes a promising salvage therapy. However, it is not recommended for first-line therapy, since the long-term side effects associated with mediastinal irradiations may be significant. Patients with stage I seminomas must be observed carefully for at least 5 years, as late retroperitoneal recurrence is possible (Fig. 31.19).

31.3.4.3 Embryonal Carcinoma

Embryonal carcinoma is usually seen in postpubertal males with testicular germ cell tumors as part of a mixed tumor. In postpubertal males, an increased percentage of embryonal carcinoma histology in a mixed tumor correlates with worse prognosis and possibly suggests a need for chemotherapy. The infrequent incidence of this histology in prepubertal males makes conclusions difficult.

31.3.5 Prognosis

Patients with mature and immature teratomas will have an EFS of near 100% with surgery alone (Mann et al. 2008b). With a multidisciplinary approach, boys with malignant testicular GCT have an outstanding prognosis. In the US intergroup studies, boys (pre- and postpubertal) with stage I, II, and III testicular GCT had an overall survival rate of 100% (Schlatter et al. 2003; Cushing et al. 2004c; Rogers et al. 2004c). Other pediatric groups have reported similar results (Göbel et al. 1990; Baranzelli and Patte

1998; Mann et al. 2000b; Göbel et al. 2002a; Lopes et al. 2009b; Terenziani et al. 2018). The US trial included boys up to age 18 years. Overall survival rates for boys <15 and >15 years were 100% and 84%, respectively (Cushing et al. 2004c). It must be noted that most of the boys >15 had pure yolk sac histology.

31.4 Germ Cell Tumors of the Ovary

31.4.1 Introduction

The general aspects common to all germ cell tumors occurring at different sites have been previously discussed in the general gonadal chapter. Ovarian tumors are rare, accounting for only about 1% of childhood malignancies (Bernstein et al. 1999). The incidence increases after 8 years and peaks at 19 years. Ovarian germ cell tumor development parallels gonadotropin release (Cronen and Nagaraj 1988; Walker et al. 1988; dos Santos and Swerdlow 1991). In contrast to adult ovarian tumors, most pediatric ovarian tumors are of germ cell origin. Few children present with tumors of epithelial and stromal origin, as seen in adult patients (Lovvorn 3rd et al. 1998; Young Jr et al. 2003). Approximately 5% of ovarian germ cell tumors develop bilaterally. Thus, bilateral tumors may be present at diagnosis (synchronous manifestation) or develop during follow-up (metachronous manifestation).

31.4.2 Ovarian Tumors GCT in Adolescents and Adults: Genetics

The genetic biology of ovarian germ cell tumors is more complex than that of testicular germ cell tumors and is considered separately for mature teratomas, immature teratomas, and malignant ovarian germ cell tumors. There is a considerable association with sex-chromosomal abnormalities such as Ullrich-Turner syndrome and testicular feminization (Sect. 31.1.1).

31.4.2.1 Teratomas

Mature teratomas demonstrate karyotypically balanced cytogenetics (95%), with only 5% showing gains of single whole chromosomes (Parrington et al. 1984; Surti et al. 1990). Characteristically, they may show an isodisomic karyotype (23,X × 2). A methylation profile of imprinted genes (e.g., hypermethylation of SNRPN), also consistent with a postmeiotic origin, is often seen in ovarian teratomas (Schneider et al. 2001g).

31.4.2.2 Immature Teratomas

Ovarian immature teratomas are heterogeneous with evidence of a meiotic stem cell origin or mitotic origins. This suggests failure of early meiotic arrest (Ohama et al. 1985). Immature and mature teratomas may represent different biologic entities, rather than simply a spectrum of maturation. Chromosomal abnormalities are more common in immature teratoma. Patients with cytogenetically abnormal immature teratomas often develop recurrence. In contrast, patients with karyotypically normal immature teratomas do not (Ohama et al. 1985; King et al. 1990; Gibas et al. 1993).

31.4.2.3 Malignant Ovarian Germ Cell Tumors

Malignant ovarian germ cell tumors in postpubertal girls have similar genetic findings when compared to testicular malignant germ cell tumors, including presence of i (12p) (75%), gains of chromosomes 21 and 1q (42% and 32% respectively), and loss of chromosomes 13 and 8 (25% and 42%, respectively) (Speleman et al. 1990; Hoffner et al. 1994; Thompson et al. 1994; Riopel et al. 1998; Bussey et al. 1999a, b). Although malignant ovarian germ cell tumors appear to be equivalent to their adolescent testicular counterparts, immature and mature ovarian teratomas remain as unique subcategories of germ cell tumors likely to have a different mechanism of origin. The analysis of bilateral ovarian germ cell tumors demonstrates a high proportion of sex chromosomal abnormalities, even clinically inapparent (Hennes et al. 2012).

31.4.3 Histopathology

Pathologic characteristics are described in Sect. 31.1.1. The majority of ovarian germ cell tumors are either mature teratomas or immature teratomas. Significant distribution differences do not exist in pre- and postpubertal females. Yolk sac tumor is the most common malignant element seen in mixed germ cell tumors. It is often associated with immature teratoma.

31.4.4 Clinical Diagnosis

Clinical features of ovarian germ cell tumors are detailed in Table 31.16. Abdominal pain is the most common presenting symptom (80%) (Cronen and Nagaraj 1988; Gribbon et al. 1992; Lovvorn 3rd et al. 1998; Schultz et al. 2005). The pain is usually chronic but some patients present with an acute abdomen, often secondary to torsion. Other signs and symptoms include a palpable or even visible abdominal mass (Fig. 31.21), abdominal distension, fever, constipation, amenorrhea, vaginal bleeding, and rarely frequency and dysuria (Harris and Boles Jr 1974; Lovvorn 3rd et al. 1998). Precocious puberty can be seen in some malignant germ cell tumors, though it is more frequent in ovarian sex cord stromal tumors. AFP levels are increased in patients with yolk sac tumors. Mixed ovarian germ cell tumors with elevated AFP are usually composed of immature teratoma and varying amounts of yolk sac tumor elements. Of note, also Sertoli-Leydig cell tumors may be associated with AFP production. Specific diagnostic strategies for ovarian tumors are described in Table 31.17.

Table 31.16 Ovarian cell tumor—characteristic clinical presentation

– Teratoma	Palpable mass, abdominal pain
Mature	15%, bilateral
Immature	Implants
– Dysgerminoma	Pain, rapid growth, ovarian torsion
– Yolk sac tumor	Pain, mass, torsion
– Embryonal carcinoma	Rare, precocious puberty
– Choriocarcinoma	Part of mixed tumor
– Mixed germ cell tumor	30% precocious puberty
– Gonadoblastoma	Dysgenetic ovaries, bilateral

31.4.5 Staging

Ultrasound is most often used for the initial evaluation of patients with abdominal or pelvic masses and will differentiate cystic from solid masses (Surratt and Siegel 1991). Although the presence of a solid ovarian mass raises the suspicion of malignancy, the majority are benign teratomas (Cronen and Nagaraj 1988). Computed tomography (CT) is helpful in identifying the site of origin, the extent of tumor, the presence of calcifications or fat, and metastatic disease. Many children with teratomas do not have evidence of fat on CT scan (Jabra et al. 1993). Neuroglial implants, containing mature or immature teratomatous elements, may be identified. They do not usually affect prognosis. Figures 31.22, 31.23, and 31.24 show CT findings of ovarian teratoma, yolk sac tumor, and dysgerminoma, respectively, illustrating that tumors are hardly distinguishable by imaging. Staging evaluation should include a chest CT and bone scan, though metastases to bones are rare. Central nervous system metastasis is unusual, and routine imaging of central nervous system is not indicated (Göbel et al. 2010, 2013a, b).

Serum tumor markers AFP and β-HCG are essential because the majority of pediatric patients with ovarian germ cell tumors have a yolk sac tumor component, and mixed malignant germ cell tumors may also include significant choriocarcinoma components (Mann et al. 1989b; Marina et al. 1992). In some histologically pure immature teratomas, moderately elevated AFP levels have been documented, although a clear cutoff value is not yet clearly defined. Of note, Sertoli-Leydig cell tumors may also be associated with moderately elevated AFP levels.

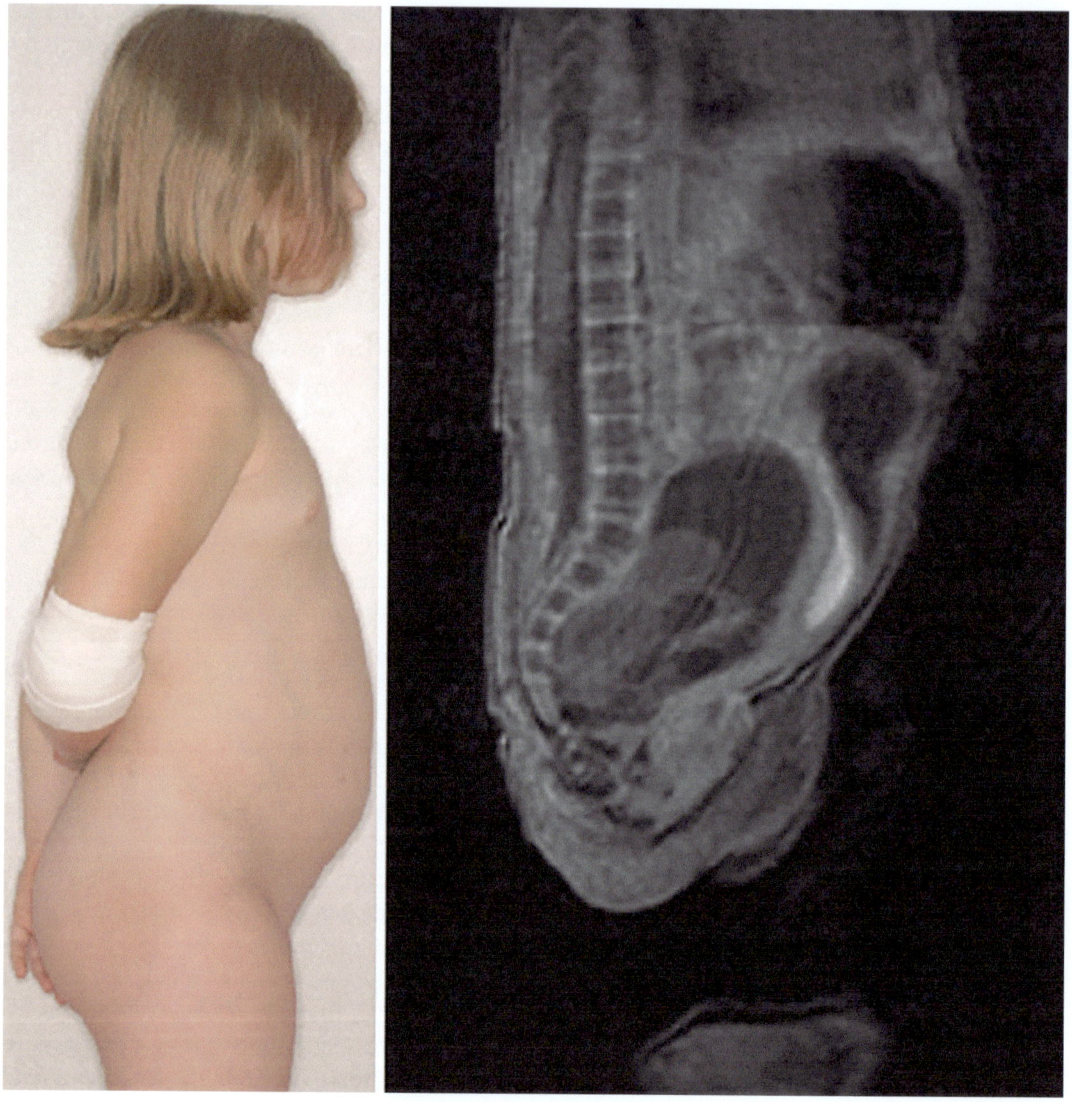

Fig. 31.21 11-year-old girl presenting with a large abdominal teratoma

Staging systems modeled after the recently updated FIGO system (Table 31.18) may be the most useful because different strategies must be followed for different histologies (Cannistra 1993; Meinhold-Heerlein et al. 2016). This system includes cytological examination of any thoracic or peritoneal fluid. The FIGO staging system has been used in several international pediatric germ cell studies. The US intergroup study used a surgicopathologic system to refine the FIGO system. In the US staging system, strict guidelines are required for an ovarian tumor to be categorized as stage I. Unless all surgical guidelines are followed or in the event of peritoneal contamination, such as seen in rupture, the patient will be upstaged to stage III and receive chemotherapy, while being stage Ic according to FIGO.

31.4.6 Therapy

The background for treatment of ovarian germ cell tumors can be informed from previous discussions in general gonadal chapter. There are

Table 31.17 Specific diagnostic strategy in ovarian tumors

Procedure	Specific questions
Clinical assessment	
Phys. examination	Abdominal pain (acute or chronic), rapidly developing abdominal mass, sexual precocious
Laboratory assessment	
– AFP (β-HCG)	Malignant GCT with yolk sac tumor—consider age-related reference range (or choriocarcinoma); note: moderate AFP may also be seen on Sertoil-Leydig cell tumors
– Catecholamines	Exclusion of neuroblastoma
– LDH	May have prognostic significance
– Inhibin, sex hormones	May indicate an ovarian sex cord stromal tumor
– CA125	Tumor marker for(epithelial) ovarian tumors; valuable for follow-up if elevated at diagnosis
Radiographic assessment	
Abdominal ultrasound	Examination of both ovaries, presence of cysts or solid components
CT chest, abdomen, pelvis	Site, size, organ of origin, cystic structures, calcification, metastases
Bone scan	Rare
Histologic assessment	
H&E	Classification according to WHO
AFP	Yolk sac tumor (microfoci in teratoma)
β-HCG	Exclusion of choriocarcinoma
CD-30	Exclusion of embryonal carcinoma
(OCT3/4)	Exclusion of dysgerminoma (embryonal carcinoma)
(Inhibin)	Exclusion of sex cord stromal tumor

features that are unique to ovarian tumors. Most recommendations relate to surgical options based on distinct histology. Surgery has a prominent role in the treatment of patients with ovarian tumors. However, since malignant germ cell tumors are very chemosensitive, primary excision should be attempted only when the surgeon thinks a complete resection can be obtained without a mutilating procedure (Billmire et al. 2004b; Billmire 2006b). If imaging shows invasion of other structures (i.e., bladder, uterus, vagina) or bilateral ovarian involvement, a tumor biopsy is the best option. The biopsy may be "open" or with a tru-cut needle. Under ultrasound guidance, multiple biopsies should be obtained from different sites for histologic diagnosis and collection of material for biology studies. If AFP and β-HCG are elevated, biopsy may not be necessary. After neoadjuvant chemotherapy, the patient will undergo delayed surgery.

Primary excision of ovarian tumors can be approached from a Pfannenstiel incision, an infraumbilical transverse incision, or a midline approach. Since malignant tumors and benign tumors cannot be distinguished based on gross features alone, all tumors should be staged according to current staging principles (Göbel et al. 1998d; Billmire 2006b).

- Aspiration of ascitis, if present, or peritoneal washing for histology.
- Examination of omentum and removal of suspected nodules.
- Inspection of peritoneum and abdominal organs, with biopsy of abnormal areas. Peritoneal implants (gliomatosis peritonei) may be associated with mature and immature teratomas.
- Examination and palpation of contralateral ovary with biopsy of suspicious areas.
- Complete removal of involved ovary, avoiding spillage. Ipsilateral fallopian tube may be spared if not adherent to mass.
- Inspection of iliac and aorto-caval nodes with biopsy of suspicious nodes. Nodal dissection should be carried out only when there is evidence of nodal abnormalities at preoperative CT scan or after surgery.

Laparoscopy is usually discouraged for removal of malignant tumors, as the violation of capsule or rupture can result in upstaging the tumor. Secondary excision should be done if the initial approach was a biopsy followed by chemotherapy (Schmidt et al. 2002b). Most authors recommend a conservative approach for bilateral tumors (if

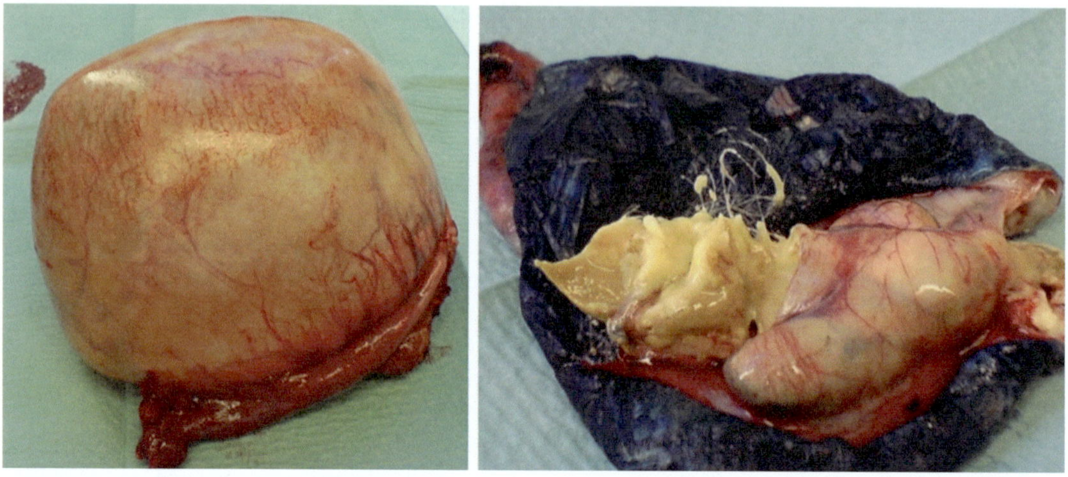

Fig. 31.22 Macroscopic presentation of a 2-kg cystic ovarian teratoma prior to and after ink impragnation and opening of the cyst

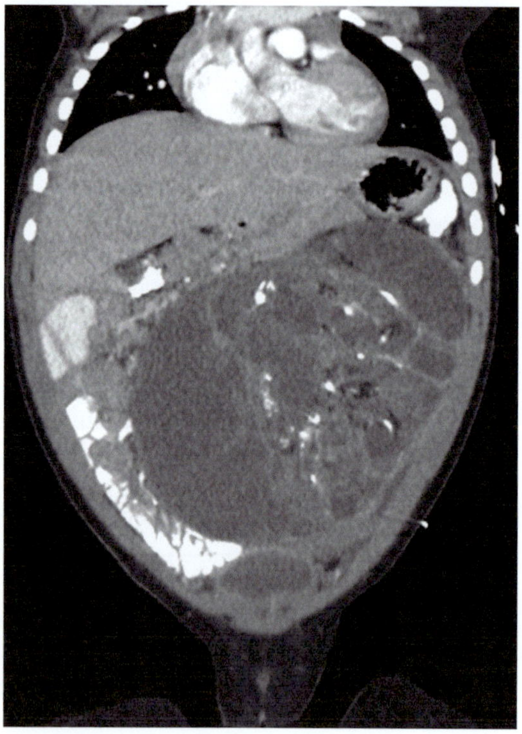

Fig. 31.23 Ovarian teratoma in a 2-year-old

possible on the least affected side) to preserve ovarian function. Bilateral oophorectomies and other extensive surgeries should be reserved when tumors do not respond to chemotherapy.

Special mention should be made concerning ovarian torsion. Approximately 10% of ovarian

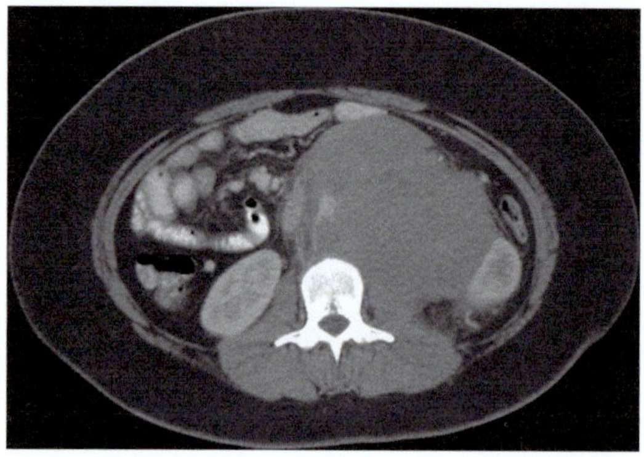

Fig. 31.24 Large ovarian yolk sac tumor involving retroperitoneal nodes. After chemotherapy, second surgery revealed only scar and no residual tumor

tumors present as acute abdomen secondary to torsion or rupture of tumor. Most ovarian masses associated with torsion are benign (Pienkowski et al. 2004). Ovarian torsion is an emergency and laparoscopy is preferred. If a tumor is suspected, immediate oophorectomy should be done. If a mass is found incidentally, a thorough abdominal inspection must be done (Hayes-Jordan 2005).

31.4.6.1 Teratoma and Immature Teratoma

The majority of ovarian germ cell tumors are either mature teratomas or immature teratomas. In the first months of life, most ovarian tumors are benign (Bagolan et al. 1992). Most teratomas

Table 31.18 Ovarian germ cell tumor—staging according to FIGO (updated in 2013)

Stage	extent of disease	
I		Limited to the ovaries
	Ia	To one ovary, no ascites. No tumor on external surface, capsule intact
	Ib	Both ovaries, no ascites. No tumor on external surface, capsule intact
	Ic	One or both ovaries but with tumor on surface of one or both ovaries, or capsule ruptured, or positive ascites or positive peritoneal washings
	Ic1	Intraoperative spillage
	Ic2	Preoperative tumor rupture or malignant cells on surface of ovary or fallopian tube
	Ic3	Malignant cells in ascites or peritoneal washings
II		Tumor involving one or both ovaries with pelvic extension
	IIa	Extension and/or metastases to uterus and/or tubes only
	IIb	Extension to other pelvic tissues
	IIc	As in IIa or IIb but with positive ascites or positive peritoneal washings, or with capsule ruptured
III		Tumor involving one or both ovaries with peritoneal implants outside the pelvis and/or positive retroperitoneal or inguinal lymph nodes, extension to small bowel or omentum, superficial liver metastases
	IIIa	Limited to true pelvis grossly with negative nodes but histologically confirmed microscopic seeding of abdominal peritoneal surfaces
	IIIb	Limited to one or both ovaries with negative nodes but histologically confirmed implants of abdominal peritoneal surfaces, not <2 cm diameter
	IIIc	Abdominal implants >2 cm diameter and/or positive retroperitoneal or inguinal nodes
IV		Tumor of one or both ovaries with distant metastases outside of peritoneal cavity, parenchymal liver metastases; pleural effusion, if present, must have positive cytology

(but also some mixed malignant germ cell tumors) are cystic and may present with considerable size (Fig. 31.25). Some may present as either syn- or metachronous bilateral tumors. Surgery is the treatment of choice, whether or not they contain malignant elements (Templeman and Fallat 2005). The procedure often requires oophorectomy due to size and pathologic uncertainty. However, in selected case, tumor enucleation may be possible. Every effort should be made to preserve hormonal and reproductive function in patients with bilateral benign germ cell tumors. Several authors recommend ovary-sparing procedures in patients with unilateral appearing lesions (Cass et al. 2001; Pienkowski et al. 2004). However, since many ovarian germ cell tumors have mixed histology, the approach should be cautious. If suspicion for malignancy is low and a pediatric surgeon is expert in minimal invasive surgery, a laparoscopic approach may be considered for benign lesions (Templeman and Fallat 2005; Ehrlich et al. 2007). In general, immature teratomas in children do not respond to chemotherapy (Mann et al. 2008c), so an attempt at complete resection should be undertaken. Figure 31.22 shows a large ovarian teratoma in a 2-year-old. A complete resection was accomplished. There have been reports that high-grade immature teratomas in postpubertal women may respond to chemotherapy (Norris et al. 1976). In a pediatric study of teratomas, gliomatosis peritonei was not associated with poor outcome (Göbel et al. 1998d). Any laparoscopic surgery should be done with the tumor in a bag during the removal, without rupture or morcellation of the specimen. Moreover a full exploration of the peritoneal cavity should be done. Fluid aspiration or intraabdominal spillage from prominent cystic components of the mass is often associated with minimal invasive techniques and presents the risk of tumor spread. This point represents a matter of discussion among surgeons with different experiences. An interesting surgical technique to prevent spillage of fluid during operation for huge

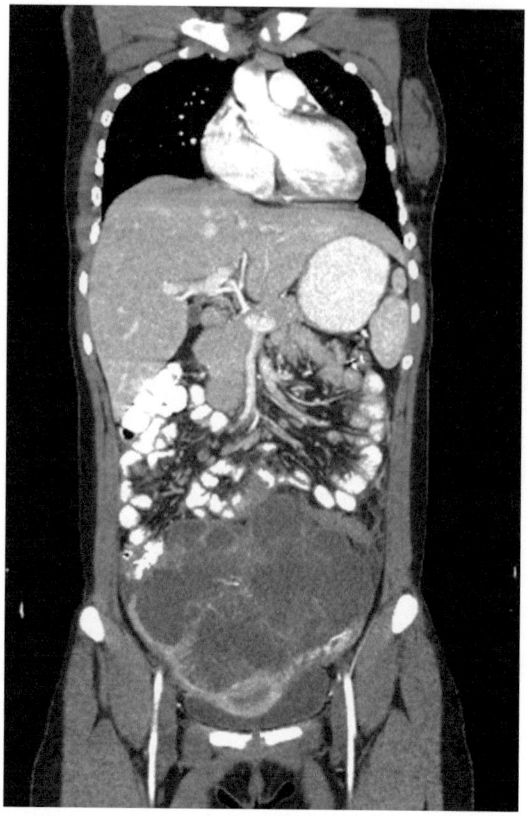

Fig. 31.25 Large ovarian dysgerminoma in an adolescent with retroperitoneal lymph node metastases

cystic tumors and to remove conservatively the mass was described by Watanabe: through a small Pfannenstiel incision maintained enlarged with a retractor, a surgical sheet is attached on the surface of the cyst to avoid fluid spread, and then the cyst is punctured and aspirated with a suction tube through the sheet, it shrinks, is brought outside, and finally a conservative resection is performed (Watanabe et al. 2013).

31.4.6.2 Yolk Sac Tumor and Embryonal Carcinoma of the Ovary

One difficulty in treating ovarian germ cell tumors is that delay in diagnosis may lead to higher-stage disease at presentation. The most common sites of metastases are lymph nodes, the peritoneal cavity, and the lungs. Patients identified as stage I may be managed with surgery and observation. This should be done under the auspices of a clinical trial. In this case overall survival should be the clinical endpoint, rather than event-free survival (tumor events to be specific). In this context, the most immanent question is, what would be an acceptable recurrence rate. In the treatment of many adults with a wide range of cancers, where observation is an option, most patients would choose as much as a 50% chance of recurrence, as a determining factor in deciding to receive chemotherapy. Are parents willing to use the same determination for their daughters? If the salvage rate is greater than 95%, observation would make sense. In this way at least 50% patients would not require toxic chemotherapy (Fig. 31.26).

The definition of stage I is important. Surgical guidelines are very specific and require careful attention to the other ovary, integrity of the capsule, spillage, and peritoneal washings. However, these strict guidelines for assessing surgical pathologic stage are often violated. This has been documented in a pediatric study (Billmire et al. 2004b). Chemotherapy was administered to all stage I and II patients and 100% survived. If chemotherapy is to be omitted, surgical guidelines as described above are an issue and should be followed. The strategy of observation with stage I ovarian tumors should be evaluated in clinical trials. Current experience of the MAKEI and the Italian studies indicates that with a watch-and-wait strategy, progression rate is approximately 20–30%, but overall survival after cisplatin combination chemotherapy is higher than 95% (Billmire et al. 2014; Terenziani et al. 2017).

If imaging studies show disease beyond the ovary, neoadjuvant chemotherapy must be administered. Subsequent surgery may be required to resect residual disease. This may be important in girls where malignant tumors are often part of a mixed tumor, containing mature or immature teratoma. Surgery is the only effective treatment for residual mature or immature teratoma. Surgery is often not required for residual gliomatosis peritonei.

Chemotherapy, as previously described in Fig. 31.6 from gonadal chapter, should be administered to all patients with stage II–IV ovarian

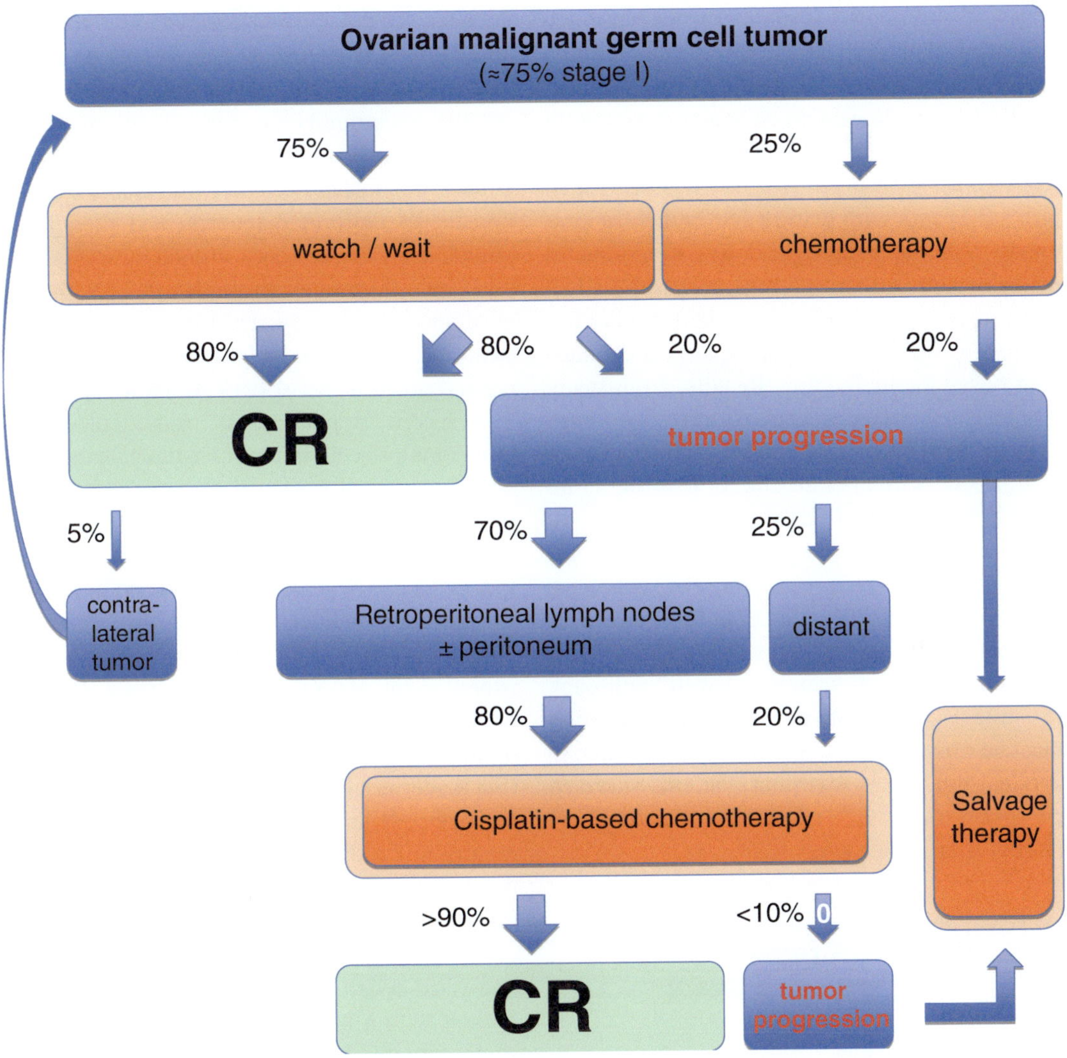

Fig. 31.26 Treatment of ovarian malignant germ cell tumors

germ cell tumor. A large ovarian yolk sac tumor with retroperitoneal nodal metastases is shown in Fig. 4. This patient responded to PEB, and a second-look surgery showed no viable tumor.

31.4.6.3 Dysgerminomas

Stage I ovarian dysgerminomas may be treated with surgery alone. Dysgerminomas of the ovary are very sensitive to chemotherapy and radiation therapy. However, radiation therapy should be avoided due to significant toxicities. It can be used in salvage strategies for recurrence. Chemotherapy regimens have been previously described in Sect. 31.1.1.

31.4.7 Prognosis

Mann et al. reported a 97% 5-year event-free survival rate in girls <15 years of age with mature teratoma and immature teratoma (Mann et al. 2008c). Patients were treated with surgery alone, and no mature or immature teratoma showed any response to chemotherapy. It is recommended that mature teratomas and immature teratomas, in girls less than 15 years of age, be managed without chemotherapy. The management of gliomatosis peritonei is less clear, and in many cases it does require resection only in case of clinical symptoms. Of note, the cellular origin of gliomatosis is distinct from teratoma, indicating that gliomatosis is rather a reactive lesion (Ferguson et al. 2001). The German MAKEI study showed no clear association with prognosis (Göbel et al. 2006). The Italian group reported a 5-year event-free survival of 91% in girls <20 years with mature and immature teratoma, with one relapse and five contralateral metachronous tumors (Terenziani et al. 2015). The prognosis of ovarian germ cell tumors has improved significantly with the advent of platinum-based chemotherapy. Results, from many international pediatric groups, have been very encouraging (Baranzelli et al. 2000b; Mann et al. 2000c; Göbel et al. 2002b; Cushing et al. 2004d; Rogers et al. 2004d; Terenziani et al. 2017). In a US intergroup study, which did not include lymph node sampling or extensive mutilating surgery, greater than 90% EFS was obtained in all stages (stages I–IV). However, if one is to attempt a "watch-and-wait" approach to stage I ovarian germ cell tumors, caution must be observed. In that US trial, adherence to surgical guidelines was poor. Patients survived because they all received chemotherapy (Billmire et al. 2004b).

31.5 Sex Cord Stromal Tumors of the Testis and Ovary

Dominik T. Schneider

Giovanni Cecchetto, and Thomas A. Olson

31.5.1 Introduction

Sex cord stromal tumors are a heterogeneous group of rare gonadal tumors. Overall, sex cord stromal tumors represent approximately 10% of all gonadal tumors during childhood. However, the true incidence of sex cord stromal tumors may be underestimated, most likely as a result of incomplete tumor registration. In the Pediatric Tumor Registry of the German Society of Pediatric Oncology and Hematology, sex cord stromal tumors contribute almost 20% to all testicular and ovarian tumors (Schneider et al. 2003b). Accordingly, a continuous rise in the registration rate of ovarian and testicular sex cord stromal tumors has been observed after the development of uniform diagnostic and therapeutic guidelines. Thus, sex cord stromal tumors constitute an illustrative example that with the development of study structures, more patients with rare tumors can be integrated into the clinical and scientific network of pediatric oncology.

Sex cord stromal tumors, in particular, juvenile granulosa cell tumors, constitute characteristic tumors of childhood. Ovarian sex cord stromal tumors may contribute up to one third of all ovarian tumors in early childhood, mainly due to the low incidence of germ cell tumors and in particular epithelial tumors in this age group. In the German MAKEI studies (children ≤5 years registered to the MAKEI studies between 1983 and 2000), there were 18 ovarian sex cord stromal tumors compared to 35 ovarian germ cell tumors (Schneider et al. 2003b). Therefore, the clinical management and scientific evaluation of these tumors in children and adolescents belong into the hands of pediatric oncologists and not to other subspecialists.

Sex cord stromal tumors develop from the non-germ-cell component of the ovary and may present with a histologic differentiation that, in some tumors, may be paradox for the host. Cellular elements, characteristic of the testis, may be seen in ovarian sex cord stromal tumors and vice versa (Young 2005c). The rarity of tumors, the heterogeneity, and the difficulty in the correct histopathologic classification of these tumors leave a significant uncertainty with regard to the correct clinical approach to patients with testicular and ovarian sex cord stromal tumors.

31.5.2 Biology

During early embryonic development (fourth week of development), the sex cords arise from the primitive genital ridge or coelomic epithelium. During female gonadal development, the germ cells retain at the periphery of the gonad, enter meiosis, and are surrounded by granulosa cells. The sex cords ultimately develop into ovarian follicles. The development of granulosa cells is dependent on the expression of the winged-helix transcription factor *FOXL2* (Schmidt et al. 2004). In male embryos, sex cords give rise to the rete testis cords that later develop into the seminiferous tubules, thus accompanying the germ cells that further migrate into the gonadal stroma and are surrounded by Sertoli cells. Sertoli cell differentiation and survival depends on the expression of the microRNA processing enzyme *DICER1* (Kim et al. 2010).

Thus, sex cord stromal tumors may develop from sex cord cells or from ovarian stromal cells of the developing gonad. Accordingly, they are histologically heterogeneous and include granulosa cell tumors, Sertoli-Leydig cell tumors, pure Sertoli cell and Leydig cell tumors, as well as theca and granulosa-theca tumors, sclerosing stromal tumors, sex cord stromal tumors with annular tubules, and gynandroblastomas with simultaneous Sertoli and granulosa cell differentiation.

Sex cord stromal tumors may develop in the context of several defined hereditary disorders. Juvenile granulosa cell tumors may be associated with multiple enchondromatosis, syn. Ollier's disease (Clement et al. 1991; Plantaz et al. 1992; Young et al. 1984a). The pathogenetic mechanism has not yet been elucidated to date. In the German series of now more than 250 sex cord stromal tumors, only three patients with Ollier's disease and juvenile granulosa cell tumor have been reported. Adult granulosa cell tumors consistently show mutations of the *FOXL2* gene, a key regulator of granulosa cell development. However, *FOXL2* mutations are only rarely found in juvenile granulosa cell tumors (Shah et al. 2009; Al-Agha et al. 2011). Notably, aberrant *FOXL2* expression may also be observed in some testicular granulosa cell tumors, although no adult but only juvenile granulosa cell tumors are observed in the testis (Kalfa et al. 2008). Otherwise, no pathognomic genetic aberration has been defined for juvenile granulosa cell tumors, but approximately one third of tumors may show point mutations of stimulatory G proteins (Kalfa et al. 2006). Moreover, the development of juvenile granulosa cell tumors appears to be associated with aberrations in wnt signaling (Boyer et al. 2009).

Genetic analysis of sporadic ovarian juvenile granulosa cell tumors with comparative genomic hybridization has not revealed frequent or characteristic chromosomal imbalances. The majority of tumors show balanced karyotypes. In approx. 25% of patients, chromosomal imbalances, such as gain of the whole chromosome 12, can be found. This analysis has not revealed any correlation between karyotype and clinical outcome (Schneider et al. 2005b). This finding is in line with a previous DNA ploidy analysis of juvenile granulosa cell tumors. In this study, almost half of the tumors showed aneuploid DNA indices. However, no correlation with clinical stage was observed (Jacoby et al. 1992).

In the last decade, it has been revealed that the second most frequent group of ovarian sex cord stromal tumors, the Sertoli-Leydig cell tumors, are consistently associated with mutations of the *DICER*1 gene, in particular, in the context of familial multinodular goiter (Rio Frio et al. 2011; Slade et al. 2011). *DICER*1 mutations are associated with pleuropulmonary blastoma (Hill et al. 2009). Of note, a significant proportion of Sertoli-Leydig cell tumor patients suffer from familial multinodular goiter (Whitcomb et al. 1986) or rarely even thyroid cancer (Poiana et al. 2010). In the German series of sex cord stromal tumors, approximately one third of patients with Sertoli-Leydig cell tumors show thyroid disease, and three have developed differentiated thyroid cancer during follow-up of Sertoli-Leydig cell tumor. A report from the US Ovarian and Testicular Sex Cord Stromal Tumor registry found germline *DICER1* mutations in approximately half of patients with Sertoli-Leydig cell tumors. In this group, a spectrum of other cancers has been reported, of which thyroid cancer was seen in 4/25 patients. Of note, thyroid cancer was also observed in two patients with DICER1 mosaicism (Schultz et al. 2017). These findings have significant impact on long-term follow-up of these patients and the surveillance of potentially affected family members (Schultz et al. 2018).

There is a pronounced association of Peutz-Jeghers syndrome with sex cord stromal tumors with annular tubules (SCTAT) of both the testis and ovary (Young et al. 1982; Young 2005b; Chang et al. 1998). Approximately one third of SCTAT appear to develop in the context of Peutz-Jeghers syndrome. These tumors usually develop at a younger age than in otherwise healthy patients, and they may develop bilaterally. In contrast, predominantly large cell calcifying Sertoli cell tumors can be found in boys with Peutz-Jeghers syndrome.

31.5.3 Pathology

Testicular and ovarian sex cord stromal tumors present as solid, sometimes lobulated, and partly cystic masses. Tumors are commonly encapsulated, and in the majority of patients, tumors do not grow beyond the gonadal capsule. Thus, testicular sex cord stromal tumors virtually always present as stage I tumors, without local or distant spread. The size of testicular sex cord stromal tumors is low and rarely exceeds 5 cm in diameter. In contrast, ovarian sex cord stromal tumors may present with considerable size. Diameters of more than 20 cm are not uncommon. Some of these large tumors may rupture spontaneously, with tumor spread within the peritoneal cavity. Approximately 5% of ovarian sex cord stromal tumors may develop bilaterally, either as simultaneous or metachronous contralateral tumors. In the context of germ line *DICER1* mutation, the risk of metachronous contralateral ovarian Sertoli Leydig cell tumor may be 10–15% (Schneider et al. 2015; Schultz et al. 2017). Some tumors may locally infiltrate the Fallopian tube. If tumor spread occurs, it is most commonly observed within the pelvis and the peritoneal cavity and to the locoregional lymph nodes. Hematogenic metastases may develop to the liver, most commonly in relapse situations. In the German MAKEI series of now more than 250 patients, apart from one patient no metastases to lungs, central nervous system, or the skeletal system have been observed. This single exception was a young adult with recurrent metastatic testicular Sertoli cell tumor.

Since no specific staging system has been developed for sex cord stromal tumors, they are usually staged according to the corresponding germ cell tumors and epithelial cancers (see Sect. 31.1). Testicular tumors are staged either according to the Lugano or COG staging system. Ovarian tumors should be staged according to the updated FIGO staging system.

Histologically, sex cord stromal tumors are categorized according to the predominant cell type of the tumor (Table 31.19) (Young 2005a, b). Of note, the histologic differentiation does not follow sex differentiation. Thus, some paradoxical differentiation patterns can be found. Characteristically, sex cord stromal tumors stain positive for inhibin, indicating that these are hormone-producing tumors (Schneider et al. 2003b). Therefore, the immunohistochemical detection of inhibin constitutes a reliable diagnostic marker that distinguishes sex cord stromal tumor from the more frequent germ cell tumors, ovarian carcinoma, or other tumors of different cellular origin (Distelmaier et al. 2006a). Tumors may also stain positive for cytokeratins and vimentin.

Granulosa cell tumors constitute the most frequent subtype of sex cord stromal tumors during childhood. In the ovary, adult and juvenile granulosa cell tumors are distinguished by their histologic appearance. Adult granulosa cell tumors only develop within the ovary. These tumors grow slowly, are diagnosed most frequently after the third decade of life, and may develop late recurrences even later than 10 years after diagnosis. In the literature, Call-Exner bodies, formed by a ring of granulosa cells with grooved nuclei

Table 31.19 Histologic differentiation of testicular and ovarian sex cord stromal tumors and their relative frequencies and characteristic age at presentation

Histology	Testis	Ovary	Age at presentation
Juvenile granulosa cell tumor (JGCT)	+++	+++	Childhood
Adult granulosa cell tumor (AGCT)	–	++	Adulthood
Sertoli-Leydig cell tumor (SLCT)	–	+++	Adolescence
Sertoli cell tumor	+++	(+)	Childhood/adulthood
Large cell calcifying Sertoli cell tumor	+++	–	Childhood
Sclerosing stroma tumor (SCLER)	–	+	Adolescence
Sex cord tumor with annular tubules (SCTAT)	–	+	Adolescence/adulthood
Steroid tumor (STER)	–	+	Adolescence/adulthood
Thecoma (THEC)	–	++	Adolescence

and central eosinophilic material, have been often considered the morphologic hallmark of these tumors. Mitotic activity is usually low, and if elevated, has been associated with higher aggressiveness of the tumor. In contrast, juvenile granulosa cell tumors do not display such Call-Exner bodies. They commonly show microfollicular structures with follicle-like structures of variable sizes that are filled with homogeneous eosinophilic material (Young et al. 1984a). Juvenile granulosa cell tumors may show nuclear atypia and high mitotic activity which may sometimes be pronounced. In tumor stage beyond Ia, high mitotic rate (≥20/10 high power fields) correlates with adverse outcome (Schneider et al. 2003a, 2004d). Juvenile granulosa cell tumors of the testis are undistinguishable from their ovarian counterparts. As they are almost exclusively diagnosed at birth or the neonatal period, it could be speculated, whether these tumors develop in the environment of female sex hormonal stimulation by the mother.

Sertoli cells constitute the characteristic component of testicular sex cord stromal tumor. Sertoli cell tumors have a peak frequency in the fourth decade of life. However, they may also be diagnosed in childhood. They present with a high variability of well, or poorly tubular, Sertoli cell aggregates. Sertoli cell tumors of childhood are well differentiated and show a favorable outcome. Large cell calcifying Sertoli cell tumors of the testis are characterized by a pronounced fibrosis that may separate the tumor cells into thin cords. Approximately, one fifth of these tumors may develop bilaterally. These tumors are typically associated with Carney's complex (Young 2005b).

Comparable tumors with pure Sertoli cell differentiation are only rarely observed in the ovary. Here, Sertoli cell differentiation is characteristically seen only within Sertoli-Leydig cell tumors, which include both cellular components (Young and Scully 1985). Of note, this tumor type is not observed within the testis. s may show a highly variable grade of differentiation. In highly differentiated s, tubular structures with Sertoli cells predominate and are accompanied by sheets of Leydig cells. As a result of hormone production, the ovarian stroma may show luteinization. Tubular structures are lost with lower grade of differentiation. Retiform and microtubular differentiation may be described, and by some authors, are considered distinct histopathologic patterns (Young et al. 1984b). In some tumors, heterologous differentiation, e.g., with intestinal epithelium, may develop. These histologic features, low differentiation, retiform pattern, and heterologous differentiation, have all been associated with adverse outcome (Young and Scully 1985).

Other very rare sex cord stromal tumors include sex cord stromal tumors with annular tubules, sclerosing stroma tumors, thecomas, and steroid cell tumors. Considering the heterogeneity of these tumors and the difficulties in distinguishing them from germ cell tumors or small cell ovarian carcinomas, a reference pathologic evaluation at an experienced paidopathologic or gynecopathologic center is strongly recommended.

Characteristic histologic samples of juvenile granulosa cell tumors are demonstrated in Figs. 31.27 and 31.28.

31.5.3.1 Clinical Presentation

Testicular sex cord stromal tumors typically present as an indolent scrotal mass. Since juvenile granulosa cell tumors often develop within the first months of life, these tumors may be present at birth. In contrast, only one in four ovarian sex cord stromal tumors are apparent as a large indolent mass (Fig. 31.29). Almost half of the patients have abdominal pain. Approximately 10% of patients present with an acute abdomen, caused either by spontaneous tumor rupture or ovarian torsion. Two thirds of ovarian sex cord stromal tumors were associated with clinical symptoms related to production of sex hormones by the tumor (Schneider et al. 2003a). Characteristically, infants and children may present with signs of isosexual precocity, including breast enlargement, pubarche, and vaginal bleeding. In postpubertal girls, tumors may lead to primary or secondary amenorrhea and unspecific signs of virilization such as pronounced acne. These are characteristic signs of Sertoli-Leydig cell tumors (Schneider et al. 2003a; Schneider et al. 2015).

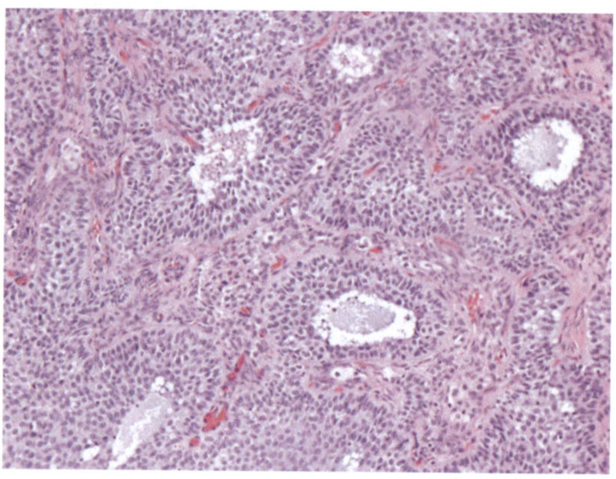

Fig. 31.27 Histologic samples from juvenile granulosa cell tumors (H+E)

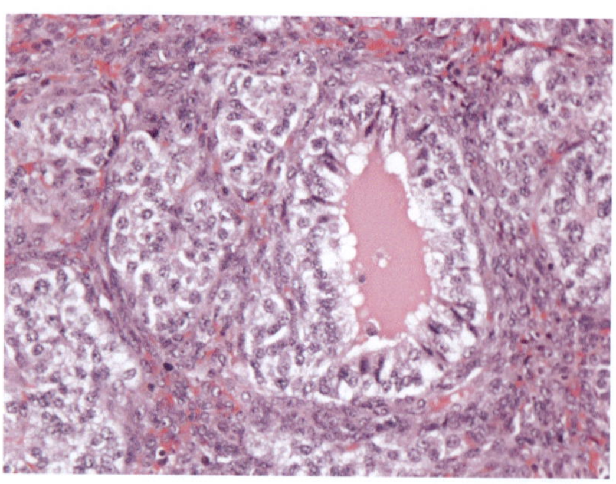

Fig. 31.28 Histologic samples from juvenile granulosa cell tumors (H+E)

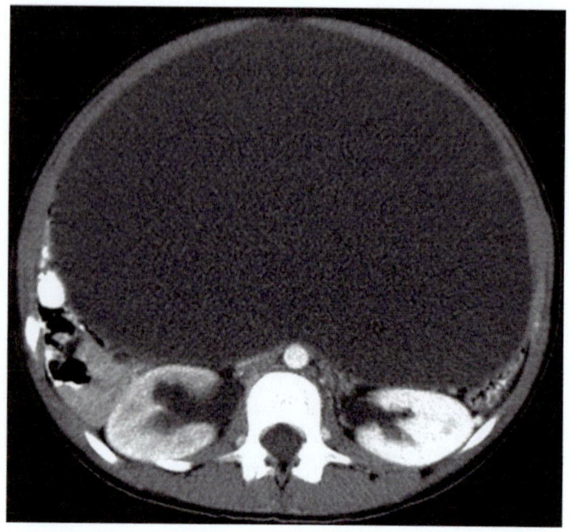

Fig. 31.29 CT scan of a large cystic juvenile granulosa cell tumor

As other steroid hormone–producing cells, sex cord stromal tumors may also produce inhibin. Free inhibin can be measured in the serum and may serve as a serological tumor marker during follow-up. However, the diagnostic value may sometimes be hampered by the physiologically broad normal range in healthy prepubertal children (Crofton et al. 2002a, b).

In some rare patients, Sertoli-Leydig cell tumors may produce AFP, which can be detected serologically. Histologically, most of these tumors resemble Sertoli-Leydig cell tumors with retiform, often hepatoid, differentiation and heterologous elements (Young et al. 1984b; Schneider et al. 2015).

31.5.4 Diagnostic Assessment and Differential Diagnosis

Due to the rarity of sex cord stromal tumors, in most patients the diagnosis of sex cord stromal tumor will not be anticipated until histologic confirmation. Nevertheless, in particular, in young children, with tumor marker (AFP, βHCG) negative gonadal tumors, sex cord stromal tumors should be considered. The diagnostic and radiographic assessment is almost identical to that of gonadal germ cell tumors (Table 31.20). Since these tumors do not metastasize beyond the abdomen, whole-body staging is not required.

Ovarian sex cord stromal tumors have to be distinguished from ovarian germ cell tumors, epithelial ovarian cancer, the rare small cell carcinoma of the hypercalcemic type, and gonadal tumors of different histogenesis, such as leukemia/lymphoma or sarcoma. Tumors presenting with vaginal bleeding in infants must be discriminated from the rare vaginal yolk sac tumors. Clinically, the evaluation of serologic tumor markers alpha-fetoprotein (AFP) and β-human chorionic gonadotropin helps in the differential diagnosis of secreting malignant germ cell tumors. Therefore, it is mandatory to measure these tumor markers preoperatively (Schneider et al. 2001h).

In some rare patients, the distinction of juvenile granulosa cell tumors from small cell ovarian carcinoma of the hypercalcemic type may be particularly difficult, since the latter may mimic the pseudofollicular growth pattern characteristic of JGCTs (Distelmaier et al. 2006b). In these situations, the immunohistochemical detection of inhibin constitutes an important diagnostic hallmark of ovarian sex cord stromal tumors. Inhibin positivity has not been observed in small cell ovarian carcinoma, while virtually all sex cord stroma tumors stain positive (Schneider et al. 2003b); in addition, SMARCA4 expression is a reliable immunohistochemical marker of ovarian small cell carcinoma (Conlon et al. 2016).

Lastly, mutation testing for *DICER1* should be performed in Sertoli-Leydig cell tumors within clinical studies. The prognostic impact of germline or somatic *DICER1* mutation on the individual tumor is unclear. However, germline or mosaic mutation of *DICER1* is associated with the risk of metachronous contralateral tumors, thyroid disease, thyroid cancer, and other tumors of the *DICER1* spectrum (Rio Frio et al. 2011; Slade et al. 2011; Schultz et al. 2017). Thus, the mutational status has significant impact on the surveillance of patients and potentially affected family members (Schultz et al. 2018).

31.5.5 Treatment and Prognostic Markers: Review of the Literature

The current literature includes only a few and mostly retrospective series of patients with testicular sex cord stromal tumors. Most publications focus on adult patients with sex cord stromal tumors or represent case reports and small patient cohorts, collected at single centers. This may be explained by the lack of cooperative study structures for sex cord stromal tumors, as have successfully been established for germ cell tumors. Thus, many patients have been registered on either the corresponding national germ cell tumor trial or the national rare tumor study group.

The largest series of ovarian sex cord stromal tumors has been reported by the German MAKEI study group and from the European Cooperative Study Group on Pediatric Rare Tumors (EXPeRT) (Schneider et al. 2003a, b, 2015). These series have focused on the pathologic differential diagnosis and prognostic factors (Schneider et al. 2003b) and the prognostic impact of staging (Schneider et al. 2003a, 2004d, 2015). In this and other studies, the favorable outcome of completely resected stage I ovarian sex cord stromal tumors has been demonstrated (Cecchetto et al. 2011; Kalfa et al. 2005). In stage Ic or higher (i.e., microscopic tumor spread), prognosis was inferior if tumors ruptured spontaneously (FIGO stage Ic2) or showed malignant ascites (FIGO stage Ic3) compared to those with only intraoperative tumor violation, e.g., during laparoscopic surgery (FIGO stage Ic1) (Schneider et al. 2004d). In stage Ic or higher, pronounced mitotic activity (>20 mitoses per 10 high power

Table 31.20 Specific diagnostic strategy in testicular or ovarian sex cord stromal tumors

Procedure	Specific questions
Clinical assessment	
Medical history	Gynecological and pubertal history? Vaginal bleeding, breast development, etc.? Thyroid disease? Inherited syndromes (Mb. Ollier's, Peutz-Jeghers, etc.)? Family history: tumors if the DICER1 spectrum? Thyroid disease? Multinodular goiter?
Phys. examination	Pubertal status, goiter, abdominal pain
Laboratory assessment	
AFP, β-HCG	Malignant germ cell tumor with yolk sac tumor (consider age-related reference values) or choriocarcinoma.
	Note: Approx. 10% of Sertoli-Leydig cell tumors may show AFP levels up to 1000 μg/L
Inhibin	Serological marker of hormone-secreting sex cord stromal tumors
Estrogen, DHEAS, LH, FSH	Endocrinological assessment
Clinical chemistry incl. calcium	Calcium may be elevated in ovarian small cell carcinoma (but also in rare germ cell or sex cord stromal tumors)
Creatinine clearance/cystatin c	Assessment of renal function (in case of chemotherapy)
Radiographic assessment	
Ultrasound	Tumor size and extension in three dimensions, anatomical relation to ovary/testis and fallopian tube/spermatic cord, lymph node, or liver metastases
Abdominal and pelvic MRI	Tumor size and extension in three dimensions, anatomical relation to ovary/testis and fallopian tube/spermatic cord, lymph node, or liver metastases
Chest X-ray	Lung metastases (extremely unlikely)
Note: Metastases beyond the abdomen are exceedingly rare. Therefore, extended radiographic assessment is required in case of clinical symptoms only	
Histologic assessment	
H&E	Classification and grading of differentiation according to WHO
Mitotic rate per 10 HPF	Prognostic assessment (in particular, juvenile granulose cell tumors)
Inhibin	Positive for sex cord stromal tumors
AFP	Yolk sac tumor, may also be positive in retiform Sertoli-Leydig cell tumors

fields) was also associated with adverse outcome, at least for juvenile granulosa cell tumors. In Sertoli Leydig cell tumors, histological grade of differentiation correlated with outcome. Thus, patients with poor differentiation, retiform pattern, or presence of heterologous elements had an event-free survival below 50% (Schneider et al. 2015). In this group, stage Ic1 was also associated with poor outcome. In stages II–III, the impact of cisplatin-based chemotherapy in accordance to current germ cell tumor protocols has been demonstrated (Schneider et al. 2002c, 2015; Cecchetto et al. 2011; Schultz et al. 2017).

This experience is further supported by case reports that argue for adjuvant chemotherapy in advanced stage juvenile granulosa cell tumors. Colombo reported on a girl with a stage III juvenile granulosa cell tumor that achieved complete remission for at least 7 months after PVB chemotherapy (Colombo et al. 1986). Powell reported on a 13-year-old primigravida with a stage IIIb juvenile granulosa cell tumor that was successfully treated with a combination of methotrexate, actinomycin, and chlorambucil. The patient has remained in complete remission for 7 years, during which time, she gave birth to further children. The same authors reported on two stage III tumors successfully treated with surgical debulking and carboplatin and etoposide. In addition, a patient with recurrent juvenile granulosa cell tumor with liver metastases achieved complete remission for 44 months after surgery and six cycles of bleomycin and Taxol (Powell and Otis 1997; Powell et al. 1993, 2001).

The largest published series, focusing specifically on ovarian juvenile granulosa cell tumors, analyzed 125 adolescent and adult patients, with follow-up data in 83 patients (Young et al. 1984a). In this series, there were only two relapses among 80 stage I tumors, but all three stage II tumors were fatal. Additional clinical and histologic parameters did not contribute to the prognostic assessment. The largest series of Sertoli-Leydig cell tumors has been reported by the same study group and included 207 patients. Follow-up information was available in 164 patients (Young and Scully 1985). Outcome correlated with both stage and histologic differentiation, and both parameters closely correlated with each other. All well-differentiated Sertoli-Leydig cell tumors behaved clinically benign, whereas 11% of Sertoli-Leydig cell tumors with intermediate differentiation and 59% of poorly differentiated Sertoli-Leydig cell tumors (all stages II-III) showed a malignant course. In particular, those tumors with retiform differentiation and/or heterologous elements were unfavorable.

Two significant studies by the French Pediatric Oncology Group each report on 40 ovarian juvenile granulosa cell tumors treated between 1965 and 1990, and 1990 and 2004, respectively (Kalfa et al. 2005; Plantaz et al. 1992). The authors report that young (prepubertal) age appears to correlate with more favorable diagnosis, in particular, if early diagnosis is established based on assessment of isosexual precocity. However, delayed diagnosis is associated with a higher risk of tumor ruptures and higher tumor stage. Thus, manifestation with acute abdominal pain correlated with adverse outcome, both in prepubertal children and in postpubertal adolescents.

Data on pediatric Sertoli-Leydig cell tumors in children and adolescents are even more limited. Recently an international cooperative analysis of EXPeRT has been performed, which included 44 patients from Poland, Italy, France, and Germany (Schneider et al. 2015). In this analysis, event-free survival was 0.7 and overall survival 0.87, which is inferior to that observed in juvenile granulosa cell tumors. Again, outcome was excellent in completely resected (stage Ia) tumors. Four metachronous contralateral tumors have been reported in this cohort. In contrast, almost half of patients with microscopic spread (e.g., malignant ascites, preoperative rupture) or even only intraoperative tumor rupture relapsed. Metastases are rare at diagnosis, and are found in approximately 10% of patients. Metastatic disease can successfully be managed with cisplatin-based chemotherapy (e.g., PEI).

Current literature indicates that the prognosis of testicular sex cord stromal tumors is excellent (Cecchetto et al. 2011; Harms and Kock 1997). Virtually, no patients develop metastases. If they do, these tumors show poorly differentiated histology and require aggressive therapy, comparable to that for metastatic germ cell tumors (Ross et al. 2002). Thus, if a metastatic testicular sex cord stromal tumor is diagnosed, the histopathologic diagnosis should first be questioned and be specified by reference evaluation. In the German series and in all currently published pediatric series, only very rare recurrences or fatal outcomes have been reported.

31.5.6 Proposed Therapeutic Strategy

It should be considered that the following recommendation is not based on prospective randomized trials but represents the experience gained in comparably small prospective series of patients. Basically, the following strategy is based on the concept of the MAKEI study, which has also been adopted as a consensus and guidance for the US ovarian and testicular sex cord stromal tumor registry (Table 31.21). The therapeutic algorithm separates patients by tumor site, stage, and histologic parameters. The uniform treatment stratification, the incorporation of uniform central pathology review, and the central evaluation and documentation of clinical data may hopefully facilitate validation and further optimization of therapy of these rare tumors.

31.5.6.1 Testicular Sex Cord Stromal Tumors

Since virtually all tumors present as localized stage I tumors, resection will constitute the only therapy of these tumors (Cecchetto et al. 2010). In principle, orchiectomy after high inguinal

Table 31.21 Proposed therapeutic algorithm in testicular and ovarian sex cord stromal tumors

Site	Stage	Histology	Neoadjuvant chemotherapy	Surgical therapy	Adjuvant chemotherapy
Testis	I	All	–	Inguinal orchiectomy	Watch & wait
	>I	All	–	Inguinal orchiectomy	≥4 × PEI/BEP
Ovary	Ia	All	–	Ovariectomy	Watch & wait
	Ic1-Ic3	Sertoli-Leydig	–		4 × PEI/BEP
	Ic1	JGCT, others	–		Watch & wait
	Ic2, Ic3		–		3-4 × PEI/BEP
	II–III	All	PEI/BEP	Adenectomy	>4 × PEI/BEP[a]

[a]A total of 5–6 cycles of chemotherapy including preoperative chemotherapy is recommended

incision and ligation of the spermatic cord constitutes the gold standard. Considering the overall favorable diagnosis, there has been some debate as to whether tumor excision after scrotal excision and even organ sparing surgery (e.g., enucleation of the tumor) may also be appropriate. However, it should be noted that this strategy has not been validated prospectively. Moreover, it remains questionable whether organ-sparing surgery may indeed contribute to further reproductive function and quality of life (Tröbs et al. 2007). The extremely rare metastatic tumor should be treated according to the corresponding concept for ovarian sex cord stromal tumors.

31.5.6.2 Ovarian Sex Cord Stromal Tumors

In all patients, the tumor resection (tumor ovariectomy/tumor adenectomy) constitutes both a diagnostic and therapeutic procedure. The surgical resection should follow the same principles as that for malignant germ cell tumors. The MAKEI data do not indicate that radical retroperitoneal lymph node resection or extended lymph node sampling is required in all ovarian sex cord stromal tumors, because lymph node metastases have been observed only rarely and most commonly in (extended) relapse situations. However, if lymph node metastases are detected (e.g., in relapse situations), all visible metastases should be resected. Ideally, this should be done after preoperative chemotherapy. The German, French, Italian, and US data presented above suggest that no adjuvant therapy is necessary in stage Ia tumors.

The data reported by the German MAKEI study group represents the first cohort of patients prospectively registered and treated according to a uniform strategy. Based on these data, a risk stratification for adjuvant chemotherapy can be proposed for patients with stage Ic, II, or III tumors:

31.5.6.3 Stage Ic

In stage Ic, the decision to add adjuvant chemotherapy is most difficult. Tumors in which a microscopic tumor spread is suspected or proven (but no pathologic evidence of peritoneal metastases) are classified as stage Ic. According to FIGO, tumors may be classified as stage Ic for several reasons: A preoperative tumor rupture may have occurred (Ic2), and in others the cytological analysis of peritoneal washings or ascites provides evidence of malignant tumor cells (Ic3). In contrast, a tumor may also be classified stage Ic if the tumor has been punctured or the capsule has otherwise been violated in situ (Ic1). In this case the tumor capsule must be intact prior to surgery (intraoperative violation of tumor capsule).

The previous analysis of a cohort of patients, which predominantly included juvenile granulosa cell tumors, has demonstrated that intraoperative violation of the tumor capsule (Ic1) does not increase risk of recurrence. In contrast, a high relapse rate (comparable to stages II–III) has been observed in those patients whose tumor has been ruptured prior to surgery or if the ascites contain malignant cells (Ic2, 3).

This observation indicates that thorough documentation and critical evaluation of the clinical and surgical report are mandatory. Cytological analysis of ascites/peritoneal washings is indispensable. In cases with incomplete documentation or missing cytological evaluation, the assessment of the proliferative activity of the tumors may help with regard to risk assessment, but nevertheless a higher grade of uncertainty remains. In the current experience of the MAKEI study, the application of four cycles of cisplatin-based chemotherapy is sufficient to control microscopic tumor spread. In Germany, PEI (see Sect. 31.1, Table 31.4) is recommended. In other countries, PEB is applied according to the respective national germ cell tumor protocol. There are no data supporting which regimen is more effective. Data on carboplatin are limited.

As mentioned above, this experience is based on the analysis of cohorts that predominantly included juvenile granulosa cell tumors. The most current analysis, specifically focusing on Sertoli-Leydig cell tumors, has demonstrated that these may develop recurrences even after only minute intraoperative tumor violation (Schneider et al. 2015). Most of these recurrent tumors show additional prognostically unfavorable features such as low histologic differentiation, retiform pattern, or heterologous elements. Thus, the decision in favor of or against chemotherapy remains individual; however, the approach for these tumors obviously has to be more aggressive than that for juvenile granulosa cell tumors.

31.5.6.4 Stages II–III

In stages II–III, micro- or macroscopic spread with peritoneal or lymph node metastases has occurred. It is very obvious that surgical treatment alone will not be curative but must be supplemented with adjuvant chemotherapy. In the past, cure of ovarian sex cord stromal tumors has been reported in single cases only (Kudelka et al. 1998; Powell and Otis 1997; Powell et al. 1993, 2001). The MAKEI study group was the first to report a series of patients with advanced tumor stage, who were treated with adjuvant cisplatin-based combination chemotherapy (Calaminus et al. 1997b; Wessalowski et al. 1995; Schneider et al. 2002c). In these series on advanced juvenile granulosa cell tumors, high proliferative activity distinguishes patients with poor prognosis. In addition to proliferative index, age also appears prognostic (Schneider et al. 2003a; Kalfa et al. 2005; Plantaz et al. 1992).

There are several issues that remain to be addressed critically. The indication for chemotherapy and the minimum amount of chemotherapy necessary in stage Ic tumors are ill-defined. The German data suggest that among stage Ic patients, a subgroup of patients at high risk can be identified through histologic assessment. These patients may be suitable for adjuvant chemotherapy. In the French study group, all patients with stage Ic1 or higher received adjuvant chemotherapy, also juvenile granulosa cell tumors stage Ic1, which would be followed expectantly in Germany. Moreover, the limited data available from our analysis does not allow definition of the required amount of chemotherapy for tumors at stage Ic or higher. In the Germany study, all patients with stage II to III tumors received at least four cycles. Considering other studies with less favorable outcome, we would not advocate less but rather argue for extension to six cycles. Although to a certain extent, chemotherapeutic regimens varied with the consecutive MAKEI protocols. All but one patient received chemotherapy that included cisplatin and etoposide, mostly as part of three-agent regimens. Therefore, it appears meaningful to include these two drugs into a three-agent combination regimen such as cisplatin, etoposide, and ifosfamide (PEI).

Lastly, alternative strategies must be developed for refractory tumors. In our experience, regional deep hyperthermia has resulted in complete remissions in recurrent or refractory OSCST, although experience with this approach is limited and responses did not translate into durable remissions longer than 2 years (Wessalowski et al. 1995).

31.5.7 A Call for International Collaboration

Sex cord stromal tumors are currently registered to germ cell tumor trials or rare tumor registries in a minority of countries. However, these tumors constitute a potentially deadly threat. It is mandatory to develop international networks for counseling, scientific evaluation, and validation of therapeutic concepts. The authors have been continuously contacted for consultation on a significant numbers of patients. However, if the data of these patients are not collected centrally and if the involved requesting partner does not provide follow-up data, this valuable clinical information will be lost to the scientific community. Future patients will not benefit from the experience gained in other patients in comparable, rare situations.

31.6 Ovarian Adenomas, Ovarian Carcinoma, and Ovarian Small Cell Carcinoma

Dominik T. Schneider

dominik.schneider@klinikumdo.de and Thomas A. Olson

thomas.olson@choa.orgKlinik für Kinder- und Jugendmedizin, Clinic of Pediatrics

DortmundGermanyDivision Pediatric Hematology/Oncology

Children's Healthcare of Atlanta at Egleston

AtlantaGAUSA

31.6.1 Introduction

In addition to the more common ovarian germ cell tumors and sex cord stromal tumors, there are several less frequent and poorly studied pediatric epithelial ovarian tumors. Their clinical spectrum varies from benign adenomas and borderline tumors to adenocarcinoma and highly aggressive tumors, such as ovarian small cell carcinoma of the hypercalcemic type (OSCCHT). The latter was first defined as a distinct entity 30 years ago (Dickersin et al. 1982). It may be the most aggressive ovarian tumor during childhood and adolescence. Until recently, OCCCHT has been considered almost inevitably fatal.

All these tumors usually fail to be identified in tumor registries. A remarkable gap between true incidence and registration exists. An epidemiological analysis of the North American Association of Cancer Registries revealed that in children younger than 15 years, ovarian carcinomas are three times more common than sex cord stromal tumors. In adolescents from 15 to 19 years of age, they were almost as common as germ cell tumors (Young Jr. et al. 2003). These epidemiologic data stand in contrast to the little experience reported in the literature. To a certain degree, this discrepancy can be attributed to the circumstance that epithelial ovarian tumors are not routinely registered on pediatric prospective studies of gonadal tumors, where the main focus is germ cell tumors. Even in a large pediatric oncologic ovarian tumor registry, the German MAKEI registry, an average of two to three epithelial or carcinomatous ovarian tumors is reported per year. This compares to more than ten sex cord stromal tumors. Moreover, with the implementation of the German Rare Tumor Registry (STEP), reporting of epithelial cancers has increased significantly. Other international pediatric study groups that register ovarian tumors experience comparably low registration rates, too. This observation can be explained by the circumstance that these children and adolescents are seen, treated, and followed up by gynecologists. As a result, they are not evaluated by pediatric oncologists. Nevertheless, pediatric oncologists are often consulted, in particular, when these patients present with advanced or recurrent disease. It is clearly important to early identify those patients that are at the highest risk to develop fatal disease. The best example might be OSCCHT, since these patients have to be treated intensively at any stage of disease.

31.6.2 Clinical Presentation and Diagnostic Assessment

Ovarian cystadenomas, borderline tumors, and most ovarian carcinomas present with local symptoms such as local swelling, obstipation, dysuria, or abdominal pain. Ovarian torsion or spontaneous rupture may mimic acute abdomen, necessitating emergency procedures. Paraneoplastic symptoms are rarely observed. Approximately, two thirds of OSCCHT may present with significant hypercalcemia, sometimes leading to renal failure. However, other ovarian neoplasms, such as dysgerminoma, may also be associated with hypercalcemia, though less frequently (Young et al. 1994) (Table 31.22).

On histopathologic examination, most epithelial tumors present as cystic adenomas (cystadenomas) or borderline tumors. True classical ovarian carcinomas may be diagnosed, too. The majority of these tumors present at a low local stage. In contrast, OSCCHT may present with extensive intra-abdominal metastases. Two thirds of patients with OSCCHT may exhibit a paraneoplastic hypercalcemia. OSCCHT is predominantly a unilateral tumor that most commonly affects young women in the second and third decade of life. Less than 30% of tumors develop in patients younger than 20 years of age and less than 1% in children. The youngest patient, reported to date, has been 14 months (Florell et al. 1999; Young et al. 1994).

The diagnostic work-up is comparable to ovarian germ cell tumors and sex cord stromal tumors (see Sect. 31.1.4, Table 31.17; Sect. 31.1.5, Table 31.19). The immunohistochemical evidence of loss or SMARCA4 (and SMARCA2) protein expression is helpful in identifying OSCCHT (N. Conlon et al. 2016). It should be followed by genetic counseling and mutation analysis of SMARCA4, both in the tumor and the germ line. The latter could be associated with

Table 31.22 Diagnostic assessment in ovarian epithelial tumors and ovarian small cell carcinoma, hypercalcemic type

Procedure	Specific questions
Clinical assessment:	
Medical history	Gynecological and pubertal history? Vaginal bleeding, breast development, etc.? Familial cancer (ovary, breast)? Other OSCCHT?
Phys. examination	Pubertal status, abdominal pain
Laboratory assessment:	
– AFP, ß-HCG	Malignant germ cell tumor with yolk sac tumor (consider age-related reference values) or choriocarcinoma;
	Note: Some Sertoli-Leydig cell tumors may show AFP levels up to 1000 µg/L
– Inhibin	Serological marker of hormone secreting sex cord stromal tumors
– Estrogen, DHEAS, LH, FSH	Endocrinological assessment
– Clinical chemistry incl. calcium	Calcium may be elevated in ovarian small cell carcinoma (but also in rare germ cell or sex cord stromal tumors)
– Creatinine clearance/cystatin c	Assessment of renal function (in case of chemotherapy, renal impairment may occur as a complication of hypercalcemia)
Radiographic assessment:	
Ultrasound	Tumor size and extension in three dimensions, anatomical relation to ovary/testis and fallopian tube/spermatic cord, lymph node, or liver metastases
Abdominal and pelvic MRI	Tumor size and extension in three dimensions, anatomical relation to ovary/testis and fallopian tube/spermatic cord, lymph node, or liver metastases
Chest X-ray	Lung metastases (extremely unlikely)
Note: OSCCHT may show metastases beyond the abdomen. Therefore, extended radiographic assessment is required in case of clinical symptoms	
Histologic assessment:	
H&E	Classification and grading according to WHO
Vimentin, cytokeratin SMARCA2, SMARCA4	Double positive in OSCCHT Loss of protein expression
Inhibin	Positive for sex cord stromal tumors, negative in ov. carcinomas
AFP, β-HCG *Genetic assessment: SMARCA4*	Exclusion of secreting germ cell tumors Mutation (tumor, potentially germ line)

familial cases of OSCCHT (A. Berchuck et al. 2015; Distelmaier et al. 2006b).

Tumor markers AFP and β-HCG serve to help exclude the diagnosis of malignant nondysgerminomatous germ cell tumors. Inhibin, androgens, and estrogens are within the normal range in epithelial tumors. CA125 is the characteristic tumor marker and can be utilized for follow-up monitoring. However, CA125 elevation may also be observed in germ cell tumors and sex cord stromal tumors (personal observation) or in benign conditions such as pregnancy, endometriosis, or Crohn's disease (Robertson et al. 2002).

Radiographic assessment includes abdominal ultrasound, supplemented with magnetic resonance tomography. The pattern of lymph node metastases may vary by site. Left ovarian tumors primarily metastasize to lymph nodes in the renal hilum, whereas right ovarian tumors metastasize to paracaval lymph nodes. A chest X-ray is indicated to exclude rare lung metastases. In OSCCHT, a brain MRI and bone scan should be performed if patients show clinical signs of skeletal or neurological involvement. The role of PET-CT in OSCCHT is unclear.

In case of classical ovarian carcinoma, the family history should specifically focus on a history of breast cancer. Genetic counseling and testing for BRCA gene mutations should be considered. However, one should be aware that OSCCHT might also occur in families without evidence of BRCA mutations (Distelmaier et al. 2006b) (Lamovec et al. 1995; Longy et al. 1996). In the German pediatric series, two pairs of siblings have been observed among a total of currently 18 patients.

The differential diagnosis of pelvic masses includes benign ovarian cysts, other ovarian tumors, and benign or malignant masses that develop from the bowel, urinary tract, or other pelvic structures. The most difficult diagnosis of cystadenomas may be benign ovarian cysts. Ovarian cysts are often asymptomatic and are detected accidentally during ultrasound. In a large series including more than 1800 prepubertal patients, ovarian cysts were detected in 5% of patients (Millar et al. 1993). However, benign cysts rarely exceed 5 cm in diameter and often show spontaneous regression during follow-up. In contrast, ovarian tumors are most commonly diagnosed with a diameter of greater than 10. The spectrum of differential diagnoses of ovarian cysts in postpubertal adolescents is broader and includes pregnancy, tubal lesions, and genital obstruction, such as imperforate hymen.

Pathologic examination follows the same principles as for ovarian germ cell and sex cord stromal tumors. It should be noted that prior to the availability of SMARCA4 immunohistochemistry and genetic testing, the majority of OSCCHTs have first been misdiagnosed (Distelmaier et al. 2006b). Therefore, consultation with a reference pathologist should be considered for all ovarian tumors, ideally prior to the start of chemotherapy.

On histopathologic examination, OSCCHTs show a solid growth pattern with admixed pseudofollicular structures and occasional areas of necrosis and hemorrhage (Fig. 31.30). The mitotic rate is usually high with an average of 23 mitoses of 10 high power fields (range 17–29/10 HPF) in the German series. Some tumors are classified as a large cell variant. Others may show a pronounced hemangiopericytic growth pattern or pronounced rhabdoid features. The most important and difficult histopathologic differential diagnosis is juvenile granulosa cell tumor, which in contrast to OSCCHT, shows inhibin positivity (Schneider et al. 2003c). All OSCCHT centrally examined at the German Childhood Tumor Registry stained negative for inhibin, alpha-fetoprotein, human placental like alkaline phosphatase, and beta-human chorionic gonadotropin upon immunohistochemical examination. Characteristically, the tumors show co-expression of cytokeratins and vimentin, and loss of expression of SMARCA4 protein.

Fig. 31.30 Ovarian small cell carcinoma of the hypercalcemic type in a 16-year-old girl (H&E, 400×). Histologically, the tumor is characterized by sheets of closely packed, small cells with scanty cytoplasm forming scattered follicle-like structures, and the morphologic similarity to sex cord stromal and germ cell tumors may pose significant problems in establishing the correct diagnosis

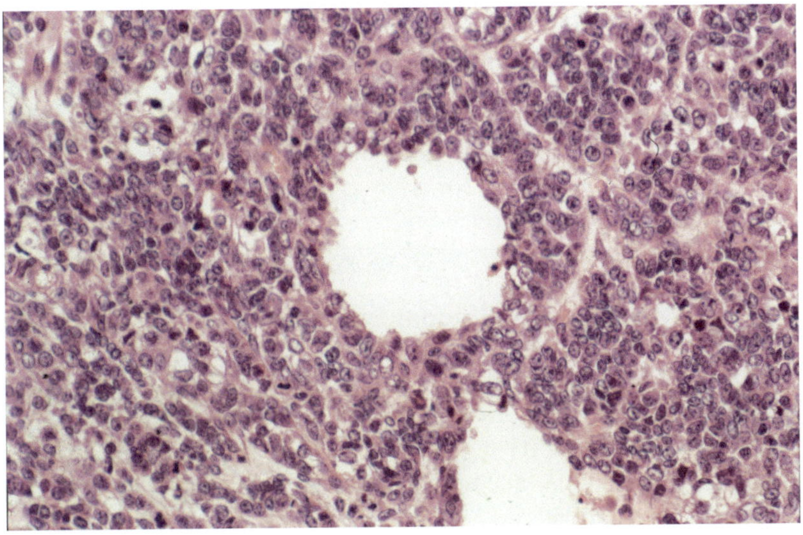

Fig. 31.30 Ovarian small cell carcinoma of the hypercalcemic type in a 16-year-old girl (H&E, 400×). Histologically, the tumor is characterized by sheets of closely packed, small cells with scanty cytoplasm forming scattered follicle-like structures, and the morphologic similarity to sex cord stromal and germ cell tumors may pose significant problems in establishing the correct diagnosis

Tumors are staged according to the International Federation of Gynecology and Obstetrics (FIGO) staging system (Benedet et al. 2000; Prat and FIGO COGO 2015) (see Sect. 31.1.4, Table 31.18).

31.6.3 Therapy

In cystadenomas, borderline tumors, and carcinomas, complete tumor resection constitutes the cornerstone of treatment. In most gynecology-oncology centers, tumor resection is done laparoscopically. However, this technique has not been validated in children and adolescents with ovarian tumors. No prospective studies have compared conservative and laparoscopic approaches in children and adolescents. The tumor-bearing ovary is removed in most patients. Again, organ-sparing surgery is not validated in children and adolescents. However, in bilateral tumors, it remains the only (but still experimental) approach to conserve fertility. During surgery, it must be decided whether the fallopian tube has to be removed, too. Since most tumors are limited to the ovary, routine adenectomy and hysterectomy are not justified. Given the perspective of chemosensitive tumors, hysterectomy is obsolete in children and adolescents; however, it is still within the range of recommendations for OSCCHT.

Normalization of renal function must be the first therapeutic intervention when OSCCHT presents with hypercalcemia. This can be achieved with aggressive hydration and diuretic therapy with furosemide. In OSCCHT, complete resection is a prerequisite for cure. However, resection alone is often not sufficient for definite cure: In the German series, all four stage I patients, followed according to a watch-and-wait strategy, relapsed (Distelmaier et al. 2006b). In the report by Young, less than 10% of adolescent stage I patients survived (Young et al. 1994). Given the poor prognosis of OSCCHT and the fact that to date, no published patients with successful pregnancy have been presented, radical surgery is still advocated. In SMARCA4 germline mutated OSCCHT, there is also some debate on the need of prophylactic removal of the contralateral ovary, both in index patients and in affected family members. However, the optimal age for prophylactic removal is still unclear. Therefore, a combined therapy including oophorectomy and oocyte preservation has been proposed (Berchuck et al. 2015).

Ovarian cystadenomas and borderline tumors usually present as stage I tumors and require no additional adjuvant therapy. Metastatic ovarian carcinomas are most commonly treated with a combination of carboplatin and Taxol, in accordance to current gyne-oncology protocols. The pediatric experience in these tumors is limited. During the last decade, nine cystadenomas and borderline tumors as well as two ovarian carcinomas have been reported to the German study group. All were stage one and have been observed without adjuvant treatment. No relapses were reported (unpublished information).

31.6.4 Review on Multimodal Therapy of OSCHHT in Adults and Children

The prognosis of OSCCHT is generally believed to be poor and almost inevitably fatal. In the largest series reported to date, event-free survival was 33% in stage Ia, 10% in stage Ic, and 6.5% in stages II–IV. Notably, half the registered patients showed abdominal or peritoneal tumor spread, corresponding to FIGO stages II–III. In addition, young age was associated with a particularly poor prognosis, even in low-stage tumors. Less than 10% of children and adolescents with stage IA OSCCHT survived (Young et al. 1994).

The ideal multimodal treatment for OSCCHT has not yet been defined. However, it is apparent from the abovementioned data that treatment of this tumor type requires a multimodal aggressive approach.

Senekjian et al. first reported on five patients with ovarian small cell carcinomas treated with a combination of vinorelbine, cisplatin, cyclophosphamide, bleomycin, Adriamycin, and etoposide (Senekjian et al. 1989). Despite initial promising responses to chemotherapy, four of five patients died of disease.

In the largest series on OSCCHT, Young et al. mention that the most patients received some form of adjuvant chemotherapy (Young et al. 1994). However, detailed information on only seven patients with favorable response to therapy, either during first- or second-line therapy, is provided. As outlined in Table 31.23, patients received combination chemotherapy with various regimens that included anthracyclins, etoposide, cisplatin, and alkylating agents. Three patients had radiation therapy. One of the seven patients is in first complete remission (CR). Three are in second CR. One is alive with disease and two are dead (Table 31.23) (Young et al. 1994). However, this report includes no information regarding the single and cumulative doses of either radio- or chemotherapy. Therefore, no specific conclusions can be drawn other than that some selected patients may benefit from adjuvant therapy.

Additional detailed and more encouraging information can be retrieved from the more recent report by Harrison et al. which included 17 adult patients treated in Australia, Canada, and Europe between 1989 and 2004 (Table 31.23) (Harrison et al. 2006). Ten patients had stage I tumors, six with stage III, and one patient with an unknown tumor stage. Surgical resection included oophorectomy (six patients), unilateral adenectomy (three patients), or hysterectomy with (bilateral) adenectomy (seven patients). After surgery and prior to the start of adjuvant chemotherapy, three patients had tumor residues larger than 1 cm. In accordance with recommendation discussed above, all patients received adjuvant chemotherapy regardless of initial tumor stage. The main drugs are listed in Table 31.23. Briefly, cisplatin-based regimens, in combination with etoposide according to strategies applied in malignant germ cell tumors, were administered. Notably, Taxol-based regimens, which are commonly used in other types of ovarian carcinoma, did not prove successful. Only one of eight patients treated with Taxol remains in continuous remission. This finding is in line with the observation, from the German series, that Taxol demonstrates only limited efficacy both in first-line and salvage therapy. The authors conclude that radiotherapy has a significant therapeutic impact. In their experience, the outcome of stage I tumors was better after irradiation. However, there is one patient, who received radiation, with active disease 8 months after diagnosis. In stage III tumors, no comparable observation supporting the impact of radiotherapy has been made.

A French study group reported on 27 adolescent and adult OSCCHT patients treated with a combination of cisplatin, Adriamycin, cyclophosphamide, and etoposide, then consolidated with high-dose chemotherapy and autologous

Table 31.23 Summary of therapeutic regimen administered in series using conventional chemotherapy ± radiotherapy but without high dose chemotherapy (this table includes only drugs included in the first-line chemotherapy)

Study	No	Stage	Irradiation	Taxol	Platin derivates	VP-16	Alkylat. Agents	Anthra-cyclins	Best status	Outcome	Follow-up (months)
Young[a]	1	Ia	+	–	+	–	–	–	CR	CR-2	45
	2	Ia	–	–	+	–	–	–	CR	CR-2	53
	3	Ia	–	–	+	+	–	+	CR	DOD	81
	4	IIb	+	–	+	+	+	+	CR	CR-2	84
	5	III	+	–	–	–	–	–	CR	DOD	66
	6	III	–	–	+	+	+	+	CR	AWD	24
	7	III	–	–	+	+	–	+	CR	NED	30
Harrison	1	I	–	–	+	+	–	–	CR	NED	10
	2	Ia	45 Gy	–	+	+	–	–	CR	NED	60
	3	Ic	45 Gy	–	+	+	–	–	CR	NED	51
	4	Ic	–	–	+	–	+	+	CR	DOD	29
	5	Ic	–	+	+	+	–	–	CR	CR-2	16
	6	Ic	45 Gy	–	+	+	–	–	CR	NED	71
	7	Ic	40 Gy	+	+	+	–	–	CR	NED	59
	8	Ic	45 Gy	–	+	+	–	–	CR	NED	65
	9	Ic	50 Gy	+	+	+	–	–	PR	AWD	8
	10	Ic	–	+	+	–	–	–	CR	AWD	16
	11	III	–	+	+	+	–	–	SD	DOD	6
	12	IIIc	–	+	+	–	–	–	CR	DOD	11
	13	IIIc	50 Gy	–	+	+	–	–	CR	NED	5
	14	IIIb	–	–	+	+	–	–	CR	DOD	7
	15	IIIb	–	+	+	–	–	–	PD	DOD	3
	16	IIIc	–	–	+	–	–	–	CR	DOD	13
	17	n.d.	–	+	+	–	–	–	PD	DOD	2
Senekijan	1	Ia	–	–	+	+	+	+	CR	NED	29
	2	Ia	–	–	+	+	+	+	CR	DOD	18
	3	IIc	45 Gy	–	+	+	+	+	CR	DOD	11
	4	IIIa	45 Gy	–	+	+	+	+	PR	DOD	13
	5	IIIa	–	–	+	+	+	+	CR	DOD	15

[a]Only the patients with "favorable response" to therapy

stem cell transplantation. In this series that included four stage II, 14 stage II, and three stage IV patients, event-free survival was 34% and overall survival 49% (Pautier et al. 2007).

In the German pediatric series, the adjuvant chemotherapeutic regimens were heterogeneous and ranged from sarcoma (CEVAIE) to ovarian cancer (Carbo-Taxol) and germ cell tumor protocols (PEI). Response to chemotherapy was heterogeneous. The best results were achieved with sarcoma or germ cell tumor regimens, while classic ovarian carcinoma regimens were ineffective. Despite initial responses, six of eleven patients suffered recurrence. However, all five patients who underwent high-dose chemotherapy with autologous stem cell transplantation achieved long-term remission. The outcome of this series is comparable to that of the French series. Event-free survival is 0.28 ± 0.15 (4/11 patients), and 5-year survival is 0.49 ± 0.15 (6/11 patients) (Distelmaier et al. 2006b).

Based on this published experience, four additional patients have been treated with a combination of cisplatin, ifosfamide, and Adriamycin, followed by high-dose chemotherapy. All four currently remain in complete remission. Thus, combining all patients reported to the MAKEI registry, all nine patients treated with high-dose chemotherapy are alive and well, while all treated without high-dose chemotherapy have died from their tumor. On recurrence, OSCCHTs characteristically show a diffuse metastatic spread within the peritoneal cavity and involved abdominal and pelvic lymph nodes. A few patients may develop distant metastases to the liver and the skeletal system.

31.6.5 Approach to a Multimodal Therapy of OSCCHT of Children and Adolescents

In summary, the optimal management of OSCCHT still remains unknown. The only clear evidence is that after the diagnosis of OSCCHT, there is no role for expectant follow-up, even in completely resected stage Ia disease. Obviously, at least microscopic tumor spread has to be assumed in virtually all tumors, so that all require adjuvant therapy. It is also evident that adjuvant chemotherapy may successfully eradicate such subclinical disease, and according to the study by Harrison, Pautier, and the German series, a platin-based regimen that includes etoposide, alkylating agents, and anthracyclins currently appears to be the most promising combination regimen (Distelmaier et al. 2006b; Harrison et al. 2006; Pautier et al. 2007).

Preliminary information indicates that high-dose chemotherapy may indeed be useful in consolidating a complete clinical remission previously achieved with surgery and conventional chemotherapy. For locally intensive tumor control, either abdominal irradiation of locoregional hyperthermia may be considered (Distelmaier et al. 2006b; Harrison et al. 2006).

This positive development and the anticipation that more patients with OSCCHT will be registered in the future have encouraged the German STEP registry group to incorporate a therapeutic recommendation for patients with OSCCHT. Thus, further patients can hopefully be evaluated prospectively. This concept has been discussed intensively with representatives of the International Society of Pediatric Oncology, Europe and the European Society of Gynecooncology, specifically focusing on adolescent and young adult patients (submitted for publication). According to the STEP strategy, a timely histopathologic review of all ovarian tumors will be mandatory. In the case of an OSCCHT, all patients will receive adjuvant chemotherapy with a combination of cisplatin, ifosfamide, and Adriamycin for six cycles. Therapy will be completed with high-dose chemotherapy including carboplatin and etoposide, thus avoiding intolerably high cumulative doses of etoposide. In case of gross tumor residues after resection, a local deep hyperthermia will be discussed. The authors can be contacted for further details regarding therapy, and they would appreciate exchange of experience.

In conclusion, ovarian small cell carcinoma of the hypercalcemic type must still be considered a prognostically unfavorable disease.

However, data are accumulating, which open encouraging perspectives for cure through the use of adjuvant multiagent chemotherapy and consolidating high-dose chemotherapy. In addition, further genetic research on the biology of this neoplasm with close biological relation of rhabdoid tumors may uncover new therapeutic targets. However, these goals can only be achieved if patients are registered centrally and prospectively. The difficulty in collecting data from rare pediatric tumors must be emphasized. In the case of OSCCHT, clinicians often query experts on the appropriate treatment. Yet, scarce follow-up data are provided. These data might help inform future treatments, but the opportunity is lost without communication Thus, this rare tumor type is an ideal candidate for international cooperation in order to achieve standardization of treatment and data collection in a registry ("Get friends!").

References

Overview on Epidemiology, Biology, Histology, and Clinic

Afifi HY, Bosl GJ et al (1997) Mediastinal growing teratoma syndrome. Ann Thorac Surg 64(2):359–362

Altaras MM, Goldberg GL et al (1986) The value of cancer antigen-125 as a tumor marker in malignant germ cell tumors of the ovary. Gynecol Oncol 25(2):150–159

Angel CA, Murillo C, Mayhew J (1998) Experience with vascular control before excision of giant, highly vascular sacrococcygeal teratomas in neonates. J Pediatr Surg 33:1840–1842

Atkin NB, Baker MC (1982) Specific chromosome change, i (12p), in testicular tumours? Lancet 2(8311):1349

Baranzelli MC, Kramar A et al (1999a) Prognostic factors in children with localized malignant nonseminomatous germ cell tumors. J Clin Oncol 17(4):1212

Belchis DA, Mowry J et al (1993) Infantile choriocarcinoma. Re-examination of a potentially curable entity. Cancer 72(6):2028–2032

Billmire DF, Grosfeld JL (1986) Teratomas in childhood: analysis of 142 cases. J Pediatr Surg 21(6):548–551

Billmire DF, Cullen JW, Rescorla FJ, Davis M, Schlatter MG, Olson TA, Malogolowkin MH, Pashankar F, Villaluna D, Krailo M, Egler RA, Rodriguez-Galindo C, Frazier AL (2014) Surveillance after initial surgery for pediatric and adolescent girls with stage I ovarian germ cell tumors: report from the Children's Oncology Group. J Clin Oncol 32:465–470

Blohm ME, Vesterling-Hörner D et al (1998) Alpha 1-fetoprotein (AFP) reference values in infants up to 2 years of age. Pediatr Hematol Oncol 15(2):135–142

Bokemeyer C, Berger CC et al (1996) Evaluation of long-term toxicity after chemotherapy for testicular cancer. J Clin Oncol 14(11):2923–2932

Bosl GJ, Geller NL et al (1988) A randomized trial of etoposide + cisplatin versus vinblastine + bleomycin + cisplatin + cyclophosphamide + dactinomycin in patients with good-prognosis germ cell tumors. J Clin Oncol 6(8):1231–1238

Brock PR, Maibach R, Childs M, Rajput K, Roebuck D, Sullivan MJ, Laithier V, Ronghe M, Dall'Igna P, Hiyama E, Brichard B, Skeen J, Mateos ME, Capra M, Rangaswami AA, Ansari M, Rechnitzer C, Veal GJ, Covezzoli A, Brugières L, Perilongo G, Czauderna P, Morland B, Neuwelt EA (2018) Sodium thiosulfate for protection from cisplatin-induced hearing loss. N Engl J Med 378:2376–2385

Buetow SA (1995) Epidemiology of testicular cancer. Epidemiol Rev 17(2):433–449

Bussey KJ, Lawce HJ et al (1999a) Chromosome abnormalities of eighty-one pediatric germ cell tumors: sex-, age-, site-, and histopathology-related differences—a Children's Cancer Group study. Genes Chromosomes Cancer 25(2):134–146

Bussey KJ, Lawce HJ et al (2001) Chromosomes 1 and 12 abnormalities in pediatric germ cell tumors by interphase fluorescence in situ hybridization. Cancer Genet Cytogenet 125(2):112–118

Calaminus G, Schneider DT et al (2009) Survival after an antiangiogenetic therapy and surgery in a wide spread growing teratoma originating from a testicular mixed malignant germ cell tumor. Klin Padiatr 221(3):136–140

Calaminus G, Frappaz D, Kortmann RD, Krefeld B, Saran F, Pietsch T, Vasiljevic A, Garre ML, Ricardi U, Mann JR, Göbel U, Alapetite C, Murray MJ, Nicholson JC (2017) Outcome of patients with intracranial non-germinomatous germ cell tumors-lessons from the SIOP-CNS-GCT-96 trial. Neuro-Oncology 19:1661–1672

Carver BS, Serio AM et al (2007a) Improved clinical outcome in recent years for men with metastatic nonseminomatous germ cell tumors. J Clin Oncol 25(35):5603–5608

Calaminus G, Kortmann R, Worch J, Nicholson JC, Alapetite C, Garrè ML, Patte C, Ricardi U, Saran F, Frappaz D (2013) SIOP CNS GCT 96: final report of outcome of a prospective, multinational nonrandomized trial for children and adults with intracranial germinoma, comparing craniospinal irradiation alone with chemotherapy followed by focal primary site irradiation for patients with localized disease. Neuro-Oncology 15:788–796

Carver BS, Shayegan B et al (2007b) Incidence of metastatic nonseminomatous germ cell tumor outside the boundaries of a modified postchemotherapy retroperitoneal lymph node dissection. J Clin Oncol 25(28):4365–4369

Carver BS, Shayegan B et al (2007c) Long-term clinical outcome after postchemotherapy retroperitoneal lymph node dissection in men with residual teratoma. J Clin Oncol 25(9):1033–1037

Chaganti RS, Rodriguez E et al (1994) Origin of adult male mediastinal germ-cell tumours. Lancet 343(8906):1130–1132

Cheng L, Roth LM et al (2010) KIT gene mutation and amplification in dysgerminoma of the ovary. Cancer 117(10):2096–2103

Clement PB, Young RH et al (1987) Endometrioid-like variant of ovarian yolk sac tumor. A clinicopathological analysis of eight cases. Am J Surg Pathol 11(10):767–778

Cohen MB, Friend DS et al (1987) Gonadal endodermal sinus (yolk sac) tumor with pure intestinal differentiation: a new histologic type. Pathol Res Pract 182(5):609–616

Conlon N, Silva A, Guerra E, Jelinic P, Schlappe BA, Olvera N, Mueller JJ, Tornos C, Jungbluth AA, Young RH, Oliva E, Levine D, Soslow RA (2016) Loss of SMARCA4 expression is both sensitive and specific for the diagnosis of small cell carcinoma of ovary, hypercalcemic type. Am J Surg Pathol 40: 395–403

Cools M, Drop SL et al (2006) Germ cell tumors in the intersex gonad: old paths, new directions, moving frontiers. Endocr Rev 27(5):468–484

Cushing B, Giller R et al (2004a) Randomized comparison of combination chemotherapy with etoposide, bleomycin, and either high-dose or standard-dose cisplatin in children and adolescents with high-risk malignant germ cell tumors: a Pediatric Intergroup Study–Pediatric Oncology Group 9049 and Children's Cancer Group 888. J Clin Oncol 22(13): 2691–2700

Dal Cin P, Drochmans A et al (1989) Isochromosome 12p in mediastinal germ cell tumor. Cancer Genet Cytogenet 42(2):243–251

De Angelis R, Sant M, Coleman MP, Francisci S, Baili P, Pierannunzio D, Trama A, Visser O, Brenner H, Ardanaz E, Bielska-Lasota M, Engholm G, Nennecke A, Siesling S, Berrino F, Capocaccia R, EUROCARE-5 WG (2014) Cancer survival in Europe 1999-2007 by country and age: results of EUROCARE-5—a population-based study. Lancet Oncol 15:23–34

Dehner LP (1983a) Gonadal and extragonadal germ cell neoplasia of childhood. Hum Pathol 14(6):493–511

Doitsidou M, Reichman-Fried M et al (2002) Guidance of primordial germ cell migration by the chemokine SDF-1. Cell 111(5):647–659

Dolci S, Pesce M et al (1993) Combined action of stem cell factor, leukemia inhibitory factor, and cAMP on in vitro proliferation of mouse primordial germ cells. Mol Reprod Dev 35(2):134–139

Draper JS, Smith K et al (2004) Recurrent gain of chromosomes 17q and 12 in cultured human embryonic stem cells. Nat Biotechnol 22(1):53–54

Einhorn LH, Donohue J (1977a) Cis-diamminedichloroplatinum, vinblastine, and bleomycin combination chemotherapy in disseminated testicular cancer. Ann Intern Med 87(3):293–298

Einhorn LH, Williams SD et al (1989a) Evaluation of optimal duration of chemotherapy in favorable-prognosis disseminated germ cell tumors: a Southeastern Cancer Study Group protocol. J Clin Oncol 7(3):387–391

Einhorn LH, Williams SD et al (2007) High-dose chemotherapy and stem-cell rescue for metastatic germ-cell tumors. N Engl J Med 357(4):340–348

Faure-Conter C, Orbach D, Cropet C, Baranzelli MC, Martelli H, Thebaud E, Vérité C, Rome A, Fasola S, Corradini N, Rocourt N, Frappaz D, Kalfa N, Patte C (2014) Salvage therapy for refractory or recurrent pediatric germ cell tumors: the French SFCE experience. Pediatr Blood Cancer 61:253–259

Fritsch MK, Schneider DT et al (2006) Activation of Wnt/beta-catenin signaling in distinct histologic subtypes of human germ cell tumors. Pediatr Dev Pathol 9(2):115–131

Ferguson AW, Katabuchi H, Ronnett BM, Cho KR (2001) Glial implants in gliomatosis peritonei arise from normal tissue, not from the associated teratoma. Am J Pathol 159:51–55

Gietema JA, Sleijfer DT et al (1992) Long-term follow-up of cardiovascular risk factors in patients given chemotherapy for disseminated nonseminomatous testicular cancer. Ann Intern Med 116(9):709–715

Frazier AL, Hale JP, Rodriguez-Galindo C, Dang H, Olson T, Murray MJ, Amatruda JF, Thornton C, Arul GS, Billmire D, Shaikh F, Pashankar F, Stoneham S, Krailo M, Nicholson JC (2015) Revised risk classification for pediatric extracranial germ cell tumors based on 25 years of clinical trial data from the United Kingdom and United States. J Clin Oncol 33:195–201

Gilbert DC, Chandler I et al (2009) Clinical and biological significance of CXCL12 and CXCR4 expression in adult testes and germ cell tumours of adults and adolescents. J Pathol 217(1):94–102

Gitlin D, Perricelli A et al (1972) Synthesis of -fetoprotein by liver, yolk sac, and gastrointestinal tract of the human conceptus. Cancer Res 32(5):979–982

Göbel U, Calaminus G et al (1997a) Extracranial non-testicular teratoma in childhood and adolescence: introduction of a risk score for stratification of therapy. Klin Padiatr 209(4):228–234

Göbel U, Calaminus G et al (1998a) Teratomas in infancy and childhood. Med Pediatr Oncol 31(1):8–15

Göbel U, Schneider DT et al (2000a) Germ-cell tumors in childhood and adolescence. GPOH MAKEI and the MAHO study groups. Ann Oncol 11(3):263–271

Göbel U, Schneider DT et al (2001a) Multimodal treatment of malignant sacrococcygeal germ cell tumors: a prospective analysis of 66 patients of the German cooperative protocols MAKEI 83/86 and 89. J Clin Oncol 19(7):1943–1950

Göbel U, Haas R, Calaminus G, Botorek P, Schmidt P, Teske C, Schönberger S, Schneider DT, Harms D (2013a) Testicular germ cell tumors in boys <10 years: results of the protocol MAHO 98 in respect to surgery and watch & wait strategy. Klin Padiatr 225:296–302

Göbel U, Schneider DT, Teske C, Schönberger S, Calaminus G (2010) Brain metastases in children and adolescents with extracranial germ cell tumor—data of the MAHO/MAKEI-registry. Klin Padiatr 222:140–144

Göbel U, von Kries R, Teske C, Schneider DT, Beyerlein A, Bernbeck B, Calaminus G (2013b) Brain metastases during follow-up of children and adolescents with extracranial malignant germ cell tumors: risk adapted management decision tree analysis based on data of the MAHO/MAKEI-registry. Pediatr Blood Cancer 60:217–223

Godin I, Deed R et al (1991) Effects of the steel gene product on mouse primordial germ cells in culture. Nature 352(6338):807–809

Gonzalez-Crussi F, Winkler RF et al (1978) Sacrococcygeal teratomas in infants and children: relationship of histology and prognosis in 40 cases. Arch Pathol Lab Med 102(8):420–425

Group, I. G. C. C. C (1997a) International germ cell consensus classification: a prognostic factor-based staging system for metastatic germ cell cancers. J Clin Oncol 15(No:2 (February)):594–603

Güler S, Demirkaya M, Balkan E, Kırıştıoğlu İ, Kılıç N, Sevinir B (2018) Late effects in patients with sacrococcygeal teratoma: a single center series. Pediatr Hematol Oncol 35:208–217

Harms D, Janig U (1986) Germ cell tumours of childhood. Report of 170 cases including 59 pure and partial yolk-sac tumours. Virchows Arch A Pathol Anat Histopathol 409(2):223–239

Harms D, Zahn S et al (2006a) Pathology and molecular biology of teratomas in childhood and adolescence. Klin Padiatr 218(6):296–302

Hartmann JT, Nichols CR et al (2000) Hematologic disorders associated with primary mediastinal nonseminomatous germ cell tumors. J Natl Cancer Inst 92(1):54–61

Hasle H, Mellemgaard A et al (1995) Cancer incidence in men with Klinefelter syndrome. Br J Cancer 71(2):416–420

Hawkins E, Perlman EJ (1996a) Germ cell tumors in childhood: morphology and biology. In: Parham DM (ed) Pediatric neoplasia: morphology and biology. Raven, New York, p 297

Hawkins EP (1990) Pathology of germ cell tumors in children. Crit Rev Oncol Hematol 10(2):165–179

Hawkins EP, Finegold MJ et al (1986) Nongerminomatous malignant germ cell tumors in children. A review of 89 cases from the Pediatric Oncology Group, 1971–1984. Cancer 58(12):2579–2584

Hennes E, Zahn S, Lopes LF, Schönberger S, Leuschner I, Göbel U, Calaminus G, Schneider DT (2012) Molecular genetic analysis of bilateral ovarian germ cell tumors. Klin Padiatr 224:359–365

Ho DM, Liu HC (1992) Primary intracranial germ cell tumor. Pathologic study of 51 patients. Cancer 70(6):1577–1584

Hoei-Hansen CE, Sehested A et al (2006) New evidence for the origin of intracranial germ cell tumours from primordial germ cells: expression of pluripotency and cell differentiation markers. J Pathol 209(1):25–33

Honecker F, Stoop H, de Krijger RR, Lau Y-FC, Bokemeyer C, Looijenga LHJ (2004) Pathobiological implications of the expression of markers of testicular carcinoma in situ by fetal germ cells. J Pathol 203:849–857

Jenderny J, Koster E et al (1995) Detection of chromosome aberrations in paraffin sections of seven gonadal yolk sac tumors of childhood. Hum Genet 96(6):644–650

Kaatsch P (2004a) German childhood cancer registry and its favorable setting. Bundesgesundheitsblatt Gesundheitsforschung Gesundheitsschutz 47(5):437–443

Kaatsch P, Häfner C, Calaminus G, Blettner M, Tulla M (2015) Pediatric germ cell tumors from 1987 to 2011: incidence rates, time trends, and survival. Pediatrics 135:e136–e143

Kaplan CG, Askin FB et al (1979a) Cytogenetics of extragonadal tumors. Teratology 19(2):261–266

Kaushik A, Bhartiya D (2018) Pluripotent very small embryonic-like stem cells in adult testes—an alternate premise to explain testicular germ cell tumors. Stem Cell Rev 14:793–800

Knight KR, Kraemer DF et al (2005) Ototoxicity in children receiving platinum chemotherapy: underestimating a commonly occurring toxicity that may influence academic and social development. J Clin Oncol 23(34):8588–8596

Koshida K, Nishino A et al (1991) The role of alkaline phosphatase isoenzymes as tumor markers for testicular germ cell tumors. J Urol 146(1):57–60

Kurman RJ, Norris HJ (1976a) Malignant mixed germ cell tumors of the ovary. A clinical and pathologic analysis of 30 cases. Obstet Gynecol 48(5):579–589

Lawrence NJ, Chan H, Toner G, Stockler MR, Martin A, Yip S, Wong N, Yeung A, Mazhar D, Pashankar F, Frazier L, McDermott R, Walker R, Tan H, Davis ID, Grimison P, ANZUP (2018) Protocol for the P3BEP trial (ANZUP 1302): an international randomised phase 3 trial of accelerated versus standard BEP chemotherapy for adult and paediatric male and female patients with intermediate and poor-risk metastatic germ cell tumours. BMC Cancer 18:854

Lee SH, Appleby V et al (2010) Variable methylation of the imprinted gene, SNRPN, supports a relationship between intracranial germ cell tumours and neural stem cells. J Neuro-Oncol 101(3):419–428

Li Y, Womer RB et al (2004) Predicting cisplatin ototoxicity in children: the influence of age and the cumulative dose. Eur J Cancer 40(16):2445–2451

Logothetis CJ, Samuels ML et al (1985) Chemotherapy of extragonadal germ cell tumors. J Clin Oncol 3(3):316–325

Looijenga LH, Stoop H et al (2003) POU5F1 (OCT3/4) identifies cells with pluripotent potential in human germ cell tumors. Cancer Res 63(9):2244–2250

Mann JR, Pearson D et al (1989a) Results of the United Kingdom Children's Cancer Study Group's malignant germ cell tumor studies. Cancer 63(9):1657–1667

Mann JR, Raafat F et al (2000) The United Kingdom Children's Cancer Study Group's second germ cell tumor study: carboplatin, etoposide, and bleomycin are effective treatment for children with malignant extracranial germ cell tumors, with acceptable toxicity. J Clin Oncol 18(22):3809–3818

Marina NMM, London WB, Frazier AJ, Rescorla F, Billmire DF, Davis M, Perlman E, Giller R, Lauer S (2003) Amifostine does not protect against the ototoxicity associated with high-dose cisplatin, etoposide, and bleomycin (HD-PEB) in pediatric germ cell tumors (Abstract # 798). In: Proceedings ASCO, American Society of Clinical Oncology

Marina N, London WB et al (2006a) Prognostic factors in children with extragonadal malignant germ cell tumors: a pediatric intergroup study. J Clin Oncol 24(16):2544–2548

Marina NM, Cushing B et al (1999a) Complete surgical excision is effective treatment for children with immature teratomas with or without malignant elements: a Pediatric Oncology Group/Children's Cancer Group Intergroup Study. J Clin Oncol 17(7):2137–2143

Mauz-Körholz C, Harms D et al (2000a) Primary chemotherapy and conservative surgery for vaginal yolk-sac tumour. Maligne Keimzelltumoren Study Group. Lancet 355(9204):625

Mayer F, Stoop H et al (2003a) Molecular determinants of treatment response in human germ cell tumors. Clin Cancer Res 9(2):767–773

McIver SC, Roman SD, Nixon B, Loveland KL, McLaughlin EA (2013) The rise of testicular germ cell tumours: the search for causes, risk factors and novel therapeutic targets. F1000Res:2:55

Meinhold-Heerlein I, Fotopoulou C, Harter P, Kurzeder C, Mustea A, Wimberger P, Hauptmann S, Sehouli J (2016) The new WHO classification of ovarian, fallopian tube, and primary peritoneal cancer and its clinical implications. Arch Gynecol Obstet

Molyneaux KA, Zinszner H et al (2003) The chemokine SDF1/CXCL12 and its receptor CXCR4 regulate mouse germ cell migration and survival. Development 130(18):4279–4286

Mostert M, Rosenberg C et al (2000) Comparative genomic and in situ hybridization of germ cell tumors of the infantile testis. Lab Investig 80(7):1055–1064

Motzer RJ, Mazumdar M et al (2000) Sequential dose-intensive paclitaxel, ifosfamide, carboplatin, and etoposide salvage therapy for germ cell tumor patients. J Clin Oncol 18(6):1173–1180

Murray MJ, Bailey S, Heinemann K, Mann J, Göbel U, Saran F, Hale JP, Calaminus G, Nicholson JC (2017) Treatment and outcomes of UK and German patients with relapsed intracranial germ cell tumors following uniform first-line therapy. Int J Cancer 141:621–635

Nakashima N, Fukatsu T et al (1987) The frequency and histology of hepatic tissue in germ cell tumors. Am J Surg Pathol 11(9):682–692

Nettersheim D, Jostes S, Schneider S, Schorle H (2016) Elucidating human male germ cell development by studying germ cell cancer. Reproduction 152:R101–R113

Nichols CR, Heerema NA et al (1987a) Klinefelter's syndrome associated with mediastinal germ cell neoplasms. J Clin Oncol 5(8):1290–1294

Oing C, Alsdorf WH, von Amsberg G, Oechsle K, Bokemeyer C (2017) Platinum-refractory germ cell tumors: an update on current treatment options and developments. World J Urol 35:1167–1175

Oldenburg J, Kraggerud SM et al (2007) Cisplatin-induced long-term hearing impairment is associated with specific glutathione s-transferase genotypes in testicular cancer survivors. J Clin Oncol 25(6): 708–714

Oosterhuis JW, Looijenga LH (2005a) Testicular germ-cell tumours in a broader perspective. Nat Rev Cancer 5(3):210–222

Oosterhuis JW, Rammeloo RH et al (1990) Ploidy of malignant mediastinal germ-cell tumors. Hum Pathol 21(7):729–732

Oosterhuis JW, Stoop H et al (2007) Why human extragonadal germ cell tumours occur in the midline of the body: old concepts, new perspectives. Int J Androl 30(4):256–263; discussion 263–264

Orazi A, Neiman RS et al (1993) Hematopoietic precursor cells within the yolk sac tumor component are the source of secondary hematopoietic malignancies in patients with mediastinal germ cell tumors. Cancer 71(12):3873–3881

Orth JM, Qiu J et al (1997) Expression of the c-kit gene is critical for migration of neonatal rat gonocytes in vitro. Biol Reprod 57(3):676–683

Osanto S, Bukman A et al (1992) Long-term effects of chemotherapy in patients with testicular cancer. J Clin Oncol 10(4):574–579

Palmer RD, Foster NA et al (2007) Malignant germ cell tumours of childhood: new associations of genomic imbalance. Br J Cancer 96(4):667–676

Palmer RD, Barbosa-Morais NL et al (2008) Pediatric malignant germ cell tumors show characteristic transcriptome profiles. Cancer Res 68(11):4239–4247

Palmer RD, Murray MJ et al (2010) Malignant germ cell tumors display common microRNA profiles resulting in global changes in expression of messenger RNA targets. Cancer Res 70(7):2911–2923

Pashankar F, Hale JP, Dang H, Krailo M, Brady WE, Rodriguez-Galindo C, Nicholson JC, Murray MJ, Bilmire DF, Stoneham S, Arul GS, Olson TA, Stark D, Shaikh F, Amatruda JF, Covens A, Gershenson DM, Frazier AL (2016) Is adjuvant chemotherapy indicated in ovarian immature teratomas? A combined data analysis from the Malignant Germ Cell Tumor International Collaborative. Cancer 122:230–237

Perlman EJ, Cushing B et al (1994a) Cytogenetic analysis of childhood endodermal sinus tumors: a Pediatric Oncology Group study. Pediatr Pathol 14(4): 695–708

Perlman EJ, Valentine MB et al (1996) Deletion of 1p36 in childhood endodermal sinus tumors by two-color fluorescence in situ hybridization: a pediatric oncology group study. Genes Chromosomes Cancer 16(1):15–20

Perlman EJ, Hu J et al (2000) Genetic analysis of childhood endodermal sinus tumors by comparative genomic hybridization. J Pediatr Hematol Oncol 22(2):100–105

Poynter JN, Amatruda JF et al (2010) Trends in incidence and survival of pediatric and adolescent patients with germ cell tumors in the United States, 1975 to 2006. Cancer 116(20):4882–4891

Prall JA, McGavran L et al (1995) Intracranial malignant germ cell tumor and the Klinefelter syndrome. Case report and review of the literature. Pediatr Neurosurg 23(4):219–224

Prat J, FIGO COGO (2015) Abridged republication of FIGO's staging classification for cancer of the ovary, fallopian tube, and peritoneum. Cancer 121:3452–3454

Rapley EA, Hockley S et al (2004) Somatic mutations of KIT in familial testicular germ cell tumours. Br J Cancer 90(12):2397–2401

Riedemann L, Lanvers C et al (2008) Megalin genetic polymorphisms and individual sensitivity to the ototoxic effect of cisplatin. Pharmacogenomics J 8(1):23–28

Ries LAG, Smith MA, Gurney JG, Linet M, Tamra T, Young JL, Bunin GR (eds) (1999a) Cancer incidence and survival among children and adolescents: United States SEER program 1975–1995. National Cancer Institute, Bethesda, SEER Program. NIH Publication No. 99-4649

Rodriguez E, Mathew S et al (1992) Cytogenetic analysis of 124 prospectively ascertained male germ cell tumors. Cancer Res 52(8):2285–2291

Rogers PC, Olson TA et al (2004a) Treatment of children and adolescents with stage II testicular and stages I and II ovarian malignant germ cell tumors: a Pediatric Intergroup Study–Pediatric Oncology Group 9048 and Children's Cancer Group 8891. J Clin Oncol 22(17):3563–3569

Rossi UG, Cariati M, Tomà P (2013) Giant sacrococcygeal teratoma embolization. Indian J Radiol Imaging 23:145–147

Samaniego F, Rodriguez E et al (1990) Cytogenetic and molecular analysis of human male germ cell tumors: chromosome 12 abnormalities and gene amplification. Genes Chromosomes Cancer 1(4):289–300

Schmoll HJ, Kollmannsberger C, Metzner B, Hartmann JT, Schleucher N, Schoffski P, Schleicher J, Rick O, Beyer J, Hossfeld D, Kanz L, Berdel WE, Andreesen R, Bokemeyer C (2003a) Long-term results of first-line sequential high-dose etoposide, ifosfamide, and cisplatin chemotherapy plus autologous stem cell support for patients with advanced metastatic germ cell cancer: an extended phase I/II study of the German Testicular Cancer Study Group. J Clin Oncol 21:4083–4091

Schneider DT, Hilgenfeld E et al (1999) Acute myelogenous leukemia after treatment for malignant germ cell tumors in children. J Clin Oncol 17(10): 3226–3233

Schneider DT, Calaminus G et al (2000a) Primary mediastinal germ cell tumors in children and adolescents: results of the German cooperative protocols MAKEI 83/86, 89, and 96. J Clin Oncol 18(4):832–839

Schneider DT, Calaminus G et al (2001a) Diagnostic value of alpha 1-fetoprotein and beta-human chorionic gonadotropin in infancy and childhood. Pediatr Hematol Oncol 18(1):11–26

Schneider DT, Schuster AE et al (2001b) Genetic analysis of childhood germ cell tumors with comparative genomic hybridization. Klin Padiatr 213(4):204–211

Schneider DT, Schuster AE et al (2001c) Multipoint imprinting analysis indicates a common precursor cell for gonadal and nongonadal pediatric germ cell tumors. Cancer Res 61(19):7268–7276

Schneider DT, Wessalowski R et al (2001d) Treatment of recurrent malignant sacrococcygeal germ cell tumors: analysis of 22 patients registered in the German protocols MAKEI 83/86, 89, and 96. J Clin Oncol 19(7):1951–1960

Schneider DT, Schuster AE et al (2002a) Genetic analysis of mediastinal nonseminomatous germ cell tumors in children and adolescents. Genes Chromosomes Cancer 34(1):115–125

Schneider DT, Calaminus G et al (2004a) Epidemiologic analysis of 1,442 children and adolescents registered in the German germ cell tumor protocols. Pediatr Blood Cancer 42(2):169–175

Schneider DT, Calaminus G et al (2005a) Ovarian sex cord-stromal tumors in children and adolescents. J Reprod Med 50(6):439–446

Schneider DT, Zahn S et al (2006) Molecular genetic analysis of central nervous system germ cell tumors with comparative genomic hybridization. Mod Pathol 19(6):864–873

Schneider DT, Orbach D, Cecchetto G, Stachowicz-Stencel T, Brummel B, Brecht IB, Bisogno G, Ferrari A, Reguerre Y, Godzinski J, Bien E, Calaminus G, Göbel U, Patte C (2015) Ovarian Sertoli Leydig cell tumours in children and adolescents: an analysis of the European Cooperative Study Group on Pediatric Rare Tumors (EXPeRT). Eur J Cancer 51:543–550

Schultz KAP, Harris AK, Finch M, Dehner LP, Brown JB, Gershenson DM, Young RH, Field A, Yu W, Turner J, Cost NG, Schneider DT, Stewart DR, Frazier AL, Messinger Y, Hill DA (2017) DICER1-related Sertoli-Leydig cell tumor and gynandroblastoma: clinical and genetic findings from the International Ovarian and Testicular Stromal Tumor Registry. Gynecol Oncol 147:521–527

Schultz KAP, Williams GM, Kamihara J, Stewart DR, Harris AK, Bauer AJ, Turner J, Shah R, Schneider

K, Schneider KW, Carr AG, Harney LA, Baldinger S, Frazier AL, Orbach D, Schneider DT, Malkin D, Dehner LP, Messinger YH, Hill DA (2018) DICER1 and Associated Conditions: identification of at-risk individuals and recommended surveillance strategies. Clin Cancer Res 24:2251–2261

Schwartz PE, Morris JM (1988) Serum lactic dehydrogenase: a tumor marker for dysgerminoma. Obstet Gynecol 72(3 Pt 2):511–515

Shaikh F, Nathan PC, Hale J, Uleryk E, Frazier L (2013) Is there a role for carboplatin in the treatment of malignant germ cell tumors? A systematic review of adult and pediatric trials. Pediatr Blood Cancer 60: 587–592

Shalaby MS, Walker G, O'Toole S, Hammond P, Carachi R (2014) The long-term outcome of patients diagnosed with sacrococcygeal teratoma in childhood. A study of a national cohort. Arch Dis Child 99:1009–1013

Sievers S, Alemazkour K et al (2005a) IGF2/H19 imprinting analysis of human germ cell tumors (GCTs) using the methylation-sensitive single-nucleotide primer extension method reflects the origin of GCTs in different stages of primordial germ cell development. Genes Chromosomes Cancer 44(3):256–264

Silver SA, Wiley JM et al (1994) DNA ploidy analysis of pediatric germ cell tumors. Mod Pathol 7(9): 951–956

Skakkebaek NE (2004) Testicular dysgenesis syndrome: new epidemiological evidence. Int J Androl 27(4):189–191

Skakkebaek NE, Holm M et al (2003) Association between testicular dysgenesis syndrome (TDS) and testicular neoplasia: evidence from 20 adult patients with signs of maldevelopment of the testis. APMIS 111(1):1–9; discussion 9–11

Skakkebaek NE (2016) A brief review of the link between environment and male reproductive health: lessons from studies of testicular germ cell cancer. Horm Res Paediatr 86:240–246

Talerman A (1987) Germ cell tumors of the ovary. In: Kurman RJ (ed) Blaustein's pathology of female genital tract. Springer, New York, p 659

Teilum G, Albrechtsen R et al (1975a) The histogenetic-embryologic basis for reappearance of alpha-fetoprotein in endodermal sinus tumors (yolk sac tumors) and teratomas. Acta Pathol Microbiol Scand A 83(1):80–86

Terenziani M, Bisogno G, Boldrini R, Cecchetto G, Conte M, Boschetti L, De Pasquale MD, Biasoni D, Inserra A, Siracusa F, Basso ME, De Leonardis F, Di Pinto D, Barretta F, Spreafico F, D'Angelo P (2017) Malignant ovarian germ cell tumors in pediatric patients: the AIEOP (Associazione Italiana Ematologia Oncologia Pediatrica) study. Pediatr Blood Cancer 64

Terenziani M, D'Angelo P, Inserra A, Boldrini R, Bisogno G, Babbo GL, Conte M, Dall'Igna P, De Pasquale MD, Indolfi P, Piva L, Riccipetitoni G, Siracusa F, Spreafico F, Tamaro P, Cecchetto G (2015) Mature and immature teratoma: a report from the second Italian pediatric study. Pediatr Blood Cancer 62:1202–1208

Terenziani M, De Pasquale MD, Bisogno G, Biasoni D, Boldrini R, Collini P, Conte M, Dall'Igna P, Inserra A, Melchionda F, Siracusa F, Spreafico F, Barretta F, D'Angelo P (2018) Malignant testicular germ cell tumors in children and adolescents: the AIEOP (Associazione Italiana Ematologia Oncologia Pediatrica) protocol. Urol Oncol 36:502.e7–502.e13

Thomson JA, Itskovitz-Eldor J et al (1998) Embryonic stem cell lines derived from human blastocysts. Science 282(5391):1145–1147

Thurlbeck WM, Scully RE (1960) Solid teratoma of the ovary. A clinicopathological analysis of 9 cases. Cancer 13:804–811

Ulbright TM, Michael H et al (1990) Spindle cell tumors resected from male patients with germ cell tumors. A clinicopathologic study of 14 cases. Cancer 65(1):148–156

Ulbright TM, Roth LM (1987) Recent developments in the pathology of germ cell tumors. Semin Diagn Pathol 4(4):304–319

van den Belt-Dusebout AW, Nuver J et al (2006) Long-term risk of cardiovascular disease in 5-year survivors of testicular cancer. J Clin Oncol 24(3):467–475

van der Gaast A, Kok TC et al (1991) Growing teratoma syndrome successfully treated with lymphoblastoid interferon. Eur Urol 19(3):257–258

van Echten J, Sleijfer DT et al (1997a) Cytogenetics of primary testicular nonseminoma, residual mature teratoma, and growing teratoma lesion in individual patients. Cancer Genet Cytogenet 96(1):1–6

van Echten J, van der Vloedt WS et al (1997b) Comparison of the chromosomal pattern of primary testicular nonseminomas and residual mature teratomas after chemotherapy. Cancer Genet Cytogenet 99(1):59–67

Van Mieghem T, Al-Ibrahim A, Deprest J, Lewi L, Langer JC, Baud D, O'Brien K, Beecroft R, Chaturvedi R, Jaeggi E, Fish J, Ryan G (2014) Minimally invasive therapy for fetal sacrococcygeal teratoma: case series and systematic review of the literature. Ultrasound Obstet Gynecol 43:611–619

Vogelzang NJ, Lange PH et al (1982) Acute changes of alpha-fetoprotein and human chorionic gonadotropin during induction chemotherapy of germ cell tumors. Cancer Res 42(11):4855–4861

Watanabe E, Tanaka K, Takeda N, Takayasu H, Yokota K, Watanabe M (2013) Surgical technique to prevent spillage of cyst fluid during operation for cystic ovarian tumors. Pediatr Surg Int 29:645–649

Wessalowski R, Blohm M et al (1997a) Treatment results in children and adolescents with loco-regional recurrences of abdominal germ cell tumors (GCTs): a pilot-study with PEI chemotherapy and regional deep hyperthermia (RHT) in comparison to a matched cohort. Klin Padiatr 209(4):250–256

Wessalowski R, Schneider DT et al (2003a) An approach for cure: PEI-chemotherapy and regional deep hyperthermia in children and adolescents with unresectable malignant tumors. Klin Padiatr 215(6):303–309

Wessalowski R, Schneider DT, Mils O, Friemann V, Kyrillopoulou O, Schaper J, Matuschek C, Rothe

K, Leuschner I, Willers R, Schönberger S, Göbel U, Calaminus G, Makei SG (2013) Regional deep hyperthermia for salvage treatment of children and adolescents with refractory or recurrent non-testicular malignant germ-cell tumours: an open-label, non-randomised, single-institution, phase 2 study. Lancet Oncol 14:843–852

Williamson SR, Delahunt B, Magi-Galluzzi C, Algaba F, Egevad L, Ulbright TM, Tickoo SK, Srigley JR, Epstein JI, Berney DM (2016) The WHO 2016 classification of testicular germ cell tumours: a review and update from the ISUP testis consultation panel. Histopathology

Young R, Scully R (1990a) Germ cell tumors: nonseminomatous tumors, occult tumors, effects of chemotherapy in testicular tumors. ASCP Press, Chicago

Young JL Jr, Cheng W, Roffers SD, Howe HL, Correa C, Weinstein R (2003) Ovarian cancer in children and young adults in the United States, 1992-1997. Cancer 97:2694–2700

Yu IT, Griffin CA et al (1995) Numerical sex chromosomal abnormalities in pineal teratomas by cytogenetic analysis and fluorescence in situ hybridization. Lab Investig 72(4):419–423

Zahn S, Sievers S et al (2006) Imbalances of chromosome arm 1p in pediatric and adult germ cell tumors are caused by true allelic loss: a combined comparative genomic hybridization and microsatellite analysis. Genes Chromosomes Cancer 45(11): 995–1006

Extragonadal Germ Cell Tumors

Alapetite C, Ricardi U, Saran F, Kortmann RD, Garre ML, Nicholson JC, Frappaz D, Göbel U, Patte C, Calaminus G (2002) Whole ventricular irradiation in combination with chemotherapy in intracranial germinoma: the consensus of the SIOP CNS GCT Study Group. Med Pediatr Oncol 39:O114

Alapetite C, Brisse H, Patte C, Raquin MA, Gaboriaud G, Carrie C, Habrand JL, Thiesse P, Cuilliere JC, Bernier V, Ben-Hassel M, Frappaz D, Baranzelli MC, Bouffet E (2010) Pattern of relapse and outcome of non-metastatic germinoma patients treated with chemotherapy and limited field radiation: the SFOP experience. Neuro-Oncology 12(12):1318–1325

Altman P, Randolph JG, Lilly JR (1974a) Sacrococcygeal teratoma: American Academy of Pediatrics surgical section survey-1973. J Pediatr Surg 9:389–398

Balmaceda C, Finlay J (2004) Current advances in the diagnosis and management of intracranial germ cell tumors. Curr Neurol Neurosci Rep 4:253–262

Balmaceda C, Heller G, Rosenblum M, Diez B, Villablanca JG, Kellie S, Maher P, Vlamis V, Walker RW, Leibel S, Finlay JL (1996) Chemotherapy without irradiation–a novel approach for newly diagnosed CNS germ cell tumors: results of an international cooperative trial. The first international central nervous system germ cell tumor study. J Clin Oncol 14:2908–2915

Bamberg M, Kortmann RD, Calaminus G, Becker G, Meisner C, Harms D, Göbel U (1999) Radiation therapy for intracranial germinoma: results of the German cooperative prospective trials MAKEI 83/86/89. J Clin Oncol 17:2585–2592

Baranzelli MC, Kramar A, Bouffet E, Quintana E, Rubie H, Edan C, Patte C (1999b) Prognostic factors in children with localized malignant nonseminomatous germ cell tumors. J Clin Oncol 17:1212–1219

Baranzelli MC, Bouffet E, Quintana E, Portas M, Thyss A, Patte C (2000a) Non-seminomatous ovarian germ cell tumours in children. Eur J Cancer 36:376–383

Bernbeck B, Schneider DT, Bernbeck B, Koch S, Teske C, Lentrodt J, Harms D, Göbel U, Calaminus G (2009b) Germ cell tumors of the head and neck: report from the MAKEI Study Group. Pediatr Blood Cancer 52:223–226

Billmire D, Vinocur C, Rescorla F, Colombani P, Cushing B, Hawkins E, Davis M, London WB, Lauer S, Giller R (2003) Malignant retroperitoneal and abdominal germ cell tumors: an intergroup study. J Pediatr Surg 38:315–318

Billmire D, Vinocur C, Rescorla F, Cushing B, London W, Schlatter M, Davis M, Giller R, Lauer S, Olson T (2004a) Outcome and staging evaluation in malignant germ cell tumors of the ovary in children and adolescents: an intergroup study. J Pediatr Surg 39: 424–429

Bokemeyer C, Schleucher N, Metzner B, Thomas M, Rick O, Schmoll HJ, Kollmannsberger C, Boehlke I, Kanz L, Hartmann JT (2003) First-line sequential high-dose VIP chemotherapy with autologous transplantation for patients with primary mediastinal nonseminomatous germ cell tumours: a prospective trial. Br J Cancer 89:29–35

Bryant WP, O'Marcaigh AS, Ledger GA, Zimmerman D (1994) Aqueous vasopressin infusion during chemotherapy in patients with diabetes insipidus. Cancer 74:2589–2592

Calaminus G, Vesterling-Hörner D, Bökkerink JP, Gadner H, Günther G, Haas HJ, Jürgens H, Teske C, Göbel U (1991) The prognostic significance of serum alpha 1-fetoprotein in children and adolescents with malignant extracranial non- testicular germ cell tumors. Klin Padiatr 203:246–250

Calaminus G, Bamberg M, Baranzelli MC, Benoit Y, Di MLC, Fossati-Bellani F, Jürgens H, Kühl HJ, Lenard HG, Lo CM, Göbel U (1994) Intracranial germ cell tumors: a comprehensive update of the European data. Neuropediatrics 25:26–32

Calaminus G, Andreussi L, Garre ML, Kortmann RD, Schober R, Göbel U (1997a) Secreting germ cell tumors of the central nervous system (CNS). First results of the cooperative German/Italian pilot study (CNS sGCT). Klin Padiatr 209:222–227

Calaminus G, Nicholson JC, Alapetite C, Bamberg M, Baranzelli MC, Frappaz D, Garre ML, Göbel U, Hale J, Kortmann RD, Mann JR, Patte C, Punt J, Ricardi U, Saran F, Harms D (2002) Malignant CNS Germ

Cell Tumors (GCTs): interim analysis after 5 Years of SIOP CNS GCT 96. Med Pediatr Oncol 39:O030

Calaminus G, Schneider DT, Bökkerink JP, Gadner H, Harms D, Willers R, Göbel U (2003) Prognostic value of tumor size, metastases, extension into bone, and increased tumor marker in children with malignant sacrococcygeal germ cell tumors: a prospective evaluation of 71 patients treated in the German cooperative protocols Maligne Keimzelltumoren (MAKEI) 83/86 and MAKEI 89. J Clin Oncol 21: 781–786

Calaminus G, Bamberg M, Harms D, Jürgens H, Kortmann RD, Sörensen N, Wiestler OD, Göbel U (2005) AFP/beta-HCG secreting CNS germ cell tumors: long-term outcome with respect to initial symptoms and primary tumor resection. Results of the cooperative trial MAKEI 89. Neuropediatrics 36:71–77

Chang CH, Housepian EM, Herbert CJ (1969) An operative staging system and a megavoltage radiotherapeutic technic for cerebellar medulloblastomas. Radiology 93:1351–1359

Cho BK, Wang KC, Nam DH, Kim DG, Jung HW, Kim HJ, Han DH, Choi KS (1998) Pineal tumors: experience with 48 cases over 10 years. Childs Nerv Syst 14:53–58

Currarino G, Coln D, Votteler T (1981) Triad of anorectal, sacral, and presacral anomalies. AJR Am J Roentgenol 137:395–398

Cushing B, Giller R, Cullen JW, Marina NM, Lauer SJ, Olson TA, Rogers PC, Colombani P, Rescorla F, Billmire DF, Vinocur CD, Hawkins EP, Davis MM, Perlman EJ, London WB, Castleberry RP (2004b) Randomized comparison of combination chemotherapy with etoposide, bleomycin, and either high-dose or standard-dose cisplatin in children and adolescents with high-risk malignant germ cell tumors: a pediatric intergroup study–Pediatric Oncology Group 9049 and Children's Cancer Group 888. J Clin Oncol 22:2691–2700

da Silva NS, Cappellano AM, Diez B, Cavalheiro S, Gardner S, Wisoff J, Kellie S, Parker R, Garvin J, Finlay J (2010) Primary chemotherapy for intracranial germ cell tumors: results of the third international CNS germ cell tumor study. Pediatr Blood Cancer 54:377–383

Dehner LP (1983b) Gonadal and extragonadal germ cell neoplasia of childhood. Hum Pathol 14:493–511

Diez B, Balmaceda C, Matsutani M, Weiner HL (1999) Germ cell tumors of the CNS in children: recent advances in therapy. Childs Nerv Syst 15:578–585

Draper H, Chitayat D, Ein SH, Langer JC (2009) Long-term functional results following resection of neonatal sacrococcygeal teratoma. Pediatr Surg Int 25: 243–246

Egler RA, Gosiengfiao Y, Russell H, Wickiser JE, Frazier AL (2017) Is surgical resection and observation sufficient for stage I and II sacrococcygeal germ cell tumors? A case series and review. Pediatr Blood Cancer 64

Esik O, Nemeth G, Szepeshazi K (1994) Calcitonin-secreting ovarian strumal carcinoid. Eur J Gynaecol Oncol 15:211–216

Frazier AL, Rumcheva P, Olson T, Giller R, Cushing B, Cullen J, Marina N, London WB (2008) Application of the adult international germ cell classification system to pediatric malignant non-seminomatous germ cell tumors: a report from the Children's Oncology Group. Pediatr Blood Cancer 50:746–751

Ganjoo KN, Rieger KM, Kesler KA, Sharma M, Heilman DK, Einhorn LH (2000) Results of modern therapy for patients with mediastinal nonseminomatous germ cell tumors. Cancer 88:1051–1056

Garre ML, El-Hossainy MO, Fondelli P, Göbel U, Brisigotti M, Donati PT, Nantron M, Ravegnani M, Garaventa A, De BB (1996) Is chemotherapy effective therapy for intracranial immature teratoma? A case report. Cancer 77:977–982

Göbel U, Calaminus G, Blohm M, Booss D, Felberbauer F, Hofmann U, Holschneider AM, Willnow U, Harms D (1997b) Extracranial non-testicular teratoma in childhood and adolescence: introduction of a risk score for stratification of therapy. Klin Padiatr 209: 228–234

Göbel U, Calaminus G, Waag K, Jonat W, Harms D (1998b) Extracranial non-testicular teratoma in childhood and adolescents-the German experience. Germ Cell Tumors IV:233–236

Göbel U, Calaminus G, Engert J, Kaatsch P, Gadner H, Bökkerink JP, Hass RJ, Waag K, Blohm ME, Dippert S, Teske C, Harms D (1998c) Teratomas in infancy and childhood. Med Pediatr Oncol 31:8–15

Göbel U, Gutjahr P, Jürgens H, Kabisch H, Lampert F, Spaar H-J, Sternschulte W (1999) Die kooperative Therapiestudie für nichttestikuläre Keimzelltumoen MAKEI83 der GPO: analyse nach 3 Jahren. Klin Padiatr 198:237–244

Göbel U, Schneider DT, Calaminus G, Haas RJ, Schmidt P, Harms D (2000b) Germ-cell tumors in childhood and adolescence. Ann Oncol 11:263–271

Göbel U, Schneider DT, Calaminus G, Jurgens H, Spaar HJ, Sternschulte W, Waag K, Harms D (2001b) Multimodal treatment of malignant sacrococcygeal germ cell tumors: a prospective analysis of 66 patients of the German cooperative protocols MAKEI 83/86 and 89. J Clin Oncol 19:1943–1950

Hale J, Dang H, Krailo M, Olson T, Donachie P, Nicholson J, Billmire D, Thornton C, Frazier L (2010) Mediastinal germ cell tumors—are all patients high risk? Pediatr Blood Cancer 55:804

Harms D, Jänig U (1986) Germ cell tumours of childhood. Report of 170 cases including 59 pure and partial yolk-sac tumours. Virchows Arch A Pathol Anat Histopathol 409:223–239

Hieda S, Fukui T (2008) Germinoma presenting with personality and socio-behavioral abnormalities may challenge differential diagnoses. Brain Nerve 60:949–953

International-Germ-Cell-Cancer-Collaborative--Group (1997) International Germ Cell Consensus Classification: a prognostic factor- based staging system for metastatic germ cell cancers. International Germ Cell Cancer Collaborative Group. J Clin Oncol 15:594–603

Jelin E, Jelin AC, Lee H (2009) Sacrococcygeal teratoma with spinal canal invasion prenatally diagnosed. J Pediatr Surg 44:E9–E11

Kapoor G, Advani SH, Nair CN, Pai K, Kurkure PA, Nair R, Saikia TK, Vege D, Desai PB (1995) Pediatric germ cell tumor. An experience with BEP. J Pediatr Hematol Oncol 17:318–324

Kellie SJ, Boyce H, Dunkel IJ, Diez B, Rosenblum M, Brualdi L, Finlay JL (2004) Primary chemotherapy for intracranial nongerminomatous germ cell tumors: results of the second international CNS germ cell study group protocol. J Clin Oncol 22:846–853

Khatua S, Dhall G, O'Neil S, Jubran R, Villablanca JG, Marachelian A, Nastia A, Lavey R, Olch AJ, Gonzalez I, Gilles F, Nelson M, Panigrahy A, McComb G, Krieger M, Fan J, Sposto R, Finlay JL (2010) Treatment of primary CNS germinomatous germ cell tumors with chemotherapy prior to reduced dose whole ventricular and local boost irradiation. Pediatr Blood Cancer 55:42–46

Kleihues P, Burger PC, Scheithauer BW (1993) The new WHO classification of brain tumours. Brain Pathol 3:255–268

Lam SK, Cheung LP (1996) Inappropriate ADH secretion due to immature ovarian teratoma. Aust N Z J Obstet Gynaecol 36:104–105

Lindahl H (1988) Giant sacrococcygeal teratoma: a method of simple intraoperative control of hemorrhage. J Pediatr Surg 23:1068–1069

Lopes LF, Chazan R, Sredni ST, de Camargo B (1999) Endodermal sinus tumor of the vagina in children. Med Pediatr Oncol 32:377–381

Lopes LF, Sonaglio V, Ribeiro KC, Schneider DT, de Camargo B (2008) Improvement in the outcome of children with germ cell tumors. Pediatr Blood Cancer 50:250–253

Lopes LF, Macedo CR, Pontes EM, Dos Santos AS, Mastellaro MJ, Melaragno R, Vianna SM, Lopes PA, Mendonca N, de Assis Almeida MT, Sonaglio V, Ribeiro KB, Santana VM, Schneider DT, de Camargo B (2009) Cisplatin and etoposide in childhood germ cell tumor: brazilian pediatric oncology society protocol GCT-91. J Clin Oncol 27:1297–1303

Mann JR, Pearson D, Barrett A, Raafat F, Barnes JM, Wallendszus KR (1989b) Results of the United Kingdom Children's Cancer Study Group's malignant germ cell tumor studies. Cancer 63:1657–1667

Mann JR, Raafat F, Robinson K, Imeson J, Gornall P, Phillips M, Sokal M, Gray E, McKeever P, Oakhill A (1998) UKCCSG's germ cell tumour (GCT) studies: improving outcome for children with malignant extracranial non-gonadal tumours—carboplatin, etoposide, and bleomycin are effective and less toxic than previous regimens. United Kingdom Children's Cancer Study Group. Med Pediatr Oncol 30: 217–227

Mann JR, Raafat F, Robinson K, Imeson J, Gornall P, Sokal M, Gray E, McKeever P, Hale J, Bailey S, Oakhill A (2000a) The United Kingdom Children's Cancer Study Group's Second Germ Cell Tumor Study: carboplatin, etoposide, and bleomycin are effective treatment for children with malignant extracranial germ cell tumors, with acceptable toxicity. J Clin Oncol 18:3809–3818

Mann JR, Gray ES, Thornton C, Raafat F, Robinson K, Collins GS, Gornall P, Huddart SN, Hale JP, Oakhill A (2008a) Mature and immature extracranial teratomas in children: the UK Children's Cancer Study Group Experience. J Clin Oncol 26: 3590–3597

Marina NM, Cushing B, Giller R, Cohen L, Lauer SJ, Ablin A, Weetman R, Cullen J, Rogers P, Vinocur C, Stolar C, Rescorla F, Hawkins E, Heifetz S, Rao PV, Krailo M, Castleberry RP (1999b) Complete surgical excision is effective treatment for children with immature teratomas with or without malignant elements: a Pediatric Oncology Group/Children's Cancer Group Intergroup Study. J Clin Oncol 17:2137

Mauz-Körholz C, Harms D, Calaminus G, Göbel U (2000b) Primary chemotherapy and conservative surgery for vaginal yolk-sac tumour. Maligne Keimzelltumoren Study Group Lancet 355:625

Mayer F, Stoop H, Scheffer GL, Scheper R, Oosterhuis JW, Looijenga LH, Bokemeyer C (2003b) Molecular determinants of treatment response in human germ cell tumors. Clin Cancer Res 9:767–773

Mostofi FK, Sobin LH (1993) Histopathological typing of testis tumors. World Health Organization, Geneva

Nichols CR, Heerema NA, Palmer C, Loehrer PJ Sr, Williams SD, Einhorn LH (1987b) Klinefelter's syndrome associated with mediastinal germ cell neoplasms. J Clin Oncol 5:1290–1294

Nicholson JC, Punt J, Hale J, Saran F, Calaminus G (2002) Neurosurgical management of paediatric germ cell tumours of the central nervous system–a multidisciplinary team approach for the new millennium. Br J Neurosurg 16:93–95

Oosterhuis JW, Looijenga LH (2005b) Testicular germ-cell tumours in a broader perspective. Nat Rev Cancer 5:210–222

Rescorla FJ (2008) Malignant germ cell tumors. In: Carachi R, Grosfeld JL, Azmy AF (eds) The surgery of childhood tumors. Springer, New York, pp 261–273

Ribeiro PR, Guys JM, Lena G (1999) Sacrococcygeal teratoma with an intradural and extramedullary extension in a neonate: case report. Neurosurgery 44:398–400

Rogers PC, Olson TA, Cullen JW, Billmire DF, Marina N, Rescorla F, Davis MM, London WB, Lauer SJ, Giller RH, Cushing B (2004b) Treatment of children and adolescents with stage II testicular and stage I and II ovarian malignant germ cell tumors: a Pediatric Intergroup Study–Pediatric Oncology Group 9048 and Children's Cancer Group 8891. J Clin Oncol 22:3563–3569

Schmoll HJ, Kollmannsberger C, Metzner B, Hartmann JT, Schleucher N, Schoffski P, Schleicher J, Rick O, Beyer J, Hossfeld D, Kanz L, Berdel WE, Andreesen R, Bokemeyer C (2003b) Long-term results of first-line sequential high-dose etoposide, ifosfamide, and cisplatin chemotherapy plus autologous stem cell support for patients with advanced metastatic germ cell cancer: an extended phase I/II study of the German Testicular Cancer Study Group. J Clin Oncol 21:4083–4091

Schneider DT, Calaminus G, Reinhard H, Gutjahr P, Kremens B, Harms D, Göbel U (2000b) Primary mediastinal germ cell tumors in children and adolescents: results of the German cooperative protocols MAKEI 83/86, 89, and 96. J Clin Oncol 18:832–839

Schneider DT, Calaminus G, Göbel U (2001e) Diagnostic value of alpha1-fetoprotein and human chorionic gonadotropic hormone in infancy and childhood. Pediatr Hematol Oncol 18:11–26

Schneider DT, Wessalowski R, Calaminus G, Pape H, Bamberg M, Engert J, Waag K, Gadner H, Göbel U (2001f) Treatment of recurrent malignant sacrococcygeal germ cell tumors: analysis of 22 patients registered in the German protocols makei 83/86, 89, and 96. J Clin Oncol 19:1951–1960

Schneider DT, Schuster AE, Fritsch MK, Calaminus G, Göbel U, Harms D, Lauer S, Olson T, Perlman EJ (2002b) Genetic analysis of mediastinal nonseminomatous germ cell tumors in children and adolescents. Genes Chromosomes Cancer 34:115–125

Schneider DT, Calaminus G, Koch S, Teske C, Schmidt P, Haas RJ, Harms D, Göbel U (2004b) Epidemiologic analysis of 1,442 children and adolescents registered in the German germ cell tumor protocols. Pediatr Blood Cancer 42:169–175

Schwabe J, Francke A, Gerharz CD, Willnow U, Schneider DT, Nürnberger W (2000) Immature teratoma arising from an intra-abdominal testis in a 5-month-old boy. Med Pediatr Oncol 35:140–141

Serov SF, Scully RE (1973) Histological typing of ovarian tumors. World Health Organization, Geneva

Teilum G, Albrechtsen R, Norgaard-Pedersen B (1975b) The histogenetic-embryologic basis for reappearance of alpha-fetoprotein in endodermal sinus tumors (yolk sac tumors) and teratomas. Acta Pathol Microbiol Scand A 83:80–86

Wessalowski R, Blohm M, Calaminus G, Engert J, Harms D, Krause I, Kruck H, Grüttner HP, Pape H, Göbel U (1997b) Treatment results in children and adolescents with loco-regional recurrences of abdominal germ cell tumors (GCTs): a pilot-study with PEI chemotherapy and regional deep hyperthermia (RHT) in comparison to a matched cohort. Klin Padiatr 209:250–256

Wessalowski R, Schneider DT, Mils O, Hannen M, Calaminus G, Engelbrecht V, Pape H, Willers R, Engert J, Harms D, Göbel U (2003b) An approach to cure: PEI chemotherapy and regional deep hyperthermia in children and adolescents with unresectable malignant tumors. Klin Padiatr 215:303–309

Yassa L, Sadow P, Marqusee E (2008) Malignant struma ovarii. Nat Clin Pract Endocrinol Metab 4:469–472

Young RH (2005a) A brief history of the pathology of the gonads. Mod Pathol 18(Suppl 2):S3–S17

Testicular Germ Cell Tumors

Altman RP, Randolph JG et al (1974b) Sacrococcygeal teratoma: American Academy of Pediatrics Surgical Section Survey-1973. J Pediatr Surg 9(3): 389–398

Atkin NB, Baker MC (1992) X-chromatin, sex chromosomes, and ploidy in 37 germ cell tumors of the testis. Cancer Genet Cytogenet 59(1):54–56

Baranzelli MC, Patte C (1998) The french experience in paediatric malignant germ cell tumours. In: Jones WG, Appleyard I, Harnden P, Joffe JK (eds) Germ cell tumours IV. John Libbey and Co. Ltd, London, pp 219–226

Baranzelli MC, Kramar A et al (1999c) Prognostic factors in children with localized malignant nonseminomatous germ cell tumors. J Clin Oncol 17(4):1212

Billmire DF (2006a) Malignant germ cell tumors in childhood. Semin Pediatr Surg 15(1):30–36

Bussey KJ, Lawce HJ et al (1999b) Chromosome abnormalities of eighty-one pediatric germ cell tumors: sex-, age-, site-, and histopathology-related differences—a Children's Cancer Group study. Genes Chromosomes Cancer 25(2):134–146

Carver BS, Motzer RJ et al (2005) Late relapse of testicular germ cell tumors. Urol Oncol 23(6):441–445

Carver BS, Shayegan B et al (2007d) Long-term clinical outcome after postchemotherapy retroperitoneal lymph node dissection in men with residual teratoma. J Clin Oncol 25(9):1033–1037

Cushing B, Giller R et al (2004c) Randomized comparison of combination chemotherapy with etoposide, bleomycin, and either high-dose or standard-dose Cisplatin in children and adolescents with high-risk malignant germ cell tumors: a Pediatric Intergroup Study–Pediatric Oncology Group 9049 and Children's Cancer Group 888. J Clin Oncol 22(13): 2691–2700

Einhorn LH, Donohue J (1977b) Cis-diamminedichloroplatinum, vinblastine, and bleomycin combination chemotherapy in disseminated testicular cancer. Ann Intern Med 87(3):293–298

Einhorn LH, Williams SD et al (1989b) Evaluation of optimal duration of chemotherapy in favorable-prognosis disseminated germ cell tumors: a Southeastern Cancer Study Group protocol. J Clin Oncol 7(3): 387–391

El-Naggar AK, Ro JY et al (1992) DNA ploidy in testicular germ cell neoplasms. Histogenetic and clinical implications. Am J Surg Pathol 16(6):611–618

Giwercman A, Grindsted J et al (1987) Testicular cancer risk in boys with maldescended testis: a cohort study. J Urol 138(5):1214–1216

Göbel U, Calaminus G et al (2002a) Management of germ cell tumors in children: approaches to cure. Onkologie 25(1):14–22

Göbel U, Calaminus G, Haas R, Teske C, Schönberger S, Schneider DT, Leuschner I, Harms D (2014) Testicular germ cell tumors in adolescents - results of the protocol MAHO 98 and the identification of good risk patients. Klin Padiatr 226:316–322

Göbel U, Haas RJ et al (1990) Treatment of germ cell tumors in children: results of European trials for testicular and non-testicular primary sites. Crit Rev Oncol Hematol 10(2):89–98

Group, I. G. C. C. C (1997b) International germ cell consensus classification: a prognostic factor-based staging system for metastatic germ cell cancers. J Clin Oncol 15(2):594–603

Haas RJ, Schmidt P et al (1999) Testicular germ cell tumors, an update. Results of the German cooperative studies 1982–1997. Klin Padiatr 211(4):300–304

Harms D, Zahn S et al (2006b) Pathology and molecular biology of teratomas in childhood and adolescence. Klin Padiatr 218(6):296–302

Hawkins E, Perlman EJ (1996b) Germ cell tumors in childhood: morphology and biology. In: Parham DM (ed) Pediatric neoplasia: morphology and biology. Raven, New York, p 297

Kaatsch P (2004b) German Childhood Cancer Registry and its favorable setting. Bundesgesundheitsblatt Gesundheitsforschung Gesundheitsschutz 47(5):437–443

Kaplan CG, Askin FB et al (1979b) Cytogenetics of extragonadal tumors. Teratology 19(2):261–266

Kurman RJ, Norris HJ (1976b) Malignant mixed germ cell tumors of the ovary. A clinical and pathologic analysis of 30 cases. Obstet Gynecol 48(5):579–589

Lo Curto M, Lumia F et al (2003) Malignant germ cell tumors in childhood: results of the first Italian cooperative study "TCG 91". Med Pediatr Oncol 41(5):417–425

Looijenga LH, Gillis AJ et al (1993) In situ numeric analysis of centromeric regions of chromosomes 1, 12, and 15 of seminomas, nonseminomatous germ cell tumors, and carcinoma in situ of human testis. Lab Investig 68(2):211–219

Lopes LF, Macedo CR et al (2009b) Cisplatin and etoposide in childhood germ cell tumor: Brazilian pediatric oncology society protocol GCT-91. J Clin Oncol 27(8):1297–1303

Mann JR, Gray ES et al (2008b) Mature and immature extracranial teratomas in children: the UK Children's Cancer Study Group Experience. J Clin Oncol 26(21):3590–3597

Mann JR, Raafat F et al (2000b) The United Kingdom Children's Cancer Study Group's second germ cell tumor study: carboplatin, etoposide, and bleomycin are effective treatment for children with malignant extracranial germ cell tumors, with acceptable toxicity. J Clin Oncol 18(22):3809–3818

Marina N, Chang KW et al (2005) Amifostine does not protect against the ototoxicity of high-dose cisplatin combined with etoposide and bleomycin in pediatric germ-cell tumors: a Children's Oncology Group study. Cancer 104(4):841–847

Marina NM, Cushing B et al (1999c) Complete surgical excision is effective treatment for children with immature teratomas with or without malignant elements: a Pediatric Oncology Group/Children's Cancer Group Intergroup Study. J Clin Oncol 17(7): 2137–2143

Marina N, London WB et al (2006b) Prognostic factors in children with extragonadal malignant germ cell tumors: a pediatric intergroup study. J Clin Oncol 24(16):2544–2548

Mostert MM, van de Pol M et al (1996) Comparative genomic hybridization of germ cell tumors of the adult testis: confirmation of karyotypic findings and identification of a 12p-amplicon. Cancer Genet Cytogenet 89(2):146–152

Oosterhuis JW, Castedo SM et al (1988) Karyotyping and DNA flow cytometry of an orchidoblastoma. Cancer Genet Cytogenet 36(1):7–11

Oosterhuis JW, Castedo SM et al (1989) Ploidy of primary germ cell tumors of the testis. Pathogenetic and clinical relevance Lab Invest 60(1):14–21

Ozols RF, Ihde DC et al (1988) A randomized trial of standard chemotherapy v a high-dose chemotherapy regimen in the treatment of poor prognosis nonseminomatous germ-cell tumors. J Clin Oncol 6(6):1031–1040

Perlman EJ, Cushing B et al (1994b) Cytogenetic analysis of childhood endodermal sinus tumors: a Pediatric Oncology Group study. Pediatr Pathol 14(4): 695–708

Ries LAG, Smith M, Gurney JG, Linet M, Tamra T, Young JL, Bunin GR (eds) (1999b) Cancer incidence and survival among children and adolescents: United States SEER program 1975–1995. National Cancer Institute, Bethesda, National Cancer Institute, SEER Program. NIH Publication No. 99-4649

Rodriguez E, Houldsworth J et al (1993) Molecular cytogenetic analysis of i (12p)-negative human male germ cell tumors. Genes Chromosomes Cancer 8(4):230–236

Rogers PC, Olson TA et al (2004c) Treatment of children and adolescents with stage II testicular and stages I and II ovarian malignant germ cell tumors: a Pediatric Intergroup Study–Pediatric Oncology Group 9048 and Children's Cancer Group 8891. J Clin Oncol 22(17):3563–3569

Schlatter M, Rescorla F et al (2003) Excellent outcome in patients with stage I germ cell tumors of the testes: a study of the Children's Cancer Group/Pediatric Oncology Group. J Pediatr Surg 38(3):319–324; discussion 319–324

Schmidt P, Haas RJ et al (2002a) Results of the German Studies (MAHO) for treatment of Testicular Germ

Cell Tumors in Children—an update. Klin Padiatr 214(4):167–172
Schneider DT, Calaminus G et al (2004c) Epidemiologic analysis of 1,442 children and adolescents registered in the German germ cell tumor protocols. Pediatr Blood Cancer 42(2):169–175
Sievers S, Alemazkour K et al (2005b) IGF2/H19 imprinting analysis of human germ cell tumors (GCTs) using the methylation-sensitive single-nucleotide primer extension method reflects the origin of GCTs in different stages of primordial germ cell development. Genes Chromosomes Cancer 44(3):256–264
Stock C, Ambros IM et al (1994) Detection of numerical and structural chromosome abnormalities in pediatric germ cell tumors by means of interphase cytogenetics. Genes Chromosomes Cancer 11(1):40–50
van Gurp RJ, Oosterhuis JW et al (1994) Biallelic expression of the H19 and IGF2 genes in human testicular germ cell tumors. J Natl Cancer Inst 86(14):1070–1075
Young R, Scully R (1990b) Germ cell tumors: nonseminomatous tumors, occult tumors, effects of chemotherapy in testicular tumors. ASCP Press, Chicago

Germ Cell Tumors of the Ovary

Bagolan P, Rivosecchi M et al (1992) Prenatal diagnosis and clinical outcome of ovarian cysts. J Pediatr Surg 27(7):879–881
Baranzelli MC, Bouffet E et al (2000b) Non-seminomatous ovarian germ cell tumours in children. Eur J Cancer 36(3):376–383
Bernstein L, Smith MA et al (1999) Germ cell, trophoblastic and other gonadal neoplasms. In: Ries LAG SM, Gurney JG, Linet M, Tamra T, Young JL, Bunin GR (eds) Cancer incidence and survival among children and adolescents: United States SEER Program 1975–1995. National Cancer Institute, Bethesda, Cancer Statistics Bran, Cancer Surveillance Research Program, Division of Cancer Control and Population Sciences, National Cancer Institute. NIH Pub. No. 99–4649, pp 125–138
Billmire D, Vinocur C et al (2004b) Outcome and staging evaluation in malignant germ cell tumors of the ovary in children and adolescents: an intergroup study. J Pediatr Surg 39(3):424–429; discussion 424–429
Billmire DF (2006b) Malignant germ cell tumors in childhood. Semin Pediatr Surg 15(1):30–36
Cannistra SA (1993) Cancer of the ovary. N Engl J Med 329:1550
Cass DL, Hawkins E et al (2001) Surgery for ovarian masses in infants, children, and adolescents: 102 consecutive patients treated in a 15-year period. J Pediatr Surg 36(5):693–699
Cronen PW, Nagaraj HS (1988) Ovarian tumors in children. South Med J 81(4):464–468
Cushing B, Giller R et al (2004d) Randomized comparison of combination chemotherapy with etoposide, bleomycin, and either high-dose or standard-dose cisplatin in children and adolescents with high-risk malignant germ cell tumors: a Pediatric Intergroup Study–Pediatric Oncology Group 9049 and Children's Cancer Group 888. J Clin Oncol 22(13): 2691–2700
dos Santos SI, Swerdlow AJ (1991) Ovarian germ cell malignancies in England: epidemiological parallels with testicular cancer. Br J Cancer 63(5):814–818
Ehrlich PF, Teitelbaum DH et al (2007) Excision of large cystic ovarian tumors: combining minimal invasive surgery techniques and cancer surgery–the best of both worlds. J Pediatr Surg 42(5):890–893
Gibas Z, Talerman A et al (1993) Cytogenetic analysis of an immature teratoma of the ovary and its metastasis after chemotherapy-induced maturation. Int J Gynecol Pathol 12(3):276–280
Göbel U, Calaminus G et al (1998d) Teratomas in infancy and childhood. Med Pediatr Oncol 31(1):8–15
Göbel U, Calaminus G et al (2002b) Management of germ cell tumors in children: approaches to cure. Onkologie 25(1):14–22
Göbel U, Calaminus G et al (2006) The malignant potential of teratomas in infancy and childhood: the MAKEI experiences in non-testicular teratoma and implications for a new protocol. Klin Padiatr 218(6):309–314
Gribbon M, Ein SH et al (1992) Pediatric malignant ovarian tumors: a 43-year review. J Pediatr Surg 27(4):480–484
Harris BH, Boles ET Jr (1974) Rational surgery for tumors of the ovary in children. J Pediatr Surg 9(3):289–293
Hayes-Jordan A (2005) Surgical management of the incidentally identified ovarian mass. Semin Pediatr Surg 14(2):106–110
Hoffner L, Deka R et al (1994) Cytogenetics and origins of pediatric germ cell tumors. Cancer Genet Cytogenet 74(1):54–58
Jabra AA, Fishman EK et al (1993) Primary ovarian tumors in the pediatric patient: CT evaluation. Clin Imaging 17(3):199–203
King ME, DiGiovanni LM et al (1990) Immature teratoma of the ovary grade 3, with karyotype analysis. Int J Gynecol Pathol 9(2):178–184
Lovvorn HN 3rd, Tucci LA et al (1998) Ovarian masses in the pediatric patient. AORN J 67(3):568–576; quiz 577, 580–84
Mann JR, Raafat F et al (2000c) The United Kingdom Children's Cancer Study Group's second germ cell tumor study: carboplatin, etoposide, and bleomycin are effective treatment for children with malignant extracranial germ cell tumors, with acceptable toxicity. J Clin Oncol 18(22):3809–3818
Mann JR, Gray ES et al (2008c) Mature and immature extracranial teratomas in children: the UK Children's Cancer Study Group Experience. J Clin Oncol 26(21):3590–3597
Marina NM, Pratt CB et al (1992) Improved prognosis of children with osteosarcoma metastatic to the lung (s) at the time of diagnosis. Cancer 70(11): 2722–2727

Norris HJ, Zirkin HJ et al (1976) Immature (malignant) teratoma of the ovary: a clinical and pathologic study of 58 cases. Cancer 37(5):2359–2372

Ohama K, Nomura K et al (1985) Origin of immature teratoma of the ovary. Am J Obstet Gynecol 152(7 Pt 1):896–900

Parrington JM, West LF et al (1984) The origin of ovarian teratomas. J Med Genet 21(1):4–12

Pienkowski C, Baunin C et al (2004) Ovarian masses in adolescent girls. Endocr Dev 7:163–182

Riopel MA, Spellerberg A et al (1998) Genetic analysis of ovarian germ cell tumors by comparative genomic hybridization. Cancer Res 58(14): 3105–3110

Rogers PC, Olson TA et al (2004d) Treatment of children and adolescents with stage II testicular and stages I and II ovarian malignant germ cell tumors: a Pediatric Intergroup Study–Pediatric Oncology Group 9048 and Children's Cancer Group 8891. J Clin Oncol 22(17):3563–3569

Schmidt P, Haas RJ et al (2002b) Results of the German Studies (MAHO) for treatment of Testicular Germ Cell Tumors in Children—an update. Klin Padiatr 214(4):167–172

Schneider DT, Schuster AE et al (2001g) Multipoint imprinting analysis indicates a common precursor cell for gonadal and nongonadal pediatric germ cell tumors. Cancer Res 61(19):7268–7276

Schultz KA, Sencer SF et al (2005) Pediatric ovarian tumors: a review of 67 cases. Pediatr Blood Cancer 44(2):167–173

Speleman F, De Potter C et al (1990) i (12p) in a malignant ovarian tumor. Cancer Genet Cytogenet 45(1):49–53

Surratt JT, Siegel MJ (1991) Imaging of pediatric ovarian masses. Radiographics 11(4):533–548

Surti U, Hoffner L et al (1990) Genetics and biology of human ovarian teratomas. I. Cytogenetic analysis and mechanism of origin. Am J Hum Genet 47(4):635–643

Templeman CL, Fallat ME (2005) Benign ovarian masses. Semin Pediatr Surg 14(2):93–99

Thompson FH, Emerson J et al (1994) Clonal chromosome abnormalities in 54 cases of ovarian carcinoma. Cancer Genet Cytogenet 73(1):33–45

Walker AH, Ross RK et al (1988) Hormonal factors and risk of ovarian germ cell cancer in young women. Br J Cancer 57(4):418–422

Sex Cord Stromal Tumors of the Testis and Ovary

Al-Agha OM, Huwait HF, Chow C, Yang W, Senz J, Kalloger SE, Huntsman DG, Young RH, Gilks CB (2011) FOXL2 is a sensitive and specific marker for sex cord-stromal tumors of the ovary. Am J Surg Pathol 35:484–494

Boyer A, Paquet M, Lague MN, Hermo L, Boerboom D (2009) Dysregulation of WNT/CTNNB1 and PI3K/AKT signaling in testicular stromal cells causes granulosa cell tumor of the testis. Carcinogenesis 30:869–878

Calaminus G, Wessalowski R, Harms D, Göbel U (1997b) Juvenile granulosa cell tumors of the ovary in children and adolescents: results from 33 patients registered in a prospective cooperative study. Gynecol Oncol 65:447–452

Cecchetto G, Alaggio R, Bisogno G, Virgone C, Dall'Igna P, Terenziani M, Boldrini R, D'Onofrio V, Ferrari A, Bernini G (2010) Sex cord-stromal tumors of the testis in children. A clinicopathologic report from the Italian TREP project. J Pediatr Surg 45:1868–1873

Cecchetto G, Ferrari A, Bernini G, Alaggio R, Collini P, Virgone C, Terenziani M, Dall'Igna P, Cozza R, Conte M, Bisogno G (2011) Sex cord stromal tumors of the ovary in children: a clinicopathological report from the Italian TREP project. Pediatr Blood Cancer 56(7):1062–1067

Chang B, Borer JG, Tan PE, Diamond DA (1998) Large-cell calcifying Sertoli cell tumor of the testis: case report and review of the literature. Urology 52:520–522

Clement PB, Young RH, Scully RE (1991) Clinical syndromes associated with tumors of the female genital tract. Semin Diagn Pathol 8:204–233

Colombo N, Sessa C, Landoni F, Sartori E, Pecorelli S, Mangioni C (1986) Cisplatin, vinblastine, and bleomycin combination chemotherapy in metastatic granulosa cell tumor of the ovary. Obstet Gynecol 67: 265–268

Crofton PM, Evans AE, Groome NP, Taylor MR, Holland CV, Kelnar CJ (2002a) Dimeric inhibins in girls from birth to adulthood: relationship with age, pubertal stage, FSH and oestradiol. Clin Endocrinol 56:223–230

Crofton PM, Evans AE, Groome NP, Taylor MR, Holland CV, Kelnar CJ (2002b) Inhibin B in boys from birth to adulthood: relationship with age, pubertal stage, FSH and testosterone. Clin Endocrinol 56:215–221

Distelmaier F, Calaminus G, Harms D, Sträter R, Cordes U, Fleischhack G, Göbel U, Schneider DT (2006a) Ovarian small cell carcinoma of the hypercalcemic type in children and adolescents: a prognostically unfavorable but curable disease. Cancer 107(9):2298–2306

Harms D, Kock LR (1997) Testicular juvenile granulosa cell and Sertoli cell tumours: a clinicopathological study of 29 cases from the Kiel Paediatric Tumour Registry. Virchows Arch 430:301–309

Hill DA, Ivanovich J, Priest JR, Gurnett CA, Dehner LP, Desruisseau D, Jarzembowski JA, Wikenheiser-Brokamp KA, Suarez BK, Whelan AJ, Williams G, Bracamontes D, Messinger Y, Goodfellow PJ (2009) DICER1 mutations in familial pleuropulmonary blastoma. Science 325:965

Jacoby AF, Young RH, Colvin RB, Flotte TJ, Preffer F, Scully RE, Swymer CM, Bell DA (1992) DNA content in juvenile granulosa cell tumors of the ovary: a study of early and advanced stage disease. Gynecol Oncol 46:97–103

Kalfa N, Patte C, Orbach D, Lecointre C, Pienkowski C, Philippe F, Thibault E, Plantaz D, Brauner R, Rubie H, Guedj AM, Ecochard A, Paris F, Jeandel C, Baldet P, Sultan C (2005) A nationwide study of granulosa cell tumors in pre- and postpubertal girls: missed diagnosis of endocrine manifestations worsens prognosis. J Pediatr Endocrinol Metab 18:25–31

Kalfa N, Ecochard A, Patte C, Duvillard P, Audran F, Pienkowski C, Thibaud E, Brauner R, Lecointre C, Plantaz D, Guedj AM, Paris F, Baldet P, Lumbroso S, Sultan C (2006) Activating mutations of the stimulatory g protein in juvenile ovarian granulosa cell tumors: a new prognostic factor? J Clin Endocrinol Metab 91:1842–1847

Kalfa N, Fellous M, Boizet-Bonhoure B, Patte C, Duvillard P, Pienkowski C, Jaubert F, Ecochard A, Sultan C (2008) Aberrant expression of ovary determining gene FOXL2 in the testis and juvenile granulosa cell tumor in children. J Urol 180:1810–1813

Kim GJ, Georg I, Scherthan H, Merkenschlager M, Guillou F, Scherer G, Barrionuevo F (2010) Dicer is required for Sertoli cell function and survival. Int J Dev Biol 54:867–875

Kudelka AP, Vasuratna A, Edwards CL, Augustine K, Benjapibal M, Verschraegen CF, Kavanagh JJ (1998) Gemcitabine after bone marrow transplantation for refractory juvenile granulosa cell tumor. Anti-Cancer Drugs 9:621–623

Plantaz D, Flamant F, Vassal G, Chappuis JP, Baranzelli MC, Bouffet E, Dyon JF, Armari C, Bost M (1992) Granulosa cell tumors of the ovary in children and adolescents. Multicenter retrospective study in 40 patients aged 7 months to 22 years. Arch Fr Pediatr 49:793–798

Poiana C, Virtej I, Carsote M, Banceanu G, Sajin M, Stanescu B, Ioachim D, Hortopan D, Coculescu M (2010) Virilising Sertoli-Leydig cell tumour associated with thyroid papillary carcinoma: case report and general considerations. Gynecol Endocrinol 26: 617–622

Powell JL, Otis CN (1997) Management of advanced juvenile granulosa cell tumor of the ovary. Gynecol Oncol 64:282–284

Powell JL, Johnson NA, Bailey CL, Otis CN (1993) Management of advanced juvenile granulosa cell tumor of the ovary. Gynecol Oncol 48:119–123

Powell JL, Connor GP, Henderson GS (2001) Management of recurrent juvenile granulosa cell tumor of the ovary. Gynecol Oncol 81:113–116

Rio Frio T, Bahubeshi A, Kanellopoulou C, Hamel N, Niedziela M, Sabbaghian N, Pouchet C, Gilbert L, O'Brien PK, Serfas K, Broderick P, Houlston RS, Lesueur F, Bonora E, Muljo S, Schimke RN, Bouron-Dal Soglio D, Arseneau J, Schultz KA, Priest JR, Nguyen VH, Harach HR, Livingston DM, Foulkes WD, Tischkowitz M (2011) DICER1 mutations in familial multinodular goiter with and without ovarian Sertoli-Leydig cell tumors. JAMA 305:68–77

Ross JH, Rybicki L, Kay R (2002) Clinical behavior and a contemporary management algorithm for prepubertal testis tumors: a summary of the Prepubertal Testis Tumor Registry. J Urol 168:1675–1678

Schneider DT, Calaminus G, Göbel U (2001h) Diagnostic value of alpha_1_-fetoprotein and human chorionic gonadotropic hormone in infancy and childhood. Pediatr Hematol Oncol 18:11–26

Schneider DT, Calaminus G, Wessalowski R, Pathmanathan R, Harms D, Göbel U (2002c) Therapy of advanced ovarian juvenile granulosa cell tumors. Klin Padiatr 214:173–178

Schneider DT, Calaminus G, Wessalowski R, Pathmanathan R, Selle B, Sternschulte W, Harms D, Göbel U (2003a) Ovarian sex cord-stromal tumors in children and adolescents. J Clin Oncol 21:2357–2363

Schneider DT, Jänig U, Calaminus G, Göbel U, Harms D (2003b) Ovarian sex cord—stromal tumors—a clinicopathologic study of 72 cases from the Kiel Pediatric Tumor Registry. Virchows Arch 443:549–560

Schmidt D, Ovitt CE, Anlag K, Fehsenfeld S, Gredsted L, Treier AC, Treier M (2004) The murine winged-helix transcription factor Foxl2 is required for granulosa cell differentiation and ovary maintenance. Development 131:933–942

Schneider DT, Calaminus G, Göbel U (2004d) Tumor rupture and mitotic index in pediatric sex cord-stromal tumors. J Clin Oncol 22:2033–2035

Schneider DT, Calaminus G, Harms D, Göbel U (2005b) Ovarian sex cord-stromal tumors in children and adolescents. J Reprod Med 50:439–446

Shah SP, Kobel M, Senz J, Morin RD, Clarke BA, Wiegand KC, Leung G, Zayed A, Mehl E, Kalloger SE, Sun M, Giuliany R, Yorida E, Jones S, Varhol R, Swenerton KD, Miller D, Clement PB, Crane C, Madore J, Provencher D, Leung P, DeFazio A, Khattra J, Turashvili G, Zhao Y, Zeng T, Glover JN, Vanderhyden B, Zhao C, Parkinson CA, Jimenez-Linan M, Bowtell DD, Mes-Masson AM, Brenton JD, Aparicio SA, Boyd N, Hirst M, Gilks CB, Marra M, Huntsman DG (2009) Mutation of FOXL2 in granulosa-cell tumors of the ovary. N Engl J Med 360:2719–2729

Slade I, Bacchelli C, Davies H, Murray A, Abbaszadeh F, Hanks S, Barfoot R, Burke A, Chisholm J, Hewitt M, Jenkinson H, King D, Morland B, Pizer B, Prescott K, Saggar A, Side L, Traunecker H, Vaidya S, Ward P, Futreal PA, Vujanic G, Nicholson AG, Sebire N, Turnbull C, Priest JR, Pritchard-Jones K, Houlston R, Stiller C, Stratton MR, Douglas J, Rahman N (2011) DICER1 syndrome: clarifying the diagnosis, clinical features and management implications of a pleiotropic tumour predisposition syndrome. J Med Genet 48(4):273–278

Tröbs RB, Krauss M, Geyer C, Tannapfel A, Körholz D, Hirsch W (2007) Surgery in infants and children with testicular and paratesticular tumours: a single centre experience over a 25-year-period. Klin Padiatr 219:146–151

Wessalowski R, Spaar HJ, Pape H, Willers R, Harms D, Göbel U (1995) Successful liver treatment of a juvenile granulosa cell tumor in a 4-year-old child by regional deep hyperthermia, systemic chemotherapy, and irradiation. Gynecol Oncol 57: 417–422

Whitcomb RW, Calkins JW, Lukert BP, Kyner JL, Schimke RN (1986) Androblastomas and thyroid disease in postmenopausal sisters. Obstet Gynecol 67:89S–91S

Young RH (2005b) A brief history of the pathology of the gonads. Mod Pathol 18(Suppl 2):S3–S17

Young RH (2005c) Sex cord-stromal tumors of the ovary and testis: their similarities and differences with consideration of selected problems. Mod Pathol 18(Suppl 2):S81–S98

Young RH, Scully RE (1985) Ovarian Sertoli-Leydig cell tumors. A clinicopathological analysis of 207 cases. Am J Surg Pathol 9:543–569

Young RH, Welch WR, Dickersin GR, Scully RE (1982) Ovarian sex cord tumor with annular tubules: review of 74 cases including 27 with Peutz-Jeghers syndrome and four with adenoma malignum of the cervix. Cancer 50:1384–1402

Young RH, Dickersin GR, Scully RE (1984a) Juvenile granulosa cell tumor of the ovary. A clinicopathological analysis of 125 cases. Am J Surg Pathol 8:575–596

Young RH, Perez-Atayde AR, Scully RE (1984b) Ovarian Sertoli-Leydig cell tumor with retiform and heterologous components. Report of a case with hepatocytic differentiation and elevated serum alpha-fetoprotein. Am J Surg Pathol 8:709–718

Ovarian Adenomas, Ovarian Carcinoma, and Ovarian Small Cell Carcinoma

Benedet JL, Bender H, Jones H III, Ngan HY, Pecorelli S (2000) FIGO staging classifications and clinical practice guidelines in the management of gynecologic cancers. FIGO Committee on Gynecologic Oncology. Int J Gynaecol Obstet 70:209–262

Berchuck A, Witkowski L, Hasselblatt M, Foulkes WD (2015) Prophylactic oophorectomy for hereditary small cell carcinoma of the ovary, hypercalcemic type. Gynecol Oncol Rep 12:20–22

Bernbeck B, Schneider DT et al (2009a) Germ cell tumors of the head and neck: report from the MAKEI Study Group. Pediatr Blood Cancer 52(2):223–226

Dickersin GR, Kline IW, Scully RE (1982) Small cell carcinoma of the ovary with hypercalcemia: a report of eleven cases. Cancer 49:188–197

Distelmaier F, Calaminus G, Harms D, Sträter R, Cordes U, Fleischhack G, Göbel U, Schneider DT (2006b) Ovarian small cell carcinoma of the hypercalcemic type in children and adolescents: a prognostically unfavorable but curable disease. Cancer 107(9):2298–2306

Florell SR, Bruggers CS, Matlak M, Young RH, Lowichik A (1999) Ovarian small cell carcinoma of the hypercalcemic type in a 14 month old: the youngest reported case. Med Pediatr Oncol 32:304–307

Harrison ML, Hoskins P, du Bois A, Quinn M, Rustin GJ, Ledermann JA, Baron-Hay S, Friedlander ML (2006) Small cell of the ovary, hypercalcemic type—analysis of combined experience and recommendation for management. A GCIG study. Gynecol Oncol 100: 233–238

Lamovec J, Bracko M, Cerar O (1995) Familial occurrence of small-cell carcinoma of the ovary. Arch Pathol Lab Med 119:523–527

Longy M, Toulouse C, Mage P, Chauvergne J, Trojani M (1996) Familial cluster of ovarian small cell carcinoma: a new Mendelian entity? J Med Genet 33:333–335

Millar DM, Blake JM, Stringer DA, Hara H, Babiak C (1993) Prepubertal ovarian cyst formation: 5 years' experience. Obstet Gynecol 81:434–438

Pautier P, Ribrag V, Duvillard P, Rey A, Elghissassi I, Sillet-Bach I, Kerbrat P, Mayer F, Lesoin A, Brun B, Crouet H, Barats JC, Morice P, Lhomme C (2007) Results of a prospective dose-intensive regimen in 27 patients with small cell carcinoma of the ovary of the hypercalcemic type. Ann Oncol 18:1985–1989

Robertson DM, Stephenson T, Pruysers E, Burger HG, McCloud P, Tsigos A, Groome N, Mamers P, McNeilage J, Jobling T, Healy D (2002) Inhibins/activins as diagnostic markers for ovarian cancer. Mol Cell Endocrinol 191:97–103

Schneider DT, Jänig U, Calaminus G, Göbel U, Harms D (2003c) Ovarian sex cord—stromal tumors—a clinicopathologic study of 72 cases from the Kiel Pediatric Tumor Registry. Virchows Arch 443:549–560

Senekjian EK, Weiser PA, Talerman A, Herbst AL (1989) Vinblastine, cisplatin, cyclophosphamide, bleomycin, doxorubicin, and etoposide in the treatment of small cell carcinoma of the ovary. Cancer 64: 1183–1187

Young RH, Oliva E, Scully RE (1994) Small cell carcinoma of the ovary, hypercalcemic type. A clinicopathological analysis of 150 cases. Am J Surg Pathol 18:1102–1116

Young JL Jr, Cheng WX, Roffers SD, Howe HL, Correa C, Weinstein R (2003) Ovarian cancer in children and young adults in the United States, 1992–1997. Cancer 97:2694–2700

32 Rare Tumors of the Urinary Tract

Filippo Spreafico and Norbert Graf

32.1 Differential Diagnosis of Urinary Tract Tumors

Malignant renal tumors cover 6% of all childhood cancers (Pastore et al. 2006). Wilms tumor or nephroblastoma is largely the most common type of cancer in the kidney of children Graf and Bergeron 2012), accounting for more than 90% of primary renal tumors. Other tumors, like clear cell sarcoma of the kidney (CCSK), rhabdoid tumor of the kidney (RTK), renal cell carcinoma (RCC), renal medullary carcinoma, congenital mesoblastic nephroma (CMN), primitive neuroectodermal tumor of the kidney, adenoma of the kidney, and others, are much rarer. As their treatment and prognosis is quite different from Wilms tumor, an early timely diagnosis is crucial to deliver the best treatment to patients.

The typical presentation of a child with a kidney tumor is a painless mass in the abdomen. Other complaints are found in <20% of children (Graf and Wilms-Tumoren 2003; Brok et al. 2016), and may include hematuria and hypertension. It is well known that Wilms tumor may be associated with different syndromes (Scott et al. 2006; Srinivasan et al. 2019), and such syndromes can guide the way to a correct diagnosis. Children with tuberous sclerosis or von Hippel–Lindau disease are at risk for developing RCC or angiomyolipoma (Sausville et al. 2009). Cystic tumors, like cystic nephroma, may be encountered in children with DICER1-related syndrome (Schultz et al. 2018). Renal medullary carcinoma, a highly malignant tumor of the epithelial origin, occurs almost exclusively in adolescents and young adults with sickle cell trait or sickle cell disease (Swartz et al. 2002). Altogether there are no typical clinical signs or symptoms in children suffering from a specific renal tumor. Furthermore, there are no specific tumor markers available.

Imaging studies are important, although none of these rare tumors show a specific appearance in ultrasound, computed tomography (CT) scan, or magnetic resonance imaging (MRI), compared to nephroblastoma (Brisse et al. 2020; Watson et al. 2020). Even if RTKs are more lobulated, often showing peripheral subcapsular bleedings, more lymph node involvement, and more often lung metastases, they cannot be clearly distinguished from other renal neoplasm by imaging studies alone (Schenk et al. 2004, 2005; Watson et al. 2020). Only in addition with further information like the knowledge of lung metastasis in a small infant having a renal mass

F. Spreafico (✉)
Pediatric Oncology Unit, Fondazione IRCCS Istituto Nazionale dei Tumori, Milan, Italy
e-mail: filippo.spreafico@istitutotumori.mi.it

N. Graf
Department Pediatric Oncology and Hematology, Saarland University, Medical School, Homburg, Germany
e-mail: graf@uks.eu

D. T. Schneider et al. (eds.), *Rare Tumors in Children and Adolescents*, Pediatric Oncology,
https://doi.org/10.1007/978-3-030-92071-5_32

makes the diagnosis of a specific neoplasm more likely as RTK in the above case. However, abdominal cross-sectional imaging is key important: despite not being able to differentiate between the tumor types, it helps diagnosing tumor thrombus in the vessels (renal or Cava veins), the presence of abdominal metastases (lymph nodes, liver, peritoneum), or the presence of lesions in the contralateral kidneys. In all cases of a renal mass, a chest X-ray or computed tomography (CT) scan of the torax is needed for staging. Further staging procedures are mandatory in patients with specific diagnoses, and for this reason they should be performed after the histologic diagnosis is clear. In case of CCSK and RTK, an MRI of the brain should be performed as these tumors may develop brain metastasis in some patients (Smets and de Kraker 2010). Radioisotope bone scan (99 m-technetium-methylene diphosphonate) is recommended only in cases of CCSK and RCC to exclude bone metastasis (Smets and de Kraker 2010; Schenk et al. 2005).

Important to note, when the radiological and clinical picture cannot be orientative of a given tumor type or exclude a Wilms tumor, a percutaneous co-axial tru-cut biopsy is the most effective and safe method to reach a diagnosis (Irtan et al. 2019).

Diffusion-weighted MRI (DWI) may help in distinguishing between necrotic and vital tumor areas, above all after chemotherapy in cases of Wilms tumor, and in the follow-up of patients in defining response to treatment (Watson et al. 2020), but more research is needed to clarify their role in the diagnostic workup of rare kidney tumors in children (van den Heuvel-Eibrink et al. 2017). Experience with new imaging methods in non-Wilms tumors of the kidney is even more limited.

A correct diagnosis can only be done by histopathology (Vujanić et al. 2018). In case of a biopsy, one should send tumor material not only for pathological analysis but also for genetics as specific genetic aberrations can be found confirming the diagnosis (Vujanić et al. 2018).

Important to note, there are childhood malignancies that can arise close to the kidney or as primary renal lesion, and may mimic primitive renal tumors, like neuroblastoma, PNET, soft tissue sarcomas, and non-Hodgkin lymphomas.

32.2 Rare Kidney Tumors

Primary non-Wilms renal tumors represent a heterogeneous, although clinically relevant, group of malignancies accounting for <1% of pediatric tumors (Pastore et al. 2006; Ahmed et al. 2007; Magnani et al. 2001; Vujanić et al. 2018) (Fig. 32.1). Most of them are especially diagnosed in children aged <6 months or >12 years. The major histological groups include RCC, CCSK, and RTK. Renal primitive neuroectodermal tumor (PNET), desmoplastic small round cell tumor, anaplastic sarcoma of the kidney, and renal medullary carcinoma represent other clinically significant types of malignant tumors. The most frequent benign lesion is angiomyolipoma, while oncocytoma is extremely rare in children and adolescents (Ciftci et al. 2000). Lesions with low to borderline malignant potential are mesoblastic nephroma, cystic nephroma (to be distinguished from a cystic appearance of a Wilms tumor), and metanephric tumors. The group of metanephric neoplasms has been more recently described; basing on the extent/appearance of epithelium or stroma, the WHO recognizes three members of a family of metanephric neoplasms of the kidney: metanephric stromal tumor (pure stromal), metanephric adenoma (pure epithelial), and metanephric adenofibroma (biphasic, stromal-epithelial) (Arroyo et al. 2001). Metanephric neoplasms have an unclear etiology but have been postulated by many researchers to potentially represent the differentiated end of the Wilms tumor spectrum, based primarily upon overlapping morphologic features (including rare composite cases with features of metanephric neoplasms and Wilms tumor) and overlapping immunohistochemical profiles (specifically, WT-1 immunoreactivity). More recently, mutations in the BRAF gene (specifically V600E) have been identified in over 90% of MA cases (including pediatric MA cases) (Argani et al. 2016), while, importantly, the BRAF V600E mutation has not been identified in prior

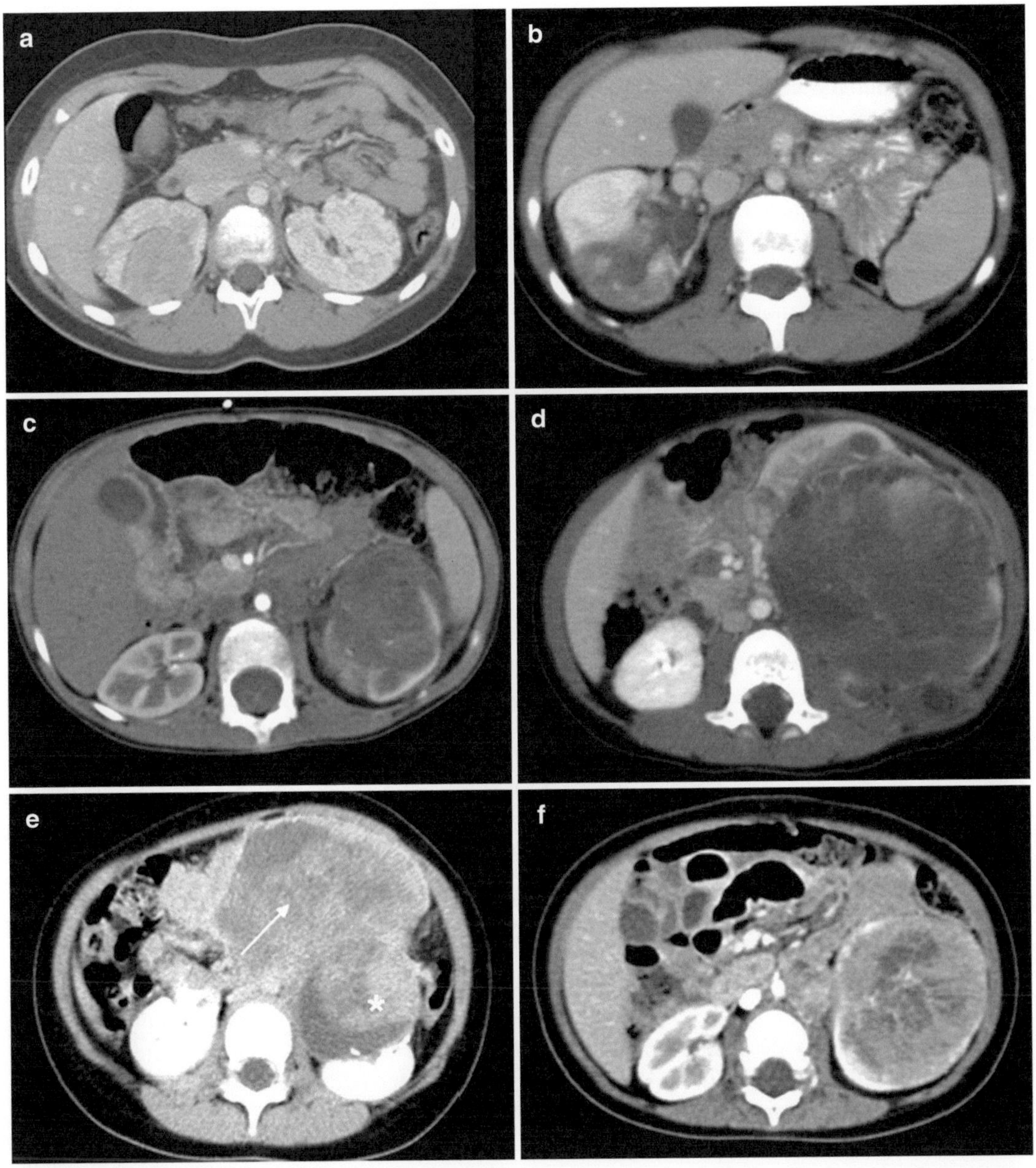

Fig. 32.1 Post-contrast CT imaging of (**a**) angiomyolipoma (male, 13-year-old); (**b**) primitive neuroectodermal tumor (female, 15-year-old); (**c**) Wilms tumor (male, 4-year-old); (**d**) clear cell sarcoma (male, 3-year-old); (**e**) 6-year-old female who displayed two rather distinct nodules that at microscopic examination turned out to be MiTF+RCC (*) and concomitant Wilms tumor (*arrow*); (**f**) Xp11.2 translocation carcinoma (female, 9-month-old)

sequencing analyses of Wilms tumor. The relationship—and sometime the association—between metanephric tumors and Wilms tumor or papillary RCC has been described and warrants further study to better elucidate potential common etiopathogenesis.

Other tumors, like non-Hodgkin lymphoma (mainly Burkitt lymphoma) or neuroblastoma, may secondarily affect the kidney, but sometimes they are the only clinical disease manifestation.

Renal medullary carcinoma was originally described in 1995 and affects young adults (mean age is 20 years) of a Black ethnicity who have a sickle cell nephropathy (Davis et al. 1995). It is a rapidly growing tumor of the renal medulla, regarded as an aggressive variant of collecting duct carcinoma (Lopez-Beltran et al. 2009).

Angiomyolipoma most likely presents in children who carry a known diagnosis of the tuberous sclerosis complex. Although benign, these tumors may cause substantial morbidity if they increase in size or if cause hemorrhage. For this reason, careful imaging examination is recommended, either with computed tomography or MRI, in order to balance the proper time for surgery (conservative whenever possible) versus a wait-and-see approach. Sometimes the low burden of fat tissue (or even absence) renders the differential diagnosis with other malignant renal tumors (like Wilms tumor) very challenging.

PNET has been documented with increasing frequency in the kidney in the last decade (Findlay et al. 2019). PNET of the kidney is clinically aggressive and requires therapeutic approach like other tumors of the Ewing sarcoma family. Noteworthy, PNET is frequently misdiagnosed as Wilms tumor, both being monotonous round cell tumors (Shet and Viswanathan 2009).

While imaging has no specific radiological features that can reliably distinguish between the histological types of renal tumors (Srinivasan et al. 2019; Watson et al. 2020; Brisse et al. 2020), one useful criterion for suspecting among the types of tumor is the age of the children. More than 50% of children with RCC are diagnosed after the age of 15 years, whereas >80% of patients with CCSK and RTK are younger than 4 years at diagnosis (Zhuge et al. 2010). CMN is the primary diagnostic consideration for a renal mass in the neonate, and its incidence decreases quickly with advancing age (van den Heuvel-Eibrink et al. 2008). RTK represents the primary diagnostic consideration for a metastatic renal tumor in children <7 months of age.

Non-Wilms tumors tend to affect more boys under the age of 5 years while more girls above the age of 15 years (Zhuge et al. 2010).

Consistent with their rarity, there is a paucity of published reports of these tumors. The rarity of the different types of primary non-Wilms renal tumors and the importance of prescribing the correct type-specific adjuvant therapy—if any—render central pathology review fundamental for the correct and modern clinical assessment of pediatric renal tumors (Vujanić et al. 2009; Vujanić et al. 2018). A comprehensive analysis of the SEER registry pointed out that patients diagnosed with a non-Wilms tumor after 1989 had much improved survival compared with those diagnosed prior to 1989, likely reflecting improvement in the diagnosis and/or treatment (Zhuge et al. 2010). Entering homogeneous groups of tumors into centralized histological database facilitates the description and classification of new entities.

Molecular biology studies have helped us in recognizing that some renal tumors are identical to tumors of other sites (such as cellular mesoblastic nephroma and infantile fibrosarcoma of soft tissue, renal and extra-renal rhabdoid tumor) as well as that some tumors of other sites may also occur in the kidney (PNET, desmoplastic small round cell tumor, synovial sarcoma). These molecular new findings are helping researchers to move from a "kidney-oriented" classification to a classification system whose fulcrum is the tissue origin of the tumor, and or related biological driver pathways, more than the fact that they are in the kidney.

32.3 Renal Cell Carcinoma (RCC)

RCC is rare in the first two decades of life and accounts for only approximately 2–5% of pediatric renal tumors (Selle et al. 2006; Pastore et al. 2006; Silberstein et al. 2009; Argani and Ladanyi 2003a, b; Geller et al. 2018; Rialon et al. 2015; Spreafico et al. 2010). Important studies have suggested that the epidemiological and histological characteristics of pediatric RCC differ from their adult counterparts. The big discovery regarding pediatric RCC has been the characterization of the translocation RCCs (Argani and Ladanyi 2003a, b; Argani and Ladanyi 2005, 2006). Since 2004, this is acknowledged by the WHO, which officially classified the translocation-type RCC (MiT-RCC), which mainly occurs in pediatric and young adult patients, as a specific entity (Cajaiba et al. 2018). MiT-RCC is characterized by translocations involving the *TFE3-gene* located on chromosome Xp11.2 and less frequently the *TFEB-gene* on 6p21, representing translocations of the microphthalmia transcription factor (MiT) family genes (Argani et al. 2005, 2006). It is likely that a large proportion of RCC in children (approximately one-third to two-thirds) belong to the translocation RCC (Argani and Ladanyi 2005, 2006; Sausville et al. 2009).

While much information is now available as far as the complementary treatment for RCC in adults, studies on children dealt with retrospective case reports, or mono- and pauci-institute series (Baek et al. 2010; Estrada et al. 2005; Geller and Dome 2004; Geller et al. 2009; Indolfi et al. 2003; Ramphal et al. 2006; Selle et al. 2006; Rao et al. 2009). The prognostic value and specific consequences for optimal treatment approach for these different histological subtypes remain however debatable. The potential bias inherent in non-consecutive case series and reports prevents a definitive formulation of standard therapeutic guidelines for RCC in children and adolescents (Spreafico et al. 2010), despite a recent study from the Children's Oncology Group reported on an extensive analysis of homogeneously and prospectively followed patients in the USA (Geller et al. 2015).

Radical nephrectomy is most important for therapy, while the role of extensive lymph node (LN) dissection—in the absence of LN spread—and of partial nephrectomy till remain clue issues for children as well.

Overall survival rates for childhood RCC are in the range of 50–60%, with outcomes worsening with advancing stages (Indolfi et al. 2003; Carcao et al. 1998; Geller and Dome 2004; Ahmed et al. 2007; Silberstein et al. 2009; Selle et al. 2006; Geller et al. 2015). Patients with tumor localized in the kidney with or without regional LN spread generally have a favorable prognosis, while outcome remains dismal for patients with distant hematogenous metastases. In the extensive review by Geller and Dome, stage-adapted survival rates for pediatric RCC were 92.5%, 84.6%, 72.7%, and 12.7% for modified Robson stages I to IV, respectively (Geller and Dome 2004). Children with LN+ M0 RCCs are likely to have an intermediate prognosis, with survival rate around 50–70% (Geller and Dome 2004, 2009; Geller et al. 2008; Indolfi et al. 2003; Selle et al. 2006: Rialon et al. 2015; Geller et al. 2015).

32.3.1 Epidemiology

The overall annual age-adjusted incidence is 0.01/100,000 children. Median age at diagnosis is 9–12 years, with equal prevalence in boys and girls (Geller and Dome 2004; Selle et al. 2006; Pastore et al. 2006; Silberstein et al. 2009; Indolfi et al. 2003; Ramphal et al. 2006). Despite RCC mostly occurs as a primitive renal tumor, it has been also recognized as a second neoplasm arising in children treated with chemotherapy (Schafernak et al. 2007; Argani et al. 2006). The association between RCC and neuroblastoma has been specifically described as a unique one, so that post-neuroblastoma RCC has been included in the 2004 WHO renal tumor classification as a distinct new category (Eble et al. 2004).

The strong association with the von Hippel–Lindau gene, known for adults (Rini et al. 2009), rarely occurs in children (Rao et al. 2011).

32.3.2 Diagnosis

Children with RCC may present with local or systemic symptoms, although current prevalent use of ultrasound and cross-sectional imaging is associated with an increasing incidental detection of asymptomatic small renal tumors (Estrada et al. 2005; Cook et al. 2006; Geller et al. 2015). Local signs and symptoms include gross hematuria, flank pain, or a palpable abdominal mass. Rarely children present with the full abovementioned clinical triad (Indolfi et al. 2003; Geller and Dome 2004). Systemic symptoms may be due to metastases or paraneoplastic syndromes, such as hypercalcemia, fever, or hypertension, which are rarely diagnosed in children.

A 30% rate of metastatic disease has been reported in the pediatric population (Geller and Dome 2004; Silberstein et al. 2009). About 5–10% of adult RCCs extend into the venous vessels as tumor thrombi, often ascending the inferior cava vein (Rini et al. 2009), and this situation, which has important surgical implications, can be encountered in children as well despite no incidence estimation is available.

Similar to adults, tumor stage in pediatric RCC represents a good prognostic indicator. The TNM system is the more frequently adopted staging classification system, while stage designation according to modified Robson system (Carcao et al. 1998) is rarely adopted. Geller and Dome reported stage-specific incidence as follows: 43.2% low-stage tumors (stage I and II) and 56.8% high-stage tumors (stage III and IV). Such advanced presentation is probably reflective of LN+M0 status (modified Robson stage IIIb; TNM stage III or IV) (Geller and Dome 2004) (Fig. 32.2).

32.3.3 Pathology and Classification

Overall, the clear-cell type of RCC, predominant in adults, is much less frequent in children, where in turn the papillary forms are much more frequent (Bruder et al. 2004; Argani and Ladanyi 2003a, b; Sebire and Vujanic 2009; Cajaiba et al. 2018).

A large part of RCCs in children and young adults show peculiar morphology, immunophenotype and genetic alterations, and belong to the group of translocation RCCs (Argani and Ladanyi 2003a, b, 2005; Camparo et al. 2008; Cajaiba et al. 2018). It is realistic to presume that many RCCs reported as papillary or clear cell in previous pediatric series would turn on contemporary examination to be translocation RCCs.

32.3.4 TFE3/MiTF Translocation Family of RCCs

Translocations involving the TFE3 gene at Xp11.2 with varying partners (Argani and Ladanyi 2005) or the TFEB gene (at 6p21) in the translocation t(6;11)(q21;q13) (Argani et al. 2001) characterize these tumors. Fusion targets for TFE3 include PRCC in 1q21 (Argani et al. 2007), ASPL of alveolar soft part sarcoma in 17q25 (Argani et al. 2001, 2007), PSF in 1p34

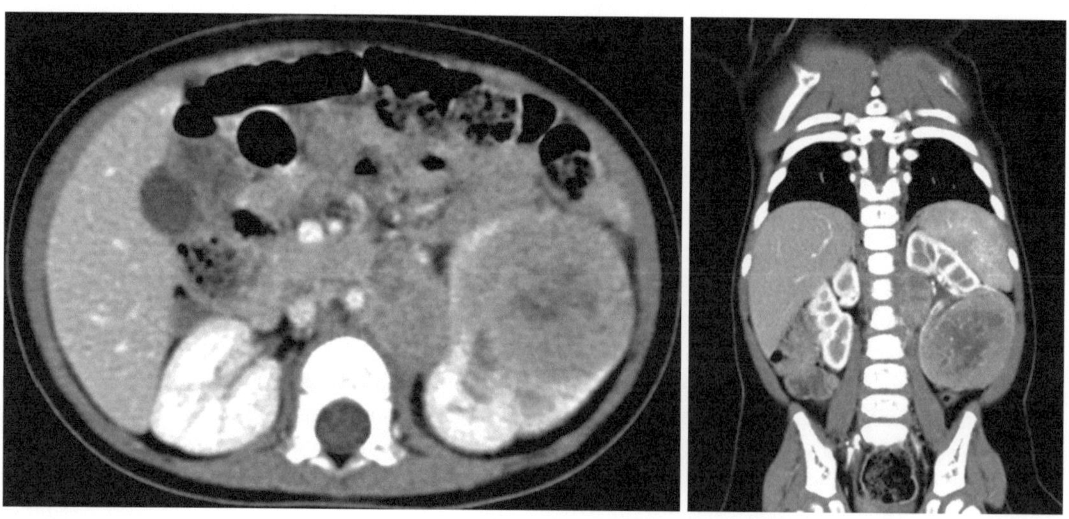

Fig. 32.2 Post-contrast CT scan of a Xp11.2 translocation carcinoma in a 9-month-old baby girl

(Argani et al. 2005), and CLTC in 17q23 (Argani and Ladanyi 2003a, b). TFE3 and TFEB are members of the microphthalmia transcription factor (MiTF) family (a subfamily of basic helix-loop-helix-leucine zipper transcription factors), together with MiTF and TFEC.

Many of these tumors show a high-grade (Fuhrman grade 3), type 2 papillary morphology and are made up by voluminous, large oxyphilic cells (Argani and Ladanyi 2005; Camparo et al. 2008; Ramphal et al. 2006). Cases with a solid, alveolar, nested, paraganglioma-like, or tubulo-papillary pattern are reported as well. The immunophenotype is distinct and quite different from the adult-type RCCs. There is a variable, usually very low or even absent expression of epithelial markers, i.e., keratins 8, 18 (CAM5.2); keratin 7; and EMA. CD10 and racemase are usually expressed. Some cases express melanocytic markers, i.e., HMB-45 and Melan-A. In addition, there is nuclear reactivity for TFE3 or TFEB.

32.4 Principles of Treatment

The differences between childhood and adulthood RCC likely prevent a direct and consistent application and translation of therapies that have been validated for adults to children.

Because RCC is among the most resistant of tumors to systemic therapy and radiotherapy, the cornerstone of therapy for RCC in children remains surgery. Radical nephrectomy represents the standard surgical approach. Since nephron-sparing approaches that preserve healthy renal parenchyma are advocated for adults and demonstrated good long-term oncologic outcome for low-volume tumors (Ficarra 2007; Touijer et al. 2010), it is reasonable to consider them in children and adolescents as well (Cook et al. 2006), at least in cases carefully selected by experienced surgeons.

Question as to what is the more adequate extension of retroperitoneal LN dissection remains relatively unanswered (John et al. 2019). To our knowledge, no formal guidelines currently exist regarding the extent of LN dissection in adults as well (Margulis and Wood 2008; Blom et al. 2009). Nevertheless, while in adults lymphatic spread by RCC, and mostly by clear-cell RCC, certainly decreases outcome, it is likely not the same for children (Geller and Dome 2004; Geller et al. 2008; Selle et al. 2006; Renshaw 2005; Geller et al. 2015). From the available experiences, children with clinical evidence of regional LN metastases derive therapeutic benefit from involved LN dissection. It remains less clear, but worth to be analyzed thoroughly, whether children with clinically normal LNs can be targeted for lymphadenectomy as an adjunct to radical nephrectomy. Patients with unsuspected LN spread, in whom LNs randomly sampled turn out to be metastatic at microscopic examination, raise the dilemma of second-look lymphadenectomy.

Overall, chemotherapy has little to no role in the treatment of RCC (Escudier 2010, b), pending new insights on similarities between childhood RCC and alveolar soft part sarcoma, in which some chemotherapy agents may be effective (such as doxorubicin). Despite no result data have been published so far, it is worth to be mentioned that pediatric oncologists have used doxorubicin, gemcitabin, oxaliplatin, and irinotecan as isolated experience, with anecdotal responses in translocation RCCs.

Until 2005, only high-dose interleukin-2 (IL-2) had been approved by the Food and Drug Administration for the treatment of RCC in adults, and this approval was based on durable complete responses obtained in only 7–8% of patients with metastatic RCC. Thereafter, the landscape of systemic therapies in metastatic or advanced-stage RCC has been changed by the introduction of drugs designed to target tumor-related angiogenesis and signal transduction (Sun et al. 2010; Brugarolas 2007; Gulati and Vaishampayan 2020). These are the multitargeted receptor tyrosine kinase inhibitors (sorafenib, sunitinib, pazopanib, axitinib), the inhibitors of the mTOR pathway (temsirolimus, everolimus), and the anti-angiogenic monoclonal antibody bevacizumab (Gulati and Vaishampayan 2020). When used as first- and second-line therapies for metastatic RCC, these agents have demonstrated previously unprecedented response rates and improvements in time to progression in phase III trials (Escudier et al. 2007; Escudier 2009, 2010; Motzer and Basch 2007; Motzer and Molina 2009; Hudes et al. 2007; Bellmunt and Guix 2009; Soulières 2009; Bukowski 2010). Systemic frontline therapy options now include immune checkpoint inhibitor-based combination therapies such as pembrolizumab/axitinib, nivolumab/ipilimumab, and avelumab/axitinib (Tenold et al. 2020; Thana and Wood 2020; Rassy et al. 2020; Gulati and Vaishampayan 2020). Despite the established efficacy of frontline immune checkpoint inhibitor-based combination, most patients will ultimately require additional lines of therapy, and oncologists must think carefully when switching to another therapy, particularly in situations of drug intolerance or apparent disease progression. Systemic therapy options after immune checkpoint inhibitor-based combination are generally tyrosine kinase inhibitor-based, and ongoing clinical trials will help optimize the treatment algorithm further. On the other hand, the utility of the abovementioned therapies in the adjuvant setting remains unproven.

Despite these several targeted therapies available for RCC, each with different profile of risk versus benefit, at the time of this writing, no prospective data have been published for pediatric age.

Many of the pediatric RCC series covered a very long time span—institutional and population-based reports may need as long as 20–40 years to accrue a significant number of children with this uncommon tumor—and mostly discussed results obtained prior to the more recently introduced targeted therapies (Geller and Dome 2004; Indolfi et al. 2003; Baek et al. 2010). Currently, the role of targeted agents such as tyrosine kinase inhibitors should be reserved to children with unresectable metastatic or advanced-stage RCC (Ambalavanan and Geller 2019; Geller et al. 2018; Craig and Poppas 2019). What might be recommended for metastatic pediatric RCCs is to adopt sequential treatment with VEGF pathway-targeted therapies, optimizing efficacy and safety results; however we are conscious that guidelines may rapidly change, basing on new data acquired in adults. The uncertain benefit of these therapies, together with their toxicity and the relatively better outlook for children and adolescents with completely resected LN+M0 RCC, support not currently using any adjuvant therapies in such pediatric RCCs (Escudier and Kataja 2010; Geller et al. 2018).

A further element which complicates the potential translation of therapeutic findings from adult to pediatric RCC relays in that a major proportion of RCCs included in adult clinical trials are clear-cell RCCs. On the other hand, the optimal therapy for the Xp11.2 translocation RCCs remains to be proven, but case report describing significant response to anti-angiogenics have been described (Joshi and Banerjee 2008; Malouf et al. 2010).

32.5 Rhabdoid Tumor of the Kidney (RTK)

Rhabdoid tumors of the kidney (RTKs) are rare and extremely aggressive malignancies that generally occur in infants and young children. These tumors tend to develop early metastasis. Besides the kidney, these tumors can arise in the CNS, the soft tissues, the liver, and at different sites in a single patient. This suggests a common genetic development including germline mutations (Schneppenheim et al. 2010; Kordes et al. 2014). They usually share biallelic SMARCB1 or rarely SMARCA4 inactivation (Versteege et al. 1998; Schneppenheim et al. 2010; Nemes and Frühwald 2018) and are characterized by a common histology and usually the loss of INI1 expression in immunostaining (Hoot et al. 2004; Hasselblatt et al. 2011).

The first description of this tumor entity was done by Haas et al. in 1981 (Haas et al. 1981). Despite a multitude of case series and single reports, much needs to be learned about this tumor as the prognosis remains dismal, with many relapses occurring early, often shortly after the end of treatment or even during treatment. Standard high-risk renal tumor regimens as well as regimens usually adopted for non-rhabdomyosarcoma soft tissue sarcomas have been unsatisfactory so far, resulting in 20–40%

OS (van den Heuvel-Eibrink et al. 2011; Tomlinson et al. 2005). Noteworthy, in vitro testing, case reports, and small series suggested sensitivity of RTK to anthracyclins (Waldron et al. 1999; Wagner et al. 2002; Lünenbürger et al. 2010; Furtwängler et al. 2014), alkylating agents, such as platinum derivates and oxazophosphorines (Gururangan et al. 1993), and radiation therapy (Furtwängler et al. 2014; Tomlinson et al. 2005; Palmer and Sutow 1983). A positive contribution of high dose chemotherapy with autologous hemopoietic stem cell rescue (HDSCT) has been reported in case series only (Koga et al. 2009), whereas comparable outcomes for patients with and without HDSCT could be shown in a retrospective analysis of 58 patients from Germany, Austria, and Switzerland, if patients were adjusted for early disease progression (Furtwängler et al. 2018).

Today, common therapeutic regimens include intensive anthracycline-based polychemotherapy and aggressive local therapy (Chi et al. 2009; Squire et al. 2007; Wagner et al. 2002; Waldron et al. 1999; Zimmerman et al. 2005). While there are multiple in vitro tests evaluating therapeutic targets for the treatment of malignant rhabdoid tumors, there is a paucity of phase I/II trials combining conventional chemotherapy with selective experimental agents (Nemes and Frühwald 2018; Bourdeaut et al. 2014).

32.5.1 Molecular Genetics

Common to rhabdoid tumors of any anatomical site are alterations in chromosome 22. The biallelic inactivation of SMARCB1 in chromosome 22q.11.23, or rarely (2–3%) SMARCA4 in chromosome 19p13.2, is rather typical of rhabdoid tumors. Apart from these mutations, no other genetic alterations that may explain clinical heterogeneity have been identified (Frühwald et al. 2016). Loss of genetic material from chromosome 22q11 in rhabdoid tumors has been demonstrated by molecular genetic analyses, fluorescence in situ hybridization, and loss of heterozygosity studies (Biegel et al. 1996; Rickert and Paulus 2004). The tumor suppressor gene SMARCB1 (hSNF5/INI1) resides on the long arm of chromosome 22. Versteege et al. isolated the gene SMARCB1 (hSNF5/INI1) from chromosome 22q11.2. SMARCB1 is a member of the SWI/SNF complex (Versteege et al. 1998). The gene contributes to gene transcription through chromatin remodeling (Zhang et al. 2002). Defects may cause a loss of function of the SWI/SNF-complex in chromatin compaction. This presumably causes easier access of polymerases to chromosomes and thus a non-specific activation of many downstream pathways involving among others sonic hedgehog pathways, Wnt-pathway, aurora-kinase pathway, and cell-cycle controls, e.g., cyclin D1, p16, and p14 (Venkataraman et al. 2012; Venneti et al. 2011; Smith et al. 2011; Algar et al. 2009). This is in contrast to the genetic stability of rhabdoid tumors, which harbor only very few mutations as compared to other tumors (Hasselblatt et al. 2013; Lee et al. 2012; McKenna et al. 2008) and show no oncogenic canonical pathway mutations (Kieran et al. 2012).

Transgenic mice heterozygous for SMARCB1 develop rhabdoid tumors and T-cell lymphomas (Roberts et al. 2000, 2002). SMARCB1 mutations have been detected in all nine exons (Biegel et al. 2002b) and show a broad mutational spectrum across tumors from different anatomical sites (Kordes et al. 2010). Today mutations can be detected at least in about 80% of cases on chromosome 22q11.2 (Biegel et al. 2002a; Jackson et al. 2009; Versteege et al. 1998). An additional 20–25% of tumors have reduced expression at the RNA or protein level, indicative of a loss-of-function event. It is unclear if this mutation indicates a common histogenesis of rhabdoid tumors (Parham et al. 1994; Weeks et al. 1989; Wick et al. 1995). Rarely (2–3%) biallelic SMARCA4 inactivation causes the lack of BRG1, another crucial subunit of the SWI/SNF complex.

Germline mutations in SMARCB1 do occur, and families are reported with more than one affected member, as well as patients with synchronous rhabdoid tumors of the CNS and the kidney (Proust et al. 1999; Sevenet et al. 1999; Taylor et al. 2000). Familial cases are summarized under the term "rhabdoid tumor predisposition syndrome"—RTPS (Kordes et al. 2010; Louis et al. 2007). While the majority of the patients affected by the rhabdoid tumor predisposition syndrome are characterized by SMARCB1 mutations, one report describes a family with two affected children without mutation of SMARCB1 (Frühwald et al. 2006). Furthermore, there are family members described who carried a germline mutation and who did not develop any tumor (Ammerlaan et al. 2007; Janson et al. 2006). Nevertheless, genetic counseling appears mandatory in families with RTPS. In case of a mutation in SMARCB1 within the tumor, analysis of constitutional DNA from the blood of the patient needs to be done. If a germline mutation is detected, parents have to be informed about the potential risk in siblings of the affected patient (Fig. 32.3). A correlation between the mutational status of certain nucleotides and the clinical course of the disease has not been demonstrated. However, reports from the literature suggest that

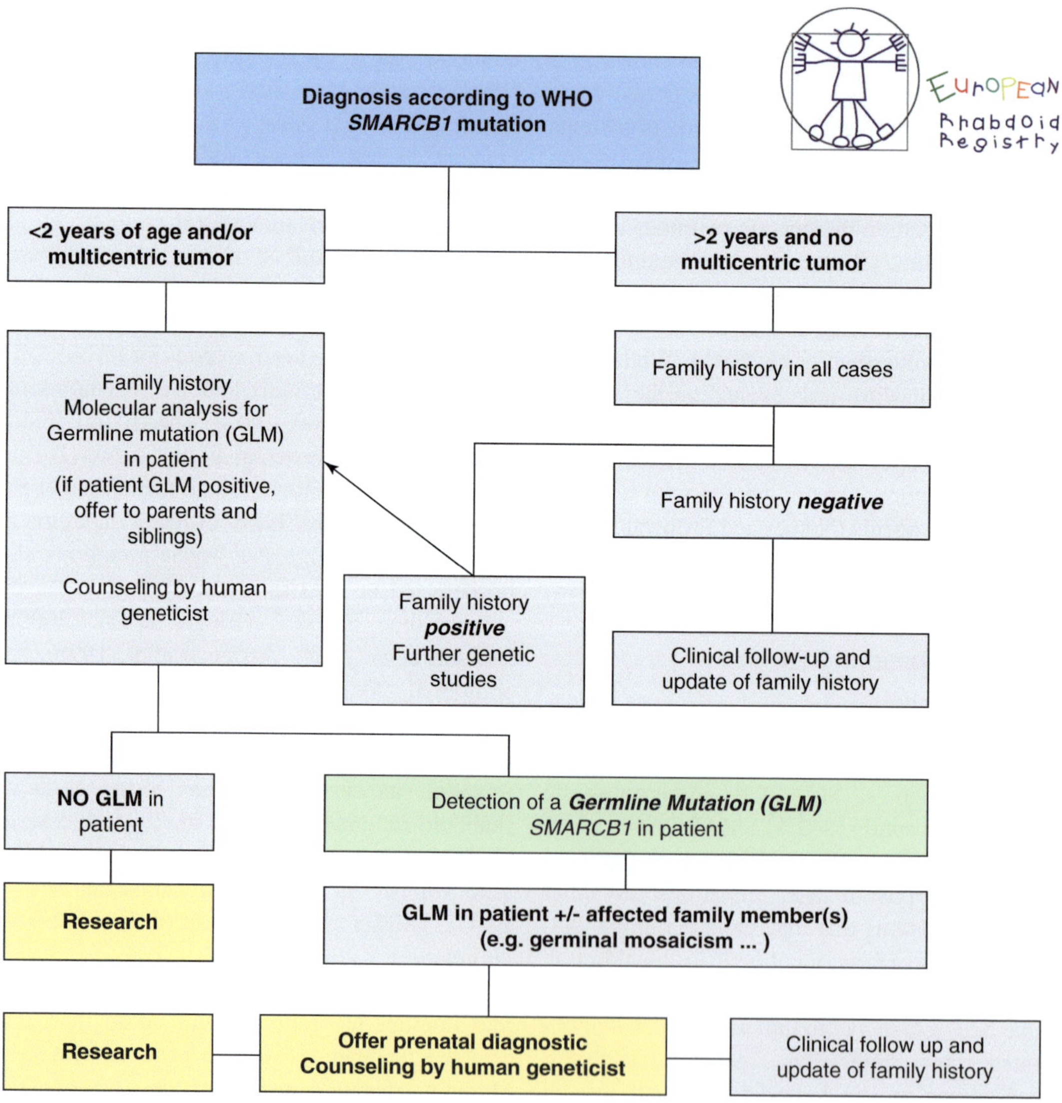

Fig. 32.3 Flow chart for genetic counseling of patients with suspected rhabdoid tumor predisposition. (From: Frühwald, M European Rhabdoid Registry protocol 2010)

patients with germline mutations are younger and are characterized by an almost inevitably fatal course (Kordes et al. 2010).

32.5.2 Diagnosis

RTKs constitute 2% of all kidney tumors in infants and children. Fever and hematuria in a young patient (mean age 11 months) with a high tumor stage should suggest the diagnosis of RTK. Tumor staging system is the same as in nephroblastoma but with a higher incidence of metastatic disease even in young infants. Among 639 cases of kidney tumors in the first 7 months of life with specified histology and stage, 9/11 stage IV tumors were RTKs, as reported by van den Heuvel-Eibrink et al. (2008). RTK tends to metastasize to the lungs and the brain. Up to 15% of patients with RTK also have brain lesions. Because of the coincidence with brain metastasis, a cerebral MRI is always indicated.

The diagnosis of RTK can only be done by histology. Today the diagnosis of RTK needs to be confirmed by immunohistochemical and/or molecular genetic techniques showing the loss of INI1 protein expression resulting from SMARCB1 mutations (Judkins 2007). In every case, tumor material should be stored for research to perform gene array and other experiments for gaining further knowledge (Huang et al. 2006).

32.5.3 Histopathology

Histopathologically, RTKs are characterized by cells with an eccentric nucleus and prominent nucleolus, abundant cytoplasm with eosinophilic inclusion bodies, and distinct cellular membranes, somewhat resembling the rhabdomyoblastic differentiation of rhabdomyosarcomas (Sotelo-Avila et al. 1986a, b). Rhabdoid differentiation may also be seen in a variety of other entities such as meningioma, melanoma, and lymphoma. Rhabdoid cells are characterized by expression of vimentin, EMA (epithelial membrane antigen), and cytokeratins, less commonly by SMA (smooth muscle actin) (Louis et al. 2007; Jackson et al. 2009; Tomlinson et al. 2005). The loss of INI1 protein confirms the diagnosis of rhabdoid tumors.

32.5.4 Treatment and Prognosis of RTK

Until now no randomized study comparing regimens has been conducted. However, several hints concerning the effect of specific drugs have been published. Waldron, Wagner, and colleagues reported three stage IV patients successfully treated with combinations of doxorubicin, cyclophosphamide, vincristine, ifosfamide, and etoposide (Waldron et al. 1999; Wagner et al. 2002). Anthracyclin-based treatment showed promising results in AT/RT in a report given by Chi et al. (2009), and anthracyclines have shown to induce volume decrease in the preoperative setting of MRTK (van den Heuvel-Eibrink et al. 2011; Furtwängler et al. 2014). However, Tomlinson et al. (2005) did not find a difference in survival based on the use of doxorubicin. The report fails to give details on the different cohorts to rule out a selection bias due to probable accumulation of higher stages in the doxorubicin receiving cohort. Alkylating agents, especially ifosfamide, seem to be important in the treatment of extracranial RT. In a series of 13 children from St. Judes, only those receiving ifosfamide survived (Gururangan et al. 1993).

Between 1984 and 1999, 70 children with rhabdoid tumors of any anatomical site were diagnosed in Germany. 35 children were below 1 year of age, 10 between 1 and 2 years, and 9 between 2 and 3 years. Only 10 children were older than 4 years. 32 tumors were localized in the kidneys, 25 in soft tissue (MRT), and 13 in the CNS (AT/RT). 20% of AT/RT and 40% of RTK patients demonstrated metastases at diagnosis. Treatment was according to the respective available protocols at that time (HIT, SIOP, CWS). Twenty-eight patients received radiotherapy (at a dose ranging between 30 and 40 Gy) in addition to surgery and chemotherapy. Of the 70 registered patients, 46 died within 2 years of diagnosis. Two additional patients succumbed to the disease until the fourth year after diagnosis. More follow-up data are currently not available. The prognosis was dismal regardless of site of the primary tumor or the protocol used. The only statistically relevant negative prognostic factor was metastatic disease (Reinhard et al. 2008). The same risk factor could be shown in larger cohort of 58 patients with RTK from Austria, Switzerland, and Germany (Furtwängler et al. 2018) (Fig. 32.4).

In the United Kingdom, patients with RTK have been treated according to the Wilms tumor studies UKW2 and UKW3, containing a combination of vincristine, actinomycin-D, and doxorubicin (Grundy et al. 2004; Mitchell et al. 2006). The survival rate of 21 patients was 35% (SD ± 9%). All deaths occurred within 13 months following diagnosis. Two stage I patients survived; three patients with stage III died. Four of nine patients with stage III survived. Of seven patients with stage IV disease, there was only one survivor. Two of the stage III patients received radiotherapy.

In the United States, patients with RTK were enrolled into the National Wilms Tumor Studies (NWTS) until recently. These studies employed a drug regimen with vincristine, actinomycin-D, and doxorubicin with or without cyclophosphamide (D'Angio et al. 1989; Tomlinson et al. 2005). Despite high therapy intensity, the survival rate remained unsatisfactory with 4-year overall survival (OS) for stage I patients of 33%, stage II of 47%, stage III of 22%, and stage IV of 8% (Tomlinson et al. 2005). Similar results have been reported by the International Society of Paediatric Oncology (Vujanic et al. 1996) and the United Kingdom group (Grundy et al. 2004). To improve these results, the National Wilms Tumor Study-5 enhanced treatment by using carboplatinum and etoposide with cyclophosphamide (regimen RTK). This trial arm was preliminary closed because of poor outcome (26% survival rate). In a review of 142 patients from NWTS-1 through NWTS-5, stage and age were significant prognostic factors. Patients with stage I and stage II disease had an OS rate of 42%; higher stage was associated with a 16% OS. Infants younger than 6 months at diagnosis demonstrated a 4-year OS of 9%, whereas OS in patients aged 2 years and older was 41%. All except one patient with a central nervous system lesion died (Tomlinson et al. 2005).

Between December 2005 and June 2014, 100 patients from 12 countries with a diagnosis of

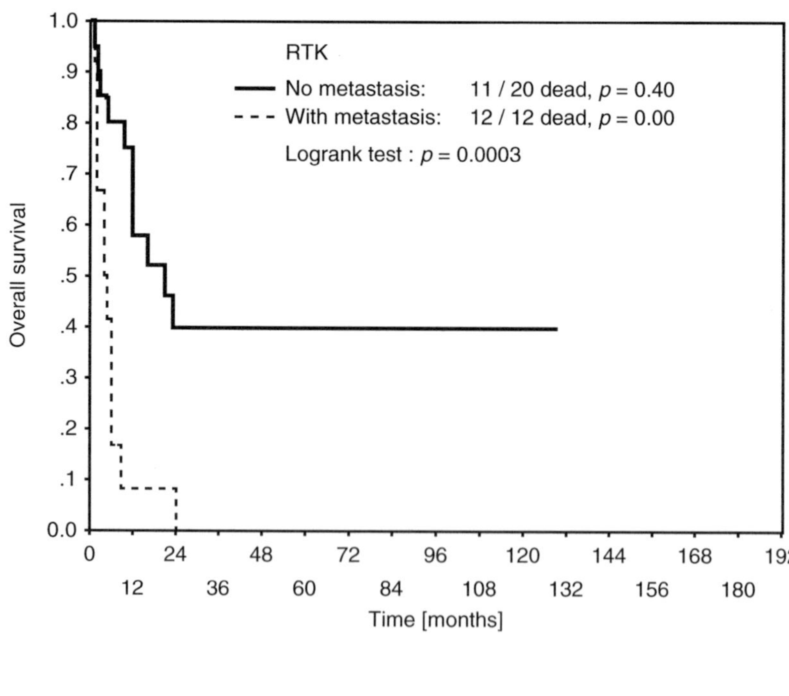

Fig. 32.4 Event-free survival (EFS) rates of patients suffering from localized, multifocal, or metastatic/stage IV disease, including one patient who did not receive any treatment. Note: Stage IV is defined as metastasis to the lungs or mediastinum (n = number of events/ number of patients, x-axis in years) (Furtwängler et al. 2018)

rhabdoid tumors at an extracranial site were prospectively registered on the EpSSG Non-Rhabdomyosarcoma Soft Tissue Sarcoma 2005 Study (NRSTS 2005). They were all treated on a standard multimodal protocol of surgery, radiotherapy, and cyclophosphamide, carboplatin, and etoposide (CyCE) alternatively. Radiotherapy was recommended for all primary tumor sites and all sites of metastatic disease. For the whole cohort, the 3-year event-free survival (EFS) was 32.3% with a 3-year overall survival (OS) of 38.4%. Disclosed risk factors for death are patients ≤1 year of age and metastatic disease (Brennan et al. 2016).

Based on the currently available data, the role of radiotherapy in the treatment of RTK seems to be beneficial (Furtwängler et al. 2019, personal communication), but because of the rarity of the disease, the young age at diagnosis and the rapid progress of the tumor in many patients, conclusive results are not available. Sultan and colleagues, reporting on SEER data, showed a significant impact of RT on survival (HR 1.89; 1.29–2.78 95%CI; $p = 0.0012$) in multivariate analysis adjusted for age and stage, both being of significant influence too. But in 229 patients analyzed, only 45 had MRTK and the remaining patients AT/RT or MRT (Sultan et al. 2010).

32.6 European Rhabdoid Registry (EU-RHAB)

As prognosis of children with rhabdoid tumors is dismal, new diagnostic and therapeutic strategies are demanding. In Europe a European Rhabdoid Registry (EU-RHAB) has been launched as a registry for all rhabdoid tumors regardless of site. The EU-RHAB hopefully will build the basis for future therapeutic trials by contributing to improvements in the diagnostic and eventually therapeutic management of affected patients. The EU-RHAB contains treatment recommendations, which were generated from data derived from the current literature and the investigators' clinical experience. The EU-RHAB aims at giving a standardized therapeutic approach. A patient with RTK should be referred to a center for pediatric oncology and enrolled in a prospective trial or registry. Treatment planning by a multidisciplinary team of cancer specialists (pediatric surgeon or pediatric urologist, pediatric radiation oncologist, and pediatric oncologist) with experience treating renal tumors is required to determine and implement optimum treatment. Patients diagnosed with a RTK and registered in the UMBRELLA protocol for kidney tumors in children adolescents and young adults of the SIOP Renal Tumour Study Group are to be included into EU-RHAB to gain more knowledge about this tumor in many more patients around the world and thus being able to faster improve outcome in RTK.

32.7 Clear Cell Sarcoma of the Kidney (CCSK)

CCSK is an important primary renal tumor representing one of the most common unfavorable kidney tumors in childhood comprising 3–5% of all primary renal tumors in children (Argani et al. 2000; Ahmed et al. 2007). CCSK was initially recognized as a distinct clinicopathologic entity with a high propensity to metastasize to bone (Kidd 1970). Marsden and Lawler noted osseous metastases in 60% of patients with CCSK and coined the term "bone-metastasizing renal tumor" (Marsden and Lawler 1980). In addition to pulmonary and bone metastases, CCSK may also spread to brain and soft tissue. CCSK is associated with a significantly higher rate of relapse, even late relapse (Kusumakumary et al. 1997; Gooskens et al. 2012) and death than Wilms tumor. The prognosis for CCSK improved after the introduction of anthracyclines to modern treatment regimens, with survival rates approaching 90% for non-metastatic tumors (Gooskens et al. 2012, 2014; Furtwängler et al. 2013).

32.7.1 Molecular Genetics

Despite the fact that several chromosomal translocations and genetic alterations are described in

CCSK, the pathogenesis of this tumor remains unknown. There is no predisposition syndrome reported that occur in patients with germline genetic mutations explaining why familial cases of CCSK are not seen (Sotelo-Avilla et al. 1986a, b; Argani et al. 2000). In addition, correlations between gene mutations and outcome are not described.

Huang et al. (2006) could show that the most common malignant tumors arising in the kidney (Klatte et al. 2009) have distinct and different gene expression profiles despite their frequent histologic similarities, helping to provide much greater diagnostic confidence than only routine pathologic examination. The top eight upregulated genes they did find in CCSK are forkhead box F1 (FOXF1), tumor suppressor homeobox HB9 (HLXB9), DNA segment chromosome 4 (D4S234E), neuronal pentraxin I (NPTX1), forkhead box F2 (FOXF2), protocadherin 11 X-linked (PCDH11), engrailed homolog 2 (EN2), and neuronal pentraxin receptor (NPTXR) (Huang et al. 2006).

Cytogenetic studies of CCSK have repeatedly reported balanced translocations t(10;17)(q22;p13), t(10;17)(q11;p12), and del(14)(q24.1q31.1) (O'Meara et al. 2008). Although the tumor suppressor gene p53 is located at the chromosome 17p13 breakpoint, p53 abnormalities are rarely present in these tumors why p53 and abnormalities are controversially discussed (Argani et al. 2000; Brownlee et al. 2007). The t(10;17) breakpoint and deletion of chromosome 14q24 suggest that other genes are involved in tumor pathogenesis (Brownlee et al. 2007; O'Meara et al. 2008). O'Meara et al. (2008) found a rearrangement of YWHAE on chromosome 17 and FAM22 on chromosome 10 in 6 of 50 CCSKs tested. A study done by Gooskens et al. (2016) did not identify an explicit clinical phenotype of CCSK cases harboring the YWHAE-NUTM2B/E fusion transcript. Another recurring cytogenetic lesion in CCSK is an interstitial deletion of chromosome 14q (Punnett et al. 1989; Brownlee et al. 2002; Douglass et al. 1985). Also, t(1;6)(p32.3;q21) and t(2;22) have been reported (Taguchi et al. 2008; Kaneko et al. 1991).

Comparative genomic hybridization (CGH) studies revealed an absence of consistent genetic gains or losses in CCSK. Such analysis done by Schuster et al. revealed quantitative abnormalities in only 4 of 30 CCSKs. Two of them showed gain of 1q, one showed loss of 10q, and the other showed loss of terminal 4p. The remaining two cases demonstrated chromosome 19 loss and chromosome 19p gain, respectively. All 22 cases in their series informative for 11p15 showed retention of both alleles. Of 14 CCSKs informative for IGF2, 6 showed biallelic expression (Schuster et al. 2003). The high frequency of LOI for IGF2 in CCSKs (43%) is comparable to that reported in Wilms tumors. This suggests that IGF2, a potent growth factor, may play a role in the development or progression of CCSK (Schuster et al. 2003).

Cutcliffe et al. found in gene expression profiles of CCSK differentially expressed genes which they grouped into four categories: (a) a wide variety of neural markers, (b) members of the Sonic hedgehog pathway, (c) members of the phosphoinositide 3-kinase/Akt cell proliferation pathway, and (d) known therapeutic targets. In particular, they found that CD 117—an epidermal growth factor receptor—is upregulated at the protein level in many CCSKs, providing potential therapeutic targets. In addition, they claimed that nerve growth factor receptor represents a promising diagnostic tool for CCSK (Cutcliffe et al. 2005).

32.7.2 Diagnosis

CCSK constitutes about 4% of all kidney tumors in children. A male predominance has been noted in all large CCSK reports (average male to female ratio of about 2:1) (Argani et al. 2000; Gooskens et al. 2012, Graf et al. 2011). There is no distinct clinical presentation to differentiate it from nephroblastoma. Tumor staging is the same as in nephroblastoma. Only 2% of kidney tumors in the first 7 months of life are CCSKs (van den Heuvel-Eibrink et al. 2008). In a series of 50 patients from GPOH, the median age at diagnosis was 2.4 years, ranging from 2 months to 19.2 years with an excess of boys (male to female

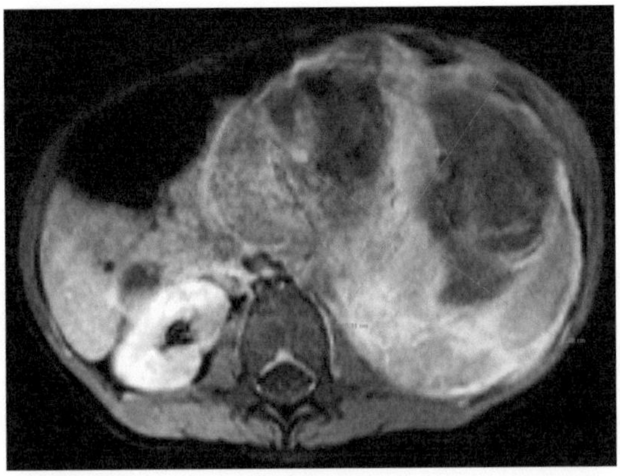

Fig. 32.5 MRI at the time of diagnosis in a 9-year-old girl with CCSK. Tumor volume at the time of diagnosis: 1370 mL with no regression after 4 weeks of preoperative chemotherapy according to the SIOP Wilms tumor protocol with vincristine and actinomycin-D

1.6:1) (Graf et al. 2011). This is in accordance with the findings of Argani et al. who found a male to female ratio of 2:1 and a mean age of 36 months in a series of 351 cases (Argani et al. 2000). Staging procedures have to be done as for nephroblastoma, with the addition of a bone scan and an MRI to the brain, as CCSKs do metastasize to the bone, lungs, and the brain. Imaging studies cannot differentiate between nephroblastoma, CCSK, and other renal tumors (Fig. 32.5).

32.7.3 Histopathology

Histologically, this tumor exhibits a great diversity of morphologic patterns that can mimic most other pediatric renal neoplasms, often leading to confusion and misdiagnosis (Kenny et al. 2016). Until recently, adjunct immunohistochemical and molecular genetic tests to support the diagnosis were lacking. The presence of internal tandem duplications in BCL-6 coreceptor (*BCOR*) and a translocation t(10;17) creating the fusion gene *YWHAE-NUTM2B/E* have now been well accepted (Aldera and Pillay 2020).

The classic pattern of CCSK is defined by nests or cords of cells separated by regularly spaced fibrovascular septa (Argani et al. 2000). Typical gross features included large size, a mucoid texture, foci of necrosis, and prominent cyst formation. Nine major histologic patterns were identified (classic, myxoid, sclerosing, cellular, epithelioid, palisading, spindle, storiform, and anaplastic) (Argani et al. 2000). Traditionally, the role of immunohistochemistry in the diagnosis of CCSK has largely been to exclude other pediatric renal tumors. Only vimentin is consistently immunoreactive in immunohistochemical stains. CCSK is consistently negative for epithelial markers (cytokeratins, epithelial membrane antigen), neural markers (synaptophysin, S100), vascular markers (CD34), muscle markers (desmin), membranous CD99, and WT1. The p53 gene product is rarely overexpressed in non-anaplastic CCSKs but strikingly overexpressed in anaplastic CCSKs (Argani et al. 2000).

Recently, diffuse strong nuclear staining with a commercially available BCL-6 coreceptor (BCOR) antibody has been shown to be highly sensitive and specific for the diagnosis of CCSK in the context of pediatric renal neoplasia (Kao et al. 2016; Argani et al. 2018). BCOR-related sarcomas, such as soft tissue undifferentiated small cell tumor of infancy and primitive mesenchymal myxoid tumor of infancy, also show diffuse, strong nuclear expression with BCOR immunohistochemistry. In the context of pediatric renal neoplasms, strong, diffuse nuclear staining with BCOR is a specific marker that can be useful in distinguishing CCSK from its mimics.

32.7.4 Treatment and Prognosis of CCSK

After the introduction of anthracyclines to the treatment protocol, the prognosis of CCSK has changed. Previously, relapses have occurred in long intervals after the completion of chemotherapy (up to 10 years). However, with current therapy, relapses after 3 years are uncommon (Seibel et al. 2004). An additional benefit could be found with the addition of alkylating agents, carboplatin and etoposide (Tournade et al. 2001; Furtwängler et al. 2013; Gooskens et al. 2018). Today 5-year overall survival rates are approaching 90% in localized diseases in all study groups as shown in Table 32.1. Even in patients with initial

Table 32.1 Treatment and outcome of CCSK in different study groups

Report	Study	Treatment		EFS	OS
		Chemotherapy	Radiotherapy		
Green et al. (1994)	NWTS 1-2	AMD/VCR (8 pt) AMD/VCR/DOX (58 pt)	0–37.8 Gy	25% (6y) 63.5% (6y)	25% (6y) 71.9% (6y)
Green et al. (1994)	NWTS 3	AMD/VCR/DOX (43 pt) AMD/VCR/DOX/CPM (30 pt)	0–37.8 Gy	64.4% (6y) 58.2% (6y)	71.3% (6y) 60.8% (6y)
Seibel et al. (2004)	NWTS 4	6m CT (AMD/VCR/DOX) (23 pt) 15m CT (AMD/VCR/DOX) (17 pt)	10.8 Gy	65.2% (5y) 87.8% (5y)	95.5% (5y) 87.5% (5y)
Seibel et al. (2006)	NWTS 5	VCR/DOX/CPM/VP-16 (110 pt)	Stage I–IV 10.8 Gy	79% (5y)	89% (5y)
Tournade et al. (2001)	SIOP 09	AMD/VCR/EPI(DOX)/IFO (16 pt)	Stage II/III 30 Gy	75% (2y)	88% (5y)
Furtwängler et al. (2013)	SIOP 93-01	St I-IV: VP-16/CARBO/IFO/EPI	Stage II/III 25.2–30 Gy	78% (5y)	86% (5y)
	SIOP 2001	St I: AMD/VCR/DOX St II-IV: VP-16/CARBO/CPM/DOX			
Mitchell (2000)	UKWT2	AMD/VCR/DOX (16 pt)	≥Stage III 30 Gy	82% (4y)	88% (4y)
Spreafico et al. (2014)	AIEOP-TW-2003	St I-IV: AMD/VCR/DOX; AMD/IFO; VP-16/CARBO	Stage I–III 25.2 Gy if <30 m, 34.2 Gy if >30 m	84% (5y)	91% (5y)

Abbreviations: *NWTS* National Wilms' Tumor Study Group; *SIOP* International Society of Pediatric Oncology; *GPOH* German Society of Pediatric Oncology and Hematology; *UKWT* United Kingdom Wilms Tumour Study Group; *AMD* actinomycin-D; *VCR* vincristine; *DOX* doxorubicin; *CPM* cyclophosphamide; *VP-16* etoposide; *IFO* ifosfamide; *CAR* carboplatin; *pt* patients; *EFS* event-free survival; *OS* overall survival; *y* year metastasis 5-year EFS and OS is about 70% as shown for patients treated according to SIOP 93-01 1nd SIOP 2001 (Furtwängler et al. 2013). In comparison the estimated 5-year EFS and OS for the seven patients with stage IV disease in NWTS 5 were only 29% (95% CI: 0%–76%) and 36% (95% CI: 0%–75%), which may be attributed to a treatment protocol without carboplatin and the low number of stage IV patients also shown by the large confidence interval (Seibel et al. 2019).

Most remarkable is the relapse pattern that is seen today after multimodal treatment and high cure rates. In the largest series of relapsed CCSK patients (37 out of 236 CCSK patients) (Gooskens et al. 2014), 13 patients relapsed in the brain as the most common relapse site that was not seen before. Such a relapse pattern in the brain is reported by many other groups as well (Seibel et al. 2006; Radulescu et al. 2008), underlining that the brain is a frequent site of recurrent disease in CCSK and demanding brain scans at diagnosis and follow-up of patients with CCSK. Independent of the relapse site outcome of patients with a relapse is still poor with a 5-year EFS of 18% and a 5-year OS of 25% (Gooskens et al. 2014).

As prognosis of patients with CCSK in general is excellent today, if they receive adequate therapy, all patients with this tumor have to be referred to a center of pediatric oncology, and late effects of treatment (cardiomyopathy [anthracyclines], nephrotoxicity [ifosfamide, carboplatin], infertility [alkylating agents], and second malignancies [etoposide] need to be taken into consideration to improve future treatments. An excellent overview on the rationale for the treatment of children with CCSK in the UMBRELLA SIOP–RTSG 2016 protocol is given in a paper by Gooskens et al. (2018) in Nature Reviews Urology.

32.8 Differential Diagnosis and Treatment of Urothelial and Bladder Tumors

Pediatric tumors of the lower urinary tract are extremely rare and comprise dissimilar histological subtypes. Noteworthy, bladder tumor occurrence and histological subtypes differ considerably between adults and children (Gripp 2005).

Tumors arising from the bladder can originate from any of its four histological layers (urothelium, lamina propria, detrusor, and adventitia) and are divided into tumors that have an epithelial origin (arising from the urothelium) and those that have a non-epithelial origin (mesenchymal neoplasms) (Shelmerdine et al. 2017). Bladder tumors are usually of mesodermal origin in children <10 years, and tumor of the epithelial origin are extremely rare, above all below the age of 10 years (Alanee and Shukla 2010; Lopes et al. 2020). Papillary urothelial neoplasms of low malignant potential (PUNLMPs) and rhabdomyosarcoma (RMS) are the most common bladder malignancies in the pediatric population.

Macroscopic hematuria and symptoms of urinary tract infections often represent the initial presentation (Lerena et al. 2010; Fine et al. 2005; Dénes et al. 2013), but a significant proportion of these tumors are detected incidentally at imaging (Lopes et al. 2020). Boys are generally more affected than girls regardless of the histology (2–3:1).

With the exception of RMS, pediatric neoplasms of the bladder are associated with favorable benign behavior and outcomes after adequate therapy.

Urinalysis and urinary culture are mandatory to exclude or confirm concomitant urinary tract infection. Owing to the low sensitivity (low cell turnover related to the benign nature of many pediatric bladder lesions) and the absence of experience of pediatric pathologists in such situations, urinary cytology is rarely useful (Dénes et al. 2013). Ultrasonography is the most common initial examination: a full bladder during examination is advisable to avoid missing small lesions or making a misinterpretation (Mbeutcha et al. 2016). If malignancy is suspected, pelvic CT scan or—preferably—MRI is performed for better characterization of the location and extent of disease. Definitive diagnosis for pediatric tumors of the lower urinary tract is usually performed by cystoscopy, which also allows evaluation of tumor extensions, excision, or biopsy. Transurethral resection represents the treatment of choice for papillary urothelial neoplasms. Interval cystoscopy has been advocated as the best method to follow these patients; however, while only cystoscopy allows for histological diagnosis, the need for general anesthesia and the risk of urethral manipulation make its limited use preferable, with ultrasound as a complementary imaging method. Work-up includes hemoglobin quantification in case of hematuria, assessment of inflammatory marker levels if suspicion of infection, and determining renal function if bladder tumor is associated with hydronephrosis.

The rarity of bladder tumors in children makes it very difficult to estimate their incidence and survival. A paper from the Surveillance, Epidemiology, and End Results (SEER) database focused on the incidence of pediatric bladder tumors. Among 140 identified cases of bladder neoplasms in children aged <18 years (over a 30 years time frame, between 1973 and 2003), PUNLMPs and embryonal RMS comprised 50.7% and 36.4% of the tumors, and transitional cell carcinoma (TCC) accounted for 9.3% (Alanee and Shukla 2010). Noteworthy, the incidence of a given histological subtype was related to the age at presentation. Embryonal RMS was the predominant type in children aged <12 years, being TCC extremely rare. It was around puberty when TCC was more common and overcame the other subtypes. The incidence of pediatric bladder tumors significantly increased over the period of the study; however, the authors warn that this can be due to the improved reporting to the SEER database more than to an actual increase. Survival calculated at 1 and 2 years after initial diagnosis was 93.6% and 97.5%.

Mesenchymal bladder tumors may exceptionally include, other than RMS, leiomyosarcoma, inflammatory myofibroblastic tumor (Berger et al. 2007; Houben et al. 2007; Lopes et al. 2020), leiomyoma, hemangioma (Wiygul and Palmer 2010), lymphangioma (Niu et al. 2010), and neuroendocrine tumors (pheochromocytoma, paraganglioma, neurofibroma) (Mou et al. 2008).

Inflammatory myofibroblastic tumors of the bladder (IMTBs) are rare (a quarter of these neoplasms occur in children) and are characterized by a benign and reactive proliferation of myofibroblasts. A review of 42 reported cases of pediatric IMTB showed equal prevalence in males and females. Clinical presentation includes hematuria, dysuria, or abdominal pain, and mean age at presentation is 7.5 years (range of 2–15 years). The etiology of IMTB is poorly understood and is attributed to infectious or traumatic causes or a possible clonal lesion mainly involving the anaplastic lymphoma kinase gene (*ALK-1*) or *NTRK*, *ROS1*, *PDGFR*, and *NTRK*, which are far more common in children and young adults (Martelli et al. 2016).

Urothelial neoplasms in children are rare and predominantly non-invasive. Lesions are classified in accordance with the 2004 WHO/International Society of Urological Pathology criteria as urothelial papillomas, PUNLMPs, low-grade urothelial carcinomas, and high-grade urothelial carcinomas. At presentation, the most common symptom is painless hematuria. In the presence of hematuria, ultrasound must be performed. If a bladder lesion is identified, transurethral resection of the bladder should be performed. The lesions are usually solitary, non-muscle invasive, and of low grade (mainly urothelial papilloma and PUNLMPs). There is no standard ideal follow-up protocol for these tumors, basing on the rarity of the disease. Recurrence or progression is uncommon in patients younger than 20 years, the reported recurrence rate is 7%, and a single case of progression has been reported so far (Lopes et al. 2020; Saltsman et al. 2018).

PUNLMPs are normally solitary and small (1–2 cm) lesions, commonly occur at the posterior lateral walls and ureteric orifices of the bladder, are non-invasive, and do not metastasize. About 35% of PUNLMPs reportedly recur after complete resection, and around 10% of them increase in size if they are not treated; therefore, regular imaging surveillance is advocated (Saltsman et al. 2018). PUNLMP seems to have excellent long-term survival (Fine et al. 2005; Alanee and Shukla 2010).

TCC of the bladder has a high incidence in adults, but it is uncommon in children and adolescents, and only small case series have been described in children (Lerena et al. 2010; Yossepowitch and Dalbagni 2002). Apart from the SEER report, there are about 125 cases of patients <20 years of age reported in the literature, with only 20 of them in patients <10 years of age (reviewed in Lerena et al. 2010). Despite some genetic conditions seem to increase the risk of TCC of the bladder in adults, such as Cowden disease, hereditary non-polyposis colon cancer, and familial increased risk, none of these have been reported to be related to this cancer in children (Giedl et al. 2006). Adolescents and young adults with Costello syndrome are at higher risk of TCC of the bladder (Gripp 2005). A known past history of smoking in adolescents has been advocated as a possible risk factor. Hematuria is the most common symptom of presentation. This finding emphasizes the need to exclude urothelial tumors in all young patients who present with painless hematuria (Hoenig et al. 1996), even though gross hematuria in children most often has a benign cause. Urine cytology has a good sensitivity and specificity only in high-grade tumors, and since the great majority of TCC in children are well differentiated, urine cytology is not recommended for diagnosis and or follow-up in children.

Fine et al. reported on a relatively large series of patients younger than 20 years with urothelial neoplasms, diagnosed following modern clinicopathological classification (Fine et al. 2005; Eble et al. 2004). This analysis confirmed that these tumors are more common in males, are likely to manifest as hematuria, occur as solitary lesions, and are generally of low-grade histology, with low recurrence potential. Cystoscopically, the majority of the lesions were described as papillary. Lesions ranged between urothelial papilloma (2 cases), PUNLMP (10 cases), noninvasive low-grade papillary urothelial cancer (8 cases), and noninvasive high-grade papillary urothelial cancer (3 cases).

References

Ahmed HU, Arya M, Levitt G, Duffy PG, Mushtaq I, Sebire NJ (2007) Part I: Primary malignant non-Wilms' renal tumours in children. Lancet Oncol 8:730–737

Alanee S, Shukla AR (2010 Aug) Bladder malignancies in children aged <18 years: results from the Surveillance, Epidemiology and End Results database. BJU Int. 106(4):557–560. https://doi.org/10.1111/j.1464-410X.2009.09093.x. Epub 2009 Dec 14

Aldera AP, Pillay K (2020) Clear cell sarcoma of the kidney. Arch Pathol Lab Med 144(1):119–123. https://doi.org/10.5858/arpa.2018-0353-RS

Algar EM, Muscat A, Dagar V, Rickert C, Chow CW, Biegel JA, Ekert PG, Saffery R, Craig J, Johnstone RW, Ashley DM (2009) Imprinted CDKN1C is a tumor suppressor in rhabdoid tumor and activated by restoration of SMARCB1 and histone deacetylase inhibitors. PLoS One 4:e4482

Ambalavanan M, Geller JI (2019) Treatment of advanced pediatric renal cell carcinoma. Pediatr Blood Cancer 66(8):e27766

Ammerlaan AC, Ararou A, Houben MP, Baas F, Tijssen CC, Teepen JL, Wesseling P, Hulsebos TJ (2007) Long-term survival and transmission of INI1-mutation via nonpenetrant males in a family with rhabdoid tumour predisposition syndrome. Br J Cancer 18:18

Argani P, Antonescu CR, Illei PB, Lui MY, Timmons CF, Newbury R, Reuter VE, Garvin AJ, Perez-Atayde AR, Fletcher JA, Beckwith JB, Bridge JA, Ladanyi M (2001a Jul) Primary renal neoplasms with the ASPL-TFE3 gene fusion of alveolar soft part sarcoma: a distinctive tumor entity previously included among renal cell carcinomas of children and adolescents. Am J Pathol. 159(1):179–192. https://doi.org/10.1016/S0002-9440(10)61684-7

Argani P, Hawkins A, Griffin CA, Goldstein JD, Haas M, Beckwith JB, Mankinen CB, Perlman EJ (2001b Jun) A distinctive pediatric renal neoplasm characterized by epithelioid morphology, basement membrane production, focal HMB45 immunoreactivity, and t(6;11)(p21.1;q12) chromosome translocation. Am J Pathol 158(6):2089–2096. https://doi.org/10.1016/S0002-9440(10)64680-9

Argani P, Ladanyi M (2003a Sep) Recent advances in pediatric renal neoplasia. Adv Anat Pathol. 10(5):243–260. https://doi.org/10.1097/00125480-200309000-00001

Argani P, Ladanyi M (2003b Dec) Distinctive neoplasms characterised by specific chromosomal translocations comprise a significant proportion of paediatric renal cell carcinomas. Pathology. 35(6):492–498. https://doi.org/10.1080/00313020310001619901

Argani P, Ladanyi M (2005 Jun) Translocation carcinomas of the kidney. Clin Lab Med. 25(2):363–378. https://doi.org/10.1016/j.cll.2005.01.008

Argani P, Laé M, Ballard ET, Amin M, Manivel C, Hutchinson B, Reuter VE, Ladanyi M (2006 Apr 1) Translocation carcinomas of the kidney after chemotherapy in childhood. J Clin Oncol. 24(10):1529–1534. https://doi.org/10.1200/JCO.2005.04.4693

Argani P, Laé M, Hutchinson B, Reuter VE, Collins MH, Perentesis J, Tomaszewski JE, Brooks JS, Acs G, Bridge JA, Vargas SO, Davis IJ, Fisher DE, Ladanyi M (2005 Feb) Renal carcinomas with the t(6;11)

(p21;q12): clinicopathologic features and demonstration of the specific alpha-TFEB gene fusion by immunohistochemistry, RT-PCR, and DNA PCR. Am J Surg Pathol. 29(2):230–240. https://doi.org/10.1097/01.pas.0000146007.54092.37

Argani P, Lee J, Netto GJ, Zheng G, Tseh-Lin M, Park BH (2016) Frequent BRAF V600E mutations in metanephric stromal tumor. Am J Surg Pathol 40(5):719–722. https://doi.org/10.1097/PAS.0000000000000603

Argani P, Olgac S, Tickoo SK, Goldfischer M, Moch H, Chan DY, Eble JN, Bonsib SM, Jimeno M, Lloreta J, Billis A, Hicks J, De Marzo AM, Reuter VE, Ladanyi M (2007 Aug) Xp11 translocation renal cell carcinoma in adults: expanded clinical, pathologic, and genetic spectrum. Am J Surg Pathol. 31(8):1149–1160. https://doi.org/10.1097/PAS.0b013e318031ffff

Argani P, Pawel B, Szabo S, Reyes-Múgica M, Timmons C, Antonescu CR (2018) Diffuse strong BCOR immunoreactivity is a sensitive and specific marker for clear cell sarcoma of the kidney (CCSK) in pediatric renal neoplasia. Am J Surg Pathol 42(8):1128–1131

Argani P, Perlman EJ, Breslow NE, Browning NG, Green DM, D'Angio GJ, Beckwith JB (2000) Clear cell sarcoma of the kidney: a review of 351 cases from the National Wilms Tumor Study Group Pathology Center. Am J Surg Pathol 24:4–18

Arroyo MR, Green DM, Perlman EJ, Beckwith JB, Argani P (2001 Apr) The spectrum of metanephric adenofibroma and related lesions: clinicopathologic study of 25 cases from the National Wilms Tumor Study Group Pathology Center. Am J Surg Pathol. 25(4):433–444. https://doi.org/10.1097/00000478-200104000-00002

Baek M, Jung JY, Kim JJ, Park KH, Ryu DS (2010 Aug) Characteristics and clinical outcomes of renal cell carcinoma in children: a single center experience. Int J Urol. 17(8):737–740. https://doi.org/10.1111/j.1442-2042.2010.02588.x. Epub 2010 Jun 29

Bellmunt J, Guix M (2009 Mar) The medical management of metastatic renal cell carcinoma: integrating new guidelines and recommendations. BJU Int. 103(5):572–577. https://doi.org/10.1111/j.1464-410X.2008.08336.x

Berger A, Kim C, Hagstrom N, Ferrer F (2007 Aug) Successful preoperative treatment of pediatric bladder inflammatory myofibroblastic tumor with anti-inflammatory therapy. Urology. 70(2):372.e13–372.e15. https://doi.org/10.1016/j.urology.2007.04.047

Biegel JA, Allen CS, Kawasaki K, Shimizu N, Budarf ML, Bell CJ (1996) Narrowing the critical region for a rhabdoid tumor locus in 22q11. Genes Chromosomes Cancer 16:94–105

Biegel JA, Kalpana G, Knudsen ES, Packer RJ, Roberts CW, Thiele CJ, Weissman B, Smith M (2002a) The role of INI1 and the SWI/SNF complex in the development of rhabdoid tumors: meeting summary from the workshop on childhood atypical teratoid/rhabdoid tumors. Cancer Res 62:323–328

Biegel JA, Tan L, Zhang F, Wainwright L, Russo P, Rorke LB (2002b) Alterations of the hSNF5/INI1 gene in central nervous system atypical teratoid/rhabdoid tumors and renal and extrarenal rhabdoid tumors. Clin Cancer Res 8:3461–3467

Blom JH, van Poppel H, Maréchal JM, Jacqmin D, Schröder FH, de Prijck L, Sylvester R, EORTC Genitourinary Tract Cancer Group (2009) Radical nephrectomy with and without lymph-node dissection: final results of European Organization for Research and Treatment of Cancer (EORTC) randomized phase 3 trial 30881. Eur Urol. 55(1):28–34. https://doi.org/10.1016/j.eururo.2008.09.052. Epub 2008 Oct 1

Bourdeaut F, Chi SH, Frühwald MC (2014) Rhabdoid tumors: integrating biological insights with clinical success. A report from the SMARCB1 and Rhabdoid Tumor Symposium, Paris, December 12-14, 2013. Cancer Genet 207:346–351

Brennan B, De Salvo GL, Orbach D, De Paoli A, Kelsey A, Mudry P, Francotte N, Van Noesel M, Bisogno G, Casanova M, Ferrari A (2016) Outcome of extracranial malignant rhabdoid tumours in children registered in the European Paediatric Soft Tissue Sarcoma Study Group Non-Rhabdomyosarcoma Soft Tissue Sarcoma 2005 Study-EpSSG-NRSTS 2005. Eur J Cancer 60:69–82

Brisse HJ, de la Monneraye Y, Cardoen L, Schleiermacher G (2020) From Wilms to kidney tumors: which ones require a biopsy? Pediatr Radiol. https://doi.org/10.1007/s00247-020-04660-x

Brok J, Treger TD, Gooskens SL, van den Heuvel-Eibrink MM, Pritchard-Jones K (2016 Nov) Biology and treatment of renal tumours in childhood. Eur J Cancer 68:179–195. https://doi.org/10.1016/j.ejca.2016.09.005

Brownlee NA, Hazen-Martin DJ, Garvin AJ, Re GG (2002) Functional and gene expression analysis of the p53 signalling pathway in clear cell sarcoma of the kidney and congenital mesoblastic nephroma. Pediatr Dev Pathol 5:257–268

Brownlee NA, Perkins LA, Stewart W, Jackle B, Pettenati MJ, Koty PP, Iskandar SS, Garvin AJ (2007) Recurring translocation (10;17) and deletion (14q) in clear cell sarcoma of the kidney. Arch Pathol Lab Med 131:446–451

Bruder E, Passera O, Harms D, Leuschner I, Ladanyi M, Argani P, Eble JN, Struckmann K, Schraml P, Moch H (2004 Sep) Morphologic and molecular characterization of renal cell carcinoma in children and young adults. Am J Surg Pathol. 28(9):1117–1132. https://doi.org/10.1097/01.pas.0000131558.32412.40

Brugarolas J (2007 Jan 11) Renal-cell carcinomaDOUBLEHYPHENmolecular pathways and therapies. N Engl J Med. 356(2):185–187. https://doi.org/10.1056/NEJMe068263

Bukowski RM (2010 Mar 26) Metastatic clear cell carcinoma of the kidney: therapeutic role of bevacizumab. Cancer Manag Res. 2:83–96. https://doi.org/10.2147/cmar.s7540

Cajaiba MM, Dyer LM, Geller JI, Jennings LJ, George D, Kirschmann D et al (2018) The classification of pediatric and young adult renal cell carcinomas registered on the children's oncology group (COG) protocol AREN03B2 after focused genetic testing. Cancer 124(16):3381–3389

Camparo P, Vasiliu V, Molinie V, Couturier J, Dykema KJ, Petillo D, Furge KA, Comperat EM, Lae M, Bouvier R, Boccon-Gibod L, Denoux Y, Ferlicot S, Forest E, Fromont G, Hintzy MC, Laghouati M, Sibony M, Tucker ML, Weber N, Teh BT, Vieillefond A (2008 May) Renal translocation carcinomas: clinicopathologic, immunohistochemical, and gene expression profiling analysis of 31 cases with a review of the literature. Am J Surg Pathol. 32(5):656–670. https://doi.org/10.1097/PAS.0b013e3181609914

Carcao MD, Taylor GP, Greenberg ML, Bernstein ML, Champagne M, Hershon L, Baruchel S (1998 Sep) Renal-cell carcinoma in children: a different disorder from its adult counterpart? Med Pediatr Oncol. 31(3):153–158. https://doi.org/10.1002/(sici)1096-911x(199809)31:3<153::aid-mpo5>3.0.co;2-a

Chi SN, Zimmerman MA, Yao X, Cohen KJ, Burger P, Biegel JA, Rorke-Adams LB, Fisher MJ, Janss A, Mazewski C, Goldman S, Manley PE, Bowers DC, Bendel A, Rubin J, Turner CD, Marcus KJ, Goumnerova L, Ullrich NJ, Kieran MW (2009) Intensive multimodality treatment for children with newly diagnosed CNS atypical teratoid rhabdoid tumor. J Clin Oncol 8:8–14

Ciftci AO, Talim B, Senocak ME, Kaymaz F, Cağlar M, Büyükpamukçu N (2000 Sep) Renal oncocytoma: diagnostic and therapeutic aspects. J Pediatr Surg. 35(9):1396–1398. https://doi.org/10.1053/jpsu.2000.9351

Cook A, Lorenzo AJ, Salle JL, Bakhshi M, Cartwright LM, Bagi D, Farhat W, Khoury A (2006 Apr) Pediatric renal cell carcinoma: single institution 25-year case series and initial experience with partial nephrectomy. J Urol. 175(4):1456–1460.; discussion 1460. https://doi.org/10.1016/S0022-5347(05)00671-3

Craig KM, Poppas DP (2019 Sep) Akhavan A Pediatric renal cell carcinoma. Curr Opin Urol 29(5):500–504. https://doi.org/10.1097/MOU.0000000000000656

Cutcliffe C, Kersey D, Huang CC, Zeng Y, Walterhouse D, Perlman EJ, Renal Tumor Committee of the Children's Oncology Group (2005) Clear cell sarcoma of the kidney: up-regulation of neural markers with activation of the sonic hedgehog and Akt pathways. Clin Cancer Res 11:7986–7994

D'Angio GJ, Breslow N, Beckwith JB, Evans A, Baum H, de Lorimier A, Fernbach D, Hrabovsky E, Jones B, Kelalis P et al (1989) Treatment of Wilms' tumor. Results of the Third National Wilms' Tumor Study. Cancer 64:349–360

Davis CJ Jr, Mostofi FK, Sesterhenn IA (1995 Jan) Renal medullary carcinoma. The seventh sickle cell nephropathy. Am J Surg Pathol. 19(1):1–11. https://doi.org/10.1097/00000478-199501000-00001

Dénes FT, Duarte RJ, Cristófani LM et al (2013) Pediatric genitourinary oncology. Front Pediatr 1:48

Douglass EC, Green AA, Hayes FA, Etcubanas E, Horowitz M, Wilimas JA (1985) Chromosome 1 abnormalities: a common feature of pediatric solid tumors. J Natl Cancer Inst 75:51–54

Escudier B (2009 Aug) New therapies after failure of angiogenesis inhibitors. Clin Adv Hematol Oncol. 7(8):512–514

Escudier BJ (2010 Oct) Combination therapy in patients with metastatic renal cell carcinoma. Clin Adv Hematol Oncol. 8(10):665–666

Escudier B, Kataja V (2010 May) ESMO Guidelines Working Group. Renal cell carcinoma: ESMO Clinical Practice Guidelines for diagnosis, treatment and follow-up. Ann Oncol. 21(Suppl 5):v137–v139. https://doi.org/10.1093/annonc/mdq206

Escudier B, Pluzanska A, Koralewski P, Ravaud A, Bracarda S, Szczylik C, Chevreau C, Filipek M, Melichar B, Bajetta E, Gorbunova V, Bay JO, Bodrogi I, Jagiello-Gruszfeld A, Moore N (2007 Dec 22) AVOREN Trial investigators. Bevacizumab plus interferon alfa-2a for treatment of metastatic renal cell carcinoma: a randomised, double-blind phase III trial. Lancet. 370(9605):2103–2111. https://doi.org/10.1016/S0140-6736(07)61904-7

Estrada CR, Suthar AM, Eaton SH, Cilento BG Jr (2005 Dec) Renal cell carcinoma: Children's Hospital Boston experience. Urology. 66(6):1296–1300. https://doi.org/10.1016/j.urology.2005.06.104

Ficarra V (2007 Mar) Open radical nephrectomy versus open partial nephrectomy: is it still an issue? Eur Urol. 51(3):593–595. https://doi.org/10.1016/j.eururo.2006.11.031. Epub 2006 Nov 20

Findlay BL, Shinder BM, Fatima A, Sadimin E, Drachtman R, Parikh RR, Singer EA (2019) Primary renal ewing sarcoma: a case report and review of the literature. J Ren Cancer 2(1):15–19

Fine SW, Humphrey PA, Dehner LP, Amin MB, Epstein JI (2005 Nov) Urothelial neoplasms in patients 20 years or younger: a clinicopathological analysis using the world health organization 2004 bladder consensus classification. J Urol. 174(5):1976–1980. https://doi.org/10.1097/01.ju.0000176801.16827.82

Frühwald MC, Biegel JA, Bourdeaut F, Roberts CW, Chi SN (2016) Atypical teratoid/rhabdoid tumors-current concepts, advances in biology, and potential future therapies. Neuro-Oncology 18:764–778

Frühwald MC, Hasselblatt M, Wirth S, Köhler G, Schneppenheim R, Subero JI, Siebert R, Kordes U, Jürgens H, Vormoor J (2006) Non-linkage of familial rhabdoid tumors to SMARCB1 implies a second locus for the rhabdoid tumor predisposition syndrome. Pediatr Blood Cancer 47:273–278

Furtwängler R, Gooskens SL, van Tinteren H, de Kraker J, Schleiermacher G, Bergeron C, de Camargo B, Acha T, Godzinski J, Sandstedt B, Leuschner I, Vujanic GM, Pieters R, Graf N, van den Heuvel-Eibrink MM (2013) Clear Cell Sarcomas of the Kidney (CCSK) registered on SIOP 93-01 and SIOP 2001 protocols: a report of the SIOP Renal Tumour Study Group. Eur J Cancer 49(16):3497–3506

Furtwängler R, Kager L, Melchior P, Rübe C, Ebinger M, Nourkami-Tutdibi N, Niggli N, Warmann S, Hubertus J, Amman G, Leuschner I, Vokuhl C, Graf N, Frühwald MC (2018) High Dose Treatment for Malignant Rhabdoid Tumor of the Kidney: no evidence for improved survival—the Gesellschaft für Pädiatrische Onkologie und Hämatologie (GPOH) experience. Pediatr Blood Cancer 65(1):e26746

Furtwängler R, Nourkami-Tutdibi N, Leuschner I, Vokuhl C, Niggli F, Kager L, Ebinger M, Frühwald MC, Graf N (2014) Malignant Rhabdoid Tumor of the Kidney: significantly improved response to preoperative treatment intensified with doxorubicin. Cancer Genet 207(9):434–436

Geller JI, Argani P, Adeniran A, Hampton E, De Marzo A, Hicks J, Collins MH (2008 Apr 1) Translocation renal cell carcinoma: lack of negative impact due to lymph node spread. Cancer. 112(7):1607–1616. https://doi.org/10.1002/cncr.23331

Geller JI, Dome JS (2004 Oct 1) Local lymph node involvement does not predict poor outcome in pediatric renal cell carcinoma. Cancer. 101(7):1575–1583. https://doi.org/10.1002/cncr.20548

Geller JI, Dome JS (2009 Mar) Retroperitoneal lymph node dissection for pediatric renal cell carcinoma. Pediatr Blood Cancer. 52(3):430. https://doi.org/10.1002/pbc.21853

Geller JI, Ehrlich PF, Cost NG, Khanna G, Mullen EA, Gratias EJ et al (2015) Characterization of adolescent and pediatric renal cell carcinoma: a report from the Children's Oncology Group study AREN03B2. Cancer 121(14):2457–2464

Geller JI, Fox E, Turpin BK, Goldstein SL, Liu X, Minard CG et al (2018) A study of axitinib, a VEGF receptor tyrosine kinase inhibitor, in children and adolescents with recurrent or refractory solid tumors: a Children's Oncology Group phase 1 and pilot consortium trial (ADVL1315). Cancer 124(23):4548–4555

Giedl J, Wild PJ, Stoehr R, Junker K, Boehm S, van Oers JM, Zwarthoff EC, Blaszyk H, Fine SW, Humphrey PA, Dehner LP, Amin MB, Epstein JI, Hartmann A (2006) Urotheltumoren bei Kindern und Jugendlichen (< 20 Jahre) haben nur selten molekulare Veränderungen und eine gute Prognose [Urothelial neoplasms in individuals younger than 20 years show very few genetic alterations and have a favourable clinical outcome]. Verh Dtsch Ges Pathol 90:253–263. German.

Gooskens SL, Furtwängler R, Spreafico F, van Tinteren H, de Kraker J, Vujanic G, Leuschner I, Coulomb-L'Herminé A, Godzinski J, Schleiermacher G, Stoneham S, Bergeron C, Pritchard-Jones K, Graf N, van den Heuvel-Eibrink MM (2014) Outcome of patients with relapsed Clear Cell Sarcoma of the Kidney (CCSK) registered on recent SIOP, UK-CCLG and AIEOP study. Br J Cancer 111:227–233

Gooskens S, Furtwängler R, Vujanic GM, Dome J, Graf N, Van den Heuvel-Eibrink M (2012) Clear cell sarcoma of the kidney: a review. Eur J Cancer 48:2219–2226

Gooskens SL, Graf N, Furtwangler R, Spreafico F, Bergeron C, Ramirez-Villar GL, Godzinski J, Rübe C, Janssens GO, Vujanic G, Leuschner I, Coulomb-L'Herminé A, Smets AM, de Camargo B, Stoneham S, van Tinteren H, Pritchard-Jones K, van den Heuvel-Eibrink MM (2018) Rational for the treatment of children with CCSK in the UMBRELLA SIOP-RTSG 2016 protocol. Nat Rev Urol 15:309–319

Gooskens SL, Kenny C, Lazaro A, O'Meara E, van Tinteren H, Spreafico F, Vujanic G, Leuschner I, Coulomb-L'Herminé A, Perotti D, de Camargo B, Bergeron C, Acha García T, Tanaka M, Pieter R, Pritchard-Jones K, Graf N, van den Heuvel-Eibrink MM, O'Sullivan MJ (2016) The clinical phenotype of the YWHAE-NUTM2B/E fusion transcript in paediatric Clear Cell Sarcoma of the Kidney. Genes Chromosom Cancer 55:143–147

Graf N, Bergeron C (2012) Wilms and other renal tumors. In: Stevens MCG, Caron HN, Biondi A (eds) Cancer in children, 6th edn. Oxford University Press, pp 312–327. ISBN 978-0-19-959941-7

Graf N, Wilms-Tumoren RH (2003 Mar) Diagnostik und Therapie [Wilms tumors. Diagnosis and therapy]. Urologe A (3):42, W391–W407. quiz W408-9. German

Green DM, Breslow NE, Beckwith JB, Moksness J, Finklestein JZ, D'Angio GJ (1994) Treatment of children with clear-cell sarcoma of the kidney: a report from the National Wilms' Tumor Study Group. J Clin Oncol 12:2132–2137

Gripp KW (2005) Tumor predisposition in Costello syndrome. Am J Med Genet C Semin Med Genet. 137C(1):72–77. https://doi.org/10.1002/ajmg.c.30065

Grundy RG, Hutton C, Middleton H, Imeson J, Pritchard J, Kelsey A, Marsden HB, Vujanic GM, Taylor RE, United Kingdom Children's Cancer Study Group (2004) Outcome of patients with stage III or inoperable WT treated on the second United Kingdom WT protocol (UKWT2); a United Kingdom Children's Cancer Study Group (UKCCSG) study. Pediatr Blood Cancer 42:311–319

Gulati S, Vaishampayan U (2020) Current state of systemic therapies for advanced renal cell carcinoma. Curr Oncol Rep 22(3):26. https://doi.org/10.1007/s11912-020-0892-1

Gururangan S, Bowman LC, Parham DM, Wilimas JA, Rao B, Pratt CB, Douglass EC (1993) Primary extracranial rhabdoid tumors: clinicopathologic features and response to ifosfamide. Cancer 71:2653–2659

Haas JE, Palmer NF, Weinberg AG, Beckwith JB (1981) Ultrastructure of malignant rhabdoid tumor of the kidney. A distinctive renal tumor of children. Hum Pathol 12:646–657

Hasselblatt M, Gesk S, Oyen F, Rossi S, Viscardi E, Giangaspero F, Giannini C, Frühwald MC, Obser T, Schneppenheim R, Siebert R, Paulus W (2011) Nonsense mutation and inactivation of SMARCA4 (BRG1) in an atypical teratoid/rhabdoid tumor showing retained SMARCB1 (INI1) expression. Am J Surg Pathol 35:933–935

Hasselblatt M, Isken S, Linge A, Eikmeier K, Jeibmann A, Oyen F, Nagel I, Richter J, Bartelheim K, Kordes U,

Schneppenheim R, Frühwald M, Siebert R, Paulus W (2013) High-resolution genomic analysis suggests the absence of recurrent genomic alterations other than SMARCB1 aberrations in atypical teratoid/rhabdoid tumors. Genes Chromosomes Cancer 52:185–190

van den Heuvel-Eibrink MM, Grundy P, Graf N, Pritchard-Jones K, Bergeron C, Patte C, van Tinteren H, Rey A, Langford C, Anderson JR, de Kraker J (2008) Characteristics and survival of 750 children diagnosed with a renal tumor in the first seven months of life: a collaborative study by the SIOP/GPOH/SFOP, NWTSG, and UKCCSG Wilms tumor study groups. Pediatr Blood Cancer 50:1130–1134

van den Heuvel-Eibrink MM, Hol JA, Pritchard-Jones K, van Tinteren H, Furtwängler R, Verschuur AC, Vujanic GM, Leuschner I, Brok J, Rübe C, Smets AM, Janssens GO, Godzinski J, Ramírez-Villar GL, de Camargo B, Segers H, Collini P, Gessler M, Bergeron C, Spreafico F, Graf N (2017) International Society of Paediatric Oncology—Renal Tumour Study Group (SIOP–RTSG). Position paper: rationale for the treatment of Wilms tumour in the UMBRELLA SIOP-RTSG 2016 protocol. Nat Rev Urol 14(12):743–752. https://doi.org/10.1038/nrurol.2017.163

van den Heuvel-Eibrink MM, van Tinteren H, Rehorst H, Coulombe A, Patte C, de Camargo B, de Kraker J, Leuschner I, Lugenberg R, Pritchard-Jones K, Sandstedt B, Spreafico F, Graf N, Vujanic GM (2011) Malignant rhabdoid tumours of the kidney (MRTKs), registered on recent SIOP protocols from 1993 to 2005: a report of the SIOP renal tumour study group. Pediatr Blood Cancer 56:733–737

Hoenig DM, McRae S, Chen SC, Diamond DA, Rabinowitz R, Caldamone AA (1996 Jul) Transitional cell carcinoma of the bladder in the pediatric patient. J Urol. 156(1):203–205

Hoot AC, Russo P, Judkins AR, Perlman EJ, Biegel JA (2004) Immunohistochemical analysis of hSNF5/INI1 distinguishes renal and extra-renal malignant rhabdoid tumors from other pediatric soft tissue tumors. Am J Surg Pathol 28(11):1485–1491

Houben CH, Chan A, Lee KH, Tam YH, To KF, Cheng W, Yeung CK (2007 Aug) Inflammatory myofibroblastic tumor of the bladder in children: what can be expected? Pediatr Surg Int. 23(8):815–819. https://doi.org/10.1007/s00383-007-1885-y. Epub 2007 Apr 19

Huang CC, Cutcliffe C, Coffin C, Sorensen PH, Beckwith JB, Perlman EJ, Renal Tumor Committee of the Children's Oncology Group (2006) Classification of malignant pediatric renal tumors by gene expression. Pediatr Blood Cancer 46:728–738

Hudes G, Carducci M, Tomczak P, Dutcher J, Figlin R, Kapoor A, Staroslawska E, Sosman J, McDermott D, Bodrogi I, Kovacevic Z, Lesovoy V, Schmidt-Wolf IG, Barbarash O, Gokmen E, O'Toole T, Lustgarten S, Moore L, Motzer RJ, Trial GARCC (2007 May 31) Temsirolimus, interferon alfa, or both for advanced renal-cell carcinoma. N Engl J Med. 356(22):2271–2281. https://doi.org/10.1056/NEJMoa066838

Indolfi P, Terenziani M, Casale F, Carli M, Bisogno G, Schiavetti A, Mancini A, Rondelli R, Pession A, Jenkner A, Pierani P, Tamaro P, De Bernardi B, Ferrari A, Santoro N, Giuliano M, Cecchetto G, Piva L, Surico G, Di Tullio MT (2003 Feb 1) Renal cell carcinoma in children: a clinicopathologic study. J Clin Oncol. 21(3):530–535. https://doi.org/10.1200/JCO.2003.02.072

Irtan S, Van Tinteren H, Graf N, van den Heuvel-Eibrink MM, Heij H, Bergeron C, de Camargo B, Acha T, Spreafico F, Vujanic G, Powis M, Okoye B, Wilde J, Godzinski J, Pritchard-Jones K (2019) Evaluation of needle biopsy as a potential risk factor for local recurrence of Wilms tumour in the SIOP WT 2001 trial. Eur J Cancer 116:13–20. https://doi.org/10.1016/j.ejca.2019.04.027

Jackson EM, Sievert AJ, Gai X, Hakonarson H, Judkins AR, Tooke L, Perin JC, Xie H, Shaikh TH, Biegel JA (2009) Genomic analysis using high-density single nucleotide polymorphism-based oligonucleotide arrays and multiplex ligation-dependent probe amplification provides a comprehensive analysis of INI1/SMARCB1 in malignant rhabdoid tumors. Clin Cancer Res 15:1923–1930

Janson K, Nedzi LA, David O, Schorin M, Walsh JW, Bhattacharjee M, Pridjian G, Tan L, Judkins AR, Biegel JA (2006) Predisposition to atypical teratoid/rhabdoid tumor due to an inherited INI1 mutation. Pediatr Blood Cancer 47:279–284

John NT, Blum KA, Hakimi AA (2019) Role of lymph node dissection in renal cell cancer. Urol Oncol 37(3):187–192. https://doi.org/10.1016/j.urolonc.2018.03.006

Joshi DD, Banerjee T (2008 Apr) Vascular endothelial growth factor (VEGF) receptor antibody bevacizumab (avastin) induces regression of renal cell carcinoma in an adolescent resulting in residual tumorectomy. Pediatr Blood Cancer. 50(4):903–904. https://doi.org/10.1002/pbc.21243

Judkins AR (2007) Immunohistochemistry of INI1 expression: a new tool for old challenges in CNS and soft tissue pathology. Adv Anat Pathol 14:335–339

Kaneko Y, Homma C, Maseki N, Sakurai M, Hata J (1991) Correlation of chromosome abnormalities with histological and clinical features in Wilms' and other childhood renal tumors. Cancer Res 51:5937–5942

Kao YC, Sung YS, Zhang L et al (2016) BCOR overexpression is a highly sensitive marker in round cell sarcomas with BCOR genetic abnormalities. Am J Surg Pathol 40(12):1670–1678

Kenny C, Bausenwein S, Lazaro A, Furtwängler R, Gooskens SL, van den Heuvel-Eibrink M, Vokuhl C, Leuchner I, Graf N, Gessler M, O'Sullivan MJ (2016) Mutually exclusive BCOR internal tandem duplications and YWHAE-NUTM2 fusions in clear cell sarcoma of kidney: not the full story. J Pathol 238(5):617–620

Kidd JM (1970) Exclusion of certain renal neoplasms from the category of Wilms tumor [abstract]. Am J Pathol 58:16a

Kieran MW, Roberts CW, Chi SN, Ligon KL, Rich BE, Macconaill LE, Garraway LA, Biegel JA (2012) Absence of oncogenic canonical pathway mutations in aggressive pediatric rhabdoid tumors. Pediatr Blood Cancer 59:1155–1157

Klatte T, Rao PN, de Martino M, LaRochelle J, Shuch B, Zomorodian N, Said J, Kabbinavar FF, Belldegrun AS, Pantuck AJ (2009 Feb 10) Cytogenetic profile predicts prognosis of patients with clear cell renal cell carcinoma. J Clin Oncol. 27(5):746–753. https://doi.org/10.1200/JCO.2007.15.8345. Epub 2009 Jan 5

Koga Y, Matsuzaki A, Suminoe A, Hatano M, Saito Y, Kinoshita Y, Tajiri T, Taguchi T, Kohashi K, Oda Y, Tsuneyoshi M, Hara T (2009) Long-term survival after autologous peripheral blood stem cell transplantation in two patients with malignant rhabdoid tumor of the kidney. Pediatr Blood Cancer 52:888–890

Kordes U, Bartelheim K, Modena P, Massimino M, Biassoni V, Reinhard H, Hasselblatt M, Scheppenheim R, Frühwald MC (2014) Favorable outcome of patients affected by rhabdoid tumors due to rhabdoid tumor predisposition syndrome (RTPS). Pediatr Blood Cancer 61:919–921

Kordes U, Gesk S, Frühwald MC, Graf N, Leuschner I, Hasselblatt M, Jeibmann A, Oyen F, Peters O, Pietsch T, Siebert R, Schneppenheim R (2010) Clinical and molecular features in patients with rhabdoid tumor predisposition syndrome. Genes Chromosomes Cancer 49:176–181

Kusumakumary P, Chellam VG, Rojymon J, Hariharan S, Krishnan NM (1997) Late recurrence of clear cell sarcoma of the kidney. Med Pediatr Oncol 28:355–357

Lee RS, Stewart C, Carter SL, Ambrogio L, Cibulskis K, Sougnez C, Lawrence MS, Auclair D, Mora J, Golub TR, Biegel JA, Getz G, Roberts CW (2012) A remarkably simple genome underlies highly malignant pediatric rhabdoid cancers. J Clin Invest 122:2983–2988

Lerena J, Krauel L, García-Aparicio L, Vallasciani S, Suñol M, Rodó J (2010 Oct) Transitional cell carcinoma of the bladder in children and adolescents: six-case series and review of the literature. J Pediatr Urol. 6(5):481–485. https://doi.org/10.1016/j.jpurol.2009.11.006. Epub 2010 Jan 18

Lopes RI, Mello MF, Lorenzo AJ (2020) Recent advances in pediatric bladder malignancies. F1000Res 9:F1000 Faculty Rev-147. https://doi.org/10.12688/f1000research.19396.1. eCollection 2020

Lopez-Beltran A, Carrasco JC, Cheng L, Scarpelli M, Kirkali Z, Montironi R (2009 May) 2009 update on the classification of renal epithelial tumors in adults. Int J Urol. 16(5):432–443. https://doi.org/10.1111/j.1442-2042.2009.02302.x. Epub 2009 Apr 20

Louis DN, Ohgaki H, Wiestler OD, Cavenee WK, Burger PC, Jouvet A, Scheithauer BW, Kleihues P (2007) The 2007 WHO classification of tumours of the central nervous system. Acta Neuropathol 114:97–109

Lünenbürger H, Lanvers-Kaminsky C, Lechtape B, Frühwald MC (2010) Systematic analysis of the antiproliferative effects of novel and standard anticancer agents in rhabdoid tumor cell lines. Anti-Cancer Drugs 21(5):514–522

Magnani C, Pannelli F, Mosciatti P, Viscomi S, Rosso S, Spitale AB, Pastore G (2001) Survival analysis of childhood tumours: data from the Italian cancer registries. Epidemiol Prev 25(3 Suppl):347–353. English, Italian

Malouf GG, Camparo P, Oudard S, Schleiermacher G, Theodore C, Rustine A, Dutcher J, Billemont B, Rixe O, Bompas E, Guillot A, Boccon-Gibod L, Couturier J, Molinié V, Escudier B (2010 Sep) Targeted agents in metastatic Xp11 translocation/TFE3 gene fusion renal cell carcinoma (RCC): a report from the Juvenile RCC Network. Ann Oncol. 21(9):1834–1838. https://doi.org/10.1093/annonc/mdq029. Epub 2010 Feb 12

Margulis V, Wood CG (2008 Sep-Oct) The role of lymph node dissection in renal cell carcinoma: the pendulum swings back. Cancer J. 14(5):308–314. https://doi.org/10.1097/PPO.0b013e31818675eb

Marsden HB, Lawler W (1980) Bone metastasizing renal tumor of childhood. Histopathological and clinical review of 38 cases. Virchows Arch A Pathol Anat Histol 387:341–351

Martelli H, Borrego P, Guérin F et al (2016) Quality of life and functional outcome of male patients with bladder-prostate rhabdomyosarcoma treated with conservative surgery and brachytherapy during childhood. Brachytherapy 15(3):306–311

Mbeutcha A, Lucca I, Mathieu R et al (2016) Current status of urinary biomarkers for detection and surveillance of bladder cancer. Urol Clin North Am 43(1):47–62

McKenna ES, Sansam CG, Cho YJ, Greulich H, Evans JA, Thom CS, Moreau LA, Biegel JA, Pomeroy SL, Roberts CW (2008) Loss of the epigenetic tumor suppressor snf5 leads to cancer without genomic instability. Mol Cell Biol 28:6223–6233

Mitchell C, Pritchard-Jones K, Shannon R, Hutton C, Stevens S, Machin D, Imeson J, Kelsey A, Vujanic GM, Gornall P, Walker J, Walker J, Taylor R, Sartori P, Hale J, Levitt G, Messahel B, Middleton H, Grundy R, Pritchard J, United Kingdom Cancer Study Group (2006) Immediate nephrectomy versus preoperative chemotherapy in the management of non-metastatic Wilms' tumour: results of a randomised trial (UKW3) by the UK Children's Cancer Study Group. Eur J Cancer 42:2554–2562

Motzer RJ, Basch E (2007 Dec 22) Targeted drugs for metastatic renal cell carcinoma. Lancet. 370(9605):2071–2073. https://doi.org/10.1016/S0140-6736(07)61874-1

Motzer RJ, Molina AM (2009 Jul 10) Targeting renal cell carcinoma. J Clin Oncol. 27(20):3274–3276. https://doi.org/10.1200/JCO.2009.21.8461. Epub 2009 May 18

Mou JW, Lee KH, Tam YH, Cheung ST, Chan KW, Thakre A (2008 Apr) Urinary bladder pheochromocytoma, an extremely rare tumor in children: case report and review of the literature. Pediatr Surg Int.

24(4):479–480. https://doi.org/10.1007/s00383-007-2013-8. Epub 2007 Sep 9

Nemes K, Frühwald MC (2018) Emerging therapeutic targets for the treatment of malignant rhabdoid tumors. Expert Opin Ther Targets 22:365–379

Niu ZB, Yang Y, Hou Y, Chen H, Liu X, Wang CL (2010 Oct) Lymphangioma of bladder. Urology. 76(4):955–957. https://doi.org/10.1016/j.urology.2010.03.050. Epub 2010 May 21

O'Meara E, Stack D, Lee CH, Garvin AJ, Morris T, Argani P, Han JS, Karlsson J, Gisselson D, Leuschner I, Gessler M, Graf N, Fletcher JA, O'Sullivan MJ (2008) Characterisation of the chromosomal translocation t(10;17)(q22;p13) in clear cell sarcoma of kidney. J Pathol 227:72–80

Palmer NF, Sutow W (1983) Clinical aspects of the rhabdoid tumor of the kidney: a report of the national Wilms' tumor study group. Med Ped Oncol 11:242–245

Parham DM, Weeks DA, Beckwith JB (1994) The clinicopathologic spectrum of putative extrarenal rhabdoid tumors. An analysis of 42 cases studied with immunohistochemistry or electron microscopy. Am J Surg Pathol 18:1010–1029

Pastore G, Znaor A, Spreafico F, Graf N, Pritchard-Jones K, Steliarova-Foucher E (2006 Sep) Malignant renal tumours incidence and survival in European children (1978-1997): report from the Automated Childhood Cancer Information System project. Eur J Cancer. 42(13):2103–2114. https://doi.org/10.1016/j.ejca.2006.05.010

Proust F, Laquerriere A, Constantin B, Ruchoux MM, Vannier JP, Freger P (1999) Simultaneous presentation of atypical teratoid/rhabdoid tumor in siblings. J Neuro-Oncol 43:63–70

Punnett HH, Halligan GE, Zaeri N, Karmazin N (1989) Translocation 10;17 in clear cell sarcoma of the kidney: a first report. Cancer Genet Cytogenet 41:123–128

Radulescu VC, Gerrard M, Moertel C, Grundy PE, Mathias L, Feusner J, Diller L, Dome JS (2008) Treatment of recurrent clear cell sarcoma of the kidney with brain metastasis. Pediatr Blood Cancer 50:246–249

Ramphal R, Pappo A, Zielenska M, Grant R, Ngan BY (2006 Sep) Pediatric renal cell carcinoma: clinical, pathologic, and molecular abnormalities associated with the members of the mit transcription factor family. Am J Clin Pathol. 126(3):349–364. https://doi.org/10.1309/98YE9E442AR7LX2X

Rao Q, Chen JY, Wang JD, Ma HH, Zhou HB, Lu ZF et al (2011) Renal cell carcinoma in children and young adults: clinicopathological, immunohistochemical, and VHL gene analysis of 46 cases with follow-up. Int J Surg Pathol 19(2):170–179

Rassy E, Flippot R, Albiges L (2020) Tyrosine kinase inhibitors and immunotherapy combinations in renal cell carcinoma. Ther Adv Med Oncol 12:1758835920907504. https://doi.org/10.1177/1758835920907504

Reinhard H, Reinert J, Beier R, Furtwängler R, Alkasser M, Rutkowski S, Frühwald M, Koscielniak E, Leuschner I, Kaatsch P, Graf N (2008) Rhabdoid tumors in children: prognostic factors in 70 patients diagnosed in Germany. Oncol Rep 19:819–823

Rialon KL, Gulack BC, Englum BR, Routh JC, Rice HE (2015) Factors impacting survival in children with renal cell carcinoma. J Pediatr Surg 50(6):1014–1018

Rickert CH, Paulus W (2004) Chromosomal imbalances detected by comparative genomic hybridisation in atypical teratoid/rhabdoid tumours. Childs Nerv Syst 20:221–224. Epub 2004 Feb 4

Rini BI, Campbell SC, Escudier B (2009 Mar 28) Renal cell carcinoma. Lancet. 373(9669):1119–1132. https://doi.org/10.1016/S0140-6736(09)60229-4. Epub 2009 Mar 5

Roberts CW, Galusha SA, McMenamin ME, Fletcher CD, Orkin SH (2000) Haploinsufficiency of Snf5 (integrase interactor 1) predisposes to malignant rhabdoid tumors in mice. Proc Natl Acad Sci U S A 97:13796–13800

Roberts CW, Leroux MM, Fleming MD, Orkin SH (2002) Highly penetrant, rapid tumorigenesis through conditional inversion of the tumor suppressor gene Snf5. Cancer Cell 2:415–425

Saltsman JA, Malek MM, Reuter VE et al (2018) Urothelial neoplasms in pediatric and young adult patients: a large single-center series. J Pediatr Surg 53(2):306–309

Sausville JE, Hernandez DJ, Argani P, Gearhart JP (2009 Aug) Pediatric renal cell carcinoma. J Pediatr Urol. 5(4):308–314. https://doi.org/10.1016/j.jpurol.2009.04.007. Epub 2009 May 14

Schafernak KT, Yang XJ, Hsueh W, Leestma JL, Stagl J, Goldman S (2007 Dec) Pediatric renal cell carcinoma as econd malignancy: reports of two cases and a review of the literature. Can J Urol. 14(6):3739–3744

Schenk JP, Engelmann D, Rohrschneider W, Zieger B, Semler O, Graf N, Tröger J (2004 Jul) Rhabdoidtumoren der Niere im Kindesalter DOUBLEHYPHEN Eine retrospektive radiomorphologische Analyse von 22 im Rahmen der Nephroblastomstudie SIOP 93/01-GPOH registrierten Fällen [Rhabdoid tumors of the kidney in childhood]. Rofo 176(7):965–971. German. https://doi.org/10.1055/s-2004-813030

Schenk JP, Engelmann D, Zieger B, Semler O, Wühl E, Furtwängler R, Graf N, Tröger J (2005 Feb) Bildgebende Differenzierung des Rhabdoidtumors vom Nephroblastom und mesoblastischen Nephrom [Radiologic differentiation of rhabdoid tumor from Wilms' tumor and mesoblastic nephroma]. Urologe A 44(2):155–161. German. https://doi.org/10.1007/s00120-004-0751-y

Schneppenheim R, Fruhwald MC, Gesk S, Hasselblatt M, Jeibmann A, Kordes U, Kreuz M, Leuschner I, Martin Subero JI, Obser T, Oven F, Vater I, Siebert R (2010) Germline nonsense mutation and somatic inactivation of SMARCA4/BRG1 in a family with rhabdoid tumor predisposition syndrome. Am J Hum Genet 86:279–284

Schultz KAP, Williams GM, Kamihara J, Stewart DR, Harris AK, Bauer AJ, Turner J, Shah R, Schneider K, Schneider KW, Carr AG, Harney LA, Baldinger S, Frazier AL, Orbach D, Schneider DT, Malkin D, Dehner LP, Messinger YH, Hill DA (2018) DICER1 and associated conditions: identification of at-risk individuals and recommended surveillance strategies. Clin Cancer Res 24(10):2251–2261. https://doi.org/10.1158/1078-0432.CCR-17-3089

Schuster AE, Schneider DT, Fritsch MK, Grundy P, Perlman EJ (2003) Genetic and genetic expression analyses of clear cell sarcoma of the kidney. Lab Investig 83:1293–1299

Scott RH, Walker L, Olsen ØE, Levitt G, Kenney I, Maher E, Owens CM, Pritchard-Jones K, Craft A, Rahman N (2006) Surveillance for Wilms tumour in at-risk children: pragmatic recommendations for best practice. Arch Dis Child 91(12):995–999. https://doi.org/10.1136/adc.2006.101295. Epub 2006 Jul 20

Sebire NJ, Vujanic GM (2009 Apr) Paediatric renal tumours: recent developments, new entities and pathological features. Histopathology. 54(5):516–528. https://doi.org/10.1111/j.1365-2559.2008.03110.x. Epub 2008 Aug 11

Seibel NL, Chi YY, Perlman EJ, Tian J, Sun J, Anderson JR, Ritchey ML, Thomas PR, Miser J, Kalapurakal JA, Grundy PE, Green DM (2019) Impact of cyclophosphamide and etoposide on outcome of clear cell sarcoma of the kidney treated on the National Wilms Tumor Study-5 (NWTS-5). Pediatr Blood Cancer 66:e27450

Seibel NL, Li S, Breslow NE, Beckwith JB, Green DM, Haase GM, Ritchey ML, Thomas PR, Grundy PE, Finklestein JZ, Kim T, Shochat SJ, Kelalis PP, D'Angio GJ (2004) Effect of duration of treatment on treatment outcome for patients with clear-cell sarcoma of the kidney: a report from the National Wilms' Tumor Study Group. J Clin Oncol 22:468–473

Seibel NL, Sun J, Anderson JR, Breslow NE, Perlamn EJ, Ritchey ML, Thomas R, Coppes MJ, Grundy PE, Green DM (2006) Outcome of clear cell sarcoma of the kidney (CCSK) treated on the National Wilms Tumor Study-5 (NWTS). J Clin Oncol 24(18S):9000

Selle B, Furtwängler R, Graf N, Kaatsch P, Bruder E, Leuschner I (2006 Dec 15) Population-based study of renal cell carcinoma in children in Germany, 1980-2005: more frequently localized tumors and underlying disorders compared with adult counterparts. Cancer. 107(12):2906–2914. https://doi.org/10.1002/cncr.22346

Sevenet N, Sheridan E, Amram D, Schneider P, Handgretinger R, Delattre O (1999) Constitutional mutations of the hSNF5/INI1 gene predispose to a variety of cancers. Am J Hum Genet 65:1342–1348

Shelmerdine SC, Lorenzo AJ, Gupta AA et al (2017) Pearls and pitfalls in diagnosing pediatric urinary bladder masses. Radiographics 37(6):1872–1891

Shet T, Viswanathan S (2009 Nov) The cytological diagnosis of paediatric renal tumours. J Clin Pathol. 62(11):961–969. https://doi.org/10.1136/jcp.2009.064659. Epub 2009 Aug 20

Silberstein J, Grabowski J, Saltzstein SL, Kane CJ (2009 Feb) Renal cell carcinoma in the pediatric population: Results from the California Cancer Registry. Pediatr Blood Cancer. 52(2):237–241. https://doi.org/10.1002/pbc.21779

Smets AM, de Kraker J (2010 Jun) Malignant tumours of the kidney: imaging strategy. Pediatr Radiol 40(6):1010–1018. https://doi.org/10.1007/s00247-010-1584-z. Epub 2010 Apr 30

Smith ME, Cimica V, Chinni S, Jana S, Koba W, Yang Z, Fine E, Zagzag D, Montagna C, Kalpana GV (2011) Therapeutically targeting cyclin D1 in primary tumors arising from loss of Ini1. Proc Natl Acad Sci U S A 108:319–324

Sotelo-Avila C, Gonzalez-Crussi F, deMello D, Vogler C, Gooch WM III, Gale G, Pena R (1986b) Renal and extrarenal rhabdoid tumors in children: a clinicopathologic study of 14 patients. Semin Diagn Pathol 3:151–163

Sotelo-Avila C, Gonzalez-Crussi F, Sadowinski S, Gooch WM, Pena R (1986a) Clear cell sarcoma of the kidney: a clinicopathologic study of 21 patients with long-term follow-up evaluation. Hum Pathol 16:1219–1230

Soulières D (2009 May) Review of guidelines on the treatment of metastatic renal cell carcinoma. Curr Oncol 16(Suppl 1):S67–S70

Spreafico F, Collini P, Terenziani M, Marchiano A, Piva L (2010) Renal cell carcinoma in children and adolescents. Expert Rev Anticancer Ther 10(12):1967–1978

Spreafico F, Gandola L, Melchionda F (2014) Stage I clear cell sarcoma of the kidney: is it the time for a less intensive adjuvant treatment? Translational Pediatrics 3:1–3

Squire SE, Chan MD, Marcus KJ (2007) Atypical teratoid/rhabdoid tumor: the controversy behind radiation therapy. J Neuro-Oncol 81:97–111

Srinivasan AS, Saade-Lemus S, Servaes SE, Acord MR, Reid JR, Anupindi SA, States LJ (2019) Imaging surveillance for children with predisposition to renal tumors. Pediatr Radiol 49(11):1453–1462. https://doi.org/10.1007/s00247-019-04432-2

Sultan I, Qaddoumi I, Rodriguez-Galindo C, Nassan AA, Ghandour K, Al-Hussaini M (2010) Age, stage, and radiotherapy, but not primary tumor site, affects the outcome of patients with malignant rhabdoid tumors. Pediatr Blood Cancer 54(1):35–40

Sun M, Shariat SF, Karakiewicz PI (2010 Sep) Factors affecting outcome in renal cell carcinoma. Curr Opin Urol. 20(5):355–360. https://doi.org/10.1097/MOU.0b013e32833c7b19

Swartz MA, Karth J, Schneider DT, Rodriguez R, Beckwith JB, Perlman EJ (2002 Dec) Renal medullary carcinoma: clinical, pathologic, immunohistochemical, and genetic analysis with pathogenetic implications. Urology. 60(6):1083–1089. https://doi.org/10.1016/s0090-4295(02)02154-4

Taguchi K, Okada A, Kamiya H, Yamada Y, Tozawa K, Kohri K (2008) Clear cell sarcoma of the kidney: a case report of an 11-year-old boy and a review of 11 cases in Japan. J Rural Med 3:19–22

Taylor MD, Gokgoz N, Andrulis IL, Mainprize TG, Drake JM, Rutka JT (2000) Familial posterior fossa brain tumors of infancy secondary to germline mutation of the hSNF5 gene. Am J Hum Genet 66:1403–1406. Epub 2000 Mar 14

Tenold M, Ravi P, Kumar M, Bowman A, Hammers H, Choueiri TK, Lara PN Jr (2020) Current approaches to the treatment of advanced or metastatic renal cell carcinoma. Am Soc Clin Oncol Educ Book 40:1–10. https://doi.org/10.1200/EDBK_279881

Thana M, Wood L (2020) Immune checkpoint inhibitors in genitourinary malignancies. Curr Oncol 27(Suppl 2):S69–S77. https://doi.org/10.3747/co.27.5121. Epub 2020 Apr 1

Tomlinson GE, Breslow NE, Dome J, Guthrie KA, Norkool P, Li S, Thomas PR, Perlman E, Beckwith JB, D'Angio GJ, Green DM (2005) Rhabdoid tumor of the kidney in the National Wilms' tumor study: age at diagnosis as a prognostic factor. J Clin Oncol 23:7641–7645

Touijer K, Jacqmin D, Kavoussi LR, Montorsi F, Patard JJ, Rogers CG, Russo P, Uzzo RG, Van Poppel H (2010 Feb) The expanding role of partial nephrectomy: a critical analysis of indications, results, and complications. Eur Urol. 57(2):214–222. https://doi.org/10.1016/j.eururo.2009.10.019. Epub 2009 Oct 20

Tournade MF, Com-Nougué C, de Kraker J, Ludwig R, Rey A, JMB B, Sandstedt B, Godzinski J, Carli M, Potter R, JZucker JM for the International Society of Pediatric Oncology Nephroblastoma Trial and Study Committee (2001) Optimal duration of preoperative therapy in unilateral and nonmetastatic Wilms' tumor in children older than 6 months: results of the Ninth International Society of Pediatric Oncology Wilms' Tumor Trial and Study. J Clin Oncol 19:488–500

Venkataraman S, Alimova I, Tello T, Harris PS, Knipstein JA, Donson AM, Foreman NK, Liu AK, Vibhakar R (2012) Targeting Aurora Kinase A enhances radiation sensitivity of atypical teratoid rhabdoid tumor cells. J Neuro-Oncol 107:517–526

Venneti S, Le P, Martinez D, Eaton KW, Shyam N, Jordan-Sciutto KL, Pawel B, Biegel JA, Judkins AR (2011) P16INK4A and p14ARF tumor suppressor pathways are deregulated in malignant rhabdoid tumors. J Neuropathol Exp Neurol 70:596–609

Versteege I, Sévenet N, Lange J, Rousseau-Merck MF, Ambros P, Handgretinger R, Aurias A, Delattre O (1998) Truncating mutations of hSNF5/INI1 in aggressive paediatric cancer. Nature 394(6689):203–206

Vujanić GM, Gessler M, Ooms AHAG, Collini P, Coulomb-l'Hermine A, D'Hooghe E, de Krijger RR, Perotti D, Pritchard-Jones K, Vokuhl C, van den Heuvel-Eibrink MM, Graf N, International Society of Paediatric Oncology–Renal Tumour Study Group (SIOP–RTSG) (2018) The UMBRELLA SIOP-RTSG 2016 Wilms tumour pathology and molecular biology protocol. Nat Rev Urol 15(11):693–701. https://doi.org/10.1038/s41585-018-0100-3

Vujanic GM, Sandstedt B, Harms D, Boccon-Gibod L, Delemarre JF (1996) Rhabdoid tumour of the kidney: a clinicopathological study of 22 patients from the International Society of Paediatric Oncology (SIOP) nephroblastoma file. Histopathology 28:333–340

Vujanić GM, Sandstedt B, Kelsey A, Sebire NJ (2009 May 1) Central pathology review in multicenter trials and studies: lessons from the nephroblastoma trials. Cancer. 115(9):1977–1983. https://doi.org/10.1002/cncr.24214

Wagner L, Hill DA, Fuller C, Pedrosa M, Bhakta M, Perry A, Dome JS (2002) Treatment of metastatic rhabdoid tumor of the kidney. J Pediatr Hematol Oncol 24:385–388

Waldron PE, Rodgers BM, Kelly MD, Womer RB (1999) Successful treatment of a patient with stage IV rhabdoid tumor of the kidney: case report and review. J Pediatr Hematol Oncol 21:53–57

Watson T, Oostveen M, Rogers H, Pritchard-Jones K, Olsen Ø (2020) The role of imaging in the initial investigation of paediatric renal tumours. Lancet Child Adolesc Health 4(3):232–241. https://doi.org/10.1016/S2352-4642(19)30340-2

Weeks DA, Beckwith JB, Mierau GW (1989) Rhabdoid tumor. An entity or a phenotype? Arch Pathol Lab Med 113:113–114

Wick MR, Ritter JH, Dehner LP (1995) Malignant rhabdoid tumors: a clinicopathologic review and conceptual discussion. Semin Diagn Pathol 12:233–248

Wiygul JB, Palmer L (2010 Aug) Isolated hemangioma causing gross painless hematuria in an adolescent male. Urology. 76(2):463–464. https://doi.org/10.1016/j.urology.2009.11.055. Epub 2010 Feb 16

Yossepowitch O, Dalbagni G (2002 Jul) Transitional cell carcinoma of the bladder in young adults: presentation, natural history and outcome. J Urol. 168(1):61–66

Zhang F, Tan L, Wainwright LM, Bartolomei MS, Biegel JA (2002) No evidence for hypermethylation of the hSNF5/INI1 promoter in pediatric rhabdoid tumors. Genes Chromosomes Cancer 34:398–405

Zhuge Y, Cheung MC, Yang R, Perez EA, Koniaris LG, Sola JE (2010 Oct) Pediatric non-Wilms renal tumors: subtypes, survival, and prognostic indicators. J Surg Res. 163(2):257–263. https://doi.org/10.1016/j.jss.2010.03.061. Epub 2010 Apr 21

Zimmerman MA, Goumnerova LC, Proctor M, Scott RM, Marcus K, Pomeroy SL, Turner CD, Chi SN, Chordas C, Kieran MW (2005) Continuous remission of newly diagnosed and relapsed central nervous system atypical teratoid/rhabdoid tumor. J Neuro-Oncol 72:77–84

33 Breast Cancer

Dominik T. Schneider

Breast cancer during adolescents and in particular childhood is exceedingly rare. While breast cancer constitutes the most frequent malignancy in women, epidemiological data from the SEER registry indicate that by far less than 1% of breast cancers develop in children and adolescents (Gutierrez et al. 2008). Over a 31-year period, 134 patients up to the age of 19 years have been identified with malignant breast tumors (Westfal et al. 2019). In this analysis, 20 carcinomas of the breast have been diagnosed in the age group 0–14 years and 114 among adolescents of 15–19 years of age, respectively (see Chap. 2). Based on these data, approximately three to four children and adolescents with breast cancer can be expected per year in the USA. In this study, the median age of patients was 17 years, demonstrating a sharp rise of incidence with the onset of puberty. Thirty-one patients died during follow-up, and among these, death was related to breast cancer in 22 patients (Westfal et al. 2019).

The vast majority of breast masses in children and adolescents are benign, ranging from the frequent postnatal breast hypertrophy to peripubertal changes. Nevertheless, the detection of a "lump in the breast" may be disconcerting for the patients and their parents, given their knowledge of the high overall frequency of breast cancer in adults. In this situation, the pediatric oncologist may also be involved in the diagnostic considerations and should be aware about the most important differential diagnoses. Considering the rarity of true epithelial breast cancer in children, the diagnosis and treatment of truly malignant breast cancer should be planned in a multidisciplinary setting that might include experienced breast cancer surgeon or gynecology oncologist, a pediatric oncologist, and medical oncologist who specializes in treatment of breast cancer.

33.1 Breast Lesions in Children and Adolescents: Clinical Approach and Differential Diagnosis

The clinical assessment and examination in case of breast enlargement may be difficult due to a broad variability of the glandular size during childhood and puberty. In general, breast masses in boys mostly represent gynecomastia, benign tumors, mesenchymal tumors arising from the chest wall, or metastatic tumors (Welch et al. 2004). Tumors arising from the glandular tissue predominantly occur in girls.

History and examination should include time of onset, signs of infection, pain, discharge, and uni-/bilateral presentation. Postnatal breast hypertrophy and, in rare cases, mastitis are easy

D. T. Schneider (✉)
Klinik für Kinder- und Jugendmedizin, Klinikum Dortmund, University Witten/Herdecke, Dortmund, Germany
e-mail: dominik.schneider@klinikumdo.de

D. T. Schneider et al. (eds.), *Rare Tumors in Children and Adolescents*, Pediatric Oncology,
https://doi.org/10.1007/978-3-030-92071-5_33

to diagnose and are usually not associated with significant complications (Stricker et al. 2005).

In contrast, the differential diagnosis of breast changes in pubertal girls is more complicated and should be evaluated in the light of physiological breast development (e.g., Tanner stages). The most frequent reasons for uni- or bilateral breast enlargement are premature (prior to the eighth year of life) or mature thelarche, which presents as enlargement of the glandular tissue below the areola. Thelarche may be earlier in association with obesity and ethnic background (Rosenfield et al. 2009). Premature thelarche may occur during toddler age. Estrogens are normal, and children do not show additional signs of pubertal development such as adrenarche or increased growth velocity. Thus, premature thelarche should be distinguished from true precocious puberty by the presence of additional signs of pubertal development. In the latter, a diagnostic work-up that includes endocrinologic testing and abdominal and pelvic ultrasound is indicated to exclude endocrinologic or ovarian disorders (e.g., juvenile granulosa cell tumor, sex cord stromal tumor with annular tubules, steroid cell tumor; see Chap. 39).

During infancy and early childhood, subcutaneous breast tumors may represent vascular tumors such as lymphangiomas and hemangiomas (Nagar et al. 1992; Welch et al. 2004). These tumors do not show a female sex restriction. They can be distinguished from glandular tumors with ultrasound (and in rare cases MRI). In the upper lateral quadrant and close to the axilla, enlarged lymph nodes may present as palpable tumors (Gao et al. 2015). Furthermore, leukemic or lymphoma infiltrates, neurofibromas, mesenchymal tumors (such as rhabdomyosarcoma), or bone tumors of the ribs (e.g., Ewing sarcoma in older children and adolescents) may develop in close proximity, but rarely within the breast (Bongiorno et al. 2010; Conter et al. 1992; Chung et al. 2009; Chateil et al. 1998; Gao et al. 2015). More commonly, these tumors are located outside and not restricted to the glandular tissue. These entities will be distinguished histopathologically.

With the onset of puberty, cysts, fibrocystic mastopathy, fibroadenoma, papilloma, hamartoma, breast trauma, and infection are the most frequent causes of a breast mass (Chung et al. 2009; Gao et al. 2015). The most common differential diagnoses are listed in Table 33.1. In most cases, diagnosis may be established based on medical history and clinical appearance. Of note, mammography has only low diagnostic impact due to dense glandular tissue in adolescents (Brand et al. 1993; Chateil et al. 1998). Therefore, the use of mammography should be very restrictive in (pre-)/pubertal girls (Ashley et al. 1989). Instead, ultrasound or MRI is required and provides good diagnostic assessment (Gao et al. 2015). Fine needle aspiration (FNA) for cytologic evaluation is often done and may show superior sensitivity compared to imaging only (Ashley et al. 1989). While this method is sufficient for most breast carcinomas, it is not adequate for sarcomas, such as angiosarcoma, which is easily missed. The value of FNA has also not been confirmed in children and adolescents, in whom adenocarcinoma is more infrequent, and therefore, differential diagnosis is different than in adults. Thus, a fine-needle biopsy may show better sensitivity and specificity than a punctate that is evaluated cytologically only. However, a recent analysis has shown that both needle aspiration and biopsy may be misleading, with 9/70 patients having discordant diagnoses on needle and final histology (Zmora et al. 2020). Therefore, at least in equivocal cases, histologic examination of an open biopsy is required for diagnostic assessment (e.g., angiosarcoma). Only in some very rare cases (e.g., intraductal papilloma), diagnosis can be established through cytologic evaluation of nipple discharge.

Some of these disorders are related to the pubertal and hormone-sensitive breast development. Thus, fibrocystic changes are commonly observed in adolescents and women of reproductive age (Greydanus et al. 2006; Neinstein et al. 1993). They present as ill-defined fibrotic hardening of the breast, most commonly in the outer upper quadrant. Lesions are usually painless, but during the late menstrual cycle, they may be painful. Pain usually responses well to ibuprofen. These changes are thought to be the

Table 33.1 Differential diagnosis of breast lesions according to age

Age	Diagnosis	Clinical hallmarks and diagnostic assessment
Neonate	Breast hypertrophy	Medical history
	Mastitis	Medical history, signs of local infection
	Hemangioma, lymphangioma	Clinical appearance. Ultrasound (Doppler)
Prepubertal	(Pre-) mature thelarche	Medical history, uni- or bilateral breast enlargement below the areola. Ultrasound
	Mesenchymal tumors	Not restricted to breast gland. Ultrasound, biopsy
Pubertal	Fibrocystic mastopathy	Painful breast during menses, improvement during menstruation, sometimes discharge. Ultrasound
	Fibroadenoma (juvenile)	Asymptomatic circumscribed, rubbery, and mobile breast lump in upper outer quadrant. Ultrasound: avascular echo, biopsy, excision in case of giant fibroadenoma (>5 cm)
	Intraductal papilloma	Bloody nipple discharge, well-circumscribed nodule. Ultrasound, cytology of nipple discharge
	Cystosarcoma phyllodes	Painless mass, sometimes with nipple discharge. Ultrasound: lobulation, heterogeneous echo, no calcification, excision
	Montgomery tubercles	Obstruction and/or inflammation of periareolar glands
	Duct ectasia	Distention of subareolar ducts, nipple discharge, sometimes blueish discolored subareolar lump
	Fat necrosis	Most commonly posttraumatic, fibrotic nodule
	Neurofibroma	Other diagnostic signs of NF-1: neurofibroma, café-au-lait spots, freckling, etc.
	Metastases	For example, leukemia, Hodgkin's lymphoma/NHL, neuroblastoma, rhabdomyosarcoma
	Primary breast cancer	Irregular mass, indolent, fixed or not, nipple discharge, peau d'orange, enlarged axillary lymph nodes. Ultrasound, MRI, biopsy

result of endocrinologic imbalances between estrogens and progesterones. Treatment may also include contraceptive drugs with estrogen component. There is a chance for resolution of these fibrocystic changes over time (Neinstein et al. 1993).

Fibroadenoma (juvenile) constitutes the most prevalent tumor lesion of the breast in adolescents (Chung et al. 2009; Greydanus et al. 2006; Simmons 1992; Gao et al. 2015; Doğan et al. 2017; Zmora et al. 2020). It may present as well-circumscribed masses of rubber consistency. Most tumors are asymptomatic and reach a size of 2–3 cm, but some of these estrogen sensitive tumors may grow to "giant fibroadenoma," causing local pain. Fibroadenomas present as solid non-vascular masses on ultrasound (Gao et al. 2015). Histologically, these tumors consist of densely proliferating glandular stroma. Of note, a significant proportion of fibroadenoma during puberty shows spontaneous regression over time, and only a few fibroadenomas may transform into malignant tumors (Carty et al. 1995; Tea et al. 2009). Therefore, smaller juvenile fibroadenoma may be followed for 2–3 menstrual cycles. However, if they continuously grow, surgical resection should be considered, since the surgical therapy may be more extensive if the tumors are larger (Greydanus et al. 2006). In general, if tumors are larger than 5 cm at diagnosis, symptomatic, continuously growing, or persisting into adulthood, excision is justified.

Other genuine breast tumors, such as phyllodes tumor (syn. Cystosarcoma phyllodes) and intraductal papilloma, more commonly develop during adulthood but may rarely arise in adolescents or children. Diagnostic assessment and treatment should be managed with an interdisciplinary approach that includes the gynecologist and pediatrician. In the SEER survey of malignant breast cancers, phyllodes tumors contributed half of the malignant primary breast tumors (Gutierrez et al. 2008). These tumors are biphasic tumors that include both an epithelial and a stromal component. They commonly present in the upper outer quadrant and may develop a considerably size (in average 8–10 cm) (Greydanus et al. 2006; Zmora et al. 2020). They frequently present with a leaf-like lobulated structure. The local relapse rate is low (approx. 10%), provided that the lobulated tumor is excised completely. The frequency of metastases is low (<5%) (Chen et al. 2005; Zmora et al. 2020).

"True" primary breast cancer in children and adolescents is exceedingly rare compared to these benign lesions (Gutierrez et al. 2008; Tea et al. 2009; Westfal et al. 2019). The most common clinical finding is a hard, often (but not always) fixed, indolent, and irregular mass. If the tumor grows subcutaneously, the skin may show a peau d'orange appearance. Nipple discharge may result from intraductal or subareolar growth. The clinical examination must always include the axillary lymph nodes to exclude lymph node metastases. Again, mammography is not indicated due to its diagnostic inaccuracy. Radiographic imaging includes imaging and MRI. Lungs must be screened for metastases with CT. Moreover, abdominal ultrasound, bone scintigraphy, and cranial MRI (in case of neurological signs) are indicated (Table 33.2).

The most difficult decision is whether to perform diagnostic and/or therapeutic maneuvers in children and adolescents with breast mass. In most small asymptomatic breast masses, lesions can be observed for at least two menstrual cycles (Templeman and Hertweck 2000; Zmora et al. 2020). They may also be evaluated with fine needle aspiration (FNA) or needle core biopsy, however, being aware of the diagnostic failures these techniques may be associated with (Zmora et al. 2020). However, needle puncture may even be therapeutic in cystic lesions. Surgical resection or biopsy may be indicated if the lesions are suspicious of malignancy (e.g., based on physical examination (skin or nipple changes, etc.), medical history of previous chest irradiation, or familial breast cancer at young age), or if lesions continuously grow beyond 5 cm in diameter. If a solid lesion persists (longer than two menstrual cycles) and shows no signs of regression, histologic verification is indicated (Ashley et al. 1989).

Table 33.2 Diagnostic assessment in primary breast cancer

Procedure	Specific question
Medical history	Duration of symptoms, nipple discharge, pubertal and medical history
	Family history of breast and ovarian cancer
	Previous malignancy, in particular irradiation to chest
Physical examination	Location, consistency, size, mobility, pain, inflammation, skin changes, nipple discharge, nipple appearance
	Axillary lymphadenopathy
	Hepatomegaly
Blood count	Signs of bone marrow failure/metastases
Liver enzymes, AP, LDH	Signs of liver metastases, bone metastases, unspecific tumor marker. Other tumor markers are not required (ASCO 1998)
Ultrasound	Cystic vs. solid, size, vascularity, lymph nodes, etc.
MRI	Cystic vs. solid, size, vascularity, lymph nodes, contralateral breast, etc.
CT thorax	Lung metastases
Bone scintigraphy	Skeletal metastases
Abdom. ultrasound	Liver metastases
Biopsy/excision	FNA or biopsy. Histology, hormone receptor status (ER, PR), HER2 expression and/or *HER2* amplification, Ki67 proliferation index

Mammography is not recommended

33.2 Breast Cancer in Adults: Current Concepts

In adult women, breast cancer is the most frequent cancer and the second most common cause of cancer death in women in western countries.

The median age at diagnosis is approximately 60 years. The risk of women to develop breast cancer during their lifetime is approximately 5–15%. During the fifth and sixth decade of life, breast cancer is the most frequent cause of death in western countries, making this cancer a major issue in clinical care, cancer research, and health policy. The incidence of breast cancer has been rising since 1970, while the mortality is slowly declining. Clinical and epidemiological studies indicate that age constitutes an independent prognostic factor, with young patients being at a higher risk.

Approximately 5–10% of all breast cancers are based on hereditary predisposition. Among these, mutations of *BRCA1* and *BRCA2* are most frequent. However, they are found in only 40–50% of patients with familial breast cancer. In patients with proven BRCA1/2 mutations, self-examination and early onset of clinical and sonographic screening are advocated starting in early adulthood (Antoniou et al. 2003; Ashley et al. 1989).

Data from long-term survivors of childhood cancer indicate that the risk of breast cancer is increased after irradiation to the thorax, e.g., for Hodgkin's lymphoma (Henderson et al. 2010; Moskowitz et al. 2014; Schellong et al. 2014). There is an obvious correlation between radiation dose to the breasts and the risk of later breast cancer. The risk does not plateau over time.

33.3 Diagnosis and Treatment

Detailed guidelines for diagnosis and treatment of breast cancer are beyond the scope of this chapter. Sufficient guidelines are available from several international and national oncology groups. Examples include the guidelines published by the American Society of Clinical Oncology (ASCO) or the European Society of Medical Oncology (ESMO), which are both updated on a regular basis (https://www.asco.org/research-guidelines/quality-guidelines/guidelines/breast-cancer; https://www.esmo.org/guidelines/breast-cancer). Briefly, standard diagnostic studies for potential breast cancer include both mammography (in adults >40 years), ultrasound, and MRI. Diagnosis is most often confirmed by ultrasound- (or MRI-) guided needle core biopsy or vacuum assisted biopsy (Fig. 33.1). During biopsy, it shall be ensured that the site of biopsy is marked, e.g., by clips. Molecular studies and endocrine receptor studies will help inform treatment strategy in particular with regard to targeted and endocrinologic treatment. Sentinel node lymph node biopsy constitutes an integral part of treatment planning. Serological tumor marker evaluation is not recommended.

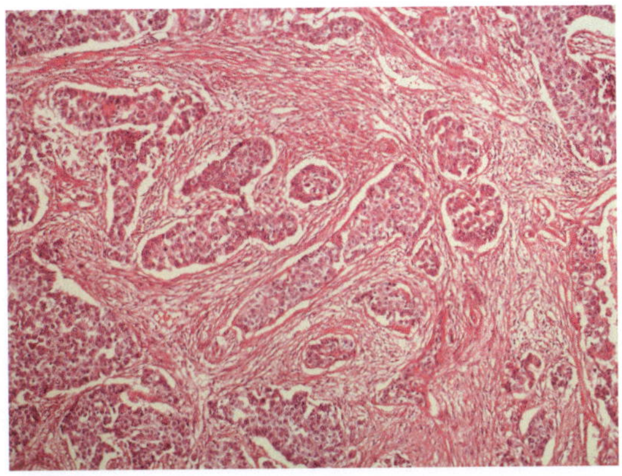

Fig. 33.1 Poorly differentiated invasive ductal carcinoma in a 35-year-old female (H&E) (Provided by Professor Lorenzen, Dortmund)

Modern surgical therapy of breast cancer aims for breast conserving local tumor resection. However, according to an analysis of two-pooled European studies, premenopausal patients tend to have a higher risk of local recurrence after breast conserving resection than postmenopausal patients. In addition, extensive intraductal growth was also associated with increased risk of local recurrence after breast conserving surgery. Thus, resection of ductal carcinoma in situ should aim for a security margin of at least 2 mm, even if adjuvant radiotherapy is planned. The risk of local recurrence did not correlate with age if mastectomy was performed. Nevertheless, conservative surgery does not show an adverse effect on survival (Voogd et al. 2001). In case of carcinoma in situ, axillary dissection is not required. In contrast, axillary lymph node staging is mandatory part of any surgical therapy of invasive breast cancer. This includes biopsy of the sentinel node as well of any suspicious nodes. Adjuvant treatment includes radiotherapy, chemotherapy, and endocrinologic and targeted therapy.

A study focusing on patients younger than 21 years reported more frequent undifferentiated histology and a higher proportion of positive lymph nodes, however, no significant differences in overall survival compared to older adults (Richards et al. 2017). The risk of distant recurrence correlates with age < 35 years, increasing tumor size, low histologic differentiation, vascular invasion, resection margins, and nodal status (Voogd et al. 2001). Based on these and comparable data from other study groups, risk groups for treatment stratification have been defined during the St. Gallen consensus conferences on early breast cancer (Goldhirsch et al. 2007, 2009). Considering the high risk of recurrence even in stage I, almost all patients younger than 35 years are eligible for adjuvant therapy—even despite the risk of long-term sequelae such as early menopause, impaired fertility, osteoporosis, and secondary cancers.

Radiotherapy serves to reduce the risk of locoregional recurrences, including lymph node metastases, and is mostly indicated after breast conserving therapy. The mode of adjuvant systemic treatment depends on the immunohistochemical and molecular profile of the tumor. In estrogen-receptor-negative tumors, chemotherapy, most commonly including an anthracycline and a taxane, is administered. In receptor-positive tumors, tamoxifen (+/− chemotherapy) significantly reduces the risk of relapse. New perspectives have been opened by the introduction of epidermal growth factor receptor antibodies (e.g., trastuzumab, Herceptin®) that target tumors with *HER2* overexpression, caused by *HER2* amplification. Bone targeted treatment (e.g., bisphosphonates or denosumab) shall help to reduce cancer treatment induced bone loss, improve bone metastases-free survival, and in case of bone metastases prevent skeletal-related events.

33.4 Management of Breast Cancer in Children and Adolescents

The clinical picture of breast cancer in children and adolescents differs from that in adults (Richards et al. 2017; Westfal et al. 2019). Carcinoma in situ is exceedingly rare, while the most common type in childhood is the "secretory carcinoma." In the SEER data, females less than 19 years of age had 15% carcinoma in situ, 55% carcinomas, and 45% sarcomas (Gutierrez et al. 2008). Most of the sarcomas were phyllodes tumors (syn. Cystosarcoma phyllodes). The choice of FNA or biopsy should be carefully considered in these young patients, since even FNA may sometimes result in cosmetic damage to the developing breast (Greydanus et al. 2006). Most phyllodes tumors in children and adolescents (provided the small data of patients reported to date) are characterized by indolent clinical behavior, even if they present with considerable size, a low tendency to develop distant metastases, and hence, they have a more favorable prognosis in respect to survival.

If true invasive ductal carcinoma is diagnosed, prognosis is more unfavorable, since these tumors may often show poor histologic differentiation, high proliferative activity, and a tendency to lymphovascular invasion. In large historic studies, young age (i.e., younger than 35 years) is an independent adverse prognostic factor (de la Rochefordiere et al. 1993). In a more recent study that included patients up to the age of 21 years, 21.6% of patients presented with stage III/IV disease, compared to 14.9% in patients older than 21 years (Richards et al. 2017). Perhaps, this may be explained by the lack of self-examination in this age group. In some studies, overall survival has been reported to be poorer than in older patients (de la Rochefordiere et al. 1993); in other studies, survival was comparable for pediatric cohorts compared to adults; however, children were treated more aggressively than adult patients (Richards et al. 2017). Of note, breast cancer in young patients may show different immunohistochemical and genetic profiles compared to older patients—however, given the little pediatric cohorts that have been studied so far, data are in part conflicting. Tumors in younger patients are more often estrogen receptor-negative, grade 3, while the frequency of *HER2* overexpression appears to be comparable. However, even in case of positive receptor status, response to treatment and prognosis in young patients may be worse than in older patients (>35 years) (Colleoni et al. 2006).

Therefore, therapy of breast carcinoma includes wide excision and assessment of axillary lymph nodes, as discussed above. In young patients, prognosis in stage I breast cancer is not satisfactory. If young patients are treated according to a "watch-and-wait" strategy, half of patients show tumor progression. Therefore, adjuvant treatment should be considered for almost all patients under the age of 35 years (Goldhirsch et al. 2007); see also current guidelines of ASCO or ESMO.

Therapeutic decisions regarding hormonal, targeted, and cytostatic treatment should be made after interdisciplinary consultation and under consideration of the pathologic stage, immunohistochemical, and genetic profile of the tumor. Anthracycline-based combination regimens, often in combination with cyclophosphamide, currently constitute the most commonly applied chemotherapy regimen. Since the 1990s of the last century, taxane-based regimens have also been evaluated and have also proven effective (e.g., combination of anthracycline, cyclophosphamide, and taxan) (Bria et al. 2006). They are currently considered standard therapy for nodal positive breast cancer. Endocrinologic treatment typically utilizes tamoxifen. The introduction of the *HER*2 inhibitor trastuzumab constitutes one of the most significant therapeutic progress in the last decade. Since the St. Gallen conference in 2009, trastuzumab in combination with chemotherapy is recommended for HER2 positive tumors larger than 1 cm (Goldhirsch et al. 2009). Of note, patient selection and stratification of trastuzumab have continuously been evaluated and slightly modified. Optimal results have been obtained so far, if trastuzumab has been applied in combination with anthracyclines, cyclophosphamide, and taxan and if administration of trastuzumab was concurrent to taxan. Last, bone targeted therapy constitutes an important adjuvant and supportive therapeutic concept.

Since the field of cytostatic, endocrinologic, and targeted treatment of breast cancer is rapidly developing, it is recommended that the therapy of children and adolescents be planned and performed by a multidisciplinary team, including a gynecooncologic breast surgeon, gynecooncologist, radiotherapist, medical oncologist, and pediatric oncologist. Currently, using such an interdisciplinary approach, a 5-year survival rate greater than 70% can be expected for adolescents and young adults with stage I/II breast cancer, while 5-year survival drops to approx. 20% for stage IV tumors (Richards et al. 2017).

References

American Society of Clinical Oncology (ASCO) (1998) 1997 update of recommendations for the use of tumor markers in breast and colorectal cancer. Adopted on November 7, 1997 by the American Society of Clinical Oncology. J Clin Oncol 16:793–795

Antoniou A, Pharoah PD, Narod S, Risch HA, Eyfjord JE, Hopper JL, Loman N, Olsson H, Johannsson O, Borg A, Pasini B, Radice P, Manoukian S, Eccles DM, Tang N, Olah E, Anton-Culver H, Warner E, Lubinski J, Gronwald J, Gorski B, Tulinius H, Thorlacius S, Eerola H, Nevanlinna H, Syrjakoski K, Kallioniemi OP, Thompson D, Evans C, Peto J, Lalloo F, Evans DG, Easton DF (2003) Average risks of breast and ovarian cancer associated with BRCA1 or BRCA2 mutations detected in case Series unselected for family history: a combined analysis of 22 studies. Am J Hum Genet 72:1117–1130

Ashley S, Royle GT, Corder A, Herbert A, Guyer PB, Rubin CM, Taylor I (1989) Clinical, radiological and cytological diagnosis of breast cancer in young women. Br J Surg 76:835–837

Bongiorno MR, Doukaki S, Arico M (2010) Neurofibromatosis of the nipple-areolar area: a case series. J Med Case Rep 4:22

Brand IR, Sapherson DA, Brown TS (1993) Breast imaging in women under 35 with symptomatic breast disease. Br J Radiol 66:394–397

Bria E, Nistico C, Cuppone F, Carlini P, Ciccarese M, Milella M, Natoli G, Terzoli E, Cognetti F, Giannarelli D (2006) Benefit of taxanes as adjuvant chemotherapy for early breast cancer: pooled analysis of 15,500 patients. Cancer 106:2337–2344

Carty NJ, Carter C, Rubin C, Ravichandran D, Royle GT, Taylor I (1995) Management of fibroadenoma of the breast. Ann R Coll Surg Engl 77:127–130

Chateil JF, Arboucalot F, Perel Y, Brun M, Boisserie-Lacroix M, Diard F (1998) Breast metastases in adolescent girls: US findings. Pediatr Radiol 28:832–835

Chen WH, Cheng SP, Tzen CY, Yang TL, Jeng KS, Liu CL, Liu TP (2005) Surgical treatment of phyllodes tumors of the breast: retrospective review of 172 cases. J Surg Oncol 91:185–194

Chung EM, Cube R, Hall GJ, Gonzalez C, Stocker JT, Glassman LM (2009) From the archives of the AFIP: breast masses in children and adolescents: radiologic-pathologic correlation. Radiographics 29:907–931

Colleoni M, Rotmensz N, Peruzzotti G, Maisonneuve P, Orlando L, Ghisini R, Viale G, Pruneri G, Veronesi P, Luini A, Intra M, Cardillo A, Torrisi R, Rocca A, Goldhirsch A (2006) Role of endocrine responsiveness and adjuvant therapy in very young women (below 35 years) with operable breast cancer and node negative disease. Ann Oncol 17:1497–1503

Conter V, D'Angelo P, Rovelli A, Uderzo C, Jankovic M, Bratina G, Masera G (1992) Isolated breast relapse after allogeneic bone marrow transplantation for childhood acute lymphoblastic leukemia. Med Pediatr Oncol 20:165–168

de la Rochefordiere A, Asselain B, Campana F, Scholl SM, Fenton J, Vilcoq JR, Durand JC, Pouillart P, Magdelenat H, Fourquet A (1993) Age as prognostic factor in premenopausal breast carcinoma. Lancet 341:1039–1043

Doğan G, Soyer T, Ekinci S, Karnak İ, Çiftçi AÖ, Tanyel FC (2017) Evaluation of surgically treated breast masses in children. Turk J Pediatr 59:177–183

Gao Y, Saksena MA, Brachtel EF, terMeulen DC, Rafferty EA (2015) How to approach breast lesions in children and adolescents. Eur J Radiol 84:1350–1364

Goldhirsch A, Wood WC, Gelber RD, Coates AS, Thurlimann B, Senn HJ (2007) Progress and promise: highlights of the international expert consensus on the primary therapy of early breast cancer 2007. Ann Oncol 18:1133–1144

Goldhirsch A, Ingle JN, Gelber RD, Coates AS, Thurlimann B, Senn HJ (2009) Thresholds for therapies: highlights of the St Gallen International Expert Consensus on the primary therapy of early breast cancer 2009. Ann Oncol 20:1319–1329

Greydanus DE, Matytsina L, Gains M (2006) Breast disorders in children and adolescents. Prim Care 33:455–502

Gutierrez JC, Housri N, Koniaris LG, Fischer AC, Sola JE (2008) Malignant breast cancer in children: a review of 75 patients. J Surg Res 147:182–188

Henderson TO, Amsterdam A, Bhatia S, Hudson MM, Meadows AT, Neglia JP, Diller LR, Constine LS, Smith RA, Mahoney MC, Morris EA, Montgomery LL, Landier W, Smith SM, Robison LL, Oeffinger KC (2010) Systematic review: surveillance for breast cancer in women treated with chest radiation for childhood, adolescent, or young adult cancer. Ann Intern Med 152(444–455):W144–W154

Moskowitz CS, Chou JF, Wolden SL, Bernstein JL, Malhotra J, Novetsky Friedman D, Mubdi NZ, Leisenring WM, Stovall M, Hammond S, Smith SA, Henderson TO, Boice JD, Hudson MM, Diller LR, Bhatia S, Kenney LB, Neglia JP, Begg CB, Robison LL, Oeffinger KC (2014) Breast cancer after chest radiation therapy for childhood cancer. J Clin Oncol 32:2217–2223

Nagar H, Marmor S, Hammar B (1992) Haemangiomas of the breast in children. Eur J Surg 158:503–505

Neinstein LS, Atkinson J, Diament M (1993) Prevalence and longitudinal study of breast masses in adolescents. J Adolesc Health 14:277–281

Richards MK, Goldin AB, Beierle EA, Doski JJ, Goldfarb M, Langer M, Nuchtern JG, Vasudevan S, Gow KW, Javid SH (2017) Breast malignancies in children: presentation, management, and survival. Ann Surg Oncol 24:1482–1491

Rosenfield RL, Lipton RB, Drum ML (2009) Thelarche, pubarche, and menarche attainment in children with normal and elevated body mass index. Pediatrics 123:84–88

Schellong G, Riepenhausen M, Ehlert K, Brämswig J, Dörffel W, German WGOTL-TSOHD, Schmutzler RK, Rhiem K, Bick U, German CFHBAOC (2014) Breast cancer in young women after treatment for Hodgkin's disease during childhood or adolescence—an observational study with up to 33-year follow-up. Dtsch Arztebl Int 111:3–9

Simmons PS (1992) Diagnostic considerations in breast disorders of children and adolescents. Obstet Gynecol Clin N Am 19:91–102

Stricker T, Navratil F, Sennhauser FH (2005) Mastitis in early infancy. Acta Paediatr 94:166–169

Tea MK, Asseryanis E, Kroiss R, Kubista E, Wagner T (2009) Surgical breast lesions in adolescent females. Pediatr Surg Int 25:73–75

Templeman C, Hertweck SP (2000) Breast disorders in the pediatric and adolescent patient. Obstet Gynecol Clin N Am 27:19–34

Voogd AC, Nielsen M, Peterse JL, Blichert-Toft M, Bartelink H, Overgaard M, van Tienhoven G, Andersen KW, Sylvester RJ, van Dongen JA (2001) Differences in risk factors for local and distant recurrence after breast-conserving therapy or mastectomy for stage I and II breast cancer: pooled results of two large European randomized trials. J Clin Oncol 19:1688–1697

Welch ST, Babcock DS, Ballard ET (2004) Sonography of pediatric male breast masses: gynecomastia and beyond. Pediatr Radiol 34:952–957

Westfal ML, Chang DC, Kelleher CM (2019) A population-based analysis of pediatric breast cancer. J Pediatr Surg 54:140–144

Zmora O, Klin B, Iacob C, Meital A, Mendlovic S, Karni T (2020) Characterizing excised breast masses in children and adolescents-Can a more aggressive pathology be predicted. J Pediatr Surg 55:2197–2200

Part VIII

Rhabdoid Tumors

Extracranial Rhabdoid Tumours

34

Michael C. Frühwald, Franck Bourdeaut, and Rhoikos Furtwängler

34.1 Introduction

Malignant rhabdoid tumours (MRT) are rare, highly aggressive malignancies at high risk of taking a dismal clinical course. As an entity morphologically distinct from Wilms tumours, MRT were first described by Beckwith and Palmer in 1978 (Beckwith and Palmer 1978). Later in 1981 Haas and Palmer characterized a series of 11 kidney tumours by a particular histological appearance as an individual anatomic identity, which they termed rhabdoid (Haas et al. 1981). Subsequently Rorke et al. defined the CNS tumour entity atypical teratoid/rhabdoid tumour (ATRT) in a series of 52 consecutive cases (Rorke et al. 1996). In 2006 Oda reviewed a series of atypical sarcomas and termed them extracranial, extrarenal malignant rhabdoid tumours (eMRT). Unifying feature of all entities regardless of anatomical origin are rhabdoid cells thus designated due to a resemblance to rhabdomyoblasts (Biegel et al. 1990; Judkins et al. 2004). However, a distinct histologic variability may be misleading. Only following introduction of INI1 immunohistochemistry may the diagnosis be made more reliable (Vujanic et al. 2018). By convention the intracranial manifestation of RT has been labelled ATRT (atypical teratoid rhabdoid tumour), originating from the kidney as (M)RTK (malignant rhabdoid tumour of the kidney) and extracranial, extrarenal as eMRT (extracranial malignant rhabdoid tumours) (Fig. 34.1). The most common location of MRT is the central nervous system (65%) followed by the kidneys (~10%) and other various soft tissues (~25%) (e.g., head and neck, liver, thorax, retroperitoneum, pelvis, heart; Fig. 34.2; German Childhood Cancer Registry 2018 http://www.kinderkrebsregister.de last accessed 2019_06_20 or (Dho et al. 2015; Uwineza et al. 2014)).

34.2 Epidemiology

In the UK and in Germany the age standardized annual incidence rate of extracranial rhabdoid tumours is 5–5.7 per million in the first year of life and decreases with age to 0.6–0.7 per million at age 1–4 years and eventually to 0.1–0.2 at 5 years (see http://www.kinderkrebsregister.de/dkkr/ergebnisse/jahresberichte/jahresbericht-2017.html and (Brennan et al. 2013)).

M. C. Frühwald (✉)
Swabian Children's Cancer Center, University Hospital Augsburg, Augsburg, Bavaria, Germany
e-mail: michael.fruehwald@uk-augsburg.de

F. Bourdeaut
PSL Research University, Pediatric Care and Research Center, Institute Curie, Paris, France

R. Furtwängler
Department of Pediatric Oncology and Hematology, Saarland University of Hospital Saarland, Homburg, Saarland, Germany

D. T. Schneider et al. (eds.), *Rare Tumors in Children and Adolescents*, Pediatric Oncology,
https://doi.org/10.1007/978-3-030-92071-5_34

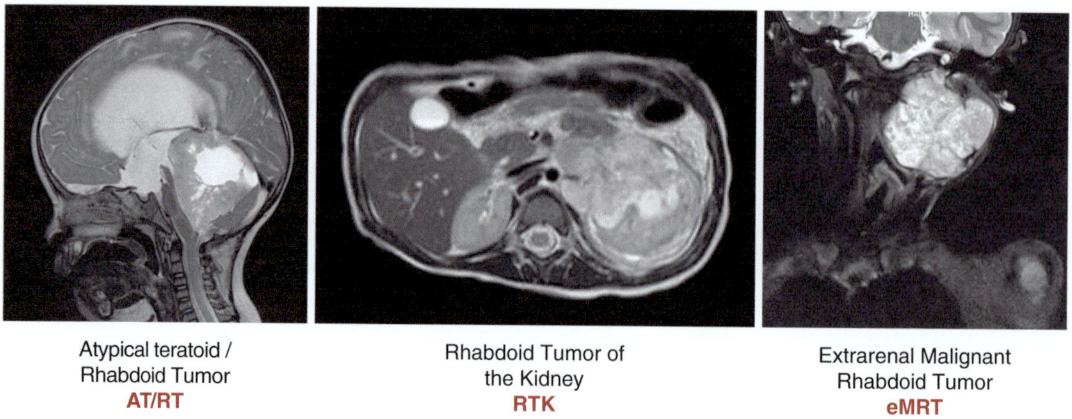

Fig. 34.1 Proposed nomenclature of malignant rhabdoid tumours (MRT). Depicted are three representative MRI of patients with MRT. As a group the term MRT applies while tumours of the CNS are labelled ATRT, those in the kidneys RTK (rhabdoid tumours of the kidneys) and those of extracranial, extrarenal sites as eMRT

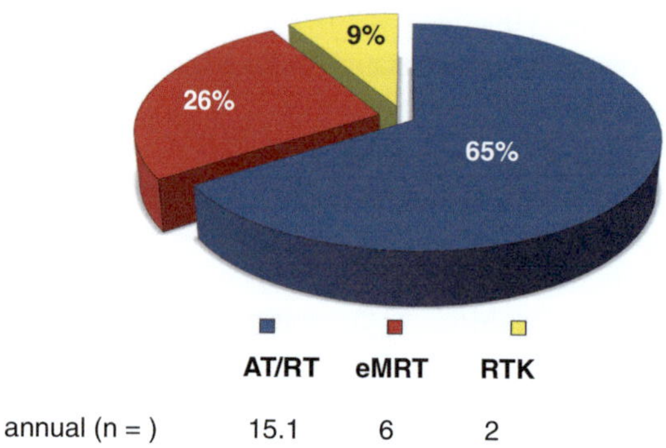

Fig. 34.2 Distribution of rhabdoid tumours according to the anatomic region of origin. A total of 65% of all MRT are derived from the CNS and thus termed ATRT, up to 26% from extracranial, extrarenal sites (eMRT) and up to 9% from renal sites (RTK). Data from the population-based German Childhood Cancer Registry (German Childhood Cancer Registry 2018 http://www.kinderkrebsregister.de last accessed 2019_08_10)

In the USA the annual incidence of eMRT among children less than 15 years is 0.32 per million and 0.19 per million for RTK (Heck et al. 2013). Of the first 4000 patients enrolled on the trial AREN03B2, extracranial rhabdoid tumours (RTK and eMRT) accounted for 3.71% (Geller 2016). RTK and eMRT accounted for 1.6% and 2.5%, respectively, among childhood tumours in the UK between 2003 and 2012 (http://www.ncin.org.uk/view?rid=329).

34.3 Age and Gender

Malignant rhabdoid tumours predominantly but not exclusively arise in infants and young children below the age of 3 years. Depending on the series at hand, patients with MRT demonstrate median ages at diagnosis in the range of 10–33 months (Reinhard et al. 2008; Morgenstern et al. 2010). In the group of extracranial RT registered to the EpSSG, the median age was 1.4 years (3 days to 10.9 years) (Brennan et al. 2016). A total of 10/100 patients had tumours of the kidney (RTK). Among 384 patients (ATRT = 244, RTK = 34, eMRT = 89 and synchronous tumours = 17) registered to the European Rhabdoid Registry (EU-RHAB), median ages were as follows:

ATRT: 18 (0–211) months
eMRT: 13.5 (0–207) months
RTK: 13 (2–166) months
Synch: 3 (0–23) months

All series report a male predominance with 1.3–1.5 male: 1 female.

34.4 Location

Over the last 25 years, MRT have been described in almost any anatomic location. In their cohort of 100 MRT, Brennan et al. identi-

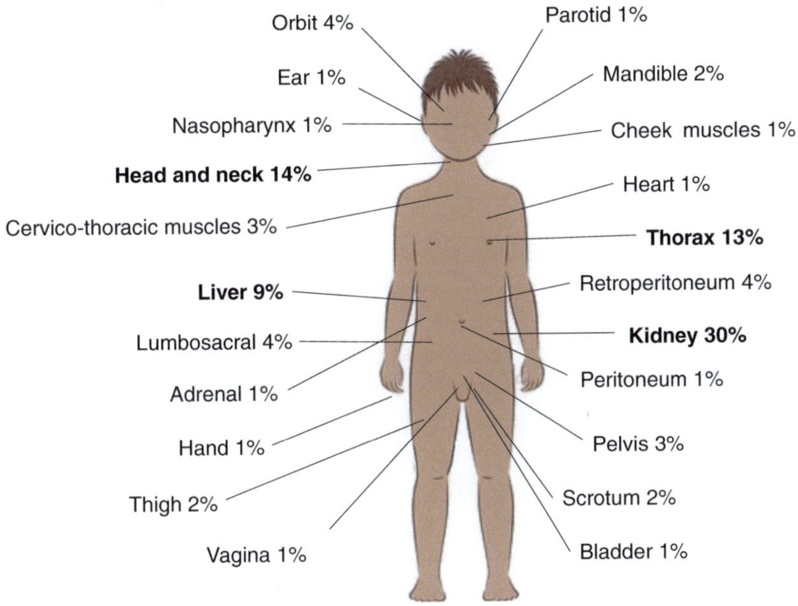

Fig. 34.3 Organ of origin in 100 cases of eMRT registered within the EU-RHAB registry

fied the kidneys, liver (17 and 15%, respectively), head and neck (12%) and paraspinal (14%) location as most frequently affected (Brennan et al. 2016). In the series of the EU-RHAB registry, kidney (30%), head and neck (14%), thorax (13%) and liver (9%) locations predominated (Fig. 34.3). Since none of the trials were epidemiologically representative and both ran simultaneously with overlapping recruiting areas, it is likely that the respective frequencies were biased by selection of the local treating institution.

Rhabdoid tumours may occur syn- or metachronous in two or more locations (Benesch et al. 2014; Szymanski et al. 2013; Pohl et al. 2010; Giunti et al. 2006; Litman et al. 1993). In most instances one of the synchronous anatomic locations is the CNS. This may not be mistaken for metastatic disease, which in most series ranges from 23 to 50% (Reinhard et al. 2008; Brennan et al. 2016; Madigan et al. 2007; Bourdeaut et al. 2008; Furtwangler et al. 2018). In certain risk groups such as patients diagnosed perinatal (congenital MRT) or patients with germline mutations, the rate of metastases may be as high as 50% (Nemes et al. 2018).

34.5 Signs and Symptoms

Presenting symptoms of MRT depend on location of the primary and metastatic sites. Rather limited data has been published on this subject. In a single-institution experience of 14 patients collected over a 20-year span, Madigan et al. describe a visible or palpable mass, fever, back pain or signs of spinal compression as most common (Madigan et al. 2007). Interestingly signs of marrow stress (haemoglobin <11 g/dL, thrombocytosis >450,000/mm^3) and an elevated LDH (>1000 U/L) were commonly noted. A large series of case reports demonstrates that patients may present with a range of symptoms from subtle to life-threatening (Tang et al. 2015; Kelly et al. 1998). When comparing symptoms at presentation in children with Wilms tumours or RTK (*n* = 50), Amar et al. detected a significantly higher rate of gross or microscopic haematuria (59 vs. 18%), fever (44 vs. 22%) and hypercalcaemia (26% of RTK) in RTK. This was mainly due to a higher stage at diagnosis for RTK (75% of RTK stage III or higher) and also to a higher incidence of metastatic disease (27.1% bone, 8.3% each brain and liver) (Amar et al. 2001). In the series of the EU-RHAB Registry metastases to the bone affected less than 5% of patients. Due to the aggressive biology of MRT, the duration of presenting symptoms is expected to be rather short as has been described by Lafay-Cousin and colleagues (median of 3 weeks) for ATRT (Lafay-Cousin et al. 2012).

34.6 Pathology

Rhabdoid tumours of childhood are prototypes of a group of cancers characterized by the loss of the gene *SMARCB1* (Agaimy 2019) or rarely *SMARCA4* (Schneppenheim et al. 2010). Extra- and intracranial rhabdoid tumours are indistinguishable by morphologic or phenotypic features alone. Distinguishing synchronous rhabdoid tumours from metastatic disease in the context of a germline mutation may be close to impossible.

On histology rhabdoid cells are characterized by heaps of cells with a large eccentric nucleus and prominent eosinophilic nucleoli, abundant eosinophilic cytoplasm with large oval hyaline inclusion bodies and distinct cellular membranes. These features might only be focal and should be specifically looked for in case of an undifferentiated childhood tumour of the kidney or soft tissue. By immunohistochemistry, rhabdoid tumour cells are characterized by expression of vimentin (a rather non-specific marker), EMA (epithelial membrane antigen) and cytokeratins, less commonly by SMA (smooth muscle actin). The combined presence of EMA and SMA in the tumour of a newborn, an infant or very young child is fairly suspicious of MRT (Judkins et al. 2005).

The defining immunohistochemical feature of MRT is the absence of SMARCB1 (INI1, BAF47) staining in tumour cells (Fig. 34.4) (Judkins et al. 2005; Winger et al. 2006; Judkins 2007). Thus, other immunohistochemistry than INI1 is not needed to confirm the diagnosis. Differential diagnosis in children older than 5 years include medullary renal cell carcinoma, which however is usually linked to a sickle cell trait, undifferentiated chordoma in vertebral and paravertebral sites and epithelioid sarcoma (Agaimy 2014; Hasselblatt et al. 2016) (Table 34.1). Loss of genetic material from chromosome 22q11 has been demonstrated by molecular genetic analyses, fluorescence in situ hybridization (FISH) and loss of heterozygosity studies (Biegel et al. 1996; Rickert and Paulus 2004). Versteege et al. isolated the gene *SMARCB1 (hSNF5/INI1)* from chromosome 22q11.2 by positional cloning. The gene fulfils the criteria of a tumour suppressor gene. Mutations of *SMARCB1* were detected in 51 of 76 RTK and in 25 of 29 extrarenal rhabdoid tumours (ATRT and eMRT) (Biegel 2006). Some authors claim that rhabdoid tumours of the CNS (ATRT) are characterized by a predominance of

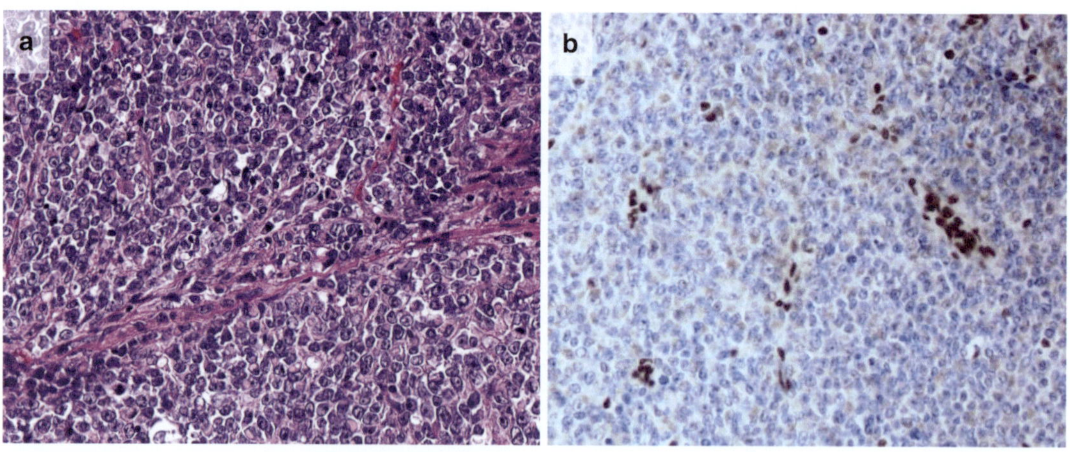

Fig. 34.4 Immunohistochemistry of rhabdoid tumours. (**a**) H&E staining demonstrating typical rhabdoid tumours with abundant cytoplasm and prominent nuclei. (**b**) INI1 staining of an eMRT. While tumour cells are negative (absence of the tumour suppressor SMARCB1/INI1), endothelial cells of blood vessels stain positive

Table 34.1 Differential diagnoses of eMRT

Entity	Site	Imaging	Typical age	Distant metastasis	INI1-IHC	Other
Rhabdoid tumour	Kidney, liver, soft tissue	Extensively infiltrating growth, lymph nodes often involved (kidney)	3–18 months (median 10–11 months)	50% at diagnosis	Negative (with the exception of mutated in SMARCA4)	Multifocal and synchronous including CNS possible
Renal tumours						
Nephroblastoma	Kidney	Unspecific, usually pseudocapsule	1.5–4 years	10–20% (older age > 3 years)— -usually lung metastases, rarely liver and other sites	Retained	Blastemal type and diffuse anaplasia
Clear cell sarcoma of the kidney (CCSK)	Kidney	Unspecific. Poor response to preoperative treatment	2–4 years	Possible—lungs and frequently bones	Retained	BCOR internal tandem duplication or rarely YWHAE-NUTM2 (t(10;17)(q22;p13))
Medullary renal cell carcinoma	Kidney	Usually locally progressed	Second and third decade	Possible	Negative	HbS
Anaplastic sarcoma of the kidney	Kidney	Unspecific, but often cystic	2–15 years	N.d. Pleuropulmonary blastomas possible	No data—should be retained	DICER1 (possibly germline), frequently TP53 mutation
Mesoblastic nephroma	Kidney	Finger-shaped infiltration of adjacent structures, rarely pseudocapsule, no lymph node involvement	<6 months typically within the first 2 months of life Antenatal diagnosis possible Median 18 days	No distant metastasis	Retained	MN cellular subtype, frequently NTRK3-ETV6 translocation
Soft-part tumours						
Rhabdomyosarcoma	Soft tissue	Predominantly head and neck and/or genito-urinary-tract location	2–4 years	10–20%, lungs, bones	Retained	Alveolar: PAX3/7-FOXO1
Infantile fibrosarcoma	Soft tissue	Predominantly limbs	<6 months, median 44 days. Not older than 1 year. Prenatal diagnosis possible	No distant metastasis	Retained	NTRK3–ETV6 translocation
Epithelioid sarcoma	Soft tissue	Typically superficial distal location. 10% lymph node metastases	Rare in children. Second and third decade of life	Rarely (<10%)	Negative	Typically hands, fingers, distal extremities

(continued)

Table 34.1 (continued)

Entity	Site	Imaging	Typical age	Distant metastasis	INI1-IHC	Other
Synovial sarcoma	Soft tissue	Predominantly extremities	13–15 years	Rarely	Possibly negative (>20%)	SYT-SSX1/2/4
Chordoma	Axial spine/clivus	Usually involving or adjacent to clivus	>10 years (typically >30)	Rarely lungs and bones	Negative	Usually poorly differentiated type
Hepatic tumours						
Hepatoblastoma	Liver	Large tumours	80% < 3 years	Lungs and CNS	Retained	WNT mutation
Hepatoblastoma, small cell undifferentiated	Liver	Large tumours	Mainly newborns and infants	Lungs and CNS	Possibly negative	No distinct entity but likely eMRT (Vokuhl et al. 2016)
Peripheral nerves						
Vestibular schwannomas	VIIIth cranial nerve	Typical anatomic region	>10 years		Retained	NF2
Malignant peripheral nerve sheet tumour (MNPST)	Soft tissue	Close proximity to peripheral nerves, <10% lymph node involvement	>10 years (second–fifth decade)	<10%	Possibly negative (>50%)	S100 positive, NF1 (20%)
eMPNST (epithelioid MPNST)	Peripheral nerve	Mostly lower limbs	5–73 years	Up to 50%	Possibly negative	NF1

mutations in exons 5 and 9. Newer reports contradict this view and show a broad mutational spectrum of *SMARCB1* across tumours from different anatomical locations (Kordes et al. 2010).

The identification of *SMARCB1* and *SMARCA4* mutations as a hallmark of MRT has also led to the reclassification of entities such as small cell undifferentiated variant of haepatoblastoma and small cell carcinoma of the ovary hypercalcaemic type (SCCOHT) (Vokuhl et al. 2016; Trobaugh-Lotrario et al. 2009). While some authors claim that these are variants of the entity of rhabdoid tumours, others favour the term SMARCB1 deficient soft tissue neoplasm with rhabdoid/epithelioid morphology (Agaimy 2019; Vokuhl et al. 2016; Witkowski et al. 2016).

34.7 Molecular Genetics

34.7.1 The SWI/SNF Complex in Rhabdoid Tumours

All rhabdoid tumours share mutations of epigenetic regulators, i.e. the core protein of the chromatin remodelling complex SWI/SNF, SMARCB1. The SWI/SNF complex plays an important role in the regulation of critical cellular processes such as cell cycle progression, programmed cell death, differentiation, gene transcription and DNA-repair (Biegel et al. 2014; Helming et al. 2014; Kadoch and Crabtree 2015; St Pierre and Kadoch 2017). Murine knockout models of *SMARCB1* demonstrated embryonic lethality in homozygous deleted animals and a predisposition to aggressive tumours including those with a classic rhabdoid phenotype (Roberts et al. 2000, 2002; Klochendler-Yeivin et al. 2000; Guidi et al. 2001; Tsikitis et al. 2005), consistent with its role as a tumour suppressor gene in heterozygous animals. Interestingly mice with a conditional biallelic inactivation of *SMARCB1* employing a Mx1-Cre transgene construct develop tumours very rapidly (median of 11 weeks, compared to *TP53* with 20 weeks) (Roberts et al. 2002). Recently Han et al. developed a mouse model of AT/RT, which provided conditional inactivation of *Smarcb1* using the Rosa26Cre^{ERT2} system. *Smarcb1* inactivation in adult mice led to T-cell lymphomas, while neonatal inactivation led to hepatic disorders; by contrast, inactivation of *Smarcb1* between E6 and E10 induced aggressive tumours, mainly in the CNS but also in soft parts, resembling human MRT, with a full penetrance and within a short time frame (median 2.5 months) (Han et al. 2016).

On average malignant tumours in children display fewer mutations than in adults. Notable extremes are on one end of the spectrum, melanomas and lung cancer ($\leq$ 200 non-synonymous mutations per tumour), and on the other, rhabdoid tumours, which exhibit far fewer point mutations (Vogelstein et al. 2013). Employing SNP-based oligonucleotide arrays, multiplex ligation-dependent probe amplification (MLPA), FISH and sequence analysis, biallelic alterations of *SMARCB1* located in chromosome 22q11.2 were detected in 50 of 51 rhabdoid tumours (Rickert and Paulus 2004). *SMARCB1* inactivation was due to deletions, SNVs and loss of heterozygosity (LOH) making it the single most important recurrent potentially driving mutation in ATRT and other rhabdoid tumours (Jackson et al. 2009). By molecular inversion probe single-nucleotide polymorphism (MIP SNP) assay, whole exome sequencing and OncoMap, a mass spectrometric method for allele detection, the absence of recurrent genomic alterations other than in *SMARCB1* was determined in a combined number of 76 ATRT (Hasselblatt et al. 2013; Lee et al. 2012; Kieran et al. 2012); on exome sequencing of a series of eMRT, Chun et al. also reported absence of recurrent genomic alterations other than in SMARCB1 (Chun et al. 2016).

The report of a family with hereditary rhabdoid tumours but no detectable mutation in *SMARCB1* suggested the presence of a second genomic locus distinct from *SMARCB1* (Fruhwald et al. 2006). Subsequent reports and candidate gene analyses led to the discovery of *SMARCA4* as a tumour suppressor in MRT (Schneppenheim et al. 2010; Hasselblatt et al. 2014). Genetically engineered homozygous mice with knockout of *SMARCA4* are lethal at an embryonal stage (Bultman et al. 2000).

Table 34.2 Hereditary syndromes associated with mutations in the SWI/SNF associated genes *SMARCB1* and *SMARCA4*

Syndrome	SWI/SNF gene	GLM frequency	OMIM # phenotype *genotype	Associated histology
RTPS 1	*SMARCB1*	~30%	#609322 *601607	MRT incl. ATRT, eMRT, RTK, eMPNST (Rekhi et al. 2017)
RTPS 2	*SMARCA4*	~40%	#613325 *603245	MRT and SCCOHT, potentially infantile pulmonary teratoid tumour (de Kock et al. 2018)
Familial schwannomatosis	*SMARCB1*	~10%	#162091 *601607	Overrepresentation of neuroblastoma-like variants; rarely with MRT
Multiple familial spinal meningiomas	*SMARCE1*	Likely major	#607174 *603111	Clear cell meningiomas
Hereditary RCC	*PBRM1*	No data	#144700 *606083	Clear cell renal cell carcinoma
SWI/SNF related meningiomas	*SMARCB1*	~5%	#607174 *601607	No distinctive histology

Heterozygous mice do not develop rhabdoid tumours but instead develop gynaecologic and pulmonary neoplasms (Bultman et al. 2008). Whether *SMARCB1* and *SMARCA4* constitute the only mutated members of the chromatin machinery in rhabdoid tumours and which other associated factors are needed for a penetrant phenotype warrants further investigation. Table 34.2 offers a list of tumour syndromes caused by mutation of genes within the SWI/SNF complex.

34.7.2 Molecular Subgroups of Extracranial Rhabdoid Tumours

As mutations of genes other than *SMARCB1/SMARCA4* are exceedingly rare in ATRT scanning, approaches have been employed to detect further genomic, epigenomic and transcriptional changes.

DNA methylation and gene expression analyses (Han et al. 2016; Chun et al. 2016; Johann et al. 2016; Torchia et al. 2016) have recently demonstrated the presence of at least three epigenetically distinct ATRT subgroups (ATRT-TYR, -MYC and -SHH) with distinguishing features such as anatomic site within the CNS, age, lineage-enriched methylation, transcriptional signatures and *SMARCB1*-specific genotypes (Torchia et al. 2016). Similar analyses for extracranial RT are limited to rather few studies.

Birks et al. analysed the microarray expression profiles of 42 ATRT and 10 RTK and compared them to other entities affecting the CNS and kidneys (Birks et al. 2013). On unsupervised hierarchical clustering three major subsets clearly separating ATRT and RTK were identified. A total of only 14 genes were dysregulated across all subtypes while thousands of differentially expressed genes indicated that factors apart from SMARCB1 contribute to pathogenesis in MRT.

Chun et al. constructed a genomic reference landscape for extracranial rhabdoid tumours employing whole genome, miRNA-Seq, RNA-Seq, DNA-Methylation and ChIP-Seq Analyses (Chun et al. 2016). Especially miRNA-Seq differentiated extracranial RT into two subgroups. One clustered with sarcomas such as synovial sarcomas also affected by SMARCB1 dysregulation. The other (larger) subgroup demonstrated overlap with pheochromocytomas and normal cerebella indicating a neural crest origin. DNA-methylation analyses confirmed the presence of at least two subgroups. It appears that extracranial RT most commonly share features of the ATRT-MYC DNA-methylation subclass (Kool M. personal communication).

Pinto et al. analysed intra- and extracranial MRT often including synchronous lesions (Pinto et al. 2018). They demonstrated a significant different pattern of genome-wide DNA methylation and/or copy number alterations among intra- and extracranial tumours of the same patient suggestive of non-clonal origin.

Thus, the clinical and molecular characteristics of extracranial MRT are heterogeneous calling for further comprehensive genetic analyses and a correlation with clinical data sets.

34.8 Genetic Predisposition to Rhabdoid Tumours

A genetic predisposition to rhabdoid tumours has to be ruled out in any child with a rhabdoid tumour and/or a family history of a rhabdoid tumour or schwannomatosis and/or synchronous, multifocal *SMARCA4*- or *SMARCB1*-deficient tumours.

Affected children present earlier in life than those with sporadic rhabdoid tumours and often display congenital, synchronous, multifocal lesions (Sredni and Tomita 2015; Nemes et al. 2017). A genetic predisposition to rhabdoid tumours caused by a germline mutation in *SMARCB1* has been termed RTPS 1, while in case of a germline mutation in *SMARCA4* it is called RTPS 2 (rhabdoid tumour predisposition syndrome) (Schneppenheim et al. 2010; Bourdeaut et al. 2011). Germline deletions of *SMARCB1* are always *de novo*, and inherited mutations in *SMARCB1* and pedigrees with transmission across generations are rare. Gonadal mosaicism has also been reported in families with multiple affected siblings and unaffected parents who have a negative screening test using peripheral blood (Hasselblatt et al. 2013). In contrast, germline mutations of *SMARCA4* are inherited from a parent in more than 50% of cases (Schneppenheim et al. 2010; Hasselblatt et al. 2014).

A heterozygous germline mutation or deletion of *SMARCB1* or *SMARCA4* commonly works as a first inactivating event. The second somatic event is characteristically a deletion or loss of heterozygosity, although second somatic mutations have also been documented.

Typical clinical scenarios comprise:

- Prenatal discovery of synchronous MRT.
- Diagnosis before or at birth or within first 28 days of life. Presentation at a median age of 4–7 months (range: prenatally–60 months) compared to sporadic rhabdoid tumours at a median age of 13–30 months (range: age 1 day to 228 months) (Nemes et al. 2017; Bruggers et al. 2011; Geller et al. 2015; Fruhwald et al. 2016).
- Individuals with genetic predisposition have a higher incidence of multiple MRT (Eaton et al. 2011).
- A family history of MRT, cribriform neuroepithelial tumour (CRINET) and/or distinct combinations of MRT with one of the following: schwannoma, malignant peripheral nerve sheath tumour, meningioma or CRINET (van den Munckhof et al. 2012).
- Clinically very aggressive MRT. Tumour progression at the time of follow-up was identified in 91% of individuals. Progression occurred in 58% of individuals while on chemotherapy (Sredni and Tomita 2015).
- A rhabdoid tumour with syndromic features suggestive of 22q11.2 distal deletion syndrome [OMIM 611867].

Prolonged survival has been documented in some patients despite the presence of germline mutations (Seeringer et al. 2014a; Kordes et al. 2014).

Surveillance of affected patients should follow a structured plan which deserves continuous evaluation and adaptation according to increasing knowledge (Table 34.3) (Nemes et al. 2017; Foulkes et al. 2017). Further analyses are needed to base guidelines on larger numbers of affected individuals.

Table 34.3 Suggested screening for patients with predisposition to rhabdoid tumours. Recommendation derived from currently available evidence (Teplick et al. 2011; Foulkes et al. 2017; Nemes et al. 2017)

	Primary site	Screening according to type of germline alteration		
		Predicted inactivating variant		Missense variant[b]
SMARCB1 association	ATRT	**<1 year**	**1–4(5) years**	Very low risk clinical examination every 3–6 months
		Monthly head ultrasound plus every 1–(2–3) months abdominal and pelvic ultrasound[a,c]	Brain, spine and whole body MRI every 3 months	
	Abdomen	**<1 year**	**1–4(–5) years**	Currently insufficient data
		Monthly abdominal, pelvic and head ultrasound, alternatively MRI every 2–3 months[c]	Every 3 months abdominal and pelvic ultrasound; if available whole body MRI incl. CNS	
SMARCA4 association	AT/RT	Currently insufficient data[b]		
	Abdomen	Currently insufficient data		

[a]If ultrasound is not sufficient, consider MRI at least every 2–3 months
[b]One in ten patients with AT/RT had a missense variant
[c]Prefer ultrasound, weigh risk of sedation/anaesthesia for MRT against risk of disease

34.9 Imaging and Other Staging Procedures

Due to the vast array of affected organs and anatomic regions, it appears difficult to identify definitive features on imaging. In a retrospective series of nine patients with extracranial RT aged 1–11 months at diagnosis, imaging features using ultrasound, MRI, CT and bone scan were rather unspecific with non-specific hypointensity on T1 and heterogenous hyperintensity on T2 (Garces-Inigo et al. 2009). In a detailed analysis of 22 RTK, Schenk and colleagues analysed 10 MRI, 15 CT and 14 ultrasound image series (Schenk et al. 2004). Characteristic features were a rather high tumour volume in relation to patient's age (mean of 238 mL), central localization with involvement of the hilus and areas of necrosis (detected in 19 of 22). A lobulated appearance, calcifications and subcapsular fluid were noted in about a quarter of cases. A total of nine cases demonstrated locoregional, 8 pulmonary and 3 CNS metastases. Children younger than 18 months suffering from a kidney tumour with metastasis are very likely to have RTK.

Due to the propensity to metastasize at an early stage and the potentially multifocal initial presentation at any site of the body, whole-body imaging technique including the CNS is indicated such as whole-body MRI as an initial screening tool, followed by focused high resolution MRI.

Functional imaging in extracranial RT has been limited to case reports rather than larger studies or clinical trials. In two cases of recurrent extra-renal, extra-cranial RT, FDG-PET was able to visualize tumour masses (Howman-Giles et al. 2012). However, the limited spatial resolution of FDG-PET-CT combined with high costs in comparison to other modalities makes it a tool for rather specific questions.

Whether PET-MRI or other functional imaging techniques will expand our armamentarium depends on future studies. Factors such as imaging time and radiation exposure always have to be considered in patients who need anaesthesia for prolonged imaging times and who are rather vulnerable due to a developing organism.

Extremity or trunk MRT are usually amenable to cutting-needle- or open biopsy. Also, retroperitoneal RTK can be biopsied using a cutting-needle, without jeopardizing the patient or causing upstaging (Irtan et al. 2015). The access route in eMRT should be discussed in a multidisciplineary panel prior to the procedure. The pathologist should be informed about the suspicion of MRT; thus he can directly include BAF47 IHC in a first panel (Vujanic et al. 2018).

As sampling of tissue for diagnosis may be rather difficult in the youngest and sickest patients, alternative avenues of approach have been tried. Thomson and colleagues demonstrated fine needle aspiration as an alternative method for tissue diagnosis in 12 of 13 cases of extracranial MRT (RTK = 7) (Thomson et al. 2011). Kerl et al. employed MLPA and DNA sequencing of cells derived from ascites in an infant which at the time of diagnosis was in no condition to undergo a surgical procedure due to life-threatening intraabdominal haemorrhage (Kerl et al. 2015). Mutant *SMARCB1* may also be detected in the form of ctDNA in CSF or plasma by PCR methods (Vu-Han et al. 2014).

34.10 Differential Diagnosis

The group of SMARCB1 (INI1) negative tumours is an expanding family of neoplasm (Agaimy 2019; Kohashi and Oda 2017). As some suggestive, but not pathognomonic, imaging features have been described, MRT is a differential diagnosis for most highly cellular tumours in infants and young children, including (blastemal predominant) nephroblastoma, clear cell sarcoma of the kidney, cellular type mesoblastic nephroma, haepatoblastoma, infantile fibrosarcoma, embryonal rhabdomyosarcoma and other rarer sarcomas.

Table 34.1 offers a list of neoplasms that may be considered in the differential diagnosis of rhabdoid tumours.

34.11 Treatment and Risk Factors

Unfortunately, little survival improvement has been achieved for MRT over recent years. In the UK the National Registry of Childhood Tumours (1993–2000) reported a 31% 1-year overall survival only. This poor survival is reflected in the NWTSG, COG trials and SEER programme; the 4-year overall survival has remained at approximately 20–33% over the years (Geller 2016). Similarly Reinhard et al. indicated in their population-based analysis (1984–1999) of German Rhabdoid Tumours registered in the German Childhood Cancer Registry a 24% 5-year overall survival for RTK and 30% for eMRT (Reinhard et al. 2008). Brennan et al. reported 3-year OS rates of 38% in a series of 74 patients with extracranial RT (1998–2008) who had completed protocol treatment according to an EpSSG study (Brennan et al. 2016).

Due to the rarity of extracranial rhabdoid tumours, and a dearth of controlled clinical trials, large data sets of uniformly treated patients are currently unavailable confounding potential stratification markers. Furthermore, the significance of clinical and genetic (type of *SMARCB1* mutation, germ-line mutation) factors has not been comprehensively assessed in well-defined cohorts. Classic risk factors for relapse include higher local stages as well as distant metastases, the worst survival being associated with multifocal disease. The GPOH reported a 2-year EFS of 58%, 18% and 8% for localized, metastatic and multifocal RTK, respectively. Survival of patients with stage I tumours was particularly favourable (83%) (Furtwangler et al. 2018). One patient survived after preoperative treatment and tumour-nephrectomy without any further treatment. Similarly, 142 patients treated on the consecutive NWTSG trials 1–5 reached 41.8% for stages I and II, while it was only 15.9% for stages III and IV[85]. In both trials younger age was associated with inferior survival, a finding consistently demonstrated throughout various series from SIOP, GPOH, EU-RHAB, EpSSG and COG (Brennan et al. 2016; Furtwangler et al. 2018; Nemes et al. 2018; Tomlinson et al. 2005; van den Heuvel-Eibrink et al. 2011). Whether this is due to a more aggressive behaviour or selection bias due to reduced use of intensive treatment, especially radiotherapy, in a very young cohort remains to be determined. The protective value of radiotherapy as a modality (Sultan et al. 2010) and higher doses of radiotherapy (≥30 Gy) (Tomlinson et al. 2005) has been discussed based on retrospective data from NWTSG and SEER, but a definitive conclusion may not be drawn due to the same age bias (i.e. for radiotherapy) as discussed above. Anatomic site of the rhabdoid tumour has not been consistently shown to be a risk factor. Recently the EpSSG demonstrated a trend to inferior survival in a set of 77 extracranial RT for unfavourable compared to favourable site (49% vs. 36%, $p = 0.28$) (Brennan et al. 2016). However, liver and kidney seem to be associated with a slightly inferior survival compared to other sites, for example, extremities or orbit, following standard soft tissue risk stratification concepts (Brennan et al. 2013; Dantonello et al. 2009).

34.11.1 Rhabdoid Tumours of the Kidney (RTK)

RTK had been treated uniformly according to high-risk strata in Europe and Brazil from 1993 on. The treatment always included an anthracycline (epirubicin or doxorubicin), oxazaphosphorine (ifosfamide or cyclophosphamide), etoposide and carboplatin. Flank radiotherapy with a cumulative dose of up to 30 Gy was recommended for local stage II or III and in case of metastases to the metastatic site(s), achieving 5-year overall survival of 26% (van den Heuvel-Eibrink et al. 2011). In the UK patients with RTK have previously been treated according to Wilms tumour studies UKW2 and 3 containing a combination of vincristine, actinomycin-D and doxorubicin. The survival rate of 21 patients was 35% (SD ± 9%). All deaths occurred within 13 months following diagnosis. One patient with a stage IV survived.

The 2-year overall survival of 58 RTK treated in consecutive SIOP and GPOH trials in Austria, Germany and Switzerland (1991–2013) was 38% (Furtwangler et al. 2018). Survival for stage IV patients was significantly inferior with only three survivors out of 17 patients, all treated by pulmonary and local radiotherapy.

In the USA patients with RTK were previously enrolled into the NWTS studies employing compounds such as vincristine, actinomycin-D and doxorubicin with or without cyclophosphamide (Tomlinson et al. 2005; D'Angio et al. 1989). Despite a high intensity of therapy, the survival within these strata was unsatisfactory. Comparable survival rates have been reported by the SIOP (Vujanic et al. 1996). To improve results, NWTS5 employed a strategy using carboplatin and etoposide with cyclophosphamide (Regimen RTK). Survival was disappointing around 26%. Due to a lack of improvement in comparison to the previous study, this arm was closed preliminarily. Little can be said about the value of single drugs as randomized trials comparing the influence of a specific drug on survival are missing. The combination of oxazaphosphorines, carboplatin, etoposide and doxorubicin has been most commonly used (Brennan et al. 2016; Nemes et al. 2018; van den Heuvel-Eibrink et al. 2011; Venkatramani et al. 2014; Seeringer et al. 2014b). In a retrospective comparison of the responses to preoperative treatment of 15 metastatic RTK treated including doxorubicin and 19 localized RTK treated only with actinomycin-D and vincristine, a significantly increased response rate was presented (Furtwangler et al. 2014). A recent window study for RTK using irinotecan in induction was prematurely closed after three enrolled patients due to inefficiency (COG AREN0321). Based on the currently available data, the role of radiotherapy in the treatment of RTK may not be judged conclusively (Reinhard et al. 2008; Tomlinson et al. 2005).

34.11.2 Extracranial, Extrarenal Malignant Rhabdoid Tumours (eMRT)

Clinical data regarding patients with extracranial, extrarenal rhabdoid tumours are rather sparse in the literature. In a retrospective analysis of the IRS3 trial only 26 cases among 3000 were compatible with the diagnosis of a rhabdoid tumour. These 26 cases were located in the extremities, soft tissue of the trunk, retroperitoneum, abdomen and pelvis. Only 5 of 26 patients survived between 2 and 13 years (Kodet et al. 1991). Within the same time frame, 22 children with extracranial/extrarenal rhabdoid tumours were enrolled into the British UKW2 and 3 studies. Of these, only one patient is alive, who was treated with vincristine, etoposide, epirubicin, actinomycin-D, ifosfamide and carboplatin. Histopathologic evaluation of *SMARCB1* was not yet possible at the time of recording.

In an institutional report from the Children's Hospital of Los Angeles, nine patients with extracranial/extrarenal rhabdoid tumours were diagnosed. At the time of publication three of the nine patients were without evidence of disease at 26, 33 and 104 months after diagnosis. The time to disease progression in the remainder was rapid (mean 3.6 months). No recurrence or death were recorded beyond 10 months following diagnosis. All survivors received multimodal therapy, including chemotherapy, surgery and in two patients radiotherapy. One patient received high-dose chemotherapy. There were no survivors after disease recurrence or progression (Madigan et al. 2007). Similar dismal results are reported in an even larger series of extracranial MRT by Bourdeaut et al. (2008).

In their comprehensive study NRSTS 2005 including renal and extrarenal, extracranial RT the EpSSG was able to evaluate alternating courses of VDCy and CyCE in 100 patients from 12 countries (Brennan et al. 2016). Only 43 patients completed the protocol treatment. A total of 23 patients demonstrated metastases at the time of diagnosis and 41% were below 1 year at diagnosis. The 3-year EFS and OS were 32.3% (CI 23.2–41.6%) and 38.4% (CI 28.8–47.9%). The most prevalent high-risk factor was age below 1 year at diagnosis (4-year EFS and OS 17.2% and 20.1%, respectively). Furthermore, males with M + -disease had a higher risk of failure.

In two subsequent studies on rhabdoid tumours in patients below 1 year at diagnosis and those with congenital MRT (i.e. diagnosed within

28 days from birth) Seeringer et al. and Nemes et al. demonstrated that multimodal therapy is feasible in the youngest and potentially efficacious (Nemes et al. 2018; Seeringer et al. 2014b).

34.11.3 High-Dose Chemotherapy Approaches

In 2003 Katzenstein et al. reported on a 21-month-old patient with a malignant rhabdoid tumour of the liver, local lymph node metastases and distant lung metastases (Katzenstein et al. 2003). As the lesions were deemed inoperable, treatment consisted of chemotherapy using cisplatin, amifostine, vincristine, 5-FU, ifosfamide, carboplatin, etoposide, cyclophosphamide and doxorubicin. Subsequent to this induction high-dose chemotherapy employing a tandem approach with etoposide, carboplatin and cyclophosphamide for the first cycle and melphalan and cyclophosphamide for the second cycle was applied. Despite these aggressive measures the tumour progressed and the patient died 9 months following diagnosis. Sahdev et al. published a report on identical twins both suffering from rhabdoid tumours of the kidney (Sahdev et al. 2003). The first patient was diagnosed at the age of 5 months. Following complete resection of the tumour, metastases to the lung and brain were demonstrated. Despite chemotherapy using carboplatin, etoposide and cyclophosphamide, the disease progressed. The patient received two cycles of taxol, but died at the age of 12 months. The second child became symptomatic at the age of 2 years. He also suffered from metastases to the lung and brain. Following subtotal resection and six cycles of chemotherapy using cisplatin, doxorubicin, vincristine, cyclophosphamide, actinomycin-D, etoposide and ifosfamide, the tumour demonstrated response. Due to chemosensitivity high-dose therapy using etoposide, thiotepa and cyclophosphamide was performed. At the time of publication, the patient was alive without evidence of disease at 6 years. In 2005 Fujita et al. published the case of a newborn with a tumour of the orbit (Fujita et al. 2005). At the age of 10 months the eye was enucleated and histologically proven to be affected by MRT. On imaging a further lesion was found in the fourth ventricle of the CNS. This lesion was completely resected. The patient received induction chemotherapy using cisplatin, etoposide, ifosfamide, carboplatin, vincristine and nimustine. Consolidation consisted of thiotepa, melphalan, followed by autologous stem cell rescue. At the time of publication the patient was alive without evidence of disease 24 months following surgery. In 2006 Watanabe et al. reported on another boy with MRT of the orbit (Watanabe et al. 2006). Following subtotal resection induction chemotherapy was applied, consisting of cisplatin, etoposide and vincristine. As there was no response, therapy was augmented with doxorubicin and ifosfamide. After two cycles clinical and radiological response was demonstrated. As the parents refused radical surgery, gamma-knife-surgery was applied in addition to high-dose chemotherapy. A first cycle of high-dose chemotherapy consisted of melphalan and cyclophosphamide, the second of ifosfamide and thiotepa. At the time of publication the patient was alive 4 years following diagnosis.

Madigan et al. report on a series of 14 patients with extracranial rhabdoid tumours treated between the years 1983 and 2003 (Madigan et al. 2007). Among these 14 patients five long-term survivors are described. All of these had radical surgery and chemotherapy with or without RT. Two of the surviving patients received high-dose chemotherapy followed by stem cell rescue in addition to induction chemotherapy. The first patient is a 6-month-old boy with a rhabdoid tumour of the kidney. Following total resection and chemotherapy with vincristine, adriamycin, cyclophosphamide, cisplatin and etoposide, high-dose chemotherapy using carbo-platinum, etoposide and melphalan was performed. The patient did not receive RT and was alive 34 months following diagnosis at the time of publication. The second patient was a 30-month-old girl with a rhabdoid tumour of the neck. She received a subtotal resection followed by induction chemotherapy using vincristine, actinomycin-D, cyclophosphamide and ifosfamide/adriamycin. She then received carboplatin, etoposide and melphalan in myeloablative doses as consolidative treatment. She furthermore received 45 Gy of local RT. This patient is without evidence of disease 104 months following diagnosis at the time of publication.

In a retrospective analysis of 58 patients with RTK recruited in the SIOP studies SIOP9/GPOH, SIOP93-01, SIOP2001 and the EU-RHAB registry, only 11 underwent HDCT (Furtwangler et al. 2018). After excluding selection bias such as time lag to diagnosis, stem cell harvest or to reach HDCT, survival was equivalent among patients with or without HDCT (60 ± 16% vs. 62 ± 11%).

34.11.4 Treatment of Recurrence and Experimental Approaches

At present systematic analyses of relapses in larger series of MRT are missing. In a preliminary evaluation of 69 relapsed patients derived from the EU-RHAB cohort (19 extracranial RT), approximately 80% of relapses were local, 10% combined and another 10% disseminated only. A total of 44% (30/69) of the patients relapsed (CR was achieved by surgery or chemotherapy) or progressed before the end of intensive therapy, while another 39% (27/69) occurred in the first 6 months after finishing intensive treatment. The median survival for all patients with relapse was only 3.5 months. The 6-months OS was 28%, 1-year OS was 16%, and the 24-months OS was a dismal 6% (EU-RHAB unpublished).

As MRT commonly affect very young children, aggressive treatment approaches (including radiotherapy) may impede development of rather vulnerable organ systems and entail significant short- and long-term side effects (Roddy and Mueller 2016). Current relapse strategies aim at aggressive local approaches such as surgery and (re)-irradiation. For those patients not amenable to local therapy, experimental phase I and II trials specifically designed for patients with resistant, or relapsed, MRT have been developed. Most of these trials are targeted at the pathways previously described as defective in MRT and specifically in ATRT (Fruhwald et al. 2016). A few examples of current strategies are described herein.

A phase I trial of the cell cycle CDK4/6 inhibitor ribociclib (NCT017747876) in rhabdoid tumours, neuroblastomas and other *CDK4*-amplified malignancies has demonstrated tolerable safety and favourable pharmacokinetics in children. Fifteen patients with RT (n = 13 AT/RT, *n* = 2 eMRT) received ribociclib orally (3 weeks on/1 week off). The maximum tolerated dose (470 mg/m^2) and recommended phase II dose (350 mg/m^2) were equal to those in adults. Two patients with AT/RT achieved prolonged disease stabilization. The majority of adverse events were hematologic (Geoerger et al. 2017). Further investigations of ribociclib in combination with topotecan and temozolomide (ARM A), and with everolimus (ARM B) in children with refractory or recurrent malignancies are ongoing (NCT02813135). A phase I study of the selective CDK4/6 inhibitor abemaciclib (LY2835219) is specifically recruiting patients with newly diagnosed diffuse intrinsic pontine glioma and children with recurrent and refractory solid tumours, including rhabdoid tumours (NCT02644460).

Epigenetic targeting is one of the most active areas of research in drug development especially for children with high-risk malignancies. The inhibition of enzymatic activities involved in epigenetic silencing by histone deacetylases (HDACs), DNA methyltransferases (DNMTs) and enhancer of zeste homologue 2 (EZH2) is tested in active clinical trials. The antagonistic relationship between SWI/SNF and the polycomb repressive complex 2 (PRC2) plays a critical role in gene transcription and makes it an attractive target for therapy in MRT (Margueron and Reinberg 2011). Preclinical studies have reported elevated expression of EZH2 in SMARCB1-deficient cells and determined apoptosis in EZH2-depleted rhabdoid tumour cell lines (Wilson et al. 2010). Further analyses revealed upregulation of EZH2 following SMARCB1 loss. This was accompanied by widespread trimethylation of histone H3K27 and repression of p16^{INK4} [105]. Effective, selective EZH2 inhibitors have been developed. One of these, tazemetostat (EPZ-6438), is a selective orally bio-available inhibitor of EZH2's enzymatic activity (Knutson et al. 2014). In a phase I trial of tazemetostat (EPZ-6438) in 30 adult patients with solid tumours (including 5 patients with malignant rhabdoid tumour) and 21 patients with B-cell non-Hodgkin's lymphoma, one patient with MRT achieved a complete response. There were also two patients with stable disease, one patient with a partial response and one with progressive disease (http://www.epizyme.com/wp-content/uploads/2015/09/Tazemetostat-ESMO-Phase-1-Trial-September-26-2015.pdf). A paediatric clinical phase I/II trial employing tazemetostat for patients with rhabdoid tumours and other INI-deficient tumours finished recruiting in 2021 following a dose expansion phase (NCT02601937, NCT02601950).

Immunotherapy is an attractive tool in tumours with resistance to conventional drugs and may be of value in difficult-to-treat solid tumours such as relapsed MRT. Congress reports and individual cases of relapsed MRT indicate activity of checkpoint inhibitors such as atezolizumab and pembrolizumab (Henon et al. 2019). A comprehensive review of experimental approaches for MRT is given among others in (Nemes and Fruhwald 2018).

References

Agaimy A (2014) The expanding family of SMARCB1(INI1)-deficient neoplasia: implications of phenotypic, biological, and molecular heterogeneity. Adv Anat Pathol 21:394–410

Agaimy A (2019) SWI/SNF complex-deficient soft tissue neoplasms: a pattern-based approach to diagnosis and differential diagnosis. Surg Pathol Clin 12:149–163

Amar AM, Tomlinson G, Green DM, Breslow NE, de Alarcon PA (2001) Clinical presentation of rhabdoid tumors of the kidney. J Pediatr Hematol Oncol 23:105–108

Beckwith JB, Palmer NF (1978) Histopathology and prognosis of Wilms tumors: results from the First National Wilms' Tumor Study. Cancer 41:1937–1948

Benesch M, Bartelheim K, Fleischhack G et al (2014) High-dose chemotherapy (HDCT) with auto-SCT in children with atypical teratoid/rhabdoid tumors (AT/RT): a report from the European Rhabdoid Registry (EU-RHAB). Bone Marrow Transplant 49:370–375

Biegel JA (2006) Molecular genetics of atypical teratoid/rhabdoid tumor. Neurosurg Focus 20:E11

Biegel JA, Rorke LB, Packer RJ, Emanuel BS (1990) Monosomy 22 in rhabdoid or atypical tumors of the brain. J Neurosurg 73:710–714

Biegel JA, Allen CS, Kawasaki K, Shimizu N, Budarf ML, Bell CJ (1996) Narrowing the critical region for a rhabdoid tumor locus in 22q11. Genes Chromosomes Cancer 16:94–105

Biegel JA, Busse TM, Weissman BE (2014) SWI/SNF chromatin remodeling complexes and cancer. Am J Med Genet C Semin Med Genet 166C:350–366

Birks DK, Donson AM, Patel PR et al (2013) Pediatric rhabdoid tumors of kidney and brain show many differences in gene expression but share dysregulation of cell cycle and epigenetic effector genes. Pediatr Blood Cancer 60:1095–1102

Bourdeaut F, Freneaux P, Thuille B et al (2008) Extra-renal non-cerebral rhabdoid tumours. Pediatr Blood Cancer 51:363–368

Bourdeaut F, Lequin D, Brugieres L et al (2011) Frequent hSNF5/INI1 germline mutations in patients with rhabdoid tumor. Clin Cancer Res 17:31–38

Brennan B, Stiller C, Bourdeaut F (2013) Extracranial rhabdoid tumours: what we have learned so far and future directions. Lancet Oncol 14:e329–e336

Brennan B, De Salvo GL, Orbach D et al (2016) Outcome of extracranial malignant rhabdoid tumours in children registered in the European Paediatric Soft Tissue Sarcoma Study Group Non-Rhabdomyosarcoma Soft Tissue Sarcoma 2005 Study-EpSSG NRSTS 2005. Eur J Cancer 60:69–82

Bruggers CS, Bleyl SB, Pysher T et al (2011) Clinicopathologic comparison of familial versus sporadic atypical teratoid/rhabdoid tumors (AT/RT) of the central nervous system. Pediatr Blood Cancer 56:1026–1031

Bultman S, Gebuhr T, Yee D et al (2000) A Brg1 null mutation in the mouse reveals functional differences among mammalian SWI/SNF complexes. Mol Cell 6:1287–1295

Bultman SJ, Herschkowitz JI, Godfrey V et al (2008) Characterization of mammary tumors from Brg1 heterozygous mice. Oncogene 27:460–468

Chun HJ, Lim EL, Heravi-Moussavi A et al (2016) Genome-wide profiles of extra-cranial malignant rhabdoid tumors reveal heterogeneity and dysregulated developmental pathways. Cancer Cell 29:394–406

D'Angio GJ, Breslow N, Beckwith JB et al (1989) Treatment of Wilms' tumor. Results of the Third National Wilms' Tumor Study. Cancer 64:349–360

Dantonello TM, Int-Veen C, Harms D et al (2009) Cooperative trial CWS-91 for localized soft tissue sarcoma in children, adolescents, and young adults. J Clin Oncol 27:1446–1455

de Kock L, Fahiminiya S, Fiset PO et al (2018) Infantile Pulmonary Teratoid Tumor. N Engl J Med 378:2238–2240

Dho YS, Kim SK, Cheon JE et al (2015) Investigation of the location of atypical teratoid/rhabdoid tumor. Childs Nerv Syst 31:1305–1311

Eaton KW, Tooke LS, Wainwright LM, Judkins AR, Biegel JA (2011) Spectrum of SMARCB1/INI1 mutations in familial and sporadic rhabdoid tumors. Pediatr Blood Cancer 56:7–15

Foulkes WD, Kamihara J, Evans DGR et al (2017) Cancer surveillance in gorlin syndrome and rhabdoid tumor predisposition syndrome. Clin Cancer Res 23:e62–e67

Fruhwald MC, Hasselblatt M, Wirth S et al (2006) Non-linkage of familial rhabdoid tumors to SMARCB1 implies a second locus for the rhabdoid tumor predisposition syndrome. Pediatr Blood Cancer 47:273–278

Fruhwald MC, Biegel JA, Bourdeaut F, Roberts CW, Chi SN (2016) Atypical teratoid/rhabdoid tumors-current concepts, advances in biology, and potential future therapies. Neuro-Oncology 18:764–778

Fujita M, Sato M, Nakamura M et al (2005) Multicentric atypical teratoid/rhabdoid tumors occurring in the eye and fourth ventricle of an infant: case report. J Neurosurg 102:299–302

Furtwangler R, Nourkami-Tutdibi N, Leuschner I et al (2014) Malignant rhabdoid tumor of the kidney: significantly improved response to pre-operative treatment intensified with doxorubicin. Cancer Genet 207:434–436

Furtwangler R, Kager L, Melchior P et al (2018) High-dose treatment for malignant rhabdoid tumor of the kidney: no evidence for improved survival-The Gesellschaft fur Padiatrische Onkologie und Hamatologie (GPOH) experience. Pediatr Blood Cancer 65(1)

Garces-Inigo EF, Leung R, Sebire NJ, McHugh K (2009) Extrarenal rhabdoid tumours outside the central nervous system in infancy. Pediatr Radiol 39:817–822

Geller JI (2016) Current standards of care and future directions for "high-risk" pediatric renal tumors: Anaplastic Wilms tumor and Rhabdoid tumor. Urol Oncol 34:50–56

Geller JI, Roth JJ, Biegel JA (2015) Biology and treatment of rhabdoid tumor. Crit Rev Oncog 20:199–216

Geoerger B, Bourdeaut F, DuBois SG et al (2017) A phase I study of the CDK4/6 inhibitor ribociclib (LEE011) in pediatric patients with malignant rhabdoid tumors, neuroblastoma, and other solid tumors. Clin Cancer Res 23:2433–2441

Giunti L, Bernini G, Forni M, Tucci F, Wheeler E, Sardi I (2006) Clonality analysis of pediatric multiple tumors: two case reports and laboratory investigation. J Pediatr Hematol Oncol 28:241–248

Guidi CJ, Sands AT, Zambrowicz BP et al (2001) Disruption of Ini1 leads to peri-implantation lethality and tumorigenesis in mice. Mol Cell Biol 21:3598–3603

Haas JE, Palmer NF, Weinberg AG, Beckwith JB (1981) Ultrastructure of malignant rhabdoid tumor of the kidney. A distinctive renal tumor of children. Hum Pathol 12:646–657

Han ZY, Richer W, Freneaux P et al (2016) The occurrence of intracranial rhabdoid tumours in mice depends on temporal control of Smarcb1 inactivation. Nat Commun 7:10421

Hasselblatt M, Isken S, Linge A et al (2013) High-resolution genomic analysis suggests the absence of recurrent genomic alterations other than SMARCB1 aberrations in atypical teratoid/rhabdoid tumors. Genes Chromosomes Cancer 52:185–190

Hasselblatt M, Nagel I, Oyen F et al (2014) SMARCA4-mutated atypical teratoid/rhabdoid tumors are associated with inherited germline alterations and poor prognosis. Acta Neuropathol 128:453–456

Hasselblatt M, Thomas C, Hovestadt V et al (2016) Poorly differentiated chordoma with SMARCB1/INI1 loss: a distinct molecular entity with dismal prognosis. Acta Neuropathol 132:149–151

Heck JE, Lombardi CA, Cockburn M, Meyers TJ, Wilhelm M, Ritz B (2013) Epidemiology of rhabdoid tumors of early childhood. Pediatr Blood Cancer 60:77–81

Helming KC, Wang X, Roberts CW (2014) Vulnerabilities of mutant SWI/SNF complexes in cancer. Cancer Cell 26:309–317

Henon C, Blay JY, Massard C et al (2019) Long lasting major response to pembrolizumab in a thoracic malignant rhabdoid-like SMARCA4-deficient tumor. Ann Oncol

Howman-Giles R, McCowage G, Kellie S, Graf N (2012) Extrarenal malignant rhabdoid tumor in childhood application of 18F-FDG PET/CT. J Pediatr Hematol Oncol 34:17–21

Irtan S, Jitlal M, Bate J et al (2015) Risk factors for local recurrence in Wilms tumour and the potential influence of biopsy—the United Kingdom experience. Eur J Cancer 51:225–232

Jackson EM, Sievert AJ, Gai X et al (2009) Genomic analysis using high-density single nucleotide polymorphism-based oligonucleotide arrays and multiplex ligation-dependent probe amplification provides a comprehensive analysis of INI1/SMARCB1 in malignant rhabdoid tumors. Clin Cancer Res 15:1923–1930

Johann PD, Erkek S, Zapatka M et al (2016) atypical teratoid/rhabdoid tumors are comprised of three epigenetic subgroups with distinct enhancer landscapes. Cancer Cell 29:379–393

Judkins AR (2007) Immunohistochemistry of INI1 expression: a new tool for old challenges in CNS and soft tissue pathology. Adv Anat Pathol 14:335–339

Judkins AR, Mauger J, Ht A, Rorke LB, Biegel JA (2004) Immunohistochemical analysis of hSNF5/INI1 in pediatric CNS neoplasms. Am J Surg Pathol 28:644–650

Judkins AR, Burger PC, Hamilton RL et al (2005) INI1 protein expression distinguishes atypical teratoid/rhabdoid tumor from choroid plexus carcinoma. J Neuropathol Exp Neurol 64:391–397

Kadoch C, Crabtree GR (2015) Mammalian SWI/SNF chromatin remodeling complexes and cancer: mechanistic insights gained from human genomics. Sci Adv 1:e1500447

Katzenstein HM, Kletzel M, Reynolds M, Superina R, Gonzalez-Crussi F (2003) Metastatic malignant rhabdoid tumor of the liver treated with tandem high-dose therapy and autologous peripheral blood stem cell rescue. Med Pediatr Oncol 40:199–201

Kelly DM, Jones M, Humphreys S, Howard ER (1998) Spontaneous rupture of a malignant rhabdoid tumour of the liver. Pediatr Surg Int 14:111–112

Kerl K, Oyen F, Leuschner I et al (2015) Detection of SMARCB1 loss in ascites cells in the diagnosis of an abdominal rhabdoid tumor. Pediatr Blood Cancer

Kieran MW, Roberts CW, Chi SN et al (2012) Absence of oncogenic canonical pathway mutations in aggressive pediatric rhabdoid tumors. Pediatr Blood Cancer 59:1155–1157

Klochendler-Yeivin A, Fiette L, Barra J, Muchardt C, Babinet C, Yaniv M (2000) The murine SNF5/INI1 chromatin remodeling factor is essential for embryonic development and tumor suppression. EMBO Rep 1:500–506

Knutson SK, Kawano S, Minoshima Y et al (2014) Selective inhibition of EZH2 by EPZ-6438 leads to potent antitumor activity in EZH2-mutant non-Hodgkin lymphoma. Mol Cancer Ther 13:842–854

Kodet R, Newton WA Jr, Sachs N et al (1991) Rhabdoid tumors of soft tissues: a clinicopathologic study of 26 cases enrolled on the Intergroup Rhabdomyosarcoma Study. Hum Pathol 22:674–684

Kohashi K, Oda Y (2017) Oncogenic roles of SMARCB1/INI1 and its deficient tumors. Cancer Sci 108:547–552

Kordes U, Gesk S, Fruhwald MC et al (2010) Clinical and molecular features in patients with atypical teratoid rhabdoid tumor or malignant rhabdoid tumor. Genes Chromosomes Cancer 49:176–181

Kordes U, Bartelheim K, Modena P et al (2014) Favorable outcome of patients affected by rhabdoid tumors due to rhabdoid tumor predisposition syndrome (RTPS). Pediatr Blood Cancer 61:919–921

Lafay-Cousin L, Hawkins C, Carret AS et al (2012) Central nervous system atypical teratoid rhabdoid tumours: the Canadian Paediatric Brain Tumour Consortium experience. Eur J Cancer 48:353–359

Lee RS, Stewart C, Carter SL et al (2012) A remarkably simple genome underlies highly malignant pediatric rhabdoid cancers. J Clin Invest 122:2983–2988

Litman DA, Bhuta S, Barsky SH (1993) Synchronous occurrence of malignant rhabdoid tumor two decades after Wilms' tumor irradiation. Am J Surg Pathol 17:729–737

Madigan CE, Armenian SH, Malogolowkin MH, Mascarenhas L (2007) Extracranial malignant rhabdoid tumors in childhood: the Childrens Hospital Los Angeles experience. Cancer 110:2061–2066

Margueron R, Reinberg D (2011) The polycomb complex PRC2 and its mark in life. Nature 469:343–349

Morgenstern DA, Gibson S, Brown T, Sebire NJ, Anderson J (2010) Clinical and pathological features of paediatric malignant rhabdoid tumours. Pediatr Blood Cancer 54:29–34

Nemes K, Fruhwald MC (2018) Emerging therapeutic targets for the treatment of malignant rhabdoid tumors. Expert Opin Ther Targets 22:365–379

Nemes K, Bens S, Bourdeaut F et al (2017) Rhabdoid tumor predisposition syndrome. In: Adam MP, Ardinger HH, Pagon RA et al (eds) . GeneReviews((R)), Seattle, WA

Nemes K, Clement N, Kachanov D et al (2018) The extraordinary challenge of treating patients with congenital rhabdoid tumors-a collaborative European effort. Pediatr Blood Cancer

Pinto EM, Hamideh D, Bahrami A et al (2018) Malignant rhabdoid tumors originating within and outside the central nervous system are clinically and molecularly heterogeneous. Acta Neuropathol

Pohl U, Dean AF, Ichimura K et al (2010) Genomic analysis of chromosome 22 in synchronous and histologically distinct intracranial tumours in a child. Neuropathol Appl Neurobiol 36:359–363

Reinhard H, Reinert J, Beier R et al (2008) Rhabdoid tumors in children: prognostic factors in 70 patients diagnosed in Germany. Oncol Rep 19:819–823

Rekhi B, Kosemehmetoglu K, Tezel GG, Dervisoglu S (2017) Clinicopathologic features and immunohistochemical spectrum of 11 cases of epithelioid malignant peripheral nerve sheath tumors, including INI1/SMARCB1 results and BRAF V600E analysis. APMIS 125:679–689

Rickert CH, Paulus W (2004) Chromosomal imbalances detected by comparative genomic hybridisation in atypical teratoid/rhabdoid tumours. Childs Nerv Syst 20:221–224. Epub 2004 Feb 2004

Roberts CW, Galusha SA, McMenamin ME, Fletcher CD, Orkin SH (2000) Haploinsufficiency of Snf5 (integrase interactor 1) predisposes to malignant rhabdoid tumors in mice. Proc Natl Acad Sci U S A 97:13796–13800

Roberts CW, Leroux MM, Fleming MD, Orkin SH (2002) Highly penetrant, rapid tumorigenesis through conditional inversion of the tumor suppressor gene Snf5. Cancer Cell 2:415–425

Roddy E, Mueller S (2016) Late effects of treatment of pediatric central nervous system tumors. J Child Neurol 31:237–254

Rorke LB, Packer RJ, Biegel JA (1996) Central nervous system atypical teratoid/rhabdoid tumors of infancy and childhood: definition of an entity. J Neurosurg 85:56–65

Sahdev I, James-Herry A, Scimeca P, Parker R (2003) Concordant rhabdoid tumor of the kidney in a set of identical twins with discordant outcomes. J Pediatr Hematol Oncol 25:491–494

Schenk JP, Engelmann D, Rohrschneider W et al (2004) Rhabdoid tumors of the kidney in childhood. Rofo 176:965–971

Schneppenheim R, Fruhwald MC, Gesk S et al (2010) Germline nonsense mutation and somatic inactivation of SMARCA4/BRG1 in a family with rhabdoid tumor predisposition syndrome. Am J Hum Genet 86:279–284

Seeringer A, Reinhard H, Hasselblatt M et al (2014a) Synchronous congenital malignant rhabdoid tumor of the orbit and atypical teratoid/rhabdoid tumor—feasibility and efficacy of multimodal therapy in a long-term survivor. Cancer Genet 207:429–433

Seeringer A, Bartelheim K, Kerl K et al (2014b) Feasibility of intensive multimodal therapy in infants affected by rhabdoid tumors—experience of the EU-RHAB registry. Klin Padiatr 226:143–148

Sredni ST, Tomita T (2015) Rhabdoid tumor predisposition syndrome. Pediatr Dev Pathol 18:49–58

St Pierre R, Kadoch C (2017) Mammalian SWI/SNF complexes in cancer: emerging therapeutic opportunities. Curr Opin Genet Dev 42:56–67

Sultan I, Qaddoumi I, Rodriguez-Galindo C, Nassan AA, Ghandour K, Al-Hussaini M (2010) Age, stage, and radiotherapy, but not primary tumor site, affects the outcome of patients with malignant rhabdoid tumors. Pediatr Blood Cancer 54:35–40

Szymanski KM, Tabib CH, Idrees MT, Cain MP (2013) Synchronous perivesical and renal malignant rhabdoid tumor in a 9-year-old boy: a case report and review of literature. Urology 82:1158–1160

Tang Y, Li S, Qu J, Zhou Y, Xiao J (2015) Malignant rhabdoid tumor with cervical vertebra involvement in a teenage child: case report and review of the literature. Pediatr Neurosurg 50:173–178

Teplick A, Kowalski M, Biegel JA, Nichols KE (2011) Educational paper: screening in cancer predisposition syndromes: guidelines for the general pediatrician. Eur J Pediatr 170(3):285–294

Thomson TA, Klijanienko J, Couturier J et al (2011) Fine-needle aspiration of renal and extrarenal rhabdoid tumors: the experience of the Institut Curie regarding 20 tumors in 13 patients. Cancer Cytopathol 119:49–57

Tomlinson GE, Breslow NE, Dome J et al (2005) Rhabdoid tumor of the kidney in the National Wilms' Tumor Study: age at diagnosis as a prognostic factor. J Clin Oncol 23:7641–7645

Torchia J, Golbourn B, Feng S et al (2016) Integrated (epi)-genomic analyses identify subgroup-specific therapeutic targets in CNS rhabdoid tumors. Cancer Cell 30:891–908

Trobaugh-Lotrario AD, Tomlinson GE, Finegold MJ, Gore L, Feusner JH (2009) Small cell undifferentiated variant of hepatoblastoma: adverse clinical and molecular features similar to rhabdoid tumors. Pediatr Blood Cancer 52:328–334

Tsikitis M, Zhang Z, Edelman W, Zagzag D, Kalpana GV (2005) Genetic ablation of Cyclin D1 abrogates genesis of rhabdoid tumors resulting from Ini1 loss. Proc Natl Acad Sci U S A 102:12129–12134

Uwineza A, Gill H, Buckley P et al (2014) Rhabdoid tumor: the Irish experience 1986-2013. Cancer Genet 207:398–402

van den Heuvel-Eibrink MM, van Tinteren H, Rehorst H et al (2011) Malignant rhabdoid tumours of the kidney (MRTKs), registered on recent SIOP protocols from 1993 to 2005: a report of the SIOP renal tumour study group. Pediatr Blood Cancer 56:733–737

van den Munckhof P, Christiaans I, Kenter SB, Baas F, Hulsebos TJ (2012) Germline SMARCB1 mutation predisposes to multiple meningiomas and schwannomas with preferential location of cranial meningiomas at the falx cerebri. Neurogenetics 13:1–7

Venkatramani R, Shoureshi P, Malvar J, Zhou S, Mascarenhas L (2014) High dose alkylator therapy for extracranial malignant rhabdoid tumors in children. Pediatr Blood Cancer 61:1357–1361

Vogelstein B, Papadopoulos N, Velculescu VE, Zhou S, Diaz LA Jr, Kinzler KW (2013) Cancer genome landscapes. Science 339:1546–1558

Vokuhl C, Oyen F, Haberle B, von Schweinitz D, Schneppenheim R, Leuschner I (2016) Small cell undifferentiated (SCUD) hepatoblastomas: all malignant rhabdoid tumors? Genes Chromosomes Cancer 55:925–931

Vu-Han TL, Fruhwald MC, Hasselblatt M et al (2014) Identifying molecular markers for the sensitive detection of residual atypical teratoid rhabdoid tumor cells. Cancer Genet 207:390–397

Vujanic GM, Sandstedt B, Harms D, Boccon-Gibod L, Delemarre JF (1996) Rhabdoid tumour of the kidney: a clinicopathological study of 22 patients from the International Society of Paediatric Oncology (SIOP) nephroblastoma file. Histopathology 28:333–340

Vujanic GM, Gessler M, Ooms A et al (2018) The UMBRELLA SIOP-RTSG 2016 Wilms tumour pathology and molecular biology protocol. Nat Rev Urol 15:693–701

Watanabe H, Watanabe T, Kaneko M et al (2006) Treatment of unresectable malignant rhabdoid tumor of the orbit with tandem high-dose chemotherapy and gamma-knife radiosurgery. Pediatr Blood Cancer 47:846–850

Wilson BG, Wang X, Shen X et al (2010) Epigenetic antagonism between polycomb and SWI/SNF complexes during oncogenic transformation. Cancer Cell 18:316–328

Winger DI, Buyuk A, Bohrer S et al (2006) Radiology-Pathology Conference: rhabdoid tumor of the kidney. Clin Imaging 30:132–136

Witkowski L, Goudie C, Foulkes WD, McCluggage WG (2016) Small-cell carcinoma of the ovary of hypercalcemic type (malignant rhabdoid tumor of the ovary): a review with recent developments on pathogenesis. Surg Pathol Clin. 9:215–226

Part IX

Rare Tumors of the Peripheral Nervous System

35

Rare Tumours of the Peripheral Nervous System: Intra-adrenal (Phaeochromocytoma) and Extra-adrenal Paraganglioma

Bernadette Brennan

35.1 Introduction

The WHO in 2004 reclassified endocrine tumours and redefined phaeochromocytoma as intra-adrenal paraganglioma and those tumours of extra-adrenal sympathetic or para-sympathetic paraganglia as extra-adrenal paragangliomas (Pacak et al. 2007). Although these entities are often described as a single tumour, their different clinical behaviour, genetic background and malignant potential suggest they are considered as distinct entities. Although rare in children, they are the commonest paediatric endocrine tumour with an instance of 1–2 per million (Stringel et al. 1980). The majority of paragangliomas arise in the adrenal medulla (Lenders et al. 2002), but when they arise in extra-adrenal sites, they occur in decreasing order of frequency in the abdomen—in the organ of Zuckerkandl, pelvis, mediastinum and the head and neck (Pacak et al. 2001). In the head and neck they are mainly para-sympathetic and non-secreting with a specific entity arising in the carotid body—carotid body tumour—which is extremely rare in childhood (Deal et al. 1990). In childhood they are often multiple or bilateral with 40% probably associated with an underlying genetic condition and very rarely are malignant (de Krijger et al. 2006).

35.2 Phaeochromocytomas in the United Kingdom National Registry of Childhood Tumours 1971–2002 (Spoudeas and Harrison 2005)

The registration of non-malignant tumours has clearly been incomplete, especially before 1981. Detailed data therefore only covers the period 1981–2000 only (Spoudeas and Harrison 2005) (Tables 35.1 and 35.2).

Table 35.1 Numbers of registrations by calendar period and tumour behaviour

	Benign and unspecified	Malignant	Total
1971–1980	6	2	8
1981–1990	11	4	15
1991–2002	20	1	21

Unspecified are regarded as benign in ICD-O

B. Brennan (✉)
Department Paediatric Oncology, Royal Manchester Children's Hospital, Manchester, UK
e-mail: bernadette.brennan@mft.nhs.uk

D. T. Schneider et al. (eds.), *Rare Tumors in Children and Adolescents*, Pediatric Oncology,
https://doi.org/10.1007/978-3-030-92071-5_35

Table 35.2 Numbers of registrations by age and sex 1981–2002

	0–4 years	5–9 years	10–14 years	Male	Female	Total
Benign and unspecified	1	13	17	19	12	31
Malignant	0	2	3	3	2	5

Phaeochromocytoma was more common in older children, with boys more frequently affected (1.5:1)
Incidence of malignant phaeochromocytoma was 0.02 per million children
For benign and unspecified, a minimum estimate of incidence is 0.11 per million
Among 31 children with benign or unspecified tumours, 3 were diagnosed at post mortem; no other deaths have been recorded
Of 5 children registered with malignant phaeochromocytoma, 2 died at intervals of 2 days and 14 months after diagnosis; the other 3 are alive with survival times between 3 and 22 years

35.3 Clinical Presentation

In children the presentation can be very variable, but symptoms are mainly due to the excess catecholamine secretion (Pham et al. 2006; Waguespack et al. 2010). Twice as many cases occur in boys than girls with a mean age of about 11 years at presentation, the majority presenting with hypertension which may be intermittent and not present in all cases (Barontini et al. 2006; Beltsevich et al. 2004; Waguespack and Ying 2014). Other symptoms of catecholamine excess include the classic triad of headache, palpitations, excess sweatiness, also weight loss, vomiting, anxiety and behavioural problems (Haws et al. 2007).

Rarely when paragangliomas occur in the bladder, they can present with haematuria and symptoms during micturition.

Probably in nearly half of paragangliomas in childhood, there will be a hereditary basis (Barontini et al. 2006; Dahia 2014; de Krijger et al. 2006; Waguespack and Ying 2014) so where there is a clinical suspicion of paragangliomas, a detailed family history and clinical examination for the physical characteristics of the following familial/genetic syndromes should be undertaken. Hereditary paragangliomas are often multifocal and in the cases of phaeochromocytomas bilateral.

Von Hippel–Lindau (VHL) is responsible for the majority of childhood cases—retinal haemangiomas, CNS haemangioblastoma (mainly cerebellar) and renal carcinoma (usually in adult life).

Familial paraganglioma syndrome (SDH mutation) is the second commonest cause—head and neck paragangliomas, intra-adrenal paragangliomas and extra-adrenal paragangliomas.

Neurofibromatosis type 1 (NF-1)—Café au lait patches, axillary freckling, neurofibromas, macrocephaly and Lisch nodules of iris.

Multiple endocrine neoplasia type 2B (MEN2B)—marfanoid habitus, ganglioneuromatosis of bowel, neuromas of tongue and lips and hyperplasia of nerves of conjunctiva.

Multiple endocrine neoplasia type 2A (MEN2A)—thyroid mass, Hirschsprung's disease and cutaneous lichen amyloidosis.

Rarely tuberose sclerosis complex is implicated.

35.4 Diagnostic Investigations

35.4.1 Biochemical

The diagnosis of paragangliomas should be confirmed by the measurement of at least two 24-h urine samples for metanephrines (normetanephrine or metanephrine), and for superior diagnostic accuracy, measurement of plasma free metanephrine and normetanephrine (Lenders et al. 2002; Pacak et al. 2007; Waguespack et al. 2010; Weise et al. 2002).

35.4.2 Imaging/Localising Investigations

Tumour localising investigations should be performed once a biochemical diagnosis has been made. However, where there is a hereditary or genetic predisposition, imaging investigations may be used for screening. Magnetic resonance imaging (MRI) of the abdomen and pelvis should be performed avoiding the radiation exposure of computed tomography (CT) scan. The MRI scan clearly helps to localise site of the tumour, assess its size and look at its relationships to major vessels (Pacak et al. 2001). Functional imaging is required, however, using I^{123} metaiodobenzylguanidine (MIBG) scintigraphy to confirm the diagnosis, detect multiple synchronous primaries and possible malignant disease (Ilias and Pacak 2004; Velchik et al. 1989). This may necessitate further cross-sectional imaging. It should be noted that malignant paragangliomas lose the ability to accumulate MIBG and hence may not detect all sites of metastatic disease. Further imaging that may be useful in this situation, and indeed superior, includes [^{18}F]—fluorodeoxyglucose positron emission tomography (FDG-PET) (Timmers et al. 2007a; Fottner et al. 2010).

35.4.3 Other Investigations

Echocardiography and ECG for longstanding evidence of hypertension.

35.5 Pre-operative Medical Management

Definitive treatment for phaeochromocytoma is surgical resection but only after there has been effective blockade of catecholamines for at least 10–14 days prior to surgery. If there is adequate pre-operative α-adrenergic blockade with phenoxybenzamine, as the usual agent, the risk of intra-operative complications is significantly reduced (Goldstein et al. 1999). Doxazosin could be considered if phenoxybenzamine is poorly tolerated. Beta blockers for tachycardia should only be used after adequate α-adrenergic blockade has been achieved. Adequate hydration is necessary to support the relatively reduced circulating blood volume resulting from the α-blockade (Hack 2000).

35.6 Operative Management

The preferred approach to resection is laparoscopic, but open resection is acceptable, particularly with invasive or metastatic disease (Brunt et al. 2002; Waguespack and Ying 2014). If there are multiple tumours, there should be an attempt to remove all tumours at the same time, and in children with bilateral adrenal involvement, cortical-sparing adrenalectomies should be considered to avoid the difficulties of cortical steroid replacement during adolescence. Post operatively patients should be monitored for the complications of hypotension and hypoglycaemia. Steroid replacement may be required for bilateral disease even in adrenal sparing surgery for the immediate perioperative period.

35.7 Malignant Paragangliomas

The incidence of malignancy is probably low at about 12% in childhood paragangliomas (Barontini et al. 2006; Chrisoulidou et al. 2007; Pham et al. 2006). Malignancy cannot be diagnosed by histology alone but by the presence of local invasion and/or metastatic disease usually in bone, lung or liver. Although generally incurable, some patients can survive for many years (Havekes et al. 2007). There is little or no literature on children with malignant paragangliomas, but individual cases are included in adult series (Gonias et al. 2009; Havekes et al. 2007). Unresectable tumours can be managed symptomatically in order to improve the quality of life of the child with either phenoxybenzamine or doxazosin, as per the preoperative use. Following debulking surgery MIBG therapy may be effective either alone (Loh et al. 1997) or in association with chemotherapy (Sisson et al. 1999) usually a combination of vincristine, cyclophosphamide and dacarbazine or doxorubicin (Auerbach et al. 1988; Berruti et al. 2012)· In a recent study, including small numbers of children, high-dose MIBG therapy was used with stem cell support producing an improved 5-year survival rate of 64% but with significant toxicities (Gonias et al. 2009).

Targeted oral agents such as sunitinib may have a palliative role (Ayala-Ramirez et al. 2012).

35.8 Carotid Body Tumours

Carotid body tumours (CBT) are a distinct clinical group of extra-adrenal paragangliomas which arise in the chemoreceptive tissue located in the carotid bifurcation or glomus body and hence also described as glomus body tumours. Certainly, in adults, CBT is the most frequent paraganglioma in the head and neck (Dardik et al. 2002; Pellitteri et al. 2004); however, data in children is lacking with only case reports or cases in adults series (Dickinson et al. 1986; Shamblin et al. 1971) and small paediatric paraganglioma series (Gounot et al. 1990; Takautz et al. 2003). Carotid body tumours are often bilateral (Dardik et al. 2002; Dickinson et al. 1986), can be multicentric, the most common association between an intravagal paraganglioma and CBTs (Beltsevich et al. 2004). Carotid body tumours are usually sporadic but rarely can have a familial inheritance associated with paraganglioma syndromes due to mutations in the succinate dehydrogenase (SDH) genes (Benn et al. 2006). Presentation is usually as a slowly enlarging pulsatile mass in the upper neck, often misdiagnosed as cervical lymphadenopathy, neurofibromas or brachial cysts. Later, cranial nerve or adjacent pharynx may be involved (Gujrathi and Donald 2005; Takautz et al. 2003). Less than 10% are secretory with sympathetic involvement (Kuchakulla et al. 2018).

Malignancy is rare in CBTs (Shamblin et al. 1971), and as with paragangliomas arising at other sites, it is defined by metastatic spread, usually to cervical lymph nodes but infrequently to distant organs. The risk of malignancy is probably greatest in younger patients with familial paraganglioma syndrome associated with SDH mutations (Timmers et al. 2007b). There is only one report, however, of a child with distant metastatic disease from a CBT, and only 5% had metastases in the only paediatric series (Hajnzic et al. 1999; Kuchakulla et al. 2018).

Once CBTs are suspected, ultrasound studies can help exclude other causes of neck masses such as lymph nodes, thyroid or brachial cysts with Doppler studies evaluating the hypervascularity of the tumour. MRI scanning, however, usually reveals a well-defined carotid space lesion (van der Mey et al. 2001). ^{111}In octreotide scintigraphy can detect metastases in patients with malignant tumours with a role for PET scanning (Gujrathi and Donald 2005). Complete surgical resection is usually curative for the majority of patients with prior tumour embolisation only being reported in one child (Waguespack and Ying 2014) although there is still a risk of stroke or cranial nerve palsies. Larger and more invasive CBTs in children may require carotid shunting and vascular reconstruction (Thompson and Cohen 1989). The treatment of malignant CBTs remains, as for other paragangliomas, surgical, though as non-secreting tumours they don't respond to α-adrenergic blockade with phenoxybenzamine.

35.9 Genetic Management

Following the diagnosis of paraganglioma in childhood, referral for genetic testing should be done in all cases as approximately nearly half of paragangliomas in children will have an underlying genetic or hereditary basis (de Krijger et al. 2006). The absence of a family history does not preclude the patient having a mutation; indeed childhood paragangliomas can be considered a probable genetic disease requiring lifelong follow-up (Ein et al. 1990). It is important when taking a history and examining patients with paragangliomas to consider a diagnosis of the following hereditary syndromes.

35.9.1 Multiple Endocrine Neoplasia Type 2 (MEN 2)

This autosomal dominant tumour syndrome is a result of a mutation in the *RET* (rearranged during transfection) proto-oncogene in an autosomal dominant pattern. There is a high percentage of bilateral paragangliomas in more than 50% of cases, but malignant paragangliomas are rare (Waguespack and Ying 2014).

35.9.2 Von Hippel–Lindau (VHL) Disease

This autosomal dominant disease is due to a mutation in the *VHL* gene on chromosome 3p25-26 with paragangliomas developing in 10–20% of patients (Ong et al. 2007). Though the paragangliomas mainly develop in adulthood, they have been reported in children with VHL and are often bilateral but malignant disease is rare (de Krijger et al. 2006; Pham et al. 2006; Waguespack et al. 2010).

35.9.3 Neurofibromatosis Type 1 (NF 1)

This distinctive clinical syndrome occurs from a mutation in the *NF1* gene on chromosome 17q11.2. Paragangliomas only occur in a small percentage of patients.

35.9.4 Paraganglioma Syndrome (SDH)

Mutations in sub-units of the succinic dehydrogenase enzyme complex gene in the mitochondrial respiratory chain are associated with familial paragangliomas. Two particular sub-units, SDH and SDHB, are most likely to be associated with childhood with paragangliomas (Stringel et al. 1980). Patients with SDHD mutation are more likely to have head and neck paragangliomas, multi-focal disease and a small chance of developing malignant tumours (Benn et al. 2006; Havekes et al. 2007). Patients with SDHB mutations are more likely to present at a younger age with paragangliomas in extra-adrenal sites with a higher chance of metastatic disease (Benn et al. 2006; Timmers et al. 2007b; Waguespack et al. 2010).

The genetic causes are rapidly expanding, and newer genes associated include KIF1B, TMEM127, EGLN1, MAX and HIF2A (Dahia 2014).

35.10 Conclusions

The management and diagnosis of paragangliomas in childhood has improved over time with better preparation prior to surgery, increasing use of laparoscopic techniques and potentially newer imaging studies to detect metastatic disease. The outcome is generally excellent for children, but genetic testing is paramount to determine the lifelong risk for further disease and malignancy.

References

Auerbach SD, Steakley LS, Rc Y et al (1988) Malignant phaeochromocytoma: effective treatment with a combination of cyclophosphamide, vincristine and decarbazine. Internal Med 109:267–273

Ayala-Ramirez M, Chougnet CN, Habra MA et al (2012) Treatment with sunitinib for patients with progressive metastatic pheochromocytomas and sympathetic paragangliomas. J Clin Endocrinol Metab 97: 4040–4050

Barontini M, Levin G, Sanso G (2006) Characteristics of pheochromocytoma in a 4- to 20-year-old population. Ann N Y Acad Sci 1073:30–37

Beltsevich DG, Kuznetsov NS, Kazaryan AM et al (2004) Pheochromocytoma surgery: epidemiologic peculiarities in children. World J Surg 28:592–596

Benn DE, Gimenez-Roqueplo AP, Reilly JR et al (2006) Clinical presentation and penetrance of pheochromocytoma/paraganglioma syndromes. J Clin Endocrinol Metab 91:827–836

Berruti A, Baudin E, Gelderblom H et al (2012) Adrenal cancer: ESMO Clinical Practice Guidelines for diagnosis, treatment and follow-up. Ann Oncol 23: 131–138

Brunt LM, Lairmore TC, Doherty GM et al (2002) Adrenalectomy for familial pheochromocytoma in the laparoscopic era. Ann Surg 235:713–720

Chrisoulidou A, Kaltsas G, Ilias I et al (2007) The diagnosis and management of malignant phaeochromocytoma and paraganglioma. Endocr Relat Cancer 14:569–585

Dahia PL (2014) Pheochromocytoma and paraganglioma pathogenesis: learning from genetic heterogeneity. Nat Rev Cancer 14:108–119

Dardik A, Eisele DW, Williams GM et al (2002) A contemporary assessment of carotid body tumor surgery. Vasc Endovasc Surg 36:277–283

de Krijger RR, Petri BJ, van Nederveen FH et al (2006) Frequent genetic changes in childhood pheochromocytomas. Ann N Y Acad Sci 1073:166–176

Deal JE, Sever PS, Barratt TM et al (1990) Pheochromocytoma—investigation and management of 10 cases. Arch Dis Child 65:269–274

Dickinson PH, Griffin SM, Guy AJ et al (1986) Carotid body tumor: 30 years experience. Br J Surg 73:14–16

Ein SH, Standling WD et al (1990) Recurrent phaeochromocytomas in children. J Pediatr Surg 25:1063–1065

Fottner C, Helisch A, Anlauf M et al (2010) 6-18F-fluoro-L-dihydroxyphenylalanine positron emission tomography is superior to 123Imetaiodobenzyl-guanidine scintigraphy in the detection of extraadrenal and hereditary pheochromocytomas and paragangliomas: correlation with vesicular monoamine transporter expression. J Clin Endocrinol Metab 95: 2800–2810

Goldstein RE, O'Neill JA Jr, Holcomb GW III et al (1999) Clinical experience over 48 years with pheochromocytoma. Ann Surg 229:755–764

Gonias S, Goldsby R, Matthay KK et al (2009) Phase II study of high-dose [131I]metaiodobenzylguanidine therapy for patients with metastatic pheochromocytoma and paraganglioma. J Clin Oncol 27(25):4162–4168

Gounot E, Couillault G, Maingueneau C et al (1990) Paraganglioma of the carotid body. A propos of a case in a 14-year-old child. Chir Pediatr 31:125–126

Gujrathi CS, Donald PJ (2005) Current trends in the diagnosis and management of the head and neck paragangliomas. Curr Opin OtolaryngoHead Neck Surg 13:339–342

Hack HA (2000) The perioperative management of children with phaeochromocytoma. Paediatr Anaesth 10:463–476

Hajnzic TF, Kruslin B, Belicza M (1999) Carotid body paraganglioma in a 9-year-old boy with extensive pulmonary metastases. Med Pediatr Oncol 32:399–400

Havekes B, Corssmit EP, Jansen JC et al (2007) Malignant paragangliomas associated with mutations in the succinate dehydrogenase D gene. J Clin Endocrinol Metab 92:1245–1248

Haws R, Joseph M, Adelman R (2007) Two cases of pheochromocytoma presenting with ADHD (attention deficit hyperactivity disorder)-like symptoms. Pediatr Nephrol 23:473–475

Ilias I, Pacak K (2004) Current approaches and recommended algorithm for the diagnostic localization of pheochromocytoma. J Clin Endocrinol Metab 89:479–491

Kuchakulla M, Shah AH, Armstrong V, J et al. (2018) Multimodal management of pediatric carotid body tumors: a systematic review and case illustrations. J Neurosurg Pediatr 23:325–332

Lenders JW, Pacak K, Walther MM et al (2002) Biochemical diagnosis of pheochromocytoma: which test is best? JAMA 287:1427–1434

Loh KC, Fitzgerald PA, Matthay KK et al (1997) The treatment of malignant phaeochromocytoma with iodine- 131 metaiodobenzylguanidine (131 I-MIBG): a comprehensive review of 116 reported patients. J Endocrinol Investig 29:648–658

Ong KR, Woodward ER, Killick P et al (2007) Genotype-phenotype correlations in von Hippel-Lindau disease. Hum Mutat 28:143–149

Pacak K, Linehan WM, Eisenhofer G et al (2001) Recent advances in genetics, diagnosis, localization, and treatment of pheochromocytoma. Ann Intern Med 134:315–329

Pacak K, Eisenhofer G, Ahlman H et al (2007) Pheochromocytoma: recommendations for clinical practice from the First International Symposium. October 2005. Nat Clin Pract Endocrinol Metab 3:92–102

Pellitteri PK, Rinaldo A, Myssiorek D et al (2004) Paragangliomas of the head and neck. Oral Oncol 40:563–575

Pham TH, Moir C, Thompson GB et al (2006) Pheochromocytoma and paraganglioma in children: a review of medical and surgical management at a tertiary care center. Pediatrics 118:1109–1117

Shamblin WR, ReMine WH, Sheps SG et al (1971) Carotid body tumor (chemodectoma). Clinicopathologic analysis of ninety cases. Am J Surg 122:732–739

Sisson JC, Shapiro B, Shulkin BL et al (1999) The treatment of malignant phaeochromocytoma with 131-I metaiodobenzylguanidine and chemotherapy. Am J Clin Oncol 22:364

Spoudeas HA, Harrison B. (2005) Paediatric endocrine tumours. The British Society of Paediatric Endocrinology and Diabetes and the UK Children's Cancer Study Group

Stringel G, Ein SH, Creighton R et al (1980) Pheochromocytoma in children-an update. J Pediatr Surg 15:496–500

Takautz TM, Pratt CB, Jenkins JJ et al (2003) Pediatric extraadrenal paragaglioma. J Pediatr Surg 38:1317–1321

Thompson JW, Cohen SR (1989) Management of bilateral carotid body tumors and a glomus jugulare tumor in a child. Int J Pediatr Otorhinolaryngol 17:75–87

Timmers HJ, Kozupa A, Chen CC et al (2007a) Superiority of fluorodeoxyglucose positron emission tomography to other functional imaging techniques in the evaluation of metastatic SDHB-associated pheochromocytoma and paraganglioma. J Clin Oncol 25:2262–2269

Timmers HJ, Kozupa A, Eisenhofer G et al (2007b) Clinical presentations, biochemical phenotypes, and genotype-phenotype correlations in patients with succinate dehydrogenase subunit B-associated pheochromocytomas and paragangliomas. J Clin Endocrinol Metab 92:779–786 van der Mey AG, Jansen JC, van Baalen JM (2001) Management of carotid body tumors. Otolaryngol Clin N Am 34:907–924

Velchik M, Alavi A, Kresse LH (1989) Localisation of phaeochromocytoma. MIBG, CT and MR correlation. J Nucl Med 30:328–336

Waguespack S, Ying AK (2014) Phaeochromocytoma and multiple endocrine neoplasia syndromes. In: Sperling MA (ed) Pediatric endocrinology, 4th edn. Elsevier Sounders, Philadelphia. PA, pp 533–568

Waguespack SG, Rich T, Grubbs E et al (2010) A current review of the etiology, diagnosis, and treatment of pediatric pheochromocytoma and paraganglioma. J Clin Endocrinol Metab 95:2023–2037

Weise M, Merke DP, Pacak K et al (2002) Utility of plasma free metanephrines for detecting childhood pheochromocytoma. J Clin Endocrinol Metab 87:1955–1960

36 Adrenocortical Tumors in Children

Carlos Rodriguez-Galindo

Adrenocortical tumors (ACT) encompass a spectrum of diseases with often seamless transition from benign (adenoma) to malignant (carcinoma) behavior. Their incidence in children is extremely low (only 0.2% of pediatric cancers) (Bernstein and Gurney 1999), and most pediatric oncologists see few cases or none. Little is known about these tumors, and most available information has been learned from their more frequent adult counterpart. In recent years, an international registry has provided insight into the clinical characteristics and relevant management issues regarding pediatric ACT and tumor tissue for biological studies (Ribeiro et al. 2001). These studies have resulted in the discovery of a novel mechanism of tumorigenesis (Wooten and King 1993).

36.1 Epidemiology of Adrenocortical Cancer

ACT appear to follow a bimodal distribution, with peaks during the first and fourth decades (Figueiredo et al. 2006). In children, 25 new cases are expected to occur annually in the United States, for an estimated annual incidence of 0.2–0.3 cases per million. Internationally, however, the incidence of ACT appears to vary substantially. The incidence of ACT is particularly high in Southern Brazil, where it is approximately 10–15 times that observed in the United States. Most cases occur in the contiguous states of Sao Paulo, Paraná, and Santa Catarina (Pianovski et al. 2006; Ribeiro and Figueiredo 2004; Rodriguez-Galindo et al. 2005).

Predisposing genetic factors have been implicated in >50% of the cases in North America and Europe and in 95% of the Brazilian cases. Germline *TP53* mutations are almost always the predisposing factors (Mastellaro et al. 2017; Wasserman et al. 2015). In the non-Brazilian cases, relatives of children with ACT often, though not invariably, have a high incidence of other non-adrenal cancers (Li-Fraumeni syndrome), and germline mutations usually occur within the region coding for the *TP53* DNA-binding domain (exons 5–8, primarily at highly conserved amino acid residues) (Wasserman et al. 2015). In the Brazilian cases, in contrast, the patients' families do not exhibit a high incidence of cancer, and a single, unique mutation at codon 337 in exon 10 of the *TP53* gene is consistently observed (see below).

Patients with Beckwith-Wiedemann and hemihypertrophy syndromes have a predisposition to cancer, and as many as 16% of their neoplasms are ACT (Hoyme et al. 1998). However, less than 1% of children with ACT have these syndromes (Steenman et al. 2000). ACT have also been reported in association with other

C. Rodriguez-Galindo (✉)
Department of Global Pediatric Medicine, St. Jude Children's Research Hospital, Memphis, TN, USA
e-mail: carlos.rodriguez-galindo@stjude.org

D. T. Schneider et al. (eds.), *Rare Tumors in Children and Adolescents*, Pediatric Oncology,
https://doi.org/10.1007/978-3-030-92071-5_36

genetic diseases such as congenital adrenal hyperplasia (Varan et al. 2000).

The differential diagnosis of ACT includes other diseases characterized by adrenal hormone hyperproduction. ACTH-independent macronodular adrenal hyperplasia (AIMAH) is a benign proliferative disorder of the adrenal cortex that presents with ACTH-independent Cushing syndrome. The majority of patients with AIMAH present in the fifth decade of life with sporadic isolated disease; however, in children, AIMAH can be associated with the McCune-Albright syndrome (Sutter and Grimberg 2006). A similar macronodular adrenocortical hyperplasia is seen in up to one-third of patients with multiple endocrine neoplasia type 1 (MEN1) syndrome, and although rare, adrenocortical carcinomas have been described in this population, usually in adult age (Langer et al. 2002). Primary pigmented nodular adrenocortical disease (PPNAD) is a benign bilateral proliferative disorder characterized by small hyperpigmented nodules, usually associated with the Carney complex. This is an autosomal dominant syndrome that includes lentiginosis (perioral, ocular, or genital), cardiac and peripheral myxomas, melanotic schwannomas, and endocrine over-activity. Clinically evident PPNAD is seen in up to 30% of patients with the Carney complex and usually presents in childhood, late adolescence, or early adulthood (Sutter and Grimberg 2006).

36.2 Biology of ACT

The molecular mechanisms of tumorigenesis of the adrenal cortex are not well understood (Kirschner 2002; Stojadinovic et al. 2002; Barlaskar and Hammer 2007). Carcinogenesis is a multistep process, and the pathogenesis of ACT may combine dedifferentiation and unchecked proliferation induced through the activation of hormonal or growth factor signaling receptors. The insulin-like growth factor (IGF) system is well characterized for its contribution to normal and pathological adrenocortical growth. Clues to the role of this pathway in the development of ACC also came through the recognition of the increased incidence of ACC in children with Beckwith-Wiedemann syndrome (BWS) (Steenman et al. 2000). Genetic alterations associated with BWS are mapped to regions of chromosome band 11p15 designated BWS chromosomal regions (*BWSCR*) 1, 2, and 3 (Steenman et al. 2000). *IGF2* is mapped to *BWSCR1*. The strong association of BWS, *IGF2*, and ACC suggests that IGF2 participates in tumorigenesis, and studies have shown increased IGF2 protein and mRNA in ACC (Ilvesmaki et al. 1993; Boulle et al. 1998). Sporadic ACT also show striking overexpression of *IGF2*, and studies in adults have documented >100-fold higher expression levels in carcinomas in comparison to adenomas and normal adrenal tissue (Gicquel et al. 2001). This differential *IGF2* expression between adenomas and carcinomas doesn't seem to be observed in pediatric tumors (see below) (Almeida et al. 2008; West et al. 2007). Interestingly, the antiproliferative effect of ACTH is blunted in ACT cell lines overexpressing *IGF1R* (Weber et al. 2000). Further, transgenic mice expressing *IGF2* postnatally develop adrenal hyperplasia (although not frank malignancy) (Weber et al. 1999). Taken together, the evidence strongly suggests that the IGF system is involved in adrenal growth and tumorigenesis. High local IGF2 levels combined with elevated *IGF1R* expression would provide a significant growth advantage, but additional steps are required for neoplastic transformation (Kirschner 2002; Barlaskar and Hammer 2007; Weber et al. 2000). Studies in several model organisms indicate the presence of undifferentiated multipotent adrenocortical cells, and a few molecular studies have implicated Wnt signaling pathway activation in ACC (Tissier et al. 2005). Further investigations are necessary to elucidate the contributions of developmental signaling pathways like Wnt in adrenal tumorigenesis.

The hypothetical multistep transformation process also requires intracellular signaling abnormalities other than dedifferentiation- and proliferation-inducing signals. *TP53* mutations appear to underlie such abnormalities in most cases, and ACT are strongly associated with germline *TP53* mutations (Wasserman et al. 2015). ACT are among the tumors most increased in frequency in families with Li-Fraumeni syndrome (Birch et al. 2001; Kleihues et al. 1997; Gonzalez et al. 2009), suggesting that germline *TP53* mutations exert tissue-specific effects. The diagnosis of ACT in a young patient should be considered a strong indicator of a germline *TP53* mutation, regardless of the family history (Gonzalez et al. 2009). A wide spectrum of germline *TP53* alterations have been described in ACT, and these mutations may contribute to the etiology of more than 80% of cases in children (Varley et al. 1999; Wagner et al. 1994). Consistent with the presence of a germline *TP53* mutation, relatives of children with ACT often have a high incidence of cancer; however, the lack of family history should not preclude investigation of *TP53* germline status (Varley et al. 1999; Wagner et al. 1994). In North American children, the spectrum of germline *TP53* mutations in ACT is quite diverse, although germline mutations occur primarily in the *TP53* DNA-binding domains (exons 4–8) (Wagner et al. 1994; Ariffin et al. 2008; Khayat and Johnston 2004). In the Brazilian cases, by contrast, a single mutation in exon 10 of the *TP53* gene is consistently observed, and it is associated with a cumulative incidence of cancer of approximately 20% at 45 years of age (Rossbach et al. 2008). This mutation encodes an arginine in place of histidine at codon 337 (*TP53*-R337H) within the tetramerization domain. Functional analyses have shown that the mutant TP53 retains transactivation function and can induce apoptosis (Wooten and King 1993). However, the mutant tetramerization domain is less stable than the wild-type domain and is sensitive to slightly increased pH, suggesting that a unique physiological condition within adrenocortical cells may contribute to the observed tissue-restricted pathogenesis (Reincke et al. 1994). Thus, this inherited unique *TP53* mutation represents a low-penetrant, hypomorphic allele that contributes to the development of ACT in a tissue-specific manner (Wooten and King 1993). Other *TP53* mutations, such as the *TP53*R157L, with sufficient activity to suppress Li-Fraumeni syndrome but not ACC, have been described (DiGiammarino et al. 2001), thus the importance of in-depth evaluation and genetic counseling of children with ACT and their families.

The molecular characteristics of childhood ACC have been recently described by Pinto et al. (2015). The most common genomic alteration, present in approximately 90% of cases, was copy number loss of heterozygosity for 11p15 with retention of the paternal allele resulting in *IGF2* overexpression. *TP53* mutations were also commonly observed. Twelve of 71 cases had the Brazilian founder R337H *TP53* germline mutation. Excluding the Brazilian founder mutation cases, *TP53* germline mutations were observed in approximately one-third of cases, with somatic *TP53* mutations observed in approximately 10% of the remaining cases, such that approximately 40% of non-Brazilian cases had *TP53* mutations (Mastellaro et al. 2017). Among cases with *TP53* mutations, chromosome 17 loss of heterozygosity with selection against wild-type *TP53* was present in virtually all cases. *ATRX* genomic alterations (primarily structural variants) were present in approximately 20% of cases. All *ATRX* alterations occurred in the presence of *TP53* alterations. The co-occurrence of *TP53* and *ATRX* mutations correlated with advanced stage, large tumor size, increased telomere length, and poor prognosis. Activating *CTNNB1* mutations were found in approximately 20% of cases and were mutually exclusive with *TP53* germline alterations.

36.3 Clinical Characteristics of Pediatric ACT

The clinical characteristics, treatment, and outcome of ACT have been described mainly in adults; because there are few reports about pediatric ACT, it is difficult to discriminate features unique to either age group. The degree and type of endocrine disturbance appear to be related to patient age (Dohna et al. 2000). Older patients tend to have a much higher incidence of nonfunctional tumors, whereas more than 90% of childhood ACT are functional (Dohna et al. 2000; Figueiredo et al. 1999). Adults usually have mixed virilization-hypercortisolism syndromes, whereas virilization syndrome is the most common presentation in children (Dohna et al. 2000).

Data from the International Pediatric Adrenocortical Tumor Registry (IPACTR) has characterized its biology, clinical features, and prognostic factors (Ribeiro et al. 2001).

Childhood ACT typically present during the first 5 years of life (median age, 3–4 years), although there is a second, smaller peak during adolescence (Ribeiro et al. 2001; Figueiredo et al. 1999; Loncarevic et al. 2008; Doghman et al. 2007; Wajchenberg et al. 2000; Ribeiro et al. 1990). Female sex is consistently predominant in most studies, with a female-to-male ratio of 1.6:1(Wajchenberg et al. 2000; Ribeiro et al. 1990; Ciftci et al. 2001). According to the IPACTR data, the female predominance is more significant for patients younger than 3 years of age (1.7:1) and for patients older than 13 years (6.2:1), but not for patients between 3 and 12 years (Ribeiro et al. 2001; Ribeiro et al. 1990). Because pediatric ACT are almost universally functional, they cause endocrine disturbances, and a diagnosis is usually made 5–8 months after the first signs and symptoms emerge (Ribeiro et al. 1990, 2001; Figueiredo et al. 1999; Doghman et al. 2007). Virilization (pubic hair, accelerated growth, enlarged penis, clitoromegaly, hirsutism, and acne) due to excess of androgen secretion is seen, alone or in combination with hypercortisolism, in more than 80% of patients (Fig. 36.1). Isolated Cushing syndrome is very rare (5% of patients), and it appears to occur more frequently in older children (median age 12.6 years in the IPACTR) (Ribeiro et al. 1990, 2001; Figueiredo et al. 1999; Doghman et al. 2007). Likewise, nonfunctional tumors are rare (less than 10%) and tend to occur in older children (Ribeiro et al. 1990). Half of the patients have severe hypertension at presentation, and hypertensive crisis resulting in seizures is the presenting feature in 10% of cases (Ribeiro et al. 1990; Driver et al. 1998). However, isolated Conn syndrome with hypertension, hypokalemia, and pseudoparalysis resulting from hyperproduction of aldosterone or deoxycorticosterone is extremely rare (less than 1% in the IPACTR data) but has been described (Ribeiro et al. 1990, 2001; Wieneke et al. 2003) An abdominal mass can be palpated in approximately half of the patients (Doghman et al. 2007).

At the time of diagnosis, two-thirds of pediatric patients have limited disease (tumors are completely resected), and the remaining patients have either unresectable or metastatic disease (Ribeiro et al. 1990, 2001). In up to 20% of the cases, intracaval extension of the tumor is present (Ribeiro et al. 1990; Sandrini et al. 1997). Unlike adult ACT, histologic differentiation of adenomas and carcinomas is difficult. However, approximately 10–20% of pediatric cases are adenomas (Ribeiro et al. 1990, 2001; Figueiredo et al. 1999)

36.4 Diagnosis

Children with ACT usually present with striking endocrine syndromes, most commonly virilization, and thus are usually diagnosed earlier than adults. Because of the hormone hypersecretion, it is possible to establish an endocrine profile for each particular tumor, which may facilitate the evaluation of response to treatment and monitor for tumor recurrence. Laboratory evaluation can also help distinguish physiological adrenarche or congenital adrenal hyperplasia from ACC. Patients with adrenarche have elevated basal concentration of DHEAS and androstenedione, while those with congenital adrenal hyperplasia may show increased basal or ACTH-stimulated peak concentration of 17-OH-progesterone (Bugg et al. 1994). While the diagnosis of ACC is usually clinical, imaging studies are important to complete staging and for surgical planning. Magnetic resonance imaging (MRI) and computed tomography (CT) are needed for the evaluation of the size and location of the primary tumor, the degree of invasion to surrounding structures, the presence of metastases, and the involvement of venous structures. Although bone metastases at diagnosis are extremely rare, scintigraphic studies are recommended. On CT, large tumors usually have a central area of stellate appearance caused by hemorrhage, necrosis, and fibrosis; this central

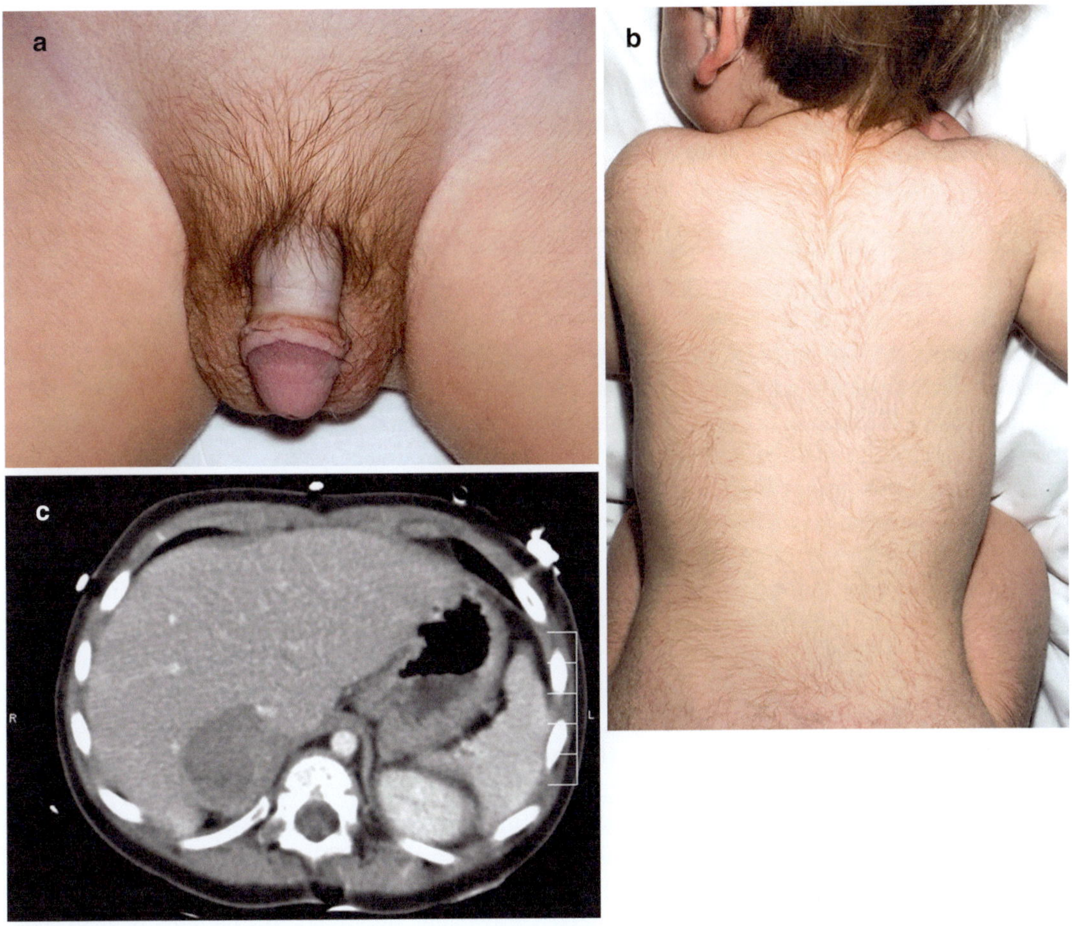

Fig. 36.1 A 2-year-old boy presenting with virilization (**a**, **b**). CT scan demonstrated a right adrenal mass (**c**)

area is usually hyperintense on T2-weighted MRI and STIR images. Calcifications are also common (Teinturier et al. 1999). In order to evaluate tumor extension into the vena cava, ultrasound or MRI is always recommended, and a careful evaluation of the presence of a tumor thrombus must always be performed prior to surgery (Sandrini et al. 1997). Because ACT are metabolically active whole-body fluorodeoxyglucose (FDG), positron emission tomography (PET) is being increasingly used. Although the experience in pediatrics is limited, available information suggests that this may be a very useful technique in the imaging of the regional and metastatic extension and in the diagnosis of recurrences in areas not typically imaged (Michalkiewicz et al. 2004; Narasimhan et al. 2003).

The distinction between benign (adenomas) and malignant (carcinomas) tumors can be problematic. In fact, adenoma and carcinoma appear to share multiple genetic aberrations and may represent points on a continuum of cellular transformation (Hanna et al. 2008; Wang et al. 2007). Macroscopically, adenomas tend to be well defined and spherical, and they never invade surrounding structures. They are typically small (usually <200 cm^3), and some studies have included size as a criterion for adenoma. Microscopically, they may resemble normal adrenal cortex. By contrast, carcinomas have macroscopic features suggestive of malignancy; they are larger, and they show marked lobulation with extensive areas of hemorrhage and necrosis. Microscopically, carcinomas comprise larger cells with eosinophilic cytoplasm, arranged in alveolar clusters. Several authors have proposed histologic criteria that may help to distinguish the two types of neoplasm (Tucci et al. 2005; Ribeiro et al. 2000). However, morphologic criteria may not allow reliable distinction of benign and malignant ACC. Mitotic rate is consistently reported as the most important determinant of aggressive behavior (Tucci et al. 2005; Mackie et al. 2006; Murphy et al. 2008; Weiss 1984). *IGF*2 expression also appears to discriminate between carcinomas and adenomas in adults, but not in children (Slooten et al. 1985; Weiss et al. 1989) Other histopathologic variables are also important, and risk groups may be identified on the basis of a score derived from characteristics, such as venous, capsular, or adjacent organ invasion; tumor necrosis; mitotic rate; and the presence of atypical mitoses (Murphy et al. 2008). Two retrospective studies have investigated histological criteria of malignancy in pediatric ACT. Bugg et al. analyzed histology, ploidy, proliferative index, and tumor size in 54 cases (Bugg et al. 1994). The histologic criteria for malignant tumors were the mitotic index, the presence of confluent necrosis and atypical mitoses, and the nuclear grade, as previously defined by Weiss (Weiss 1984; Weiss et al. 1989). The most statistically significant predictors of outcome were tumor histology and tumor weight (<100 g vs. >100 g). Ploidy and proliferative index were not predictive of outcome (Kendrick et al. 2001). More recently, Wieneke et al. analyzed features associated with increased probability of a malignant behavior in a series of 83 pediatric ACC (Wieneke et al. 2003). Tumor weight >400 g; tumor size >10.5 cm in the largest diameter; vena cava, capsular, or vascular invasion; extension into periadrenal soft tissues; confluent necrosis; presence of severe nuclear atypia; atypical mitoses; and presence of >15 mitotic figures per 20 high-power field were all associated with adverse outcome. However, on multivariate analysis, only vena cava invasion, presence of necrosis, and high mitotic rate retained prognostic significance. Recently, DNA methylation analysis has proven to identify two subgroups that segregate with *CTNNB1* and *TP53* variants; this technology can provide additional support in diagnosis and prognostication when combined with standard histological evaluation (Harrison et al. 1999).

36.5 Prognostic Factors

In an analysis of 40 cases in Southern Brazil, Ribeiro et al. (1990) found tumor volume >200 mL or weight >80 g, and age >3.5 years, to be associated with worse outcome, although only tumor size was independently predictive. In the IPACTR data, several clinical features, including age, sex, clinical syndrome, interval between first symptoms and diagnosis, blood pressure, disease stage, tumor spillage, tumor thrombus, and tumor weight, were examined for their association with outcome. In patients with localized disease, age between 0 and 3 years, virilization alone, normal blood pressure, disease stage I, absence of spillage during surgery, and tumor weight ≤200 g were associated with a greater probability of survival. In a Cox regression model analysis, only stage I, virilization alone, and age 0–3 years were independently associated with a better outcome (Ribeiro et al. 1990) (Figs. 36.2 and 36.3).

Thus, available data suggest that tumor size is especially important in children; patients with small tumors have an excellent outcome with surgery alone, regardless of histologic features (Ribeiro et al. 1990). A staging system based on disease extent and tumor size has been proposed on the basis of these findings (Table 36.1) (Wajchenberg et al. 2000). Low stage and complete resection are the most important prognostic factors (Rosati et al. 2008; Cecchetto et al. 2016; Ribeiro et al. 1990) more than 90% of patients with small localized tumors are long-term survivors, compared with 10% of those with metastatic disease (Ribeiro et al. 2001; Rosati et al. 2008) (Fig. 36.3). Determining the prognosis of patients with intermediate-stage disease is much more difficult. Despite complete tumor resection, disease recurs in 50% of patients with large localized tumors (Ribeiro et al. 2001). The reason for this increased risk of recurrence is not well understood; tumor spillage is common, and studies in adults have suggested that retroperitoneal

Fig. 36.2 Probability of 5-year event-free survival according to age at the time of diagnosis in 254 children with ACT. (From Michalkiewicz et al. 2004 with permission)

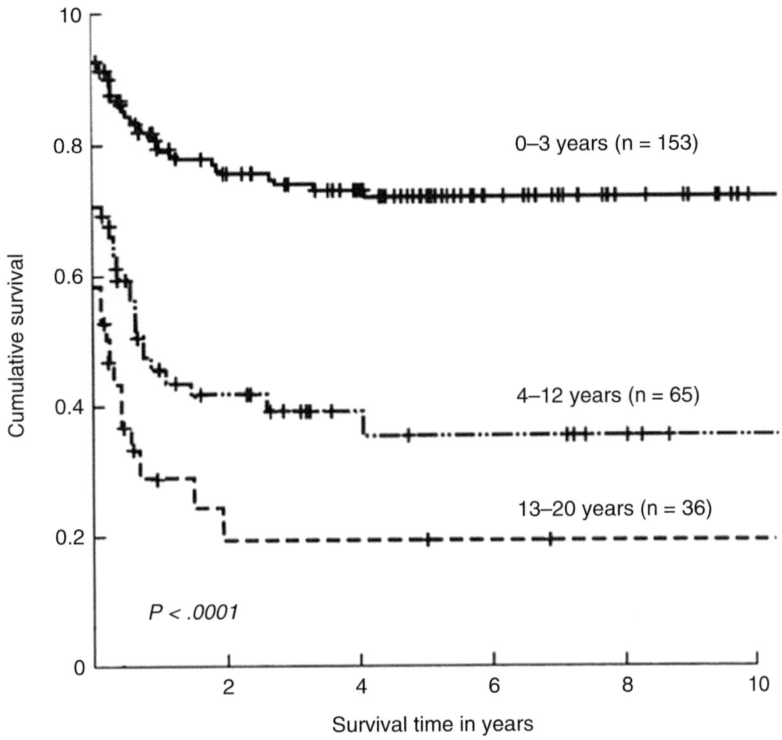

Fig. 36.3 Probability of 5-year event-free survival according to disease stage at the time of diagnosis in 254 children with ACT. (From Michalkiewicz et al. 2004 with permission)

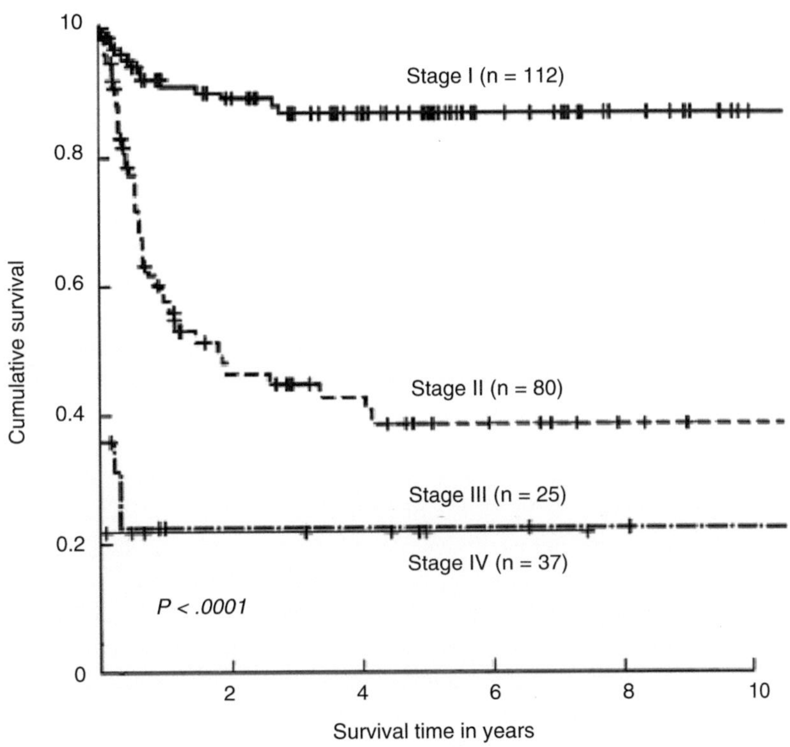

Table 36.1 Proposed staging of adrenocortical tumors in children (modified from Sandrini et al. (1997))

• **Stage I**
– Completely resected, small tumors (<100 g and <200 cm^3) with normal post-operative hormone levels
• **Stage II**
– Completely resected, large tumors (≥100 g or ≥200 cm^3) with normal post-operative hormone levels
• **Stage III**
– Unresectable, gross, or microscopic residual disease
– Tumor spillage
– Patients with stage I and II tumors who fail to normalize hormone levels after surgery
– Patients with retroperitoneal lymph node involvement
• **Stage IV**
– Presence of distant metastases

lymph node involvement may play a role (Erickson et al. 2001).

36.6 Treatment of Pediatric ACT

The principles of therapy have been adapted from those established for adults (de Reynies et al. 2009; Fassnacht et al. 2020). Surgery is the mainstay of therapy, and for children with advanced disease, chemotherapy and mitotane have been proposed. An aggressive surgical approach of the primary tumor and all metastatic sites is recommended when feasible (Sandrini et al. 1997; Michalkiewicz et al. 1997). Because of tumor friability, rupture of the capsule with resultant tumor spillage is frequent (approximately 20% of initial resections and 43% of resections after recurrence) (Wajchenberg et al. 2000; Ribeiro et al. 1990). In fact, spontaneous tumor rupture resulting in acute abdomen as presentation of a pediatric ACT has been described (Zancanella et al. 2006). When the diagnosis of ACT is suspected, laparotomy and a curative procedure are recommended rather than a biopsy, to avoid the risk of tumor rupture and spillage (Hovi et al. 2003). Laparoscopic resection is associated with a high risk of rupture and peritoneal carcinomatosis; thus, open adrenalectomy remains the standard of care (Stewart et al. 2004). The lymph node drainage of the adrenal gland is complex. There is an extensive subserosal network of lymphatic channels around the gland, crossing several levels in different directions inside the fascia and connective tissue involving the adrenal gland. The incidence of lymph node involvement is not known, although some studies report it to be between 25% and 40% in adults (Erickson et al. 2001; Leung et al. 2002; Kardar 2001). Whether ipsilateral retroperitoneal lymph node dissection may improve, local control is a matter of debate, although the results of the ARAR0332 from the Children's Oncology Group seem to suggest that extended surgery may not play a role in childhood ACC (see below).

Chemotherapeutic regimens used for patients with advanced disease have been derived from the standard treatments used in adults. A cisplatin-based combination, usually incorporating doxorubicin and etoposide, is most commonly used. Because of cisplatin's renal dose-limiting toxicity, Ayass and coworkers substituted carboplatin for cisplatin given in combination with etoposide to a 17-month-old boy with ACT that had metastasized to the brain and chest. After complete resection of the primary tumor and eight cycles of etoposide and carboplatin, the metastatic disease responded completely, and the patient survived long-term (Gonzalez et al. 2005).

Little information is available about the use of mitotane in children, although response rates appear to be similar to those in adults (Crucitti et al. 1996). Compliance with mitotane administration is a limitation, and monitoring for neurotoxicity is particularly important as mitotane has been associated with motor and speech developmental delays (Lee et al. 1995). There have been several reports of complete responses in children with advanced or metastatic ACT, but these appear to be rare events. In a review of 11 children with advanced ACT treated with mitotane and a cisplatin-based chemotherapeutic regimen, measurable responses were seen in 7 patients. The mitotane daily dose required for therapeutic levels was around 4 g/m^2, and therapeutic levels were achieved after 4–6 months of therapy (Crucitti et al. 1996). Compliance with daily mitotane administration is a major limitation to therapy in young children; nausea, vomiting, diarrhea, and neurologic alterations are common (Crucitti et al. 1996). Monitoring for neurotoxicity is particularly important in young patients as the use of mitotane has been associated with motor and speech developmental delays (Lee et al. 1995).

The use of radiotherapy in pediatric ACT has not been consistently investigated. ACT are generally considered to be radioresistant (Dohna et al. 2000). Furthermore, because many children with ACT carry germline *TP53* mutations that predispose to cancer, radiation may increase the incidence of secondary tumors. Driver et al. reported that three of five long-term survivors of pediatric ACT died of secondary sarcoma that arose within the radiation field (Ayass et al. 1991). For most patients with metastatic or recurrent disease that is unresponsive to mitotane and chemotherapy, repeated surgical resection is the only alternative. However, given the infiltrative nature of the disease, complete resection is difficult to achieve. Image-guided tumor ablation with radiofrequency currently offers a valid alternative for these patients. Radiofrequency ablation is a minimally invasive and safe treatment for patients in whom surgery may not be possible. Data regarding the use of this treatment modality in children is limited; however, it appears to offer a valid alternative for children with unresectable ACT (Coelho Netto et al. 1963).

Finally, advances in our understanding of ACT biology may lead to the identification of new molecular targets. In a pan-genomic characterization of adult ACC, at least one alteration of potential driver genes was found in 69% of tumors, with 51 potentially actionable alterations (Ostuni and Roginsky 1975). Tumor-infiltrating lymphocytes have been correlated with improved outcomes in adult ACC (De Leon et al. 2002; Landwehr et al. 2020), and checkpoint inhibitors have shown potential, with response rates ranging from 6% to 23% (Wood et al. 2003; Hoffer et al. 2009; Kirschner 2006; Barlaskar et al. 2009; Carneiro et al. 2019; Raj et al. 2020). We have previously reported the association of MHC class expression with outcome, suggesting that immune responses modulate tumorigenesis and may help identify those who could benefit from checkpoint inhibitors (Pinto et al. 2016). Responses to pembrolizumab have been reported in children (Geoerger et al. 2020).

36.7 A Collaborative Research Initiative for Childhood ACT

Cooperative multi-institutional efforts have been pivotal in the advancement of pediatric oncology during the past several decades (Ribeiro et al. 2012, Virgone et al. 2021). Rare pediatric tumors, however, have remained research orphans, and children with these rare malignancies have yet to benefit from group-wide initiatives. In recent years, the Children's Oncology Group (COG) has made a commitment to develop research programs in rare childhood malignancies. Part of this effort is a collaboration between COG and Brazilian institutions to develop a study protocol for childhood ACC (ARAR0332) (Table 36.2). This protocol investigated three main clinical questions: (1) the efficacy of surgery alone for stage I tumors; (2) the role of retroperitoneal lymph node resection in reducing local recurrence of stage II tumors; and (3) the impact of mitotane and cisplatin-based chemotherapy for unresectable and metastatic disease.

The analysis of the results of this study has been recently completed (Rodriguez-Galindo et al. 2021). Between 9/2006 and 5/2013, 78 patients (77 eligible, 51 females) were enrolled. The 5-year EFS estimates for stages I (24 patients), II (15 patients), III (24 patients), and IV

Table 36.2 Treatment on the COG ARAR 0332 protocol

Stage	Treatment
Stage I	• Surgery alone
Stage II	• Surgery
	• RPLN dissection
Stage III	• Mitotane
	• CDDP/ETO/DOX
	• Surgery + RPLN dissection
Stage IV	• Mitotane
	• CDDP/ETO/DOX
	• Surgery + RPLN dissection

Abbreviations: *RPLN* retroperitoneal lymph node, *CDDP* cisplatin, *ETO* etoposide, *DOX* doxorubicin

(14 patients) were 86.2%, 53.3%, 81%, and 7.1%, respectively. The corresponding 5-year OS estimates were 95.2%, 78.8%, 94.7%, and 15.6%, respectively. On univariate analysis, age, stage, presence of virilization, Cushing syndrome, or hypertension, germline *TP53* status, and presence of a somatic *ATRX* mutation were associated with outcome. On multivariable analysis, only stage and age were significantly associated with outcome. The probabilities of mitotane and chemotherapy feasibility events were 10.5% and 31.6%, respectively. The results of this study suggest that the outcome for children with stage I ACC is excellent with surgery. Outcome for patients with stage II disease is inferior despite RPLND. Patients with stage III ACC have an excellent outcome combining surgery and chemotherapy. Patients with stage IV ACC are older and have a poor outcome; new treatments should be explored for this high-risk group. The combination of mitotane and chemotherapy as prescribed in ARAR0332 resulted in significant toxicity; one-third of patients with advanced disease could not complete the scheduled treatment.

References

Almeida MQ, Fragoso MCBV, Lotfi CFP et al (2008) Expression of insulin-like growth factor-II and its receptor in pediatric and adult adrenocortical tumors. J Clin Endocrinol Metab 93:3524–3531

Ariffin H, Martel-Planche G, Daud SS, Ibrahim K, Hainaut P (2008) Li-Fraumeni syndrome in a Malaysian kindred. Cancer Genet Cytogenet 186:49–53

Ayass M, Gross S, Harper J (1991) High-dose carboplatinum and VP-16 in treatment of metastatic adrenal carcinoma. Am J Pediatr Hematol Oncol 13:470–472

Barlaskar FM, Hammer GD (2007) The molecular genetics of adrenocortical carcinoma. Rev Endocr Metab Disord 8:343–348

Barlaskar FM, Spalding AC, Heaton JH et al (2009) Preclinical targeting of the type I insulin-like growth factor receptor in adrenocortical carcinoma. J Clin Endocrinol Metab 94:204–212

Bernstein L, Gurney JG (1999) Carcinomas and other malignant epithelial neoplasms. In: Ries LAG, Smith MA, Gurney JG et al (eds) Cancer and survival among children and adolescents: United States SEER program 1975–1995. National Cancer Institute, SEER Program, Bethesda, MD, pp 139–147

Birch J, Alston RD, McNally RJQ et al (2001) Relative frequency and morphology of cancers in carriers of germline TP53 mutations. Oncogene 20: 4621–4628

Boulle N, Logie A, Gicquel C, Perin L, Le Bouc Y (1998) Increased levels of insulin-like growth factor II (IGF-II) and IGF binding protein-2 are associated with malignancy in sporadic adrenocortical tumors. J Clin Endocrinol Metab 83:1713–1720

Bugg MF, Ribeiro RC, Roberson PK et al (1994) Correlation of pathologic features with clinical outcome in pediatric adrenocortical neoplasia. Am J Clin Pathol 101:625–629

Carneiro BA, Konda B, Costa RB et al (2019) Nivolumab in metastatic adrenocortical carcinoma: results of a phase 2 trial. J Clin Endocrinol Metab 104: 6193–6200

Cecchetto G, Ganarin A, Bien E et al (2016) Outcome and prognostic factors in high-risk childhood adrenocortical carcinomas: a report from the European Cooperative Study Group on Pediatric Rare Tumors (EXPeRT). Pediatr Blood Cancer. https://doi.org/10.1002/pbc.26368

Ciftci AO, Senocak ME, Tanyel FC, Buyukpamukcu N (2001) Adrenocortical tumors in children. J Pediatr Surg 36:549–554

Coelho Netto AS, Wajchenberg BL, Ravaglia C et al (1963) Treatment of adrenocortical cancer with o,p′-DDD. Ann Intern Med 59:74–78

Crucitti F, Bellantone R, Ferrante A, Boscherini M, Crucitti P (1996) The Italian Registry for Adrenal Cortical Carcinoma: analysis of a multiinstitutional series of 129 patients. The ACC Italian Registry Study Group. Surgery 119:161–170

De Leon DD, Lange BJ, Walterhouse D, Moshang T (2002) Long-term (15 years) outcome in an infant with metastatic adrenocortical carcinoma. J Clin Endocrinol Metab 87:4452–4456

de Reynies A, Assie G, Rickman DS et al (2009) Gene expression profiling reveals a new classification of adrenocortical tumors and identifies molecular predictors of malignancy and survival. J Clin Oncol 27:1108–1115

DiGiammarino EL, Lee AS, Cadwell C et al (2001) A novel mechanism of tumorigenesis involving pH-dependent destabilization of a mutant p53 tetramer. Nat Struct Biol 9:12–16

Doghman M, Karpova T, Rodrigues GA et al (2007) Increased steroidogenic factor-1 dosage triggers adrenocortical cell proliferation and cancer. Mol Endocrinol 21:2968–2987

Dohna M, Reincke M, Mincheva A, Allolio B, Solinas-Toldo S, Lichter P (2000) Adrenocortical carcinoma is characterized by a high frequency of chromosomal gains and high-level amplifications. Genes Chromosomes Cancer 28:145–152

Driver CP, Birch J, Gough DCS, Bruce J (1998) Adrenal cortical tumors in childhood. Pediatr Hematol Oncol 15:527–532

Erickson LA, Jin L, Sebo TJ et al (2001) Pathologic features and expression of insulin-like growth factor-2 in adrenocortical neoplasms. Endocr Pathol 12:429–435

Fassnacht M, Assie G, Baudin E et al (2020) Adrenocortical carcinomas and malignant phaeochromocytomas: ESMO-EURACAN Clinical Practice Guidelines for diagnosis, treatment and follow-up. Ann Oncol 31:1476–1490

Figueiredo BC, Stratakis CA, Sandrini R et al (1999) Comparative genomic hybridization analysis of adrenocortical tumors of childhood. J Clin Endocrinol Metab 84:1116–1121

Figueiredo BC, Sandrini R, Zambetti GP et al (2006) Penetrance of adrenocortical tumours associated with the germline *TP53* R337H mutation. J Med Genet 43:91–96

Geoerger B, Kang HJ, Yalon-Oren M et al (2020) Pembrolizumab in paediatric patients with advanced melanoma or a PD-L1-positive, advanced, relapsed, or refractory solid tumour or lymphoma (KEYNOTE-051): interim analysis of an open-label, single-arm, phase 1–2 trial. Lancet Oncol 21: 121–133

Gicquel C, Bertagna X, Gaston V et al (2001) Molecular markers and long-term recurrences in a large cohort of patients with sporadic adrenocortical tumors. Cancer Res 61:6762–6767

Gonzalez RJ, Shapiro S, Sarlis N et al (2005) Laparoscopic resection of adrenal cortical carcinoma: a cautionary note. Surgery 138:1078–1086

Gonzalez KD, Noltner KA, Buzin CH et al (2009) Beyond Li Fraumeni syndrome: clinical characteristics of families with p53 germline mutations. J Clin Oncol 27:1250–1256

Habra MA, Stephen B, Campbell M et al (2019) Phase II clinical trial of pembrolizumab efficacy and safety in advanced adrenocortical carcinoma. J Immunother Cancer 7:253

Hanna AM, Pham TH, Skegard-Giesmann JR et al (2008) Outcome of adrenocortical tumors in children. J Pediatr Surg 43:843–849

Harrison LE, Gaudin PB, Brennan MF (1999) Pathologic features of prognostic significance for adrenocortical carcinoma after curative resection. Arch Surg 134:181–185

Hoffer FA, Daw NC, Xiong X et al (2009) A phase 1/pilot study of radiofrequency ablation for the treatment of recurrent pediatric solid tumors. Cancer 115:1328–1337

Hovi L, Wikström S, Vettenrante K, Heikkilä P, Saarinen-Pihkala UM (2003) Adrenocortical carcinoma in children: a role for etoposide and cisplatin adjuvant therapy? Preliminary report. Med Pediatr Oncol 40:324–326

Hoyme HE, Seaveer LH, Jones KL, Procopio F, Crooks W, Feingold M (1998) Isolated hemihyperplasia (Hemihypertrophy): report of a prospective multicenter study of the incidence of neoplasia and review. Am J Med Genet 79:274–278

Ilvesmaki V, Kahri AI, Miettinen PJ, Voutilainen R (1993) Insulin-like growth factors (IGFs) and their receptors in adrenal tumors: high IGF-II expression in functional adrenocortical carcinomas. J Clin Endocrinol Metab 77:852–858

Kardar AH (2001) Rupture of adrenal carcinoma after biopsy. J Urol 166:984

Kendrick ML, Lloyd R, Erickson L et al (2001) Adrenocortical carcinoma: surgical progress or status quo? Arch Surg 136:543–549

Khayat CM, Johnston DL (2004) Rhabdomyosarcoma, osteosarcoma, and adrenocortical carcinoma in a child with a germline p53 mutation. Pediatr Blood Cancer 43:683–686

Kirschner LS (2002) Signaling pathways in adrenocortical cancer. Ann N Y Acad Sci 968:222–239

Kirschner LS (2006) Emerging treatment strategies for adrenocortical carcinoma: a new hope. J Clin Endocrinol Metab 91:14–21

Kleihues P, Schäuble B, zur Hausen A, Estève J, Ohgaki H (1997) Tumors associated with *p53* germline mutations. A synopsis of 91 families. Am J Pathol 150:1–13

Landwehr LS, Altieri B, Schreiner J et al (2020) Interplay between glucocorticoids and tumor-infiltrating lymphocytes on the prognosis of adrenocortical carcinoma. J Immunother Cancer 8:e000469

Langer P, Cupisti K, Bartsch DK et al (2002) Adrenal involvement in multiple endocrine neoplasia type 1. World J Surg 26:891–896

Lee JE, Berger DH, el-Naggar AK et al (1995) Surgical management, DNA content, and patient survival in adrenal cortical carcinoma. Surgery 118:1090–1098

Leung LYJ, Leung WY, Chan KF, Fan TW, Chung KW, Chan CHS (2002) Ruptured adrenocortical carcinoma as a cause of paediatric acute abdomen. Pediatr Surg Int 18:730–732

Loncarevic IF, Herin A, Pososrki N, Linden T, Hoyer H, Bucksy P (2008) Number of genomic imbalances correlates with the overall survival for adrenocortical cancer in childhood. Pediatr Blood Cancer 51:356–362

Mackie GC, Shulkin BL, Ribeiro RC et al (2006) Use of [18F]fluorodeoxyglucose positron emission tomography in evaluating locally recurrent and metastatic adrenocortical carcinoma. J Clin Endocrinol Metab 91:2665–2671

Mastellaro MJ, Seidinger AL, Kang G et al (2017) Contribution of the TP53 R337H mutation to the cancer burden in southern Brazil: insights from the study of 55 families of children with adrenocortical tumors. Cancer 123:3150–3158

Michalkiewicz EL, Sandrini R, Bugg MF et al (1997) Clinical characteristics of small functioning adrenocortical tumors in children. Med Pediatr Oncol 28:175–178

Michalkiewicz E, Sandrini R, Figueiredo B et al (2004) Clinical and outcome characteristics of children with adrenocortical tumors. An analysis of 254 cases from the International Pediatric Adrenocortical Tumor Registry. J Clin Oncol 22:838–845

Murphy JJ, Tawfeeq M, Chang B, Nadel H (2008) Early experience with PET/CT scan in the evaluation of pediatric abdominal neoplasms. J Pediatr Surg 43:2186–2192

Narasimhan KL, Samujh R, Bhansali A et al (2003) Adrenocortical tumors in childhood. Pediatr Surg Int 19:432–435

Ostuni JA, Roginsky MS (1975) Metastatic adrenal cortical carcinoma: documented cure with combined chemotherapy. Arch Intern Med 135:1257–1258

Pianovski MAD, Maluf EMCP, de Carvalho DS et al (2006) Mortality rate of adrenocortical tumors in children under 15 years of age in Curitiba, Brazil. Pediatr Blood Cancer 47:56–60

Pinto EM, Chen X, Easton J et al (2015) Genomic landscape of paediatric adrenocortical tumours. Nat Commun 6:6302

Pinto EM, Rodriguez-Galindo C, Choi JK et al (2016) Prognostic significance of major histocompatibility complex class II expression in pediatric adrenocortical tumors: a St. Jude and Children's Oncology Group Study. Clin Cancer Res 22:6247–6255

Raj N, Zheng Y, Kelly V et al (2020) PD-1 blockade in advanced adrenocortical carcinoma. J Clin Oncol 38:71–80

Reincke M, Karl M, Travis WH et al (1994) p53 mutations in human adrenocortical neoplasms: immunohistochemical and molecular studies. J Clin Endocrinol Metab 78:790–794

Ribeiro RC, Figueiredo B (2004) Childhood adrenocortical tumours. Eur J Cancer 40:1117–1126

Ribeiro RC, Sandrini Neto R, Schell MJ, Lacerda L, Sambaio GA, Cat I (1990) Adrenocortical carcinoma in children: a study of 40 cases. J Clin Oncol 8:67–74

Ribeiro J, Ribeiro RC, Fletcher BD (2000) Imaging findings in pediatric adrenocortical carcinoma. Pediatr Radiol 30:45–51

Ribeiro RC, Sandrini F, Figueiredo B et al (2001) An inherited p53 mutation that contributes in a tissue-specific manner to pediatric adrenal cortical carcinoma. Proc Natl Acad Sci U S A 98:9330–9335

Ribeiro RC, Pinto EM, Zambetti GP et al (2012) The International Pediatric Adrenocortical Tumor Registry initiative: contributions to clinical, biological, and treatment advances in pediatric adrenocortical tumors. Mol Cell Endocrinol 351:37–43

Rodriguez-Galindo C, Figueiredo BC, Zambetti GP, Ribeiro RC (2005) Biology, clinical characteristics, and management of adrenocortical tumors in children. Pediatr Blood Cancer 45:265–273

Rodriguez-Galindo C, Krailo M, Pinto E et al (2021) Treatment of pediatric adrenocortical carcinoma with surgery, retroperitoneal lymph node dissection and chemotherapy: the Children's Oncology Group ARAR0332 protocol. J Clin Oncol 39(22):2463–2473

Rosati R, Cerrato F, Doghman M et al (2008) High frequency of loss of heterozygosity at 11p15 and IGF2 overexpression are not related to clinical outcome in childhood adrenocortical tumors positive for the R337H TP53 mutation. Cancer Genet Cytogenet 186:19–24

Rossbach H-C, Baschinsky D, Wynn T, Obzut D, Sutcliffe M, Tebbi C (2008) Composite adrenal anaplastic neuroblastoma and virilizing adrenocortical tumor with germline TP53 R248W mutation. Pediatr Blood Cancer 50:681–683

Sandrini R, Ribeiro RC, DeLacerda L (1997) Childhood adrenocortical tumors. J Clin Endocrinol Metab 7:2027–2031

Slooten HV, Schaberg A, Smeenk D, Moolenaar AJ (1985) Morphologic characteristics of benign and malignant adrenocortical tumors. Cancer 55:766–773

Steenman M, Westerveld A, Mannens M (2000) Genetics of Beckwith-Wiedeman syndrome-associated tumors: common genetic pathways. Genes Chromosomes Cancer 28:1–13

Stewart JN, Flageole H, Kavan P (2004) A surgical approach to adrenocortical tumors in children: the mainstay of treatment. J Pediatr Surg 39:759–763

Stojadinovic A, Ghossein RA, Hoos A et al (2002) Adrenocortical carcinoma: clinical, morphologic, and molecular characterization. J Clin Oncol 20:941–950

Sutter JA, Grimberg A (2006) Adrenocortical tumors and hyperplasias in childhood - etiology, genetics, clinical presentation and therapy. Pediatr Endocrinol Rev 4:32–39

Teinturier C, Pauchard MS, Brugieres L, Landais P, Chaussain JL, Bougneres PF (1999) Clinical and prognostic aspects of adrenocortical neoplasms in childhood. Med Pediatr Oncol 32:106–111

Tissier F, Cavard C, Groussin L et al (2005) Mutations of {beta}-catenin in adrenocortical tumors: activation of the Wnt signaling pathway is a frequent event in both benign and malignant adrenocortical tumors. Cancer Res 65:7622–7627

Tucci JR, Martins ACP, Suaid HJ, Cologna AJ, Reis RB (2005) The impact of tumor stage on prognosis in children with adrenocortical carcinoma. J Urol 174:2338–2342

Varan A, Unal S, Ruacan S, Vidinlisan S (2000) Adrenocortical carcinoma associated with adrenogenital syndrome in a child. Med Pediatr Oncol 35:88–90

Varley JM, McGown G, Thorncroft M et al (1999) Are there low-penetrance *TP53* alleles? Evidence from childhood adrenocortical tumors. Am J Hum Genet 65:995–1006

Virgone C, Roganovic J, Redlich A, et al (2021) The Paediatric Rare Tumours Network - European Registry (PARTNER) Consortium Project, Adrenocortical tumours in children and adolescents: The EXPeRT/PARTNER diagnostic and therapeutic recommendations, 68 (S4).

Wagner J, Portwine C, Rabin K, Leclerc J-M, Narod SA, Malkin D (1994) High frequency of germline p53 mutations in childhood adrenocortical cancer. J Natl Cancer Inst 86:1707–1710

Wajchenberg BL, Pereira MAA, Medonca BB et al (2000) Adrenocortical carcinoma: clinical and laboratory observations. Cancer 88:711–736

Wang X, Liang L, Jiang Y (2007) Nine cases of childhood adrenal tumour presenting with hypertension and a review of the literature. Acta Paediatr 96:930–934

Wasserman JD, Novokmet A, Eichler-Jonsson C et al (2015) Prevalence and functional consequence of TP53 mutations in pediatric adrenocortical carcinoma: a Children's Oncology Group Study. J Clin Oncol 33:602–U107

Weber MM, Fottner C, Schmidt P et al (1999) Postnatal overexpression of insulin-like growth factor II in transgenic mice is associated with adrenocortical hyperplasia and enhanced steroidogenesis. Endocrinology 140:1537–1543

Weber MM, Fottner C, Wolf E (2000) The role of the insulin-like growth factor system in adrenocortical tumorigenesis. Eur J Clin Invest 30(Suppl 3):69–75

Weiss LM (1984) Comparative histologic study of 43 metastasizing and nonmetastasizing adrenocortical tumors. Am J Surg Pathol 8:163–169

Weiss LM, Medeiros LJ, Vickery AL (1989) Pathologic features of prognostic significance in adrenocortical carcinoma. Am J Surg Pathol 13:202–206

West AN, Neale GA, Pounds S et al (2007) Gene expression profiling of childhood adrenocortical tumors. Cancer Res 67:600–608

Wieneke JA, Thompson LDR, Heffess CS (2003) Adrenal cortical neoplasms in the pediatric population: a clinicopathologic and immunophenotypic analysis of 83 patients. Am J Surg Pathol 27:867–881

Wood BJ, Abraham J, Hvizda JL, Alexander HR, Fojo T (2003) Radiofrequency ablation of adrenal tumors and adrenocortical carcinoma metastases. Cancer 97:554–560

Wooten MD, King DK (1993) Adrenal cortical carcinoma. Epidemiology and treatment with mitotane and a review of the literature. Cancer 72:3145–3155

Zancanella P, Pianovski MAD, Oliveira BH et al (2006) Mitotane associated with cisplatin, etoposide, and doxorubicin in advanced childhood adrenocortical carcinoma. Mitotane monitoring and tumor regression. J Pediatr Hematol Oncol 28:513–524

Medulloepithelioma

37

Gianni Bisogno

Medulloepithelioma (MEP) is a rare tumor derived from the primitive neuroepithelium that forms the ciliary body of the eye, iris, retina, or optic nerve head. It usually arises from the non-pigmented ciliary body of the eye; however, tumors arising from the optic nerve, retina, or central nervous system have also been described (Vajaranant et al. 2005; Molloy et al. 1996).

It represents the second most common intraocular tumor in childhood after retinoblastoma, with 75–90% of cases occurring in children aged less than 10 years (Tadepalli et al. 2019). Very rarely, these tumors can affect adults, in some cases as a late malignant transformation of a benign asymptomatic MEP arisen in childhood (Husain et al. 1998).

MEP is a locally aggressive tumor that may extend anteriorly into the iris or posteriorly into the vitreous cavity, involving the retina, with the entire globe filled with tumor similar to retinoblastoma. In advanced cases, it may present with extraocular extension and involve the regional lymph nodes. Distant metastasis to the lungs and parotid gland has been rarely described (Broughton and Zimmerman 1978; Viswanathan et al. 2008). There is no racial or gender predilection, and both eyes are equally affected, but it is commonly unilateral (Tadepalli et al. 2019).

G. Bisogno (✉)
Department for the Women's and Children Health, University of Padova, Padova, Italy
e-mail: gianni.bisogno@unipd.it

MEP can be associated with central nervous system malignancies (i.e., pinealoblastoma) or malformations (i.e., corpus callosum agenesis, schizencephaly) (Vajaranant et al. 2005). In addition, MEP has been found associated with pleuropulmonary blastoma (Priest et al. 2011) as part of the DICER1 familiar tumor predisposition syndrome. It has been reported that 5% of patients with MEP have a history of pleuropulmonary blastoma but the risk for MEP in pleuropulmonary blastoma patients is low (<1%) (Kaliki et al. 2013). Recently, somatic mutations of the KMT2D gene have been found, but their role in MEP needs to be further elucidated (Sahm et al. 2016).

37.1 Clinical Presentation

MEP is characterized by a slow growth, and it is often asymptomatic until it is large enough to be seen through the pupil. The most common presenting symptoms are pain and poor vision, related to secondary lens subluxation, glaucoma, or cataract formation. Leukocoria, strabismus, and the evidence of a mass in the iris or ciliary body are also part of the initial signs (Chung et al. 2007; Tadepalli et al. 2019).

On fundoscopic examination, the tumor presents an irregular surface with characteristic cystic lesions (Fig. 32.3 1a). In up to 60% of patients, cysts break off the surface and float freely in

D. T. Schneider et al. (eds.), *Rare Tumors in Children and Adolescents*, Pediatric Oncology,
https://doi.org/10.1007/978-3-030-92071-5_37

aqueous or vitreous humor. Retinal detachment is seen in many cases (Chung et al. 2007). On ultrasound, MEP appears as an echogenic irregular mass with a cystic structure and calcifications in some cases. Ultrasound biomicroscopy is more precise to define tumor dimensions and internal characteristics (Bianciotto et al. 2011). CT scan shows a dense irregular mass in the region of the ciliary body with marked to moderate enhancement after contrast, but MRI is preferred to investigate MEP. On MRI, the mass shows both solid and cystic components and appears moderately hyperintense compared to vitreous on T1-weighted images and hypointense on T2-weighted images with marked enhancement after gadolinium administration (Fig. 42.3.1b). Invasion of the sclera or optic nerve can also be identifiable (Sansgiri et al. 2013).

37.2 Diagnosis

The diagnosis requires a histopathologic examination. MEP is characterized by proliferating folded and multilayered sheets and cords of poorly differentiated neuroepithelium, resembling the primitive medullary plate and neural tube. Cystic spaces full of hyaluronic acid are present. MEP has been classified as nonteratoid (approximately two-thirds of cases) and teratoid type, and both types can be benign or malignant. The nonteratoid MEP is a pure proliferation of cells of the medullary epithelium, and it is typically positive for vimentin and neuron-specific enolase. The teratoid subtype includes also heteroplastic elements, such as cartilage, skeletal muscle, and brain-like tissue, and accounts for 30–50% of cases.

The histopathological criteria for malignancy are the presence of frequent mitotic figures or nuclear pleomorphism, poor cellular differentiation with or without rosettes, sarcomatous changes, and invasion of surrounding ocular tissues with or without extrascleral extension (Broughton and Zimmerman 1978).

When MEP is very extended and includes calcification, it may be difficult to distinguish it from an anteriorly located retinoblastoma. Differential diagnosis should also include benign conditions such xanthogranuloma, a cyst of the ciliary body, or the persistence and hyperplasia of the primary vitreous (Vajaranant et al. 2005; Chung et al. 2007).

A recent study investigating for MEP biomarkers found that EZH2, an epigenetic enzyme that regulates tumor suppressor genes or oncogene expression, is strongly positive in moderate to poorly differentiated primitive/neuroblastic MEP cells and negative in the surrounding nonneoplastic tissues. EZH2 positivity has been observed in other forms of cancer including retinoblastoma, and this limits its diagnostic utility (Avedschmidt et al. 2016). More interesting may be the role of LIN28A, a miRNA binding protein, able to downregulate tumor suppressing microRNAs of the let-7 family. LIN28A is positive in all tumors showing the tendency to form rosettes and tubules, but it is negative in retinoblastoma, showing a potential role to differentiate MEP from retinoblastoma and representing a possible therapeutic target (Stagner and Jakobiec 2016).

37.3 Treatment and Prognosis

MEP treatment is usually based on the surgical removal of the tumor. Enucleation may be necessary in larger lesions and exenteration when there is evidence of extraocular extension. Limited local resection has been used in small tumors, but the risk of recurrence is high. The successful use of brachytherapy after conservative surgery has also been reported, and cryotherapy has been used in recurrent tumors (Tadepalli et al. 2019; Cassoux et al. 2010). The prognosis is less favorable for tumor with extraocular extension. In these cases, chemotherapy and radiotherapy have been adopted. Recent reports have showed tumor response after chemotherapy including vincristine, carboplatin, cyclophosphamide, and etoposide underlining the possible use of preoperative chemotherapy to limit the aggressiveness of surgery (Meel et al. 2010) or for metastatic tumors (Hellman et al. 2018).

Prognosis is excellent (5-year survival of 90–95%) for patients with MEP without extraocular extension treated with enucleation (Vajaranant et al. 2005). When extraocular extension is evident, the prognosis is poor (Broughton and Zimmerman 1978) although a report exists of a metastatic MEP long-term survivor after multimodality treatment (Hellman et al. 2018).

References

Avedschmidt SE, Stagner AM, Eagle RC, Harocopos GJ, Dou Y, Rao RC (2016) The targetable epigenetic tumor protein EZH2 is enriched in intraocular medulloepithelioma. Invest Ophthalmol Vis Sci 57:6242–6246

Bianciotto C, Shields CL, Guzman JM, Romanelli-Gobbi M, Mazzuca D Jr, Green WR et al (2011) Assessment of anterior segment tumors with ultrasound biomicroscopy versus anterior segment optical coherence tomography in 200 cases. Ophthalmology 118:1297–1302

Broughton WL, Zimmerman LE (1978) A clinicopathologic study of 56 cases of intraocular medulloepitheliomas. Am J Ophthalmol 85(3):407–418

Cassoux N, Charlotte F, Sastre X, Orbach D, Lehoang P, Desjardins L (2010) Conservative surgical treatment of medulloepithelioma of the ciliary body. Arch Ophthalmol 128(3):380–381

Chung EM, Specht CS, Schroeder JW (2007) From the archives of the AFIP: pediatric orbit tumors and tumorlike lesions: neuroepithelial lesions of the ocular globe and optic nerve. Radiographics 27(4):1159–1186

Hellman JB, Harocopos GJ, Lin LK (2018) Successful treatment of metastatic congenital intraocular medulloepithelioma with neoadjuvant chemotherapy, enucleation and superficial parotidectomy. Am J Ophthalmol Case Rep 11:124–127

Husain SE, Husain N, Boniuk M, Font RL (1998) Malignant nonteratoid medulloepithelioma of the ciliary body in an adult. Ophthalmology 105:596–599

Kaliki S, Shields CL, Eagle RC Jr, Vemuganti GK, Almeida A, Manjandavida FP, Mulay K, Honavar SG, Shields JA (2013) Ciliary body medulloepithelioma: analysis of 41 cases. Ophthalmology 120(12):2552–2559

Meel R, Chawla B, Mohanti BK, Kashyap S, Bakhshi S (2010) Ocular medulloepithelioma chemosensitivity. Ophthalmology 117(12):2440.e1–2440.e2

Molloy PT, Yachnis AT, Rorke LB et al (1996) Central nervous system medulloepithelioma: a series of eight cases including two arising in the pons. J Neurosurg 84:430–436

Priest JR, Williams GM, Manera R, Jenkinson H, Bründler MA, Davis S, Murray TG, Galliani CA, Dehner LP (2011) Ciliary body medulloepithelioma: four cases associated with pleuropulmonary blastoma—a report from the International Pleuropulmonary Blastoma Registry. Br J Ophthalmol 95(7):1001–1005

Sahm F, Jakobiec FA, Meyer J, Schrimpf D, Eberhart CG, Hovestadt V et al (2016) Somatic mutations of DICER1 and KMT2D are frequent in intraocular medulloepitheliomas. Genes Chromosomes Cancer 55:418–427

Sansgiri RK, Wilson M, McCarville MB, Helton KJ (2013) Imaging features of medulloepithelioma: report of four cases and review of the literature. Pediatr Radiol 43:1344–1356

Stagner AM, Jakobiec FA (2016) Updates on the molecular pathology of selected ocular and ocular adnexal tumors: potential targets for future therapy. Semin Ophthalmol 31(1–2):188–196

Tadepalli SH, Shields CL, Shields JA, Honavar SG (2019) Intraocular medulloepithelioma—a review of clinical features, DICER 1 mutation, and management. Indian J Ophthalmol 67(6):755–762

Vajaranant TS, Mafee MF, Kapur R, Rapoport M, Edward DP (2005) Medulloepithelioma of the ciliary body and optic nerve: clinicopathologic, CT, and MR imaging features. Neuroimaging Clin N Am 15(1):69–83

Viswanathan S, Mukul S, Qureshi S, Ramadwara M, Arora B, Kane SV (2008) Orbital medulloepitheliomas—with extensive local invasion and metastasis: a series of three cases with review of literature. Int J Pediatr Otorhinolaryngol 72:971–975

38 Chordoma

Gianni Bisogno

Chordoma is a rare but aggressive tumor that occurs in the spine. It is believed to arise from notochord remnants located along the craniovertebral axis. The notochord develops during the third week of gestation and is located in the central portion of the future vertebral bodies. When vertebrae develop, the notochord cells form the nucleus pulposus of the intervertebral discs. It has never been shown that intravertebral discs are the site of origin of chordoma, but the fact that this tumor most frequently arises in the sacrococcygeal and sphenooccipital regions, where ectopic notochord remnants are most often found in fetuses along with the morphological similarities between notochord and chordoma cells, supports this view. But probably the most compelling evidence of notochord origin is given by the positivity of chordomas for brachyury, a transcription factor required for notochord development during embryogenesis (Beccaria et al. 2015; Vujovic et al. 2006).

It has been estimated that about 300 new cases of chordoma/year occur in the United States, and this corresponds to an incidence of approximately 1 case per million people/year (McMaster et al. 2001). The median age at presentation is 60 years. It is extremely rare in children and young adults where it represents less than 5% of all chordomas. Among children, the average age at diagnosis is among 10 years. No sex predisposition has been described (Beccaria et al. 2015; McMaster et al. 2001).

Chordoma etiology is unknown. Rarely, families with multiple affected members have been reported, suggesting an inherited predisposing condition possibly due to a gene duplication in the transcription factor T gene (brachyury) (Walcott et al. 2012). Childhood chordoma has been associated with the tuberous sclerosis complex. In these patients, the sacral location is more frequent, and mutations of tumor suppressor genes TSC1 and TSC2 are found. Prognosis seems satisfactory (McMaster et al. 2011).

Although extremely rare, chordoma in children and young adults presents distinctive clinical and pathological characteristics and in general a better prognosis in comparison to adults (Beccaria et al. 2015).

38.1 Clinical Characteristics

Chordoma is a rare but aggressive tumor that most frequently occurs in the mobile spine and sacrum. However, in younger patients, especially in children and adolescents, intracranial manifestations, in particular at the clivus are diagnosed more frequently. It is believed to arise from the notochord remnants located along the craniovertebral axis. Very rarely, chordoma can occur outside the spine and other midline sites.

G. Bisogno (✉)
Department for the Women's and Children Health, University of Padova, Padova, Italy
e-mail: gianni.bisogno@unipd.it

D. T. Schneider et al. (eds.), *Rare Tumors in Children and Adolescents*, Pediatric Oncology,
https://doi.org/10.1007/978-3-030-92071-5_38

The tumor tends to remain localized, but the risk of distant dissemination seems to be higher in children under 5 years with metastasis occurring more frequently in the lungs but also in the lymph nodes, bone, liver, kidney, adrenal gland, and heart (Beccaria et al. 2015).

Chordoma is generally a slowly growing neoplasm and causes symptoms invading the nearby structures. Pain and neurological signs are more often reported: skull base tumors may cause headache, cranial nerve palsy, and torticollis, while chordoma of the spine may cause alteration of bowel and/or bladder function, pain, tingling, and numbness or weakness of the arms and legs.

38.2 Diagnosis

Chordoma usually presents as a soft tissue mass associated with bone destruction and may extend into the intracranial compartment and sphenoid bone and sphenoid sinus. Both MRI and CT scan are employed to have a clear picture of tumor extension and bone involvement. CT shows an enhancing soft tissue mass with internal densities thought to represent fragments of bone and invasion of surrounding structures. On MRI, the lesion presents variable intensity on T1-weighted images and hyperintense with lobulated appearance and multiple hypointense septae on T2-weighted images (Walcott et al. 2012; Lui et al. 2010).

A total body CT scan is also indicated to exclude distant metastasis. Fine needle aspiration or a trucut biopsy is recommended to establish the diagnosis (Walcott et al. 2012). Three histological variants have been described: classical (conventional), chondroid, or dedifferentiated. Classic chordoma is characterized by a lobular pattern of growth with epithelioid cells arranged in nests, sheets, and syncytial cords in an abundant mucoid matrix. The cells show an abundant vacuolated (physaliphorous) cytoplasm, the number of mitosis is usually low, and some degree of nuclear atypia and necrosis may be present. The chondroid chordoma may contain elements that resemble neoplastic hyaline cartilage. It may behave less aggressively than the conventional type. Finally, the dedifferentiated chordoma, characterized by the presence of undifferentiated spindle cells or cells resembling osteosarcoma, is rarely encountered in children. Immunohistochemistry of conventional and chondroid chondromas usually results positive for cytokeratin, epithelial membrane antigen (EMA), vimentin, S-100 protein, and specially brachyury that is considered fundamental to make a diagnosis of chordoma and to distinguish it from chondrosarcoma (Walcott et al. 2012). Two more subtypes have been described in pediatric age: (a) the cellular chordoma, possibly a conventional chordoma that lacks stroma, and (b) the poorly differentiated chordoma composed of sheets of epithelioid cells tightly packed with high nuclear/cytoplasmic ratio and distinct nucleoli. This latter variant affects very young children, behaving aggressively, tending to grow rapidly, and is often associated with metastasis (Hoch et al. 2006).

38.3 Treatment

Due to the small number of cases described in the literature, the management of pediatric cases of chordoma mainly derives from the experience gathered with adults.

Surgery has an established role, and complete tumor resection at diagnosis with an en bloc excision of the tumor without violation of the capsule provides the best chances for local control and long-term survival (Tzortzidis et al. 2006; Stacchiotti et al. 2015). Unfortunately, aggressive surgery is often required with a high risk of post-operative death (Borba et al. 1996) and significant morbidity (Sekhar et al. 2001).

In most cases, and especially in children where clival chordomas are more frequent, only partial tumor resection is possible, and high-dose radiotherapy is administered. Doses in excess of 60 Gy are required, and this represents a major limitation in children in consideration of the possible late toxic effects. Techniques to maximize the dose of radiation to the tumor, while sparing adjacent critical structures, have been used including intensity-modulated radiation therapy (IMRT) and especially proton or carbon ion radiotherapy. A limited number of patients have been treated so far, but results seem promising: an overall survival of 81% has been reported in a series of 73 children and adolescents treated with proton beam radiotherapy after surgery. This compares favorably with a 55% 5-year survival described in adults with chordoma treated at the same institution (Hoch et al. 2006). A more recent study including 106 patients reported a 5-year survival of 88.3% using a combined photon and proton irradiation strategy (Fung et al. 2018).

Chordomas are generally reputed resistant to chemotherapy with only few reports describing a response to antineoplastic regimens including alkylating agents (ifosfamide or cyclophosphamide) combined with doxorubicin or etoposide and other agents (Walcott et al. 2012).

Molecular biology investigations have opened the possibility to investigate target agents. In consideration of the overexpression of platelet-derived growth factor receptors (PDGFR) and KIT receptors, imatinib has been studied in adults with some evidence of activity: among 50 patients, 1 partial response and 28 stable diseases at 6 months have been reported (Stacchiotti et al. 2012).

Very few children have been treated with imatinib. In a study including among various tumors three patients with chordoma, only one of them showed a temporary metabolic response to imatinib on PET scan (Geoerger et al. 2009).

The use of other targeted therapies such as cetuximab, gefitinib, erlotinib, and sirolimus has been reported (Hof et al. 2006; Stacchiotti et al. 2009). A phase I trial testing brachyury vaccine is ongoing. Finally, the presence of *SMARCB1* mutation in some patients with chordoma may offer them the possibility to be included in ongoing trials with tazemetostat. The role of target therapy needs to be further elucidated, and at the moment, its use is limited to patients with inoperable, metastatic, and relapsed disease. In addition, the response is often difficult to evaluate, and a combination of clinical (symptoms relief), radiological, and metabolic changes should be taken into account (Meng et al. 2019).

38.4 Prognosis and Survival

The overall survival rates obtained in the United States in adult patients with chondroma are 68% at 5 years and 40% at 10 years, with a median survival of about 7 years (McMaster et al. 2001), but results seem more satisfying in pediatric studies (Beccaria et al. 2015; Hoch et al. 2006; Fung et al. 2018).

Recent reports of pediatric patients treated at single institutions showed a better outcome with four of six patients alive at a median follow-up of 9 years described by Dhall et al. (2011) and an overall survival rate of 81% (median follow-up of 7.2 years) in a cohort of patients with skull base chordoma referred to the Boston Massachusetts General Hospital for proton beam radiotherapy (Hoch et al. 2006). Complete tumor resection (Hug 2001) and histological subtype (Hoch et al. 2006) seem to be the major prognostic determinants. Patients with conventional chordoma have the best prognosis, while the chance of survival in the case of the poorly differentiated subtype remains very low: a retrospective series of seven children showed a median survival of 9 months; all tumors showed loss of *SMARCB1* expression by immunohistochemistry (Hasselblatt et al. 2016). Other prognostic factors seem to be the tumor localization and age at diagnosis. Intracranial chordomas have a better outcome in comparison with those arising in the spine which have a better prognosis in comparison to those arising in the sacral region. Children less than 5 years have a lower chance of cure, and this may be partially explained by the higher incidence of dedifferentiated forms and sacrococcygeal location in this age (Beccaria et al. 2015).

References

Beccaria K, Sainte-Rose C, Zerah M et al (2015) Paediatric chordomas. Orphanet J Rare Dis 10(1):116

Borba LA, Al-Mefty O, Mrak RE, Suen J (1996) Cranial chordomas in children and adolescents. J Neurosurg 84(4):584–591

Dhall G, Traverso M, Finlay JL, Shane L, Gonzalez-Gomez I, Jubran R (2011) The role of chemotherapy in pediatric clival chordomas. J Neurooncol 103(3):657–662

Fung V, Calugaru V, Bolle S, Mammar H, Alapetite C, Maingon P, De Marzi L, Froelich S, Habrand JL, Dendale R, Noël G, Feuvret L (2018) Proton beam therapy for skull base chordomas in 106 patients: a dose adaptive radiation protocol. Radiother Oncol 128(2):198–202

Geoerger B, Morland B, Ndiaye A, Doz F, Kalifa G, Geoffray A, et al, Innovative Therapies for Children with Cancer European Consortium (2009) Target-driven exploratory study of imatinib mesylate in children with solid malignancies by the Innovative Therapies for Children with Cancer (ITCC) European Consortium. Eur J Cancer 45:2342–2351

Hasselblatt M, Thomas C, Hovestadt V et al (2016) Poorly differentiated chordoma with SMARCB1/INI1 loss: a distinct molecular entity with dismal prognosis. Acta Neuropathol 132(1):149–151

Hoch BL, Nielsen GP, Liebsch NJRA (2006) Base of skull chordomas in children and adolescents: a clinicopathologic study of 73 cases. Am J Surg Pathol 30(7):811–818

Hof H, Welzel T, Debus J (2006) Effectiveness of cetuximab/gefitinib in the therapy of a sacral chordoma. Onkologie 29:572–574

Hug EB (2001) Review of skull base chordomas: prognostic factors and long-term results of proton-beam radiotherapy. Neurosurg Focus 10:E11

Lui YW, Dasari SB, Young RJ (2010) Sphenoid masses in children: radiologic differential diagnosis with pathologic correlation. AJNR Am J Neuroradiol 32(4):617–626

McMaster ML, Goldstein AM, Bromley CM et al (2001) Chordoma: incidence and survival patterns in the United States, 1973–1995. Cancer Causes Control 12:1–11

McMaster ML, Goldstein AM, Parry DM (2011) Clinical features distinguish childhood chordoma associated with tuberous sclerosis complex (TSC) from chordoma in the general paediatric population. J Med Genet 48(7):444–449

Meng T, Jin J, Jiang C et al (2019) Molecular targeted therapy in the treatment of chordoma: a systematic review. Front Oncol 9:30

Sekhar LN, Pranatartiharan R, Chanda A et al (2001) Chordomas and chondrosarcomas of the skull base: results and complications of surgical management. Neurosurg Focus 10(3):E2

Stacchiotti S, Marrari A, Tamborini E et al (2009) Response to imatinib plus sirolimus in advanced chordoma. Ann Oncol 20(11):1886–1894

Stacchiotti S, Longhi A, Ferraresi V et al (2012) Phase II study of imatinib in advanced chordoma. J Clin Oncol 30(9):914–920

Stacchiotti S, Sommer J, Chordoma Global Consensus Group (2015) Building a global consensus approach to chordoma: a position paper from the medical and patient community. Lancet Oncol 16(2):e71–e83

Tzortzidis F, Elahi F, Wright D, Natarajan SK, Sekhar LN (2006) Patient outcome at long-term follow-up after aggressive microsurgical resection of cranial base chordomas. Neurosurgery 59:230–237

Vujovic S, Henderson S, Presneau N et al (2006) Brachyury, a crucial regulator of notochordal development, is a novel biomarker for chordomas. J Pathol 209(2):157–165

Walcott BP, Nahed BV, Mohyeldin A, Coumans JV, Kahle KT, Ferreira MJ (2012) Chordoma: current concepts, management, and future directions. Lancet Oncol 13(2):e69–e76

Part X

Rare Tumors of the Skin and Subcutaneous Tissue

Epidemiology and Differential Diagnosis of Cutaneous Tumors

39

Andrea Ferrari and Paola Collini

Cutaneous malignant tumors rarely occur in children and adolescents. Skin carcinomas are exceedingly rare. Only 49 cases are registered in the Surveillance, Epidemiology, and End Results (SEER 9 database, accessed March 26, 2018): from this source, the incidence rate is 0.9 per 100,000 in general population (all ages), while it is 0.0077 per 100,000 in the population less than 20 years old.

Melanoma is less uncommon: in a study of 7814 cases of primary skin cancers in patients under 30 years of age, melanoma was the most common malignancy accounting for 83% of the cases. The second most common cutaneous cancers were soft tissue sarcomas, the most common being dermatofibrosarcoma protuberans. The third most common cutaneous malignancies were lymphomas, with the mature T cell and NK cell subtypes comprising 80% of the cases (Senerchia et al. 2014).

Melanoma in children and adolescents accounts for only 0.7% of cancers in patients under 10 years of age and for 5.3% of all cancers in 10–19 years old (Fig. 39.1). The peak incidence is reached between 20 and 29 years when melanoma is diagnosed in 12.4% of all cancer patients (Leiter et al. 2014). The melanoma age-adjusted-specific incidence rate in patients under 20 years is 5.8 per million, and current estimates suggest that there are approximately 427 new cases of melanoma diagnosed each year in the United States in patients under the age of 20 (Bleyer et al. 2006). Melanoma is more common in young females, while its incidence among adolescents and young adults (AYAs) is generally higher in males than in females (9.5 per 100,000 in males vs. 6.2 per 100,000 in females) (Leiter et al. 2014). In a review by Strouse, the incidence of pediatric melanoma was reported to have increased at a rate of 2.9% per year over a 28-year period after adjusting for age, race, sex, and ambient UV radiation (Strouse et al. 2005). In this study, AYAs had increased incidence rates when compared to younger patients. Epidemiological studies report that melanoma incidence increases with age: over 90% of cases occur in patients older than 10 years of age, and 74% are seen in those aged 15–19 years (Bleyer et al. 2006). Looking at survival curves for melanoma patients according to the age groups, the SEER database reported similar outcome, with the exception of 15–39-year subgroup, for which females have significantly better survival, with around 9% gap, which is not seen in other age groups: 5-year overall survival (OS) was 89.6% and 89.1% in males and females, respectively, aged 0–14 years old; 84.1% and 93.4% in patients

A. Ferrari (✉)
Pediatric Oncology Unit, Fondazione IRCCS Istituto Nazionale Tumori, Milan, Italy
e-mail: andrea.ferrari@istitutotumori.mi.it

P. Collini
Department of Pathology, Fondazione IRCCS Istituto Nazionale Tumori, Milan, Italy

D. T. Schneider et al. (eds.), *Rare Tumors in Children and Adolescents*, Pediatric Oncology,
https://doi.org/10.1007/978-3-030-92071-5_39

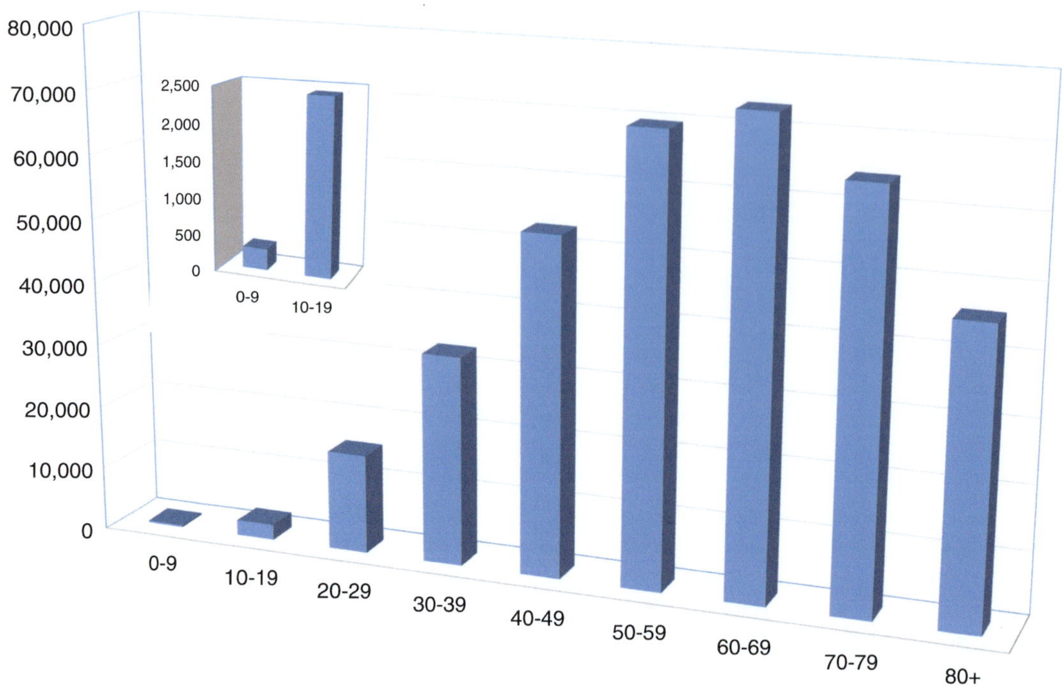

Fig. 39.1 Number of cases of cutaneous melanoma registered in the Surveillance, Epidemiology, and End Results (SEER) 9 database (accessed 26 Mar 2018)

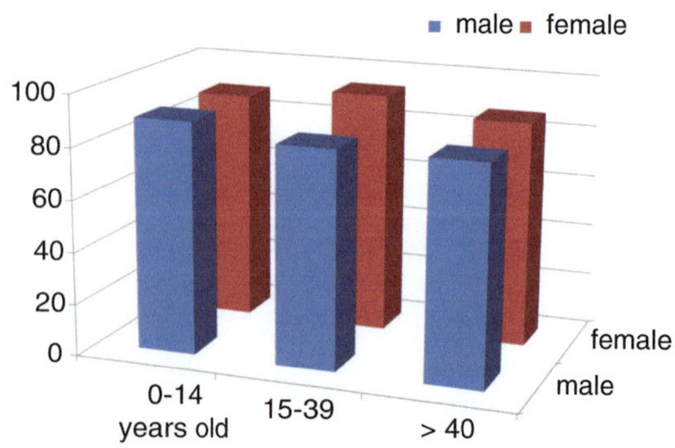

Fig. 39.2 Overall survival of melanoma cases according to age group, i.e., 0–14 years old, 15–59 years old, and over 40 years old. (From the Surveillance, Epidemiology, and End Results (SEER) 9 database (accessed 26 Mar 2018))

aged 15–59 years old; and 84.2% and 87.1% in patients over 40 years old (Fig. 39.2).

A study from the Italian TREP project (Tumori Rari in Età Pediatrica [*Rare Tumors in Pediatric Age*]) analyzed the incidence of rare tumors included in the TREP list (Ferrari et al. 2014). Using data from the population-based cancer registries AIRTUM (that covers 33% of the Italian resident population in the 0–14-year-old age group and 27% of the 15–19-year-old age group), this study reported an annual incidence of less than 2 per million population for melanoma among 0–10-year-olds (0.64 for 1–4- and 0.30 for 5–9-year-olds), but higher than 2 cases per million population in the age ranges over 10 years, being in particular 2.38 for 10–14- and 8.78 for 15–17-year-olds. Thus, according to the definition for rare tumors in children stated by the TREP and the European Cooperative Study Group for Pediatric Rare Tumors (EXPeRT) (i.e., an annual incidence of less than two cases per million population), melanoma is to be considered a rare tumor in children, but not in adolescents and young adults (Ferrari et al. 2013, 2017).

Noteworthy, a recent European study from the Joint Action on Rare Cancers (JARC) in cooperation with the European Cooperative Study Group for Pediatric Rare Tumors (EXPeRT) reported an incidence rate of 1.3 per million in 0–14-year-old population, but of 4.5 if we consider cases of 0–19-year-olds, suggesting that melanoma is definitely rare in children, but maybe not in adolescents (Ferrari et al. 2019).

The clinical diagnosis of cutaneous tumors in a child may be a challenge, due to the rarity of the diseases, but also because benign lesions may have alarmingly malignant tumor-like features, as well as malignant neoplasms may present with benign characteristics (i.e., pedunculated or amelanotic melanoma simulating a pyogenic granuloma). The same can be said for the pathological diagnosis. For some histotypes, the histological diagnosis of a tumor of the skin in a child can be very difficult for many reasons. For example, the diagnosis of melanoma in pediatric age is near always a problem for pathologists. Melanoma is a very rare evenience in children, so pathologists are always psychologically tempted to find an alternative diagnosis. Actually, pediatric melanomas do exist and deserve a distinct treatment. In pediatric age, the histological characteristics of melanoma are mimicked by other more frequent neoplasms, i.e., Spitz tumors, for which a spectrum of aggressiveness is reported from benign lesions (Spitz nevi) through the so-called atypical lesions (atypical Spitz tumors, with a risk ranging from low to high) up to the Spitzoid melanoma. Moreover, the borders between these entities are not so sharply defined. Referring suspected cases to expert physicians who are professionally dedicated to skin tumors is of critical importance, also in the light that early diagnosis remains the most reliable way to cure melanoma and other cutaneous tumors. The creation of panel of experts, the building of network of cooperation, the centralized review, and the option of second opinion are possible suggestion to improve the quality of pathological diagnosis of childhood skin tumors (Ferrari et al. 2021).

References

Bleyer A, O'Leary M, Barr R, Ries LA (2006) Cancer epidemiology in older adolescents and young adults 15 to 29 years of age including SEER incidence and survival: 1975–2000. National Cancer Institute, Bethesda, MD

Ferrari A, Schneider DT, Bisogno G (2013) The founding of the European Cooperative Study Group on Pediatric Rare Tumors – EXPeRT. Expert Rev Anticancer Ther 13(1):1–3

Ferrari A, Bisogno G, Cecchetto G et al (2014) Cutaneous melanoma in children and adolescents: the Italian Rare Tumors in Pediatric Age Project Experience. J Pediatr 164:375–382

Ferrari A, Schneider DT, Bisogno G et al (2017) The challenge of very rare childhood cancer in developed and developing countries. Expert Opin Orphan Drugs 5(4):331–341

Ferrari A, Brecht IB, Gatta G et al (2019) Defining and listing very rare cancers of pediatric age: consensus of the Joint Action on Rare Cancers (JARC) in cooperation with the European Cooperative Study Group for Pediatric Rare Tumors (EXPeRT). Eur J Cancer 110:120–126. https://doi.org/10.1016/j.ejca.2018.12.031

Ferrari A, Lopez Almaraz R, Reguerre Y, et al (2021). Cutaneous melanoma in children and adolescents: the EXPeRT/PARTNER diagnostic and therapeutic recommendations. Pediatr Blood Cancer 68:e28992

Leiter U, Eigentler T, Garbe C (2014) Epidemiology of skin cancer. Adv Exp Med Biol 810:120–140

Senerchia AA, Ribeiro KB, Rodriguez-Galindo C (2014) Trends in incidence of primary cutaneous malignancies in children, adolescents, and young adults: a population-based study. Pediatr Blood Cancer 61(2):211–216

Strouse JJ, Fears TR, Tucker MA, Wayne AS (2005) Pediatric melanoma: risk factor and survival analysis of the surveillance, epidemiology and end results database. J Clin Oncol 23:4735–4741

Cutaneous Melanoma

40

Alice Indini, Alberto S. Pappo,
Thomas K. Eigentler, Paola Collini,
and Andrea Ferrari

Melanoma is rare in children, and little information is available on clinical and biological features of childhood melanoma, as compared to the large amount of data arising every day on the adult counterpart. However, epidemiological studies suggested that its incidence rapidly increases with age and melanoma needs to be considered rare in children but not in adolescents (Ferrari et al. 2014, 2019).

40.1 Risk Factors

Similar to other cancers, cutaneous melanoma is a multifactorial disease. Several phenotypic traits that are associated with a higher risk of melanoma in the adulthood have been observed in children, specifically fair skin, hair, and eyes, freckles, poor tanning ability, dysplastic nevi, and numerous melanocytic nevi (Strouse et al. 2005). Given that most cases of melanoma in young people are sporadic (Pappo 2003), a subset of pediatric patients have unique risk factors that predispose them to the development of malignant melanoma, and these include:

1. Xeroderma pigmentosum. This autosomal recessive disorder is characterized by extreme photosensitivity to UV radiation and mutations of the nucleotide excision repair complementation groups. Most skin cancers develop during the first decade of life and preferentially affect the head and neck area. Early recognition of sun sensitivity with molecular testing is essential in establishing the diagnosis (Mocellin et al. 2009).
2. Retinoblastoma. Survivors of hereditary retinoblastoma are at increased risk for developing melanoma, and this risk is seen in both irradiated and non-irradiated patients (Kleinerman et al. 2005).
3. Werner syndrome. Patients with Werner syndrome are at increased risk for developing various malignancies including melanoma (Lauper et al. 2013). This autosomal recessive syndrome is characterized by the onset of premature features associated with aging and is due to mutations of the

A. Indini (✉)
Medical Oncology Unit, Department of Internal Medicine, Fondazione IRCCS Ca' Granda Ospedale Maggiore Policlinico, Milan, Italy

A. S. Pappo
Department of Oncology, St. Jude Children's Research Hospital, Memphis, TN, USA

T. K. Eigentler
Sektion Dermatologische Onkologie, University Hospital Tübingen, Tübingen, Germany

P. Collini
Department of Pathology, Fondazione IRCCS Istituto Nazionale Tumori, Milan, Italy

A. Ferrari
Pediatric Oncology Unit, Fondazione IRCCS Istituto Nazionale Tumori, Milan, Italy

D. T. Schneider et al. (eds.), *Rare Tumors in Children and Adolescents*, Pediatric Oncology,
https://doi.org/10.1007/978-3-030-92071-5_40

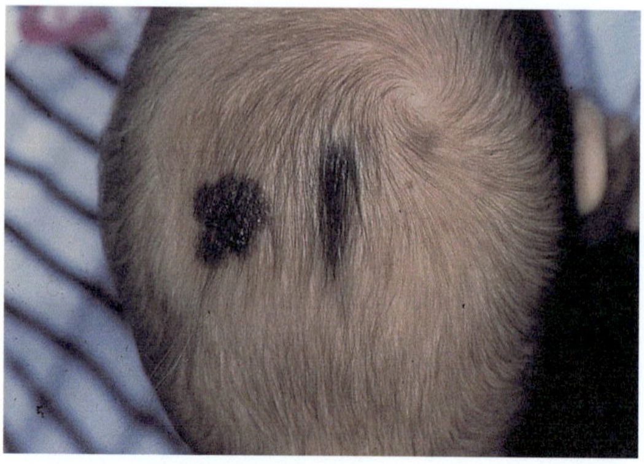

Fig. 40.1 Congenital melanoma arising in a medium-sized nevus

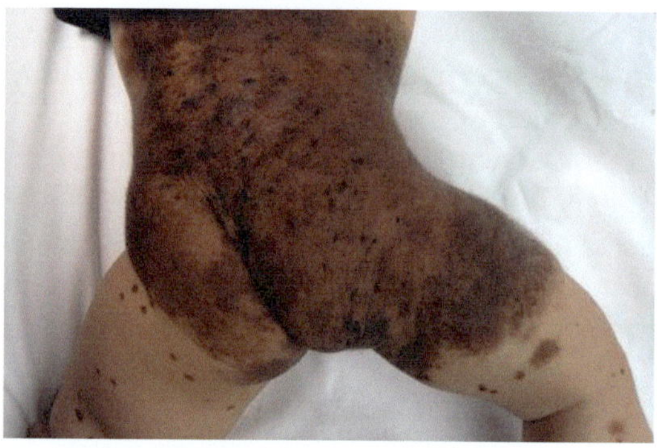

Fig. 40.2 Giant congenital melanocytic nevi

WRN gene, a member of the human RecQ family of DNA helicases (Muftuoglu et al. 2008).

4. Melanoma is the most common transplacentally acquired malignancy. So far, six cases of congenital melanoma have been reported in literature, with only one of them being a long-term survivor. It is recommended that all neonates from women with suspected diagnosis of melanoma are screened for signs of disease for up to 24 months postpartum (Alexander et al. 2003).
5. Melanoma can arise from medium-sized and large congenital nevi, which more commonly involve the scalp (Fig. 40.1). The overall risk for developing melanoma in a congenital nevus is only 0.7%, and this risk can rise with the size of the nevus and is highest in the presence of those designated as "garment" nevi.
6. Giant congenital melanocytic nevi (Fig. 40.2) affect less than 1 in 20,000 newborns. Patients with these lesions have about a 5% lifetime risk of developing melanoma, and most develop early in life (Margaryan et al. 2016). Patients with larger size nevi and increased numbers of satellite nevi are at increased risk for developing melanoma.
7. Neurocutaneous melanosis is an extremely rare disorder, characterized by the presence of large or multiple congenital nevi in association with meningeal melanoma or melanosis (Makkar and Frieden 2004). The risk of developing neurocutaneous melanosis in the context of large congenital giant nevi ranges from 2.5% to 12%, with larger nevus size and the presence of multiple satellites being favoring conditions (Ceballos et al. 1995). Most symptomatic patients present with neurological manifestations such as increased intracranial pressure within the first 2 years of life. Central nervous system (CNS) melanoma develops in up to 64% of patients with symptomatic disease, and the prognosis is extremely poor with a median survival of about 6 months. Approximately 25% of asymptomatic patients with large congenital nevi have magnetic resonance imaging (MRI) evidence of CNS melanosis: in 1 case series, only 1 out of 20 children developed symptomatic disease (Ceballos et al. 1995).
8. Immunosuppression. Patients with immune deficiencies and those who have undergone solid organ and bone marrow transplantation are at increased risk for developing melanoma (Curtis et al. 1997; Euvrard et al. 2003). Survivors of childhood cancer also have an increased risk of developing melanoma (Friedman et al. 2010).
9. Genetic factors. It is estimated that about 8–10% of cases have a family history of melanoma. Germline mutations in CDKN2A and CDK4 susceptibility genes have been identified in only 10–25% of these familial melanoma cases, suggesting the role of other high-penetrance predisposition genes (e.g., the locus on chromosome band 1p22) (Hayward 2003; Whiteman et al. 1997).

10. Environmental factors. A history of sunburns in early life and tanning bed exposure also confers an increased risk for developing melanoma (Lazovich et al. 2010; Melanoma Treatment (PDQ®): Health Professional Version n.d.). The incidence of melanoma in pediatric age varies also with latitude, with an increased incidence in the Northern Europe (Pearce et al. 2003) and particularly in Australia (Milton et al. 1997). The great awareness of physicians and parents and the improved accuracy in histological diagnosis (e.g., diagnosis of melanoma versus atypical Spitz nevus) may play a role, but the main reason for the higher incidence lies in the cumulative UV exposure during childhood and adolescence (Printz 2015).

40.2 Genomic Subtypes of Melanoma

In adults, there are four major genomic types of melanomas: (1) those with BRAF activating mutations, (2) those with RAS activating mutations such as NRAS, (3) those with NF1 mutations, and (4) those which are triple negative and have an increased copy number and complex rearrangements (Cancer Genome Atlas Network 2015). Genetic analysis of the three most common pediatric melanoma subtypes (conventional melanoma, Spitzoid melanoma, large congenital melanocytic nevi) revealed that every subtype has distinct molecular characteristics (Lu et al. 2015): conventional melanoma shows a high burden of single-nucleotide variations and most of the genomic alterations observed in adults (i.e., activating BRAF V600 mutations, PTEN loss of functions) as well as TERT promoter mutations and a UV-induced signature; Spitzoid melanomas are characterized by kinase gene fusions involving several genes such as RET, ROS1, NTRK1, ALK, MET, and BRAF; and melanomas arising in large congenital melanocytic nevi have activating NRASQ61 mutations and TERT promoter upregulation through aberrant promoter methylation.

Whole genome sequencing analysis of adolescent and young adult (AYA) melanoma patients (onset 10–30 years, median 20) showed that the frequencies of somatic mutations in BRAF (96%) and PTEN (36%) in AYA cohort were double the rates observed in adult melanomas. Furthermore, AYA melanomas contained a higher proportion of non-UVR-related mutation signatures than mature adult melanomas as a proportion of total mutation burden. Germline variants that may have conferred disease susceptibility correlated with somatic mutation signatures in a subset of AYA melanomas (Wilmott et al. 2019). Other specific molecular features described in young patients are c-Kit gene alterations and a dysregulated expression of microRNA targeting proliferation (Daniotti et al. 2009; Tricoli et al. 2016). In AYA patients with melanoma, genetic and epigenetic alterations of *TERT* leading to *TERT* upregulation and mRNA expression are associated with an inferior clinical outcome (Seynnaeve et al. 2017). It has also been suggested that extreme telomere shortening and dysfunction in the cancer cells might be associated with favorable biologic behavior (Barhami and Barnhill 2018).

40.3 Clinical Manifestations

Diagnosing melanoma in pre-pubertal children is a challenge even for clinicians who see pigmented skin lesions in children on a daily basis. This is partly due to the alarming melanoma-like features of some benign nevi (e.g., Spitz, Reed, and junctional nevi) and to the appearance of some pre-pubertal melanomas which may differ from the typical appearance of adult forms. The cutaneous lesion often presents as nodular, or raised, and/or amelanotic, sometimes simulating pyogenic granulomas (Ferrari et al. 2005; Handfield-Jones and Smith 1996; Mones and Ackerman 2003; Zuckerman et al. 2001). The ABCDE clinical rule commonly applied to adults (Asymmetry—Border irregularity—Color variability—Diameter > 6 mm—Evolution) may be useless and even misleading in childhood melanoma (Cordoro et al. 2013; Ferrari et al. 2005). Nodular melanoma may lack these signs and should be considered in any skin lesion that presents EFG features (i.e., evolution, firmness to touch, and growth) (Wouters et al. 2018). Regarding tumor size, it is noteworthy that benign nevi normally grow up to relatively large size as the child grows, whereas at the same time melanomas may be frequently detected at a very small size (Bono and Ferrari 2005). When melanoma arises in a congenital nevus (particularly in the case of "bathing trunk nevus," which is congenital and often disfiguring darkly pigmented melanocytic lesion, sometimes associated with neurofibromatosis, lipomas, and spina bifida), diagnosis is even more difficult, because malignant transformation often evolves in its deeper components, and surface alterations may be a late manifestation.

Cutaneous melanoma in young patients may qualify as an "orphan" disease. In fact, there is still a lack of awareness that young people can develop melanoma, and this can lead to diagnostic delays and misdiagnosis (Ferrari et al. 2014). Clinical presentation seen in adults with bleeding, ulceration, increasing mole size, and itching is rarely present in pediatric cases (Kaste et al. 1996). In two large series of pediatric melanomas from the SEER and National Cancer Databases, two-thirds of patients presented with localized disease, and less than 5% of patients presented with distant metastatic disease (Strouse et al. 2005; Lange et al. 2007). In these series, over 90% of children were white, and the most common histologic subtype was superficial spreading melanoma; thin and intermediate thickness lesions were more commonly observed, while thick lesions (i.e., >4 mm in thickness) were seen in only 2% of cases. In both series, younger patients were more likely to present with the following characteristics: non-white ethnicity, history of family cancer, nodular histology, thick lesions, head and neck primaries, disseminated disease at presentation, and overall inferior clinical outcomes (Strouse et al. 2005; Lange et al. 2007).

40.4 Establishing the Diagnosis of Pediatric Melanoma

Back in 1948, Sophie Spitz published a landmark paper defining the term "juvenile melanoma" which described a benign nevus in childhood histologically mimicking malignant melanoma (Spitz 1948). Later on, the term "juvenile melanoma" was replaced by "Spitz nevus" to emphasize the clinical benign behavior of these lesions. Establishing the diagnosis of pediatric melanoma can be challenging, and other cutaneous lesions can be misdiagnosed in the pediatric population. Early diagnosis is crucial, and diagnostic tools as dermoscopy and serial and total body photography can be useful. However, a suspicious lesion in a child should always be referred to an experienced dermatologist: in fact, dermoscopy is of great help only when performed by trained experts. In a study reporting histopathologic diagnosis of childhood melanoma cases, a poor reliability was detected even among experts (Wechsler et al. 2002). Results of a European study showed that only 60 of 102 originally diagnosed melanoma cases were confirmed by an expert review panel and 42 of them benign lesions (Spatz et al. 1996). Additionally, it seems that in some retrospective re-evaluations of histological specimens after knowing the patients' clinical course, the initial diagnosis of melanoma had to be revised to benign melanocytic lesions (Leman et al. 2005).

Moreover, the emergence of entities such as Spitzoid melanoma, atypical Spitzoid lesions, melanocytic lesions or tumors of unknown metastatic potential (MELTUMPs), and atypical Spitz nevus has made things even more difficult for pathologists. The challenge of differential diagnosis places a significant responsibility on the treating clinician who is ultimately responsible for making therapeutic decisions such as the appropriateness of complete lymph node dissections or administration of adjuvant treatment.

Several investigators are now relying on molecular tests to better classify the diagnosis of melanocytic tumors in children. Comparative genomic hybridization (CGH) and fluorescence in situ hybridization (FISH), using a combination of probes for regions commonly affected by DNA copy number alterations in melanoma, might help in the differential diagnosis between melanomas and nevi. The chromosomal aberrations seen in melanoma, which most commonly involve regions at 6p25, 6q23, 9p, 10q, 8p 1q, and 11q13 (Gerami et al. 2009), are not seen in patients with Spitzoid lesions which usually have a normal chromosomal complement and occasional gains of chromosome 11p. In an Italian case series of 21 pediatric patients with melanoma, genetic analysis revealed CDKN2A and MC1R gene variants in 2/21 and 12/21 patients, respectively. At the somatic level, 9/14 lesions had CDKN2A locus homozygous deletions and a null p16 immunophenotype. Loss of KIT protein expression was seen in 7/14 cases, and BRAF(V600E) mutations were seen in 5/10 cases (Daniotti et al. 2009). Gene expression analysis of signatures differentiating primary melanomas and other pigmented lesions in adults (e.g., preferentially expressed antigen in melanoma [PRAME] and long intergenic non-coding RNA 518 [LINC]) has demonstrated to be applicable also for differential diagnosis of pediatric lesion. In an interesting study investigating gene expression patterns of pigmented lesions of pediatric patients, the expression of PRAME gene but not expression of LINC gene demonstrated to be a valuable molecular aid to differentiate melanomas from Spitz nevi (Jansen et al. 2018).

40.5 Histological Diagnosis

The reproducibility of histological diagnoses of melanocytic lesions is poor especially for intermediate lesions and melanocytic lesions of low malignant potential. For these diagnostically problematic lesions characterized by conflicting criteria, these terms are proposed in the 2018 WHO Classification of Skin Tumours, strongly suggesting to specify the entities included in the differential diagnosis:

- SAMPUS (superficial atypical melanocytic proliferation of uncertain significance) for lesions featuring thin non-mitogenic and non-tumorigenic radial growth phase (RGP).
- IAMPUS (intraepidermal atypical melanocytic proliferation of uncertain significance): for lesions including melanoma in situ in differential diagnosis.
- MELTUMP (melanocytic tumors of uncertain malignant potential): for tumorigenic lesions whose differential diagnosis includes vertical growth phase (VGF) melanoma.

40.6 Histological Diagnosis: MELTUMP

MELTUMP is a term proposed in 2004, which encompasses a group of lesions which definition of malignant potential is difficult as defined by the classical histological parameters. This means that the application of the histological criteria of malignancy of conventional melanocytic lesions does not carry the same risk of malignancy when applied to these lesions. MELTUMPs are a heterogeneous group including atypical Spitz tumors (AST), cellular and atypical epithelioid/spindled blue nevi (ABN), minimal deviation melanomas, and pigmented epithelioid melanocytoma. MELTUMPs should not be a waste-basket for any difficult lesion. MELTUMPs *are tumorigenic atypical deep compound and dermal melanocytic tumors*. They exhibit one or several features indicative of possible malignancy, such as nuclear atypia, macronucleoli, mitotic activity, necrosis, or ulceration, but they exhibit these features in number or degree insufficient to justify a diagnosis of malignancy. The term MELTUMP should be used to indicate "lesions that do not display all of the characteristics that permit a diagnosis of vertical growth phase melanoma and whose capacity to metastasize is indeterminate or uncertain." Histological diagnosis is challenging, and there is still no consensus on or established criteria for the histopathological diagnosis of atypical Spitz tumors, atypical blue nevi, deep penetrating nevi, and the like (Cerroni et al. 2010). Facing an atypical skin lesion in a young patient, it is therefore strongly advisable to have the histology reviewed by a pathologist expert on adult melanoma (Massi et al. 2015). Given the uncertain malignant potential of these lesions, their managements should be individualized (Cerroni et al. 2010). Over the last years, clinicians' behavior in the presence of MELTUMPs has changed: until a few years ago, borderline lesions categorized as MELTUMPs were treated considering the worst-case scenario in the differential diagnosis. Thus, in the presence of frank histological atypia, the lesion was to be treated as a melanoma of equivalent depth (Cerroni et al. 2010). Moreover, given that in approximately half of the cases patients harbor small deposits of melanocytic cells in regional lymph nodes, the general attitude was to routinely perform sentinel lymph node biopsy (SLNB) (Cerroni et al. 2010). Things have changed based on the results of a systematic review published in 2014 by Lallas et al. This analysis included 541 patients with atypical Spitz tumors: the overall prognosis was good (i.e., 99% of patients alive after a mean follow-up of 59 months [range 1–190]). More than half of the patients (56%) had SLNB, which was positive in 39% of patients; 82% of the patients with SLNB positivity underwent complete lymph node dissection, and 19% had one or more positive nodes at dissection. A relevant result emerging from this review was there was no significant difference in survival between patients having positive SLNB and those who were treated with wide local excision alone (99% vs. 98%, respectively) (Lallas et al. 2014). So, even in the absence of high-quality evidence, the prognostic benefit of SLNB remains unclear, and no definitive recommendations can be made on the need for this procedure. Overall, experts recommend excision with clear surgical margins of 1 cm at the very least and careful follow-up as the initial treatment for patients with atypical Spitz tumors (Lallas et al. 2014). On a case-by-case basis, the pros and cons of this procedure may be discussed with the patient and family. Diagnostic tools as FISH can be helpful to identify patients with more aggressive tumors, for whom SLNB might have a prognostic and therapeutic benefit (Gerami et al. 2009). TERT promoter mutations (Lee et al. 2015) and 9p loss (Gerami et al. 2013) may be of prognostic significance in atypical Spitzoid melanocytic neoplasms.

40.7 Histological Diagnosis: Melanoma

In pediatric ages, melanoma is often underdiagnosed (rarity of occurrence, particularly in prepubertal ages) or overdiagnosed (high frequency of simulants of melanoma in pediatric ages). The diagnostic criteria of pediatric melanoma are essentially the same as for adult melanomas.

Pediatric melanomas can be classified into two subtypes:

- Pre-pubertal (congenital and childhood) melanomas in children up to 10–12 years.
  This group differs from adult melanomas for:
  - The high frequency of origin from congenital nevi and Spitzoid neoplasms.
  - Increased frequency of NRAS mutations.
  - The limited role of UV radiation.
  - The limited occurrence of BRAF mutations.
- Post-pubertal (adolescent) melanomas in patients between 10–12 years and 19 years of age.
  There are four histopathological subtypes:
  - De novo melanomas: arising at birth or in mainly pre-pubertal patients. They commonly develop in the dermis with an undifferentiated or blast-like cytomorphology. They develop rapidly. The differential diagnosis is with other undifferentiated or poorly differentiated malignant neoplasms.
  - Melanomas arising in congenital nevi: arising at birth or in childhood. They often develop in the dermis or subcutis in large or giant congenital nevi.
  - Spitz melanomas: they can arise in patients of any age.
  - Conventional adult-type melanomas: they usually have an epithelioid cytomorphology and correspond to superficial spreading and nodular subtypes in adults.

As detailed before, the histological diagnosis of melanoma in childhood is difficult due to its rarity in pediatric age, to its peculiar histologic features not seen in adulthood melanoma, and to the difficulty in differential diagnosis with atypical cutaneous lesions and MELTUMPs. In the presence of a suspected diagnosis of pediatric melanoma, histological specimens must always be examined by an expert pathologist in the field of melanoma, other than by a pediatric pathologist (Woulters et al. 2018). The five major histology subtypes of adult melanoma are superficial spreading, nodular, lentigo maligna, acral lentiginous, and mucosal lentiginous melanoma. These histotypes can be found also in children, but typically with the presence of epithelioid and spindle cells with Spitzoid characteristics, requiring a careful differential diagnosis in the range of atypical Spitzoid tumors. Also, there are melanomas arising in congenital nevi that are to be carefully differentiated from proliferative nodules.

A series of features should alert the pathologist to take into consideration the diagnosis of melanoma: diameter larger than 7 mm, asymmetry, poorly defined borders, ulceration, marked pagetoid spread, pleomorphism, expansile dermal growth, high mitotic count (>4/mm^2), deep and/or atypical mitoses, absence of maturation, lymphatic/vascular invasion, and perineural diffusion. The presence of a single factor should be considered and evaluated in the context of the entire lesion and its features. Overall, a second opinion is recommended in the presence of complex melanocytic lesions of uncertain or ambiguous histopathological diagnosis (including MELTUMPs) and is highly recommended in patients younger than 19 years old (Woulters et al. 2018). Use of molecular techniques such as CGH or FISH can be considered as it might help for diagnosis and prognosis assessment in challenging cases.

When diagnosis of melanoma is made, the pathologist should apply the same histological parameters as in adult cases, following the specific tumor entities listed in the WHO classification, and must provide a complete report containing items for pathological staging and refinement of prognostic models (Gershenwald et al. 2017). In particular, a diagnosis of primary cutaneous melanoma should include histological subtype, Clark level, Breslow thickness, mitoses/mm^2, type of growth phase, presence of microscopic satellites, presence of regression, presence of ulceration, tumor-infiltrating lymphocytes (TIL), neuro- and vascular diffusion, associated nevus, and state of resection margins (Cerroni et al. 2010; Brenn and McKee 2008).

40.8 Staging

Staging guidelines for pediatric melanomas refer to the adult American Joint Committee on Cancer (AJCC) classification (Table 40.1). According to this staging system which has recently been revised in 2017 (Gershenwald et al. 2017), patients are stratified into four staging groups, and prognosis varies widely on the basis of the stage. Patients with localized disease can be classified as stages I and II, based on Breslow thickness of the primary tumor and the presence or absence of ulceration; patients with stage III disease have nodal involvement, while those with stage IV disease have distant metastases. Features such as ulceration and tumor thickness affect the risk of node involvement, and consequently patients' prognosis, as in adults (Ferrari et al. 2014; Strouse et al. 2005; Paradela et al. 2010) (Fig. 40.3).

40.9 Treatment

Melanoma in young age can be defined as an "orphan" disease, and research is difficult because of its rarity. The lack of awareness that young people can develop melanoma leads to diagnostic delays and inappropriate patients' referral to specialized oncologic centers (Ferrari et al. 2014) (Table 40.2). Little is known about the biology of melanoma in this age group. Data from the literature consist mainly in retrospective

Table 40.1 TNM classification of melanoma (according to the American Joint Committee on Cancer, AJCC VIII edition, 2017)

Stage	TNM classification	Histologic/clinical features
0	Tis N0 M0	Intraepithelial/in situ melanoma
IA	T1a N0 M0	Breslow <0.8 mm w/o ulceration
IB	T1b N0 M0 T2a N0 M0	Breslow 0.8–1 mm w/o ulceration or ≤1 mm w/ ulceration Breslow 1.1–2 mm w/o ulceration
IIA	T2b N0 M0 T3a N0 M0	Breslow 1.1–2 mm w/ ulceration Breslow 2.1–4 mm w/o ulceration
IIB	T3b N0 M0 T4a N0 M0	Breslow 2.1–4 mm w/ ulceration Breslow >4 mm w/o ulceration
IIC	T4b N0 M0	Breslow >4 mm w/ ulceration
IIIA	T1–2a N1a M0 T1–2a N2a M0	Breslow ≤1 mm or 1.1–2 mm w/o ulceration; 0–1 node, clinically occult[1], no MSI[2] Breslow ≤1 mm or 1.1–2 mm w/o ulceration; 2–3 nodes, clinically occult[1], no MSI[2]
IIIB	T0 N1b–c M0 T1–2a N1b–c M0 T1–2a N2b M0 T2b–3a N1a–2b	No evidence of primary tumor; 0–1 node, b: Clinically detected[1], no MSI[a]; c: 0 nodes, MSI present[2] Breslow ≤1 mm or 1.1–2 mm w/o ulceration; 0–1 node, b: Clinically detected[1], no MSI[2]; c: 0 nodes, MSI present[2] Breslow ≤1 mm or 1.1–2 mm w/o ulceration; 2–3 nodes clinically detected[1], no MSI[2] Breslow 1.1–2 mm w/ ulceration or 2.1–4 mm w/o ulceration; 0–1 node, clinically occult[1], no MSI[2], or 2–3 nodes clinical or occult[1], w/ or w/o MSI[2]
IIIC	T0 N2b–c M0 T0 N3b–c M0 T1a–3a N2c–3c M0 T3b–4a any N M0 T4b N1a–2c M0	No evidence of primary tumor; b: 2–3 nodes clinically detected[1], no MSI[2]; c: 1 node clinical or occult[1], MSI present[2] No evidence of primary tumor; b: >3 nodes, ≥1 clinically detected or matted[1], no MSI[2]; c: >1 nodes clinical or occult[1], MSI present[2] Breslow 0.8–4 mm w/o ulceration or 1.1–2 mm w/ ulceration; 1 node clinical or occult[1], MSI present[2], or >3 nodes, all clinically occult[1], no MSI[2], or >3 nodes, ≥1 clinically detected[1] or matted, no MSI[2] or >1 nodes clinical or occult[1], MSI present[2] Breslow 2.1–4 mm w/ ulceration or >4 mm w/o ulceration; any N Breslow >4 mm w/ ulceration; 0–1 node, clinically occult[1], no MSI[2], or 2–3 nodes clinically detected[1], no MSI[2], or 1 node clinical or occult[1], MSI present[2]
IIID	T4b N3a–c M0	Breslow >4 mm w/ ulceration; >3 nodes, all clinically occult[1], no MSI[2], or >3 nodes, ≥1 clinically detected[1] or matted, no MSI[2], or >1 nodes clinical or occult[1], MSI present[2]
IV	Any T any N M1a–d Any T any N M1a–d(0) Any T any N M1a–d(1)	Skin/subcutaneous/nodule (a), lung (b), other visceral (c), brain (d); serum LDH not assessed Skin/subcutaneous/nodule (a), lung (b), other visceral (c), brain (d); normal serum LDH Skin/subcutaneous/nodule (a), lung (b), other visceral (c), brain (d); elevated serum LDH

Abbreviations: *w/* with, *w/o* without, *LDH* lactate dehydrogenase
[a] MSI comprise any satellite, locally recurrent, or in-transit lesions
[1]Nodes are designated as “clinically detectable” if they can be palpated on physical exam and are confirmed melanoma by pathology following excision/biopsy
[2] MSI comprise any satellite, locally recurrent or in transit lesion

single-institution series: Table 40.3 lists results from the main clinical trials and reported case series of children and AYA melanomas (Mones et al. 2003; Pearce et al. 2003; Chao et al. 2005; Navid et al. 2005; Ferrari et al. 2005; Butter et al. 2005; Leman et al. 2005; Strouse et al. 2005; Jafarian et al. 2005; Daryanani et al. 2006; Shah et al. 2006; Karlsson and Fredrikson 2007; Lange

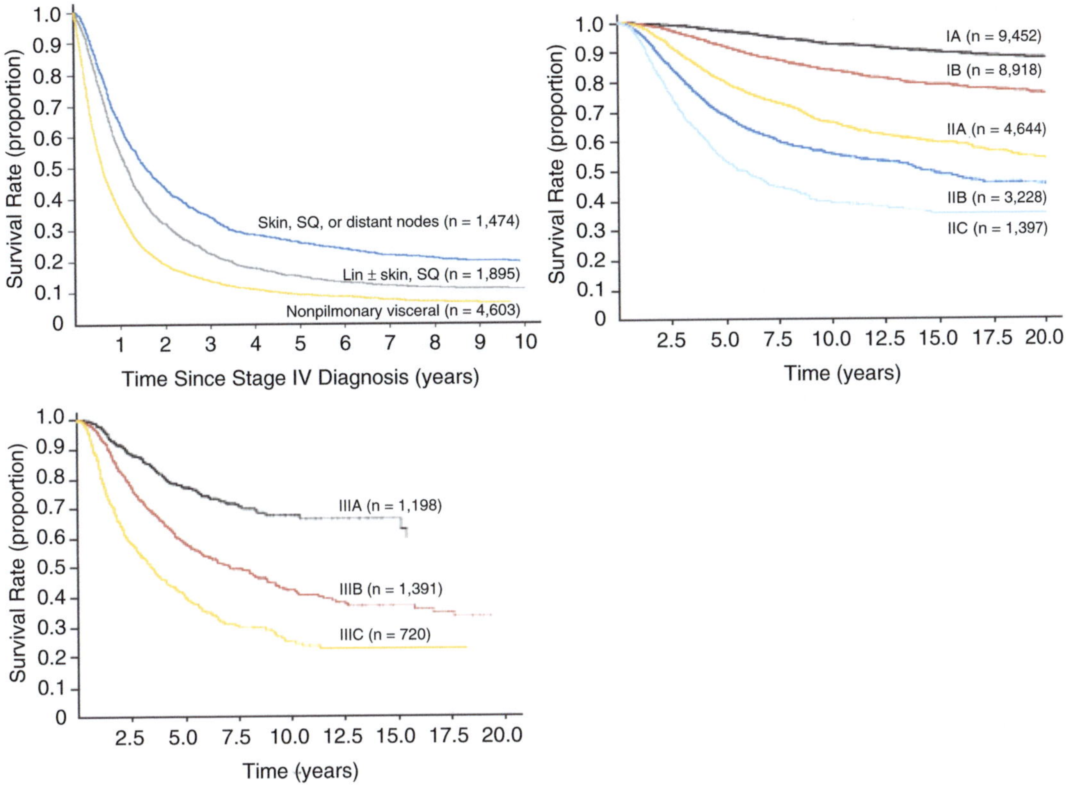

Fig. 40.3 Survival for patients with melanoma stages I–IV. (Reproduced with permission. JCO 27:6199, 2009)

et al. 2007; Livestro et al. 2007; Aldrink et al. 2009; Howman-Giles et al. 2010; Tatiana et al. 2010; Berk et al. 2010; Paradela et al. 2010; Moore-Olufemi et al. 2011; Moscarella et al. 2012; Mu et al. 2012; Han et al. 2012; Cordoro et al. 2013; Wong et al. 2013; Ferrari et al. 2014; Lam et al. 2018; Offenmueller et al. 2017; Brecht et al. 2018; Eggen et al. 2018; Bailey et al. 2018; Bartenstein et al. 2018; Réguerre et al. 2016; Chisholm et al. 2018; Geoerger et al. 2017).

To date, few prospective studies have been conducted and only on small sample of patients (Shah et al. 2006; Chisholm et al. 2018; Geoerger et al. 2017). An observational analysis from the EXPeRT recently reported data of a relatively large sample of melanoma cases (219 patients aged 0–18 years) prospectively registered and treated from 2002 to 2012 in different countries (Italy, Poland, France, Germany, Israel) (Brecht et al. 2018). Three-year overall survival (OS) and disease-free survival (DFS) rates were 91.4% and 84.0%, respectively. Sentinel lymph node biopsy (SLNB) was performed in 112 cases, while systemic therapy was given to 33 patients. Of note, survival rates of patients with stage III disease were similar with or without adjuvant therapy. Another interesting finding was that patients treated at pediatric oncology departments and registered by national cooperative pediatric oncology groups focusing on rare tumors ($n = 140$) were more likely to have advanced disease than those listed in dermatology registries ($n = 79$) (Brecht et al. 2018).

Evidences from most published studies suggest that the clinical behavior of childhood melanoma resembles that of adult disease. Since the best management approach for pediatric melanoma remains unclear, there is a general consensus that therapeutic recommendations for melanoma in the young age should remain the same as for adults. Recommendations for managing melanoma in young patients were recently

Table 40.2 Practical diagnostic and treatment guidelines for pediatric melanoma

Biopsy	When a diagnostic excision should be done in front of a suspected pigmented lesions? When (1) there is the well-founded clinical suspicion of malignancy, (2) the lesion evolves quickly, and (3) the lesion has atypical morphology Dermoscopy may reinforce the decision for biopsy In cases where a moderate perplexity remains, a short-term observation may be suggested (the removal of a pigmented lesion in a child will result in a significant cosmetic, and sometimes in a functional, impairment) When excision is justified, the surgical width should be limited (to 2 mm from lesion borders) for functional and aesthetic reasons
Diagnostic work	Comprehensive guidelines for the appropriate staging work-up for children with melanoma have not been established Chest X-ray and abdominal and regional nodal basin ultrasound are recommended for all patients. Whole-body contrast enhanced (c.e.) computed tomography (CT) scan or positron emission tomography (PET) with brain c.e. magnetic resonance imaging (MRI) could be suggested in the case of thicker lesions or according to the physician's decision on a case-by-case basis
Pathological assessment	Histological diagnosis should provide details on tumor thickness according to the Clark level and Breslow microstaging (expressed in millimeters) and the presence of ulceration. Other important features are type of growth phase, mitotic rate (mitoses/mm^2), presence of lymphatic/vascular invasion and perineural diffusion, presence of microscopic satellites, presence of regression, tumor-infiltrating lymphocytes (TIL), and state of resection margins Sentinel node biopsy in staging regional lymph nodes, to establish whether elective node dissection is warranted, is recommended for high-risk cases (thickness >0.8–1 mm without ulceration or thickness ≥1 mm with ulceration)
Staging systems	TNM AJCC system (VIII edition)
General treatment guidelines	Therapeutic recommendations for childhood melanoma should remain the same as for adults Need for referral to prime oncology center with expert physicians professionally dedicated to the management of this cancer in adults (or strict collaboration with them)
– Surgery	If the diagnosis of melanoma is confirmed at biopsy, a re-excision could be performed (at least 1 cm of surgical margin or according to tumor dimension) If the sentinel node is positive, the possibility of complete lymph node dissection versus close follow-up should be offered and shared with the patient
– Radiotherapy	No role in localized disease Palliative and curative role on oligo-metastatic sites, undergoing disease progression during systemic therapy Palliative role in metastatic disease
– Systemic treatment	Inclusion in clinical trials with immune-checkpoint inhibitors and/or targeted therapy (combined BRAF and MEK inhibitors for BRAF-mutant disease)

provided in a paper by the European Cancer Organization (ECCO) on the Essential Requirements for Quality Cancer Care (ERQCC) (Wouters et al. 2018). In pediatric age, disease prevention is paramount, and many collaborative efforts have been made to have dedicated scholar meetings recommending protection against sun UV radiation from infancy. These guidelines also stress the need for pediatric oncologists and surgeons treating children and adolescents with melanoma to cooperate closely with experts at specialist adult melanoma centers. To ensure that young patients with melanoma receive the treatment recognized as standard in adults, with adoption of the best therapeutic strategy, networks of specialists like the EXPeRT (http://www.raretumors-children.eu) are available for all experienced centers treating these patients (Leiter and Garbe 2008; Ferrari et al. 2014). Care of pediatric melanoma patients must be organized and delivered as a result of consensus among multidisciplinary teams, with significant expertise in the field (i.e., treating a sufficient number of melanoma

Table 40.3 Overview of the principal published studies on pediatric melanoma

Author, year Center	Type of study/Registry	Period	N° of patients	Age (yrs)	Aims—results
Kalani, 2019 University of Colorado, Aurora, Colorado, USA	Colorado Central Cancer Registry	1988–2015	256	<20	Girls 10–14 and 15–19 years old at increased risk of melanoma compared to boys in these age groups There are sex-specific differences in anatomic site consistent with prior literature
Georger, 2017	Phase II	2013–2016	12	12–16	At 1 year, 3 of 4 patients on 3 mg/kg and 5 of 8 patients on 10 mg/kg were alive Two patients on 10 mg/kg had partial response, and 1 on 3 mg/kg had stable disease The safety profile was consistent with that observed in the adult population The study was stopped due to slow accrual of patients
Chisholm, 2018	Phase I, open-label, dose-escalation	2011–2015	6	12–17	A recommended and effective dose of vemurafenib for patients was not identified Extremely low enrollment in this trial highlights the importance of considering the inclusion of adolescents with adult cancers in adult trials
Bartenstein, 2018 Massachusetts General Hospital, Boston, USA	Retrospective cohort study	1995–2016	32	<19	Children and adolescents present with different melanoma subtypes. Adolescents have a more aggressive disease course than children
Bailey, 2018	The University of Michigan's pediatric oncology database	2000–2013	30	<20	Importance of expert pathology review upfront Education at primary care level could minimize diagnostic delays

(continued)

Table 40.3 (continued)

Author, year Center	Type of study/Registry	Period	N° of patients	Age (yrs)	Aims—results
Eggen, 2018	Netherlands Cancer Registry	1989–2013	625	0–19	Melanoma is very rare under the age of 12, with stable incidence rates Melanoma is more common in adolescents with a decreasing trend in the past decade Male sex and increasing Breslow thickness are associated with worse survival in pediatric patients 1-year OS 98% 5-year OS 94% 10-year OS 90%
Brecht, 2018 EXPeRT	Prospective registry of cases (Italy, Poland, Germany, and France). Dermatology registries (Germany and Israel)	2002–2012	219	0–19	The clinical history of melanoma in children and adolescents might resemble that of adult counterpart. Patients treated by pediatric oncologists were more likely to have advanced disease than those treated by dermatologists. In stage III cases, similar survival rates for patients who received or not adjuvant therapy 3-year OS 94.1% (median follow-up 41.8 months)
Offenmueller, 2017	German pediatric rare tumor registry (STEP)	2006–2014	60	0–17	Patients with Spitzoid histotype (40%) did not show a significantly different outcome compared to non-Spitzoid melanomas Adjuvant therapy was used in 45% of cases 3-year OS 100%
Lam, 2018	SEER registry	2004–2008	1255	0–21	Disparities in the ≤12-year-old melanoma population, as they had later stage melanomas, less invasive surgery, and lower survival rates

Ferrari, 2014 Italian TREP project	Prospective series	2000–2012	54	<18	Variables influencing survival in children are the same as for adults. The clinical approach used in adults is feasible in children Pediatric cases are more likely to have advanced disease at diagnosis but similar survival
Wong, 2013	NCI, SEER databases	1973–2009	1230	0–19	2% per year increase of incidence Analysis on risk factors
Cordoro, 2013 University of California, San Francisco	Retrospective single-institution	1984–2009	70	<20	Modification of detection criteria
Han, 2012 Moffitt Cancer Center, Tampa, FL	Retrospective single-institution	1986–2001	127	<20	Higher risk of nodal metastases than for adults, but similar survival rates OS 84.1%
Mu, 2012	NCI, SEER databases	2003–2008	2085	<25	Thickness and ulceration were predictors of both the use of SLNB and positivity of SLNB. Children were more likely to have SLNB metastases despite similar rates of SLNB use OS 87% (in SLNB positive)
Moscarella, 2012 Medical University of Graz, Austria	Retrospective series	1998–2007	38	<20	To investigate accuracy in melanoma diagnosis
Moore, 2011 MD Anderson Cancer Center, Houston, TX	Retrospective single-institution	1992–2006	109	<18	Comparison between pre-pubescent ($n = 25$) and adolescent ($n = 84$) patients: no difference in survival by age group; younger age associated with thicker tumors and a higher risk of lymph node metastasis OS 89%

(continued)

Table 40.3 (continued)

Author, year Center	Type of study/Registry	Period	N° of patients	Age (yrs)	Aims—results
Paradela, 2010 MD Anderson Cancer Center Histologic database	Retrospective series	1992–2006	137	<18	Presence of metastases as main prognostic factor Children <11 years old had less aggressive tumor behavior OS 86.3%
Berk, 2010 Stanford University, California	Retrospective single-institution	1995–2008	13	<21	High rate of node positivity in MELTUMPs OS 92.3%
Tatiana, 2010 Hospital of Sick Children, Toronto, CA	Retrospective single-institution	2000–2008	14	<18	Melanoma is the most common malignant skin tumor in children OS 100%
Howman-Giles, 2010 Sidney University, Australia	Retrospective single-institution	1993–2008	55	<20	Young people had higher risk of SLNB positivity OS 94.1%
Aldrink, 2009 Duke University Medical Center, NC, USA	Retrospective single-institution	1973–2007	150	<20	10.7% initially incorrect diagnoses OS 84%
Livestro, 2007 Massachusetts General Hospital, Boston, USA	Retrospective single-institution	1971–2001	73	<21	Lymph node metastases were more prevalent in young patients than in adults (matched for tumor thickness) Survival rates were similar OS 89.4%
Lange, 2007	US National Cancer Database	1985–2003	3158	<20	Differences between children/adolescents and adults (demographic, presentation, survival) OS <10 years: 77% OS >10 years: 87%
Karlsson, 2007	Epidemiological study Swedish Cancer Registry	1973–2002	250	<20	Decrease in incidence in the last decades, possible result of public health prevention campaigns 90% in 1993–2002 subgroup
Shah, 2006 Hospital for Sick Children, Toronto, CA	Retrospective single-institution	1995–2005	11	<15	Feasibility of SLNB to identify patients at high risk Tolerance of high-dose IFN therapy OS 90%

Daryanani, 2006 Groningen, Netherlands	Retrospective single-institution	1965–2003	49	<20	Comparison with adult cohort (n = 900 adults): more advanced disease in adolescents, similar survival rates OS 79%
Jafarian, 2005 Sainte Justine Hospital, Montreal, CA	Retrospective single-institution	1980–2002	13	<17	Thicker lesions than in adults; delay in diagnosis OS 58.8%
Strouse, 2005	NCI, SEER databases	1973–2001	1255	<20	Increasing incidence of pediatric melanoma over the decades Analysis of risk factors and prognostic factors OS 93.6%
Leman, 2005 West of Scotland	Retrospective pathological multicentric review	1979–2002	20	<16	Overdiagnosis of pediatric melanoma OS 95%
Butter, 2005 Montreal Children's Hospital, Montreal, CA	Retrospective single-institution	1989–2004	12	<18	SLNB useful to identify high-risk patients OS stage I = 100% OS stage II = 83% OS stage III = 75%
Ferrari, 2005 Istituto Nazionale Tumori Milano, Italy	Retrospective single-institution	1975–2001	33	<14	Peculiar clinical presentation (amelanotic, raised lesion) in pre-pubertal cases Better outcome in young children OS 70%
Navid, 2005 St. Jude Children's Research Hospital, Memphis, Tennessee, USA	Prospective, single-institution	1999–2004	15	<18	Feasibility of high-dose IFN alpha-2b therapy OS for stage III: 74.1% (follow-up: 20 months)
Chao, 2005 Ann Arbor, Michigan, USA	Retrospective single-institution	1989–2003	14	<18	To assess efficacy and tolerability of high-dose IFN in high-risk pediatric patients (stages IIB, IIC, III) OS 100% (median follow-up 24 months)

(continued)

Table 40.3 (continued)

Author, year Center	Type of study/Registry	Period	N° of patients	Age (yrs)	Aims—results
Pearce, 2003	Northern Region Young Persons' Malignant Disease Registry, UK	1968–1995	138	<25	Increasing incidence of pediatric melanoma over the decades OS <14 years: 85% OS >14 years: 70%
Mones, 2003 Ackerman Academy of Dermatopathology, NY, USA	Retrospective single-institution	Unspecified	11	<10	Clinical characteristics and histopathological features peculiar to pre-pubescent melanomas OS 90%

Abbreviations: *EXPeRT* European Cooperative Study Group for Pediatric Rare Tumors, *IFN* interferon, *MELTUMPs* melanocytic lesions or tumors of unknown metastatic potential, *NCI* National Cancer Institute, *OS* overall survival, *SEER* Surveillance, Epidemiology, and End Results, *SLNB* sentinel lymph node biopsy, *yrs* years patients per year and with the possibility to access the infrastructure to treat patients with advanced loco-regional disease). The core of a multidisciplinary group should be composed of a team of dedicated dermatologists, pathologists, radiologists, surgeons, and oncologists (Wouters et al. 2018).

As in adults, most cases of melanoma arising in early age are localized at diagnosis (~75%). Therefore, surgical resection remains the mainstay of treatment for approximately 90% of patients with pediatric melanoma. The estimated 5-year OS rate for patients with disease amenable to radical excision has been reported to exceed 90% (Tricoli et al. 2016; Brecht et al. 2015). Experts recommend to follow the same surgical guidelines that have been developed for adults, when feasible: lesions ≤1 mm should be resected with a 1 cm margin, 1–4 mm lesions with a 2 cm margin, and those more than 4 cm with at least a 2 cm margin. Patients with lesions ≤1 mm and no ulceration or mitotic rate <1 mm^2 can be treated with surgical resection alone and observation. The use of SLNB for staging has become widespread, and features like Breslow thickness >0.8 mm and/or ulceration have been correlated with higher rates of nodal involvement (Mu et al. 2012). SLNB may be considered for T1a melanoma if other adverse features are present, including young age, presence of lymphovascular invasion, positive deep biopsy margin, high mitotic rate, or a combination of these factors. In the event of SLNB positivity, it is possible to consider complete lymph node dissection (CLND) (Daniotti et al. 2009; Navid et al. 2016; Chao et al. 2005). However, results of two randomized phase III trials, the MSLT2 and the DeCOG-SLT trial, demonstrated that immediate CLND increased the rate of regional disease control and provided prognostic information, but did not increase melanoma-specific survival among adult patients with melanoma and sentinel node metastases (Leiter et al. 2016; Faries et al. 2017). CLND should not be recommended in patients with melanoma with lymph node micrometastases of at least a diameter of 1 mm or smaller. Interdisciplinary collaboration involving surgical and medical oncologists is recommended for discussion on possible CLND vs. regional nodal ultrasound surveillance. CLND should be restricted to those patients with features identified in their SLNB that indicate a high risk of regional relapse (extracapsular spread, ≥3 involved sentinel nodes, multifocal or extensive disease) and for those with clinically detectable nodal disease (i.e., palpable nodes and/or radiologic evidence of nodal disease).

The prognosis for patients with nodal involvement is intermediate, with about 60% of patients expected to have a long-term survival after surgery (Tricoli et al. 2016; Mu et al. 2012). Young patients with high-risk primary cutaneous melanoma (e.g., those with regional lymph node involvement) have limited treatment options. Adjuvant therapy with interferon (IFN) alpha-2b has only a limited impact on oncologic outcomes (Shah et al. 2006; Navid et al. 2005, 2016; Chao et al. 2005): its use in this subset of adult patients is still controversial and has been rapidly replaced by novel-targeted therapy and immunotherapies. However, the use of novel therapeutic agents in this setting has not been validated for pediatric patients; thus, a valid therapeutic alternative is lacking for patients at high risk of disease relapse. Radiotherapy should not be used as adjuvant treatment for stage III disease. Rather, it can be considered as a palliative treatment for advanced disease (e.g., treatment brain metastases) or as treatment for oligo-metastatic progressive disease during systemic treatment.

Regarding advanced stages (i.e., unresectable [stage III] and/or metastatic [stage IV] melanoma), they are rare in the young and usually associated with poor prognosis (estimated 5-year OS of 12–20%) (Pappo et al. 2003). Only few reports exist in literature on systemic treatments for advanced melanoma in young people. Given the lack of a standard treatment and a limited access to clinical trials (phase III studies conducted to date have excluded patients under

18 years old), the therapeutic options used for young patients with advanced melanoma included chemotherapy, either alone or in combination with interferon (Brecht et al. 2018). However, it is well known that only a small proportion of patients with melanoma gain clinical benefit from chemotherapy, which normally achieves poor disease control and unsatisfactory survival curves (Quéreux and Dréno 2011). Loco-regional approaches such as surgical excision, electrochemotherapy, and isolated limb perfusion may apply in selected cases for the treatment of cutaneous and subcutaneous nodules and also for satellites and in-transit metastases.

In recent years, the treatment landscape of adult melanoma has significantly changed with the introduction of two classes of drugs which have dramatically improved survival outcomes. The first class of drugs target the mitogen-activated protein kinase (MAPK) pathway, which is constitutively active in melanoma harboring BRAF V600 mutations (i.e., approximately 50% of adult patients). First, two BRAF inhibitors (vemurafenib (McArthur et al. 2014) and dabrafenib (Hauschild et al. 2012)) were approved by the US Food and Drug Administration (FDA) as a monotherapy for treating BRAF-mutant advanced melanoma. Insight in the resistance mechanisms (which are mainly MEK-dependent) limiting the duration of response to this treatment (Paraiso et al. 2010) led to the development of combined BRAF + MEK inhibitor therapies (i.e., vemurafenib + cobimetinib, dabrafenib + trametinib, encorafenib + binimetinib). Evidence from phase III trials of combined targeted therapies demonstrating their superiority to BRAF inhibitors alone prompted their approval for use in the treatment of BRAF-mutant advanced melanoma (Ascierto et al. 2016; Long et al. 2015; Dummer et al. 2018).

The second therapeutic strategy involves modulation of immune system with monoclonal antibodies acting as immune checkpoint inhibitors (ICIs) (i.e., ipilimumab targeting the cytotoxic T-lymphocyte-associated antigen 4 [CTLA4]; nivolumab and pembrolizumab targeting the programmed death-1 [PD1] receptor). Based on the results of phase III randomized trials, these drugs have been approved as monotherapies for metastatic melanoma (Hodi et al. 2010; Weber et al. 2015; Ribas et al. 2015). Combination treatment with anti-PD1 and anti-CTLA4 is approved in the USA and seems to further improve the outcomes, albeit with a higher incidence of serious immune-related adverse events (Larkin et al. 2015; Wolchok et al. 2017).

Given the successful results obtained in the treatment of metastatic disease, both combo-targeted therapies and immunotherapy have been explored in the adjuvant setting (Eggermont et al. 2015; Eggermont et al. 2018; Weber et al. 2017; Long et al. 2017). In fact, the efficacy of adjuvant IFN has proved rather modest in preventing disease relapse or improving survival in stage IIIB/C melanoma and is associated with significant toxicities (especially when used at high doses) (Mocellin et al. 2010). To date, both combo-targeted therapies and immunotherapy have confirmed a recurrence-free survival improvement for adult patients with high-risk resected stage III disease (nivolumab, pembrolizumab, dabrafenib, and trametinib) and resected stage IV disease (nivolumab). At the present time, 12-month adjuvant treatment with anti-PD1 (nivolumab, pembrolizumab) is approved for resected stage III melanoma, regardless of BRAF mutational status; 12-month adjuvant treatment with dabrafenib and trametinib is approved for resected stage III BRAF-mutant melanoma. Nivolumab is the only agent approved for the treatment of resected stage IV disease with no evidence of disease (Long et al. 2017; Weber et al. 2017; Eggermont et al. 2018).

Combined together, these results have led to an overall improvement in the prognosis of patients with melanoma in the adult. For the reasons extensively detailed before, melanoma in the young shares the same unmet needs of adult melanoma in the past, even so younger patients have not gained a benefit from these recent improvements. More than one element can explain this specific situation. First of all, due to the rarity of the disease, children and adolescents may be inadequately diagnosed, referred (due to delayed access to experienced centers), and ultimately treated. A fundamental role is played by the limited access to clinical trials, which are usually for patients over 18 years (Ferrari et al. 2008). In the last years, efforts to pursue targeted therapies and immunotherapies in young patients have been made. However, the development of new drugs in this subset of patients has been hindered by the difficulty in enrolling patients even with the aid of large international projects. A phase I trial of ipilimumab in children and adolescents enrolled 12 patients with melanoma to receive treatment with 5 mg/kg or 10 mg/kg per dose every 3 weeks for four cycles (Merchant et al. 2016). The treatment demonstrated a similar toxicity profile as that seen in adults, paving the way to the subsequent steps of development. Unfortunately, the phase II study of ipilimumab in adolescents (i.e., age 12–18 years) with unresectable stage III or IV melanoma failed to achieve accrual goals. The plan had been to enroll 40 patients, but the study was prematurely closed after only 12 patients had been recruited over a 3.5-year period (Geoerger et al. 2017). Indeed, results from this trial reported clinical activity in this subset of patients: two out of eight patients who received ipilimumab 10 mg/kg had partial response, and one out of four patients who received 3 mg/kg had stable disease. At 1-year follow-up, five patients who received 10 mg/kg and three patients who received 3 mg/kg were alive. The same patient recruitment problem affected the recently published phase I, open-label, dose-escalation study on vemurafenib for pediatric, stage IIIc/IV BRAF V600 mutation-positive melanoma: the study was interrupted prematurely after it succeeded in enrolling only six patients (Chisholm et al. 2018). Unlike adult patients with BRAF V600-mutated metastatic melanoma, no objective responses were observed in the study population. However, given the small sample size and the absence of a clinical rationale to explain this inferiority of outcome, the possibility that this may have occurred by chance cannot be excluded. Because of the extremely low enrollment in this trial, a recommended and effective dose of vemurafenib for patients aged 12–17 years was not identified.

Even with the difficulty related to the relatively small number of cases, there have been reports of a positive trend in the enrollment of young patients in clinical trials in recent years: this has translated in a statistically insignificant trend toward a better 3-year OS for young patients with advanced disease who were enrolled in clinical trials than for those who were not (Sreeraman Kumar et al. 2018). Another problem is represented by legal restrictions on the development of new drugs for use in children with rare diseases. The reason for promoting the enrollment of young patients with melanoma (and in general with adult-type cancers) in clinical trials is that most drugs have similar pharmacokinetics, tolerability profiles, and recommended doses for young patients (mostly AYAs) relative to adults (Rose and Grant-Kels 2018; Momper et al. 2007). A possible strategy to overcome such difficulties lies in the collaboration between adult and pediatric cancer centers, in order to facilitate the referral of young patients to centers recruiting for such trials (Chuk et al. 2017). Among the various initiatives, it is worth to mention the ACCELERATE project—promoted by the European Society for Paediatric Oncology (SIOPE) and the *Innovative Therapies* for Children with Cancer (*ITCC*) Consortium—that proposes adult phase I/II trials to include adolescents above the age of 12 years: this approach is considered not only ethical but feasible and safe supported by similar dosing and PK parameters in adolescents and adults and no extra toxicity observed in adolescents (Gaspar et al. 2018).

40.10 Survival

The population-based analysis from the SEER reported a 5-year melanoma-specific survival of 94.5% (Strouse et al. 2005). This result is better than those reported in published hospital-based series (that can be biased by the selection of patients with more advanced disease) and is slightly better than that usually achieved in adults. Data from the literature showed a moderate improvement in melanoma 5-year from 82% in 1999–2001 to 85% in the 2000–2007 period from the EUROCARE study (Crocetti et al. 2015). Detailed information on survival by stage is limited for pediatric melanoma. In a systematic review that included studies from nine European countries, the reported 5-year overall survival rates were 95–100% (stage I), 65–92.8% (stage II), 41–71% (stage III), and 9–28% (stage IV). Authors concluded that there are large variations in stage-specific overall and recurrence-free survival by study type and by country (Svedman et al. 2016).

Long-term follow-up is required for melanoma patients to detect early recurrences, new secondary melanomas, or other related cancers. However, no definite consensus exists on optimal schedules and timing of follow-up; therefore, attention should be given in order to avoid unnecessary and costly follow-up investigations (Wouters et al. 2018) (Figs. 40.4 and 40.5).

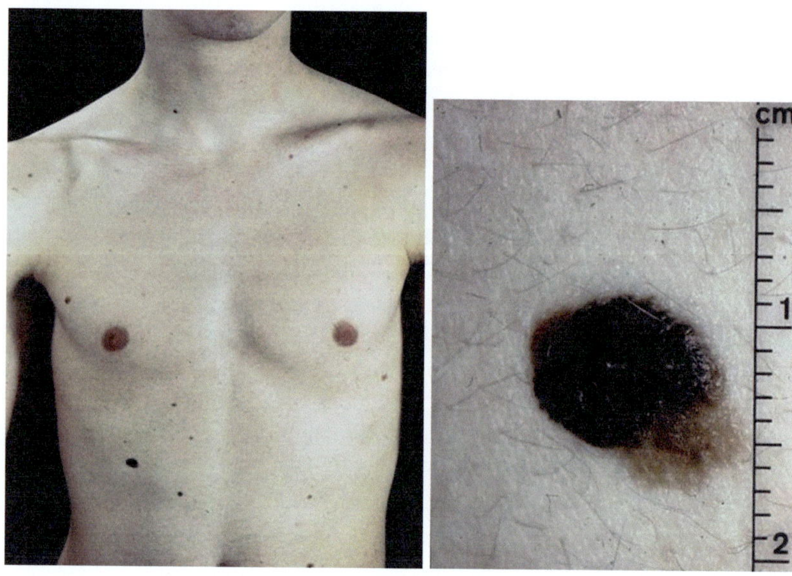

Fig. 40.4 Superficial spreading melanoma in a 17-year-old boy

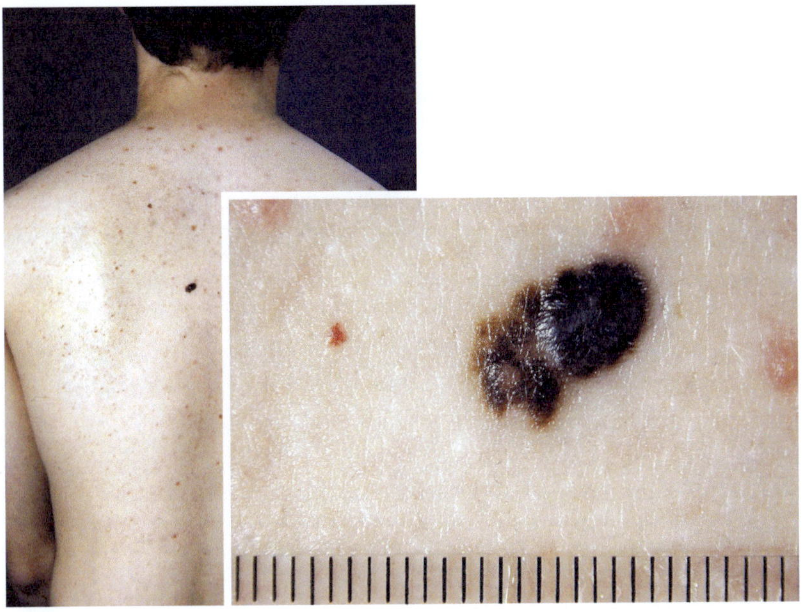

Fig. 40.5 Superficial spreading melanoma in a 18-year-old boy

References

Aldrink JH, Selim MA, Diesen DL, Johnson J, Pruitt SK, Tyler DS, Seigler HF (2009) Pediatric melanoma: a single-institution experience of 150 patients. J Pediatr Surg 44:1514–1521

Alexander A, Samlowski WE, Grossman D et al (2003) Metastatic melanoma in pregnancy: risk of transplacental metastases in the infant. J Clin Oncol 21:2179–2186

Ascierto PA, McArthur GA, Dréno B et al (2016) Cobimetinib combined with vemurafenib in advanced BRAFV600-mutant melanoma (coBRIM): updated efficacy results from a randomised, double-blind, phase 3 trial. Lancet Oncol 17(9):1248–1260

Bailey KM, Durham AB, Zhao L et al (2018) Pediatric melanoma and aggressive Spitz tumors: a retrospective diagnostic, exposure and outcome analysis. Transl Pediatr 7(3):203–210

Barhami A, Barnhill RL (2018) Pathology and genomics of pediatric melanoma: a critical reexamination and new insights. Pediatr Blood Cancer 65(2)

Bartenstein DW, Kelleher CM, Friedmann AM et al (2018) Contrasting features of childhood and adolescent melanomas. Pediatr Dermatol 35(3):354–360

Berk DR, LaBuz E, Dadras SS et al (2010) Melanoma and melanocytic tumors of uncertain malignant potential in children, adolescents and young adults - the Stanford experience 1995–2008. Pediatr Dermatol 27:244–254

Bono A, Ferrari A (2005) Early diagnosis remains the most reliable way to cure children with melanoma. Pediatr Blood Cancer 45(3):355

Brecht IB, Garbe C, Gefeller O et al (2015) 443 paediatric cases of malignant melanoma registered with the German Central Malignant Melanoma Registry between 1983 and 2011. Eur J Cancer 51(7):861–868

Brecht IB, De Paoli A, Bisogno G, Orbach D, Schneider DT, Leiter U, Offenmueller S, Cecchetto G, Godzinski J, Bien E, Stachowicz-Stencel T, Ben-Ami T, Chiaravalli S, Maurichi A, De Salvo GL, Sorbara S, Bodemer C, Garbe C, Reguerre Y, Ferrari A. Pediatric patients with cutaneous melanoma: A European study. Pediatr Blood Cancer. 2018;65(6):e26974. https://doi.org/10.1002/pbc.26974. Epub 2018 Jan 19. PMID: 29350487.

Brenn T, McKee PHM (2008) Melanoma in children and adolescents. Diagn Histopathol 14:18–27

Butter A, Hui T, Chapdelaine J, Beaunoyer M et al (2005) Melanoma in children and the use of sentinel lymph node biopsy. J Pediatr Surg 40:797–800

Cancer Genome Atlas Network (2015) Genomic classification of cutaneous melanoma. Cell 161(7):1681–1696

Ceballos PI, Ruiz-Maldonado R, Mihm MC Jr (1995) Melanoma in children. N Engl J Med 332:656–662

Cerroni L, Barnhill R, Elder D et al (2010) Melanocytic tumors of uncertain malignant potential: results of a tutorial held at the XXIX Symposium of the International Society of Dermatopathology in Graz, October 2008. Am J Surg Pathol 34:314–326

Chao MM, Schwartz JL, Wechsler DS, Thornburg CD, Griffith KA, Williams JA (2005) High-risk surgically resected pediatric melanoma and adjuvant interferon therapy. Pediatr Blood Cancer 44:441–448

Chisholm JC, Suvada J, Dunkel IJ et al (2018) BRIM-P: a phase I, open-label, multicenter, dose-escalation study of vemurafenib in pediatric patients with surgically incurable, BRAF mutation-positive melanoma. Pediatr Blood Cancer 65(5):e26947

Chuk MK et al (2017) Enrolling adolescents in disease/target-appropriate adult oncology clinical trials of investigational agents. Clin Cancer Res 23(1):9–12

Cordoro KM, Gupta D, Frieden IJ, McCalmont T, Kashani-Sabet M (2013) Pediatric melanoma: results of a large cohort study and proposal for modified ABCD detection criteria for children. J Am Acad Dermatol 68:912–925

Crocetti E, Mallone S, Robsahm TE et al (2015) Survival of patients with skin melanoma in Europe increases further: results of the EUROCARE-5 study. Eur J Cancer 51(15):2179–2190

Curtis RE, Rowlings PA, Deeg HJ et al (1997) Solid cancers after bone marrow transplantation. N Engl J Med 336:897–904

Daniotti M, Ferrari A, Frigerio S et al (2009) Cutaneous melanoma in childhood and adolescence shows frequent loss of INK4A and gain of KIT. J Invest Dermatol 129(7):1759–1768

Daryanani D, Plukker JT, Nap RE et al (2006) Adolescent melanoma: risk factors and long term survival. Eur J Surg Oncol 32(2):218–223

Dummer R, Ascierto PA, Gogas HJ et al (2018) Overall survival in patients with BRAF-mutant melanoma receiving encorafenib plus binimetinib versus vemurafenib or encorafenib (COLUMBUS): a multicentre, open-label, randomised, phase 3 trial. Lancet Oncol 19(10):1315–1327

Eggen CAM, Durgaram VVL, van Doorn R et al (2018) Incidence and relative survival of melanoma in children and adolescents in the Netherlands, 1989–2013. J Eur Acad Dermatol Venereol 32(6):956–961

Eggermont AM, Chiarion-Sileni V, Grob JJ et al (2015) Adjuvant ipilimumab versus placebo after complete resection of high-risk stage III melanoma (EORTC18071): a randomised, double-blind, phase 3 trial. Lancet Oncol 16:522–530

Eggermont AMM, Blank CU, Mandala M et al (2018) Adjuvant pembrolizumab versus placebo in resected Stage III melanoma. N Engl J Med 378(19):1789–1801

Euvrard S, Kanitakis J, Claudy A (2003) Skin cancers after organ transplantation. N Engl J Med 348:1681–1691

Faries MB, Thompson JF, Cochran AJ et al (2017) Completion dissection or observation for sentinel-node metastasis in melanoma. N Engl J Med 376(23):2211–2222. https://doi.org/10.1056/NEJMoa1613210

Ferrari A, Bono A, Baldi M, Collini P, Casanova M, Pennacchioli E et al (2005) Does melanoma behave better in younger children than in adults? A retrospective study on 33 cases of childhood melanoma from a single institution. Pediatrics 115:649–654

Ferrari A, Montello M, Budd T, Bleyer A (2008) The challenges of clinical trials for adolescents and young adults with cancer. Pediatr Blood Cancer 50(5 Suppl):1101–1104

Ferrari A, Bisogno G, Cecchetto G et al (2014) Cutaneous melanoma in children and adolescents: the Italian Rare Tumors in Pediatric Age Project Experience. J Pediatr 164:375–382

Ferrari A, Brecht IB, Gatta G et al (2019) Defining and listing very rare cancers of pediatric age: consensus of the Joint Action on Rare Cancers (JARC) in cooperation with the European Cooperative Study Group for Pediatric Rare Tumors (EXPeRT). Eur J Cancer 110:120–126. https://doi.org/10.1016/j.ejca.2018.12.031

Friedman DL, Whitton J, Leisenring W et al (2010) Subsequent neoplasms in 5-year survivors of childhood cancer: the Childhood Cancer Survivor Study. J Natl Cancer Inst 102:1083–1095

Gaspar N, Marshall LV, Binner D et al (2018) Joint adolescent–adult early phase clinical trials to improve access to new drugs for adolescents with cancer: proposals from the multi-stakeholder platform—ACCELERATE. Ann Oncol 29(3):766–771

Geoerger B, Bergeron C, Gore L et al (2017) Phase II study of ipilimumab in adolescents with unresectable stage III or IV malignant melanoma. Eur J Cancer 86:358–363

Gerami P, Jewell SS, Morrison LE et al (2009) Fluorescence in situ hybridization (FISH) as an ancillary diagnostic tool in the diagnosis of melanoma. Am J Surg Pathol 33:1146–1156

Gerami P et al (2013) Risk assessment for atypical spitzoid melanocytic neoplasms using FISH to identify chromosomal copy number aberrations. Am J Surg Pathol 37(5):676–684

Gershenwald JE, Scolyer RA, Hess KR et al (2017) Melanoma staging: evidence-based changes in the American Joint Committee on Cancer eighth edition cancer staging manual. CA Cancer J Clin 67(6):472–492

Han D, Zager JS, Han G et al (2012) The unique clinical characteristics of melanoma diagnosed in children. Ann Surg Oncol 19:3888–3895

Handfield-Jones SE, Smith NP (1996) Malignant melanoma in childhood. Br J Dermatol 134:607–616

Hauschild A, Grob J, Demidov LV et al (2012) Dabrafenib in BRAF-mutated metastatic melanoma: a multicentre, open-label, phase 3 randomised controlled trial. Lancet 380(9839):358–365

Hayward NK (2003) Genetics of melanoma predisposition. Oncogene 22:3053–3062

Hodi FS, O'Day SJ, McDermott DF et al (2010) Improved survival with ipilimumab in patients with metastatic melanoma. N Engl J Med 363:711–723

Howman-Giles R, Shaw HM, Scolyer RA et al (2010) Sentinel lymph node biopsy in pediatric and adolescent cutaneous melanoma patients. Ann Surg Oncol 17:138–143

Jafarian F, Powell J, Kokta V et al (2005) Malignant melanoma in childhood and adolescence: report of 13 cases. J Am Acad Dermatol 53:816–822

Jansen B, Hansen D, Moy R et al (2018) Gene expression analysis differentiates melanomas from Spitz nevi. J Drugs Dermatol 17(5):574–576

Kalani N, Guidry JA, Farahi JM et al (2019) Pediatric melanoma: characterizing 256 cases from the Colorado

Central Cancer Registry. Pediatr Dermatol 36(2):219–222. https://doi.org/10.1111/pde.13747

Karlsson PM, Fredrikson M (2007) Cutaneous malignant melanoma in children and adolescents in Sweden, 1993–2002: the increasing trend is broken. Int J Cancer 121:323–328

Kaste SC, Pappo AS, Jenkins JJ III, Pratt CB (1996) Malignant melanoma in children: imaging spectrum. Pediatr Radiol 26:800–805

Kleinerman RA, Tucker MA, Tarone RE et al (2005) Risk of new cancers after radiotherapy in long-term survivors of retinoblastoma: an extended follow-up. J Clin Oncol 23:2272–2279

Lallas A, Kyrgidis A, Ferrara G et al (2014) Atypical Spitz tumours and sentinel lymph node biopsy: a systematic review. Lancet Oncol 15(4):178–183

Lam PH, Obirieze AC, Ortega G et al (2018) An age-based analysis of pediatric melanoma: staging, surgery and mortality in the surveillance, epidemiology and end results database. Am Surg 84(5):739–745

Lange JR, Palis BE, Chang DC, Soong S-J, Balch CM (2007) Melanoma in children and teenagers: an analysis of patients from the National Cancer Data Base. J Clin Oncol 25:1363–1368

Larkin J, Chiarion-Sileni V, Gonzalez R et al (2015) Combined nivolumab and ipilimumab or monotherapy in untreated melanoma. N Engl J Med 373(1):23–34

Lauper JM, Krause A, Vaughan TL, Monnat RJ Jr (2013) Spectrum and risk of neoplasia in Werner syndrome: a systematic review. PLoS One 8(4):e59709

Lazovich D, Vogel RI, Berwick M, Weinstock MA, Anderson KE, Warshaw EM (2010) Indoor tanning and risk of melanoma: a case-control study in a highly exposed population. Cancer Epidemiol Biomark Prev 19:1557–1568

Lee S et al (2015) TERT promoter mutations are predictive of aggressive clinical behavior in patients with spitzoid melanocytic neoplasms. Sci Rep 5:11200

Leiter U, Garbe C (2008) Epidemiology of melanoma and nonmelanoma skin cancer - the role of sunlight. Adv Exp Med Biol 624:89–103

Leiter U, Stadler R, Mauch C et al (2016) Complete lymph node dissection versus no dissection in patients with sentinel lymph node biopsy positive melanoma (DeCOG-SLT): a multicentre, randomised, phase 3 trial. Lancet Oncol 17(6):757–767. https://doi.org/10.1016/S1470-2045(16)00141-8

Leman JA, Evans A, Mooi W, Mackie RM (2005) Outcomes and pathological review of a cohort of children with melanoma. Br J Dermatol 152(6):1321–1323

Livestro DP, Kaine EM, Michaelson JS et al (2007) Melanoma in the young: differences and similarities with adult melanoma: a case-matched controlled analysis. Cancer 110:614–624

Long GV, Stroyakovskiy D, Gogas H et al (2015) Dabrafenib and trametinib versus dabrafenib and placebo for Val600 BRAF-mutant melanoma: a multicentre, double-blind, phase 3 randomised controlled trial. Lancet 386(9992):444–451

Long GV, Hauschild A, Santinami M et al (2017) Adjuvant dabrafenib plus trametinib in stage III BRAF-mutated melanoma. N Engl J Med 377(19):1813–1823

Lu C, Zhang J, Nagahawatte P et al (2015) The genomic landscape of childhood and adolescent melanoma. J Invest Dermatol 135(3):816–823

Makkar HS, Frieden IJ (2004) Neurocutaneous melanosis. Semin Cutan Med Surg 23:138–144

Margaryan NV, Gilgur A, Seftor EA et al (2016) Melanocytes affect nodal expression and signaling in melanoma cells: a lesson from pediatric large congenital melanocytic nevi. Int J Mol Sci 17(3):418

Massi D, Tomasini C, Senetta R et al (2015) Atypical Spitz tumors in patients younger than 18 years. J Am Acad Dermatol 72(1):37–46

McArthur GA, Chapman PB, Robert C et al (2014) Safety and efficacy of vemurafenib in BRAFV600E and BRAFV600 K mutation-positive melanoma (BRIM-3): extended follow-up of a phase 3, randomised, open-label study. Lancet Oncol 15(3):323–332

Melanoma Treatment (PDQ®): Health Professional Version. (n.d.) PDQ Adult Treatment Editorial Board. PDQ Cancer Information Summaries [Internet]. Bethesda (MD): National Cancer Institute (US); 2002–2018 Feb 2

Merchant MS, Wright M, Baird K et al (2016) Phase I clinical trial of ipilimumab in pediatric patients with advanced solid tumors. Clin Cancer Res 22(6):1364–1370

Milton GW, Shaw HM, Thompson JF, McCarthy WH (1997) Cutaneous melanoma in childhood: incidence and prognosis. Australas J Dermatol 38:44–48

Mocellin S, Verdi D, Nitti D (2009) DNA repair gene polymorphisms and risk of cutaneous melanoma: a systematic review and meta-analysis. Carcinogenesis 30(10):1735–1743

Mocellin S, Pasquali S, Rossi CR, Nitti D (2010) Interferon alpha adjuvant therapy in patients with high-risk melanoma: a systematic review and meta-analysis. J Natl Cancer Inst 102:493–501

Momper JD, Mulugeta Y, Green DJ et al (2007) Adolescent dosing and labeling since the Food and Drug Administration Amendments Act of 2007. JAMA Pediatr 167:926–932

Mones JM, Ackerman AB (2003) Melanomas in prepubescent children. Review comprehensively, critique historically, criteria diagnostically, and course biologically. Am J Dermatopathol 25:223–238

Moore-Olufemi S, Herzog C, Warneke C et al (2011) Outcomes in pediatric melanoma: comparing prepubertal to adolescent pediatric patients. Ann Surg 253:1211–1215

Moscarella E, Zalaudek I, Cerroni L et al (2012) Excised melanocytic lesions in children and adolescents - a 10-year survey. Br J Dermatol 167:368–373

Mu E, Lange JR, Strouse JJ (2012) Comparison of the use and results of sentinel lymph node biopsy in children and young adults with melanoma. Cancer 118(10):2700–2707

Muftuoglu M, Oshima J, von Kobbe C, Cheng WH, Leistritz DF, Bohr VA (2008) The clinical characteristics of Werner syndrome: molecular and biochemical diagnosis. Hum Genet 124:369–377

Navid F, Furman WL, Fleming M et al (2005) The feasibility of adjuvant interferon alpha-2b in children with high-risk melanoma. Cancer 103:780–787

Navid F, Herzog CE, Sandoval J et al (2016) Feasibility of pegylated interferon in children and young adults with resected high-risk melanoma. Pediatr Blood Cancer 63(7):1207–1213

Offenmueller S, Leiter U, Bernbeck B et al (2017) Clinical characteristics and outcome of 60 pediatric patients with malignant melanoma registered with the German Pediatric Rare Tumor Registry (STEP). Klin Padiatr 229(6):322–328

Pappo AS (2003) Melanoma in children and adolescents. Eur J Cancer 39:2651–2661

Paradela S, Fonseca E, Pita-Fernandez S et al (2010) Prognostic factors for melanoma in children and adolescents: a clinicopathologic, single-center study of 137 patients. Cancer 116:4334–4344

Paraiso KHT, Fedorenko IV, Cantini LP et al (2010) Recovery of phospho-ERK activity allows melanoma cells to escape from BRAF inhibitor therapy. Br J Cancer 102(12):1724–1730

Pearce MS, Parker L, Cotterill SJ et al (2003) Skin cancer in children and young adults: 28 years' experience from the Northern Region Young Person's Malignant Disease Registry, UK. Melanoma Res 13(4):421–426

Printz C (2015) Sun behaviors and genes may affect future melanoma risk. Cancer 121(8):1157

Quéreux G, Dréno B (2011) Fotemustine for the treatment of melanoma. Expert Opin Pharmacother 12(18):2891–2904

Réguerre Y, Vittaz M, Orbach D et al (2016) Cutaneous malignant melanoma in children and adolescents treated in pediatric oncology units. Pediatr Blood Cancer 63(11):1922–1927

Ribas A, Puzanov I, Dummer R et al (2015) Pembrolizumab versus investigator-choice chemotherapy for ipilimumab-refractory melanoma (KEYNOTE-002): a randomised, controlled, phase 2 trial. Lancet Oncol 16:908–918

Rose K, Grant-Kels JM (2018) Most adolescents' melanomas are conventional malignant adult-type melanomas. Eur J Cancer 95:117–119

Seynnaeve B et al (2017) Genetic and epigenetic alterations of TERT are associated with inferior outcome in adolescent and young adult patients with melanoma. Sci Rep 7:45704

Shah NC, Gerstle JT, Start M et al (2006) Use of sentinel lymph node biopsy and high-dose interferon in pediatric patients with high-risk melanoma: the Hospital for Sick Children experience. J Pediatr Hematol Oncol 28:496–500

Spatz A, Ruiter D, Hardmeier T et al (1996) Melanoma in childhood: an EORTC-MCG multicenter study on the clinico-pathological aspects. Int J Cancer 68(3):317–324

Spitz S (1948) Melanomas of childhood. Am J Pathol 24:591–609

Sreeraman Kumar R, Thapa R, Kim Y, Khushalani NI, Sondak VK, Reed DR (2018) Higher than reported adolescent and young adult clinical trial enrollment during the "Golden Age" of melanoma clinical trials. Cancer Med 7(4):991–996

Strouse JJ, Fears TR, Tucker MA, Wayne AS (2005) Pediatric melanoma: risk factor and survival analysis of the surveillance, epidemiology and end results database. J Clin Oncol 23:4735–4741

Svedman FC, Pillas D, Taylor A et al (2016) Stage-specific survival and recurrence in patients with cutaneous malignant melanoma in Europe – a systematic review of the literature. Clin Epidemiol 8:109–122

Whiteman DC, Milligan A, Welch J et al (1997) Germline CDKN2A mutations in childhood melanoma. J Natl Cancer Inst 89:1460

Wilmott JS, Johansson PA, Newell F et al (2019) Whole genome sequencing of melanomas in adolescent and young adults reveals distinct mutation landscapes and the potential role of germline variants in disease susceptibility. Int J Cancer 144(5):1049–1060

Tricoli JV, Blair DG, Anders CK et al (2016) Biologic and clinical characteristics of adolescent and young adult cancers: acute lymphoblastic leukemia, colorectal cancer, breast cancer, melanoma, and sarcoma. Cancer 122(7):1017–1028

Zuckerman R, Maier JP, Guiney WB Jr et al (2001) Pediatric melanoma: confirming the diagnosis with sentinel node biopsy. Ann Plast Surg 46:394–399

Woulters MW, Michielin O, Bastiaannet E et al (2018) ECCO essential requirements for quality cancer care: melanoma. Crit Rev Oncol Hematol 122:164–178

Wechsler J, Bastuji-Garin S, Spatz A et al (2002) Reliability of the histopathologic diagnosis of malignant melanoma in childhood. Arch Dermatol 138(5):625–628

Tatiana KSC, Somers GR, Pope E, Zuker RM (2010) Predisposing factors and outcomes of malignant skin tumors in children. Plast Reconstr Surg 126:508–514

Weber JS, D'Angelo SP, Minor D et al (2015) Nivolumab versus chemotherapy in patients with advanced melanoma who progressed after anti-CTLA-4 treatment (CheckMate 037): a randomised, controlled, open-label, phase 3 trial. Lancet Oncol 16:375–384

Wolchok JD, Chiarion-Sileni V, Gonzalez R et al (2017) Overall survival with combined nivolumab and ipilimumab in advanced melanoma. N Engl J Med 377:1345–1356

Wong JR, Harris JK, Rodriguez-Galindo C, Johnson KJ. Incidence of childhood and adolescent melanoma in the United States: 1973-2009. Pediatrics. 2013 May;131(5):846-54.

Weber J, Mandala M, Del Vecchio M et al (2017) Adjuvant nivolumab versus ipilimumab in resected stage III or IV melanoma. N Engl J Med 377:1824–1835

Skin Carcinoma

41

Thomas K. Eigentler and Andrea Ferrari

Squamous cell carcinoma (SCC) of the skin is rarely diagnosed in childhood and adolescence (incidence rate approximately 0.0077 per 100,000 in the population less than 20 years old). It is a malignant locally destructive epithelial tumor developing from the keratinocytes of the skin which uncommonly metastasizes in non-immunosuppressed patients.

Most cases are described in children suffering from xeroderma pigmentosum, an autosomal recessive disorder with mutations in the nucleotide excision repair complementation groups resulting in extreme photosensitivity to ultraviolet radiation. It affects boys and girls in equal frequencies. In a series of 830 published cases, 45% of the patients had basal cell carcinoma or SCC. The median age of first non-melanoma skin cancer among these patients was 8 years (Kraemer et al. 1987).

Another risk factor for developing SCC is iatrogenic chronic immunosuppression, e.g., after solid organ transplantation, whereas the risk of post-transplant cutaneous SCC is related to the kind of immunosuppression (especially cyclosporine), the duration of the immunosuppressive therapy, and the amount of cumulative UV exposure (Jensen et al. 1999). Also, sporadic chronic immunosuppression, e.g., in the case of AIDS, is a risk factor for the development of SCC (Godfrey et al. 2003).

SCC is also reported to develop in children with interferon gamma receptor 2 deficiency (Toyoda et al. 2010); in patients suffering from dystrophic epidermolysis bullosa (DEB), a genodermatosis resulting from mutations in COL7A1 and encoding type VII collagen (Horn and Tidman 2002); and in children with systemic sclerosis or pansclerotic morphea (Wollina et al. 2002) or chronic infections and wounds (Kassi et al. 2010). Single cases of a SCC arising in a nevus sebaceous of Jadassohn were also reported in the literature (Ball et al. 2005).

Other risk populations comprise children with oculocutaneous albinism (OCA), a group of genetic diseases characterized by diffuse reduced pigmentation affecting melanocytes and keratinocytes of the skin, hair follicles, and eyes, accompanied by reduced visual acuity with nystagmus and photophobia (de Vijlder et al. 2013). OCA patients are very susceptible to UV-induced skin cancer. Mutations in genes coding for tyrosinase (OCA1A and OCA1B), P protein (OCA2), tyrosinase-related protein 1 (OCA3), and MATP (OCA4) have been identified as cause of the disease. Depending on the mutation, differences in sensitivity to skin cancer can be anticipated. In OCA1A, there is no melanin synthesis at all, while in all other types,

T. K. Eigentler (✉)
Department of Dermatology, Venereology and Allergology, Charité - Universitätsmedizin Berlin, corporate member of Freie Universität Berlin and Humboldt-Universität zu Berlin, Berlin, Deutschland
e-mail: thomas.eigentler@charite.de

A. Ferrari
Pediatric Oncology Unit, Fondazione IRCCS Istituto Nazionale Tumori, Milan, Italy

D. T. Schneider et al. (eds.), *Rare Tumors in Children and Adolescents*, Pediatric Oncology,
https://doi.org/10.1007/978-3-030-92071-5_41

there is some pigmentation; thus, especially the OCA1A population has an extremely elevated risk.

Treatment of choice is the complete excision of the tumor with three-dimensional histological visualization and evaluation of excision margins (Moehrle et al. 2007). In selected cases (deep-infiltrating tumors), a sentinel node biopsy can be applied.

References

Ball EA, Hussain M, Moss AL (2005) Squamous cell carcinoma and basal cell carcinoma arising in a naevus sebaceous of Jadassohn: case report and literature review. Clin Exp Dermatol 30:259–260

de Vijlder HC, de Vijlder JJM, Neumann HAM (2013) Oculocutaneous albinism and skin cancer risk. J Eur Acad Dermatol Venereol 27(3):e433–e434

Godfrey JC, Vaughan MC, Williams JV (2003) Successful Treatment of Bowenoid Papulosis in a 9-Year-Old Girl With Vertically Acquired Human Immunodeficiency Virus. Pediatrics 112(1):e73–e76. https://doi.org/10.1542/peds.112.1.e73

Horn HM, Tidman MJ (2002) The clinical spectrum of dystrophic epidermolysis bullosa. Brit Journal Dermatol 146(2):267–274. https://doi.org/10.1046/j.1365-2133.2002.04607.x

Jensen P, Hansen S, Moller B et al (1999) Skin cancer in kidney and heart transplant recipients and different long-term immunosuppressive therapy regimens. J Am Acad Dermatol 40:177–186

Kassi K, Kouame K, Allen W et al (2010) Squamous cell carcinoma secondary to Buruli ulcer: a clinical case report in a young girl. Bacteriol Virusol Parazitol Epidemiol 55:25–28

Kraemer KH, Lee MM, Scotto J (1987) Xeroderma pigmentosum. Cutaneous, ocular, and neurologic abnormalities in 830 published cases. Arch Dermatol 123:241–250

Moehrle M, Breuninger H, Rocken M (2007) A confusing world: what to call histology of three-dimensional tumour margins? J Eur Acad Dermatol Venereol 21:591–595

Toyoda H, Ido M, Nakanishi K et al (2010) Multiple cutaneous squamous cell carcinomas in a patient with interferon gamma receptor 2 (IFN gamma R2) deficiency. J Med Genet 47:631–634

Wollina U, Buslau M, Weyers W (2002) Squamous cell carcinoma in pansclerotic morphea of childhood. Pediatr Dermatol 19:151–154

42 Other Rare Tumors of the Skin and Subcutaneous Tissue

Alberto Pappo and Andrea Ferrari

42.1 Dermatofibrosarcoma Protuberans

Dermatofibrosarcoma protuberans (DFSP) is a fibrohistiocytic tumor of intermediate malignancy that accounts for about 1–2% of all soft tissue sarcomas and most commonly affects young adults (McArthur 2007; Terrier-Lacombe et al. 2003). This malignancy has been described in children and can be congenital (Checketts et al. 2000; Chien et al. 2007; Jafarian et al. 2008; Pappo et al. 1997). In one series, pediatric DFSP accounted for 6% of all of this diagnosis seen at a single institution (McKee and Fletcher 1991). This tumor most commonly affects males and typically arises in the trunk and extremities. DFSP usually presents as a slow-growing vascular-appearing macule or plaque that later develops into a nodular cutaneous mass. In a review of over 25 pediatric DFSP, the median age at presentation was 12 years. In another review of over 150 cases of pediatric DFSP, the most common sites of involvement were the trunk and extremities; the former location is preferentially seen in patients with congenital DFSP (Checketts et al. 2000; Chien et al. 2007; Jafarian et al. 2008; Pappo et al. 1997). Histologically, this tumor is characterized by a monotonous proliferation of fibroblasts arranged in a storiform pattern. A small number of DFSP have sarcomatous changes, a feature that has rarely been reported in the pediatric literature but that has been reported to carry an increased risk for the development of local recurrence and distant metastases (Abbott et al. 2006; Mentzel et al. 1998). DFSP is characterized by a common translocation t(17;22)(q22;q13) which fuses the *COL1A1* and *PDGFB* genes (McArthur 2007). This fusion protein is processed to a mature PDGFB and interacts with the PDGFB receptor present on the cell surface of DFSP in an autocrine or paracrine fashion (Rubin et al. 2002). The primary treatment of DFSP is wide surgical resection with negative margins (Fiore et al. 2005); Moh's micrographic surgery has also been used in selected cases (Sondak et al. 1999). Using this primary surgical approach, cause-specific mortality in adults has been reported to be 3% at 10 years, and local recurrence rates have been documented in less than 5% of cases (Fiore et al. 2005). For adults and children with unresectable or metastatic DFSP, the administration of imatinib mesylate has produced promising clinical responses (Rutkowski et al. 2010; Price et al. 2005; Gooskens et al. 2010). A systematic review of 9 studies and 152 patients ranging in age from 20 to 73 years who were treated with imatinib for

A. Pappo (✉)
Department of Oncology, St. Jude Children's Research Hospital, Memphis, TN, USA
e-mail: Alberto.Pappo@STJUDE.ORG

A. Ferrari
Pediatric Oncology Unit, Fondazione IRCCS Istituto Nazionale Tumori, Milan, Italy

D. T. Schneider et al. (eds.), *Rare Tumors in Children and Adolescents*, Pediatric Oncology,
https://doi.org/10.1007/978-3-030-92071-5_42

locally advanced or metastatic DFSP revealed a complete response rate of 5.2%, a partial response rate of 55.2%, and disease stabilization in 28% of patients. There were no differences in response between those patients who received 400 and 800 mg a day (Navarrete-Dechent et al. 2019).

42.2 Giant Cell Fibroblastoma

Giant cell fibroblastoma (GCF) is a rare nonmetastasizing subcutaneous fibrohistiocytic neoplasm that occurs predominately in younger patients. In 1 series of 86 GCF, the median age at diagnosis was 6 years, and nearly 2/3 of the patients were younger than 10 years of age. This tumor most commonly presents as painless mass located in the dermis or subcutis and most commonly arises in the trunk. GCF has been referred to as a juvenile form of DFSP, and both entities share the t(17;22)(q22;q13) and the *COL1A1-PDGFB* fusion (Jha et al. 2007). Histologically, GCF is characterized by the presence of spindle cells that infiltrate adnexal structures and form pseudovascular spaces that are lined with discontinuous multinucleated giant tumor cells (Billings and Folpe 2004). Although both GCF and DFSP have similar cytogenetic findings, adult DFSP is often characterized by the presence of ring chromosomes, a feature that is notably absent in pediatric GCF. The clinical behavior of GCF is similar to DFSP, and surgical resection with negative margins is the treatment of choice.

42.3 Angiomatoid Fibrous Histiocytoma

Angiomatoid fibrous histiocytoma (AFH) is a rare subcutaneous fibrohistiocytic tumor of intermediate malignancy that accounts for about 0.3% of all soft tissue sarcomas (Thway 2008). AFH was initially described by Enzinger in 1979 as a soft tissue tumor related to malignant fibrous histiocytoma that affected the superficial tissues of younger patients (Enzinger 1979). More recent studies have demonstrated that this entity has an excellent prognosis following surgical resection alone and thus the original nomenclature of "malignant" has been removed from its name (Thway 2008). In 1 series of 108 patients, the median age at presentation was 14 years, females were slightly more commonly affected, and the tumor most commonly arose in the extremities (65%) and trunk (28%) (Costa and Weiss 1990). These tumors have an indolent clinical presentation, and most are located superficially; in one series, 60% of tumors arose within areas of normal lymphoid tissue (Fanburg-Smith and Miettinen 1999; Antonescu et al. 2007). Systemic symptoms such as anemia, weight loss, and fever have been described in 14%, 4%, and 2% of patients; some of these symptoms may be related to excessive interleukin-6 production (Fanburg-Smith and Miettinen 1999). Histologically, AFH is characterized by the presence of a fibrous pseudocapsule, a round or spindled histiocyte-like proliferation of cells, a plasma lymphocytic response, and pseudovascular spaces (Antonescu et al. 2007). Cytogenetic studies have documented translocations involving the *FUS* gene on chromosome 12q13 with either the *EWSR1* gene on chromosome 22q12 or the *FUS* on 16p11. More recently, a translocation between *EWSR1* and *CREB1* on chromosome 2q34 has been identified as the predominant fusion product in AFH (Antonescu et al. 2007). The treatment of choice for this tumor is complete surgical excision. Local recurrences have been reported to occur in up to 12% of patients after incomplete excision, but reexcision often renders patients disease-free. In 1 series, 85 of 86 patients were alive and disease-free, and only 1 patient developed nodal metastases. In another series, only 1 of 94 patients developed distant metastases (Fanburg-Smith and Miettinen 1999; Antonescu et al. 2007).

42.4 Plexiform Fibrohistiocytic Tumor

Plexiform fibrohistiocytic tumor is a rare neoplasm with features that resemble fibrous histiocytoma and fibromatosis and mainly affects children and young adults. The median age at diagnosis in two large series were 14.5 and

20 years, respectively (Moosavi et al. 2007; Enzinger and Zhang 1988). This tumor occurs slightly more often in females and presents as a painless slow-growing nodule located in the dermis or subcutis (Luzar and Calonje 2010). The tumor most often involves the upper extremity with the fingers, the hands, and the wrist being more commonly affected (Taher and Pushpanathan 2007). The lesions are usually small and contain a mixture of histiocyte-like and spindle fibroblast-like cells. On low-power microscopy, the dermis and subcutaneous tissue are infiltrated with multiple nodules that contain multinucleated osteoclast-like giant cells (Luzar and Calonje 2010). Immunocytochemistry reveals CD68 positivity on the histiocyte- and osteoclast-like cells, whereas the fibroblast-like cells show focal positivity for smooth muscle actin. Cytogenetic analysis in two cases has revealed numerous deletions and a 46,XY,t(4;15)(q21;q15) translocation (Luzar and Calonje 2010). Surgical excision is the treatment of choice, but local recurrences have been documented in up 40% of cases within the first 2 years from diagnosis. Recurrences are usually successfully treated with surgical reexcision. Metastases to lymph nodes and lung have been rarely described (Salomao and Nascimento 1997).

42.5 Dermoid Cysts

Dermoid cysts are a subset of benign heterotopic neoplasms termed choristomas, probably deriving from dermal and epidermal tissues trapped in the cranial fusion lines as the neural tube closes in embryogenesis. Histologically, they may have a lining of squamous epithelium with dermal elements such as hair follicles, sebaceous glands, and sweat glands: within the cyst, mature skin completes with hair follicles and sweat glands; sometimes clumps of long hair and often pockets of sebum, blood, fat, bone, nails, teeth, eyes, cartilage, and thyroid tissue can be found.

Dermoid cysts can be deep and superficial (the former more frequent in teenagers, the latter in early childhood) and may occur as soft tissue swelling in three primary locations in the head and neck: the frontotemporal region, the periorbital region, and the nasoglabellar region.

Complete surgical excision—preferably in one piece and without any spillage of cyst contents—is curative, but dermoid cysts can recur if not completely excised. Lesions invading deeply within the orbit may require a more aggressive approach. Craniotomy and neurosurgical involvement may be required for intracranial extension (Ahuja and Azar 2006; Bartlett et al. 1993; Pryor et al. 2005).

References

Abbott JJ, Oliveira AM, Nascimento AG (2006) The prognostic significance of fibrosarcomatous transformation in dermatofibrosarcoma protuberans. Am J Surg Pathol 30:436–443

Ahuja R, Azar NF (2006) Orbital dermoids in children. Semin Ophthalmol 21:207–211

Antonescu CR, Dal Cin P, Nafa K et al (2007) EWSR1-CREB1 is the predominant gene fusion in angiomatoid fibrous histiocytoma. Genes Chromosomes Cancer 46:1051–1060

Bartlett SP, Lin KY, Grossman R, Katowitz J (1993) The surgical management of orbitofacial dermoids in the pediatric patient. Plast Reconstr Surg 91:1208–1215

Billings SD, Folpe AL (2004) Cutaneous and subcutaneous fibrohistiocytic tumors of intermediate malignancy: an update. Am J Dermatopathol 26:141–155

Checketts SR, Hamilton TK, Baughman RD (2000) Congenital and childhood dermatofibrosarcoma protuberans: a case report and review of the literature. J Am Acad Dermatol 42:907–913

Chien CR, Chang YL, Lin DT, Yang RS (2007) Excellent survival of pediatric dermatofibrosarcoma protuberans in Taiwanese. Pediatr Surg Int 23:211–214

Costa MJ, Weiss SW (1990) Angiomatoid malignant fibrous histiocytoma. A follow-up study of 108 cases with evaluation of possible histologic predictors of outcome. Am J Surg Pathol 14:1126–1132

Enzinger FM (1979) Angiomatoid malignant fibrous histiocytoma: a distinct fibrohistiocytic tumor of children and young adults simulating a vascular neoplasm. Cancer 44:2147–2121

Enzinger FM, Zhang RY (1988) Plexiform fibrohistiocytic tumor presenting in children and young adults. An analysis of 65 cases. Am J Surg Pathol 12:818–826

Fanburg-Smith JC, Miettinen M (1999) Angiomatoid "malignant" fibrous histiocytoma: a clinicopathologic study of 158 cases and further exploration of the myoid phenotype. Hum Pathol 30:1336–1343

Fiore M, Miceli R, Mussi C et al (2005) Dermatofibrosarcoma protuberans treated at a single institution: a surgical disease with a high cure rate. J Clin Oncol 23:7669–7675

Gooskens SL, Oranje AP, van Adrichem LN et al (2010) Imatinib mesylate for children with dermatofibrosarcoma protuberans (DFSP). Pediatr Blood Cancer 55:369–373

Jafarian F, McCuaig C, Kokta V, Laberge L, Ben Nejma B (2008) Dermatofibrosarcoma protuberans in childhood and adolescence: report of eight patients. Pediatr Dermatol 25:317–325

Jha P, Moosavi C, Fanburg-Smith JC (2007) Giant cell fibroblastoma: an update and addition of 86 new cases from the Armed Forces Institute of Pathology, in honor of Dr. Franz M. Enzinger. Ann Diagn Pathol 11:81–88

Luzar B, Calonje E (2010) Cutaneous fibrohistiocytic tumours – an update. Histopathology 56:148–165

McArthur G (2007) Dermatofibrosarcoma protuberans: recent clinical progress. Ann Surg Oncol 14:2876–2886

McKee PH, Fletcher CD (1991) Dermatofibrosarcoma protuberans presenting in infancy and childhood. J Cutan Pathol 18:241–246

Mentzel T, Beham A, Katenkamp D, Dei Tos AP, Fletcher CD (1998) Fibrosarcomatous ("high-grade") dermatofibrosarcoma protuberans: clinicopathologic and immunohistochemical study of a series of 41 cases with emphasis on prognostic significance. Am J Surg Pathol 22:576–587

Moosavi C, Jha P, Fanburg-Smith JC (2007) An update on plexiform fibrohistiocytic tumor and addition of 66 new cases from the Armed Forces Institute of Pathology, in honor of Franz M. Enzinger, MD. Ann Diagn Pathol 11:313–319

Navarrete-Dechent C, Mori S, Barker CA, Dickson MA, Nehal KS (2019) Imatinib treatment for locally advanced or metastatic dermatofibrosarcoma protuberans: a systematic review. JAMA Dermatol. https://doi.org/10.1001/jamadermatol.2018.4940

Pappo AS, Rao BN, Cain A, Bodner S, Pratt CB (1997) Dermatofibrosarcoma protuberans: the pediatric experience at St. Jude Children's Research Hospital. Pediatr Hematol Oncol 14:563–568

Price VE, Fletcher JA, Zielenska M et al (2005) Imatinib mesylate: an attractive alternative in young children with large, surgically challenging dermatofibrosarcoma protuberans. Pediatr Blood Cancer 44:511–515

Pryor SG, Lewis JE, Weaver AL, Orvidas LJ (2005) Pediatric dermoid cysts of the head and neck. Otolaryngol Head Neck Surg 132:938–942

Rubin BP, Schuetze SM, Eary JF et al (2002) Molecular targeting of platelet-derived growth factor B by imatinib mesylate in a patient with metastatic dermatofibrosarcoma protuberans. J Clin Oncol 20:3586–3591

Rutkowski P, Van Glabbeke M, Rankin CJ et al (2010) Imatinib mesylate in advanced dermatofibrosarcoma protuberans: pooled analysis of two phase II clinical trials. J Clin Oncol 28:1772–1779

Salomao DR, Nascimento AG (1997) Plexiform fibrohistiocytic tumor with systemic metastases: a case report. Am J Surg Pathol 21:469–476

Sondak VK, Cimmino VM, Lowe LM, Dubay DA, Johnson TM (1999) Dermatofibrosarcoma protuberans: what is the best surgical approach? Surg Oncol 8:183–189

Taher A, Pushpanathan C (2007) Plexiform fibrohistiocytic tumor: a brief review. Arch Pathol Lab Med 131:1135–1138

Terrier-Lacombe MJ, Guillou L, Maire G et al (2003) Dermatofibrosarcoma protuberans, giant cell fibroblastoma, and hybrid lesions in children: clinicopathologic comparative analysis of 28 cases with molecular data – a study from the French Federation of Cancer Centers Sarcoma Group. Am J Surg Pathol 27:27–39

Thway K (2008) Angiomatoid fibrous histiocytoma: a review with recent genetic findings. Arch Pathol Lab Med 132:273–277

Part XI

Vascular Tumors

43 Vascular Tumors Including Kaposi Sarcoma

Jochen Rössler

43.1 Introduction

Vascular tumors belong to the group of vascular anomalies as described in the classification of the International Society for the Study of Vascular Anomalies (ISSVA) (Wassef et al. 2015). It is crucial to discriminate vascular tumors from vascular malformations. In vascular tumors, endothelial cells show cell proliferation and growth (angiogenesis). In contrary, vascular malformations are inborn defects of embryonal development (vasculogenesis) with stable size or enlargement according to physiological body growth.

The latest update of the ISSVA classification from 2014 differs benign, locally aggressive or borderline, and malignant vascular tumors (Table 43.1) (Wassef et al. 2015). In addition to the ISSVA classification, the World Health Organization (WHO) included vascular tumors in their recently updated soft tissue and bone tumor chapter (Table 43.2) (Fletcher et al. 2013). However, the ISSVA classification uses more precise terminology and phenotypes.

J. Rössler (✉)
Division of Pediatric Hematology and Oncology, Department of Pediatrics, Inselspital, Bern University Hospital, University of Bern, Bern, Switzerland
e-mail: jochen.roessler@insel.ch

43.2 Infantile Hemangioma

The most frequent vascular tumor in childhood with a prevalence of 4–5% is infantile hemangioma (IH), which shows a special biology with continuous growth during the first year of life but spontaneous regression thereafter. IH can present as capillary IH, cavernous IH, segmental IH, and congenital IH. The most frequent localization of IH is the head and neck region. Superficial IH can be discriminated from deep IH or combined IH. In consequence, they can appear as bluish-red, rubbery or firm, or well-circumscribed mass or as a swelling (Chang et al. 2008; Tollefson and Frieden 2012).

Complications of IH are ulcerations, rarely hemorrhages, or in the case of localization at the larynx or mediastinum vital disturbances (Naouri et al. 2010). In most cases, IH will spontaneously regress over time; however, treatment is required when IH interferes with vision and breathing or threatens significant cosmetic injury (Haggstrom et al. 2006).

Different treatments were used over the last years, i.e., surgery, oral corticosteroids, injection of corticosteroid directly into the lesion, pulsed-dye laser, and systemic therapy with interferon and vincristine. However, since the approval of propranolol based on a large international, trans-atlantic clinical study, the pan beta-blocker is now the first-line therapy for complicated IH (Leaute-Labreze et al. 2015).

D. T. Schneider et al. (eds.), *Rare Tumors in Children and Adolescents*, Pediatric Oncology,
https://doi.org/10.1007/978-3-030-92071-5_43

Table 43.1 ISSVA classification of vascular tumors

Name	Somatic mutation
A: Benign vascular tumors	
Infantile hemangioma/hemangioma of infancy	
Congenital hemangioma	GNAQ/GNA11
– Rapid involuting (RICH)[a]	
– Non-involuting (NICH)	
– Partially involuting (PICH)	
Tufted angioma[b]	GNA14
Spindle cell hemangioma	IDH1/IDH2
Epithelioid hemangioma	FOS
Pyogenic granuloma (also known as lobular capillary hemangioma)	BRAF/RAS/GNA14
Others	
– Hobnail hemangioma	
– Microvenular hemangioma	
– Anastomosing hemangioma	
– Glomeruloid hemangioma	
– Papillary hemangioma	
– Intravascular papillary endothelial hyperplasia	
– Cutaneous epithelioid angiomatous nodule	
– Acquired elastotic hemangioma	
– Littoral cell hemangioma of the spleen	
Related lesions	
– Eccrine angiomatous hamartoma	
– Reactive angioendotheliomatosis	
– Bacillary angiomatosis	
B: Locally aggressive or borderline vascular tumors	
Kaposiform hemangioendothelioma[a,b]	GNA14
Retiform hemangioendothelioma	
Papillary intralymphatic angioendothelioma (PILA), Dabska tumor	
Composite hemangioendothelioma	
Pseudomyogenic hemangioendothelioma	FOSB
Polymorphous hemangioendothelioma	
Hemangioendothelioma no otherwise specified	
Kaposi sarcoma	
Others	
C: Malignant vascular tumors	
Angiosarcoma	(Post-radiation) MYC
Epithelioid hemangioendothelioma	CAMTA1/TFE3
Others	

Adapted from ISSVA Classification of Vascular Anomalies. ©2014 International Society for the Study of Vascular Anomalies. Available at "issva.org/classification." Accessed January 2020 (Chang et al. 2008)
[a] Some lesions may be associated with thrombocytopenia and/or coagulopathy
[b] Many experts believe that tufted angioma and kaposiform hemangioendothelioma are part of a spectrum rather than distinct entities

43.3 Congenital Hemangiomas

Congenital hemangiomas (CH) proliferate in utero, and their development is complete at birth. Histologically, these lesions are GLUT1 negative, unlike IH. They are usually cutaneous, but can be also found in organs. Complications include hemorrhage, transient heart failure, and transient coagulopathy (Vildy et al. 2015). Somatic activating mutations of GNAQ and GNA11 have been found to be associated with congenital hemangiomas (Ayturk et al. 2016).

Table 43.2 WHO classification of tumours of soft tissue and bone

Category	Vascular tumor type
Benign	Hemangioma
	Epithelioid hemangioma
	Angiomatosis
	Lymphangioma
Intermediate (locally aggressive)	Kaposiform hemangioendothelioma
Intermediate (rarely metastasizing)	Retiform hemangioendothelioma
	Papillary intralymphatic angioendothelioma
	Composite hemangioendothelioma
	Kaposi sarcoma
Malignant	Epithelioid hemangioendothelioma
	Angiosarcoma of soft tissue

Adapted from Fletcher et al. (2013)

Congenital hemangiomas are divided into the following three forms: rapidly involuting congenital hemangiomas (RICH), partially involuting congenital hemangiomas (PICH), and non-involuting congenital hemangiomas (NICH).

All CH are completely formed at birth. The RICH are large high-flow lesions that rapidly involute by 12–15 months. They can ulcerate and bleed and cause transient heart failure and mild coagulopathy. Therapy is therefore not necessary. Some residual changes in the skin can be present after involution (Maguiness et al. 2015; Scalise et al. 2014; Kumarasamy et al. 2014; Hughes et al. 2014). In contrary, PICH involute only partially (Nasseri et al. 2014). And finally, NICH never involute. Depending on the location of the lesions and whether they cause functional impairment, the lesions may need to be removed surgically (Lee et al. 2014; Enjolras et al. 2001).

43.4 Infantile Hepatic Hemangiomas

Vascular tumors of the liver are classified according to their clinical characteristics and radiologic assessment. Lesions are usually divided into the following three categories (Hsi Dickie et al. 2014): focal vascular lesions (congenital hemangiomas), multiple liver lesions (infantile hemangiomas), and diffuse liver lesions (infantile hemangiomas). They can be found in the context of disseminated or diffuse neonatal hemangiomatosis with multiple cutaneous infantile hemangioma. The clinical presentation can be asymptomatic or associated with hepatomegaly, jaundice, or liver dysfunction. Ultrasound or magnetic resonance imaging (MRI) can identify the vascular tumors with increased perfusion in the duplex ultrasound and hyperintensive signals in T2 (Fig. 43.1a–c).

The focal lesions are usually congenital hemangiomas (RICH or NICH). RICH can present with symptoms of heart failure and mild to moderate coagulopathy. Treatment can be supportive management, embolization (Kayaalp and Sabuncuoglu 2015), or surgery. Multifocal hepatic lesions are infantile hemangiomas that may not need to be treated if the patient is asymptomatic. In general, they follow the same proliferative and involution course as cutaneous hemangiomas (Hsi Dickie et al. 2014). Close monitoring is necessary, and if there is growth, propranolol therapy should be considered (Mazereeuw-Hautier et al. 2010). Finally, diffuse liver lesions can be life-threatening. Next to hypothyroidism caused by the expression of iodothyronine deiodinase, congestive heart failure and compartment syndrome can occur (Hsi Dickie et al. 2014; Rialon et al. 2015a, b; Yeh et al. 2011). Treatment options are propranolol, chemotherapy (steroids, cyclophosphamide, or vincristine), and, if there is absolutely no response and liver failure, organ transplantation.

43.5 Spindle Cell Hemangioma

Spindle cell hemangiomas often occur as superficial (skin and subcutis), painful lesions involving distal extremities in children and adults (Perkins and Weiss 1996; Fletcher et al. 1991). The tumors appear as red-brown or bluish lesions that can begin as a single nodule and develop into multifocal painful lesions over years. The lesions can be seen in Maffucci syndrome (cutaneous spindle cell hemangiomas occurring with cartilaginous tumors,

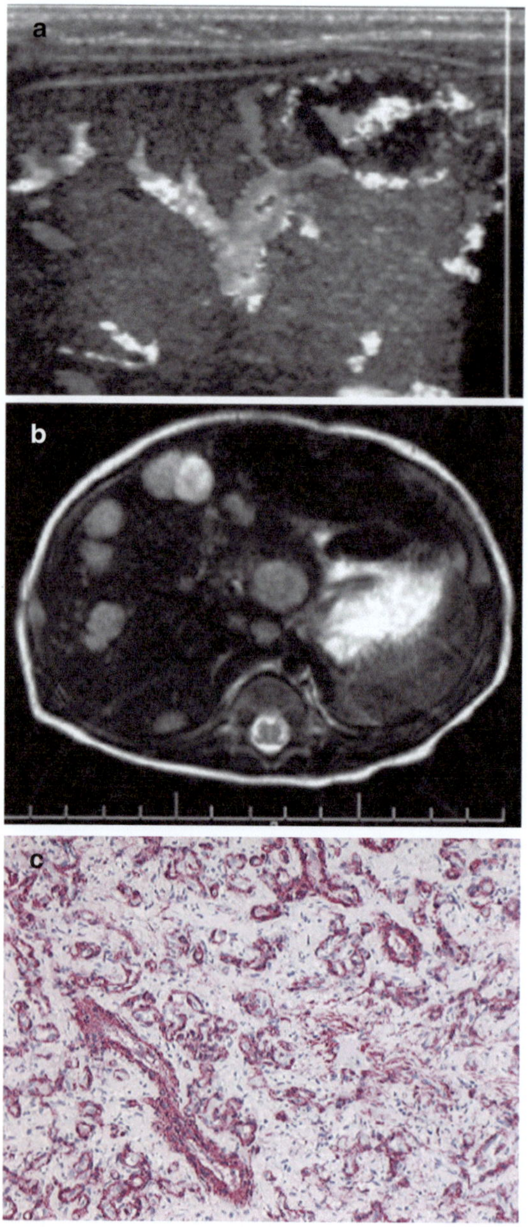

Fig. 43.1 Infantile hepatic hemangiomas in a newborn child with numerous skin hemangiomas. (**a**) Duplex ultrasound detects multiple hepatic lesions with perfusion signal. (**b**) In T2-weighted MRI, the lesions are hyperintense. (**c**) Shows an immunohistological staining of a biopsy with alpha-actin antibodies. Multiple blood vessels are seen, confirming the diagnosis of infantile hepatic hemangiomas

enchondromas), Klippel-Trenaunay syndrome (capillary/lymphatic/venous malformations), generalized lymphatic anomalies, and lymphedema. Spindle cell hemangiomas are well circumscribed, occasionally contain phleboliths, and consist of cavernous blood spaces alternating with areas of nodular spindle cell proliferation (Enjolras et al. 2013; Hoeger and Colmenero 2014).

There is no standard treatment for spindle cell hemangioma, but surgical removal is usually curative, although there is a risk of recurrence.

43.6 Epithelioid Hemangioma

Epithelioid hemangiomas are benign lesions that can be located on the skin, the subcutis, or the bone. The lesions can be isolated; however, multifocal lesions are possible (Enjolras et al. 2013; Guo and Gavino 2015). Some of the epithelioid hemangiomas can arise after traumatism or during pregnancy. Next to a local swelling and pain, lytic lesions of the skeleton can be found (Enjolras et al. 2013; O'Connell et al. 2001).

Histology shows small caliber capillaries with eosinophilic, vacuolated cytoplasm and large oval, grooved, and lobulated nuclei. The endothelial cells are plump and mature, well-formed vessels surrounded by multiple epithelioid endothelial cells within abundant cytoplasm. They lack cellular atypia and mitotic activity (Enjolras et al. 2013; Guo and Gavino 2015; O'Connell et al. 2001).

Therapy consists of surgery, endovascular embolization, cryoablation, and rarely radiation (Enjolras et al. 2013; O'Connell et al. 2001). Reports on medical management such as sirolimus or interferon are available (Liu et al. 2019).

43.7 Pyogenic Granuloma (Lobular Capillary Hemangioma)

Pyogenic granuloma (PG), also known as lobular capillary hemangioma, is a benign reactive mucocutaneous lesion that can present at any age, including infancy, although it is most common in older children and young adults. It is usually a small red, oozing, and bleeding bump (Fig. 43.2). They can present as single or multiple lesions (Wassef et al. 2010; Swerlick and Cooper 1983; Campbell et al. 1983; Mills et al. 1980). They can develop also within capillary and arteriovenous malformations.

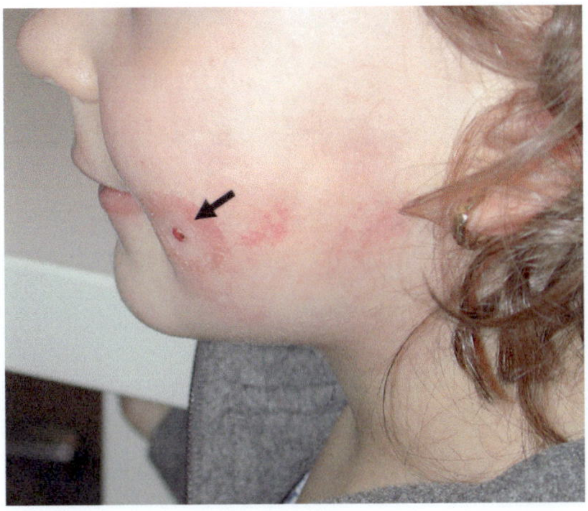

Fig. 43.2 Pyogenic granuloma at the cheek of a 4-year-old girl. The reddish nodule developed in the last 4 weeks and shows intermittent bleeding

PG appear as small or large, smooth or lobulated vascular nodules that can grow rapidly, sometimes over weeks to months, and have a tendency to bleed profusely. The localization is usually cutaneous, but deep-seated/subcutaneous pyogenic granulomas are noted and mimic other vascular lesions (Putra et al. 2017). Histologically, these lesions are composed of capillaries and venules with plump endothelial cells separated into lobules by fibromyxoid stroma.

Most PG can be removed by surgery, curettage, or laser photocoagulation, but recurrence is common (Patrizi et al. 2015).

43.8 Kaposiform Hemangioendothelioma (and Tufted Angioma)

Kaposiform hemangioendothelioma (KHE) and tufted angioma are rare vascular tumors that typically occur during infancy or early childhood but have been reported in adults. Both tumors are thought to be a spectrum of the same disease, because both can be locally aggressive and cause Kasabach-Merritt phenomenon, a serious life-threatening coagulopathy characterized by profound thrombocytopenia and hypofibrinogenemia. They are discussed here as a single entity.

KHE is characterized by sheets of spindle cells with an infiltrative pattern in the dermis, subcutaneous fat, and muscle. There are often areas of fibrosis, with dilated thin-walled vessels infiltrated around the areas of spindle cells. Nests of rounded epithelioid cells of vascular origin can be found in these areas as well as aggregates of capillaries with round or irregularly shaped lumens containing platelet-rich fibrin thrombi. Abnormal lymphatic spaces can be present, sometimes within or at the periphery of the lesion. The rate of mitosis is variable but usually low. Tufted angiomas are difficult to discriminate from KHE, but they show multiple, discrete lobules of tightly packed capillaries (tufts) scattered in the dermis and sometimes in the subcutis, so-called *cannonball* pattern (Enjolras et al. 2008).

Localization of KHE is often at the extremities. Less frequently, they involve the trunk and head and neck area (Croteau et al. 2013). Most lesions involve the skin. Deeper lesions (retroperitoneum, thoracic cavity, and muscle) can appear as a bluish-purpuric hue on the skin, whereas superficial lesions can be firm, purpuric or ecchymotic, and painful (Figs. 43.3 and 43.4). Lesions are usually unifocal, and growth is contiguous. Rare multifocal presentations have been reported mostly in the bone (Croteau et al. 2013; Rodriguez et al. 2009; Ryan et al. 2010).

The diagnosis is based on the combination of clinical, histologic, and imaging features. Seventy percent of patients with KHE develop Kasabach-Merritt phenomenon (KMP; see next chapter). Whenever possible, histologic confirmation should be obtained, because prolonged therapy is often needed. However, if clinical and imaging findings are highly suggestive of the diagnosis, deferring biopsy is an option but needs to be planned with an interdisciplinary approach.

An American and Canadian multidisciplinary expert panel published guidelines for the management of complicated kaposiform hemangioendothelioma (Drolet et al. 2013). A number of treatment therapies have been reported, but none have been uniformly effective (Haisley-Royster et al. 2002; Hauer et al. 2007). If the tumor is localized and easy accessible, surgical excision with or without embolization can be performed. Today, initial treatment is sirolimus because of the possibility of oral administration and close monitoring of plasma levels. Second-line therapy

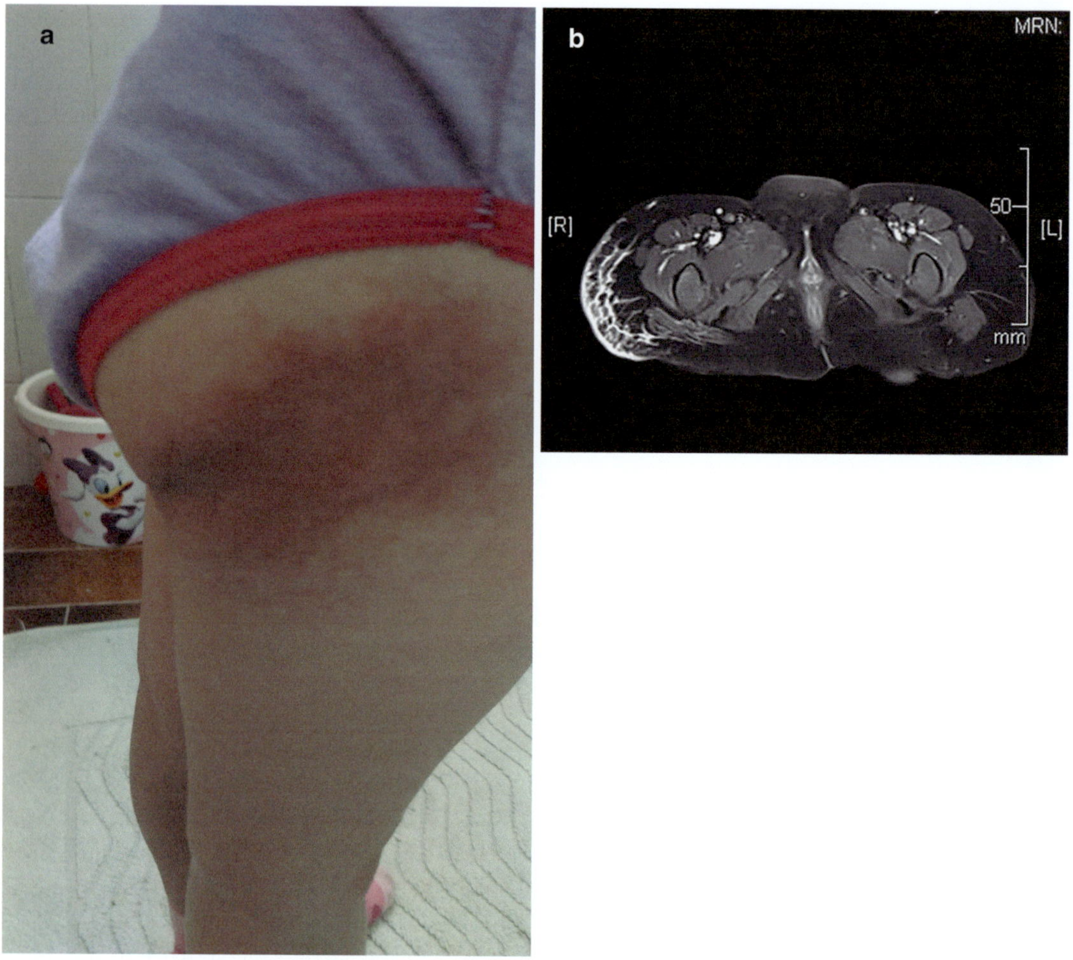

Fig. 43.3 Tufted angioma with KMP in a 3-year-old girl. (**a**) Superficial firm and purpuric lesion at the right gluteal region. (**b**) Infiltrative growth with contrast enhancement in the subcutaneous region confirmed by MRI

is steroids followed by vincristine (Hammill et al. 2011; Blatt et al. 2010; Oza et al. 2016).

43.9 Kasabach-Merritt Phenomenon

Kasabach-Merritt phenomenon (KMP) is defined as thrombocytopenia and hypofibrinogenemia with elevated fibrin split products (D-dimers), suggestive of an active consumptive coagulopathy. Thrombocytes are low, ranging from 6000 to 98,000, with fibrinogen levels less than 100 mg/dL, whereas D-dimers are elevated. Prothrombin times (PT) and activated partial thromboplastin time (PTT) can range from normal to significantly prolonged. Additionally, anemia can be present at diagnosis as a consequence of intravascular hemolysis, including red blood cell fragmentation, elevated LDH, and hyperbilirubinemia.

Successful treatment of the underlying vascular tumor is critical to the correction of KMP and to the overall survival of patients. Children with KMP can die of hemorrhage or invasion/compression of vital structures by the vascular tumor. Mortality has ranged from 10% to 30% in most series.

A curative therapy of KMP can only be achieved by the treatment of the underlying vascular tumor. However, supportive care to maintain hemostasis is necessary. Platelet transfusions

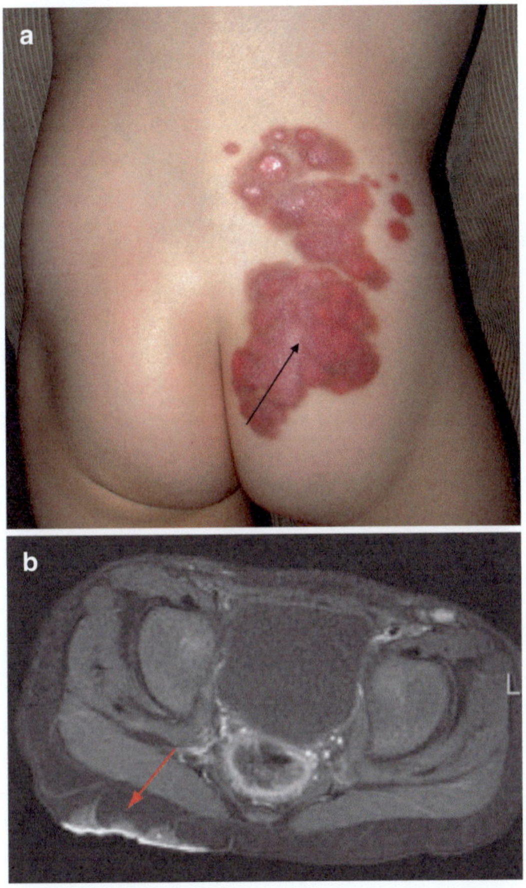

Fig. 43.4 Kaposiform hemangioendothelioma without KMP in a 3-year-old boy. (**a**) Tumor at the lumbosacral region. (**b**) Infiltrative growth in the subcutaneous region confirmed by MRI

should be reserved for active bleeding or in preparation for surgery or procedures. Aminocaproic acid and local measures may be helpful to reduce the need for platelet transfusions (Stahl et al. 1991). Antiplatelet agents, such as acetylsalicylic acid and dipyridamole, have been used to reduce platelet aggregation within the vascular tumor (Wananukul et al. 2003). Treatment of hypofibrinogenemia with cryoprecipitate and prolonged PT or PTT with fresh frozen plasma should be a clinical decision rather than correction of a laboratory result. Symptomatic anemia should be treated with red blood cell transfusions. Several drug regimens have been administered for KMP, including chemotherapeutics such as vincristine (Haisley-Royster et al. 2002). Recent reports show that the mTOR inhibitor sirolimus is very effective in KMP (Zhang et al. 2018).

43.10 Pseudomyogenic Hemangioendothelioma

Pseudomyogenic hemangioendothelioma is a rare, newly designated, distinct vascular tumor. In the ISSVA classification, it is characterized as an intermediate-grade tumor with moderately aggressive local spread and rare distant metastatic disease.

Pseudomyogenic hemangioendothelioma is characterized by loose fascicles of plump spindle and epithelioid cells with abundant eosinophils, cytoplasm, and coexpression of keratins and endothelial markers (Hornick and Fletcher 2011; Billings et al. 2003; Mirra et al. 1992). The etiology for this tumor is unclear, although a balanced translocation t(7;19) resulting in the *SERPINE1-FOSB* fusion gene was reported (Walther et al. 2014).

The tumor usually presents in young men aged 20–50 years (Hornick and Fletcher 2011; Billings et al. 2003). Multifocal disease occurs in 70% of patients. Sites of involvement include the dermis, subcutis, and bones. Patients usually present with pain or a soft tissue mass (Hornick and Fletcher 2011; Billings et al. 2003; Mirra et al. 1992; Walther et al. 2014; Amary et al. 2013).

Most patients are treated with surgery, including amputation with multifocal bony disease (Hornick and Fletcher 2011). In reported cases, chemotherapy has produced responses (Pranteda et al. 2018; Joseph et al. 2015). Recently, the mammalian target of rapamycin (mTOR) inhibitors has been considered as treatment options (Joseph et al. 2015; Ozeki et al. 2017).

43.11 Retiform Hemangioendothelioma

Retiform hemangioendotheliomas (RH) are slow-growing, exophytic, flat tumors found in young adults and occasionally children (El

Darouti et al. 2000). They are usually located in the limbs and trunk. Histologically, they are located in the dermis and subcutaneous tissue. Vessels exhibit a pattern resembling the rete testis and are lined by protruding endothelial cells. They do not express lymphatic markers but stain positive for endothelial markers. Local recurrences are common, but distinct metastases are extremely rare (Colmenero and Hoeger 2014).

Surgical excision with adequate surgical tumor margins and monitoring for local recurrence is the treatment for this tumor. There are case reports of the use of radiation therapy and chemotherapy for inoperable and recurrent tumors (Enjolras et al. 2013; Keiler et al. 2011; Hirsh et al. 2010; Tamhankar et al. 2015).

43.12 Epithelioid Hemangioendothelioma

Epithelioid hemangioendothelioma (EH) was first described in soft tissue by Weiss and Enzinger in 1982. It can occur at younger ages, but the peak incidence is in the fourth and fifth decades of life. The tumors can have an indolent or very aggressive course, with overall survival of 73% at 5 years (Mehrabi et al. 2006; Haro et al. 2015; Sardaro et al. 2014; Dong et al. 2015; Adams and Hammill 2014; Xiao et al. 2013; Reich et al. 2010). The localization is superficial or deep, arising at a variety of sites, including the skin and subcutis, the skeleton (Fig. 43.5a–c), the lung, the liver, and the central nervous system. Microscopically, it arises from a vessel and extends into the surrounding soft tissue. The tumor is composed of epithelioid endothelial cells arranged in short cords or solid nests, with a prominent myxoid-jaline matrix. The diagnostic key feature is represented by epithelioid cells with a cytoplasmic vacuole representing a miniature lumen. It shows positive staining for endothelial markers (CD31, CD34) and cytokeratin.

A *WWTR1-CAMTA1* gene fusion has been found in a large percentage of patients; less commonly, a *YAP1-TFE3* gene fusion has been reported (Mehrabi et al. 2006). These fusions are not directly targetable with current medicines. Monoclonality has been described in multiple liver lesions, suggesting a metastatic process.

Treatment options for epithelioid hemangioendothelioma can be observation, surgery, immunotherapy, targeted therapy, or chemotherapy (Sparber-Sauer et al. 2020). For indolent cases, observation is warranted. For more aggressive cases, multiple medications have been used, including interferon, thalidomide, sorafenib, pazopanib, and sirolimus (Stacchiotti et al. 2016). The most aggressive cases are treated with angiosarcoma-type chemotherapy. Surgery is used when possible. Liver transplantation has been used with aggressive liver lesions, both with and without metastases (Sardaro et al. 2014; Semenisty et al. 2015; Raheja et al. 2015; Ahmad et al. 2014; Otte and Zimmerman 2010). In a multi-institutional case series reported on 24 patients aged 2–26 years with epithelioid hemangioendothelioma, the majority presented with multi-organ disease (Cournoyer et al. 2020). Progression was seen in 63% of patients with a mean time to progression of 18.4 months (range: 0–72). Three patients treated with sirolimus achieved stable disease or partial response for >2.5 years. In children with visceral EH, complete resection achieved complete remission (Hettmer et al. 2017). However, four children experienced rapid progression and died. In six children, disease remained stable for years without therapy. Two patients died from progressive EHE 21 and 24 years after the first diagnosis.

43.13 Angiosarcoma

Angiosarcomas (AS) typically affect adult and elderly patients (it accounts for 1% of all adult soft tissue sarcomas) (Penel et al. 2011) and are extremely rare in children, representing less than 0.3% of pediatric sarcomas overall. Only two series have been reported in pediatric age, respectively (Ferrari et al. 2002).

Histology shows vascular structures with an infiltrative growth pattern and more solid areas with sheets and nests of malignant endothelial cells frequently displaying an epithelioid

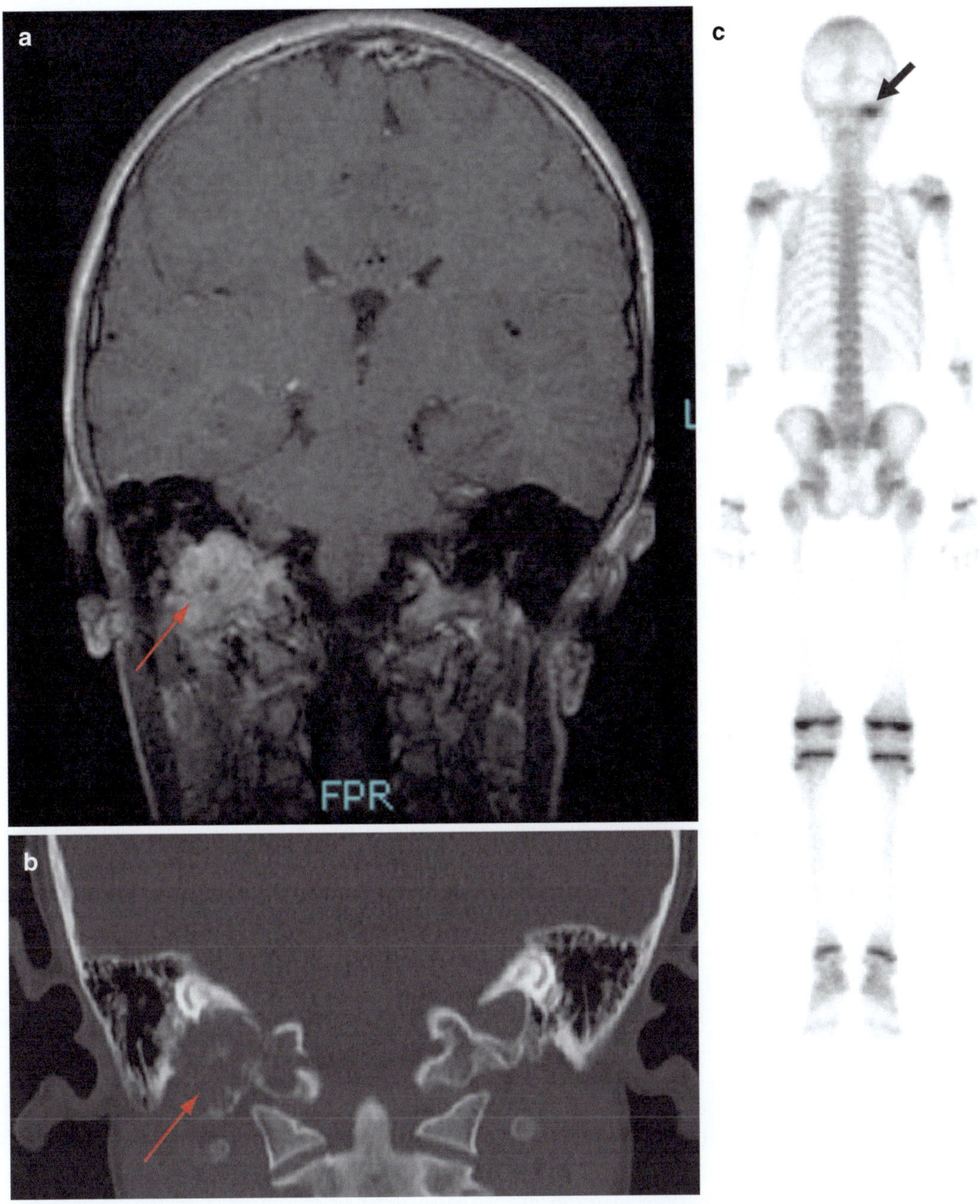

Fig. 43.5 Epithelioid hemangioendothelioma in a 12-year-old boy who presented with facial nerve paresis on the right side. (**a**) MRI of vascular lesion at the right petrosal bone with contrast enhancement in T1. (**b**) Signs of skeletal destruction at the CT scan. (**c**) Early phase of technetium-99 m scintigraphy showing a unifocal lesion at the right petrosal bone

morphology. Spindled areas can be present as well. Necrosis is found in more than 80% of cases. Tumor cells express CD31 and CD34.

In adults, the majority of AS develop as cutaneous tumors. In children, the majority of AS arise in the mediastinum and heart, but may involve also the visceral organs, breast, and deep soft tissue of the abdomen or pelvis. Two risk factors are well established: chronic lymphoedema and previous radiotherapy. Clinical presentations of AS are heterogeneous. Possible output cardiac failure can result in very young patients due to arteriovenous shunting. The lesions can appear as hemorrhagic masses. Hepatic AS are extremely rare and usually present with a rapidly enlarging liver. By the time they are diagnosed, the lesion is often unresectable. AS are highly aggressive tumors; metastases are common, frequently to the lung. The mortality rate is generally high, particularly in hepatic AS in which death usually occurs within the first 6 months. In childhood, published series reported a mortality rate ranging between 62% and 65%.

Large resection followed, if possible, by adjuvant radiotherapy is the cornerstone of curative-intent treatment of localized AS. There are no convincing data supporting the administration of adjuvant chemotherapy, but most protocols currently require adjuvant chemotherapy in high-grade (as AS is) and large tumors, even when resected. For metastatic or locally advanced AS, doxorubicin-based chemotherapy or chemotherapy based on weekly paclitaxel (Penel et al. 2011) seems to provide the longer progression-free survival. Three phase II or parts of phase II trials have been published in the adult setting, investigating weekly paclitaxel, sorafenib, and imatinib, demonstrating that clinical trials are feasible for such rare diseases. There is data on the use of anti-angiogenic agents for angiosarcoma, such as f.e. bevacizumab, a monoclonal antibody against vascular endothelial growth factor. Combination systemic chemotherapy is possible (Jeng et al. 2014; Dickson et al. 2015).

43.14 Kaposi Sarcoma

Kaposi sarcoma (KS) is rarely diagnosed in childhood and adolescence in general. It is a locally aggressive vascular neoplasm caused by the human herpesvirus 8 (HHV-8) (Jackson et al. 2016). KS can be classified into four different types: classic, iatrogenic (immunosuppression-associated), AIDS-associated, and African/endemic. The classic type predominantly affects older adults of Mediterranean or Eastern European ancestry. Only single cases have been reported in children (Byun et al. 2010; Sahin et al. 2010). The iatrogenic type is linked to immunosuppression (e.g., after solid organ transplantation) and normally resolves with immune restoration. In a series of 326 organ-transplanted pediatric patients, 6 children developed a KS (Penn 1994). In contrast to the classic form of KS which is mainly located at the extremities, AIDS-associated KS usually develops on the head, back, neck, muscular palate, and area of the gingiva and is seen in patients with low CD4-T-lymphocytes (<400/μL).

Typically, KS presents with cutaneous lesions in the form of plaques, patches, or nodules. In the classic type, purplish, reddish-blue, or dark-brown macules that can ulcerate are found. In rare cases, internal organs can be affected as well as the lymph nodes. In histopathology, the patch stage and the plaque, as well as the nodular stage, can be described. A vascular proliferation is seen with endothelial cells lining perivascular spaces, and new blood vessels can be produced in the lumen of preexisting blood vessels.

In a US series of 4954 children with AIDS, 8 developed an AIDS-associated KS (Biggar et al. 2000). In patients with AIDS-associated KS, a highly active antiretroviral therapy (HAART) has been shown to prevent or induce regression of KS. Finally, the African/endemic type can be differentiated into the cutaneous and lymphadenopathic type and is seen in pediatric populations in Africa, most of whom develop the clinical disease as a consequence of HIV infection (Ziegler and Katongole-Mbidde 1996).

As most cases of KS in children appear in relation to immunosuppression, the major goal in the treatment is to restore immune competence either by changing the immunosuppressant scheme in organ-transplanted children (e.g., to mTOR inhibitors) or by applying an antiviral therapy in the case of HIV infection.

Chemotherapy regimens, including bleomycin, vincristine, and taxanes, have been used on an individual basis. There is data from children in Malabia who showed that an overall survival rate was 71% and the event-free survival rate was 50% when treated with chemotherapy (Macken et al. 2018). Response rates to different chemotherapeutic agents can be found in a systemic review (Regnier-Rosencher et al. 2013). There are also reports on local therapies with intralesional injection of vincristine or interferon alfa-2 or radiation therapy.

References

Adams DM, Hammill A (2014) Other vascular tumors. Semin Pediatr Surg 23(4):173–177

Ahmad N, Adams DM, Wang J, Prakash R, Karim NA (2014) Hepatic epithelioid hemangioendothelioma in a patient with hemochromatosis. J Natl Compr Cancer Netw 12(9):1203–1207

Amary MF, O'Donnell P, Berisha F, Tirabosco R, Briggs T, Pollock R et al (2013) Pseudomyogenic (epithelioid sarcoma-like) hemangioendothelioma: characterization of five cases. Skelet Radiol 42(7):947–957

Ayturk UM, Couto JA, Hann S, Mulliken JB, Williams KL, Huang AY et al (2016) Somatic activating mutations in GNAQ and GNA11 are associated with congenital hemangioma. Am J Hum Genet 98(4):789–795

Biggar RJ, Frisch M, Goedert JJ (2000) Risk of cancer in children with AIDS. AIDS-Cancer Match Registry Study Group. JAMA 284(2):205–209

Billings SD, Folpe AL, Weiss SW (2003) Epithelioid sarcoma-like hemangioendothelioma. Am J Surg Pathol 27(1):48–57

Blatt J, Stavas J, Moats-Staats B, Woosley J, Morrell DS (2010) Treatment of childhood kaposiform hemangioendothelioma with sirolimus. Pediatr Blood Cancer 55(7):1396–1398

Byun M, Abhyankar A, Lelarge V, Plancoulaine S, Palanduz A, Telhan L et al (2010) Whole-exome sequencing-based discovery of STIM1 deficiency in a child with fatal classic Kaposi sarcoma. J Exp Med 207(11):2307–2312

Campbell JP, Grekin RC, Ellis CN, Matsuda-John SS, Swanson NA, Voorhees JJ (1983) Retinoid therapy is associated with excess granulation tissue responses. J Am Acad Dermatol 9(5):708–713

Chang LC, Haggstrom AN, Drolet BA, Baselga E, Chamlin SL, Garzon MC et al (2008) Growth characteristics of infantile hemangiomas: implications for management. Pediatrics 122(2):360–367

Colmenero I, Hoeger PH (2014) Vascular tumours in infants. Part II: Vascular tumours of intermediate malignancy [corrected] and malignant tumours. Br J Dermatol 171(3):474–484

Cournoyer E, Al-Ibraheemi A, Engel E, Chaudry G, Stapleton S, Adams DM (2020) Clinical characterization and long-term outcomes in pediatric epithelioid hemangioendothelioma. Pediatr Blood Cancer 67(2):e28045

Croteau SE, Liang MG, Kozakewich HP, Alomari AI, Fishman SJ, Mulliken JB et al (2013) Kaposiform hemangioendothelioma: atypical features and risks of Kasabach-Merritt phenomenon in 107 referrals. J Pediatr 162(1):142–147

Dickson MA, D'Adamo DR, Keohan ML, D'Angelo SP, Carvajal RD, Gounder MM et al (2015) Phase II trial of gemcitabine and docetaxel with bevacizumab in soft tissue sarcoma. Sarcoma 2015:532478

Dong K, Wang XX, Feng JL, Liu H, Zu KJ, Chang J et al (2015) Pathological characteristics of liver biopsies in eight patients with hepatic epithelioid hemangioendothelioma. Int J Clin Exp Pathol 8(9):11015–11023

Drolet BA, Trenor CC III, Brandao LR, Chiu YE, Chun RH, Dasgupta R et al (2013) Consensus-derived practice standards plan for complicated Kaposiform hemangioendothelioma. J Pediatr 163(1):285–291

El Darouti M, Marzouk SA, Sobhi RM, Bassiouni DA (2000) Retiform hemangioendothelioma. Int J Dermatol 39(5):365–368

Enjolras O, Mulliken JB, Boon LM, Wassef M, Kozakewich HP, Burrows PE (2001) Noninvoluting congenital hemangioma: a rare cutaneous vascular anomaly. Plast Reconstr Surg 107(7):1647–1654

Enjolras O, Soupre V, Picard A (2008) Uncommon benign infantile vascular tumors. Adv Dermatol 24:105–124

Enjolras O, Mulliken JB, Kozakewich HPW (2013) Vascular tumors and tumor-like lesions. In: Mulliken JB, Burrows PE, Fishman SJ (eds) Mulliken & Young's vascular anomalies: hemangiomas and malformations, 2nd edn. Oxford University Press, New York, pp 259–324

Ferrari A, Casanova M, Bisogno G, Cecchetto G, Meazza C, Gandola L et al (2002) Malignant vascular tumors in children and adolescents: a report from the Italian and German Soft Tissue Sarcoma Cooperative Group. Med Pediatr Oncol 39(2):109–114

Fletcher CD, Beham A, Schmid C (1991) Spindle cell haemangioendothelioma: a clinicopathological and immunohistochemical study indicative of a non-neoplastic lesion. Histopathology 18(4):291–301

Fletcher CDM, Bridge JA, Hogendoorn P, Mertens F (2013) WHO classification of tumours of soft tissue and bone, 4th edn. IARC Press, Lyon, France

Guo R, Gavino AC (2015) Angiolymphoid hyperplasia with eosinophilia. Arch Pathol Lab Med 139(5):683–686

Haggstrom AN, Lammer EJ, Schneider RA, Marcucio R, Frieden IJ (2006) Patterns of infantile hemangiomas: new clues to hemangioma pathogenesis and embryonic facial development. Pediatrics 117(3):698–703

Haisley-Royster C, Enjolras O, Frieden IJ, Garzon M, Lee M, Oranje A et al (2002) Kasabach-merritt phenomenon: a retrospective study of treatment with vincristine. J Pediatr Hematol Oncol 24(6):459–462

Hammill AM, Wentzel M, Gupta A, Nelson S, Lucky A, Elluru R et al (2011) Sirolimus for the treatment of complicated vascular anomalies in children. Pediatr Blood Cancer 57(6):1018–1024

Haro A, Saitoh G, Tamiya S, Nagashima A (2015) Four-year natural clinical course of pulmonary epithelioid hemangioendothelioma without therapy. Thorac Cancer 6(4):544–547

Hauer J, Graubner U, Konstantopoulos N, Schmidt S, Pfluger T, Schmid I (2007) Effective treatment of kaposiform hemangioendotheliomas associated with Kasabach-Merritt phenomenon using four-drug regimen. Pediatr Blood Cancer 49(6):852–854

Hettmer S, Andrieux G, Hochrein J, Kurz P, Rossler J, Lassmann S et al (2017) Epithelioid hemangioendotheliomas of the liver and lung in children and adolescents. Pediatr Blood Cancer 64(12)

Hirsh AZ, Yan W, Wei L, Wernicke AG, Parashar B (2010) Unresectable retiform hemangioendothelioma treated with external beam radiation therapy and chemotherapy: a case report and review of the literature. Sarcoma 2010:756246

Hoeger PH, Colmenero I (2014) Vascular tumours in infants. Part I: Benign vascular tumours other than infantile haemangioma. Br J Dermatol 171(3):466–473

Hornick JL, Fletcher CD (2011) Pseudomyogenic hemangioendothelioma: a distinctive, often multicentric tumor with indolent behavior. Am J Surg Pathol 35(2):190–201

Hsi Dickie B, Fishman SJ, Azizkhan RG (2014) Hepatic vascular tumors. Semin Pediatr Surg 23(4):168–172

Hughes R, McAleer M, Watson R, Collins S, Irvine A, White M (2014) Rapidly involuting congenital hemangioma with pustules: two cases. Pediatr Dermatol 31(3):398–400

Jackson CC, Dickson MA, Sadjadi M, Gessain A, Abel L, Jouanguy E et al (2016) Kaposi sarcoma of childhood: inborn or acquired immunodeficiency to oncogenic HHV-8. Pediatr Blood Cancer 63(3):392–397

Jeng MR, Fuh B, Blatt J, Gupta A, Merrow AC, Hammill A et al (2014) Malignant transformation of infantile hemangioma to angiosarcoma: response to chemotherapy with bevacizumab. Pediatr Blood Cancer 61(11):2115–2117

Joseph J, Wang WL, Patnana M, Ramesh N, Benjamin R, Patel S et al (2015) Cytotoxic and targeted therapy for treatment of pseudomyogenic hemangioendothelioma. Clin Sarcoma Res 5:22

Kayaalp C, Sabuncuoglu MZ (2015) Embolization of liver hemangiomas. Hepat Mon 15(8):e30334

Keiler SA, Honda K, Bordeaux JS (2011) Retiform hemangioendothelioma treated with Mohs micrographic surgery. J Am Acad Dermatol 65(1):233–235

Kumarasamy MT, Castrisios G, Sharma BK (2014) Rapidly involuting congenital haemangioma in a term neonate. BMJ Case Rep 2014:bcr2018224337

Leaute-Labreze C, Hoeger P, Mazereeuw-Hautier J, Guibaud L, Baselga E, Posiunas G et al (2015) A randomized, controlled trial of oral propranolol in infantile hemangioma. N Engl J Med 372(8): 735–746

Lee PW, Frieden IJ, Streicher JL, McCalmont T, Haggstrom AN (2014) Characteristics of noninvoluting congenital hemangioma: a retrospective review. J Am Acad Dermatol 70(5):899–903

Liu KX, Duggan EM, Al-Ibraheemi A, Shaikh R, Adams DM (2019) Characterization of long-term outcomes for pediatric patients with epithelioid hemangioma. Pediatr Blood Cancer 66(1):e27451

Macken M, Dale H, Moyo D, Chakmata E, Depani S, Israels T et al (2018) Triple therapy of vincristine, bleomycin and etoposide for children with Kaposi sarcoma: results of a study in Malawian children. Pediatr Blood Cancer 65(2)

Maguiness S, Uihlein LC, Liang MG, Kozakewich H, Mulliken JB (2015) Rapidly involuting congenital hemangioma with fetal involution. Pediatr Dermatol 32(3):321–326

Mazereeuw-Hautier J, Hoeger PH, Benlahrech S, Ammour A, Broue P, Vial J et al (2010) Efficacy of propranolol in hepatic infantile hemangiomas with diffuse neonatal hemangiomatosis. J Pediatr 157(2):340–342

Mehrabi A, Kashfi A, Fonouni H, Schemmer P, Schmied BM, Hallscheidt P et al (2006) Primary malignant hepatic epithelioid hemangioendothelioma: a comprehensive review of the literature with emphasis on the surgical therapy. Cancer 107(9):2108–2121

Mills SE, Cooper PH, Fechner RE (1980) Lobular capillary hemangioma: the underlying lesion of pyogenic granuloma. A study of 73 cases from the oral and nasal mucous membranes. Am J Surg Pathol 4(5):470–479

Mirra JM, Kessler S, Bhuta S, Eckardt J (1992) The fibroma-like variant of epithelioid sarcoma. A fibrohistiocytic/myoid cell lesion often confused with benign and malignant spindle cell tumors. Cancer 69(6):1382–1395

Naouri M, Schill T, Maruani A, Bross F, Lorette G, Rossler J (2010) Successful treatment of ulcerated haemangioma with propranolol. J Eur Acad Dermatol Venereol 24(9):1109–1112

Nasseri E, Piram M, McCuaig CC, Kokta V, Dubois J, Powell J (2014) Partially involuting congenital hemangiomas: a report of 8 cases and review of the literature. J Am Acad Dermatol 70(1):75–79

O'Connell JX, Nielsen GP, Rosenberg AE (2001) Epithelioid vascular tumors of bone: a review and proposal of a classification scheme. Adv Anat Pathol 8(2):74–82

Otte JB, Zimmerman A (2010) The role of liver transplantation for pediatric epithelioid hemangioendothelioma. Pediatr Transplant 14(3):295–297

Oza VS, Mamlouk MD, Hess CP, Mathes EF, Frieden IJ (2016) Role of sirolimus in advanced kaposiform hemangioendothelioma. Pediatr Dermatol 33(2):e88–e92

Ozeki M, Nozawa A, Kanda K, Hori T, Nagano A, Shimada A et al (2017) Everolimus for treatment of pseudomyogenic hemangioendothelioma. J Pediatr Hematol Oncol 39(6):e328–ee31

Patrizi A, Gurioli C, Dika E (2015) Pyogenic granulomas in childhood: new treatment modalities. Dermatol Ther 28(5):332

Penel N, Marreaud S, Robin YM, Hohenberger P (2011) Angiosarcoma: state of the art and perspectives. Crit Rev Oncol Hematol 80(2):257–263

Penn I (1994) De novo malignancy in pediatric organ transplant recipients. J Pediatr Surg 29(2):221–226; discussion 227–228

Perkins P, Weiss SW (1996) Spindle cell hemangioendothelioma. An analysis of 78 cases with reassessment of its pathogenesis and biologic behavior. Am J Surg Pathol 20(10):1196–1204

Pranteda G, Magri F, Muscianese M, Pigliacelli F, D'Arino A, Federico A et al (2018) The management of pseudomyogenic hemangioendothelioma of the foot: a case report and review of the literature. Dermatol Ther 31(6):e12725

Putra J, Rymeski B, Merrow AC, Dasgupta R, Gupta A (2017) Four cases of pediatric deep-seated/subcutaneous pyogenic granuloma: review of literature and differential diagnosis. J Cutan Pathol 44(6):516–522

Raheja A, Suri A, Singh S, Kumar R, Kumar R, Nambirajan A et al (2015) Multimodality management of a giant skull base hemangioendothelioma of the sphenopetroclival region. J Clin Neurosci 22(9):1495–1498

Regnier-Rosencher E, Guillot B, Dupin N (2013) Treatments for classic Kaposi sarcoma: a systematic review of the literature. J Am Acad Dermatol 68(2):313–331

Reich S, Ringe H, Uhlenberg B, Fischer B, Varnholt V (2010) Epithelioid hemangioendothelioma of the lung presenting with pneumonia and heart rhythm disturbances in a teenage girl. J Pediatr Hematol Oncol 32(4):274–276

Rialon KL, Murillo R, Fevurly RD, Kulungowski AM, Christison-Lagay ER, Zurakowski D et al (2015a) Risk factors for mortality in patients with multifocal and diffuse hepatic hemangiomas. J Pediatr Surg 50(5):837–841

Rialon KL, Murillo R, Fevurly RD, Kulungowski AM, Zurakowski D, Liang M et al (2015b) Impact of screening for hepatic hemangiomas in patients with multiple cutaneous infantile hemangiomas. Pediatr Dermatol 32(6):808–812

Rodriguez V, Lee A, Witman PM, Anderson PA (2009) Kasabach-merritt phenomenon: case series and retrospective review of the mayo clinic experience. J Pediatr Hematol Oncol 31(7):522–526

Ryan C, Price V, John P, Mahant S, Baruchel S, Brandao L et al (2010) Kasabach-Merritt phenomenon: a single centre experience. Eur J Haematol 84(2):97–104

Sahin G, Palanduz A, Aydogan G, Cassar O, Ertem AU, Telhan L et al (2010) Classic Kaposi sarcoma in 3 unrelated Turkish children born to consanguineous kindreds. Pediatrics 125(3):e704–e708

Sardaro A, Bardoscia L, Petruzzelli MF, Portaluri M (2014) Epithelioid hemangioendothelioma: an overview and update on a rare vascular tumor. Oncol Rev 8(2):259

Scalise R, Bolton J, Gibbs NF (2014) Rapidly involuting congenital hemangioma (RICH): a brief case report. Dermatol Online J 20(11)

Semenisty V, Naroditsky I, Keidar Z, Bar-Sela G (2015) Pazopanib for metastatic pulmonary epithelioid hemangioendothelioma-a suitable treatment option: case report and review of anti-angiogenic treatment options. BMC Cancer 15:402

Sparber-Sauer M, Koscielniak E, Vokuhl C, Schmid I, Bien E, Seitz G et al (2020) Endothelial cell malignancies in infants, children and adolescents: treatment results of three Cooperative Weichteilsarkom Studiengruppe (CWS) trials and one registry. Pediatr Blood Cancer 67(3):e28095

Stacchiotti S, Provenzano S, Dagrada G, Negri T, Brich S, Basso U et al (2016) Sirolimus in advanced epithelioid hemangioendothelioma: a retrospective case-series analysis from the Italian Rare Cancer Network Database. Ann Surg Oncol 23(9):2735–2744

Stahl RL, Henderson JM, Hooks MA, Martin LG, Duncan A (1991) Therapy of the Kasabach-Merritt syndrome with cryoprecipitate plus intra-arterial thrombin and aminocaproic acid. Am J Hematol 36(4):272–274

Swerlick RA, Cooper PH (1983) Pyogenic granuloma (lobular capillary hemangioma) within port-wine stains. J Am Acad Dermatol 8(5):627–630

Tamhankar AS, Vaidya A, Pai P (2015) Retiform hemangioendothelioma over forehead: a rare tumor treated with chemoradiation and a review of literature. J Cancer Res Ther 11(3):657

Tollefson MM, Frieden IJ (2012) Early growth of infantile hemangiomas: what parents' photographs tell us. Pediatrics 130(2):e314–e320

Vildy S, Macher J, Abasq-Thomas C, Le Rouzic-Dartoy C, Brunelle F, Hamel-Teillac D et al (2015) Life-threatening hemorrhaging in neonatal ulcerated congenital hemangioma: two case reports. JAMA Dermatol 151(4):422–425

Walther C, Tayebwa J, Lilljebjorn H, Magnusson L, Nilsson J, von Steyern FV et al (2014) A novel SERPINE1-FOSB fusion gene results in transcriptional up-regulation of FOSB in pseudomyogenic haemangioendothelioma. J Pathol 232(5):534–540

Wananukul S, Nuchprayoon I, Seksarn P (2003) Treatment of Kasabach-Merritt syndrome: a stepwise regimen of prednisolone, dipyridamole, and interferon. Int J Dermatol 42(9):741–748

Wassef M, Hunt SF, Santa Cruz DJ (2010) Vascular tumors and vascular malformations. In: Barnhi RL, Crowson AN, Magro CM et al (eds) Dermatopathology, 3rd edn. McGraw Hill Medic, New York, pp 802–856

Wassef M, Blei F, Adams D, Alomari A, Baselga E, Berenstein A et al (2015) Vascular anomalies classification: recommendations from the International Society for the Study of Vascular Anomalies. Pediatrics 136(1):e203–e214

Xiao Y, Wang C, Song Y, Wang C, Wang X, Zhang X et al (2013) Primary epithelioid hemangioendothelioma of the kidney: the first case report in a child and literature review. Urology 82(4):925–927

Yeh I, Bruckner AL, Sanchez R, Jeng MR, Newell BD, Frieden IJ (2011) Diffuse infantile hepatic hemangiomas: a report of four cases successfully managed with medical therapy. Pediatr Dermatol 28(3):267–275

Zhang G, Chen H, Gao Y, Liu Y, Wang J, Liu XY (2018) Sirolimus for treatment of Kaposiform haemangioendothelioma with Kasabach-Merritt phenomenon: a retrospective cohort study. Br J Dermatol 178(5):1213–1214

Ziegler JL, Katongole-Mbidde E (1996) Kaposi's sarcoma in childhood: an analysis of 100 cases from Uganda and relationship to HIV infection. Int J Cancer 65(2):200–203

Part XII

Rare Mesenchymal Tumors

Soft Tissue Sarcomas

44

Andrea Ferrari and Rita Alaggio

While benign neoplasms of soft tissues (i.e., lipoma, fibroma, leiomyoma, hemangioma) are relatively frequent and outnumber by 100 times malignant cases (incidence of about 300 new cases per 100,000), soft tissue sarcomas are a rare disease. They account for less than 1% of all malignant tumors and 2% of all cancer-related deaths. Data from the Surveillance, Epidemiology, and End Results (SEER) registry indicated an overall incidence of 5.9 per 100,000 persons/year. The incidence rates increased with age, rising from 0.9/100,000 in children younger than age 10 years to 18.2 for individuals older than age 70 (Ferrari et al. 2011a, b).

However, though their absolute number is lower than in adult age, in childhood and adolescence, soft part sarcomas encounter for about 8% of all malignancies and as a whole group represent the fifth most frequent childhood cancer. More than half of pediatric soft tissue sarcomas are represented by rhabdomyosarcoma, which is one of the most typical tumors of childhood. The remaining entities are usually grouped under the definition of "non-rhabdomyosarcoma soft tissue sarcomas" (NRSTS), a term that describes a heterogeneous group of mesenchymal extraskeletal malignant tumors: some of them are peculiar of infants and small children, but most of the entities included in this group are really tumors more common in adults than in children (Fig. 44.1). The term "NRSTS" (currently in widespread use) reflects the fact that these tumors have been historically managed according to the principles adopted for rhabdomyosarcoma, but, though they share some clinical characteristics, NRSTS must be considered as clearly different entities. Each NRSTS histotype should be considered a very rare tumor in childhood. As examples, Fig. 44.2 shows the age-specific incidence of some subtypes from the SEER: synovial sarcoma, dermatofibrosarcoma protuberans, and malignant peripheral nerve sheath tumors (MPNST).

NRSTS can arise anywhere in the body and can have a local invasiveness and a tendency to give distant metastases that is correlated to the different degree of malignancy along histotype and tumor grade. As a general view, borderline and low-grade tumors may be locally aggressive, but unlikely to metastasize: the growth rate may be indolent, and sometimes the diagnosis is done after removing a small swelling that has existed for several years. High-grade tumors are more aggressive and can have a strong propensity to

A. Ferrari (✉)
Pediatric Oncology Unit, Fondazione IRCCS Istituto Nazionale Tumori, Milan, Italy
e-mail: andrea.ferrari@istitutotumori.mi.it

R. Alaggio
Pathology Department, Ospedale Pediatrico Bambino Gesù IRCCS, Rome, Italy

D. T. Schneider et al. (eds.), *Rare Tumors in Children and Adolescents*, Pediatric Oncology,
https://doi.org/10.1007/978-3-030-92071-5_44

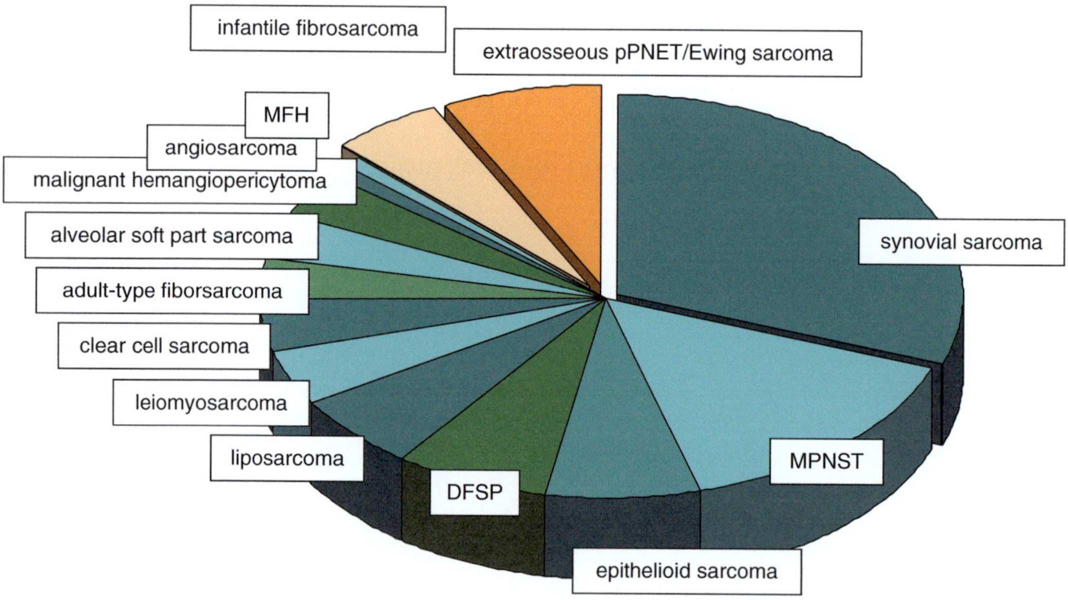

Fig. 44.1 Different non-rhabdomyosarcoma soft tissue sarcoma histotypes in the series from the Istituto Nazionale Tumori in Milan (Ferrari A, et al. J Clin Oncol 2005;23:4021–4030). In blue-green colors, the "adult-type" subtypes. *pPNET* peripheral primitive neuroectodermal tumors, *MPNST* malignant peripheral nerve sheath tumors, *DFSP* dermatofibrosarcoma protuberans, *MFH* malignant fibrous histiocytoma

metastasize, particularly to the lung. The clinical history may be very different among the different entities included under the NRSTS umbrella: e.g., MPNST are generally axial and aggressiveness diseases, characterized by poor prognosis, particularly when associated with neurofibromatosis type 1 (NF1) (Ferrari et al. 2007a, b; Carli et al. 2005); epithelioid sarcomas present typical features such as peculiar superficial distal location (i.e., hand, fingers), indolent growth, and tendency for lymph node involvement (Casanova et al. 2006; Spunt et al. 2019); infantile fibrosarcoma is a peculiar subtype that may have initial rapid growth and metastatic spread, but also indolent evolution (and also spontaneous regressions have been described) (Orbach et al. 2010, 2016); desmoplastic small round cell tumors (DSRCT) usually present as large abdominal masses generally disseminated at the time of diagnosis, with extensive spread to regional lymph nodes, peritoneal seeding, and distant metastases; the outcome is extremely poor despite intensive multimodality treatment approaches (Kushner et al. 1996; Bisogno et al. 2010).

As a preliminary statement, it could be said that the rarity and the heterogeneity of NRSTS would suggest that children and adolescents with these tumors should be referred to selected experienced institutions with multidisciplinary skills in enrolling patients in clinical trials. Tumors of intermediate malignancy are usually treated with surgery alone. For truly malignant tumors, and for high-grade sarcomas in particular, a multimodal therapy including surgery, radiotherapy, and chemotherapy needs to be considered the best approach. Most of NRSTS are usually considered scarcely chemosensitive tumors, but this is not true for all the histotypes, some of them requiring peculiar tailored approaches. In all the cases, the indication for the different treatment modalities and their intensity should be modulated according to the risk group, with the aim to give more intensive therapies to patients with less favorable prognostic factors while avoiding overtreatment and side effects (without jeopardizing the outcome) in cases with more favorable clinical features (Ferrari and Casanova 2005).

The overall cure rate for NRSTS patients, in fact, is around 70%, but this data is strictly cor-

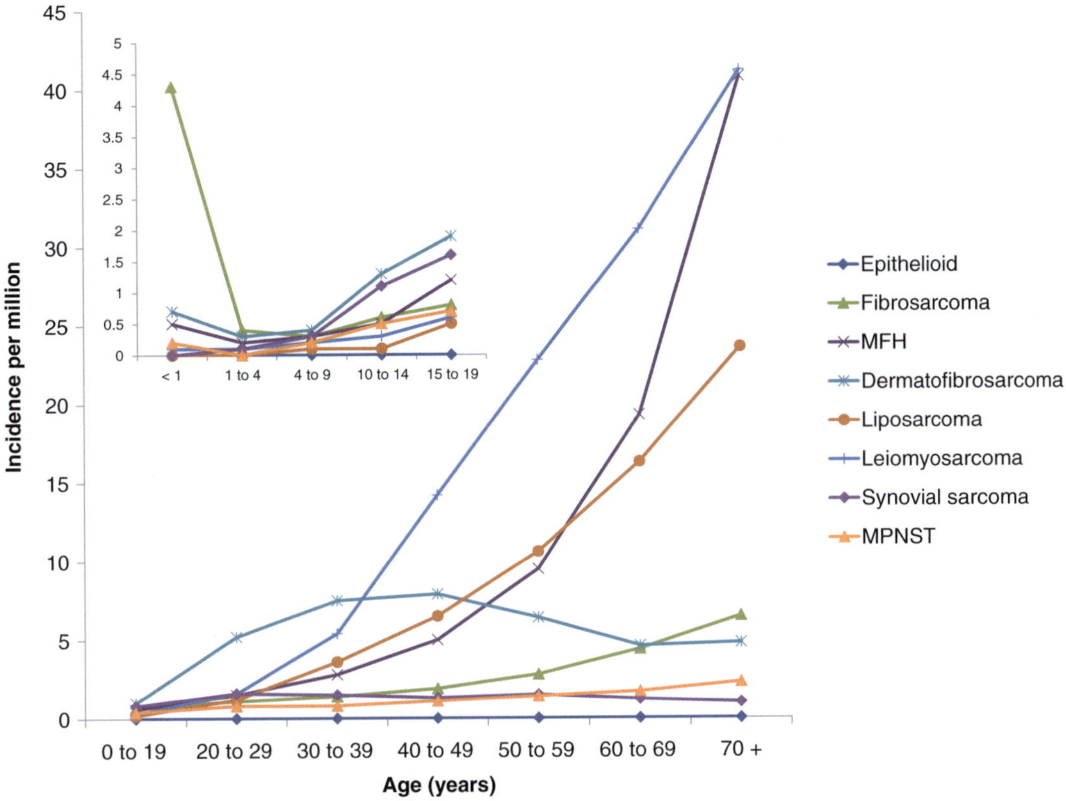

Fig. 44.2 Age-specific incidence of some non-rhabdomyosarcoma soft tissue sarcoma subtypes from the Surveillance, Epidemiology, and End Results (SEER) public-access database collected from various geographic areas in the United States (1973–2007) (www.seer.cancer.gov). (Courtesy of Dr. Iyad Sultan, King Hussein Cancer Center, Amman, Jordan)

related to the presence of the different prognostic variables. For most NRSTS, and in particular for those entities typical of adult age (adult-type NRSTS), the variables known to have a prognostic role in adults are relevant also in children (Spunt et al. 1999; Ferrari et al. 2007a, b, 2005a,b): the disease extension at onset, the degree of the initial surgery, the grade of malignancy, the tumor site (Ferrari et al. 2008, 2017a, b, c), and the tumor size (though it should be considered that the risk associated with a given tumor size may be not the same in patients with the same tumor but of different age and body size) (Ferrari et al. 2009). Patient's age is often a prognostic factor (Hayes-Jordan et al. 2000), and for many NRSTS subtypes, treatment results reported in pediatric series are significantly better than those reported in adult cohorts (Sultan et al. 2009; Ferrari et al. 2004).

While in the past children with NRSTS were often treated according to the guidelines defined for rhabdomyosarcoma, in the first decade of the new millennium, both the North American Soft Tissue Sarcoma Committee of the Children's Oncology Group (COG) and the European Paediatric Soft Tissue Sarcoma Study Group (EpSSG) developed specific multimodal risk-adapted trials focused on pediatric NRSTS, the COG ARST0332 (conducted from 2007 to 2012) (Spunt et al. 2014, 2020) and the EpSSG NRSTS 2005 (conducted from 2005 to 2017) (Ferrari et al. 2015a, b, 2017a, b, c, 2021; Orbach et al. 2016, 2017; Brennan et al. 2016, 2018). The results of the COG ARST0332 and the EpSSG NRSTS 2005 studies have been recently published and represent the present benchmark for NRSTS, defining risk-adapted standards of care.

44.1 The Pathological Characterization

The histologic classification of soft tissue tumors is based on their morphologic resemblance to one of the constituent mesenchymal tissues in the different developmental stages. Whether these tumors originate from a mesenchymal stem cell or from a less primitive precursor committed to a differentiative lineage is still unknown. For a large and heterogeneous group of soft tissue tumors, the putative cell of origin remains a mystery.

The WHO classification for soft tissue tumors (Fletcher et al. 2013) recognizes three prognostic categories: benign tumors, malignant tumors, and tumors with intermediate prognosis (locally aggressive and rarely metastasizing). In the case of benign or intermediate tumors, it is important to avoid the risk of a mutilating surgery or overtreatment, and in the case of sarcomas, the correct categorization allows the adequate treatment. Although the diagnosis is based on morphology, the widespread use of immunohistochemistry with specific lineage markers and the identification of numerous cytogenetic and molecular abnormalities are contributing to a more precise classification and to a better understanding of the mechanisms involved in tumor development, progression, and prognosis.

Genomic and expression profiling studies suggest that sarcomas can be divided into four major genetic groups: (a) sarcomas with specific translocation, (b) sarcomas with specific activating or inactivating mutations, (c) sarcomas with 12q13–15 amplification, and (d) sarcomas with a complex genomic profile (Coindre and Chibon 2010). Most of sarcomas typical of childhood fall in the first group, whereas more than 50% of the adult-type sarcomas are encompassed in the last category, together with some sarcomas arising in the context of family cancer syndromes and those arising as second tumors after radiotherapy.

Tables 44.1 and 44.2 summarize the most frequent pediatric sarcomas other than rhabdomyosarcoma in children and adolescents, the chromosomal aberrations and the associated cancer syndromes.

44.2 Soft Tissue Tumors with Intermediate Prognosis

Soft part tumors with intermediate prognosis are mostly of fibroblastic-myofibroblastic origin and include some lesions occurring in both children and adults, such as fibromatoses and inflammatory myofibroblastic tumor, and others occurring exclusively in childhood, such as infantile fibrosarcoma (Ferrari et al. 2013). This group includes also tumors of fibrohistiocytic origin (plexiform fibrohistiocytic tumor), of vascular origin (kaposiform hemangioendothelioma), or with unknown histogenesis (angiomatoid fibrous histiocytoma). Plexiform fibrohistiocytic tumor, angiomatoid fibrous histiocytoma, and *kaposiform hemangioendothelioma* are discussed in Chap. 42.

These lesions of intermediate malignancy may display a worrisome morphology mimicking highly aggressive sarcomas, and clinical features of a poorly circumscribed mass with infiltrative margins may further support this possibility. They represent a therapeutic challenge for oncologists and surgeons, in particular in the case of large unresectable lesions. Historically, surgery had been generally considered the mainstay of treatment for these tumors. However, treatment strategies are currently changing to some degree, from a strategy of aggressive surgery to a multidisciplinary approach that includes also various potentially effective systemic therapies and takes the functional and cosmetic sequelae of treatments into account too (Table 44.3).

44.2.1 Fibromatoses

The fibromatoses are benign or intermediate locally aggressive fibroblastic-myofibroblastic proliferations and may be sporadic or associated with syndromes or genetic disorders. Classically, they are divided into juvenile and adult-type fibromatoses (Allen 1977).

The great majority of *juvenile fibromatoses* are benign and include different clinicopathologic entities, some solitary and only occasionally multiple, like fibrous hamartoma of infancy, and others frequently multicentric, like

Table 44.1 Clinicopathologic features of rare soft tissue tumors with intermediate prognosis in children

Histotype	Site	Genetic alterations	Associated syndromes or malformations	Histologic key features
Superficial fibromatoses	Plantar, less frequently palmar	Autosomal dominant	Spine malformations, bifid uvula, geographic tongue, inflammatory bowel disease, and Ehlers-Danlos-like findings	Proliferation of fibroblasts and plump myofibroblasts in bundles
Desmoid-type fibromatoses	Abdominal, extra-abdominal	Mutations in APC gene in FAP CTNNB1 (exon 3) in sporadic variants	FAP/Gardner syndrome	Uniform spindle cells in fascicle with thin-walled vessels running parallely, scattered mast cells
Lipofibromatosis	Distal extremities, trunk, head	Possible deregulation of the PI3K-AKT-mTOR pathway via fusions involving RTK (BRAF, EGFR, PDGFRB, RET, ROS1) or ligands to the RTK EGFR (EGF, HBEGF, TGFA)		Mature adipose tissue traversed by fascicles of fibroblasts
Inflammatory myofibroblastic tumor	Lung, mesentery, omentum, retroperitoneum, liver, head, neck	ALK rearrangements with different partners Frequent EML4 in children Gene fusions involving ROS1, PDGFRB, RET		Fasciitis-like, fibrous histiocytoma-like, desmoid-like
Infantile fibrosarcoma family	Trunk, distal extremities	*ETV6-NTRK3* *EML4-NTRK3* Rearrangements of kinase genes (*ALK*, *BRAF*, *NTRK1*) *BRAF* intragenic deletions *TFG-MET*	–	Spindle cells with high nuclear/cytoplasm ratio and nuclear hyperchromasia, in fascicles with herringbone pattern

FAP familial adenomatous polyposis, *RTK* receptor tyrosine kinases

myofibromatosis. The clinical behavior may differ from spontaneous regression, in either solitary or multicentric variants, to lethal forms with visceral involvement (Chung and Enzinger 1981). Some other fibromatoses are hereditary, such as juvenile hyaline fibromatosis and gingival fibromatosis (Coffin and Boccon-Gibod 2004).

Lipofibromatosis is the only juvenile fibromatosis classified among the intermediate, soft tissue neoplasms, with recurrences or persistent growth observed after surgery in 72% of cases. It is typical of infants, congenital in 25% of cases, more frequent in males, and generally localized in the upper and lower distal extremities. In the past, many cases had been diagnosed as desmoid fibromatosis. The diagnostic key feature is the presence of adipose tissue traversed by fibrous septa containing fascicles of bland fibroblasts. Risk of recurrence may be associated with congenital onset, male sex, hand and feet location, incomplete surgery, and a high mitotic activity (Fetsch et al. 2000). In a recent study, fusions involving several genes encoding for receptor tyrosine kinases (RTK) or ligands to the RTK EGFR have been identified, suggesting a role of the PI3K-AKT-mTOR pathway deregulation in the pathogenesis of a large subset of

Table 44.2 Clinicopathologic features of rare malignant soft tissue tumors in children

Differentiative lineage	Histotype	Site	Genetic alterations	Associated syndromes or malformations, predisposing factors	Histologic key features
	Myofibrosarcoma	Head and neck, rarely bone	Non-specific alterations at 12p11, 12q13-q22,1p gain	–	Myofibroblastic differentiation (with EM or IHC)
	Low-grade fibromyxoid sarcoma	Superficial, head and neck, lower extremities, and trunk	FUS-CREB3L2 *FUS-CREB3L1* (mostly LGFMS/mixed) EWSR1-CREB3L1 (mostly SEF)	–	Biphasic tumor with myxoid/fibrous areas and bland spindle cells in myxoid stroma with prominent arciform vessels Mixed forms with SEF areas
	Sclerosing epithelioid fibrosarcoma (SEF)	Deep, limb, trunk, shoulder, neck		–	Carcinoma-like nests, sheets, or cords of epithelioid cells in a fibrous stroma
	Myxofibrosarcoma	Trunk, distal extremities	–	–	Low grade: Scattered spindle/stellate cells with hyperchromatic nuclei in myxoid matrix High grade: increase of cellularity and atypia
Smooth muscle	Leiomyosarcoma	Skin, superficial and deep soft tissue, bone, viscera (lung and GI tract)	Extra copies of chr 5, 18, 20, 21, and 22 in infantile form, complex structural and numerical cytogenetic alterations in others		Spindle cells with elongated, blunt-ended nuclei in interlacing bundles Variants: inflammatory and myxoid leiomyosarcoma; epithelioid and pleomorphic leiomyosarcoma exceedingly rare
	Smooth muscle tumors with uncertain malignant potential	Multifocal	–	Immunocompromised patients (associated with Epstein-Barr virus infection)	Well-differentiated mitotic activity <18/10HPF
Adipose	Liposarcoma	Lower extremities, mediastinum	MLPS *FUS-DDIT3* (most frequent) *EWSR1-DDIT3* WDLPS: *MDM2* amp MPLPS: *RB* del	Li-Fraumeni syndrome	More than 90% myxoid LPS (including pleomorphic and spindle cell variants) <5% atypical lipomatous tumors <2% pleomorphic liposarcoma

Differentiative lineage	Histotype	Site	Genetic alterations	Associated syndromes or malformations, predisposing factors	Histologic key features
Nerve sheath	MPNST		Mutation of NF1 gene in syndromic MPNST TP53, p16INK4 mutations	NF1	Classic spindle cells with weavy nuclei, nuclear palisades Variants: epithelioid, glandular, triton tumor
Uncertain differentiation	Epithelioid sarcoma	Finger, hand, wrist, forearm, lower extremities, trunk, head and neck, genital areas	INI mutation i(majority)	–	Classic: nodules of large, eosinophilic cells, central necrosis Morphologic variants: fibroma-like, dermatofibroma-like, angiomatoid Proximal-type: prominent epithelioid cells with rhabdoid cells
	Clear cell sarcoma of soft parts	Tendons, aponeuroses, distal extremities	*EWSR1-ATF1*		Fascicles/nests of pale, elongated epithelioid cells
	Alveolar soft part sarcoma		*ASPSCR1-TFE3*		Epithelioid cells in nests. PAS-positive cytoplasmic rhomboid crystals
	Desmoplastic small round cell tumor	Abdominal, pelvic cavity, other sites	*EWS-WT1*		Solid sheets, nests, or cords of small cells in a desmoplastic stroma
	Extra-renal rhabdoid tumor	Somatic soft tissues, abdomen, pelvis, retroperitoneum, liver, heart, GI tract	Deletion or mutation of hSNF5/SMARCB1/INI1	Syndrome of predisposition to rhabdoid tumor (germline mutation/deletion of INI1 gene)	Epithelioid cells, large nuclei with prominent nucleoli, cytoplasmic juxtanuclear hyaline globules
	Synovial sarcoma	Any site	*SS18-SSX1* *SS18-SSX2* *SS18-SSX4*	–	Monophasic fibrous or epithelial Biphasic (spindle and epithelioid cells) poorly differentiated

IHC immunohistochemistry, *EM* electron microscopy, *GI tract* gastrointestinal tract, *Inf LMS* inflammatory leiomyosarcoma, *MPNST* malignant peripheral nerve sheath tumors, *NF1* neurofibromatosis type 1, *LGFMS* low-grade fibromyxoid sarcoma, *SEF* sclerosing epithelioid fibrosarcoma

Table 44.3 Unclassifiable soft tissue malignancies in infants and children

	Site	Age	Histologic key features	Prognosis
Round cells/spindle cells				
CIC-DUX4	Extremities, trunk, rarely visceral, or bone		Round, spindle, epithelioid variable myxoid stromal CD99 (focal), WT1 ETV4+	Highly aggressive (5-year OS of 49% in localized forms)
BCOR-CCNB3 *BCOR-MAML4*	Bone (axial/extra-axial l). Less frequent: visceral (kidney)	Adolescent, young man	Small-/medium-sized cells with vescicular nuclei. Arciform vasculature spindle morphology in a subset of cells; immunostains: *BCOR*, *CCNB3*, cyclin D1, SATB2+	Better prognosis compared to Ewing's sarcoma and CIC-DUX4
BCOR ITD, YWHAE-NUTM2B/E (UNDS/PMMTI)	Paraspinal retroperitoneum/pelvis, head/neck, rarely extremities	Infants	Cytology, vascular pattern like in CCSK and in BCOR-CCNB3 PMMTI prominent myxoid stroma	Variable
Epithelioid spindle cell				
GLI-rearranged tumors[a,b] *GLI1-ACTB* *GLI-PTCH1* *GLI-1MALAT1* *GLI* ampl	Cervical Extremities, back, lung	1 case in 16 years/F 5–54 years	Nests/cords of epithelioid cells separated by septa, with thin capillary network S100 +/−, SOX10, SMA, EMA−	Not well defined Not well defined
Pleomorphic cells				
High-grade pleomorphic sarcoma	Site of radiation therapy, deep dermal	Older children, adolescents	Spindle cells in fascicles or sheets and storiform pattern focal pleomorphism	Better than in adults

UNDS undifferentiated sarcoma, *PMMTI* primitive myxoid mesenchymal tumor of infancy

[a] GLI1-MALAT1 reported in 15–20% of gastric plexiform fibromyxoma and 100% of gastroblastomas and benign and low-grade tumors, respectively. Plexiform fibromyxoma: report of two pediatric cases and review of the literature. (Duckworth LV, Gonzalez RS, Martelli M, Liu C, Coffin CM, Reith JD. Pediatr Dev Pathol. 2014 Jan–Feb;17(1):21–7. https://doi.org/10.2350/13-09-1373-OA.1; World J Gastroenterol. 2010 Jun 21; 16(23): 2835–2840. https://doi.org/10.3748/wjg.v16.i23.2835; World J Gastroenterol. 2017 Aug 21;23(31):5817–5822. https://doi.org/10.3748/wjg.v23.i31.5817)

[b] Antonescu CR, Agaram NP, Sung YS, Zhang L, Swanson D, Dickson BC. A Distinct Malignant Epithelioid Neoplasm With GLI1 Gene Rearrangements, Frequent S100 Protein Expression, and Metastatic Potential: Expanding the Spectrum of Pathologic Entities With ACTB/MALAT1/PTCH1-GLI1 Fusions. Am J Surg Pathol. 2018 Apr;42(4):553–560. https://doi.org/10.1097/PAS.0000000000001010

lipofibromatosis. In particular, the FN1-EGF gene fusion, typical of calcifying aponeurotic fibroma, has been found in 4 out of 20 lipofibromatosis cases, while 7 showed one each EGR1-GRIA1, TPR-ROS1, SPARC-PDGFRB, FN1-TGFA, EGFR-BRAF, VCL-RET, or HBEGF-RBM27 fusions (Al-Ibraheemi et al. 2018).

The *adult fibromatoses* include the deep-seated *desmoid fibromatosis* (aggressive fibromatosis) and *superficial palmar/plantar fibromatosis*, both representing intermediate, locally recurring soft tissue neoplasms.

Although considered adult fibromatoses, *desmoid tumors* occur in both adults and children, with an incidence of 0.2–0.4 per 100,000 population/year. It accounts for up to 60% of fibrous tumors in childhood, where up to 30% occur in the first year of life, with a peak incidence around 4.5 years. A male predominance has been observed in pediatric series.

The pathogenesis of aggressive fibromatosis is most likely multifactorial, and genetic predisposition, endocrine factors, and trauma all seem to play an important part. This neoplasm can be sporadic or arise in the setting of familial adenomatous polyposis (FAP) or the Gardner variant of the syndrome, often characterized by intra-abdominal mesenteric lesions with aggressive behavior. Syndromic desmoid may be preceded or accompanied by fibrous, plaque-like lesions called the Gardner fibroma.

Histologically, desmoid fibromatosis shows a morphologic variation in terms of cellularity and degree of collagenization. Elongated fibroblasts with dark condensed nuclear chromatin resembling the inactive fibrous tissue are embedded in the densely collagenized variants of desmoid fibromatosis. Active fibroblasts with oval nuclei, vesicular chromatin, and small nucleoli reminiscent of wound healing may be seen in other areas or in more densely cellular forms. The cells are uniform with subtle collagen bundles arranged in long fascicles. Thin-walled blood vessels are parallel to the fascicles. Nuclear hyperchromasia, cellular atypia, and pleomorphism are absent. Mitoses are rare. Mast cells may be seen, especially around blood vessels. At the periphery, desmoid fibromatosis shows an infiltrative growth with subtle bands of collagen or cell fascicles the dissecting adipose tissue or entrapping muscle fibers. Well-circumscribed lesions with rounded margins are rarely seen. Recurrent desmoid fibromatosis has similar morphology. The collagenization related to the scarring process may represent a challenge in the evaluation of surgical margins. Immunostains are positive for vimentin with variable expression of muscle-specific actin, desmin, and smooth muscle actin.

Cytogenetic investigation of desmoids in FAP has clarified the key role played by beta-catenin, a transcriptional activator involved in the promotion of mesenchymal cell proliferation. In FAP-related desmoids, germline mutations in APC gene inhibit its ability to induce the phosphorylation of beta-catenin necessary for its proteosomal degradation, and it accumulates in the cytoplasm and migrates to the nucleus with a permanent activation of genes involved in cell proliferation. In sporadic desmoids, mutations more frequently involve codons 41 (41A) and 45 (45F and 45P) of beta-catenin gene CTNNB1 resulting in a non-phosphorylated active beta-catenin. The mutated form of beta-catenin shows a positive nuclear immunostaining (Salas et al. 2010). Some studies indicate that increased nuclear expression of beta-catenin, especially if associated with p53 positivity, may be predictive of a high recurrence rate (wild-type beta-catenin tumors seem to have a better relapse-free survival) and may be potentially used as molecular biomarkers of local recurrence (Dômont et al. 2010; Lazar et al. 2008; Le Guellec et al. 2012).

In children, desmoid fibromatosis may involve the extremities, trunk, head, and neck. There is a strong tendency for local recurrence (ranging from 24% to 77%), without metastasizing to other organs (overall survival is generally over 90% at 10 years) (Meazza et al. 2010; Oudot et al. 2012).

Surgery had been generally considered the mainstay of treatment for these tumors; the goal should be a microscopically complete resection, but the influence of positive margins on local relapse is still debated; hence, a mutilating surgery should be avoided. However, treatment strategies are currently changing: On the one hand, it is clear that surgery is not resolutive in many cases and, moreover, it might be the cause of fibromatosis growth and recurrence. On the other hand, various pharmacological treatments have proved to be relatively effective (Desmoid Tumor Working Group 2020). Therapeutic options may be non-cytotoxic agents, including hormonal treatment (tamoxifen) (Skapek et al. 2013), non-steroidal anti-inflammatory drugs, and interferon-alpha, or cytotoxic agents, in particular the prolonged low-dose chemotherapy such the weekly low-dose methotrexate plus vinca alkaloid (vinblastine or vinorelbine) combination. Interesting responses have been seen also using target therapy (Sparber-Sauer et al. 2021) as imatinib (probably via a mechanism of action not involving c-kit and PDGFR receptor) (Heinrich et al. 2006; Cough et al. 2010), pazopanib (Toulmonde et al. 2018), and sorafenib (Gounder et al. 2018). The response rate to the various systemic regimens is generally around 50% (or less) (Skapek et al. 2007). The goal of systemic therapy in this disease, however, is not only the tumor shrinkage to permit a subsequent resection (as in malignant tumors) but also the induction of growth arrest and tumor stabilization (Meazza et al. 2010).

Desmoid tumors can remain stable for a long time, with or without primary treatment, and this finding has prompted the suggestion that also a "wait-and-see" strategy (clinical-radiological monitoring alone) might be suitable in cases of non-evolving disease. A watchful waiting strategy is currently suggested by many experts: therapies should be given only in the event of tumor growth (or in the case of life-threatening tumors), and first therapeutic option might be a "minimal-morbidity systemic therapy" (being the combination of low-dose methotrexate plus vinblastine/vinorelbine the first choice) rather than a surgical resection (Bonvalot et al. 2008; Fiore et al. 2009; Colombo et al. 2015; Woltsche et al. 2014; Honeyman et al. 2013).

Due to the potentially long-term cosmetic or functional morbidity in children, radiation therapy may have a role after failure to chemotherapy, in the case of progression despite multiple surgeries, or as alternative to mutilating surgery.

The EpSSG recently published the results of the prospective series enrolled in the EpSSG NRSTS 2005 study and treated according to a conservative treatment algorithm, consisting of an initial wait-and-see strategy, non-mutilating surgery, and minimal-morbidity chemotherapy (in the case of tumor progression). From 2005 to 2016, 173 pediatric patients with desmoid-type fibromatosis were registered from 57 centers (and 8 different countries): 35% of them had no immediate therapy (wait-and-see strategy), 31% had immediate surgery, and 34% had immediate chemotherapy after diagnosis (vinblastine and methotrexate were the first choice). Progression-free survival was 36.5% and did not significantly differ in the three treatment groups. Apart from one patient who died from a secondary tumor, all patients were alive at the time of analysis. The conservative strategy did not compromise outcomes and could be adopted to reduce treatment burden (8% of patients had biopsy and no further treatment, 42% had chemotherapy only, 20% had surgery only, 23% had both chemotherapy and surgery, and 6% had radiotherapy in addition to other therapies) (Orbach et al. 2017).

Another recently published interesting study reports on a case series of 16 pediatric patients with progressive or recurrent disease after at least one line of systemic therapy, treated with oral hydroxyurea (Ferrari et al. 2019). That study is of interest for the discussion regarding the evaluation of tumor response in desmoid-type fibromatosis. In such disease, in fact, assessing the antitumor activity of any medication may be a challenge. Tumor response may be underestimated using traditional dimensional criteria alone: a treatment's antitumor activity may prompt other types of radiological response, such as changes in morphology and vascularity (e.g., changes in T2-weighted signal intensity on MRI, as seen in some of our cases), that might correspond to fibrotic transformation or reduction of the amount of vital cells. In the hydroxyurea study, the response rate was 18.7% of major partial remissions, 37.5% considering any amount of shrinkage, and 68.7% considering symptom response or signs of tissue response as well. On the other hand, tumor response might be overestimated as a tumor's shrinkage or lack of growth is not necessarily due to any drug efficacy, since desmoid tumors may spontaneously regress (or remain dimensionally stable). Noteworthy, in fact, a phase III, randomized, double-blind, placebo-controlled trial on sorafenib for adult fibromatosis reported durable partial response in the placebo arm (21% versus 33% in the sorafenib arm) (Gounder et al. 2018); in other words, reductions in tumor size might be related to spontaneous shrinkage.

The *superficial fibromatoses*, including *palmar and plantar fibromatosis*, usually affect adults over the age of 40 years and are rare in children (very uncommon before the age of 5 years) (Fetsch et al. 2005; Urban et al. 1996). Both these entities have a genetic predisposition. Palmar fibromatosis involves the ulnar aspect of the palm, whereas plantar fibromatosis affects the medial plantar arch. The tumors involve the aponeuroses, and their morphology varies according to the stage of development (pediatric lesions are more cellular and show fibroblastic nodules and frequent mitoses; as the lesions evolve, they become hypocellular and collagenized).

Different from adults, in children, there is a prevalence of plantar fibromatosis with more frequent occurrence in females. Palmar and plantar fibromatosis may coexist in the same patient, may be bilateral, or may be associated with the involvement of the extensor surface of the finger joints (knuckle pads) and keloids. An association between palmar-plantar fibromatosis and fifth finger clinodactyly has been reported in about 13% of cases, as well as isolated cases of spine malformation, bifid uvula, "geographic" tongue, inflammatory bowel disease, and Ehlers-Danlos-like findings.

The recurrence rate is higher in children than in adults (about 80%). Surgery is essentially the only treatment and is recommended when the contracture is significant; however, recurrence after surgery is frequent. A wide or radical fasciectomy or dermofasciectomy is generally reserved for lesions determining functional impairment (Fetsch et al. 2005).

44.2.2 Inflammatory Pseudotumors

The umbrella term "inflammatory pseudotumors" includes reactive and neoplastic lesions characterized by a proliferation of fibroblasts and myofibroblasts with a prominent chronic inflammatory infiltrate (Gleason and Hornick 2008).

Inflammatory myofibroblastic tumor (IMT) is a distinctive neoplasm, observed mainly in children and young adults. It is a tumor of intermediate malignancy, and distant metastases occur in less than 5% of cases. Approximately 150–200 new cases are diagnosed annually in the United States (Webb et al. 2009). IMT was originally described in the lung, but it involves also the mesentery, omentum, retroperitoneum, abdominal soft tissues, liver, head, and neck. A palpable mass may be the clinical presentation, sometimes accompanied by an inflammatory syndrome, microcytic hypochromic anemia, thrombocytosis, and polyclonal hyperglobulinemia (Coffin et al. 1995, 1998).

Macroscopically, IMT are multinodular, nonencapsulated lesions, with a firm consistency, and may reach a large size, especially the intra-abdominal forms, which infiltrate the intestinal wall. Histologically, IMT are composed of myofibroblasts with scattered large, ganglion-like cells and a prominent inflammatory infiltrate containing plasma cells, lymphocytes, and eosinophils. According to the degree of cellularity, inflammatory infiltrate, and prevalence of myxoid or fibrous stroma, IMT may display different patterns varying from fasciitis-like lesions, with prominent inflammatory infiltrate and myxoid stroma, to those highly cellular fibrohistiocytoma-like or hypocellular, desmoid-like (Coffin et al. 1998) (Fig. 44.5d). The round/epithelioid cell variant is rare (Chen and Lee 2008). Immunohistochemistry shows reactivity for vimentin and variable staining for smooth muscle actin, muscle-specific actin, and desmin.

In IMT, the anaplastic lymphoma kinase (ALK) gene, located on chromosome 2p23, codifying for a tyrosine kinase receptor rearranges with a variety of gene partners (TPM3, CLTC, RANBP2, and others) (Bridge et al. 2001), resulting in a persistently activated protein and a positive immunostaining for ALK-1 in approximately 50–60% of cases (Cessna et al. 2002; Cook et al. 2001; Coffin et al. 2001). ALK-1 is more frequently positive in pediatric tumors and abdominal sites. Recent studies have contributed to expand the spectrum of genetic alterations in IMT. Gene fusions involving ROS1, PDGFRB, RET, and NTRK have been identified (Lovly et al. 2014). Additionally, Antonescu et al. in a large series including 24 pediatric cases detected an *EML4-ALK* inversion in 50% of pediatric cases (Antonescu et al. 2015).

A chimeric A2M-ALK gene fusion, previously described in *fetal lung interstitial tumor* (FLIT), has been recently reported in two infantile IMT. FLIT are infantile pulmonary mass-like lesion morphologically resembling a fetal lung with interstitial proliferation of primitive mesenchymal cells. IMT differ from FLIT for their solid appearance and the inflammatory infiltrate (Tanaka et al. 2017).

The clinical behavior of IMT varies according to the anatomical site. Extra-pulmonary IMT lesions tend to recur more frequently, with a relapse rate of 25%. Distant metastases occur in less than 5% of cases, mostly in the lung and brain. Tumor size and histologic features do not appear to influence the clinical outcome. However, aneuploidy may indicate a more aggressive potential (Hussong et al. 1999). A group of ALK-negative IMT might have a higher risk of metastasis and unfavorable prognosis (Coffin et al. 2007). Round/epithelioid cell IMT carry an ALK-RANBP2 fusion gene and behave aggressively (Chen and Lee 2008).

Surgery remains the mainstay of treatment, and the prognosis is generally good when the tumor is widely resected. Historically, radiotherapy and systemic treatments—corticosteroids and chemotherapy (anthracycline/ifosfamide chemotherapy or low-dose methotrexate and vinorelbine/vinblastine)—have been variously used in high-risk situations, but their role remains to be established yet (Alaggio et al. 2010a, b; Kube et al. 2018). In the last years, however, treatment strategy substantially changed with the evidence of the high activity of ALK inhibitors (crizotinib and ceritinib) (Butrynski et al. 2010; Brivio and Zwaan 2019). The COG crizotinib phase I/II trial (14 IMT pediatric patients) showed an overall response rate for IMT patients of 86% (5/14 complete response, 7/14 partial response) (Mossé et al. 2013, 2017). The CREATE trial, a multinational multi-tumor phase II basket study promoted by the European Organisation for Research and Treatment of Cancer (EORTC), showed objective response in 6/12 ALK-positive adult patients and in 1/7 ALK-negative adult patients (Schöffski et al. 2018). Crizotinib should be currently considered not only a new good option in the armamentarium of systemic therapies but probably the standard of care for patients with locally advanced or metastatic ALK-positive IMT (Mahajan et al. 2021). Things change rapidly, and the availability of targeted treatment also for ROS1 and NTRK translocated IMT will further modify the approach to this disease. It is worth noting that EpSSG recently reported a series of 60 IMT patients (median age 9.5 years) treated from 2005 to 2016. The lung was the primary site in 14 cases. IMT developed as a second tumor in 2 cases. Forty cases were ALK-positive, and 20 were ALK-negative. EFS and OS at 5 years were 83% and 98%, respectively. No clinical variables correlated statistically with the outcome: survival was the same for ALK-positive and ALK-negative cases. The overall response to systemic therapy in case with unresectable disease was 64%: 8/10 cases responded to vinblastine-methotrexate chemotherapy, and 5/5 to ALK-inhibitors (Casanova et al. 2020).

44.2.3 Infantile Fibrosarcoma and NTRK1 Mesenchymal Tumors

Infantile fibrosarcoma (IFS) is the most common non-benign soft tissue tumor under 1 year of age (Sultan et al. 2010). It is considered a tumor of low malignant potential, only rarely metastasizing. Near 50% of cases are diagnosed at birth (or, occasionally, in utero) (Chung and Enzinger 1976; Coffin et al. 1994).

Histologically, IFS display a wide morphologic spectrum. These tumors are generally highly cellular neoplasms, composed of spindle cells with hyperchromatic nuclei arranged in sheets, bands, or fascicles (Fig. 44.5c). A prominent hemangiopericytomatous vasculature is frequent. A focal herringbone pattern may simulate an adult fibrosarcoma. Large vascular spaces in the context of the tumor may simulate a vascular lesion either clinically/radiologically or histologically. Mitoses are frequent. Immunostains show variable expression of smooth muscle actin, less frequently desmin. IFS is characterized by the recurrent translocation t(12;15)(p13;q25) with the transcript ETV6-NTRK3, which is shared by cellular mesoblastic nephroma (Knezevich et al. 1998; Bourgeois et al. 2000). The transcript is detected in the majority of lesions histologically diagnosed as IFS by RT-PCR or FISH; however, a subset may be negative. In a recent study, 36% of IFS negative for ETV6 rearrangements by FISH revealed an ETV6-NTRK3 rearrangement with next-generation sequencing (Davis et al. 2019). In addition, IFS may have other cytogenetic abnormalities, including trisomy 11; random gains of chromosomes 8, 11, 17, and 20; and deletion of long arm of chromosome 17 (Bernstein et al. 1994; Dal Cin et al. 1991; Mandahl et al. 1989).

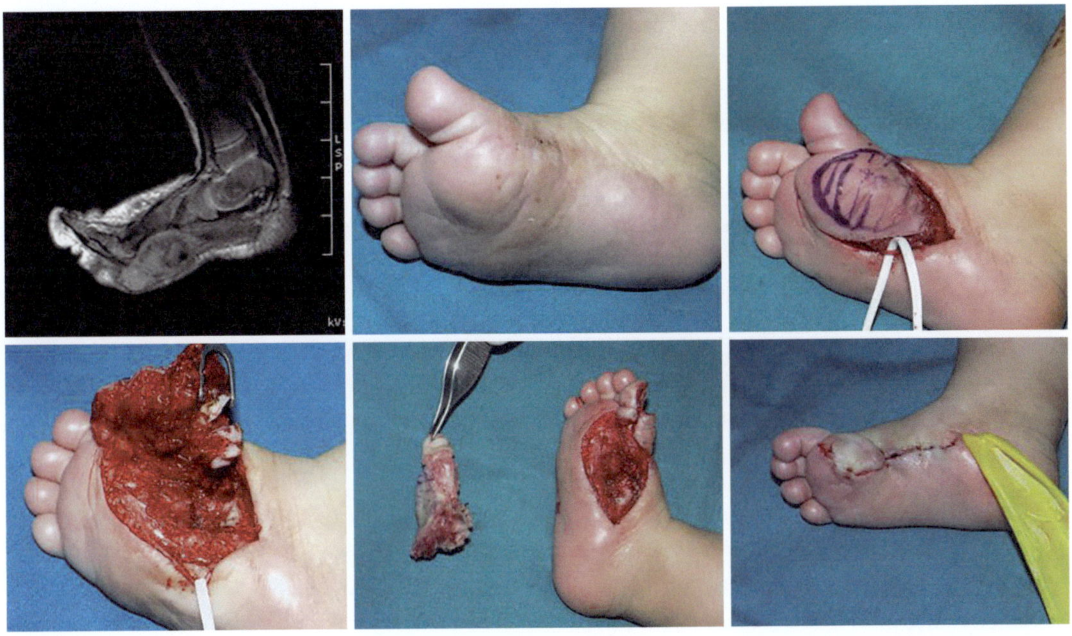

Fig. 44.3 Congenital infantile fibrosarcoma of the right foot. Wide surgical resection with amputation of the first finger. (Courtesy of Dr. Alessandro Gronchi, Melanoma Sarcoma Surgical Unit, Fondazione IRCCS Istituto Nazionale Tumori, Milano, Italy)

IFS is generally located in the deep soft tissues of distal extremities (and less frequently the trunk). Tumors usually have rapid growth and huge size, while distant metastases are rare. However, the prognosis is favorable in the majority of cases, with survival rates between 90% and 100%. Surgery is the mainstay of treatment (Fig. 44.3), but chemotherapy is effective and plays a major role in the treatment strategy, also utilizing mild alkylating/anthracycline-free regimens: the VA regimen (vincristine and actinomycin) is the chemotherapy of choice, and more intensive regimen should be considered only in the event of no response to VA chemotherapy (Orbach et al. 2010). Due to the young age of patients, radiotherapy must not be seen as an option.

In the EpSSG NRSTS 2005, 50 infants (median age 1.4 months) were prospectively treated (from 2005 and 2012) with a conservative strategy based on the VA chemotherapy. Response rate to VA was 68.0%. Event-free survival and overall survival at 3 years were 84.0% and 94.0%, respectively; only three children required mutilating surgery, and alkylating or anthracycline-based chemotherapy was avoided in 71.0% of patients needing chemotherapy (Orbach et al. 2016).

The treatment strategy may change in the near future due to the availability of very effective biologic agents, i.e., the TRK inhibitors (Orbach et al. 2020). The ETV6-NTRK3 fusion is present in around 85% of cases, but it has been described that in ETV6-NTRK3-negative tumors, other fusions involving NTRK1 or NTRK3 are present, suggesting that TRK fusions are nearly universal drivers in this disease (Pavlick et al. 2017; Wong et al. 2016). Larotrectinib is the first highly selective pan-TRK inhibitor to enter clinical development with IC_{50} values in the low nanomolar range of inhibition for all the three TRK family members. The efficacy of this drug in IFS has been clearly demonstrated (Nagasubramanian et al. 2016). The North American multicenter, open-label, phase I/II study (2015–2017) involved 24 children (17 with tumors harboring TRK fusions, 7 without a documented TRK fusion).

Among the 17 enrolled patients harboring TRK fusion-positive cancers, 8 had IFS, 7 had other soft tissue sarcomas, and 2 had papillary thyroid cancer. The drug was very well tolerated and showed encouraging antitumor activity in TRK fusion-positive tumors (objective response in 14/15 cases, 1 minor response in the other case), while none of the 7 patients with TRK fusion-negative cancers had an objective response (Laetsch et al. 2018; DuBois et al. 2018). It remains to be clarified the role of TRK inhibitor in a disease like IFS characterized by overall favorable survival when treated with mild chemotherapy as VA (though the prize of survival in terms of functional morbidity related to surgery may be sometimes severe). However, these agents may be of particular interest in other TRK fusion-positive mesenchymal or non-mesenchymal tumors (Davis et al. 2019; Laetsch and Hawkins 2018).

The biology of IFS is challenging. A subset of lesions morphologically overlapping with IFS harbor other recurrent chromosomal abnormalities including EML4-NTRK3 and rearrangements of the kinase genes ALK, BRAF, and NTRK1. Interestingly, IFS with BRAF intragenic deletions may have coexisting ETV6-NTRK3 fusions. Whether BRAF abnormalities are synergistic or secondary is object of study (Kao et al. 2018a, b).

A novel TFG-MET fusion, retaining the MET kinase domain, has been reported in a spindle cell infantile pelvic tumor. The tumor, composed of hyperchromatic spindle cells in fascicles with high mitotic rate, showed positive staining for S100 and negative staining for SOX10 and retained H3K27me3 (Flucke et al. 2017).

Most IFS-like tumors occur in the same age range as IFS and have a predilection for intra-abdominal sites. Rare cases in older children are reported. Their prognosis is still object of debate; however, a subset of NTRK1 tumors have a more aggressive clinical course compared to classic IFS and may show relapses and distant metastases (Davis et al. 2019).

In addition, the widespread use of molecular characterization has allowed the identification of a group of lesions previously classified as IFS because of their occurrence in infants and their morphologic overlap with primitive forms of IFS. These tumors, now identified as primitive myxoid mesenchymal tumor of infancy (PMMTI), are characterized by a diffuse growth of primitive spindle, polygonal, and round cells embedded in a myxoid stroma with a characteristic prominent vascular network and lack the ETV6-NTRK3 transcript. These tumors generally have an aggressive behavior: surgery is the elective treatment, being PMMTI poorly responsive to chemotherapy (Alaggio et al. 2006).

44.3 Malignant Soft Tissue Tumors

The large part of NRSTS represent the so-called adult-type sarcomas, tumor entities typically occurring in adults and elders and only occasionally in children. Most of them show an identifiable differentiative lineage and include adult fibrosarcomas, liposarcoma, leiomyosarcomas, and MPNST. A common denominator in this group of tumors (with the exclusion of MPNST) is the prognostic role of tumor grade. The two most widely used grading systems are the NCI (US National Cancer Institute) system, which has been adapted for pediatric sarcomas in the POG (Pediatric Oncology Group) system (Parham et al. 1995), and the FNCLCC (French Fédération Nationale des Centres de Lutte Contre le Cancer) system (Coindre et al. 1996; Guillou et al. 1997a, b). All have proven to be highly predictive of prognosis in this group of sarcomas. FNCLCC system identifies three grades, grade 1 the lowest, 2 intermediate, and 3 the highest, resulting from the addition of different scores given to tumor resemblance to its normal counterpart, mitotic activity, and necrosis. POG system takes into account the peculiarity of pediatric sarcomas which are considered by definition grade 1 or 3 according to histotype, whereas only adult-type sarcomas are graded according to mitotic rate and necrosis. Currently both FNCLCC and POG systems are being used in pediatric sarcomas.

Synovial sarcoma, alveolar soft part sarcoma, clear cell sarcoma of soft parts, epithelioid sarcoma, desmoplastic small round cell tumor, and rhabdoid tumor are characterized by the absence of a lineage differentiation or an identifiable normal cellular counterpart. With the partial exception of synovial sarcoma, their behavior is not influenced by tumor grade. All these tumors, but rhabdoid tumor, arise in young adults and adolescents and are less frequent in elders and children.

Dermatofibrosarcoma protuberans, *angiosarcoma*, and *epithelioid hemangioendothelioma* (this is defined by the WHO as a malignant vascular tumor because of its metastatic risk) are discussed in other chapters.

44.3.1 Treatment Strategy

The treatment management of adult-type NRSTS is complex and necessarily multidisciplinary (Table 44.4). As a general rule, these tumor types are usually considered scarcely sensitive to chemotherapy (tumor response in the range of 40% or less), and surgery thus remains the unquestionable keystone of treatment. Radiotherapy plays a well-defined role in local control, after incomplete resection and, according to adult experiences, also after wide excision, especially in the case of large tumors. However, the indications for radiotherapy are usually stricter in children, given the higher risk of severe late effects (i.e., the risk of retardation or arrest of irradiated bone growth, the risk of functional impairment, and that of second post-irradiation tumor). Aggressiveness and intensity of surgery and radiotherapy should be discussed and customized for each patient (taking into account the anatomical site, tumor size, patient's age, response to initial chemotherapy), considering the need to maximize the chances of local control, but also containing the sequelae and preserve function (Ferrari and Casanova 2005).

The role of chemotherapy as part of the multidisciplinary approach in adult-type NRSTS remains uncertain. It must be currently recognized that the more than 50 different subtypes of soft tissue sarcomas are indeed heterogeneous not only in their biology and clinical behavior but also in their therapeutic sensitivity, e.g., synovial sarcoma is far more sensitive to standard chemotherapy compared to near-resistant ones like alveolar soft part sarcoma or clear cell sarcoma. Generally, chemotherapy is usually given in frontline treatment in patients with advanced unresectable disease (and also in all cases where the surgeon is unsure of being able to achieve a complete resection at the first attempt). Neoadjuvant chemotherapy may have a role in converting these cases into conservative complete resections, but it may play an important role also in treating any micrometastases promptly (Ferrari et al. 2005a, b; Spunt et al. 2002; Pappo et al. 2005).

Noteworthy, various international research groups pooled their series on unresected NRSTS in a joint study comprising 304 patients (Ferrari et al. 2011a, b). Response rate to chemotherapy was 41% in terms of major responses, but also minor responses were seen (16%). Overall survival at 10 years was roughly 50% and was associated with patient's age, histological subtype, and tumor site and size. MPNST was the tumor type with the worst rate of response to chemotherapy and the worst outcome. Patients who respond to chemotherapy have better chances of survival, as well as those who had a complete delayed surgical resection and those treated with radiotherapy, suggesting that intensive multimodal treatment should be recommended in these patients.

A major debate concerns whether or not to provide adjuvant chemotherapy for adult-type soft tissue sarcomas, in order to prevent distant recurrences after initial surgery. Patients' outcome after initial resection is good (survival rate up to 90%) in patients with small and low-grade tumor, but the prognosis for patients with high-grade and large invasive tumors is often unsatisfactory, when treated with local therapy alone, even after initial microscopically complete resection, because of a high risk of developing lung metastases (Ferrari et al. 2005a, b). Pediatric retrospective studies confirmed that in group I–II

Table 44.4 A general view: practical diagnostic and therapeutic guidelines for pediatric soft tissue sarcomas

Physical examination	Soft tissue mass Signs of neurofibromatosis type 1, i.e., multiple café-au-lait spots, axillary or inguinal freckling, neurofibromas, Lisch nodules (iris hamartomas), plus learning disabilities
Laboratory assessment	No specific tumor markers available
Radiological assessment	
– First assessment	Ultrasonogram
– Local staging	Computed tomography (CT) scan or magnetic resonance imaging (MRI) of the primary site is mandatory for local extension assessment before any treatment. MRI is usually considered superior in defining soft tissue extension
– Diagnostic work-up	Chest CT scan to identify lung metastases, in high-grade sarcomas Abdominal ultrasound, ultrasound of regional lymph nodes Technetium bone scan and positron emission tomography (PET) are not considered a standard staging investigation (eventually in high-grade tumors)
Pathological assessment	In the case of a large and deep soft tissue mass, biopsy should be always the initial surgical procedure, in order to avoid inadequate surgery The initial biopsy (incisional biopsy or core needle biopsy) has the aim to define the diagnosis, but also should provide enough material for immunochemistry, cytogenetics, biological studies, and central pathology review for patients to be included in clinical trials Histological subtype Tumor grade
Staging systems for risk-adapted treatment strategy	**TNM classification** Based on local invasiveness, **T1** and **T2**, and tumor size, **A** or **B**, i.e., less or more than 5 cm; **N0/N1** and **M0/M1**: absence or presence of nodal and distant involvement **Intergroup Rhabdomyosarcoma Study (IRS) post-surgical grouping system** **Group I**—completely excised tumors with negative microscopic margins **Group II**—grossly resected tumors with microscopic residual disease and/or regional lymph nodal spread **Group III**—gross residual disease after incomplete resection or biopsy **Group IV**—metastases at onset
General treatment guidelines	Need for multidisciplinary approach
– Surgery	Keystone of treatment Goal: complete and non-mutilating resection Importance of the referral to specialist centers
– Radiotherapy	Well-defined role in local control, after incomplete resection or after wide excision in the case of high-grade and large tumor Indication stricter in younger children due to the higher risk of severe late effects
– Chemotherapy	Out of clinical trials, the indication to chemotherapy should be based on a shared and personalized decision-making, but also on the identification of those patients who are in much need of systemic treatment due to a high risk of metastatic failure, as well as those whose histological characteristics make them more likely to respond to chemotherapy Doxorubicin/ifosfamide-based chemotherapy in unresected or metastatic tumors (specific therapy in specific histotypes) Adjuvant chemotherapy in high-grade and large-sized sarcomas (especially in synovial sarcomas)

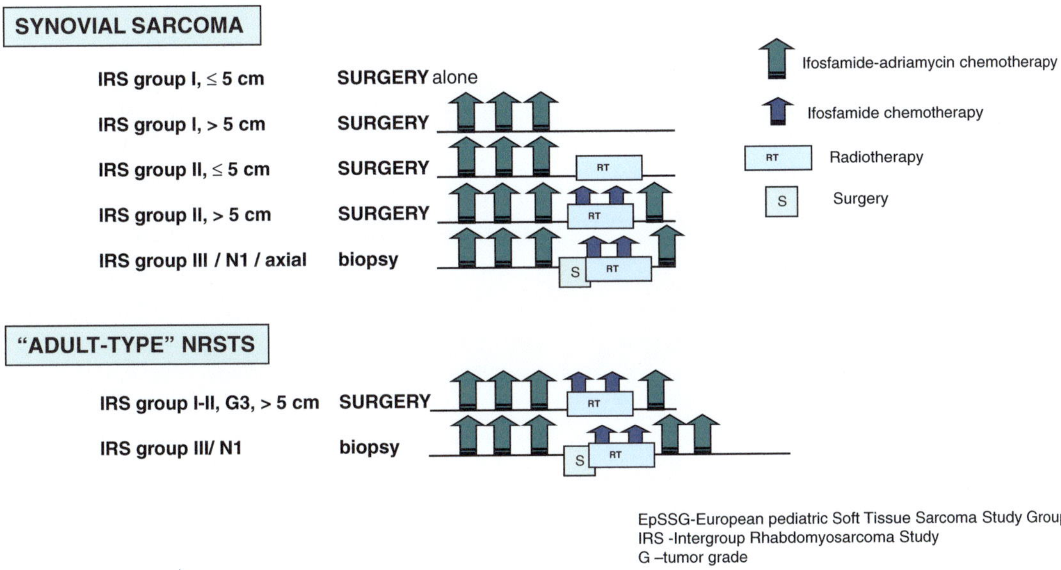

Fig. 44.4 Risk-adapted treatment strategy in the European Paediatric Soft Tissue Sarcoma Study Group (EpSSG) NRSTS 2005 protocol for synovial sarcoma and adult-type NRSTS patients

patients, the combination of two variables—high tumor grade plus large tumor size—gives rise to a very high risk of metastases (metastases-free survival around 30–40%), irrespective of the results of initial surgery, with better survival in those patients who received adjuvant chemotherapy, as compared to those who have not been given (Ferrari et al. 2005a, b).

This would suggest, in principle, the use of systemic chemotherapy to try to improve survival in those selected patients with high tumor grade and large tumor size (Ferrari 2008) (Fig. 44.4). The only randomized trial on adjuvant chemotherapy in pediatric age (conducted by the Pediatric Oncology Group POG between 1986 and 1992) failed to assess the benefits of adjuvant chemotherapy because the majority of patients refused randomization, showing how difficult it is to conduct prospective randomized studies in pediatric patients with such rare tumors, for which no standard therapy has been established (Pratt et al. 1999).

In adult oncology, the discussion on the role of adjuvant chemotherapy in soft tissue sarcomas has always been a point of controversy (Bramwell 2001): on the one hand, we know that most randomized trials performed by international collaborative groups showed no statistically significant benefit for patients given adjuvant chemotherapy (Santoro et al. 1995; Sarcoma Meta-analysis Collaboration 1997); on the other hand, it is clear that some of these negative results need to be reconsidered since these trials did not use the combinations of drugs currently recognized as the most effective in soft tissue sarcomas (ifosfamide, in particular, was not included in most of these studies), nor had they selected patients most likely to respond to chemotherapy (tumors of diverse histology, grade, and size were grouped together). When these criteria were considered (targeting a selected group of high-risk patients and delivering a regimen of full-dose ifosfamide plus anthracyclines), a more significant beneficial impact emerged: the Italian Sarcoma Group (ISG) was closed in advance (after the enrollment of 104 patients) because an interim analysis showed a clear improvement in the survival of patients receiving adjuvant chemotherapy by comparison with those given local therapy alone (Frustaci et al. 2001).

In the lack of a clear consensus (also due to the extreme heterogeneity of tumor entities), in adults, the indication to adjuvant chemotherapy should be currently based on a shared and

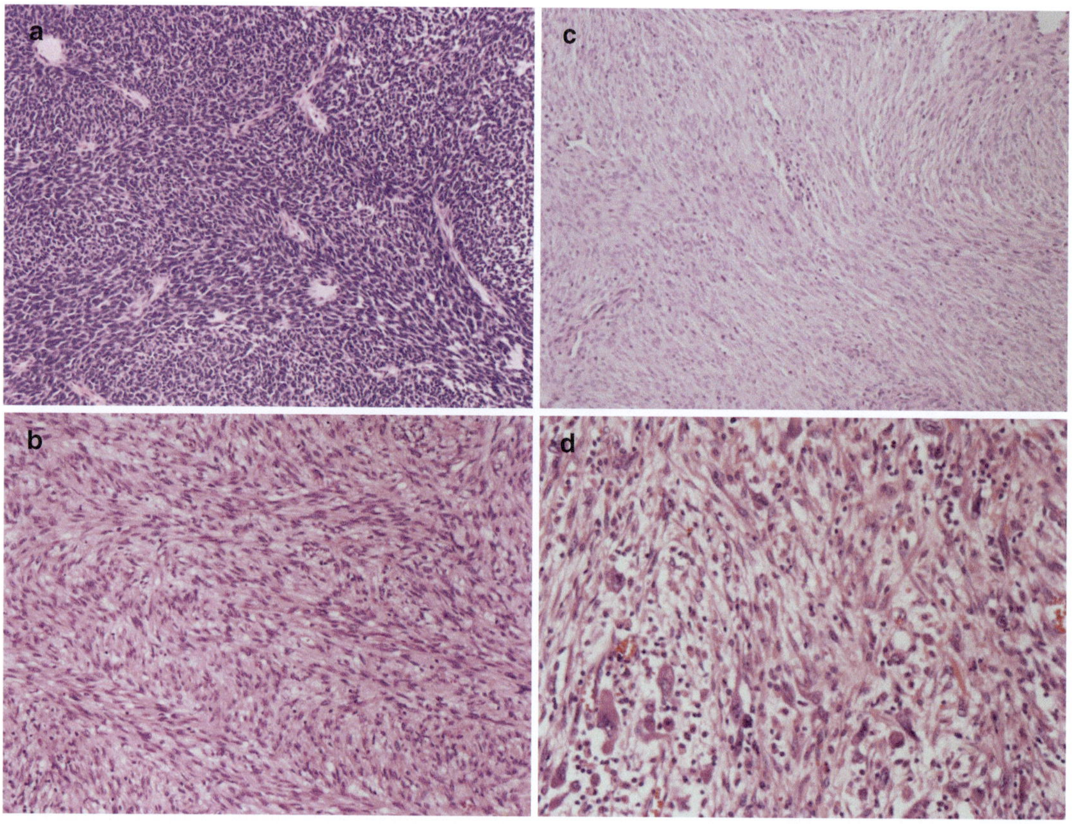

Fig. 44.5 Spindle cell sarcomas: **a** (HE staining, 100×) synovial sarcoma with the typical hemangiopericytomatous pattern; **b** (HE staining, 100×) malignant peripheral nerve sheath tumor (MPNST) showing fascicles of elongated cells with weavy nuclei; **c** (HE staining, 100×) congenital infantile fibrosarcoma with primitive elongated spindle cells; **d** (HE staining, 100×) inflammatory myofibroblastic tumor with elongated cells and scattered ganglion-like cells intermingled with lymphocytes and plasma cells

personalized decision-making, but also on an accurate identification of those patients who are in much need of systemic treatment due to a high risk of metastatic failure, as well as those whose histological characteristics make them more likely to respond to chemotherapy. The 2018 Clinical Practice Guidelines from the European Society for Medical Oncology-European Reference Network on Rare Adult Solid Cancers (ESMO-EURACAN) propose adjuvant chemotherapy as an option to the high-risk individual patient (high-grade, deep, >5 cm tumor) (Casali et al. 2018; Pasquali et al. 2019). In many adult sarcoma referral centers, chemotherapy is proposed in neoadjuvant setting (aiming also at a local benefit facilitating surgery, in addition to the systemic one): ifosfamide and anthracycline combination for three (preoperative) courses is considered the standard of care, when needed, by many experts (Gronchi et al. 2012).

44.3.2 Fibroblastic/Myofibroblastic Malignancies

Low-grade fibromyxoid sarcoma (*LGFMS*) is a slow-growing mass, deeply located in the soft tissues of lower extremities and trunk and occasionally head, neck, or spine (Evans 1987). In children, LGFMS is generally superficial and involves more frequently the head and neck region (Billings et al. 2005). Histologically, the tumors display a typical biphasic pattern, with an abrupt or gradual transition from myxoid to fibrous, heavily collagenized areas. Spindle cells with bland nuclei, lacking pleomorphism, are embedded in an abundant myxoid stroma, containing prominent vessels in an arcade-like configuration. Scattered giant rosettes, with a central zone of eosinophilic collagen surrounded by spindle and epithelioid cells, characterize the variant of LGFMS called hyalinizing spindle cell tumor with giant rosettes (Lane et al. 1997; Folpe et al. 2000a, b). Immunohistochemically LGFMS shows a positive staining for MUC4 and for EMA. LGFMS shows specific recurrent translocations involving the FUS gene: FUS-CREB3L2 transcript resulting from translocation t(7;16)(q32-34;p11) and the less frequent FUS-CREB3L1 from t(11;16)(p11;p11) (Mertens et al. 2005; Guillou et al. 2007; Prieto-Granada et al. 2015). If completely excised, LGFMS has a relapse rate of 10%. Metastases may occur even many years after the initial diagnosis in 5–26% of cases. Superficial lesions have a more favorable prognosis (Folpe et al. 2000a, b).

Sclerosing epithelioid fibrosarcoma (SEF) is an entity strictly related to LGFMS (Meis-Kindblom et al. 1995). It is typical of adults, and only 10% of patients are younger than 20 years. The tumors, often large in size, are deeply located in muscles in the lower limb, trunk, shoulder, and neck. Histologically, the tumors show epithelioid or fusiform cells with bland nuclei and clear cytoplasms arranged in carcinoma-like nests, sheets, or cords and embedded in a fibrous stroma

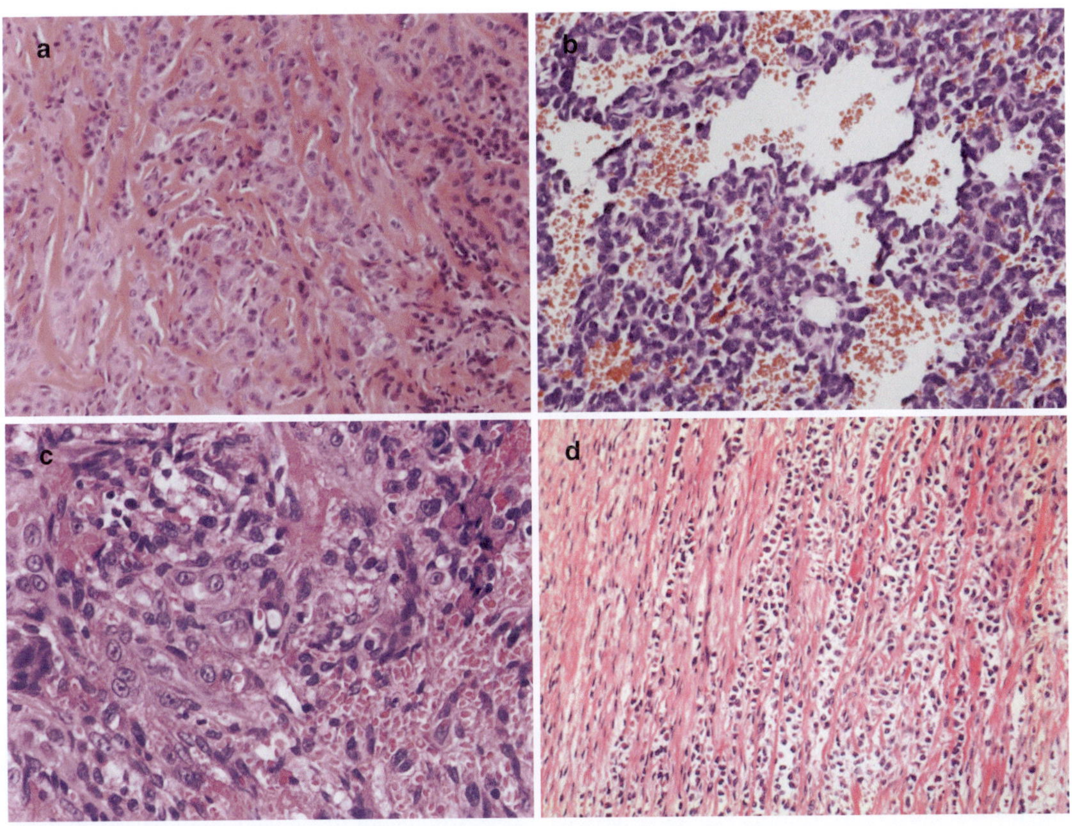

Fig. 44.6 Sarcomas with "epithelioid" cells: **a** (HE staining, 160×) epithelioid sarcoma showing large cells arranged in nests and cords embedded in a collagen stroma. **b** (HE staining, 100×) epithelioid sarcoma with vascular pattern mimicking epithelioid hemangioendothelioma. **c** (HE staining, 160×) epithelioid hemangioendothelioma with typical intracytoplasmic vacuoles, occasionally containing red cells. **d** (HE staining, 100×) sclerosing epithelioid fibrosarcoma: cords of epithelioid in a collagen stroma. Fascicles of spindle cells with typical features of fibrosarcoma on the left

or sclerotic matrix (Fig. 44.6d). Tumors with mixed features of SEF and LGFMS are frequent. Like in LGFMS, immunostain for MUC 4 is positive, and the EWS-CREB3L1/2 or FUS-CREB3L2 rearrangements are found (Guillou et al. 2007). More recently, FUS-CREM, PAX5-CREB3L1, and EWSR1-CREB3L3 transcripts have been reported mostly in SEF (Arbajian et al. 2017; Dewaele et al. 2017).

SEF may have an aggressive behavior with persistent disease or local recurrence in more than 50% of patients, with a metastatic rate between 43% and 86%, and with a mortality rate between 25% and 57% (Antonescu et al. 2001).

Myxofibrosarcoma is the commonest soft tissue sarcoma in limbs of older adults, whereas it is very rare under 20 years, with only few cases reported in children, mostly occurring in unusual sites (Denschlag et al. 2005). These tumors show a wide morphologic spectrum and include low- and high-grade forms, often coexisting. Scattered spindle or stellate tumor cells with atypical hyperchromatic nuclei embedded in an abundant myxoid matrix are found in low-grade tumors. Cellularity and atypias progressively increase in intermediate- and high-grade variants with evidence of sheets of pleomorphic cells and necrosis. The treatment is surgical resection, and myxofibrosarcoma can recur and metastasize.

Myofibrosarcomas are a controversial myofibroblastic malignancy displaying a range of appearances from low-grade lesions to high-grade forms resembling *high-grade pleomorphic sarcoma* (Fisher 2004; Montgomery et al. 2001).

Less than 10% of *low-grade myofibrosarcomas* occur in children and privilege the deep soft tissues of the head and neck (and rarely bone) (Smith et al. 1995; Keller et al. 2004). There is a slight male predominance with tumor size ranging from 1.5 to 17 cm. Tumors generally have an indolent clinical course, characterized by relapses in about 33% of cases and metastases, even after a long time, in 3–10% of cases, generally involving the lung.

44.3.3 Leiomyosarcoma

Smooth muscle tumors are rare in children and adolescents and include hamartomas, benign tumors (such as angioleiomyoma, leiomyoma, and leiomyomatosis), leiomyosarcoma, and smooth muscle tumors of uncertain malignant potential in immunocompromised individuals.

Leiomyosarcomas account for less than 4% of childhood soft tissue sarcomas, are more frequent in males, and involve the skin, superficial and deep soft tissue, bone, and viscera, such as the lung and GI tract. The mean age at diagnosis is 8–11 years and may arise as a second malignancy in patients treated with radiotherapy. Their prognosis is better than that in adults with a survival rate bigger than 70%. Late metastases in unusual sites may be seen (De Saint Aubain Somerhausen and Fletcher 1999; Ferrari et al. 2001). Macroscopically, leiomyosarcomas are large, not encapsulated nodular masses ranging from 1 to 13 cm, with frequent foci of hemorrhage and necrosis. Histologically, they are characterized by spindle cells with elongated, blunt-ended nuclei arranged in interlacing bundles. Morphologic variants include *inflammatory leiomyosarcoma*, showing a prominent mixed inflammatory infiltrate, and *myxoid leiomyosarcoma*, a low-grade variant only rarely metastasizing, with more than 50% of tumor composed of myxoid stroma. Pleomorphic and *epithelioid leiomyosarcomas* are exceptional in children. Immunohistochemistry shows reactivity for smooth muscle actin, muscle-specific actin, desmin, and h-caldesmon.

Smooth muscle tumors with uncertain malignant potential are less aggressive tumors, occurring in immunocompromised patients. They are generally visceral, often multifocal. The Epstein-Barr virus infection is involved in their pathogenesis. Compared to sporadic leiomyosarcoma, the tumors are well differentiated, with minor cytologic atypia and mitotic activity ranging from 0 to 18 mitoses per 10 high-power field (Deyrup et al. 2006).

44.3.4 Liposarcoma

Liposarcoma is the most common malignant soft tissue tumor in adults. In children, the neoplasms of adipose tissue are relatively infrequent, and liposarcomas account for less than 3% of all pediatric sarcomas (La Quaglia et al. 1993). While the anatomic distribution is similar in children and adults, being the lower extremities, especially the thigh, the most frequent site of involvement, the histotypes differ substantially. In adults, the *atypical lipomatous neoplasms* (*well-differentiated liposarcomas*) and their high-grade counterpart (*dedifferentiated liposarcoma*) account for approximately 60% of cases, the *myxoid and round cell liposarcomas* comprise about 35% of cases, and the *pleomorphic liposarcoma* comprise the remaining 5%.

In children, the conventional myxoid liposarcoma is the most frequent histotype, including around 90% of cases. Atypical lipomatous tumors and pleomorphic liposarcoma are very rare, representing less than 5% and less than 2% of cases, respectively.

Histologically, *myxoid liposarcomas* are characterized by a plexiform vascular pattern, abundant myxoid matrix, and uniform, bland, round cells with lipoblastic differentiation. Some tumors may display round cell areas. Like in older patients, pediatric myxoid liposarcomas show evidence of FUS-DDTI gene fusions, reflecting the presence of the t(12;16)(q13;p11). EWSR1-DDTI gene fusion is very rare, and its exact incidence in pediatric myxoid liposarcomas is unknown. Myxoid liposarcomas have a generally indolent clinical course. Patients' outcome, as for other adult-type soft tissue sarcomas, is correlated to the presence of metastases, tumor size, tumor respectability, and patient's age. Surgery is the cornerstone of treatment, and chemotherapy may play a role in advanced disease (Ferrari et al. 1999). Aggressive local growth and death have been reported in children affected by *pleomorphic myxoid liposarcoma*, a recently recognized variant of liposarcoma displaying mixed features of conventional and pleomorphic liposarcoma (Alaggio et al. 2009). Pleomorphic myxoid liposarcoma arising in the context of Li-Fraumeni syndrome has been reported (Sinclair et al. 2017; Debelenko et al. 2010). *Spindle cell myxoid liposarcoma* is another subtype of myxoid liposarcoma found in children. It behaves as a low-grade tumor, roughly similar to conventional myxoid liposarcoma (Alaggio et al. 2009).

In adult studies, a relatively new specific drug—i.e., trabectedin—has recently shown to be active in myxoid/round cell liposarcoma, possibly with a direct effect on the products of the histotype-specific FUS-CHOP translocation. This drug represents an alternative to the classic ifosfamide-doxorubicin chemotherapy in patients with advanced disease (Grosso et al. 2007).

44.3.5 Malignant Peripheral Nerve Sheath Tumors

Malignant peripheral nerve sheath tumors (MPNST) occur mainly in adults, and only 10–20% are diagnosed in the first two decades. Nevertheless, they represent one of the most frequent subtypes among pediatric NRSTS. In about 21–67% of cases, MPNST arise in patients affected by neurofibromatosis type 1 (NF1), by malignant transformation of pre-existing neurofibromas. The lifetime risk of developing MPNST in NF1 patients has been estimated at 8–13%, as compared to 0.001% in the general population (Evans et al. 2002). The molecular mechanisms responsible for malignant transformation of neurofibromas and those involved in tumor progression in both sporadic and NF1-associated MPNST are being progressively clarified. NF1 is caused by mutation in the NF1 suppressor gene, located in chromosome band 17q11. It encodes the neurofibromin, a protein inhibiting p21-RAS. NF1 inactivation promotes the development of neurofibromas, but it is not sufficient for malignant transformation. Further genetic alterations are needed, i.e., inducing aberrant growth factor signaling and mutations affecting the $p16^{INK4A}$-cyclin D1-CDK4-Rb and $p19^{ARF}$-Mdm2-p53 cell cycle pathways (Carroll 2016). Recently, loss-of-function mutations in SUZ12 and EED, two critical components of the polycomb repressor 2 (PRC2) complex, have been reported in 23–70% of NF1-associated MPNST, 90% of those radiotherapy-associated MPNST, and 36–92% of sporadic MPNST, but not in neurofibromas. SUZ12 and EED are chromatin-modifying proteins, which encode for zeste homolog 12 protein and embryonic ectoderm development protein, respectively. Together with EZH1 and EZH2, these PRC2 proteins establish and maintain the di- and trimethylation of lysine 27 of histone H3 (H3K27me2 and H3K27me3). Mutations in these genes seem to play a role in malignant transformation of neurofibromas (Carroll 2016).

The diagnosis of malignant peripheral nerve sheath tumor can be challenging due to morphological overlap with other histotypes as synovial sarcoma, myxofibrosarcoma, or undifferentiated spindle cell sarcoma. At least focally, the cells are arranged in sweeping fascicles, exhibit weavy nuclei typical of Schwann cells, and form palisades in about 10% of cases; other areas may be hypocellular with a myxoid stroma. Blood vessel show a hyalinized wall, which is an important diagnostic tool (Fig. 44.5b). Criteria of malignancy are necrosis and mitotic activity. Tumors with PRC2 loss, caused by mutations in SUZ12 or EED, show complete loss of positive staining for H3K27me3 in about 56% of NF1-associated malignant peripheral nerve sheath tumors and >90% of sporadic and radiotherapy-associated ones (Carroll 2016).

Morphologic variants of MPNST include epithelioid or glandular MPNST, respectively, characterized by aggregates of epithelioid cells in solid nests or foci of glandular differentiation with mucin-secreting cells; rhabdoid MPNST; *triton tumor* (a MPNST with a rhabdomyosarcomatous component); and MPNST with a perineurioma-like component, showing a prominent perineurial differentiation. Unfortunately, in sporadic MPNST, there are no histologic markers predictive of clinical behavior, and tumor grade does not appear to have a prognostic significance.

The largest published series of MPNST in children and adolescents is the one by the Italian and German cooperative groups, reporting on a series of 167 cases (17% having NF1), with a 5-year overall survival and progression-free survival of 51% and 37%, respectively. Outcome was satisfactory only for the small group of resected and small tumors. NF1 patients has a peculiar poor outcome. That series confirmed the aggressiveness of MPNST, for which complete surgical resection is the mainstay of successful treatment. MPNST is generally regarded as a tumor with poor chemoresponsiveness, but in that series, an overall response rate to primary chemotherapy of 45% was recorded (Carli et al. 2005).

A further interesting study regards relapsing patients, i.e., a series of 73 patients <21 years of age with relapsing MPNST (enrolled in Italian pediatric protocols from 1979 to 2004). The time to relapse ranged from 1 to 204 months after the first diagnosis (median 7 months), and the first relapse event was mainly local. That study confirmed the dismal prognosis of relapsing MPNST (only 9/73 patients were alive in remission at the time of the analysis, median overall survival after first relapse was 11 months, and survival rate was 15.8% at 5 years). The major variable influencing survival was the achievement of a secondary complete remission (which was related to the feasibility of radical surgery), suggesting an aggressive surgical approach as being the only effective salvage treatment (Bergamaschi et al. 2018).

44.3.6 Malignant Tumors of Uncertain Differentiation

44.3.6.1 Epithelioid Sarcoma

Epithelioid sarcoma is a distinctive lesion, generally involving the dermis or subcutaneous tissue, that may mimic clinically and morphologically a benign granulomatous process (Enzinger 1970). Peculiarly, it involves the finger, hand, wrist, and forearm of adolescents and young adults. The lower extremities, shoulder, and less frequently trunk, head, and neck can be also involved. Epithelioid sarcoma may also occur in mucosal sites including the tongue and in genital areas (Gross et al. 1996; Kodet et al. 1994). The tumors are slow-growing single or multiple ulcerating nodules of variable size. A particular tendency for lymph node involvement has been observed. The so-called “proximal-type” epithelioid sarcoma occurs in axial locations: it shares some morphological features with rhabdoid tumor, and a more aggressive clinical behavior has been reported (Guillou et al. 1997a, b).

Histologically, epithelioid sarcoma consists of nodular masses or large, eosinophilic polygonal cells imperceptibly merging with spindle cells. Cytologic atypia is minimal. Areas of central necrosis are frequent. Tumors may also show predominant spindle cells in a fibroma-like or dermatofibroma-like pattern or an angiomatoid angiosarcoma-like appearance with large epithelioid cells surrounding hemorrhagic spaces (Mirra et al. 1992; von Hochstetter et al. 1991) (Fig. 44.6a, b). Proximal-type epithelioid sarcoma shows prominent epithelioid cells with vesicular nuclei, prominent nucleoli, and eosinophilic cytoplasm.

Immunostains for low and high molecular weight keratin, epithelial membrane antigen, and vimentin are generally positive. More than 50% of tumors express CD34; CA 125 is also reported as positive. INI-1 loss of expression is reported in 76–93% of cases (Chbani et al. 2009; Hornick et al. 2009). The underlying genetic alteration of SMARCB1-INI is still incompletely explored. The genomic landscape of epithelioid sarcoma appears heterogeneous and distinct from rhabdoid tumors. The distinction between these two entities may be difficult, and immunostains are not helpful. It has been proposed that ERG 1 and SALL4 may be helpful being ERG 1 expressed mostly in ES and SALL 4 in rhabdoid tumors (Kohashi et al. 2015).

Little information is available on clinical management in children. An Italian study reported on 30 patients <18 years old (19 classic-type and 11 proximal-type), suggesting a clinical course less aggressive than that generally observed in adults. In that series, 5-year event-free survival and overall survival rates were 62% and 92%, but overall survival dropped to 87% and 72% at 10 and 15 years, respectively. Local relapse was the major cause of treatment failure. The most significant finding influencing survival was tumor site (extremity location predicting a favorable outcome). A worse outcome was associated with the proximal-type variant. A response to chemotherapy was seen in 3/7 patients with measurable disease. The tendency for lymph nodal spread described in adults would be not clearly confirmed in pediatric cases (Casanova et al. 2006).

A larger pediatric series has been recently published, merging together cases from the North American COG ARST0332 trial and from the EpSSG NRSTS 2005 protocol: 63 patients (median age 13.1 years) were treated with a risk-adapted therapy (based on tumor diameter, histologic grade, extent of surgery, and presence/absence of metastases) including surgery ± radiotherapy for all patients with the addition of ifosfamide/doxorubicin chemotherapy for intermediate-/high-risk patients. The main clinical features were as follows: 68% of cases arose from extremity, median tumor diameter was 3.5 cm, 56% had high histologic grade, and 14% showed nodal metastases and 14% distant metastases. Partial response to chemotherapy was observed in 11/22 patients receiving neoadjuvant therapy (50%). Estimated 5-year survival was 86.4% for patients with localized initially resected disease, 63.5% for those with locally advanced disease, and 0% for patients with metastatic tumors (Spunt et al. 2019).

44.3.6.2 Extrarenal Rhabdoid Tumor

Malignant rhabdoid tumor is a highly aggressive neoplasm, mostly occurring in the central nervous system and kidney of infants and young children. Less frequently, it may arise in the somatic soft tissues, abdomen, pelvis, retroperitoneum, liver, heart, and gastrointestinal tract. The histologic diagnosis is generally straightforward when the tumor shows the typical morphology characterized by large epithelioid cells, with abundant eosinophilic or amphophilic cytoplasm containing juxtanuclear hyaline-like globules, large nuclei with prominent nucleoli, and a polyphenotypic immunophenotype, with variable expression of vimentin, EMA, cytokeratins, CD99, S-100, and SMA. SMARCB1 gene biallelic inactivating mutations are present in more than 95% of rhabdoid tumors. SMARCB1 is a tumor suppressor gene located on the long arm of chromosome 22 (22q11.2). The deletion or mutation of hSNF5/SMARCB1/INI1 gene results in the loss or reduced expression of INI protein (Versteege et al. 1998; Weeks et al. 1989; Wick et al. 1995; Parham et al. 1994; Schofield et al. 1996). SMARCB1 is part of the SWI/SNF complex, composed of multiple proteins encoded by different genes. This complex acts epigenetically on the chromatin remodeling process regulating the transcription of multiple genes. Germline mutations of SMARCB1 or, rarely, SMARCA4 are found in 35% of patients affected by rhabdoid and are responsible of the rhabdoid predisposition syndrome types 1 and 2, respectively (Agaimy and Foulkes 2018).

Rhabdoid tumors are very rare and very aggressive disease. These tumors are currently treated with intensive chemotherapeutic strategy, but the outcome remains largely unsatisfactory. The difficulties to deliver optimal local therapy (since most patients are infants) remain a major problem (Kodet et al. 1991).

The EpSSG reported on 100 pediatric patients treated from 2005 to 2014 with a multimodal protocol including surgery, radiotherapy, and intensive multiagent chemotherapy over 30 weeks (using vincristine, doxorubicin, carboplatin, etoposide, and cyclophosphamide). In that series, 77 patients had localized disease and 23 metastatic disease at diagnosis. The protocol treatment was completed by 43 patients. Event-free survival at 3 years was 32.3% and overall survival 38.4%. Outcome was related to the presence of metastases and patient's age (age less than 1 year was associated with a higher risk of death) (Brennan et al. 2016). A more aggressive approach was thereafter proposed by the EpSSG, following the concept of dose density/dose compression (increasing treatment intensity by giving chemotherapy every two weeks instead of every three). The French group recently reported on 35 patients treated with the EpSSG strategy, showing overall good tolerance of such therapy and 2-year event-free survival and overall survival of 42.9% and 47.6%, respectively (Enault et al. 2022).

The dismal prognosis of rhabdoid tumors suggests developing the use of targeted therapies for future treatment strategies, also thanks to some improvements in genetic studies casting light on tumor biology. Various novel approaches may be potentially considered: (a) targeting the cell cycle control, i.e., cyclin D1 (since the crucial role of SMARCB1 in the G1-to-S transition (Alacon-Vargas et al. 2006)); (b) histone-deacetylase inhibitors (supported by the antagonist effects of PRC2 and SWI/SNF complexes on histone modifications (Watanabe et al. 2009; Fouladi et al. 2010; Muscat et al. 2016)); (c) tyrosine kinase inhibitors, e.g., aurora kinase inhibitors (Lee et al. 2011); (d) EZH2 inhibitors (tazemetostat), whose activity is related to the polycomb complex PRC2 (Wilson et al. 2010; Kia et al. 2008); and (e) DNA methylation inhibitors (e.g., azacitidine and decitabine), since various studies showed overall hypermethylated state of DNA in rhabdoid tumors (Johann et al. 2016).

44.3.6.3 Alveolar Soft Part Sarcoma

Alveolar soft part sarcoma (ASPS) represents less than 1% of soft tissue sarcomas and occurs more frequently in patients younger than 40 years, often in the extremities and trunk (Folpe and Deyrup 2006). In children, it may arise in the head and neck (Casanova et al. 2000).

ASPS is characterized by a peculiar organoid pattern showing nests of epithelioid polygonal cells with eosinophilic cytoplasms, vesicular nuclei, and prominent nucleoli. PAS-positive intracytoplasmic rhomboid crystals are virtually diagnostic of ASPS. Immunostains are not helpful for diagnosis. The ASPSCR1-TFE3 fusion gene, deriving from chromosomal rearrangement at17q25 and Xp11.2, is typical of ASPS and is associated with a positive nuclear immunostaining for TFE3 (van Echten et al. 1995; Ladanyi et al. 2001; Argani et al. 2003).

Although tumor growth is slow and asymptomatic, ASPS is highly malignant with early vascular invasion and metastatic dissemination, more frequently to the brain and lung. The elective treatment is a radical surgery that generally allows a prolonged survival (Orbach et al. 2013). The role of chemotherapy is unclear; this entity is generally considered scarcely chemosensitive (Bisogno et al. 2014a, b). The EpSSG NRSTS 2005 study enrolled 22 pediatric patients in more than 10 years. Most of them had localized disease (20 cases), resected upfront (19 cases), with small tumors excised with histologically free margins (12 cases). Of the four patients who received conventional chemotherapy (ifosfamide and doxorubicin), there were no responses. The

5-year event-free survival and overall survival of patients with localized disease were 94.7% and 100% (Brennan et al. 2018).

In patients with advanced disease and in those with metastases, however, the clinical course is often slow and indolent, but the final outcome often dismal. The indolent course of ASPS is also confirmed by the fact that metastases (to the lungs or brain) may become evident several years after the end of treatment (a very long follow-up is recommended).

Given the very poor chemosensitivity of ASPS, new effective agents are clearly needed. The ASPSCR1-TFE3 chimeric transcription factor induces the expression of numerous proteins that might represent therapeutic targets, including, among others, the Met, which is an angiogenetic factor, activating the downstream effectors AKT and MEK. Overexpression of VEGF mRNA has also been identified in gene expression profiling of ASPS samples and may be a promising therapeutic target (Lazar et al. 2009; Tsuda et al. 2007). Reports of responses to agents that target the tyrosine kinase receptors or blood vessel formation (first in adults and subsequently in children) have been published, and there are increasing evidence that biologic agents such as sunitinib, cediranib, pazopanib, tivantinib, or bevacizumab may prolong survival in ASPS (Li et al. 2016; Hilbert et al. 2012).

44.3.6.4 Clear Cell Sarcoma of Tendons and Aponeuroses

Clear cell sarcoma (CCS), also called melanoma of soft parts, has a proclivity to involve tendons and aponeuroses of distal extremities of young individuals (Enzinger 1965). It has a close resemblance to melanoma and is characterized by fascicles and nests of pale, elongated, or epithelioid cells encased by delicate fibrous septa. The cells show clear cytoplasm frequently containing melanin and nuclei with prominent nucleoli. S-100 is generally positive. The cytogenetic hallmark is t(12;22)(q13;q12), resulting in a chimeric EWS/ATF1 gene, detected in about 75% of cases; less frequently, a EWSR1-CREB1 transcript is found.

The tumor has a prolonged clinical course with multiple local recurrences, late metastases, and a high rate of tumor deaths. Radical surgery is the elective treatment. Chemotherapy is generally considered ineffective. A series of 28 pediatric patients has been reported by the Italian and German Soft Tissue Sarcoma Cooperative Group, with survival rates around 60% (Ferrari et al. 2002).

Gastrointestinal CCS-like tumor is a distinctive lesion morphologically resembling CCS, characterized by identical cytogenetic alterations and showing scattered osteoclast-like giant cells. Immunohistochemically, two groups are recognized: the **GI** *CCS-like tumor*, showing a melanocytic differentiation (S-100, HMB45, Melan-A) and related to CCS of soft parts, and the *malignant GI neuroectodermal tumor* non-expressing melanocytic markers but positive for S-100, SOX10, and vimentin (100%), CD56 (70%), synaptophysin (56%), NSE (45%), and neurofilaments (14%). The tumors reported in children are mostly of neuroectodermal type. Clinically, they are accompanied by prominent weight loss, anorexia, abdominal pain, bloody stools, and anemia and have a very aggressive course. A prior history of acute lymphoblastic leukemia has been reported in one case (Stockman et al. 2012).

44.3.7 The PEComa Family Tumors

Perivascular epithelioid cell tumors (PEComa) are a family of tumors sharing a common origin from a cell with an hybrid melanocytic and muscular phenotype, lacking a normal counterpart. The PEComa family includes *angiomyolipomas*, *lymphangioleiomyomatosis*, *clear cell "sugar" tumor of the lung*, *clear cell myomelanocytic tumor of the falciform ligament/ligamentum teres*, and *abdomino-pelvic sarcoma of perivascular epithelioid cells (PEC)*. These different morphologic entities show variation in their clinicopathologic features (Zamboni et al. 1996; Hornick and Fletcher 2006; Martignoni et al. 2007, 2008; Folpe et al. 2000a, b; Bonetti et al. 1992).

Angiomyolipomas may occur in the context of tuberous sclerosis complex (TSC) and arise in kidney, less frequently in the liver (Goodman and Ishak 1984) or other sites (Hulbert and Graf

1983; Castillenti and Bertin 1989). Classic angiomyolipomas are characterized by a variable combination of blood vessels with a hyalinized wall, smooth muscle, and mature adipose tissue, whereas epithelioid angiomyolipomas display nests and sheets of large epithelioid cells (Mai et al. 1996; Martignoni et al. 1998).

Lymphangioleiomyomatosis in children is exceptional (Nagy et al. 1998) and may occur in the context of TSC. It is characterized by multiple pulmonary nodules, composed of elongated cells surrounding small blood vessel, interstitial myoid cells, and ectatic lymphatics. The lymph nodes, retroperitoneum, and mediastinum may be also involved (Matsui et al. 2000; Torres et al. 1995). The nodules may evolve into cystic lesions with destruction of the lung and pneumothorax and pulmonary failure requiring lung transplant.

Only few *clear cell "sugar" tumors of the lung* have been reported in children with identical clinical features as in adults. They generally occur as single benign nodules, histologically composed of sheets or nests of large epithelioid cells with clear cytoplasm and a prominent vascular network (Vijayabhaskar et al. 2010; Gora-Gebka et al. 2006). Extra-pulmonary sugar tumors have been also reported in children in breast, bone, urethra. They differ from their pulmonary counterpart for the more frequent nuclear atypia, mitoses, and necrosis.

Clear cell myomelanocytic tumor (CCMMT) is a variant of PEComa with a predilection for ligaments (ligamentum teres and falciform ligament) and extremities, characterized by fascicles of spindle cells with clear to eosinophilic cytoplasms (Folpe et al. 2000a, b).

Abdominopelvic sarcoma of PEC is the malignant variant of PEComa, composed of sheets of epithelioid cells, with pleomorphism, necrosis, and vascular invasion (Bonetti et al. 2001). Immunohistochemistry plays a key role in the diagnostic work-up, disclosing the typical hybrid melanocytic (HMB45, Melan-A, tyrosinase, MiT family of transcription factors members, microphthalmia transcription factor (MiTF), and TFE3) and muscular (smooth muscle actin, muscle-specific actin, sometimes calponin or h-caldesmon, and less frequently desmin) phenotype of cells (Pea et al. 1991).

Sporadic or TSC-associated angiomyolipomas and other PEComas share common cytogenetic alterations. TSC is caused by malfunction of the TSC1/TSC2 complex, related to a somatic deletion in TSC1 gene (on chromosome 9q34) or inactivating mutations in TSC1 or TSC2 (on 16p13). In sporadic AML and PEComas, loss of heterozygosity of TSC2 gene is common (Pan et al. 2006, 2008). These genetic alterations activate the mTOR pathway promoting cell growth (Kenerson et al. 2007; Wagner et al. 2010; Weinreb et al. 2007). Other genetic alterations include deletion of 1p, deletions on cr 19, and chromosomal gain on 12q, 2q, 3q, and 5 (Pan et al. 2006). Only a minority of PEComas carry a TFE3 gene fusion, and some of them have been reported in association with neuroblastoma (Argani et al. 2010; Cho et al. 2008; Tanaka et al. 2009).

The prognosis of PEComa is influenced by the histotypes. Classic angiomyolipomas are generally benign. Epithelioid angiomyolipomas of the kidney metastasize in one third of cases. The presence of at least three unfavorable prognostic features (atypical epithelioid cells representing at least 70% of the population, 2 or more mitotic figures/10 HPF, atypical mitoses or necrosis) appears to be predictive of a malignant behavior. Hepatic epithelioid angiomyolipomas are generally benign. CCMMT showing a main diameter larger than 5 cm, infiltrative growth, hypercellularity, nuclear enlargement and hyperchromasia, high mitotic rate, atypical mitoses, and coagulative necrosis may have a more aggressive clinical behavior. PEComas are treated by complete surgical excision. Radiotherapy and chemotherapy are not effective. The use the mTOR inhibitors, such as sirolimus, may be an option in unresectable tumors (Subbiah et al. 2010; Curatolo et al. 2016; Raimondi et al. 2018).

44.3.7.1 Desmoplastic Small Round Cell Tumor

Desmoplastic small round cell tumor (DSRCT) is a rare neoplasm mainly affecting children and young adults with a male preponderance. Its classical histological appearance, represented by solid sheets, nests, or cords of small cells in a desmoplastic stroma, can show many different morphological variations. Its specific immunohistochemical profile with divergent epithelial, muscular, and neural differentiation and the recurrent translocation t (11;22)(p13;q12), which gives rise to the fusion gene EWS-WT1, represent important diagnostic tools, especially when the typical clinicopathologic features are lacking.

DSRCT occurs in the abdominal and pelvic cavity or in other sites in association with serosal surfaces such as paratesticular region and pleura. Rare examples of extra-serosal DSRCT involving the parotid gland, posterior cranial fossa, bone and soft tissue, pancreas, and kidney have been also reported. In particular when arising in abdominal cavity, the tumor is often disseminated at onset (with classic multiple peritoneal lesions) and is characterized by a dismal outcome, despite the various intensive multimodality treatment approaches (including aggressive surgery, intensive chemotherapy including also high-dose chemotherapy with autologous peripheral stem cell rescue, and whole abdomino-pelvic radiotherapy radiotherapy) attempted over the years (Ferrari et al. 2021; Kushner et al. 1996; Bisogno et al. 2010).

Hyperthermic peritoneal perfusion with cisplatin chemotherapy (HIPEC) is considered a potentially effective approach for loco-regional disease. Patients require aggressive and complete cytoreduction before HIPEC to optimize outcome. Very promising results have been reported by specific dedicated centers (Hayes-Jordan et al. 2014), though in other cases the results were less satisfactory (Honoré et al. 2017).

Various targeted therapies with monoclonal antibodies and multikinase inhibitors are under investigation, in the view of the EWS-WT1 fusion transcript upregulation of PDGFA and IGF-R1: activities were reported for imatinib, sunitinib, pazopanib, and ganitumab, but also trials with negative results have been published (Bond et al. 2008; De Sanctis et al. 2017; Italiano et al. 2013; Frezza et al. 2014; Tap et al. 2012).

44.3.7.2 Synovial Sarcoma

Synovial sarcoma is a tumor of uncertain histogenesis, accounting for 6–10% of adult soft tissue sarcomas and predominantly affecting children older than 10 years, adolescents, and young adults. It is the most frequent pediatric NRSTS (Sultan et al. 2009).

Histologically, this tumor is variously composed of spindle and epithelioid cells. Spindle cells are small, uniform, and ovoid with pale nuclei, sparse cytoplasm, and inconspicuous cell borders. Epithelioid cells exhibit the same nuclei and a more abundant cytoplasm (Fig. 44.5a). According to the different components, three major subtypes are recognized: the monophasic fibrous synovial sarcoma, composed of spindle cells with no evidence of epithelial component (the epithelial monophasic type is very rare and mimics an adenocarcinoma); the biphasic synovial sarcoma, containing spindle and epithelioid cells in variable proportions; and the poorly differentiated synovial sarcoma, a highly cellular sarcoma resembling a small round cell tumor, whose diagnosis may be challenging. Synovial sarcoma expresses cytokeratins, in particular cytokeratins 7 and 19, epithelial membrane antigen, vimentin, CD99, and bcl2. Cytogenetic studies show chromosomal translocation t(X;18)(p11.2;q11.2). The SS18 (or SYT) gene from chromosome 18 is disrupted and juxtaposed to either SSX1, SSX2, or SSX4 on chromosome X, in a mutually exclusive manner. SYT-SSX1 may be associated with a biphasic histology and higher ki67 index. SYT-SSX2 is more frequently found in monophasic fibrous type (Mancuso et al. 2000; Mezzelani et al. 2001). Some studies suggest a better prognosis for tumors bearing the SYT-SSX1 transcript, but the prognostic significance of molecular findings is controversial (Guillou et al. 2004). The proteic product of SMARCB1/INI1 gene, lost in malignant rhabdoid tumor, is reduced in the majority of synovial sarcoma with a consequent reduced immunohistochemical staining for INI. The specific molecular mechanism is not known, and a post-transcriptional interaction of SS18-SSX transcript with the chromatin remodeling pathway has been suggested. Moreover, gene expression studies are providing

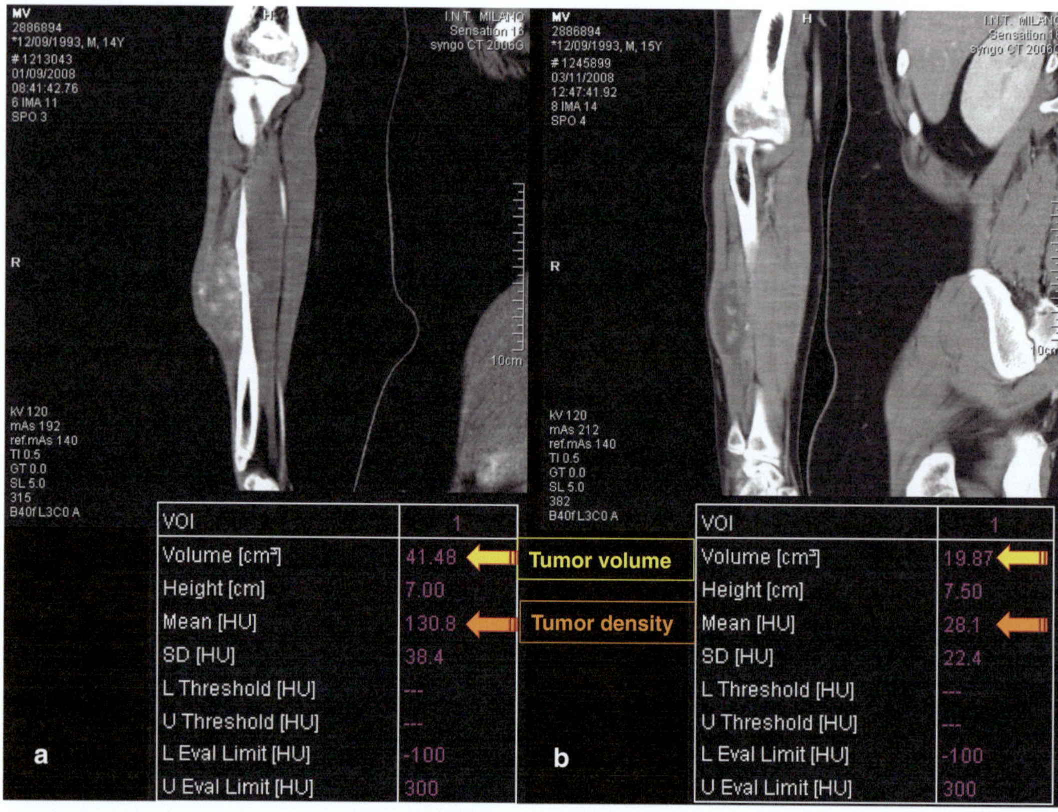

Fig. 44.7 Computed tomography scan of synovial sarcoma of the right forearm: (**a**) At onset, before chemotherapy; (**b**) after three courses of chemotherapy with ifosfamide and doxorubicin. Response to chemotherapy is shown by volume reduction as well as changes in tumor tissue characteristics (reduction of tumor density). (Courtesy of Dr. Carlo Morosi, Radiology Department, Fondazione IRCCS Istituto Nazionale Tumori, Milano, Italy)

new insights into the molecular pathways involved in tumor progression in synovial sarcoma, including Wnt, IGF, ERBB2, HGF/MET, and beta-catenin pathways, disclosing new therapeutic perspectives (Tamborini et al. 2004; Kawaguchi et al. 2005; Thomas et al. 2005).

Synovial sarcoma is the typical sarcoma subtype crosswise between the pediatric and the adult age groups (Sultan et al. 2009). However, since up to recent times, different therapeutic strategies have been developed for pediatric and adult oncology protocols dealing with this tumor, in particular concerning the use of systemic therapy (van der Graaf et al. 2017; Ferrari et al. 2018a, b). Historically, relatively high rates of response to chemotherapy were recorded in pediatric series (i.e., an approximately 60% rate, which is higher than the response rate usually reported for other adult soft tissue sarcomas, but lower than that observed in rhabdomyosarcoma) (Fig. 44.7), and therefore synovial sarcoma was traditionally considered as a "rhabdomyosarcoma-like" tumor by pediatric oncologists, particularly in Europe: children were enrolled over the years in rhabdomyosarcoma protocols, thus receiving the same chemotherapy as for rhabdomyosarcoma patients, even in the case of completely resected small tumors (Ferrari et al. 2008; Okcu et al. 2003; Brennan et al. 2010; Orbach et al. 2011; Stegmaier et al. 2017).

Differently, adult patients with synovial sarcoma were treated according to the same guidelines adopted for other soft tissue sarcomas; for

Table 44.5 Main published series on pediatric synovial sarcoma

Pediatric synovial sarcoma series	
Okcu et al. (2003) Multicenter study MDACC, SJCRH, INT Milan, CWS	219 pts <20 years 5-year OS 80% Rate of response to chemotherapy—60%
Brecht et al. (2006) CWS, AIEOP-STSC	150 pts <18 years, IRS groups I–II (initial gross resection) Nearly all patients received chemotherapy 5-year OS 89% Identification of low-risk patients (group I, ≤5 cm) for which chemotherapy might be omitted
Ferrari et al. (2009) AIEOP-STSC	115 patients <20 years 5-year OS 76.9% Worse outcome for non-extremity sites vs. limbs (OS 55.1% vs. 84.0%)
Brennan et al. (2010) UK CCLG	77 patients <18 years 5-year EFS and OS 72% and 76% Prognostic factors: T stage and IRS group
Orbach et al. (2011) SIOP-MMT	88 patients <18 years 5-year EFS 68%, OS 85% Only 32% of survivors received RT
Ferrari et al. (2015a, b) EpSSG	138 patients <21 5-year EFS 80.7%, OS 90.7% EFS particularly better for high-risk categories 76.5% (versus 41.4%) in tumors >5 cm, 77.3% (versus 44.2%) in unresected disease, 73.8% (versus 43.3%) in axial tumors Response rate to chemotherapy 55.2%
Stegmaier et al. (2017) CWS	84 patients with localized disease No prognostic significance was shown for SYT-SSX fusion status and for histological grade
Ferrari et al. (2017a, b, c) EpSSG—COG	60 low-risk patients (small tumors completely resected at diagnosis) treated with surgery alone: EFS 90% (8 local recurrences, no metastatic recurrence), OS 100% Feasibility of a "surgery-alone" strategy in low-risk cases
Comparison pediatric vs. adult series	
Ferrari et al. (2004) INT Milan	271 patients of all ages (46 <17 years) 5-year OS 64% Role of adjuvant chemotherapy Age <17 years: 78% received chemotherapy—5-year EFS 66% Age ≥17 years: <20% received adjuvant CT—5-year EFS ~35%
Sultan et al. (2009) SEER (1983–2005)	Epidemiological study 1268 cases (213 ≤18 years) No major differences in stage distribution 5-year cancer-specific survival: 83% vs. 62% ($p < 0.001$) Multivariate analysis: significantly higher mortality for adults after adjusting for other variables
Italiano et al. (2009) French Sarcoma Group	237 patients Worse outcome for patients >35 years
Vlenterie et al. (2015) Netherlands Cancer Registry	Epidemiological study 613 patients 5-year OS: 89% in patients <18 years, 73% in 18–34 years, 55% in 35–65 years, 43% in ≥65 years

(continued)

OS overall survival, *EFS* event-free survival, *IRS* Intergroup Rhabdomyosarcoma Study, *MDACC* M.D. Anderson Cancer Center, *SJCRH* St. Jude Children Research Hospital, *INT* Istituto Nazionale Tumori Milan, *CWS* Cooperative Weichteilsarkomen Studie (German Soft Tissue Sarcoma Cooperative Group), *AIEOP-STSC* Associazione Italiana Ematologia Oncologia Pediatrica-Soft Tissue Sarcoma Committee (Italian Cooperative Group), *UK CCLG* United Kingdom Children's Cancer and Leukaemia Group, *SIOP-MMT* International Society of Pediatric Oncology-Malignant Mesenchymal Tumors Working Group, *EpSSG* European Paediatric Soft Tissue Sarcoma Study Group, *COG* Children's Oncology Group, *SEER* Surveillance, Epidemiology, and End Results

instance, adjuvant chemotherapy was generally only used for those patients enrolled in randomized trials with a no-therapy control arm. Whether these different strategies produced differences in patient survival remains to be demonstrated: however, pediatric reported series showed 5-year survival rates of around 80%, which is higher than is usually reported in adult series (Lewis et al. 2000; Trassard et al. 2001). Some studies directly compared clinical outcome of children and adults (Sultan et al. 2009; Ferrari et al. 2004; Italiano et al. 2009; Vlenterie et al. 2015) (Table 44.5). A study on the large cohort of synovial sarcoma cases registered in the SEER database (1983–2005) highlighted that the cancer-specific mortality was higher in adults than in children (34% vs, 16%, respectively) and the outcome remained consistently worse for adults when the analysis was adjusted for the different prognostic variables (i.e., tumor size, site, and stage), suggesting that factors other than the possible difference in the incidence of unfavorable clinical variables might be involved in the unsatisfactory outcome for adult cases (Sultan et al. 2009). The hypothesis that the different treatment results might be related, at least in part, to the different treatment strategies adopted (i.e., the different use of chemotherapy) would be supported by the retrospective study of the Istituto Nazionale dei Tumori in Milan (on patients of all ages), in which adjuvant chemotherapy (administered to most of the children and to a minority of the older patients) seemed to improve patient outcome (Ferrari et al. 2004).

In recent years, the management of synovial sarcoma patients seems to be changing to some degree in both pediatric and adult cases, tending to converge toward a common strategy (Ferrari 2009; Ferrari et al. 2015a, b). Pediatric oncologists have taken suggestions from adult experiences and moved toward a treatment concept partially similar to that adopted in the adult setting: the ifosfamide-doxorubicin chemotherapy is currently adopted as standard regimen, and its indication is given according to the patient's risk stratification, based on tumor size and site and surgical stage; in low-risk patients (completely resected tumors under 5 cm in size), chemotherapy is omitted (Brecht et al. 2006) (Fig. 44.2). On the other hand, adult oncologists seem to be recognizing that synovial sarcoma may be quite different from other adult soft tissue sarcomas, particularly in the light of its higher chemosensitivity, probably standing midway between that of the most typical adult histotypes and that of pediatric small round cell tumors, such as rhabdomyosarcoma. Despite in the absence of a published proof of its efficacy, in day-to-day clinical practice, many adult oncologists generally recommend chemotherapy for synovial sarcoma patients, not only in cases of advance disease but also as an adjuvant treatment after surgery (Canter et al. 2008; Eilber et al. 2007).

The first results of this new pediatric oncology approach have been reported by the EpSSG. Between 2005 and 2012, 138 synovial sarcoma patients <21 years were prospectively registered and treated according to the risk-adapted program (Ferrari et al. 2015a, b). The study, first of all, demonstrated the feasibility of large prospective cooperation dedicated to rare tumors on a European scale (the EpSSG includes 15 different countries, with 131 centers). As main results, that study showed higher survival rates than those previously published by pediatric groups: 5-year event-free survival and overall survival were 80.7% and 90.7%, respectively. The survival rates were particularly better for those categories considered at higher risk, e.g., 5-year event-free survival was 76.5% (versus 41.4%) (Ferrari et al. 2008) in patients with tumors >5 cm, 77.3% (versus 44.2%) in patients with unresected disease, and 73.8% (versus 43.3%) in patients with axial tumors (Ferrari et al. 2015a, b). Overall response rate to chemotherapy was 55.2% (22.4% major remission plus 32.8% minor remission), with a 97% of "no progression." The feasibility of a "surgery-alone" strategy in low-risk cases (small tumors completely resected at diagnosis) was a major issue of that trial and was further confirmed by a subsequent joint pediatric European-North American study that pooled data from the two prospective clinical trials, the EpSSG NRSTS 2005 and the COG ARST0332: among 60 patients treated with surgery alone, only 8 recurrences were seen, and all were local, with no metastatic recurrence; all patients with recurrence were effectively salvaged, resulting in 100% overall survival (Ferrari et al. 2017a, b, c). This demonstration was of great importance since avoiding the use of adjuvant chemotherapy and radiotherapy in this low-risk patient population may decrease both short- and long-term morbidity and mortality.

In the EpSSG synovial sarcoma publication, the authors themselves emphasized the need to create larger international cooperation, in particular with adult sarcoma groups. Broader international collaborations may also be essential for promoting age-related molecular profiling studies in synovial sarcoma. In fact, recent studies have suggested that differences in genomic instability between adult and pediatric synovial sarcoma might offer a biological explanation for the reported differences in outcome. Complexity index in sarcoma ("CINSARC") is a 67-gene signature related to chromosome integrity and genomic complexity that has shown high prognostic value in adult sarcoma (and in synovial sarcoma, in particular). This biologic signature may be potentially used to better identify patients more appropriate to receive systemic therapy. While no specific gene patterns were found to discriminate between pediatric and adult tumors, chromosomal instability was reported as frequent in adult synovial sarcoma and rare in pediatric cases (Lagarde et al. 2013; Chakiba et al. 2014).

The EpSSG biologic study called SYNOBIO aimed to assess genomic index (GI)—using array comparative genomic hybridization (aCGH)—in pediatric patients with synovial sarcoma. The study included 61 patients from the EpSSG NRSTS 2005 protocol: 5-year event-free survival was 93.8% in cases with GI-1 (flat profile, no copy number alterations) versus 64.9% in those with GI-2 (rearranged profile, one or more copy number alterations) ($P < 0.006$). GI status remained an independent prognostic for EFS also in multivariate analysis, suggesting it could be a good tool to predict the metastatic behavior of pediatric synovial sarcoma (Orbach et al. 2018).

While the overall prognosis is generally quite satisfactory in children and adolescents with localized synovial sarcoma, the outcome remains poor for patients with metastatic disease at diagnosis and for those who relapse. A study from the German Cooperative Group Cooperative Weichteilsarkomen Studie (CWS) on 27 pediatric patients with initial metastases reported 5-year event-free survival and overall survival rates of 26% and 30%, respectively (Scheer et al. 2016). An Italian pediatric study on 44 relapsing synovial sarcoma showed a 21% overall survival at 10 years, with the variables influencing survival being the timing and type of relapse and the chances of a secondary remission, which correlated strongly with the feasibility of complete surgery (Ferrari et al. 2012). Based on these variables, it is possible to estimate the chances of survival and develop a sort of risk-adapted stratification to identify those patients who should be treated with standard therapy, those who need aggressive surgery, and those—unfortunately the majority—whose outcome is so poor to suggest the use of experimental therapies.

The intrinsic biological characteristics of synovial sarcoma (chromosomal translocations and fusion proteins) and the receptors overexpressed by cancer cells (EGFR, HER-2/neu, Bcl-2, NY-ESO-1) make it a potential target of novel therapies. Among tyrosine kinase inhibitors, pazopanib (Casanova et al. 2017), regorafenib, and anlotinib have been variously investigated in synovial sarcoma (Baldi et al. 2019). Innovative approaches are targeting NY-ESO-1, a hydrophobic cancer-testis antigen expressed in approximately 80% of synovial sarcoma (Lai et al. 2012). Promising results were reported with genetically modified T cells transduced with NY-ESO-1 T-cell receptor (Robbins et al. 2011, 2015). Another approach involved a lentiviral vector (LV305) targeting dendritic cells to prime NY-ESO-1-specific T cells: the CMB305 therapeutic vaccine induces NY-ESO-1-specific T-cell responses in synovial sarcoma (Pollack et al. 2017; D'Angelo et al. 2018). Various early-phase trials testing potentially effective new agents in synovial sarcoma are ongoing, but mainly of them involve adult patients.

44.3.7.3 Myoepithelial Tumors

Myoepithelial tumors of soft tissues are rare neoplasms, occurring in all ages, with more than 20% arising in children, mostly in the extremities and trunk. The morphologic features and histologic criteria of malignancy differ from their salivary gland counterpart. About 65% of pediatric myoepithelial tumors are malignant. Myoepithelial tumors are multinodular, lobulated lesions showing a wide morphologic and immunophenotypic spectrum. More than 90% of myoepithelial neoplasms show sheets or nests of epithelioid cells reminiscent of epithelioid sarcoma. Tumors with a predominant small round cells may mimic an extraskeletal myxoid chondrosarcoma. A spindle to ovoid cell component may be variously combined. A myxoid or fibrous-hyaline background is present. Immunostains for muscular and epithelial markers show a variable positivity, although a positive staining for at least one epithelial marker and GFAP or S-100 are required for the diagnosis of myoepithelial carcinoma. Cytologic atypia is associated with a malignant behavior. High mitotic rate and necrosis are frequent in myoepithelial carcinomas, but are not predictive of malignancy in the absence of atypia (Hornick and Fletcher 2003; Gleason and Fletcher 2007).

Myoepithelial neoplasms show EWSR1 rearrangements with POU5F1, PBX1, and ZNF444 in or an INI-1 deletion in a subset of benign and malignant myoepithelial tumors of the skin, soft tissue, bone, and viscera and a pleomorphic adenoma gene 1 (PLAG1) rearrangement in benign mixed tumors of the skin and soft tissues (Antonescu et al. 2010; Fletcher 2014; Jo and Fletcher 2015; Agaram et al. 2015).

Myoepithelial carcinomas are highly aggressive in children, with local recurrence reported in 39%, metastases (lungs, lymph node, bone, soft tissue, liver, brain, skin) in 52%, and death in 43% (Gleason and Fletcher 2007). In principle, the recommended treatment is the same of other highly malignant sarcomas. The chemotherapy of choice is usually the ifosfamide-doxorubicin combination, though anecdotal experiences might suggest to add also cisplatin and etoposide (Bisogno et al. 2014a, b).

44.3.8 Unclassifiable Sarcomas

The 2013 WHO classification for soft tissue tumors has recognized for the first time the category of unclassifiable sarcomas, encompassing those soft tissue sarcomas "showing no identifiable line of differentiation when analyzed by presently available technology," and divides them into round cell, spindle cell, pleomorphic cell, epithelioid cell, or not otherwise specified according to the cytologic features.

The progressive identification of homogeneous morphologic and immunophenotypic groups sharing common recurrent genetic alterations has contributed to redefine the landscape of undifferentiated tumors and shed new light on potential therapeutic targets.

Round cell undifferentiated sarcomas represent the largest group of unclassifiable sarcomas in children. Their least common denominator is represented by a morphology resembling Ewing's sarcomas. Since the publication of WHO classification in 2013, new entities were identified and isolated.

44.3.8.1 CIC-DUX4 Sarcomas

CIC-DUX4 sarcomas were identified in 2009 by Kawamura and Saito and regarded as Ewing's family tumors. The CIC-DUX4 fusion results from a t(4;19)(q35;q13) or a t(10;19)(q26;q13) translocation (Yoshimoto et al. 2009; Italiano et al. 2012; Graham et al. 2012). Although CIC-DUX4 sarcomas overexpress the PEA3 (polyomavirus enhancer activator 3) subfamily of transcription factors, they are now considered an entity distinct from Ewing's sarcoma (Kawamura-Saito et al. 2006). These tumors are more frequent in adults, with less than 22% arising in children. More than 85% of CIC-DUX4 occur in the somatic soft tissues, mostly the extremities and trunk, followed by visceral location and rarely bone (Antonescu et al. 2017). Histologically, these sarcomas show a mixture of round, spindle, and epithelioid cells in the context of a variable amount of myxoid stroma. The nuclei are larger than those in Ewing's sarcoma and more variable in shape and show vesicular chromatin and isolated prominent nucleoli. The cytoplasm is mildly eosinophilic. Immunophenotypically, CIC-rearranged tumors in contrast with Ewing's sarcomas are only focally CD99 positive, with a diffuse staining in less than 25%, and diffusely WT1 positive (Antonescu et al. 2017). CIC-rearranged sarcomas have a more aggressive clinical course compared to Ewing's sarcoma, with a 5-year OS of 49% for localized disease at diagnosis (Antonescu et al. 2017).

44.3.9 BCOR Family of Undifferentiated Sarcomas

BCOR family of undifferentiated sarcomas are characterized by genetic abnormalities involving BCOR. BCOR is a transcriptional corepressor gene, with key role in the regulation of development, hematopoiesis, and mesenchymal stem cell differentiation. Somatic BCOR mutations are found in a subset of acute myeloid leukemia, while germline mutations cause the oculo-facio-cardio-dental syndrome.

Soft tissue sarcomas in children may show internal tandem duplications (ITD) of BCOR or rearrangements such as BCOR-CCNB3 or other less frequent rearrangements. All these alterations involve the last exon of BCOR, which encodes the domain for the anchoring of C-terminal BCOR to PCGF, causing an alteration of binding affinity between BCOR and PCGF1 with modification of downstream gene regulation. BCOR gene upregulation gives a protein overexpression. Thus, immunostaining for BCOR is a reliable diagnostic tool for these tumors.

BCOR-CCNB3 sarcomas are characterized by a paracentric inversion of the X chromosome, resulting in the BCOR-CCNB3 fusion gene (Pierron et al. 2012). Histologically, BCOR-CCNB3 sarcomas are highly cellular with small-to medium-sized cells showing a more irregular appearance compared to Ewing's sarcoma. The nuclei are vesicular with finely dispersed chromatin and lack prominent nucleoli. A subtle arciform vasculature resembling that of clear cell sarcoma of the kidney is characteristic. A subset of tumors may have a prominent spindle morphology, or spindle cells may be intermingled with round cells; immunostains for BCOR or CCNB3 can be useful. These tumors are cyclin D1 positive, and 90% may express SATB2, a marker of osteosarcoma. SATB2 overexpression is related to the upregulation of the gene by the chromosomal rearrangement involving BCOR (Kao et al. 2018a, b). Alternative BCOR fusions have been reported, mostly in adults. A BCOR-MAML3 in the ilium in a 7-year-old boy (successfully treated with chemotherapy and radiotherapy) has been reported (Specht et al. 2016). These tumors show a histologic and immunohistochemical overlap with BCOR-CCNB3.

BCOR-CCNB3 sarcomas are biologically and genetically distinct from Ewing's sarcoma. They have a predilection for young males and involve more frequently bone in axial and extra-axial locations. However, visceral tumors (e.g., kidney) have been reported (Argani et al. 2017).

A study from the Société Française des Cancers de L'Enfant reported on 26 patients (age 6–25 years, median 13) with Ewing-like sarcoma harboring BCOR-CCNB3 gene fusion transcript (retrospective multicenter study on tumor samples collected between 1994 and 2012). Most patients (24/26) had localized tumors. All tumors but five were localized to the bone. Most patients received chemotherapy (15 according to protocols designed for Ewing tumors), before and/or after local treatment. Overall survival and disease-free survival at 5 years were, respectively, 76.5% and 67.9%. Induction chemotherapy and treatment according to an Ewing protocol might influence survival for patients with localized tumors (Cohen-Gogo et al. 2014).

BCOR-internal tandem duplications (ITD) sarcomas are a specific subgroup. In fact, a subset of sarcomas occurring in children in the first year of life is represented by unclassifiable sarcomas with a very primitive morphology. Recent studies have demonstrated in more than 50% of these sarcomas a recurrent BCOR exon 15 ITD or, in very rare cases, YWHAE-NUTM2B fusions. These genetic alterations are mutually exclusive and are the same found also in clear cell sarcoma of the kidney. Histologically, infantile undifferentiated sarcomas show round to ovoid cells in nests and sheets with a delicate arborizing vascular network. Cytologic details and vascular pattern have a striking resemblance to the ones found in CCSK and in BCOR-CCNB3 sarcomas, thus confirming the biologic relationship among these entities (Kao et al. 2016).

A strictly related group of tumors is represented by the so-called *primitive myxoid mesenchymal tumor of infancy* (PMMTI), an entity recognized in 2006, and histologically characterized by a prominent myxoid background with cystic areas and variable cellularity with characteristics similar to those of undifferentiated sarcomas. Fascicles of spindle cells with elongated eosinophilic cytoplasms, arranged in fascicles, may be also seen (Santiago et al. 2017). A subset of PMMTI were previously included in the category of infantile fibrosarcomas and translocation negative (Alaggio et al. 2006). PMMTI is a rare entity: about 20 cases have been reported so far, 15 with molecular characterization and all but 1 with BCOR ITD (Saeed et al. 2019).

These tumors have a predilection for males. The most frequent sites are paraspinal region and soft tissue of the trunk, less frequently retroperitoneum/pelvis and head and neck, and rarely extremities. Further studies are needed to define prognosis and the best therapeutic approach in BCOR ITD sarcomas. However, preliminary studies suggest that BCOR ITD are aggressive tumors with a poor prognosis in most of patients (Cramer et al. 2017; Foster et al. 2016).

44.3.9.1 Pleomorphic Malignant Fibrous Histiocytoma/Undifferentiated High-Grade Pleomorphic Sarcoma

Undifferentiated high-grade pleomorphic sarcoma (UHGPS), in the past called *malignant fibrous histiocytoma* (MFH), is a controversial entity characterized by pleomorphic spindle cells with fibroblastic and histiocytic differentiation. Its existence has been challenged, being the morphologic features common to a variety of poorly differentiated sarcomas (Fletcher 1992).

The diagnosis of MFH in childhood is a diagnosis of exclusion; in pre-immunohistochemistry era, it comprised about 2–6% of all pediatric sarcomas, including angiomatoid fibrous histiocytoma (now classified separately as an intermediate soft tissue neoplasm of uncertain histogenesis) (Cole et al. 1993; Corpron et al. 1996). Like their adult counterpart, pediatric high-grade pleomorphic sarcomas can arise in sites previously irradiated or as second malignancies (especially after retinoblastoma) and may be associated with a family history of cancer. Histologically, pleomorphic lesions are composed of spindle cells arranged in fascicles or sheets, displaying a focal storiform pattern and scattered pleomorphic cells with hyperchromatic nuclei and atypical mitoses or multinucleated cells. Large aggregates of polygonal/epithelioid cells may be found in more aggressive tumors. Immunostains are helpful to exclude other diagnoses, being the tumors negative for lineage-specific markers, although some may be SMA positive.

UHGPS are highly aggressive tumors with a high metastatic rate and an overall 5-year survival around 60–70%. Survival and metastases are related to tumor depth and size (Alaggio et al. 2010a, b).

44.3.9.2 Extraosseous Chondrosarcoma

Chondrosarcoma is a tumor of the bone and of adulthood and old age. *Mesenchymal chondrosarcoma* (MCS), however, should be seen as a different entity. In comparison to the most frequent classic chondrosarcoma, MCS typically occurs in young adults; it is aggressive and highly malignant (it should be always regarded as a high-grade sarcoma) and has a high proportion of extraskeletal tumors (about half of MCS occur in soft tissues, whereas extraosseous classic chondrosarcoma accounts for <1% of all cases).

MCS is characterized by a biphasic histologic pattern of small undifferentiated round cells intermixed with islands of well-differentiated cartilaginous matrix. It shows a recurrent *HEY-NCOA2* fusion and shows a biphasic appearance with a small round cell component resembling Ewing's sarcoma and chondro-osseous areas.

In the SEER database (1973–2006), only 24 children with MCS are recorded (and 142 adults). Tumor locations are the bone and joints (n = 9), soft tissue (n = 7), nose/nasal cavity (n = 2), eye/orbit (3), cranial nerves (1), lung (1), and kidney (1).

A German retrospective study reported on 15 cases aged 0–25 years, 4 osseous and 11 extraosseous. Tumor sites were the head/neck (6 cases), paravertebral (3), pelvis (3), limbs (2), and kidney (1). Actuarial 10-year event-free and overall survival rates were 53% and 67%, respectively

(Dantonello et al. 2008). Patients with MCS should be probably treated with multimodal regimens, following Ewing's sarcoma protocols.

44.3.10 Other Recently Identified Entities

44.3.10.1 Epithelioid-Spindle Cell Tissue Tumors with GLI1 Rearrangements or Amplifications

GLI1-rearranged or GLI1-amplified tumors represent a clinically and morphologically group of mesenchymal tumors. A group of malignant neoplasms with round to epithelioid morphology and S100 protein immunoreactivity with GLI1 rearrangements has been recently reported: four cases with a GLI1-ACTB fusion and one case with GLI-PTCH1 gene, all occurring in adults. A single pediatric case with GLI1-MALAT1 rearrangement arising in cervical region has been identified. MALAT1 (metastasis-associated lung adenocarcinoma transcript 1) is involved in GLI1 overexpression. Microscopically, all the tumors were composed of nests or cords of epithelioid cells separated by septa, with a thin capillary network. S100 is inconstantly positive, with SOX10, SMA, and EMA negative. Lymph nodes or distant metastases developed in three patients. GLI1 activation with PTCH1 overexpression represents a potential therapeutic target for sonic hedgehog pathway inhibitors (Antonescu et al. 2018).

Another new entity characterized by *GLI1* gene amplifications, often associated with co-amplifications of *CDK4* and *MDM2* genes, has been reported in seven patients with age range of 5–54 years. Tumors occurred in the extremities, back, and lung. Morphology was reminiscent to *GLI1* gene fusion positive, with occasional necrosis, high mitotic rate, and vascular invasion in one. The prognosis is not well defined yet (Agaram et al. 2019).

GLI1-rearranged tumors include previously reported benign and low-grade tumors. ACTB-GLI1 fusions were originally recognized in pericytomas with the t(7;12) translocation. Three out of the seven reported cases occurred in children. Peculiar sites were described, e.g., two in the tongue and one in the stomach. Morphologically, the tumors showed sheets of ovoid to spindle cells with a perivascular arrangement, SMA reactivity, and S100 and cytokeratin negativity. More recently, a recurrent GLI1-MALAT1 fusion was reported in 15–20% of gastric plexiform fibromyxoma and 100% of gastroblastomas, both rare tumors of the stomach occurring in young adults. Six plexiform fibromyxomas and three gastroblastomas have been reported in patients younger than 18 years (Duckworth et al. 2014; Szurian et al. 2017). *Plexiform fibromyxoma* is a benign multinodular myxoid gastric neoplasm composed of myofibroblastic spindle cells with a prominent capillary network. Tumor cells are smooth muscle actin positive, while S100 protein, CD117, DOG1, CD34, and EMA are negative. *Gastroblastoma* shows a biphasic morphology with epithelioid cells in gland or rosette-like structures with endoluminal secretions and spindle cells in fascicles, in whorls, or in reticular pattern. The mesenchymal component is positive for vimentin and CD10, while epithelial cells are pan-cytokeratin positive. Gastroblastomas are low-grade tumors, with an indolent clinical course, and only one showed distant metastases. The elective treatment is complete surgical resection.

44.4 Targeted Therapies

The heterogeneity and the rarity of NRSTS (and more in general of adult soft tissue sarcomas) represent a major challenge for physicians and researchers, and it remains unclear how they can continue to study all the NRSTS entities together, as a mixed bunch, or—on the other hand—how they can develop studies dedicated to single histotype (Ferrari 2008). In the last years, various drugs other than the classic ifosfamide-doxorubicin regimen have proved effective in particular histotypes ("histology-driven therapy"): e.g., taxanes in angiosarcoma (Penel et al. 2008), gemcitabine and gemcitabine ± docetaxel in leiomyosarcoma

(Hensley et al. 2002; Maki et al. 2007), and trabectedin in liposarcoma (Grosso et al. 2007; Samuels et al. 2013). However, it is important to mention the adult trial comparing preoperative chemotherapy with full-dose anthracyclines (epirubicin) plus ifosfamide (three cycles) versus a histology-driven chemotherapy, which was trabectedin for high-grade myxoid liposarcoma, gemcitabine and dacarbazine for leiomyosarcoma, high-dose ifosfamide for synovial sarcoma, etoposide and ifosfamide for MPNST, and gemcitabine plus docetaxel for undifferentiated pleomorphic sarcoma (Gronchi et al. 2017). More than histology-driven chemotherapy, sarcoma experts are awaiting for effective histology-driven target therapies. In fact, the better understanding of the molecular pathways involved in tumor growth and progression is currently leading to the identification of new potential therapeutic targets: the product of the specific chromosomal translocations occurring in NRSTS may be perfect targets for new molecular agents specifically designed to influence the tumor's biology, changing the approach to soft tissue sarcomas. Various tumor-specific genetic changes can be targeted pharmacologically: new targets can be subdivided into signaling elements involved in cell cycle regulation and apoptosis, molecules responsible of tumor neoangiogenesis, and factors providing connective tissue disruption and tumor spread. A number of new drugs have demonstrated activity in various adult subtypes, for example, pazopanib, a multi-targeted receptor tyrosine kinase inhibitor, as the main example (van der Graaf et al. 2012) and more recently olaratumab, a platelet-derived growth factor receptor (PDGFR)α inhibitor. In 2016, the US Food and Drug Administration (FDA) and the European Medicines Agency (EMA) approved olaratumab for its use in association with doxorubicin in the treatment of advanced adult soft tissue sarcomas, based on the results of a phase Ib–II trial versus doxorubicin alone (Tap et al. 2016). This approval was subject to the results of the phase III randomized trial in the same patient population. The official report of this trial is not yet available at the time of this chapter, but press release has anticipated, at the beginning of 2019, disappointing final results.

Other target agents effective in specific histotypes are imatinib in dermatofibrosarcoma protuberans (McArthur et al. 2003), sunitinib in solitary fibrous tumor and alveolar soft part sarcoma (Stacchiotti et al. 2011, 2012), cediranib in alveolar soft part sarcoma (Kummar et al. 2013), crizotinib in inflammatory myofibroblastic tumor (Butrynski et al. 2010), m-TOR inhibitors in perivascular epithelioid cell tumors (Wagner et al. 2010), and eribulin mesylate in leiomyosarcoma and adipocytic sarcomas (Schöffski et al. 2016).

However, it is important to mention that, as seen in other malignancies, the impact of targeted agents in the pediatric population has not paralleled the progress seen in adult soft tissue sarcoma patients. Various barriers still exist (e.g., the small numbers of pediatric patients even in international projects, but also law regulations that offer only limited opportunities for the development of new drugs in children and adolescents), and multilevel action is warranted to deal with this disadvantage. A key milestone in the recent history of NRSTS is the recently published COG ARST1321 study, conducted in cooperation between COG and one of the adult oncology cooperative groups of the USA National Clinical Trials Network (NCTN), NRG Oncology. A primary aim of the study was to investigate the value of the addition of pazopanib to preoperative chemoradiotherapy in advanced NRSTS. Conducted between 2014 and 2018, 81 pediatric and adult patients were randomly assigned to receive ifosfamide-doxorubicin chemotherapy and preoperative radiation with or without pazopanib. At a planned interim analysis, the study showed significant improvement in pathological response rate with the addition of pazopanib, crossing the predetermined boundary and enrollment was stopped. While data on survival outcomes requires longer follow-up and is not available at the time of this publication, it is important to underline that this was the first NRSTS clinical trial to investigate the role of a new biological targeted agent; in addition, it was the first prospective protocol co-developed by pediatric and adult consortia spanning nearly the entire age spectrum. (Vassal et al. 2017; Weiss et al. 2020).

44.5 The Challenge of Adolescents

Adolescents (and young adults) with cancer represent a particular group of patients facing particular difficulties, e.g., from the delay in diagnosis to issue related to the location of care and clinical trial enrolment, from the particular need for age-specific psychological support (just as examples, adherence to therapy, need for independence, issues related to communication, sexuality, and body image) to financial issues before, during, and after treatment (Barr et al. 2016). Soft tissue sarcomas are relatively frequent in adolescents and young adults: their clinical management is quite challenging, mainly because of different therapeutic approaches adopted by pediatric and adult oncologists (dealing with the same disease) and tumor-associated factors related to this peculiar age group. Overcoming these barriers is essential for adolescent and young adult patients, whose survival and long-term physical effects are worse than their pediatric counterparts (van der Graaf et al. 2017; Ferrari et al. 2018a, b).

Among the various studies, it is worth mentioning the analysis recently published by the EpSSG aiming to evaluate the enrolment in EpSSG protocols: the study compared the number of children (0–14-year-olds) and adolescents (15–19-year-olds) enrolled in the EpSSG trials to the number of cases expected to occur according to epidemiological data. The observed-to-expected ratio was 0.64 for among patients 0–14 and 0.30 for those 15–19 years old, confirming that adolescents were less well represented than children on the EpSSG protocols (Ferrari et al. 2017a, b, c).

Various data suggest that survival outcomes for adolescent and young adult patients with soft tissue sarcomas lag behind those of children diagnosed with histologically similar tumors (Ferrari et al. 2011a, b). The reason is certainly multifactorial, i.e., delays in diagnosis, trial availability and participation, aspects of the organization of care, national centralization of sarcoma care, international consortia, and, certainly, factors related to tumor biology. Young patients ideally should be treated in specialized cancer centers who have the resources in place to provide the highly specialized surgery required, but are also able to address the short- and long-term needs of the patients so that they can maximize their long-term outcomes and address the long-term secondary consequences of intensive chemotherapy.

Noteworthy, constant efforts from international collaborations between pediatric and adult oncologists of sarcoma groups have optioned in converging toward a common therapeutic strategy, while improving quality of treatment, as well as research advances dedicated to this at-risk age group of patients with sarcomas. While defining common therapeutic approach is of key importance, effective cooperation may be seen, however, not just as a matter of standardizing the treatment of young patients but as a challenge to see pediatric and adult oncologists pooling their resources. Both would have much to gain from cooperating with one another, and sharing their experiences and expertise would have synergistic effects. For example, the pediatric oncologists' experience of developing multidisciplinary cooperative protocols and their established national and international networks could prove very helpful for adult oncologists, while the experience adult oncologists have gained of novel therapies may help pediatric oncologists to gain access to new drugs and participate in phase I–II trials.

Better cooperation is essential to facilitate the development of biological studies that could potentially lead to the identification of specific molecular targets for novel therapeutic approaches. On the other hand, it may help in developing the ideal strategy to concentrate on specific histology-based trials rather than the traditional mixed bag of soft tissue sarcomas, acknowledging the difficulties in developing studies dedicated to single histotypes among rare tumors. Efforts should be made to overcome potential cultural and logistic problems (e.g., methods of data collection or classification systems) to overcome cooperation reluctance and to develop projects applicable to different age groups.

References

Agaimy A, Foulkes WD (2018) Hereditary SWI/SNF complex deficiency syndromes. Semin Diagn Pathol 35(3):193–198

Agaram NP, Chen HW, Zhang L et al (2015) EWSR1-PBX3: a novel gene fusion in myoepithelial tumors. Genes Chromosomes Cancer 54(2):63–71

Agaram N, Zhang L, Sung Y-S et al (2019) GLI1-amplified soft tissue neoplasm: a novel entity showing morphologic overlap with tumors with GLI1 gene fusions. USCAP 2019 National Harbour, Washington

Alacon-Vargas D, Zhang Z, Agarwal B et al (2006) Targeting cyclin D1, a downstream effector of INI1/hSNF5, in rhabdoid tumors. Oncogene 25:722–734

Alaggio R, Ninfo V, Rosolen A, Coffin CM (2006) Primitive myxoid mesenchymal tumor of infancy: a clinicopathologic report of 6 cases. Am J Surg Pathol 30:388–394

Alaggio R, Coffin CM, Weiss SW et al (2009) Liposarcomas in young patients: a study of 82 cases occurring in patients younger than 22 years of age. Am J Surg Pathol 33:645–658

Alaggio R, Cecchetto G, Bisogno G et al (2010a) Inflammatory myofibroblastic tumours in childhood: a report from the Italian Cooperative Group studies. Cancer 116:216–226

Alaggio R, Collini P, Randall RL et al (2010b) Undifferentiated high-grade pleomorphic sarcomas in children: a clinicopathologic study of 10 cases and review of literature. Pediatr Dev Pathol 13:209–217

Al-Ibraheemi A, Folpe AL, Perez-Atayde AR et al (2018) Aberrant receptor tyrosine kinase signaling in lipofibromatosis: a clinicopathological and molecular genetic study of 20 cases. Mod Pathol. https://doi.org/10.1038/s41379-018-0150-3

Allen PW (1977) The fibromatoses: a clinicopathologic classification based on 140 cases. Am J Surg Pathol 1:255–270, 305–321

Antonescu CR, Rosenblum MK, Pereira P et al (2001) Sclerosing epithelioid fibrosarcoma: a study of 16 cases and confirmation of a clinicopathologically distinct tumor. Am J Surg Pathol 25:699–709

Antonescu CR, Zhang L, Chang NE et al (2010) EWSR1-POU5F1 fusion in soft tissue myoepithelial tumors. A molecular analysis of sixty-six cases, including soft tissue, bone, and visceral lesions, showing common involvement of the EWSR1 gene. Genes Chromosomes Cancer 49(12):1114–1124

Antonescu CR, Suurmeijer AJ, Zhang L et al (2015) Molecular characterization of inflammatory myofibroblastic tumors with frequent ALK and ROS1 gene fusions and rare novel RET rearrangement. Am J Surg Pathol 39(7):957–967

Antonescu CR, Owosho AA, Zhang L et al (2017) Sarcomas with CIC-rearrangements are a distinct pathologic entity with aggressive outcome: a clinicopathologic and molecular study of 115 cases. Am J Surg Pathol 41(7):941–949

Antonescu CR, Agaram NP, Sung YS et al (2018) A distinct malignant epithelioid neoplasm with GLI1 gene rearrangements, frequent S100 protein expression, and metastatic potential: expanding the spectrum of pathologic entities with ACTB/MALAT1/PTCH1-GLI1 fusions. Am J Surg Pathol 42(4):553–560

Arbajian E, Puls F, Antonescu CR et al (2017) In-depth genetic analysis of sclerosing epithelioid fibrosarcoma reveals recurrent genomic alterations and potential treatment targets. Clin Cancer Res 23(23):7426–7434

Argani P, Lal P, Hutchinson B et al (2003) Aberrant nuclear immunoreactivity for TFE3 in neoplasms with TFE3 gene fusions: a sensitive and specific immunohistochemical assay. Am J Surg Pathol 27:750–761

Argani P, Aulmann S, Illei PB et al (2010) A distinctive subset of PEComas harbors TFE3 gene fusions. Am J Surg Pathol 34:1395–1406

Argani P, Kao YC, Zhang L et al (2017) Primary renal sarcomas with BCOR-CCNB3 gene fusion: a report of 2 cases showing histologic overlap with clear cell sarcoma of kidney, suggesting further link between BCOR-related sarcomas of the kidney and soft tissues. Am J Surg Pathol 41(12):1702–1712

Baldi GG, Orbach D, Bertulli R et al (2019) Standard treatment and emerging drugs for managing synovial sarcoma: adult's and pediatric oncologist perspective. Expert Opin Emerg Drugs. https://doi.org/10.1080/14728214.2019.1591367

Barr RD, Ferrari A, Ries L et al (2016) Cancer in adolescents and young adults: a narrative review of the current status and a view of the future. JAMA Pediatr 170(5):495–501

Bergamaschi L, Bisogno G, Manzitti C et al (2018) Salvage rates and prognostic factors after relapse in children and adolescents with malignant peripheral nerve sheath tumors. Pediatr Blood Cancer 65(2):2018

Bernstein R, Zeltzer PM, Lin F, Carpenter PM (1994) Trisomy 11 and other nonrandom trisomies in congenital fibrosarcoma. Cancer Genet Cytogenet 78:82–86

Billings SD, Giblen G, Ganburg-Smith JC (2005) Superficial low-grade fibromyxoid sarcoma (Evans tumor): a clinicopathologic analysis of 19 cases with a unique observation in the pediatric population. Am J Surg Pathol 29:204–210

Bisogno G, Ferrari A, Rosolen A et al (2010) Sequential intensified chemotherapy with stem cell rescue for children and adolescents with desmoplastic small round-cell tumor. Bone Marrow Transplant 45:907–911

Bisogno G, Ferrari A, Orbach D (2014a) Treatment options for alveolar soft part sarcoma in pediatric patients. Expert Opin Orphan Drugs 2:579–589

Bisogno G, Tagarelli A, Schiavetti A et al (2014b) Myoepithelial carcinoma treatment in children: a report from the TREP project. Pediatr Blood Cancer 61(4):643–646

Bond M, Bernstein M, Pappo A et al (2008) A phase II study of imatinib mesylate in children with refractory or relapsed solid tumors: a Children's Oncology Group study. Pediatr Blood Cancer 50:254–258

Bonetti F, Pea M, Martignoni G et al (1992) PEC and sugar tumor. Am J Surg Pathol 16:307–308

Bonetti F, Martignoni G, Colato C et al (2001) Abdominopelvic sarcoma of perivascular epithelioid cells. Report of four cases in young women, one with tuberous sclerosis. Mod Pathol 14:563–568

Bonvalot S, Eldweny H, Haddad V et al (2008) Extra-abdominal primary fibromatosis: aggressive management could be avoided in a subgroup of patients. Eur J Surg Oncol 34:462–468

Bourgeois JM, Knezevich SR, Mathers JA, Sorensen PH (2000) Molecular detection of the ETV6-NTRK3 gene fusion differentiates congenital fibrosarcoma from other childhood spindle cell tumors. Am J Surg Pathol 24:937–946

Bramwell VHC (2001) Adjuvant chemotherapy for adult soft tissue sarcoma: is there a standard of care? J Clin Oncol 19:1235–1237

Brecht IB, Ferrari A, Int-Veen C et al (2006) Grossly-resected synovial sarcoma treated by the German and Italian pediatric soft tissue sarcoma cooperative group: discussion on the role of adjuvant therapies. Pediatr Blood Cancer 46:11–17

Brennan B, Stevens M, Kelsey A, Stiller CA (2010) Synovial sarcoma in childhood and adolescence: a retrospective series of 77 patients registered by the Children's Cancer and Leukaemia Group between 1991 and 2006. Pediatr Blood Cancer 55:85–90

Brennan B, De Salvo GL, Orbach D et al (2016) Outcome of extracranial malignant rhabdoid tumours in children registered in the European Paediatric Soft Tissue Sarcoma Study Group Non-Rhabdomyosarcoma Soft Tissue Sarcoma 2005 Study-EpSSG NRSTS 2005. Eur J Cancer 60:69–82

Brennan B, Zanetti I, Orbach D et al (2018) Alveolar soft part sarcoma in children and adolescents: The European Paediatric Soft Tissue Sarcoma study group prospective trial (EpSSG NRSTS 2005). Pediatr Blood Cancer 65(4)

Bridge JA, Kanamori M, Ma Z et al (2001) Fusion of the ALK gene to the clathrin heavy chain gene, CLTC, in inflammatory myofibroblastic tumor. Am J Pathol 159:411–415

Brivio E, Zwaan CM (2019) ALK inhibition in two emblematic cases of pediatric inflammatory myofibroblastic tumor: efficacy and side effects. Pediatr Blood Cancer 66:e27645

Butrynski JE, D'Adamo DR, Hornick JL et al (2010) Crizotinib in ALK-rearranged inflammatory myofibroblastic tumor. N Engl J Med 363:1727–1733

Canter RJ, Qin LX, Maki RG et al (2008) A synovial sarcoma-specific preoperative nomogram supports a survival benefit to ifosfamide-based chemotherapy and improves risk stratification for patients. Clin Cancer Res 14:8191–8197

Carli M, Ferrari A, Mattke A et al (2005) Malignant peripheral nerve sheath tumours in pediatric age: a report from the Italian and German Soft Tissue Sarcoma Cooperative Group. J Clin Oncol 23:8422–8430

Carroll SL (2016) The challenge of cancer genomics in rare nervous system neoplasms: malignant peripheral nerve sheath tumors as a paradigm for cross-species comparative oncogenomics. Am J Pathol 186(3):464–477

Casali PG, Abecassis N, Aro HT et al (2018) Soft tissue and visceral sarcomas: ESMO-EURACAN Clinical Practice Guidelines for diagnosis, treatment and follow-up. Ann Oncol 29(Suppl_4):iv51–iv67. https://doi.org/10.1093/annonc/mdy096

Casanova M, Ferrari A, Bisogno G et al (2000) Alveolar soft part sarcoma in children and adolescents: a report from the Soft-tissue Sarcoma Italian Cooperative Group. Ann Oncol 11:1–5

Casanova M, Ferrari A, Collini P et al (2006) Epithelioid sarcoma in children and adolescents: a report from the Italian Soft Tissue Sarcoma Committee. Cancer 106:708–717

Casanova M, Basso E, Magni C et al (2017) Response to pazopanib in two pediatric patients with pretreated relapsing synovial sarcoma. Tumori 103(1):e1–e3

Casanova M, Brennan B, Alaggio R, et al. Inflammatory myofibroblastic tumor: the experience of the European paediatric Soft Tissue Sarcoma Study Group (EpSSG). Eur J Cancer 2020;127:123–129

Castillenti TA, Bertin AP (1989) Angiomyolipoma of the spermatic cord: case report and literature review. J Urol 142:1308–1309

Cessna MH, Zhou H, Sanger WG et al (2002) Expression of ALK1 and p80 in inflammatory myofibroblastic tumor and its mesenchymal mimics: a study of 135 cases. Mod Pathol 15:931–938

Chakiba C, Lagarde P, Pissaloux D et al (2014) Response to chemotherapy is not related to chromosome instability in synovial sarcoma. Ann Oncol 25:2267–2271

Chbani L, Guillou L, Terrier P (2009) Epithelioid sarcoma: a clinicopathologic and immunohistochemical analysis of 106 cases from the French sarcoma group. Am J Clin Pathol 131:222–227

Chen ST, Lee JC (2008) An inflammatory myofibroblastic tumor in liver with ALK and RANBP2 gene rearrangement: combination of distinct morphologic, immunohistochemical, and genetic features. Hum Pathol 39:1854–1858

Cho HY, Chung DH, Khurana H et al (2008) The role of TFE3 in PEComa. Histopathology 53:236–249

Chung EB, Enzinger FM (1976) Infantile fibrosarcoma. Cancer 38:729–739

Chung EB, Enzinger FM (1981) Infantile myofibromatosis. Cancer 48:1807–1818

Coffin S, Boccon-Gibod L (2004) Fibroblastic-myofibroblastic proliferations of childhood and adolescents. Ann Pathol 24:605–620

Coffin CM, Jaszcz W, O'Shea PA, Dehner LP (1994) So-called congenital-infantile fibrosarcoma: does it exist and what is it? Pediatr Pathol 14:133–150

Coffin CM, Watterson J, Priest JR, Dehner LP (1995) Extrapulmonary inflammatory myofibroblastic tumor (inflammatory pseudotumor). A clinicopathologic and immunohistochemical study of 84 cases. Am J Surg Pathol 19:859–872

Coffin CM, Dehner LP, Meis-Kindblom JM (1998) Inflammatory myofibroblastic tumor, inflammatory fibrosarcoma, and related lesions: an historical review with differential diagnostic considerations. Semin Diagn Pathol 15:102–110

Coffin CM, Patel A, Perkins S et al (2001) ALK1 and p80 expression and chromosomal rearrangements involving 2p23 in inflammatory myofibroblastic tumor. Mod Pathol 14:569–576

Coffin CM, Hornick JL, Fletcher CD (2007) Inflammatory myofibroblastic tumor: comparison of clinicopathologic, histologic, and immunohistochemical features including ALK expression in atypical and aggressive cases. Am J Surg Pathol 31:509–520

Cohen-Gogo S, Cellier C, Coindre JM et al (2014) Ewing-like sarcomas with BCOR-CCNB3 fusion transcript: a clinical, radiological and pathological retrospective study from the Société Française des Cancers de L'Enfant. Pediatr Blood Cancer 61(12):2191–2198

Coindre JM, Chibon F (2010) Grading of soft tissue sarcomas – from histologic to molecular assessment. Companion Meeting of the International Society of Bone and Soft Tissue Pathology, Washington DC, March. www.uscap.org

Coindre JM, Terrier P, Bui NB et al (1996) Prognostic factors in adult patients with locally controlled soft tissue sarcoma. A study of 546 patients from the French Federation of Cancer Centers Sarcoma Group. J Clin Oncol 14:869–877

Cole CH, Magee JF, Gianoulis M, Rogers PC (1993) Malignant fibrous histiocytoma in childhood. Cancer 71:4077–4083

Colombo C, Miceli R, Le Pechoux C et al (2015) Sporadic extra abdominal wall desmoid-type fibromatosis: surgical resection can be safely limited to a minority of patients. Eur J Cancer 51:186–192

Cook JR, Dehner LP, Collins MH et al (2001) Anaplastic lymphoma kinase (ALK) expression in the inflammatory myofibroblastic tumor: a comparative immunohistochemical study. Am J Surg Pathol 25:1364–1371

Corpron CA, Black CT, Raney RB et al (1996) Malignant fibrous histiocytoma in children. J Pediatr Surg 31:1080–1083

Cough R, Wathen JK, Patel SR et al (2010) Efficacy of imatinib in aggressive fibromatosis: results of a phase II multi-center Sarcoma Alliance for Research through Collaboration (SARC) trial. Clin Cancer Res 16:4484–4491

Cramer SL, Li R, Ali S et al (2017) Successful treatment of recurrent primitive myxoid mesenchymal tumor of infancy with BCOR internal tandem duplication. J Natl Compr Cancer Netw 15(7):868–871

Curatolo P, Bjørnvold M, Dill PE et al (2016) The role of mTOR inhibitors in the treatment of patients with tuberous sclerosis complex: evidence-based and expert opinions. Drugs 76(5):551–565

D'Angelo SP, Melchiori L, Merchant MS et al (2018) Antitumor activity associated with prolonged persistence of adoptively transferred NY-ESO-1 ^{c259}T cells in synovial sarcoma. Cancer Discov 8(8):944–957

Dal Cin P, Brock P, Casteels-Van Daele M et al (1991) Cytogenetic characterization of congenital or infantile fibrosarcoma. Eur J Pediatr 150:579–581

Dantonello T, Int-Veen C, Leuschner I et al (2008) Mesenchymal chondrosarcoma of soft tissues and bone in children, adolescents, and young adults: experiences of the CWS and COSS study groups. Cancer 112:2424–2431

Davis JL, Lockwood CM, Stohr B et al (2019) Expanding the spectrum of pediatric NTRK-rearranged mesenchymal tumors. Am J Surg Pathol 43(4):435–445

De Saint Aubain Somerhausen N, Fletcher CDM (1999) Leiomyosarcoma of soft tissue in children. Clinicopathologic analysis of 20 cases. Am J Surg Pathol 23:755–763

De Sanctis R, Bertuzzi A, Bisogno G et al (2017) Imatinib mesylate in desmoplastic small round cell tumors. Future Oncol 13(14):1233–1237

Debelenko LV, Perez-Atayde AR, Dubois SG et al (2010) p53+/mdm2− atypical lipomatous tumor/well-differentiated liposarcoma in young children: an early expression of Li-Fraumeni syndrome. Pediatr Dev Pathol 13(3):218–224

Desmoid Tumor Working Group. The management of desmoids tumors: a joint global consensus-based guideline approach for adult and pediatric patients. Eur J Cancer 2020;127:96–107

Denschlag D, Kontny U, Tempfer C et al (2005) Low-grade myxofibrosarcoma of the vulva in a 15-year-old adolescent: a case report. Int J Surg Pathol 13:117–119

Dewaele B, Libbrecht L, Levy G et al (2017) A novel EWS-CREB3L3 gene fusion in a mesenteric sclerosing epithelioid fibrosarcoma. Genes Chromosomes Cancer 56(9):695–699

Deyrup AT, Lee VK, Hill CE et al (2006) Epstein-Barr virus-associated smooth muscle tumors are distinctive mesenchymal tumors reflecting multiple infection events: a clinicopathologic and molecular analysis of 29 tumors from 19 patients. Am J Surg Pathol 30:75–82

Dômont J, Salas S, Lacroix L et al (2010) High frequency of beta-catenin heterozygous mutations in extra-abdominal fibromatosis: a potential molecular tool for disease management. Br J Cancer 102:1032–1036

DuBois SG, Laetsch TW, Federman N et al (2018) The use of neoadjuvant larotrectinib in the management of children with locally advanced TRK fusion sarcomas. Cancer 124(21):4241–4247

Duckworth LV, Gonzalez RS, Martelli M et al (2014) Plexiform fibromyxoma: report of two pediatric cases and review of the literature. Pediatr Dev Pathol 17(1):21–27

Enault M, Minard-Colin V, Corradini N et al (2022) Extracranial rhabdoid tumours: Results of a SFCE series of patients treated with a dose compression strategy according to European Paediatric Soft tissue sarcoma Study Group recommendations. Eur J Cancer 161:64–78.

Eilber FC, Brennan MF, Eilber FR et al (2007) Chemotherapy is associated with improved survival in adult patients with primary extremity synovial sarcoma. Ann Surg 246:105–113

Enzinger FM (1965) Clear cell sarcoma of tendons and aponeuroses. An analysis of 21 cases. Cancer 18:1163–1174

Enzinger FM (1970) Epithelioid sarcoma. A sarcoma simulating a granuloma or a carcinoma. Cancer 26:1029–1041

Evans HL (1987) Low-grade fibromyxoid sarcoma. A report of two metastasizing neoplasms having a deceptively benign appearance. Am J Clin Pathol 88:615–619

Evans DGR, Baser ME, McGaughran J et al (2002) Malignant peripheral nerve sheath tumours in neurofibromatosis 1. J Med Genet 39:311–314

Ferrari A (2008) Role of chemotherapy in pediatric non-rhabdomyosarcoma soft-tissue sarcomas. Expert Rev Anticancer Ther 8:929–938

Ferrari A (2009) Harmonizing adult and pediatric approaches to the treatment of soft tissue sarcoma. Expert Rev Anticancer Ther 9:1541–1543

Ferrari A, Casanova M (2005) New concepts for the treatment of pediatric non-rhabdomyosarcoma soft tissue sarcomas. Expert Rev Anticancer Ther 5:307–318

Ferrari A, Casanova M, Spreafico F et al (1999) Childhood liposarcoma: a single-institutional twenty-year experience. Pediatr Hematol Oncol 16:1–7

Ferrari A, Bisogno G, Casanova M et al (2001) Childhood leiomyosarcoma: a report from the Soft-tissue Sarcoma Italian Cooperative Group. Ann Oncol 12: 1163–1168

Ferrari A, Casanova M, Bisogno G et al (2002) Clear cell sarcoma of tendons and aponeuroses in pediatric patients: a report from the Italian and German Soft Tissue Sarcoma Cooperative Group. Cancer 94:3269–3276

Ferrari A, Gronchi A, Casanova M et al (2004) Synovial sarcoma: a retrospective analysis of 271 patients of all ages treated at a single institution. Cancer 101:627–634

Ferrari A, Casanova M, Meazza C et al (2005a) Adult-type soft tissue sarcomas in pediatric age: experience at the Istituto Nazionale Tumori in Milan. J Clin Oncol 23:4021–4030

Ferrari A, Brecht IB, Koscielniak E et al (2005b) The role of adjuvant chemotherapy in surgically-resected adult-type soft tissue sarcomas of children and adolescents. Pediatr Blood Cancer 45:128–134

Ferrari A, Bisogno G, Macaluso A et al (2007a) Soft tissue sarcomas in children and adolescents with neurofibromatosis type 1. Cancer 109:1406–1412

Ferrari A, Miceli R, Casanova M et al (2007b) Adult-type soft tissue sarcomas in pediatric age: a nomogram-based prognostic comparison with adult sarcomas. Eur J Cancer 43:2691–2697

Ferrari A, Bisogno G, Alaggio G et al (2008) Synovial sarcoma of children and adolescents: the prognostic role of axial sites. Eur J Cancer 44:1202–1209

Ferrari A, Miceli R, Meazza C et al (2009) Soft tissue sarcomas of childhood and adolescence: the prognostic role of tumour size in relation to patient body size. J Clin Oncol 27:371–376

Ferrari A, Sultan I, Rodriguez-Galindo C et al (2011a) Soft tissue sarcoma across the age spectrum: a population-based study from the surveillance epidemiology and end results database. Pediatr Blood Cancer 57(6):943–949

Ferrari A, Miceli R, Rey A et al (2011b) Non metastatic unresected pediatric non-rhabdomyosarcoma soft tissue sarcomas: results of a pooled analysis from United States and European groups. Eur J Cancer 47:724–731

Ferrari A, De Salvo GL, Dall'Igna P et al (2012) Salvage rates and prognostic factors after relapse in children and adolescents with initially localised synovial sarcoma. Eur J Cancer 48(18):3448–3455

Ferrari A, Alaggio R, Meazza C et al (2013) Fibroblastic tumors of intermediate malignancy in childhood. Expert Rev Anticancer Ther 13(2):225–236

Ferrari A, De Salvo GL, Brennan B et al (2015a) Synovial sarcoma in children and adolescents: the European pediatric Soft tissue sarcoma Study Group prospective trial (EpSSG NRSTS 2005). Ann Oncol 26(3):567–572

Ferrari A, Chiaravalli S, Casanova M et al (2015b) Considering chemotherapy in synovial sarcoma. Expert Opin Orphan Drugs 3(10):1111–1124

Ferrari A, Magni C, Bergamaschi L et al (2017a) Pediatric non-rhabdomyosarcoma soft tissue sarcomas arising at visceral sites. Pediatr Blood Cancer 64(9)

Ferrari A, Trama A, De Paoli A et al (2017b) Access to clinical trials for adolescents with soft tissue sarcomas: enrolment in European pediatric Soft tissue sarcoma Study Group (EpSSG) protocols. Pediatr Blood Cancer 64(6)

Ferrari A, Chi Y, De Salvo GL et al (2017c) Surgery alone is sufficient therapy for children and adolescents with low-risk synovial sarcoma: a joint analysis from the European paediatric Soft tissue sarcoma Study Group and the Children's Oncology Group. Eur J Cancer 78:1–6

Ferrari A, Bleyer A, Patel S et al (2018a) The challenge of the management of adolescents and young adults with soft tissue sarcomas. Pediatr Blood Cancer 65(7):e27013

Ferrari A, Gasparini P, Gill J et al (2018b) Challenges of clinical management of adolescent and young adults with bone and soft tissue sarcoma. Cancer J 24:301–306

Ferrari A, Orbach D, Affinita C et al (2019) Evidence of hydroxyurea activity in children with pre-treated desmoid-type fibromatosis: a new option in the armamentarium of systemic therapies. Pediatr Blood Cancer 66(1):e27472

Ferrari A, van Noesel MM, Brennan B, et al. Pediatric non-rhabdomyosarcoma soft tissue sarcomas: the prospective NRSTS 2005 study by the European pediatric Soft tissue sarcoma Study Group (EpSSG). Lancet Child Adolesc Health 2021;5(8):546–558

Ferrari A, Bergamaschi L, Chiaravalli S, et al. Multi-agent chemotherapy including IrIVA regimen and maintenance therapy in the treatment of desmoplastic small round cell tumor. Tumori. 2021 Feb 17:300891621995250. https://doi.org/10.1177/0300891621995250

Fetsch JF, Miettinen M, Laskin WB et al (2000) A clinicopathologic study of 45 pediatric soft tissue tumors with an admixture of adipose tissue and fibroblastic elements, and a proposal for classification as lipofibromatosis. Am J Surg Pathol 24:1491–1500

Fetsch JF, Laskin WB, Miettinen M (2005) Palmar-plantar fibromatosis in children and preadolescents: a clinicopathologic study of 56 cases with newly recognized demographics and extended follow-up information. Am J Surg Pathol 29:1095–1105

Fiore M, Rimareix F, Mariani L et al (2009) Desmoid-type fibromatosis: a front-line conservative approach to select patients for surgical treatment. Ann Surg Oncol 16:2587–2593

Fisher C (2004) Myofibrosarcoma. Virchows Arch 445:215–223

Fletcher CD (1992) Pleomorphic malignant fibrous histiocytoma: fact or fiction? A critical reappraisal based on 159 tumors diagnosed as pleomorphic sarcoma. Am J Surg Pathol 16:213–228

Fletcher CD (2014) Recently characterized soft tissue tumors that bring biologic insight. Mod Pathol 27(Suppl 1):S98–S112

Fletcher C, Bridge J, Hogendoorn PC, Mertens AC (2013) Desmoid-type fibromatosis. In: Fletcher CDM, Unni KK, Mertens F (eds) WHO classification of tumours of soft tissue and bone. International Agency for Research on Cancer, Lyon, pp 72–74

Flucke U, van Noesel MM, Wijnen M et al (2017) TFG-MET fusion in an infantile spindle cell sarcoma with neural features. Genes Chromosomes Cancer 56(9):663–667

Folpe AL, Deyrup AT (2006) Alveolar soft-part sarcoma: a review and update. J Clin Pathol 59:1127–1113

Folpe AL, Lane KL, Paull G, Weiss SW (2000a) Low-grade fibromyxoid sarcoma and hyalinizing spindle cell tumor with giant rosettes: a clinicopathologic study of 73 cases supporting their identity and assessing the impact of high-grade areas. Am J Surg Pathol 24:1353–1360

Folpe AL, Goodman ZD, Ishak KG et al (2000b) Clear cell myomelanocytic tumor of the falciform ligament/ligamentum teres: a novel member of the perivascular epithelioid clear cell family of tumors with a predilection for children and young adults. Am J Surg Pathol 24(9):1239–1246

Foster JH, Vasudevan SA, John Hicks M et al (2016) Primitive myxoid mesenchymal tumor of infancy involving chest wall in an infant: a case report and clinicopathologic correlation. Pediatr Dev Pathol 19(3):244–248

Fouladi M, Park JR, Stewart CF et al (2010) Pediatric phase I trial and pharmacokinetic study of vorinostat: a Children's Oncology Group phase I consortium report. J Clin Oncol 28:3623–3629

Frezza A, Benson C, Judson I et al (2014) Pazopanib in advanced desmoplastic small round cell tumours: a multi-institutional experience. Clin Sarcoma Res 4:7

Frustaci S, Gherlinzoni F, De Paoli A et al (2001) Adjuvant chemotherapy for adult soft tissue sarcomas of extremities and girdles: results of the Italian randomized cooperative trial. J Clin Oncol 19: 1238–1247

Gleason BC, Fletcher CD (2007) Myoepithelial carcinoma of soft tissue in children: an aggressive neoplasm analyzed in a series of 29 cases. Am J Surg Pathol 31(12):1813–1824

Gleason BC, Hornick JL (2008) Inflammatory myofibroblastic tumours: where are we now? J Clin Pathol 61:428–437

Goodman ZD, Ishak KG (1984) Angiomyolipomas of the liver. Am J Surg Pathol 8:745–750

Gora-Gebka M, Liberek A, Bako W et al (2006) The "sugar" clear cell tumor of the lung-clinical presentation and diagnostic difficulties of an unusual lung tumor in youth. J Pediatr Surg 41(6):27–29

Gounder MM, Mahoney MR, Van Tine BA et al (2018) Phase III, randomized, double blind, placebo-controlled trial of sorafenib in desmoid tumors (Alliance A091105). J Clin Oncol 36(Suppl):abstr 11500

Graham C, Chilton-MacNeill S, Zielenska M et al (2012) The CIC-DUX4 fusion transcript is present in a subgroup of pediatric primitive round cell sarcomas. Hum Pathol 43:180–189

Gronchi A, Frustaci S, Mercuri M et al (2012) Short, full-dose adjuvant chemotherapy in high-risk adult soft tissue sarcomas: a randomized clinical trial from the Italian Sarcoma Group and the Spanish Sarcoma Group. J Clin Oncol 30:850–856

Gronchi A, Ferrari S, Quagliuolo V et al (2017) Histotype-tailored neoadjuvant chemotherapy versus standard chemotherapy in patients with high-risk soft-tissue sarcomas (ISG-STS 1001): an international, open-label, randomised, controlled, phase 3, multicentre trial. Lancet Oncol 18:812–822

Gross E, Rao BN, Pappo A et al (1996) Epithelioid sarcoma in children. J Pediatr Surg 31:1663–1665

Grosso F, Jones RL, Demetri GD et al (2007) Efficacy of trabectedin (ecteinascidin-743) in advanced pretreated myxoid liposarcomas: a retrospective study. Lancet Oncol 8:595–602

Guillou L, Coindre JM, Bonichon F et al (1997a) Comparative study of the National Cancer Institute and French Federation of Cancer Centers Sarcoma Group grading systems in a population of 410 adult patients with soft tissue sarcoma. J Clin Oncol 15:350–362

Guillou L, Wadden C, Coindre JM et al (1997b) "Proximal-type" epithelioid sarcoma, a distinctive aggressive neoplasm showing rhabdoid features. Clinicopathologic, immunohistochemical, and ultrastructural study of a series. Am J Surg Pathol 21:130–146

Guillou L, Benhattar J, Bonichon F et al (2004) Histologic grade, but not SYT-SSX fusion type, is an important prognostic factor in patients with synovial sarcoma: a multicenter, retrospective analysis. J Clin Oncol 22:4040–4050

Guillou L, Benhattar J, Gengler C et al (2007) Translocation-positive low-grade fibromyxoid sarcoma: clinicopathologic and molecular analysis of a series expanding the morphologic spectrum and suggesting potential relationship to sclerosing epithelioid fibrosarcoma: a study from the French Sarcoma Group. Am J Surg Pathol 31:1387–1402

Hayes-Jordan AA, Spunt SL, Poquette CA et al (2000) Nonrhabdomyosarcoma soft tissue sarcomas in children: is age at diagnosis an important variable? J Pediatr Surg 35:948–954

Hayes-Jordan A, Green HL, Lin H et al (2014) Complete cytoreduction and HIPEC improves survival in desmoplastic small round cell tumor. Ann Surg Oncol 21:220–224

Heinrich MC, McArthur GA, Demetri GD et al (2006) Clinical and molecular studies of the effect of imatinib on advanced aggressive fibromatosis (desmoid tumor). J Clin Oncol 24:1195–1203

Hensley ML, Maki R, Venkatraman E et al (2002) Gemcitabine and Docetaxel in patients with unresectable leiomyosarcoma: results of a phase II trial. J Clin Oncol 20:2824–2831

Hilbert M, Mary P, Larroquet M et al (2012) Alveolar soft part sarcoma in childhood: is Sunitinib-Sutent(R) treatment an effective approach? Pediatr Blood Cancer 58:475–476

Honeyman JN, Theilen TM, Knowles MA et al (2013) Desmoid fibromatosis in children and adolescents: a conservative approach to management. J Pediatr Surg 48:62–66

Honoré C, Atallah V, Mir O et al (2017) Abdominal desmoplastic small round cell tumor without extraperitoneal metastases: is there a benefit for HIPEC after macroscopically complete cytoreductive surgery? PLoS One 12(2)

Hornick JL, Fletcher CD (2003) Myoepithelial tumors of soft tissue: a clinicopathologic and immunohistochemical study of 101 cases with evaluation of prognostic parameters. Am J Surg Pathol 27(9):1183–1196

Hornick JL, Fletcher CD (2006) PEComa: what do we know so far? Histopathology 48(1):75–82

Hornick JL, Dal Cin P, Fletcher CD (2009) Loss of INI1 expression is characteristic of both conventional and proximal-type epithelioid sarcoma. Am J Surg Pathol 33:542–545

Hulbert JC, Graf R (1983) Involvement of the spleen by renal angiomyolipoma: metastasis or multicentricity? J Urol 130:328–329

Hussong JW, Brown M, Perkins SL et al (1999) Comparison of DNA ploidy, histologic, and immunohistochemical findings with clinical outcome in inflammatory myofibroblastic tumors. Mod Pathol 12:279–286

Italiano A, Penel N, Robin YM et al (2009) Neo/adjuvant chemotherapy does not improve outcome in resected primary synovial sarcoma: a study of the French Sarcoma Group. Ann Oncol 20:425–430

Italiano A, Sung YS, Zhang L et al (2012) High prevalence of CIC fusion with double-homeobox (DUX4) transcription factors in EWSR1-negative undifferentiated small blue round cell sarcomas. Genes Chromosomes Cancer 51:207–218

Italiano A, Kind M, Cioffi A et al (2013) Clinical activity of sunitinib in patients with advanced desmoplastic round cell tumor: a case series. Target Oncol 8:211–213

Jo VY, Fletcher CD (2015) Myoepithelial neoplasms of soft tissue: an updated review of the clinicopathologic, immunophenotypic, and genetic features. Head Neck Pathol 9(1):32–38

Johann PD, Erkek S, Zapatka M et al (2016) Atypical teratoid/rhabdoid tumors are comprised of three epigenetic subgroups with distinct enhancer landscapes. Cancer Cell 29(3):379–393

Kao YC, Sung YS, Zhang L et al (2016) Recurrent BCOR internal tandem duplication and YWHAE-NUTM2B fusions in soft tissue undifferentiated round cell sarcoma of infancy: overlapping genetic features with clear cell sarcoma of kidney. Am J Surg Pathol 40(8):1009–1020

Kao YC, Fletcher CD, Alaggio R et al (2018a) Recurrent BRAF gene fusions in a subset of pediatric spindle cell sarcomas: expanding the genetic spectrum of tumors with overlapping features with infantile fibrosarcoma. Am J Surg Pathol 42(1):28–38

Kao YC, Owosho AA, Sung YS et al (2018b) BCOR-CCNB3 fusion positive sarcomas: a clinicopathologic and molecular analysis of 36 cases with comparison to morphologic spectrum and clinical behavior of other round cell sarcomas. Am J Surg Pathol 42(5):604–615

Kawaguchi S, Wada T, Ida K et al (2005) Phase I vaccination trial of SYT-SSX junction peptide in patients with disseminated synovial sarcoma. J Transl Med 12:1

Kawamura-Saito M, Yamazaki Y, Kaneko K et al (2006) Fusion between CIC and DUX4 up-regulates PEA3 family genes in Ewing-like sarcomas with t(4;19)(q35;q13) translocation. Hum Mol Genet 15:2125–2137

Keller C, Gibbs CN, Kelly SM et al (2004) Low-grade myofibrosarcoma of the head and neck: importance of surgical therapy. J Pediatr Hematol Oncol 26:119–120

Kenerson H, Folpe AL, Takayama TK et al (2007) Activation of the mTOR pathway in sporadic angiomyolipomas and other epithelioid cell neoplasms. Hum Pathol 38:1361–1371

Kia SK, Gorski MM, Giannakopoulos S et al (2008) SWI/SNF mediates polycomb eviction and epigenetic reprogramming of the INK4b-ARF-INK4a locus. Mol Cell Biol 28:3457–3464

Knezevich SR, Garnett MJ, Pysher TJ et al (1998) ETV6-NTRK3 gene fusions and trisomy 11 establish a histogenetic link between mesoblastic nephroma and congenital fibrosarcoma. Cancer Res 58:5046–5048

Kodet R, Newton WA, Sachs N et al (1991) Rhabdoid tumors of soft tissues: a clinicopathologic study of 26 cases enrolled on the Intergroup Rhabdomyosarcoma Study. Hum Pathol 22:674–684

Kodet R, Smelhaus V, Newton WA et al (1994) Epithelioid sarcoma in childhood: an immunohistochemical, electron microscopic, and clinicopathologic study of 11 cases under 15 years of age and review of the literature. Pediatr Pathol 14:433–451

Kohashi K, Yamada Y, Hotokebuchi Y et al (2015) ERG and SALL4 expressions in SMARCB1/INI1-deficient tumors: a useful tool for distinguishing epithelioid sarcoma from malignant rhabdoid tumor. Hum Pathol 46(2):225–230

Kube S, Vokuhl C, Dantonello T et al (2018) Inflammatory myofibroblastic tumors—a retrospective analysis of the Cooperative Weichteilsarkom Studiengruppe. Pediatr Blood Cancer 65(6):e27012

Kummar S, Allen D, Monks A et al (2013) Cediranib for metastatic alveolar soft part sarcoma. J Clin Oncol 31:2296–2302

Kushner BH, La Quaglia MP, Wollner N et al (1996) Desmoplastic small round-cell tumour: prolonged progression-free survival with aggressive multimodality therapy. J Clin Oncol 14:1526–1531

La Quaglia MP, Spiro SA, Ghavimi F et al (1993) Liposarcoma in patients younger than or equal to 22 years of age. Cancer 72:3114–3119

Ladanyi M, Lui MY, Antonescu CR et al (2001) The der(17)t(X;17)(p11;q25) of human alveolar soft part sarcoma fuses the TFE3 transcription factor gene to ASPL, a novel gene at 17q25. Oncogene 20:48–57

Laetsch TW, Hawkins DS (2018) Larotrectinib for the treatment of TRK fusion solid tumors. Expert Rev Anticancer Ther 23:1–10

Laetsch TW, DuBois SG, Mascarenhas L et al (2018) Larotrectinib for paediatric solid tumours harbouring NTRK gene fusions: phase 1 results from a multicentre, open-label, phase 1/2 study. Lancet Oncol 19(5):705–714

Lagarde P, Przybyl J, Brulard C et al (2013) Chromosome instability accounts for reverse metastatic outcomes of pediatric and adult synovial sarcomas. J Clin Oncol 31:608–615

Lai JP, Robbins PF, Raffeld M et al (2012) NY-ESO-1 expression in synovial sarcoma and other mesenchymal tumors: significant for NY-ESO-1 based targeted therapies and differential diagnosis. Mod Pathol 25(6):854–858

Lane KL, Shannon RJ, Weiss SW (1997) Hyalinizing spindle cell tumor with giant rosettes: a distinctive tumor closely resembling low-grade fibromyxoid sarcoma. Am J Surg Pathol 21:1481–1488

Lazar AJ, Tuvin D, Hajibashi S et al (2008) Specific mutations in the beta-catenin gene (CTNNB1) correlate with local recurrence in sporadic desmoid tumors. Am J Pathol 173:1518–1527

Lazar AJ, Lahat G, Myers SE et al (2009) Validation of potential therapeutic targets in alveolar soft part sarcoma: an immunohistochemical study utilizing tissue microarray. Histopathology 55:750–755

Le Guellec S, Soubeyran I, Rochaix P et al (2012) CTNNB1 mutation analysis is a useful tool for the diagnosis of desmoid tumors: a study of 260 desmoid tumors and 191 potential morphologic mimics. Mod Pathol 25:1551–1558

Lee S, Cimica V, Ramachandra N et al (2011) Aurora A is a repressed effector target of the chromatin remodeling protein INI1/hSNF5 required for rhabdoid tumor cell survival. Cancer Res 71:3225–3235

Lewis JJ, Antonescu CR, Leung DH et al (2000) Synovial sarcoma: a multivariate analysis of prognostic factors in 112 patients with primary localized tumours of the extremity. J Clin Oncol 18:2087–2094

Li T, Wang L, Wang H et al (2016) A retrospective analysis of 14 consecutive Chinese patients with unresectable or metastatic alveolar soft part sarcoma treated with sunitinib. Investig New Drugs 34(6):701–706

Lovly CM, Gupta A, Lipson D et al (2014) Inflammatory myofibroblastic tumors harbor multiple potentially actionable kinase fusions. Cancer Discov 4:889–895

Mahajan P, Casanova M, Ferrari A, et al. Inflammatory myofibroblastic tumor: molecular landscape, targeted therapeutics, and remaining challenges. Curr Probl Cancer 2021;45(4):100768

Mai KT, Perkins DG, Collins JP (1996) Epithelioid cell variant of renal angiomyolipoma. Histopathology 28:277–280

Maki R, Wathen JK, Patel SR et al (2007) Randomized phase II study of gemcitabine and docetaxel compared with gemcitabine alone in patients with metastatic soft tissue sarcomas: results of Sarcoma Alliance for Research Through Collaboration study 002. J Clin Oncol 5:2755–2763

Mancuso T, Mezzekani A, Riva C et al (2000) Analysis of SYT-SSX fusion transcripts and bcl-2 expression phosphorylation status in synovial sarcoma. Lab Investig 80:805–813

Mandahl N, Heim S, Rydholm A et al (1989) Nonrandom numerical chromosome aberrations (+8, +11, +17, +20) in infantile fibrosarcoma. Cancer Genet Cytogenet 40:137–139

Martignoni G, Pea M, Bonetti F et al (1998) Carcinoma-like monotypic epithelioid angiomyolipoma in patients without evidence of tuberous sclerosis: a clinicopathologic and genetic study. Am J Surg Pathol 22:663–672

Martignoni G, Pea M, Reghellin D et al (2007) Perivascular epithelioid cell tumor (PEComa) in the genitourinary tract. Adv Anat Pathol 14(1):36–41

Martignoni G, Pea M, Reghellin D et al (2008) PEComas: the past, the present and the future. Virchows Arch 452(2):119–132

Matsui K, Tatsuguchi A, Valencia J et al (2000) Extrapulmonary lymphangioleiomyomatosis (LAM): clinicopathologic features in 22 cases. Hum Pathol 31:1242–1248

McArthur GA, Demetri GD, van Oosterom A et al (2003) Molecular and clinical analysis of locally advanced dermatofibrosarcoma protuberans treated with imatinib: Imatinib Target Exploration Consortium Study B2225. J Clin Oncol 23:866–873

Meazza C, Bisogno G, Gronchi A et al (2010) Aggressive fibromatosis in children and adolescents: the Italian experience. Cancer 116:233–240

Meis-Kindblom JM, Kindblom LG, Enzinger FM (1995) Sclerosing epithelioid fibrosarcoma. A variant of fibrosarcoma simulating carcinoma. Am J Surg Pathol 19:979–993

Mertens F, Fletcher CD, Antonescu CR et al (2005) Clinicopathologic and molecular genetic characterization of low-grade fibromyxoid sarcoma, and cloning of a novel FUS/CREB3L1 fusion gene. Lab Investig 85:408–415

Mezzelani A, Mariani L, Tamborini E et al (2001) SYT-SSX fusion genes and prognosis in synovial sarcoma. Br J Cancer 85:1535–1539

Mirra JM, Kessler S, Bhuta S, Eckardt J (1992) The fibroma-like variant of epithelioid sarcoma. A fibrohistiocytic/myoid cell lesion often confused with benign and malignant spindle cell tumors. Cancer 69:1382–1395

Montgomery E, Goldblum JR, Fisher C (2001) Myofibrosarcoma: a clinicopathologic study. Am J Surg Pathol 25:219–228

Mossé YP, Lim MS, Voss SD et al (2013) Safety and activity of crizotinib for paediatric patients with refractory solid tumours or anaplastic large-cell lymphoma: a Children's Oncology Group phase 1 consortium study. Lancet Oncol 14:472–480

Mossé YP, Voss SD, Lim MS et al (2017) Targeting ALK with crizotinib in pediatric anaplastic large cell lymphoma and inflammatory myofibroblastic tumor: a Children's Oncology Group Study. J Clin Oncol 35:3215–3221

Muscat A, Popovski D, Jayasekara WS et al (2016) Low-dose histone deacetylase inhibitor treatment leads to tumor growth arrest and multi-lineage differentiation of malignant rhabdoid tumors. Clin Cancer Res 22:3560–3570

Nagasubramanian R, Wei J, Gordon P et al (2016) Infantile fibrosarcoma with NTRK3-ETV6 fusion successfully treated with the tropomyosin-related kinase inhibitor LOXO-101. Pediatr Blood Cancer 63(8):1468–1470

Nagy B, Nábrády Z, Nemes Z (1998) Pulmonary lymphangiomyomatosis in a preadolescent girl. N Engl J Med 338(7):473–474

Okcu MF, Munsell M, Treuner J et al (2003) Synovial sarcoma of childhood and adolescence: a multicenter, multivariate analysis of outcome. J Clin Oncol 21:1602–1611

Orbach D, Rey A, Cecchetto G et al (2010) Infantile fibrosarcoma: place of chemotherapy and treatment proposals based on the European experience. J Clin Oncol 28:318–323

Orbach D, Mc Dowell H, Rey A et al (2011) Sparing strategy does not compromise prognosis in pediatric localized synovial sarcoma: experience of the International Society of Pediatric Oncology, Malignant Mesenchymal Tumors (SIOP-MMT) Working Group. Pediatr Blood Cancer 57(7):1130–1136

Orbach D, Brennan B, Casanova M et al (2013) Paediatric and adolescent alveolar soft part sarcoma: a joint series from European cooperative groups. Pediatr Blood Cancer 60(11):1826–1832

Orbach D, Brennan B, De Paoli A et al (2016) Conservative strategy in infantile fibrosarcoma is possible: the European pediatric Soft tissue sarcoma Study Group experience. Eur J Cancer 57:1–9

Orbach D, Brennan B, Bisogno G et al (2017) Desmoid tumors in children: the experience of the European pediatric Soft tissue sarcoma Study Group (EpSSG) – NRSTS 05 study – an international prospective case series. Lancet Child & Adolescent Health 1:284–292

Orbach D, Mosseri V, Pissaloux D et al (2018) Genomic complexity in pediatric synovial sarcoma (SYNOBIO study): the European Pediatric Soft Tissue Sarcoma Group (EpSSG NRSTS 2005) experience. Cancer Med 7(4):1384–1393

Orbach D, Sparber-Sauer M, Laetsch TW, et al. Spotlight on the treatment of infantile fibrosarcoma in the era of neurotrophic tropomyosin receptor kinase inhibitors: International consensus and remaining controversies. Eur J Cancer 2020;137:183–192

Oudot C, Orbach D, Minard-Colin V et al (2012) Desmoid fibromatosis in pediatric patients: management based on a retrospective analysis of 59 patients and a review of the literature. Sarcoma 2012:475202

Pan CC, Jong YJ, Chai CY et al (2006) Comparative genomic hybridization study of perivascular epithelioid cell tumor: molecular genetic evidence of perivascular epithelioid cell tumor as a distinctive neoplasm. Hum Pathol 37(5):606–612

Pan CC, Chung MY, Ng KF et al (2008) Constant allelic alteration on chromosome 16p (TSC2 gene) in perivascular epithelioid cell tumour (PEComa): genetic evidence for the relationship of PEComa with angiomyolipoma. J Pathol 214(3):387–393

Sparber-Sauer M, Orbach D, Navid F, et al. Rationale for the use of tyrosine Kinase inhibitors in the treatment of pediatric desmoids-type fibromatosis. Br J Cancer. 2021;124(10):1637–1646

Spunt SL, Francotte N, De Salvo GL et al (2019) Clinical features and outcomes of young patients with epithelioid sarcoma: an analysis from the Children's Oncology Group (COG) and the European paediatric soft tissue Sarcoma Study Group (EpSSG) prospective clinical trials. Eur J Cancer 112:98–106

Spunt SL, Poquette CA, Hurt YS et al (1999) Prognostic factors for children and adolescents with surgically resected nonrhabdomyosarcoma soft tissue sarcoma: an analysis of 121 patients treated at St Jude Children's Research Hospital. J Clin Oncol 17:3697–3705

Sultan I, Rodriguez-Galindo C, Saab R et al (2009) Comparing children and adults with synovial sarcoma in the Surveillance, Epidemiology and End Results Program, 1983 to 2005: an analysis of 1268 patients. Cancer 115:3537–3547

Spunt SL, Million L, Anderson JR et al (2014) Risk-based treatment for nonrhabdomyosarcoma soft tissue sarcomas (NRSTS) in patients under 30 years of age: Children's Oncology Group study ARST0332. J Clin Oncol 32(15_Suppl):10008. (abstract)

Salas S, Chibon F, Noguchi T et al (2010) Molecular characterization by array comparative genomic hybridization and DNA sequencing of 194 desmoid tumours. Genes Chromosomes Cancer 49:560–568

Skapek SX, Anderson JR, Hill DA et al (2013) Safety and efficacy of high-dose tamoxifen and sulindac for desmoid tumor in children: results of a Children's Oncology Group (COG) phase II study. Pediatr Blood Cancer 60:1108–1112

Toulmonde M, Ray-Coquard IL, Pulido M et al (2018) DESMOPAZ pazopanib (PZ) versus IV methotrexate/vinblastine (MV) in adult patients with progressive desmoid tumors (DT) a randomized phase II study from the French Sarcoma Group. J Clin Oncol 36(Suppl):abstr 11501

Skapek SX, Ferguson WS, Granowetter L et al (2007) Vinblastine and methotrexate for desmoid fibromatosis in children: results of a Pediatric Oncology Group Phase II Trial. J Clin Oncol 25:501–506

Woltsche N, Gilg MM, Fraissler L et al (2014) Is wide resection obsolete for desmoid tumors in children and adolescents? Evaluation of histological margins, immunohistochemical markers, and review of literature. Pediatr Hematol Oncol 32:60–69

Urban M, Feldberg L, Janssen A, Elliot D (1996) Dupuytren's disease in children. J Hand Surg Br 21:112–116

Webb TR, Slavish J, George RE et al (2009) Anaplastic lymphoma kinase: role in cancer pathogenesis and small-molecule inhibitor development for therapy. Expert Rev Anticancer Ther 9:331–356

Tanaka M, Kohashi K, Kushitani K et al (2017) Inflammatory myofibroblastic tumors of the lung carrying a chimeric A2M-ALK gene: report of 2 infantile cases and review of the differential diagnosis of infantile pulmonary lesions. Hum Pathol 66: 177–182

Schöffski P, Sufliarsky J, Gelderblom HA et al (2018) Prospective, non-randomized, multicenter, phase 2 trial of crizotinib in patients with advanced, inoperable inflammatory myofibroblastic tumor with and without anaplastic lymphoma kinase gene alterations: EORTC study 90101 CREATE. Lancet Respir Med 6:431–441

Sultan I, Casanova M, Al Jumaily U et al (2010) Soft tissue sarcomas in the first year of life. Eur J Cancer 46(13):2449–2456

Pavlick D, Schrock AB, Malicki D et al (2017) Identification of NTRK fusions in pediatric mesenchymal tumors. Pediatr Blood Cancer 64(8)

Wong V, Pavlick D, Brennan T et al (2016) Evaluation of a congenital infantile fibrosarcoma by comprehensive genomic profiling reveals an LMNA-NTRK1 gene fusion responsive to crizotinib. J Natl Cancer Inst 108(1)

Parham DM, Webber BL, Jenkins JJ et al (1995) Nonrahbdomyosarcomatous soft tissue sarcomas of childhood: formulation of a simplified system for grading. Mod Pathol 8:705–710

Spunt SL, Ashley Hill D, Motosue AM et al (2002) Clinical features and outcome of initially unresected nonmetastatic pediatric nonrhabdomyosarcoma soft tissue sarcoma. J Clin Oncol 20:3225–3235

Spunt SL, Million L, Chi Y-Y, et al. A risk-based treatment strategy for non-rhabdomyosarcoma soft-tissue sarcomas in patients younger than 30 years (ARST0332): a Children's Oncology Group prospective study. Lancet Oncol 2020;21(1):145–161

Pappo AS, Devidas M, Jenkins J et al (2005) Phase II trial of neoadjuvant vincristine, ifosfamide, and doxorubicin with granulocyte colony-stimulating factor support in children and adolescents with advanced-stage nonrhabdomyosarcomatous soft tissue sarcomas: a Pediatric Oncology Group Study. J Clin Oncol 23:4031–4038

Pratt CB, Pappo AS, Gieser P et al (1999) Role of adjuvant chemotherapy in the treatment of surgically resected pediatric nonrhabdomyosarcomatous soft tissue sarcomas: a Pediatric Oncology Group Study. J Clin Oncol 17:1219–1226

Santoro A, Tursz T, Mouridsen H et al (1995) Doxorubicin versus CYVADIC versus doxorubicin plus ifosfamide in first-line treatment of advanced soft tissue sarcomas: a randomized study of the European Organization for Research and Treatment of Cancer Soft Tissue and Bone Sarcoma Group. J Clin Oncol 13:1537–1545

Sarcoma Meta-analysis Collaboration (1997) Adjuvant chemotherapy for localised resectable soft-tissue sarcoma of adults: meta-analysis of individual data. Lancet 350:1647–1654

Pasquali S, Pizzamiglio S, Touati et al (2019) The impact of chemotherapy on survival of patients with extremity and trunk wall soft tissue sarcoma: revisiting the results of the EORTC-STBSG 62931 randomised trial. Eur J Cancer 109:51–60

Prieto-Granada C, Zhang L, Chen HW et al (2015) A genetic dichotomy between pure sclerosing epithelioid fibrosarcoma (SEF) and hybrid SEF/low-grade fibromyxoid sarcoma: a pathologic and molecular study of 18 cases. Genes Chromosomes Cancer 54(1):28–38

Smith DM, Mahmoud HH, Jenkins JJ et al (1995) Myofibrosarcoma of the head and neck in children. Pediatr Pathol Lab Med 15:403–418

Sinclair TJ, Thorson CM, Alvarez E et al (2017) Pleomorphic myxoid liposarcoma in an adolescent with Li-Fraumeni syndrome. Pediatr Surg Int 33(5):631–635

von Hochstetter AR, Meyer VE, Grant JW et al (1991) Epithelioid sarcoma mimicking angiosarcoma: the value of immunohistochemistry in the differential diagnosis. Virchows Arch A Pathol Anat Histopathol 418:271–278

Versteege I, Sevenet N, Lange J et al (1998) Truncating mutations of hSNF5/INI1 in aggressive paediatric cancer. Nature 394:203–206

Weeks DA, Beckwith JB, Mierau GW (1989) Rhabdoid tumor. An entity or a phenotype? Arch Pathol Lab Med 113:113–114

Wick MR, Ritter JH, Dehner LP (1995) Malignant rhabdoid tumors: a clinicopathologic review and conceptual discussion. Semin Diagn Pathol 12:233–248

Parham DM, Weeks DA, Beckwith JB (1994) The clinicopathologic spectrum of putative extrarenal rhabdoid tumors. An analysis of 42 cases studied with immunohistochemistry or electron microscopy. Am J Surg Pathol 18:1010–1029

Schofield DE, Beckwith JB, Sklar J (1996) Loss of heterozygosity at chromosome regions 22q11-12 and 11p15.5 in renal rhabdoid tumors. Genes Chromosomes Cancer 15:10–17

Watanabe M, Adachi S, Matsubara H et al (2009) Induction of autophagy in malignant rhabdoid tumor cells by the histone deacetylase inhibitor FK228 through AIF translocation. Int J Cancer 124:55–67

Wilson BG, Wang X, Shen X et al (2010) Epigenetic antagonism between polycomb and SWI/SNF complexes during oncogenic transformation. Cancer Cell 18:316–328

van Echten J, van den Berg E, van Baarlen J et al (1995) An important role for chromosome 17, band q25, in the histogenesis of alveolar soft part sarcoma. Cancer Genet Cytogenet 82:57–61

Tsuda M, Davis IJ, Argani P et al (2007) TFE3 fusions activate MET signaling by transcriptional up-regulation, defining another class of tumors as candidates for therapeutic MET inhibition. Cancer Res 67:919–929

Stockman DL, Miettinen M, Suster S et al (2012) Malignant gastrointestinal neuroectodermal tumor: clinicopathologic, immunohistochemical, ultrastructural, and molecular analysis of 16 cases with a reappraisal of clear cell sarcoma-like tumors of the gastrointestinal tract. Am J Surg Pathol 36(6):857–868

Zamboni G, Pea M, Martignoni G et al (1996) Clear cell "sugar" tumor of the pancreas. A novel member of the family of lesions characterized by the presence of perivascular epithelioid cells. Am J Surg Pathol 20:722–730

Torres VE, Bjornsson J, King BF et al (1995) Extrapulmonary lymphangioleiomyomatosis and lymphangiomatous cysts in tuberous sclerosis complex. Mayo Clin Proc 70:641–648

Vijayabhaskar R, Mehta SS, Deodhar KK et al (2010) PEComa of the lung. J Cancer Res Ther 6(1):109–111

Pea M, Bonetti F, Zamboni G et al (1991) Melanocyte-marker-HMB-45 is regularly expressed in angiomyolipoma of the kidney. Pathology 23:185–188

Wagner AJ, Malinowska-Kolodziej I, Morgan JA et al (2010) Clinical activity of mTOR inhibition with sirolimus in malignant perivascular epithelioid cell tumors: targeting the pathogenic activation of mTORC1 in tumors. J Clin Oncol 28:835–840

Weinreb I, Howarth D, Latta et al (2007) Perivascular epithelioid cell neoplasms (PEComas): four malignant cases expanding the histopathological spectrum and a description of a unique finding. Virchows Arch 450(4):463–470

Tanaka M, Kato K, Gomi K et al (2009) Perivascular epithelioid cell tumor with SFPQ/PSF-TFE3 gene fusion in a patient with advanced neuroblastoma. Am J Surg Pathol 33(9):1416–1429

Subbiah V, Trent JC, Kurzrock R (2010) Resistance to mammalian target of rapamycin inhibitor therapy in perivascular epithelioid cell tumors. J Clin Oncol 28(24):415

Raimondi A, Colombo F, Pintarelli G et al (2018) Prolonged activity and toxicity of sirolimus in a patient with metastatic renal perivascular epithelioid cell tumor: a case report and literature review. Anticancer Drugs 29(6):589–595

Tap WD, Demetri G, Barnette P et al (2012) Phase II study of ganitumab, a fully human anti-type-1 insulin-like growth factor receptor antibody, in patients with metastatic Ewing family tumors or desmoplastic small round cell tumors. J Clin Oncol 30:1849–1856

Tamborini E, Bonadiman L, Greco A et al (2004) Expression of ligand-activated KIT and platelet-derived growth factor receptor β tyrosine kinase receptors in synovial sarcoma. Clin Cancer Res 10:938–943

Thomas DG, Giordano TJ, Sanders D et al (2005) Expression of receptor tyrosine kinases growth factor receptor and HER-2/neu in synovial sarcoma. Cancer 103:830–808

van der Graaf W, Orbach D, Judson J, Ferrari A (2017) Challenges to improve existing survival gaps for soft tissue sarcomas of adolescents and young adults. Lancet Oncol 18:e166–e175

Stegmaier S, Leuschner I, Poremba C et al (2017) The prognostic impact of SYT-SSX fusion type and histological grade in pediatric patients with synovial sarcoma treated according to the CWS (Cooperative Weichteilsarkom Studie) trials. Pediatr Blood Cancer 64(1):89–95

Trassard M, Le Doussal V, Hacene K et al (2001) Prognostic factors in localized primary synovial sarcoma: a multicenter study of 128 adult patients. J Clin Oncol 19:525–534

Vlenterie M, Ho VK, Kaal SE et al (2015) Age as an independent prognostic factor for survival of localised synovial sarcoma patients. Br J Cancer 113:1602–1606

Scheer M, Dantonello T, Hallmen E et al (2016) Primary metastatic synovial sarcoma: experience of the CWS Study Group. Pediatr Blood Cancer 63(7):1198–1206

Robbins PF, Morgan RA, Feldman SA et al (2011) Tumor regression in patients with metastatic synovial sarcoma and melanoma using genetically engineered lymphocytes reactive with NY-ESO-1. J Clin Oncol 29:917–924

Robbins PF, Kassim SH, Tran TL et al (2015) A pilot trial using lymphocytes genetically engineered with NY-ESO-1 reactive T-cell receptor: long-term follow-up and correlates with response. Clin Cancer Res 21(5):1019–1027

Pollack SM, Lu H, Gnjatic S et al (2017) First in human treatment with a dendritic cell targeting lenti-viral vector expressing NY-ESO-1, LV305, induces deep, durable response in refractory metastatic synovial sarcoma patient. J Immunother 40:302–306

Yoshimoto M, Graham C, Chilton-MacNeill S et al (2009) Detailed cytogenetic and array analysis of pediatric primitive sarcomas reveals a recurrent CIC-DUX4 fusion gene event. Cancer Genet Cytogenet 195:1–11

Pierron G, Tirode F, Lucchesi C et al (2012) A new subtype of bone sarcoma defined by BCOR-CCNB3 gene fusion. Nat Genet 44(4):461–466

Specht K, Zhang L, Sung YS et al (2016) Novel BCOR-MAML3 and ZC3H7B-BCOR gene fusions in undifferentiated small blue round cell sarcomas. Am J Surg Pathol 40(4):433–442

Santiago T, Clay MR, Allen SJ et al (2017) Recurrent BCOR internal tandem duplication and BCOR or BCL6 expression distinguish primitive myxoid mesenchymal tumor of infancy from congenital infantile fibrosarcoma. Mod Pathol 30(6):884–891

Saeed AA, Riaz Q, Din NU et al (2019) Primitive myxoid mesenchymal tumor of infancy with brain metastasis: first reported case. Childs Nerv Syst 35(2):363–368

Szurian K, Till H, Amerstorfer E et al (2017) Rarity among benign gastric tumors: plexiform fibromyxoma - report of two cases. World J Gastroenterol 23(31):5817–5822

Penel N, Bui B, Bay JO et al (2008) Phase II trial of weekly paclitaxel for unresectable angiosarcoma: the ANGIOTAX Study. J Clin Oncol 26:5269–5274

Samuels BL, Chawla S, Patel S et al (2013) Clinical outcomes and safety with trabectedin therapy in patients with advanced soft tissue sarcomas following failure of prior chemotherapy: results of a worldwide expanded access program study. Ann Oncol 24:1703–1709

van der Graaf WTA, Blay JY, Chawla SP et al (2012) Pazopanib for metastatic soft-tissue sarcoma (PALETTE): a randomised, double-blind, placebo controlled phase 3 trial. Lancet 379:1879–1886

Tap W, Jones RL, Van Tine AB et al (2016) Olaratumab and doxorubicin versus doxorubicin alone for treatment of soft-tissue sarcoma: an open label phase 1b and randomised phase 2 trial. Lancet 388:488–497

Stacchiotti S, Negri T, Zaffaroni N et al (2011) Sunitinib in advanced alveolar soft part sarcoma: evidence of a direct antitumor effect. Ann Oncol 22:1682–1690

Stacchiotti S, Negri T, Libertini M et al (2012) Sunitinib malate in solitary fibrous tumor (SFT). Ann Oncol 23:3171–3179

Schöffski P, Chawla S, Maki RG et al (2016) Eribulin versus dacarbazine in previously treated patients with advanced liposarcoma or leiomyosarcoma: a randomised, open-label, multicentre, phase 3 trial. Lancet 387:1629–1637

Vassal G, Kearns P, Blanc P et al (2017) Orphan drug regulation: a missed opportunity for children and adolescents with cancer. Eur J Cancer 84:149–158

Weiss AR, Chen YL, Scharschmidt TJ, et al. Pathological response in children and adults with large unresected intermediate-grade or high-grade soft tissue sarcoma receiving preoperative chemoradiotherapy with or without pazopanib (ARST1321): a multicentre, randomised, open-label, phase 2 trial. Lancet Oncol. 2020;21(8):1110–1122

Rare Bone Tumors

45

Uta Dirksen and Andrea Ferrari

Less than 0.2% of the malignant tumors are primary bone neoplasms. Though they are rare tumors, osteosarcoma and Ewing sarcoma are tumor types typical of children and adolescents. The multimodal treatment of these rare bone tumors combines multiagent systemic chemotherapy and local control modalities as surgery and/or radiotherapy. The treatment of these diseases is defined by structured treatment protocols since more than 40 years. Chondrosarcoma is typically a tumor of the adulthood and is very rare in pediatric age. A wide variety of benign or locally aggressive tumors may affect bone in children: These entities can be classified into different categories according to the matrix, or substance, that they produce: i.e., osteoid or bone-forming tumors, cartilage-forming tumors, and fibrous lesions. Many cases are discovered incidentally; in other cases, they present with localized pain, swelling, deformity, or pathologic fracture. These tumors have characteristic radiographic features (i.e., type of periosteal reaction, calcification, well-defined or sclerotic border, lack of destruction of the cortex, and soft tissue extension) and can be diagnosed with plain radiographs: The evaluation of expert radiologists may avoid in many cases unnecessary invasive diagnostic studies. It is important to refer these cases to experienced orthopedic surgeon: Most cases can be managed with observation. Curettage and bone grafting or excision may be required in more aggressive cases (Fritzsche et al. 2017; Yildiz et al. 2003). However, it is very important to consider that patients with enchondromatoses or multiple osteochondromas have a higher risk of developing chondrosarcoma.

Enchondromas are usually asymptomatic, and the incidence of the development of enchondroma in children, adolescents, and young adults is not well defined. The diagnosis is usually made after imaging for other reasons. Predilection sites are the tubular bones of the hand, where enchondroma is the most frequent bone tumor. Other preferred location is the long bones (especially the femur). Enchondroma can reach considerable extension in the major long bones and may cause pathologic fractures. The neoplasm is frequently central, sometimes eccentric, or intracortical. It is an osteolysis, with rounded, lobulated, well-defined edges with a thin rind of reactive sclerosis. Usually, the lesion contains granular, popcorn, or ring-like opacities that represent calcification and ossification at the periphery of the lobules. The computed tomography scan shows a radiodense lobular or

U. Dirksen (✉)
Pediatrics III, Hematology/Oncology, International Ewing Sarcoma Study Group, West German Cancer Centre, University Hospital Essen, Essen, Germany
e-mail: uta.dirksen@uk-essen.de

A. Ferrari
Pediatric Oncology Unit, Fondazione IRCCS Istituto Nazionale Tumori, Milan, Italy
e-mail: andrea.ferrari@istitutotumori.mi.it

D. T. Schneider et al. (eds.), *Rare Tumors in Children and Adolescents*, Pediatric Oncology,
https://doi.org/10.1007/978-3-030-92071-5_45

multi-island lesion with sharp limits and a clear lack of permeative alterations of the cortex. The pathology appearance is characterized by lobules of cartilage with the typical aspect of hyaline cartilage. The calcified areas appear as granules white-opaque. The chondrocytes are sparse, with small, round, dense nuclei, of relatively uniform size. Enchondromas harbor active hedgehog signaling, which contributes to the inhibition of the growth plate chondrocyte differentiation. Diagnosis can usually be made on the basis of the clinico-radiographic features. The majority of enchondromas do not require biopsy nor surgical treatment, and patients should be followed up by means of standard radiography (Bovee et al. 2010).

Periosteal chondroma is a benign hyaline cartilage neoplasm of bone surface that arises from the periosteum. It prefers the metaphyses of the long bones, particularly the proximal humerus. It may be painful, and some swelling can be observed. The imaging shows a superficial erosion of the bone cortex with regular borders. Such erosion is caused by a hemispherical parosteal cartilaginous mass, usually of small-to-moderate size. In the largest chondromas, the tumor often contains granular or popcorn densities. Histologically, the tumor is very similar to enchondroma, but more frequently it displays features of cell proliferation (high cellularity, nuclear plumpness, and frequent double nucleated cells). Being somewhat painful and causing some swelling in most instances, it usually requires surgical management consisting of either en bloc marginal excision or thorough curettage (Boriani et al. 1983).

45.1 Enchondromatoses (Ollier Disease, Maffucci Syndrome)

Enchondromatoses are rare skeletal disorders in which patients have multiple enchondromas. Enchondromas are defined as benign hyaline cartilage forming tumors. In 10% of patients with enchondromatoses, a mutation in the PTHLH receptor is detected in the tumor tissue. Enchondromatosis manifests itself early in childhood without any significant gender bias. Enchondromatosis encompasses several different subtypes of which Ollier disease and Maffucci syndrome are most common, while the other subtypes (metachondromatosis, genochondromatosis, spondyloenchondrodysplasia, dysspondyloenchondromatosis, and cheirospondyloenchondromatosis) are extremely rare. It has been reported that age at presentation is inversely related to the severity of the disease. *Ollier disease* is a developmental disorder characterized by failure of normal endochondral ossification and production of cartilaginous masses (enchondromas) leading to bone deformity. There is predominant unilateral involvement. About 80% of the patients diagnosed with Ollier disease harbor heterozygous somatic isocitrate dehydrogenase (IDH)1 or IDH2 mutations. In some patients, mutations on the parathyroid hormone receptor 1 are detected (Baumhoer et al. 2019). *Maffucci syndrome* is a non-hereditary disease and combines the features of Ollier disease associated with multiple soft tissue hemangiomas and to a lesser extent lymphangiomas. The lesions occur asymmetrically. In 80% of the patients, the disease develops before puberty, and in 25%, it occurs in the first year of life. The most affected bones are the small tubular bones of the hand and foot, but the enchondromas may present everywhere in the skeleton. Swelling, deformities, and lower limb length discrepancy (even >10 cm) are the dominant symptoms (Pansuriya et al. 2010). Chondrosarcomas may develop in both syndromes (in approximately 25% of cases, after the age of 20–40 years), and there is an increased risk of extraskeletal malignancies, such as breast, liver, and ovarian cancers and brain tumors. Surgical treatment is aimed to relieve symptoms, rather than excise the enchondromas. Skeletal deformities and limb length discrepancy are addressed by osteotomies and/or lengthening procedures. Prognosis is burdened by the incidence of malignant change (Edmondson and Kalish 2015; Albregts and Rapini 1995; Altay et al. 2007; Silve and Juppner 2006). Molecular pathology plays an increasing role in reaching a diagnosis in these rare tumors (Baumhoer et al. 2019).

Osteochondroma (osteocartilaginous exostosis) is a cartilage-capped bony projection arising on the external surface of the bone containing a marrow cavity that is continuous with that of the underlying bone. Osteochondroma is not a neoplasm, but, especially the poliostotic presentation, can go toward a malignant transformation. The diagnosis of osteochondroma is usually performed in the pediatric age with a prevalence for the male gender. The most frequent localization is in the metaphysic of long bones: distal femur, proximal humerus, and proximal tibia. *Multiple osteochondroma* is an autosomal dominant condition. It is genetically heterogeneous and is caused by mutations in one of the exostosin (EXT) genes, tumor suppressor genes located, respectively, at 8q24 and 11p11-p12 (Fig. 45.1). The most important complication of this condition is the malignant transformation in chondrosarcoma. A cartilage cap >1.5 cm, as evaluated by means of magnetic resonance imaging, should be regarded with caution as a possible radiographic marker of malignant transformation (Bovee et al. 2010; Ahmed et al. 2003).

Chondrosarcoma Primary chondrosarcoma is a tumor of adulthood and old age. The majority of patients are older than 50 years with a peak incidence in the fifth to the seventh decades of life. Chondrosarcomas are graded on a scale of 1–3 (based on nuclear size, nuclear staining, and cellularity), from moderately cellular tumors similar to enchondroma to pleomorphic and atypical lesion with high mitotic rate. The majority of primary chondrosarcomas are grade 1 or 2.

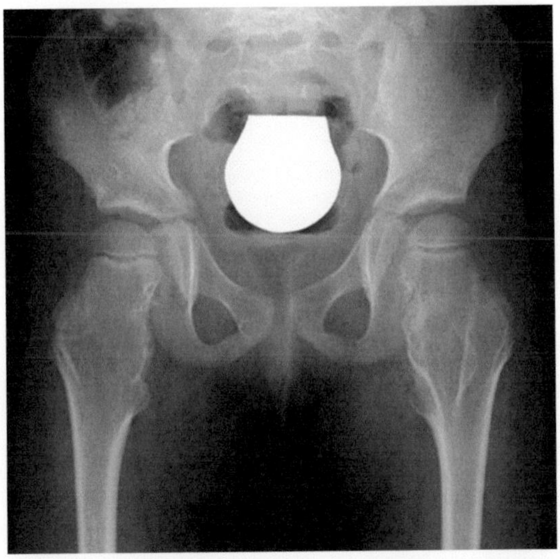

Fig. 45.1 Multiple osteochondromas in a 4-year-old girl. (Courtesy Dr. Annette Schmitz-Stolbrink, Pediatric Radiology, Dortmund, Germany)

Secondary chondrosarcoma arises from, in a benign precursor, either osteochondroma or enchondroma. The risk to develop chondorsarcoma has been reported around 2% for solitary osteochondroma and 10–25% for multiple osteochondromas 5–25%. Patients with secondary chondrosarcoma are generally younger than patients with primary tumor. The pelvic and shoulder girdle bones are frequently affected. Changes in symptoms (sudden pain, increase in swelling) and radiological findings (increased thickness of the cartilage cap, destructive permeation of bone, development of soft tissue mass) in a patient with a known precursor lesion herald the development of chondrosarcoma. Secondary chondrosarcomas are generally low-grade tumors. About 60% of chondrosarcoma harbor a IDH1 R132 or IDH2 R172 mutation and, if present, are diagnostic for chondrosarcoma; they are not detected in mesenchymal chondrosarcoma or osteosarcoma. Heterozygous somatic IDH mutations are also found in patients with Ollier disease (Baumhoer et al. 2019).

Mesenchymal Chondrosarcoma Mesenchymal chondrosarcoma (MCS) is a rare malignancy characterized by a biphasic histologic pattern of small undifferentiated round cells intermixed with islands of well-differentiated cartilaginous matrix. Because of its aggressive clinical behavior, MCS should be always regarded as a high-grade sarcoma. MCS is a rare tumor. In comparison to the most frequent classic chondrosarcoma, generally affecting patients who are >50 years old, MCS typically occurs in young adults; it is highly malignant and has a high proportion of extraskeletal tumors (about one-third of MCS occur in soft tissues, whereas extraosseous classic chondrosarcoma accounts for <1% of all cases). In the SEER database (1973–2006), only 24 children with MCS are recorded (and 142 adults). Tumor locations are bone and joints (n = 9), soft tissue (n = 7), nose/nasal cavity (n = 2), eye/orbit (3), cranial nerves (1), lung (1), and kidney (1). A German retrospective study reported on 15 cases aged 0–25 years, 4 osseous and 11 extraosseous. Tumor sites were the head/neck (6 cases), paravertebral (3), pelvis (3), limbs (2), and kidney (1). Actuarial 10-year event-free and overall survival rates were 53% and 67%, respectively (Dantonello et al. 2008). Emerging cytogenetic data have raised the idea that this tumor may be closely related to extraskeletal Ewing sarcoma; patients with MCS should be probably treated with multimodal regimens, following Ewing sarcoma protocols. The prognosis may be slightly inferior compared to Ewing sarcoma (Frank et al. 2017).

Chondroblastoma is a benign rare tumor of the second decade of life, usually epiphyseal, located distally in long bones. Pain is usually present and, relatively common, also joint effusion. The radiographic appearance is characterized by a round or oval radiolucent lesion, small-to-moderate in size within the epiphysis or an apophysis or even extending across the plate. The margins are sharp with a sclerotic rim. The cortex may be expanded but preserved in most cases. Usually no periosteal reaction can be detected. Calcification inside the defect is observed in 30–40% of cases. Histologically, chondroblastoma shows a combination of mononuclear cells and giant cell. The typical cell is uniform, round to polygonal cell with well-defined cytoplasmic borders, clear to slightly eosinophilic cytoplasm, and a round to ovoid nucleus (chondroblasts). Chondroblasts are packed in pseudo-lobulated sheets often showing a pavement-like pattern. Chondroblastoma is molecularly characterized by a H2F3 p.K36 mutation and in rare cases by a H3F3A mutation. The mutations are diagnostic. The malignant cell in this disease is the stromal mononuclear cell (Baumhoer et al. 2019). Chondroblastoma has a slow course and may be surgically treated with curettage. The incidence of local recurrence is <20% and is related to the site of the tumor. Lung metastases can exceptionally complicate the course of the disease, but they can be effectively surgically removed.

Chondromyxoid fibroma is a benign tumor made by lobulated, fibromyxoid, and chondroid tissue, typical of the second and third decades of life, arising in the metaphysis of long bones (preferred sites are the proximal tibia). Mild-to-moderate pain is generally associated with local swelling. Radiographically, it appears as a small, metaphyseal, and eccentric radiolucent defect, usually with the long axis parallel to the bone of origin, sharply marginated for a sclerotic rim. There may be cortical destruction with extension to the soft tissue with absent or minimal periosteal reaction (Fig. 45.2).

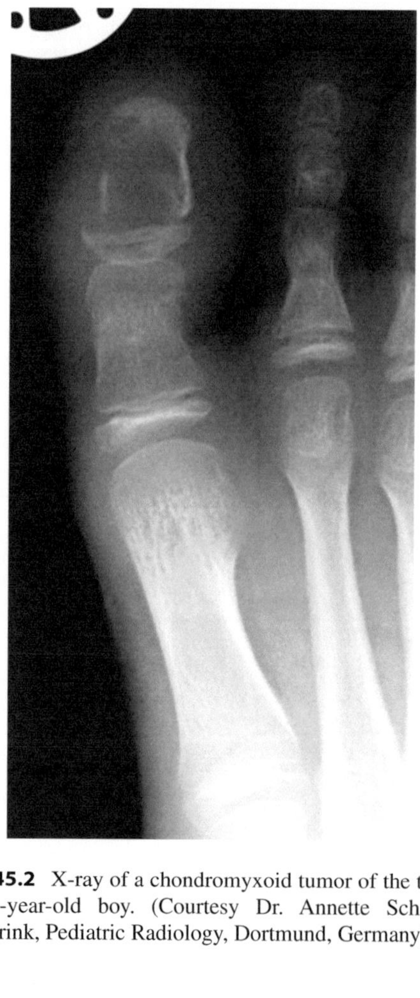

Fig. 45.2 X-ray of a chondromyxoid tumor of the toe in a 12-year-old boy. (Courtesy Dr. Annette Schmitz-Stolbrink, Pediatric Radiology, Dortmund, Germany)

Osteoblastoma is a benign tumor, made of osteoblasts producing osteoid and woven bone, arising in the second to third decades with an evident predilection for the posterior arch of the vertebral column and the sacrum. The tumor shows a rearrangement in the AP-1 transcription factor, either FOS on chromosome 14 or FOSB on chromosome 19 (Baumhoer et al. 2019). Signs of root compression may be present. Osteoblastoma is an osteolytic tumor well circumscribed and confined by a shell of reactive bone. Most of the tumors are of small size. In larger tumors, cystic spaces can be detected with radiographic appearance similar to an aneurismal bone cyst. Microscopically, the tumor consists of large osteoblasts producing osteoid and woven bone spicules and thin trabeculae. The surgical curettage is curative in most of the lesions. In selective cases, arterial embolization may be useful to reduce hemorrhage during surgery, and postoperative radiation therapy can be added to improve the local control (Greenspan 1993).

Osteoid osteoma is a small benign tumor, made of osteoid and woven bone, surrounded by reactive bone. The tumor usually affects patients in the pediatric age. It mainly occurs in the appendicular skeleton (femur in particular), while it is rare in the trunk, with the exception of the spine (mostly localized in the posterior arch). The almost constant symptom is pain, with a typical tendency to increase during the night, relieved by nonsteroidal anti-inflammatory drugs. When localized near a joint, limited motion and chronic synovitis can be observed. In the spine, it may cause muscular spasm with stiff scoliosis. The basic radiographic element is a small (1–2 cm) rounded area of osteolysis (“nidus”), surrounded by a halo of bone sclerosis. Left untreated, it increases very slowly. Surgery, up to the late 1990s, has been historically the mainstay of treatment. Nowadays, computed tomography-guided percutaneous radiofrequency or laser ablation is considered the treatment choice. Success rate of this approach is usually more than 90% based on pain relief. The main risk factor for symptomatic recurrence is female sex (Baal et al. 2019). Surgery remains an option in cases refractory to percutaneous ablation (Kaweblum et al. 1993; Kneisl and Simon 1992).

Giant cell tumor of bone is a relatively rare tumor (high incidence rates are reported in Asia) characterized by a benign but locally aggressive behavior. The tumor is molecularly characterized by a H3F3A p.G34W mutation (Baumhoer et al. 2019). Rare cases of metastases are reported, as well as transformations to a malignant sarcoma phenotype. Giant cell tumor of bone usually affects young female, arising in long bones. The tumor presents as an osteolytic lesion, characterized by the presence of multinucleated giant cells (osteoclast-like cells) and stromal cells that express RANK ligand, a key mediator of osteoclastic activation. Radiologically, the tumor may show a non-sclerotic and sharply defined border and a characteristic “soap bubble” appearance. Substantial skeletal morbidity may occur. Surgery is the treatment of choice. In unresectable cases, therapy with bisphosphonates may be used in order to induce apoptosis and prevent osteolysis. More recently, denosumab (a monoclonal antibody targeting the RANK ligand) showed to be significantly active (86% of tumor response was reported in a phase II trial on 37 patients with recurrent or unresectable disease) and may represent an important treatment option (Baal et al. 2019; Balke and Hardes 2010; Palmerini et al. 2019).

Adamantinoma is a slow-growing primary malignant tumor of the long bone. The tumor may be characterized by a wide range of morphological patterns, the most common of which consists of circumscribed masses or tubular formations of what appear to be epithelial cells surrounded by spindle-celled fibrous tissue. Immunohistochemically, the epithelial cells show co-expressions of keratin, especially basal epithelial cell keratins (CKs 5, 14, and 19) and vimentin. The cells of origin and the pathogenesis of the disease are still unknown. Adamantinoma is a very rare disease. Though the real number of cases may be underestimated in a cancer registry, only 15 cases under 20 years of age and 42 older cases are reported in the SEER database (1973–2006). A comprehensive literature review was able to identify 119 pediatric cases (Van Rijn et al. 2006). The term "adamantinoma" derives from the Greek word "adamantinos," which means "very hard." The typical presentation of adamantinoma is a painless swelling on the anterior side of the tibia. On conventional imaging, adamantinoma initially appears as a cortical lytic lesion without significant periosteal reaction, but in advanced cases, the tumor consists of a bubbly multiloculated sharply delineated lesion, with cortex disruption and soft tissue component.

Surgery is the mainstay of treatment. However, tumors may present in advanced stage, and conservative-wide resection with free margins is often unfeasible. Amputation might be required in more aggressive cases. Chemotherapy and radiotherapy do not have a role in the treatment of this tumor. The overall outcome is relatively good. In the pediatric review (Van Rijn et al. 2006), 13% of cases developed metastases (mainly in the lungs), and 10% of cases died of tumor. However, amputation was necessary in around 30% of cases.

45.2 Osteosarcoma

Although rare, osteosarcoma or osteogenic sarcoma is the most common malignant bone sarcoma. Osteosarcoma occurs most frequently in teenagers and young adults but may be diagnosed in younger children and older adults, in the latter often as secondary malignancy after previous radiotherapy. In the classical age group, there is a predominance in males. Osteosarcoma is associated with cancer predisposition syndromes, as Li-Fraumeni syndrome (mutated p53 gene), hereditary retinoblastoma (mutated RB1 gene), osteochondromatoses, Rothmund-Thomson syndrome, Bloom syndrome, Werner syndrome, and Diamond-Blackfan anemia. High-grade osteosarcoma is histologically described as osteoblastic, chondroblastic, fibroblastic, small cell, telangiectatic, or high-grade surface. Very rare are malignant soft tissue osteosarcomas. Treatment of these malignant osteosarcomas follows recommendations by specialized groups or is performed within clinical trials and consists of chemotherapy with common used agents as high-dose methotrexate, anthracyclines, cisplatin, and surgery. Radiation therapy is less effective in osteosarcoma, though the use of new improved radiation techniques, such as proton beam or heavy ion therapy, is currently studied. The clinical management is usually well known by pediatric and medical oncologists in specialized sarcoma centers. Parosteal, periosteal, and low-grade surface osteosarcoma are of low or intermediate malignancy and have thus no tendency to spread and treated by local treatment modalities only (Baumhoer et al. 2019; Bielack et al. 2016; Strauss and Whelan 2018).

45.3 Ewing Sarcoma

Ewing sarcoma is a very rare malignant bone or soft tissue sarcoma that tends to occur in children, adolescents, and young adults. It is more common in males. Risk factors for Ewing sarcoma are unknown. Interestingly, it occurs significantly more frequent in the Caucasian population. EWS is a small blue round cell sarcoma and is characterized by tumor-specific chromosomal translocations, in which ETS transcription factors are fused with a member of the FET gene family. The most common tumor-specific chimeric transcription factor EWSR1-FLI1 is composed of Ewing sarcoma breakpoint region 1 (EWSR1) protein and an ETS-family gene such as Friend leukemia integration 1 transcription factor (Fli1) (Delattre et al. 1992; Sand et al. 2015). Cooperative group clinical trials have demonstrated that multidrug treatment and treatment intensity are important factors of therapy and that intensity of chemotherapy is important for outcome. Modern protocols consist of intense induction chemotherapy with vinca alkaloids, alkylating agents, and anthracyclines. Local control in Ewing sarcoma comprises surgery and/or radiotherapy. The outcome in patients with localized disease has constantly improved over the past. In patients with disseminated disease or relapse the outcome remains poor and novel treatment approaches are needed (Grunewald et al. 2018; Pappo and Dirksen 2018).

References

Ahmed AR et al (2003) Secondary chondrosarcoma in osteochondroma: report of 107 patients. Clin Orthop Relat Res 411:193–206

Albregts AE, Rapini RP (1995) Malignancy in Maffucci's syndrome. Dermatol Clin 13(1):73–78

Altay M et al (2007) Secondary chondrosarcoma in cartilage bone tumors: report of 32 patients. J Orthop Sci 12(5):415–423

Baal JD et al (2019) Factors associated with osteoid osteoma recurrence after CT-guided radiofrequency ablation. J Vasc Interv Radiol 30(5):744–751

Balke M, Hardes J (2010) Denosumab: a breakthrough in treatment of giant-cell tumour of bone? Lancet Oncol 11(3):218–219

Baumhoer D, Amary F, Flanagan AM (2019) An update of molecular pathology of bone tumors. Lessons learned from investigating samples by next generation sequencing. Genes Chromosomes Cancer 58(2):88–99

Bielack SS et al (2016) Advances in the management of osteosarcoma. F1000Res 5:2767

Boriani S et al (1983) Periosteal chondroma. A review of twenty cases. J Bone Joint Surg Am 65(2):205–212

Bovee JV et al (2010) Cartilage tumours and bone development: molecular pathology and possible therapeutic targets. Nat Rev Cancer 10(7):481–488

Dantonello TM et al (2008) Mesenchymal chondrosarcoma of soft tissues and bone in children, adolescents, and young adults: experiences of the CWS and COSS study groups. Cancer 112(11):2424–2431

Delattre O et al (1992) Gene fusion with an ETS DNA-binding domain caused by chromosome translocation in human tumours. Nature 359(6391):162–165

Edmondson AC, Kalish JM (2015) Overgrowth syndromes. J Pediatr Genet 4(3):136–143

Frank JA et al (2017) Results for patients with sarcoma not otherwise specified and other diagnoses than Ewing sarcoma treated according to the Euro-EWING 99 trial. Pediatr Blood Cancer 64(10)

Fritzsche H, Schaser KD, Hofbauer C (2017) Benign tumours and tumour-like lesions of the bone: general treatment principles. Orthopade 46(6):484–497

Greenspan A (1993) Benign bone-forming lesions: osteoma, osteoid osteoma, and osteoblastoma. Clinical, imaging, pathologic, and differential considerations. Skelet Radiol 22(7):485–500

Grunewald TGP et al (2018) Ewing sarcoma. Nat Rev Dis Primers 4(1):5

Kaweblum M et al (1993) Diagnosis of osteoid osteoma in the child. Orthop Rev 22(12):1305–1313

Kneisl JS, Simon MA (1992) Medical management compared with operative treatment for osteoid-osteoma. J Bone Joint Surg Am 74(2):179–185

Palmerini E et al (2019) Malignancy in giant cell tumor of bone: a review of the literature. Technol Cancer Res Treat 18:1533033819840000

Pansuriya TC, Kroon HM, Bovée JVMG (2010) Enchondromatosis: insights on the different subtypes. Int J Clin Exp Pathol 3(6):557–569

Pappo AS, Dirksen U (2018) Rhabdomyosarcoma, Ewing sarcoma, and other round cell sarcomas. J Clin Oncol 36(2):168–179

Sand LG, Szuhai K, Hogendoorn PC (2015) Sequencing overview of Ewing sarcoma: a journey across genomic, epigenomic and transcriptomic landscapes. Int J Mol Sci 16(7):16176–16215

Silve C, Juppner H (2006) Ollier disease. Orphanet J Rare Dis 1:37

Strauss SJ, Whelan JS (2018) Current questions in bone sarcomas. Curr Opin Oncol 30(4):252–259

Van Rijn R et al (2006) Adamantinoma in childhood: report of six cases and review of the literature. Pediatr Radiol 36(10):1068–1074

Yildiz C et al (2003) Benign bone tumors in children. Curr Opin Pediatr 15(1):58–67

Part XIII

Tumors of Unknown Primary Site

46 Tumors of Unknown Primary Site

Thomas A. Olson

46.1 Cancers of Unknown Origin: Adult Patients

The primary site of a metastatic carcinoma is not identified in approximately 3% of patients. It has been called a CUP or occult primary malignancy (Briasoulis and Pavlidis 1997; Pavlidis 2003; Pavlidis et al. 2003). In adult patients, distribution does not match usual distribution patterns. In adults, there are several types of CUP: adenocarcinomas, poorly differentiated cancers, squamous cell carcinomas, and neuroendocrine carcinomas. The most common tumors that present as CUPs are carcinoma of the lung and pancreas. Common malignancies such as colorectal, breast, and prostate cancer are infrequently first identified as a CUP (Neumann and Nystrom 1982; Altman and Cadman 1986). The pattern of spread can usually aid in the diagnosis of a CUP. However, the pattern may differ significantly from the known primary of a similar carcinoma. The biological basis for this is unknown (Neumann and Nystrom 1982). Although few patients will have curable disease at diagnosis, it is important to employ modern imaging techniques coupled with molecular studies to identify those patients who may have a response.

46.2 Cancers of Unknown Origin: Pediatric Patients

There are few reports of malignancy of unknown primaries in children. In a retrospective review of the St. Jude's experience (over 30 years), Kuttesch Jr et al. (1995) reported on 17 patients with embryonal malignancies without an identifiable primary in children. These patients had originally been identified as CUP. After extensive studies, a primary site was identified in only five patients. Two primary sites were identified during treatment. Three were identified at autopsy. The survival was poor (median 6 months), but three patients were long-term survivors. Most patients had either rhabdomyosarcoma or neuroblastoma. The authors concluded that extensive search for the primary tumor was not indicated as long as adequate sampling could confirm the histology. This becomes more relevant in the molecular biology age, for example, the NUT Midline Carcinoma (French et al. 2004). Previously, patients were subjected to extensive studies and often repeat biopsies. Now that this entity has been identified by molecular biology techniques, perhaps a treatment solution can be obtained through further molecular studies.

T. A. Olson (✉)
Aflac Cancer and Blood Disorders Center, Children's Healthcare of Atlanta at Egleston, Atlanta, GA, USA
e-mail: thomas.olson@choa.org

D. T. Schneider et al. (eds.), *Rare Tumors in Children and Adolescents*, Pediatric Oncology,
https://doi.org/10.1007/978-3-030-92071-5_46

46.3 Diagnostic Staging

Most strategies for staging must be gleaned from the adult oncology literature. In adult oncology, there is serious debate on the value of extensive evaluations to determine the primary in these patients. The most important strategy for diagnostic staging starts with a complete medical history and thorough physical examination (Briasoulis et al. 2009). Other basic investigations are listed in Table 46.1. There are some presentations that might be gender or location specific. One example would be prostate cancer that is amenable to hormone treatment. A prostate-specific antigen (PSA) might be helpful. Obviously, in both adult and pediatric oncology, the identification of curable metastatic diseases should be pursued. Two examples, in both pediatric and adult oncology, are germ cell tumors and lymphomas. Primitive midline germ cell tumors may be identified by measuring alpha-fetoprotein (AFP) and human chorionic gonadotropin (B-HCG) levels. In adolescents and adults, isochromosome 12p (i12P) can also help establish the diagnosis of germ cell tumor (Bosl et al. 1994). For the majority of CUPs, one can question the cost/benefit ratio of extensive diagnostic studies (Maisey and Ellam 1984; Schapira and Jarrett 1995). FDG PET might provide more direction for the discovery of unknown primaries. Bohuslavizki et al. reported on 53 adult patients with tumors metastatic to lymph nodes without a known primary (Bohuslavizki et al. 2000). FDG PET detected lesions in 27/53 patients. One patient declined further studies, and in 6/27 patients, the FDG PET was a false-positive. However, in 20/27, FDG PET did identify the lesion. In several patients, the FDG PET confirmed a suspected lesion in breast and ileocolonic area, where physicians anticipated finding the primary. FDG PET was useful for unusual sites in the head and neck. They concluded that FDG PET might aid in search for CUP by identifying potential biopsy sites. There are no data on the application of FDG PET to identify tumors of unknown primary site in pediatric patients. Imaging should target areas that are suspected, given that most metastatic spread in carcinomas is nodal. Though this may not be true in pediatric embryonal cancers, strategies based on nodal location are described in Table 46.2. Axillary nodes, in women, should suggest the breast as a potential source of an adenocarcinoma. The presence of cervical adenopathy should lead to a thorough investigation of the head and neck. Two other presentations should be mentioned. Peritoneal carcinomatosis is most often associated with ovarian epithelial tumors (Strnad et al. 1989). Germ cell tumors and other childhood embryonal tumors may also present in this way. When multiple organs are involved, histological identification is paramount, and an extensive search for a primary site may not be warranted. Many metastatic pediatric embryonal tumors may respond to chemotherapy. In the case of Metastatic in front of germ cell, it is essential. Germ cell tumor, cure may be achieved with Chemotheraphy.

Table 46.1 Diagnostic strategy for CUP in pediatrics

Thorough medical history and physical examination with attention to sites of adenocarcinoma in adults (breast, head and neck, rectum) and in particular to nodal areas
Basic laboratory tests including CBC, chemistries, UA, and test for occult blood in stools. Laboratory tests that may be specific for certain tumors
Scans should be directed to suspected primary sites (CT chest/abdomen/pelvis). CT/FDG PET may be beneficial
Specific areas to be assessed according to locations of involved nodes
Specific immunochemistry
Collection of material for molecular studies
Consideration of possible resource centers outside of organization

46.4 Pathology: Cellular Classification

This book has been dedicated to the identification and treatment of rare pediatric tumors. The involvement of oncologists, surgeons, radiologists, and pathologists with interest in rare pediatric cancers is most important in tumors of unknown primaries. The pathologist has a central role in the evaluation of CUPs. As stated above,

Table 46.2 Nodal metastases

Nodal location	Possible primaries	Diagnostics
Cervical	Head/neck, salivary, thyroid, lymphoma	CT/MRI head and neck, PET, guided biopsies
Axillary (isolated)	Breast, sarcomas of upper extremity, chest wall tumors, and lymphoma	Mammogram/breast MRI, chest CT, MRI of upper extremity
Supraclavicular	Lymphomas, spread from abdominal lymphomas, carcinomas, and germ cell tumors	CT chest and abdomen, PET
Inguinal	Lymphoma, testicular tumors, and sarcomas of extremities	Careful examination of extremity, MRI extremity, testicular ultrasound
Retroperitoneal	Embryonal small, blue cell tumors (neuroblastoma; rhabdomyosarcoma, lymphoma, and primitive neuroectodermal tumors), small colonic carcinomas	CT/MRI of the abdomen, PET
Isolated node	Melanoma	Careful examination

collaboration with oncologists, surgeons, and radiologists is essential. In addition, the pathologist must be keenly aware of the difficulties that these very primitive poorly differentiated tumors present. They must distinguish tumors of epithelial, hematopoietic, or neuroectodermal origin. Cases of CUP in adults are broadly characterized by pathologists into several broad categories:

- Adenocarcinoma—well and moderately differentiated
- Adenocarcinoma—poorly differentiated
- Carcinomas—poorly differentiated
- Carcinomas with neuroendocrine features
- Squamous cell carcinomas
- Undifferentiated tumors, not otherwise specified

Immunochemistry is essential to help identify potential tumors, such as lymphoma, that may be chemosensitive (Pavlidis et al. 2010; Pavlidis and Pentheroudakis 2010). Immunostains for prostate-specific antigen (PSA) in males and estrogen and progesterone receptors (in women with axillary metastases) are advisable. In general, the ease of pathologic identification is inversely related to the degree of differentiation. Distinguishing germ cell tumors, sarcomas, or lymphomas from epithelial tumors may be easy if the tumors are well differentiated. However, if the tumor is very primitive and undifferentiated, identification may be very difficult. Some strategies to improve identification are described in Tables 46.3 and 46.4. It is crucial that both the surgeon and pathologist are in communication before the procedure, so that appropriate material can be obtained. The identification of embryonal pediatric tumors requires immunohistochemical studies and cytogenetics (Table 46.3). The identification of many specific translocations and tumor fusion genes has significantly improved our ability to discover tumor origin sites in embryonal tumors. Immunohistochemical studies and applications of newer molecular methods have been applied to the identification of carcinoma primary sites (Table 46.4). Gene profiling has recently been used to identify the tissue of origin for CUP. Molecular assays have developed that evaluated the expression of tissue-type-specific gene markers using reverse-transcriptase PCR (RT-PCR). Six specific sites—the lung, breast, colon, ovary, pancreas, and prostate—were targeted (Talantov et al. 2006). Using this technology and material from formalin-fixed paraffin-embedded (FFPE) specimens, the issue of origin was identified in 61% of CUP (Varadhachary et al. 2008). Gene expression profiling has also been used to successfully identify the site of origin of adenocarcinomas using FFPE (Horlings et al. 2008). This retrospective study was done in adult cancers and may not be applicable to pediatric cancers. Molecular gene profiling has been used to predict potential sites of unknown primaries (Hainsworth et al. 2013). But this methodology may be applied to the study of rare pediatric tumor. It must be emphasized that the cost-effectiveness of newer molecular studies, such as gene profiling,

Table 46.3 Cellular classification—pediatric tumors

Method	Specifics	Diagnoses
Immunohistochemical	Keratins, myogen, desmin, S-100, AFP, B-HCG	Epithelial tumors, rhabdomyosarcoma, melanoma, Ewing's sarcoma
Cytogenetics	Translocations EWS variety, PAX 3	Ewing's sarcoma, alveolar rhabdomyosarcoma
FISH analysis	Similar targets as above but may applicable to paraffin block material	Ewing's sarcoma, alveolar rhabdomyosarcoma
PCR	EBV, i(12p)	NPC, germ cell tumors

Table 46.4 Cellular classification—adult tumors

Site	Immunohistochemical	Molecular
Breast	Cytokeratins, ER, CK7+/CK20−	Gene expression profiling[a]
Colon	CEA, CK7−/CK20+	Gene expression profiling[a]
Lung	CK7+/CK20−	Ewing's sarcoma, alveolar rhabdomyosarcoma
Sarcoma	Vimentin, desmin	Specific translocations

[a] Horlings et al. (2008), Varadhachary et al. (2008), Varadhachary and Rabe (2009)

has not been determined (Varadhachary and Rabe 2009). However, it is critical that investigators continue these investigations, not only to help identify CUP but to eventually develop treatment strategies.

46.5 Treatment Strategy

The key strategy must be the administration of tumor-specific therapy. First, the cell of origin must be identified. Many advances have been made in pediatric embryonal tumors. However, the site of primary may significantly impact the treatment plan. Radiation is often essential for the successful treatment of solid tumors. Therefore, all tumor sites should be confirmed. However, in some cases, overall survival may be affected by the lack of information on primary site. One potential strategy, in this situation, might be a comprehensive surveillance program. It may be that the primary site may be identified later in the course of treatment, so an aggressive treatment approach to local control can be developed. Pediatric oncologists often have a different approach to "curability" because their patients have more embryonal tumors with a good prognosis. Strategies for confirmed histologies are suggested in Fig. 46.1. Embryonal pediatric tumors may be responsive to standard chemotherapy. This is especially true when histology has been confirmed. In rhabdomyosarcoma, this might preclude radiation to the primary site, resulting in relapse. The child with an adult epithelial tumor presents a different challenge. Gene profiling has helped classify adult CUP. However, CUPs in adult patients may not respond as a similar tumor of known primary. Though histologically similar, these same tumors in pediatric patients may have significantly different biologic characteristics and clinical behavior. Treatment options for unknown histology and unknown primary site are suboptimal at best. Most of these tumors are very primitive, and palliation may be the only option. Several guidelines have been published recently for the treatment of CUP in adults (Table 46.5) (Briasoulis et al. 2009; Pavlidis and Fizazi 2009; MacReady 2010; Pavlidis et al. 2010). It should be emphasized that these strategies are based on data from tumors that have an identified primary and histology.

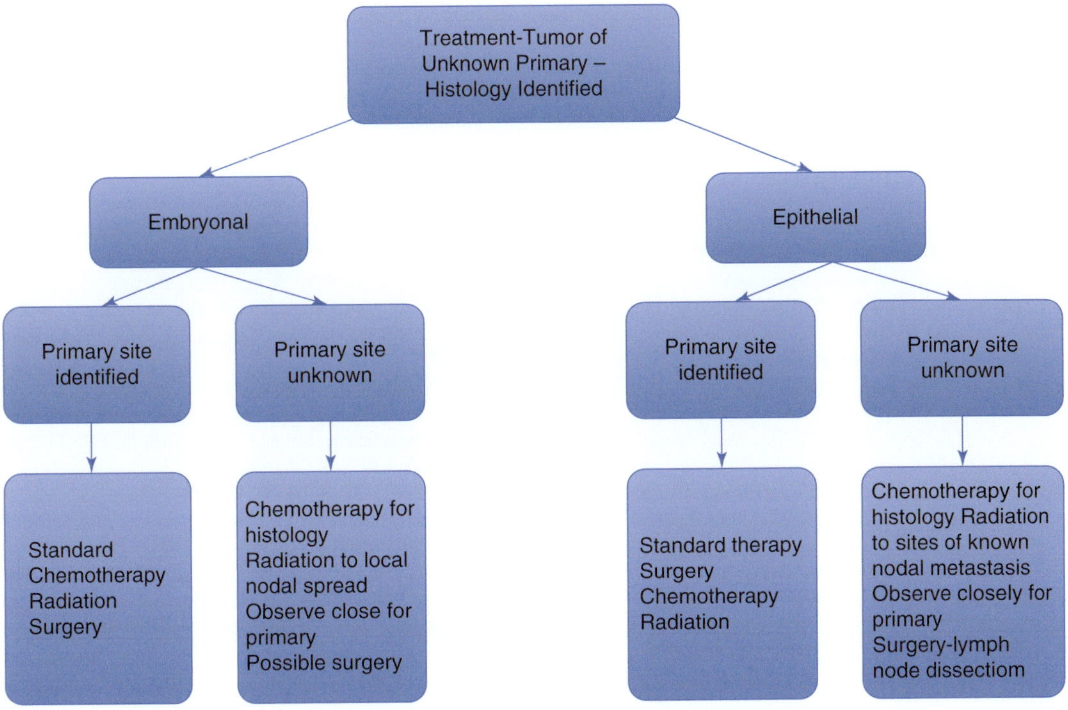

Fig. 46.1 Strategy for the treatment of tumors of unknown origin with known histology

Table 46.5 Treatment of adult CUP malignancies

Cervical adenopathy—squamous cell carcinoma	Radical neck dissection ± radiation therapy with platinum-based chemotherapy for more advanced disease
Peritoneal serous adenocarcinoma in female	Treat as ovarian cancer with platinum ± paclitaxel; response rates may approach ovarian treatment rates
Axillary adenopathy in female	Treat as node-positive breast cancer
Bone metastases and elevated PSA	Treat as prostate cancer—hormonal therapy
Adenocarcinoma—multiple metastatic sites	Palliation
Poorly differentiated carcinomas (± AFP, BHCG)	May be treated as primitive germ cell tumors with BEP. Response rate near 60%
Poorly differentiated neuroendocrine tumors	Cisplatin/doxorubicin combinations
Melanoma	Radical nodal dissection may yield survival better than in conventional stage II

References

Altman E, Cadman E (1986) An analysis of 1539 patients with cancer of unknown primary site. Cancer 57(1):120–124

Bohuslavizki KH, Klutmann S et al (2000) FDG PET detection of unknown primary tumors. J Nucl Med 41(5):816–822

Bosl GJ, Ilson DH et al (1994) Clinical relevance of the i(12p) marker chromosome in germ cell tumors. J Natl Cancer Inst 86(5):349–355

Briasoulis E, Pavlidis N (1997) Cancer of unknown primary origin. Oncologist 2(3):142–152

Briasoulis E, Pavlidis N et al (2009) Cancers of unknown primary site: ESMO clinical recommendations for diagnosis, treatment and follow-up. Ann Oncol 20(Suppl 4):154–155

French CA, Kutok JL et al (2004) Midline carcinoma of children and young adults with NUT rearrangement. J Clin Oncol 22(20):4135–4139

Hainsworth JD, Rubin MD et al (2013) Molecular gene profiling to predict the tissue of origin and to direct site-specific therapy in patients with carcinoma of unknown primary site – a prospective trial of the Sarah Cannon Research Institute. J Clin Oncol 31(2):217–223

Horlings HM, van Laar RK et al (2008) Gene expression profiling to identify the histogenetic origin of metastatic adenocarcinomas of unknown primary. J Clin Oncol 26(27):4435–4441

Kuttesch JF Jr, Parham DM et al (1995) Embryonal malignancies of unknown primary origin in children. Cancer 75(1):115–121

MacReady N (2010) NICE issues guidance on cancer of unknown primary. Lancet Oncol 11(9):824

Maisey MN, Ellam SV (1984) Investigating the adenocarcinoma of unknown origin (ACUP): a cost benefit analysis. Rev Epidemiol Sante Publique 32(1):57–61

Neumann KH, Nystrom JS (1982) Metastatic cancer of unknown origin: nonsquamous cell type. Semin Oncol 9(4):427–434

Pavlidis N (2003) Cancer of unknown primary: biological and clinical characteristics. Ann Oncol 14(Suppl 3):iii11–iii18

Pavlidis N, Fizazi K (2009) Carcinoma of unknown primary (CUP). Crit Rev Oncol Hematol 69(3):271–278

Pavlidis N, Pentheroudakis G (2010) Cancer of unknown primary site: 20 questions to be answered. Ann Oncol 21(Suppl 7):vii303–vii307

Pavlidis N, Briasoulis E et al (2003) Diagnostic and therapeutic management of cancer of an unknown primary. Eur J Cancer 39(14):1990–2005

Pavlidis N, Hansen H et al (2010) ESMO clinical practice guidelines: development, implementation and dissemination. Ann Oncol 21(Suppl 5):v7–v8

Schapira DV, Jarrett AR (1995) The need to consider survival, outcome, and expense when evaluating and treating patients with unknown primary carcinoma. Arch Intern Med 155(19):2050–2054

Strnad CM, Grosh WW et al (1989) Peritoneal carcinomatosis of unknown primary site in women. A distinctive subset of adenocarcinoma. Ann Intern Med 111(3):213–217

Talantov D, Baden J et al (2006) A quantitative reverse transcriptase-polymerase chain reaction assay to identify metastatic carcinoma tissue of origin. J Mol Diagn 8(3):320–329

Varadhachary GR, Rabe MN (2009) Gene expression profiling in cancers of unknown primary. J Clin Oncol 27(25):e85–e86, author reply e87–88

Varadhachary GR, Talantov D et al (2008) Molecular profiling of carcinoma of unknown primary and correlation with clinical evaluation. J Clin Oncol 26(27):4442–4448

Part XIV

Rare Tumors as Second Malignancies

47 Rare Subsequent Primary Cancers in Pediatric Cancer Survivors

Ann C. Mertens and Thorsten Langer

47.1 Introduction

Advances in cancer therapy during the past four decades have resulted in remarkable increases in survival for most cancers of childhood and adolescence. Data from the National Cancer Institute's Surveillance, Epidemiology, and End Results (SEER) Program show that the overall 5-year survival rate for childhood cancer has increased from 45% in 1970 to over 80% in 2005 (Ries et al. 1999). It is estimated that 1 in every 640 young adults is now a survivor of childhood cancer and that at least 328,000 persons in the USA alone have survived cancer diagnosed before the age of 20 years (Mariotto et al. 2009). Because of the relatively young age of these survivors, and their potential longevity, the delayed consequences of therapy may have a significant impact on their lives, and on society at large, over an extended period of time.

Also with this success has come the realization that a substantial proportion of childhood cancer survivors will experience late-occurring adverse health effects resulting from their disease and treatment. As pediatric cancer survivors are being followed long term, nearly 73% of adult survivors of pediatric cancer have chronic health conditions, many of which are severe or disabling (Oeffinger et al. 2006). Numerous reports and reviews of late effects of chemotherapy and radiation have been published, describing sequelae present at, or shortly following, the end of therapy, as well as the occurrence of selected late complications. Most studies of late sequelae have focused on medical outcomes (Oeffinger and Hudson 2004). These studies have shown that the type and intensity of therapy, as well as the age at therapy, are important factors in both overall survival and late effect outcomes. Children who are younger at diagnosis and treatment are more severely affected than older children, particularly if treatment is administered at a significant time of development and growth.

One of the most devastating late effects is the development of a subsequent secondary malignancy (SN) that originates in a new primary site or tissue. Over the past 30 years, numerous reports and reviews of late effects of chemotherapy and radiation have been published, describing an increased risk of developing subsequent malignant neoplasms in survivors of childhood cancers. Survivors of childhood cancers have a sixfold increased risk of developing a SN (Friedman et al. 2010; Turcotte et al. 2015). The incidence of subsequent primary cancers has

A. C. Mertens (✉)
The Mark R. Hudgens Chair for Clinical Research in Children's Cancer and Blood Disorders Aflac Cancer Center and Blood Disorders Service, Emory University, Atlanta, GA, USA
e-mail: ann.mertens@choa.org

T. Langer
Pediatric Hematology/Oncology, Universitäts-Kinderklinik, Erlangen, Germany

D. T. Schneider et al. (eds.), *Rare Tumors in Children and Adolescents*, Pediatric Oncology,
https://doi.org/10.1007/978-3-030-92071-5_47

been primarily linked to treatment, which is demonstrated in higher rates in certain types of cancer who receive these multimodal treatments (Ng et al. 2010). Other primary subsequent cancer has been linked to genetic predisposition to multiple cancers and sensitivity to radiogenic cancer, which has been demonstrated in children diagnosed with retinoblastoma (Kleinerman et al. 2005).

47.2 Study Findings

Information we have on the development of rare subsequent cancer in pediatric cancer survivors comes from two major sources: reports from the Surveillance, Epidemiology, and End Results (SEER) Program and three large studies that have followed pediatric cancer survivors into adulthood. From these studies, it is clear that the major types of subsequent cancers are due to radiation exposure and certain chemotherapies, particularly alkylating agents. Recent studies have also indicated that the incidence of basal cell carcinoma is also very high in the survivor population. However, this is more difficult to enumerate since there are no record keeping of these cancers in the general population. The more rare cancers in this pediatric cancer survivor population are described below.

47.2.1 Surveillance, Epidemiology, and End Results (SEER) Program

SEER data is a compilation of population-based registries allowing for objective assessments and now covers 26% of the US population. In a recent monograph published through SEER looking at New Malignancies Among Cancer Survivors, descriptive analysis on new malignancies following childhood cancer was highlighted (Curtis et al. 2006). This study population included 23,819 children diagnosed with cancer before the age of 18, who had survived 2 or more months following diagnosis. This population was observed for an average of 8.3 years (median, 5.8 years). Within this population, there were 12,951 5-year survivors, 8424 10-year survivors, and 2637 20-year survivors. The maximum age at the end of follow-up was 44 years.

During this follow-up period, 352 new primary cancers were diagnosed in 327 individuals, accounting for a sixfold increase in incidence relative to the general population (observed/expected (O/E) = 6.07, 95% CI = 5.45–6.74, excess absolute risk (EAR) = 15 per 10,000 person-years). Of particular concern in this cohort is the occurrence of new primary cancers in this young population of longer-term survivors. The pattern of cancer incidence in this group patterned the cancer incidence seen more commonly in older adults. The more rare but significant subsequent primary cancers were diagnosed in the buccal cavity, digestive, respiratory, male genital, urinary, and central nervous system. Within these systems, increased risk of subsequent primary cancers due to radiation exposure was noted in cancers found in the salivary gland (O/E = 27.13), stomach (O/E = 35.89), pancreas (O/E = 69.36), and lung (O/E = 14.20).

In addition, childhood cancer patients whose initial treatment included radiotherapy were at higher risk of developing a subsequent cancer than those not given radiotherapy, as reflected by the high O/E ratios and absolute risks seen (Table 47.1). Subsequent cancer sites showing the greatest increased risk following radiotherapy among 5-year survivors included the breast, brain, bone and soft tissue, thyroid gland, digestive system, and lung. Also of interest are the increased risk of melanoma and the female and male genital system in patients without radiotherapy.

47.2.2 Population-Based Studies

In the synopsis of current data on subsequent primary cancers, two large population-based studies are highlighted due to the long average follow-up period of pediatric cancer survivors into adulthood. Both studies, using age-, sex-, and calendar time-specific comparisons with the general population, demonstrate that the risk of a subsequent

Table 47.1 Risk of subsequent primary cancers following childhood cancer by initial treatment with radiation

	Any radiation (n = 9063)				No radiation (n = 13,905)			
Subsequent primary cancer	Observed	Expected	O/E	EAR	Observed	Expected	O/E	EAR
Buccal cavity, pharynx	7	0.47	15.03*	0.80	10	0.55	18.25*	0.87
Salivary gland	4	0.15	27.13*	0.47	4	0.18	22.03*	0.35
Digestive system	14	1.08	12.99*	1.59	10	1.29	7.74*	0.80
Stomach	4	0.11	35.89*	0.48	2	0.13	15.24*	0.17
Pancreas	5	0.07	69.36*	0.61	0	0.08	0.00	−0.01
Respiratory system	6	0.48	12.38*	0.68	2	0.57	3.48	0.13
Lung, bronchus	4	0.28	14.20*	0.46	1	0.32	30.9	0.06
Female breast	29	1.71	16.91*	7.14	10	2.08	4.81	1.48
Female genital system	3	2.14	1.40	0.22	7	2.56	2.73*	0.83
Male genital system	2	2.15	0.93	−0.03	10	2.24	4.46*	1.41
Urinary system	2	0.64	3.12	0.17	3	0.87	3.44	0.20
Melanoma of the skin	6	2.57	2.34	0.42	19	2.82	6.74	1.49
Brain, CNS	27	2.19	12.32*	30.5	12	3.00	4.00*	0.83
Thyroid	17	20.8	8.18*	1.83	12	2.41	4.99*	0.89
Bone, joints	23	0.80	28.83*	2.73	12	0.99	12.07*	1.02
Soft tissue	19	0.81	23.48*	2.23	7	1.09	6.45*	0.55
Hodgkin lymphoma	3	2.51	1.20	0.06	1	2.85	0.35	−0.17
Non-Hodgkin lymphoma	9	1.81	4.97*	0.88	6	2.11	2.85*	0.36
Acute lymphocytic leukemia	5	1.30	3.85*	0.45	3	2.09	1.44	0.08
Acute nonlymphocytic leukemia	12	0.72	16.66*	1.39	14	0.94	14.93*	1.21

O observed number of subsequent primary cancers, *E* expected number of subsequent primary cancers, *EAR* excess absolute risk (excess cancers per 10,000 person-years)* $p < 0.05$

cancer is substantially higher than that seen in the general population.

The first is a cohort of 16,541 3-year survivors of childhood cancer treated in Britain between 1962 and 1987 (Jenkinson et al. 2004). Within this cohort of children diagnosed before the age of 15, 245 subsequent malignancies were identified, yielding an overall standardized incidence ratio (SIR) of 6.2 (95% confidence interval = 5.5–7.1). Of note, a statistically significant excess SIR was found within each decade of follow-up, with the overall SIR declining with successive decades from diagnosis (Table 47.2).

The second population-based study reported on a cohort of 47,697 children diagnosed before the age of 20 years, from the cancer registries of the Nordic countries (Denmark, Finland, Iceland, Norway, and Sweden) during 1943–2005 (Olsen et al. 2009). Over this time period, 1180 subsequent cancers were observed in 1088 persons. The overall SIR was 3.3 (95% CI = 3.1–3.5). The relative risks were statistically significant at all ages, including cohort members up to the age of 70 years. Cohort members who were treated during the multimodal treatment era (1975–2005) had the highest age-specific incidence rate of a subsequent cancer. Among survivors, the cumulative risks for second cancers before the age of 50 were 8.6% in the 1943–1959 subcohort (pre-chemotherapy era), 12.2% for the 1960–1974 subcohort (first-generation chemotherapy era), and 13.3% for the 1975–2005 subcohort (combination chemotherapy era). The number of excess second primary cancers observed by age is shown in Fig. 47.1, demonstrating continued increased risk decades of life after the original cancer diagnosis.

Table 47.2 Risk of subsequent malignant neoplasms (SMN) after nonretinoblastoma childhood cancer by duration of follow-up from original diagnosis

	Follow-up period from diagnosis (years)			
	3–9	10–19	20–29	30 or more
Number of persons at risk	15,452	7862	2806	808
Observed number of SMN	92	64	34	11
SIR (95% CI)	10.2 (8.3–12.6)	5.7 (4.4–7.3)	3.5 (2.4–4.9)	2.4 (1.2–4.3)

SIR standardized incidence ratio, *95% CI* 95% confidence interval

47.2.3 Childhood Cancer Survivor Study (CCSS)

The CCSS is a multi-institutional study of individuals who survived for 5 or more years after treatment for cancer diagnosed during childhood or adolescence. Eligibility criteria for CCSS are diagnosis of leukemia, central nervous system (CNS) malignancies (all histologies), Hodgkin disease, non-Hodgkin lymphoma, malignant kidney tumor, neuroblastoma, soft tissue sarcoma, or bone tumor; diagnosis and initial treatment at 1 of the 26 collaborating CCSS institutions; and diagnosis between 1970 and 1986 (Robison et al. 2002).

The CCSS represents the largest cohort of relatively long-term survivors of childhood cancer and has contributed significantly because of the extensive medical record review of survivors and pathology validation of reported subsequent primary cancers. Because of the continued surveillance in this population, the 30-year cumulative incidence of the development of a subsequent primary cancer has been estimated to be 9.3% compared with the 20-year incidence in this cohort of 3.2% (Meadows et al. 2009). These data highlight the fact that the standardized incidence ratio continues to increase as this cohort ages.

A recent analysis within the CCSS cohort documented 802 subsequent malignant cancers among 732 survivors with a median time of follow-up since the primary cancer diagnosis of 22.9 years (range = 5.0–36.7 years) (Friedman et al. 2010). Associations between the primary cancer and subsequent cancers are shown in Table 47.3. The diagnosis of Hodgkin disease showed a disproportionate number of subsequent cancers, with 35% of the reported subsequent malignant cancers in this group that only

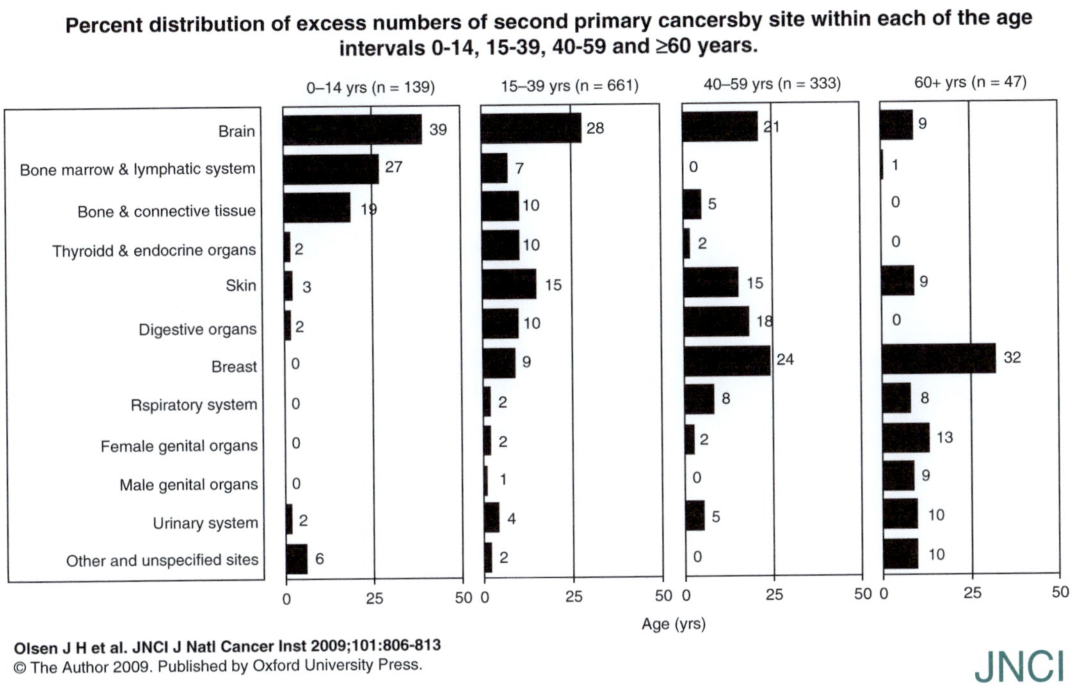

Fig. 47.1 Percent distribution of excess numbers of second primary cancers by site within each of the age intervals 0–14, 15–39, 40–59, and ≥60 years (Olsen et al. 2009)

comprises 13% of the cohort. Standardized incidence ratios, using age-, sex-, and race-specific rates, found the highest risks were observed for subsequent bone cancer, thyroid cancer, head and neck cancer, CNS malignancies, and breast cancer (Table 47.4). Of particular interest is the increased risk of solid organ malignancies typically seen in older adults, such as head and neck tumors, small intestine and colorectal cancer, cancer of the lung and bronchus, and cancer of the female genital tract.

Earlier nested case-control studies of specific subsequent cancers have yielded important information regarding the influence of radiation dose on the occurrence of the more common subsequent cancers. In a study of 69 cases with confirmed thyroid cancer, a significant dose response of radiation to the risk of thyroid cancer increases up to 20–29 Gy of radiation (odds ratio (OR) = 9.8, 95% CI = 3.2–34.8), with a fall in the dose-response relationship at greater than 30 Gy, suggesting a cell-killing effect (Sigurdson et al. 2005). In a study of subsequent CNS tumors, the dose response for excess relative risk from radiation exposure for 40 subsequent gliomas was linear and peaked for doses of 30–44.9 Gy (OR = 21.0, 95% CI = 2.1–42.3) (Neglia et al. 2006). Similarly for a study of 120 subsequent breast cancer in female survivors, the odds ratio for breast cancer increased linearly with radiation dose, with the highest at doses 40 Gy (OR = 10.9, 95% CI = 3.8–31.0) (Inskip et al. 2006). For each of these subsequent cancers, chemotherapy for the first cancer diagnosis, exposure to chemotherapy, showed no association for the observed increase in risk. Recently, CCSS reported that multiple SNs are common among aging childhood cancer survivors (Armstrong et al. 2011).

A Dutch study demonstrated increased SNs in patients with increasing doxorubicin and cyclophosphamide doses (Teepen et al. 2017). The increase in doxorubicin dose-response breast cancer was higher in patients whose cancer was in childhood Li-Fraumeni syndrome.

Table 47.3 Original and subsequent malignant neoplasm diagnoses

Subsequent diagnosis		Leukemia			Lymphoma			CNS			Solid organ					Skin
		ALL	AML	Other	HL	NHL	Other	Glial	Medullo PNET	Other	Breast	Bone	STS	Thyroid	Other	Melanoma
Primary diagnosis	Number in cohort (%)															
Leukemia	4830 (33.6)	3	6		2	3	2	30	2	8	16	4	12	28	50	20
CNS tumors	1877 (13.1)		2	1	1		2	13	1	1	4	5	12	15	22	10
Hodgkin lymphoma	1927 (13.4)		8	6		10	6	4	1	3	161	6	26	42	69	13
Non-Hodgkin lymphoma	1080 (7.5)	2	2		3	1		2		5	6	2	4	10	16	2
Kidney	1256 (8.7)	2							1		7	4	8	3	12	3
Neuroblastoma	955 (6.7)	1	3		1			2			2		5	10	17	
Soft tissue sarcoma	2434 (17.0)		1	3	2			1		5	16	13	18	8	22	8
Bone tumors	1246 (8.7)	2	2	1				2		2	35	10	7	12	22	8
Total		10	24	11	9	14	10	54	5	24	247	44	92	128	230	64

Table 47.4 Observed and expected numbers of invasive second malignant neoplasms by second malignancy diagnosis

Second malignancy diagnosis	Cases observed	Cases expected	Standardized incidence ratio (95% C.I.)	Median time to SMN occurrence (years)
All invasive second malignancies	802	130	6.2 (5.7, 6.7)	17.8
Leukemia	41	130	6.2 (4.5, 8.4)	8.9
Acute lymphoblastic leukemia	10	7	3.7 (2.0, 6.8)	11.5
Acute myeloid leukemia	21	3	9.5 (6.2, 14.5)	7.4
Central nervous system	77	7	10.6 (8.5, 13.3)	13.2
Glial	52	6	9.0 (6.9, 11.9)	11.7
Medulloblastoma, PNET	6	0.6	7.6 (3.1, 18.3)	11.6
Meningioma (malignant)	11	0.04	91.3 (27.5, 302.8)	22.9
Breast cancer	188	17	10.7 (9.1, 12.6)	21.3
Melanoma	48	14	3.4 (2.5, 4.6)	18.9
Thyroid cancer	128	11	11.2 (9.4, 13.4)	18.6
Bone cancer	45	2	19.2 (14.4, 25.7)	9.8
Osteosarcoma	35	1	30.2 (21.4, 42.4)	9.3
Ewing sarcoma	4	0.6	6.7 (2.5, 17.9)	14.0
Lymphoma	33	18	1.8 (1.3, 2.6)	18.5
Hodgkin lymphoma	9	9	1.0 (0.5, 1.9)	18.5
Non-Hodgkin lymphoma	21	8	2.6 (1.6, 4.1)	21.6
Soft tissue sarcoma	73	9	8.2 (6.5, 10.4)	15.2
Kidney cancer	20	3	7.7 (4.8, 12.1)	19.6
Head and neck cancer	38	3	11.2 (8.1, 15.5)	15.6
Small intestine and colorectal cancer	27	6	4.9 (3.3, 7.1)	23.1
Lung and bronchus cancer	11	3	2.6 (2.0, 6.5)	20.3
Female genital cancer	23	10	2.2 (1.5, 3.3)	19.5
Other cancers	50	19	2.7 (2.0, 3.5)	21.0

47.3 Synopsis of Above Data

The development of subsequent primary cancers in pediatric cancer survivors is a rare occurrence but nonetheless of particular concern to survivors and their families. The most common of these occurrences are subsequent cancers of the bone and soft tissue sarcomas, epithelial cancers (e.g., breast, head, and neck), thyroid cancer, and melanoma. Each of the studies reported above shows similar patterns, regardless of the makeup of the cohort being followed. First, exposure to radiotherapy increases the risk of certain cancers; however, chemotherapy also plays an important role. Second, the risk of the development of these subsequent cancers does not appear to diminish over the lifetime of the cancer survivor and is shown to stay increased through older adulthood. And, third, the type of subsequent cancer that develops appears to be determined by the therapeutic treatment of the original cancer and years since diagnosis.

These studies clearly indicate the need for careful surveillance and monitoring of subsequent cancers, from the time of completion of treatment through subsequent decades of life in pediatric cancer survivors. Recommendations for cancer surveillance have been outlined in the Long-Term Follow-Up Guidelines for Survivors of Childhood, Adolescent and Young Adult Cancers, a collaborative effort within the Children's Oncology Group (COG Guidelines). These evidence-based guidelines are organized by therapeutic exposure and include a cancer screening section that lists elements of the history, physical exam, radiology, and other specialized tests that are recommended to aid in the detection of subsequent cancers in survivors. It is important to point out that many adult survivors do not realize the health risks that are related to their childhood cancer and do not have regular medical follow-up or practiced recommended cancer screening (Kadan-Lottick et al. 2002). Continued education of cancer survivors and their healthcare providers is critical, to ensure this continued surveillance. Furthermore, continued follow-up of these described cohorts will continue to provide further insight into this increased risk decades after the original diagnosis.

47.4 Treatment of Rare Tumors as Secondary Tumors

The causes of SNs are multi-factorial. Most secondary tumors in survivors of childhood cancer do not occur in childhood but rather in adulthood at an earlier age. However, a few specific secondary tumors are frequently encountered in childhood. Examples include sarcomas in patients with retinoblastoma and acute myelogenous leukemia in patients treated with etoposide. In both cases, standard treatment strategies must be directed against the secondary treatment. There are some limitations. Previous treatment may reduce the ability to deliver full doses of therapy such as radiation and anthracyclines (Milano et al. 2010). Recently, analysis of SEER data showed that survivors of childhood cancer diagnosed with a second primary malignancy had poorer overall survival than did their peers (HR, 1.86; 95% Cl, 1.72–2.02) after correcting for cancer type, age, sex, race, and decade of diagnosis (Brown et al. 2019). Similar findings were reported by CCSS on breast cancer in childhood cancer survivors (Moskowitz et al. 2019). In the case of rare secondary tumors, pediatric oncologists, internal medicine oncologists, and primary physicians caring for patients who were childhood cancer survivors should be aware that tumors may occur at significant earlier ages. One goal of childhood cancer survivorship programs is education. Patients are informed of the need for close monitoring of their health. That is often not adequate as childhood cancer survivors often tend to avoid medical care. Ongoing education of the medical community is essential.

References

Armstrong GT, Liu W et al (2011) Occurrence of multiple subsequent neoplasms in long-term survivors of childhood cancer: a report from the childhood cancer survivor study. J Clin Oncol 29(22):3056–3064

Brown AL, Arroyo VM et al (2019) Survival disparities for second primary malignancies diagnosed among childhood cancer survivors: a population-based assessment. Cancer 125(20):3623–3630

Curtis RE, Freedman DM, Ron E, Ries LAG, Hacker DG, Edwards BK, Tucker MA, Fraumeni JF (eds) (2006) New malignancies among cancer survivors: SEER Cancer Registries, 1973–2000. National Cancer Institute, Bethesda

Friedman DL, Whitton J et al (2010) Subsequent neoplasms in 5-year survivors of childhood cancer: the Childhood Cancer Survivor Study. J Natl Cancer Inst 102(14):1083–1095

Inskip PD, Ries LAD, Cohen RJ, Curtis RE (2006) New malignancies following childhood cancer, in. Curtis RE, Freedman DM, Ron E, Ries LAG, Hacker DG, Edwards BK, Tucker MA, Fraumeni JF (eds). New malignancies among cancer survivors: SEER Cancer Registries, 1973–2000. National Cancer Institute, NIH Publ. No. 05-5302. Bethesda, MD, pp 465–482

Jenkinson HC, Hawkins MM et al (2004) Long-term population-based risks of second malignant neoplasms after childhood cancer in Britain. Br J Cancer 91(11):1905–1910

Kadan-Lottick NS, Robison LL et al (2002) Childhood cancer survivors' knowledge about their past diagnosis and treatment: childhood Cancer Survivor Study. JAMA 287(14):1832–1839

Kleinerman RA, Tucker MA et al (2005) Risk of new cancers after radiotherapy in long-term survivors of retinoblastoma: an extended follow-up. J Clin Oncol 23(10):2272–2279

Mariotto AB, Rowland JH et al (2009) Long-term survivors of childhood cancers in the United States. Cancer Epidemiol Biomark Prev 18(4):1033–1040

Meadows AT, Friedman DL et al (2009) Second neoplasms in survivors of childhood cancer: findings from the Childhood Cancer Survivor Study cohort. J Clin Oncol 27(14):2356–2362

Milano MT, Li H et al (2010) Long-term survival among patients with Hodgkin's lymphoma who developed breast cancer: a population-based study. J Clin Oncol 28(34):5088–5096

Moskowitz CS, Chou JF et al (2019) Mortality after breast cancer among survivors of childhood cancer: a report from the childhood cancer survivor study. J Clin Oncol 37(24):2120–2130

Neglia JP, Robison LL et al (2006) New primary neoplasms of the central nervous system in survivors of childhood cancer: a report from the Childhood Cancer Survivor Study. J Natl Cancer Inst 98(21):1528–1537

Ng AK, Kenney LB et al (2010) Secondary malignancies across the age spectrum. Semin Radiat Oncol 20(1):67–78

Oeffinger KC, Hudson MM (2004) Long-term complications following childhood and adolescent cancer: foundations for providing risk-based health care for survivors. CA Cancer J Clin 54(4):208–236

Oeffinger KC, Mertens AC et al (2006) Chronic health conditions in adult survivors of childhood cancer. N Engl J Med 355(15):1572–1582

Olsen JH, Moller T et al (2009) Lifelong cancer incidence in 47,697 patients treated for childhood cancer in the Nordic countries. J Natl Cancer Inst 101(11):806–813

Ries LAG, Smith MA, Gurney JG, Linet M, Tamra T, Young JL, Bunin GR (eds) (1999) Cancer incidence and survival among children and adolescents: United States SEER Program 1975–1995, National Cancer Institute, SEER Program. NIH Publication No. 99-4649. National Cancer Institute, Bethesda

Robison LL, Mertens AC et al (2002) Study design and cohort characteristics of the Childhood Cancer Survivor Study: a multi-institutional collaborative project. Med Pediatr Oncol 38(4):229–239

Sigurdson AJ, Ronckers CM et al (2005) Primary thyroid cancer after a first tumour in childhood (the Childhood Cancer Survivor Study): a nested case-control study. Lancet 365(9476):2014–2023

Teepen JC, van Leeuwen FE et al (2017) Long-term risk of subsequent malignant neoplasms after treatment of childhood cancer in the DCOG LATER study cohort: role of chemotherapy. J Clin Oncol 35(20):2288–2298

Turcotte LM, Whitton JA et al (2015) Risk of subsequent neoplasms during the fifth and sixth decades of life in the childhood cancer survivor study cohort. J Clin Oncol 33(31):3568–3575

MIX
Papier aus verantwortungsvollen Quellen
Paper from responsible sources
FSC® C105338

If you have any concerns about our products,
you can contact us on
ProductSafety@springernature.com

In case Publisher is established outside the EU,
the EU authorized representative is:
Springer Nature Customer Service Center GmbH
Europaplatz 3, 69115 Heidelberg, Germany

Printed by Libri Plureos GmbH
in Hamburg, Germany